Handbook of Trauma

Pitfalls and Pearls

Handbook of Trauma

Pitfalls and Pearls

Editor

Robert F. Wilson, M.D., F.A.C.S., F.C.C.M.
Professor of Surgery
Wayne State University

Vice Chief of Surgery and
Director of Trauma
Detroit Medical Center

Chief, Surgical Services
Chief, Section of Thoracic & Cardiovascular Surgery
Detroit Receiving Hospital

LIPPINCOTT WILLIAMS & WILKINS
A **Wolters Kluwer** Company
Philadelphia • Baltimore • New York • London
Buenos Aires • Hong Kong • Sydney • Tokyo

Acquisitions Editor: Lisa McAllister
Developmental Editor: Joanne Husovski
Manufacturing Manager: Kevin Watt
Production Manager: Robert Pancotti
Production Editor: Frank Aversa
Cover Designer: Patricia Gast
Indexer: Kathrin Unger
Compositor: Lippincott Williams & Wilkins Desktop Division
Printer: Transcontinental

Material adapted from *Management of Trauma: Pitfalls and Practice,* edited by Robert F. Wilson and Alexander J. Walt; 1996 Williams & Wilkins.

Printed in Canada

9 8 7 6 5 4 3

Library of Congress Cataloging-in-Publication Data

Handbook of trauma : pitfalls and pearls / edited by Robert F. Wilson.
p. cm.
Shortened version of : Management of trauma. 2nd ed / edited by Robert F. Wilson and Alexander J. Walt. 1996.
Includes bibliographical references and index.
ISBN 0-683-30672-3
1. Wounds and injuries—Handbooks, manuals, etc. I. Wilson, Robert F. (Robert Francis), 1934— . II. Management of trauma.
[DNLM: 1. Wounds and Injuries—therapy handbooks. WO 39 H2372 1999]
RD93.H36 1999
617.1—dc21
DNLM/DLC 98-52874
For Library of Congress CIP

Care has been taken to confirm the accuracy of the information presented and to describe generally accepted practices. However, the authors, editor, and publisher are not responsible for errors or omissions or for any consequences from application of the information in this book and make no warranty, expressed or implied, with respect to the contents of the publication.

The authors, editor, and publisher have exerted every effort to ensure that drug selection and dosage set forth in this text are in accordance with current recommendations and practice at the time of publication. However, in view of ongoing research, changes in government regulations, and the constant flow of information relating to drug therapy and drug reactions, the reader is urged to check the package insert for each drug for any change in indications and dosage and for added warnings and precautions. This is particularly important when the recommended agent is a new or infrequently employed drug.

Some drugs and medical devices presented in this publication have Food and Drug Administration (FDA) clearance for limited use in restricted research settings. It is the responsibility of the health care provider to ascertain the FDA status of each drug or device planned for use in their clinical practice.

DEDICATION

We dedicate this handbook to Doctor Walt, who worked at Wayne State University and Detroit Receiving Hospital with such unparalleled commitment and honor from 1961 until his death in 1996.

Alexander J. Walt, M.B., Ch.B., was born in Cape Town, South Africa, in 1926. He received his medical degree from the University of Cape Town in 1948 and completed his training at the Royal College of Surgeons, London, and the Mayo Clinic, Rochester, Minnesota. He edited two books, published more than 150 scientific papers, and held numerous editorial board positions. He was Chairman of the Department of Surgery of Wayne State University from 1966–1988, president of the American Board of Medical Specialties from 1992–1994, and president of the American College of Surgeons from 1994–1995.

Doctor Walt had a remarkable knowledge of classic literature, and one of his favorite quotes was from "Ulysees" by Alfred Lord Tennyson:

> And this . . . spirit yearning in desire
> To follow knowledge like a sinking star,
> Beyond the utmost bound of human thought.

Even after he retired from the chairmanship of the Department of Surgery, he noted, as in the last stanza of "Ulysses":

> Tho' much is taken, much abides; and tho'
> We are not now that strength which in old days
> Moved earth and heaven, that which we are, we are;
> One equal temper of heroic hearts,
> Made weak by time and fate, but strong in will
> To strive, to seek, to find, and not to yield.

And Shakespeare could have been describing Dr. Walt very well:

> *His life was gentle, and the elements*
> *So mix'd in him that Nature might stand up*
> *And say to all the world, This was a man!*

CONTENTS

PREFACE

This shortened version of the Second Edition of *Management of Trauma: Pitfalls and Practice* was written to provide a more concise guide to the treatment of injured patients and the complications that they are most likely to develop. About 50% to 70% of the tables, figures, text, and references from the Second Edition have been excluded from the handbook; however, almost all of the axioms and summary points are still present. A few of the more important articles on trauma, published in 1996 and 1997, were added in most of the chapters, in an effort to make this text as up-to-date as possible.

For those wishing to review only the most important points on each topic, one can read the "Frequent Errors" and "Summary Points" at the end of each chapter. The summary points are a sequential compilation of the "Axioms" and "Pitfalls" found on almost every page in the text. We hope that some of our readers will be stimulated to read the Second Edition of *Management of Trauma* for further details on each topic.

I hope that Doctor Walt, who died shortly before the Second Edition was printed, would have approved of this shortened version.

Robert F. Wilson

ACKNOWLEDGMENTS

I am deeply indebted to Bernadette Daley and Dana Cooley for the immense amount of work and time they put into typing and organizing the four to five revisions of each chapter. Without their dedication to the project, we would never have even come close to the publisher's deadline.

Additional thanks go to Lisa Berant, Vickie Davis, Marlene Kaniarz, Sherry Prescott, and Sheryl Wier for their assistance with the typing.

Special thanks are also necessary to Joanne Husovski from Lippincott Williams & Wilkins who, as developmental editor for the handbook, helped in developing the revisions.

Handbook of Trauma

Pitfalls and Pearls

1. PREHOSPITAL MEDICAL CARE OF THE INJURED PATIENT(1)

Emergency medical services (EMSs), in relation to trauma, refers to prehospital care of acutely injured patients at the scene of the injury and during transport to a hospital (2). Hospital personnel are notified of the incoming case, the condition of the patient, and the care provided at the scene and en route to the hospital. EMSs also includes training and certifying individuals involved in this type of care.

Each year, unintentional injuries and injuries related to violence claim more than 135,000 lives (3) and are responsible for more than one third of all emergency department (ED) visits (4). In 1995, injuries were responsible for more than $430 billion in medical expenses and economic losses (5). Approximately 50% of those who die from injuries do so before reaching the hospital (6). Of those who reach the hospital alive, 60% of the deaths occur within the first 4 hours and are usually the result of hemorrhage. Therefore, if a measurable reduction in trauma mortality is to be achieved, the necessary interventions should be provided as close to the time of injury as possible.

AXIOM A properly run air-transport system can save lives that might be lost during a long EMS run on the ground.

EMERGENCY MEDICAL SERVICE ORGANIZATION

The first goal of EMS is to make properly trained personnel and appropriate equipment rapidly available to critically ill or injured patients. To do this effectively, communication between all individuals involved is essential.

It is estimated that to achieve a 4- to 6-minute response time in an urban community, one EMS unit is required for each 50,000 of the population (2). Therefore, in a city of 600,000 people, approximately 12 units are needed on the street at all times.

In patient transport involving long distances, helicopters can be lifesaving, but such transport can be misused. Norton et al. (7) noted that an EMS system audit provided increased awareness of the proper criteria for helicopter retrievals and significantly decreased the total number of trauma scene flights in an urban trauma system.

Medical Control

Medical control of an effective EMS system is provided by physicians committed to providing optimal prehospital care (8). To do this most effectively, they must spend some time in the field observing all aspects of the system in operation along with proper medical control and quality-assurance programs. When medical control is not provided, protocols with standing orders can significantly reduce prehospital times and improve the quality of care provided.

If a licensed physician on the scene wishes to assume medical control of the patient, that physician becomes responsible for the patient until medical responsibility is assumed by another physician (2). The physician on the scene may accompany the patient to the hospital while supervising the medical care en route, or he may transfer medical control via radio to the physician at the medical command authority.

Current prehospital practice is to apply spinal immobilization liberally in case of suspected neck or back injury by using rigid cervical collars, long backboards, and straps (9). The Philadelphia and similar hard collars, however, allow approximately 60% of normal rotary and lateral head motion and 40% of normal anteroposterior cervical spine movement. Proper taping of the patient's head to sandbags and the backboard can reduce neck mobility to negligible levels.

The Pneumatic Antishock Garment (PASG) is seldom used in an urban environment, but it may be useful in

- Hypotensive patients with transport times exceeding 10 to 15 minutes;
- Patients with continuing abdominal, pelvic, or lower-extremity hemorrhage; and
- Patients with unstable fractures of the pelvis or lower extremities.

AXIOM Pulmonary edema is an absolute contraindication to inflation of a PASG.

Respiratory difficulty may be a relative contraindication to inflating the abdominal portion of the garment. In hypotensive pregnant patients, the abdominal panel should not be inflated except for control of uterine hemorrhage. Complications such as compartment syndrome are more likely to develop if the PASG is inflated to a pressure greater than 40 to 60 mm Hg for more than 2 hours, especially if the patient is hypotensive (10).

When the PASG is going to be deflated in the operating room or in the ED, it should be done gradually while the patient's blood pressure (BP) is monitored closely. With any decrease in BP of 5 mm Hg or more, deflation of the PASG should be stopped to allow further fluid to be infused as needed.

Cardiopulmonary Resuscitation

Prehospital endotracheal intubation, vigorous fluid resuscitation, and rapid transport can be effective in preventing cardiopulmonary arrest in many trauma patients (11). Maintaining an open airway with optimal oxygenation plus protecting the cervical spine is particularly important in patients with head injuries. Inserting an endotracheal tube in the field can sometimes be extremely difficult or impossible. Blostein et al. (12) reported on the use of the esophageal tracheal combitube (ETC) in trauma patients for whom orotracheal rapid-sequence intubation (RSI) fails. The ETC insertion was successful in all 10 patients in whom it was attempted. Definitive airway control was achieved later by conversion to orotracheal intubation in seven patients, ED cricothyroidotomy in one patient, and operative room tracheostomy in two patients. No patient died because of failure to control the airway.

Tension pneumothorax also can be rapidly fatal. Schmidt et al. (13) noted that chest-tube decompression of blunt chest injuries by physicians in the field is safe and effective. Nontherapeutic chest-tube placements occurred in only 15 (2.4%) of 624 patients, and missed pneumothoraces occurred in only six (less than 1%) of 624 patients.

AXIOM Transport of injured patients in an urban setting should not be delayed while multiple attempts are made to start an intravenous line.

In a frequently quoted study by Martin et al. (14) in 1991, patients with penetrating truncal trauma and a systolic BP less than 90 mm Hg were given aggressive prehospital preoperative fluid resuscitation (3,125 mL vs. 3 mL in the control group). This resulted in a decrease in survival from a predicted survival (PS) of 57% to an observed survival (OS) of 52%. In contrast, the patients with essentially no preoperative fluid resuscitation had a PS of 49% and an OS of 58%.

Triage

A major determinant of the resources required by a regional trauma system is the number of patients the system will have to manage. This is determined primarily at the prehospital level by triage criteria that identify patients who require care at a trauma center. Although all triage systems can predict death fairly accurately, predicting the presence of a major injury has a sensitivity and specificity of only about 70% (15).

Search and Rescue

Search and rescue (SAR) operations can be an important aspect of prehospital care. Eight key elements to on-scene direction and control in SAR include

1. Establish **victim-oriented** activity and operations in the field;
2. Identify all **hazards**;
3. Perform thorough **terrain analysis** (reconnaissance);
4. Protect **access** to the search base site;
5. Monitor and control **communication flow and volume**;
6. Have available **backup communication** at all times;
7. Establish **victim care** as soon as possible; and
8. Establish and **log each subject's destination** and estimated time of arrival (ETA) at a medical facility.

⊘ FREQUENT ERRORS

1. ***Inadequate medical control.***
2. ***Inadequate initial and continued EMS training.***
3. ***Failure to promptly recognize and correct esophageal intubation.***
4. ***Delay in delivery of the patient to an appropriate trauma facility because of attempts at resuscitation in the field.***
5. ***Failure to have adequate prehospital radio control or written protocols.***
6. ***Inadequate stabilization of a patient with possible spinal injuries.***
7. ***Improper use of tourniquets to control bleeding, leading to further damage or ischemia or both of the injured limb.***

SUMMARY POINTS

1. The EMS systems must work closely with the ED to assure a continuity of patient care from the time of the incident to discharge from the ED.

2. Proper communication between all involved individuals is essential for a properly functioning EMS system.

3. Adequate initial and continued training for EMT personnel is critical to providing the best care possible in the field.

4. Because of the education of nurses in pathophysiology and quality assurance, their use in prehospital EMS systems management and reviews can be of great benefit.

5. An EMS system is only as good as its medical control.

6. Standing orders, when used with proper medical control and quality-assurance programs, can significantly reduce prehospital times without reducing the quality of care provided.

7. The cervical collar is primarily a reminder to a patient not to move the neck.

8. Although there is controversy about the value of increasing BP with the PASG in hypotensive prehospital patients, there is no question that allowing an abrupt decrease in BP during deflation of the PASG can be very dangerous.

9. Providing and maintaining an adequate airway and ventilation is the single most important therapy provided to victims of severe injuries.

10. Transport of injured patients in an urban setting should not be delayed while multiple attempts are made to start an intravenous line.

11. It is important that SAR plans be developed before their actual need.

REFERENCES

1. Bock BF, Berk WA, Bonner SC, Wilson RF. Prehospital care of the injured patient. In: Wilson RF, Walt AJ, eds. *Management of trauma: pitfalls and practice.* 2nd ed. Philadelphia: Williams & Wilkins, 1996:112.

2. McSwain NE Jr. Prehospital emergency medical systems and cardiopulmonary resuscitation. In: Moore EE, Mattox KL, Feliciano DV, eds. *Trauma.* 2nd ed. Norfolk: Appleton & Lange, 1991:99.
3. Rosenberg HM, Ventura SJ, Maurer JD. Births and deaths: United States, 1995. *Month Vital Stat Rep* 1996;45(suppl 2):31.
4. Burt CW. Injury-related visits to hospital emergency departments: United States, 1992. In: *Advance data from vital and health statistics, no. 261.* Hyattsville, MD: National Center for Health Statistics, 1995:1–19.
5. National Safety Council. *Accident facts: costs of unintentional injuries by class, 1995.* Itaska, IL: National Safety Council, 1997:1–3.
6. Champion HR. Organization of trauma care. In: Kreis DJ Jr, Gomez GA, eds. *Trauma management.* Boston: Little, Brown, 1989:11–27.
7. Norton R, Wortman E, Eastes L, et al. Appropriate helicopter transport of urban trauma patients. *J Trauma* 1996;41:886.
8. McSwain NE. Medical control of prehospital care. *J Trauma* 1984;24:172.
9. De Lorenzo RA. A review of spinal immobilization techniques: selected topics: prehospital care. *J Emerg Med* 1996;14:603.
10. Bass RR, Allison EJ, Reines HD, et al. Tight compartment syndrome without lower extremity trauma following application of PASG trousers. *Ann Emerg Med* 1983;12:382.
11. Copass MK, Oreskovich MR, Bladergroen MR, et al. Prehospital cardiopulmonary resuscitation of the critically injured patient. *J Surg* 1984;148:20.
12. Blostein PA, Koestner AJ, Hoak S. Failed rapid sequence intubation in trauma patients: esophageal tracheal combitube is a useful adjunct. *J Trauma* 1998;44:534.
13. Schmidt U, Stalp M, Gerich T, et al. Chest tube decompression of blunt chest injuries by physicians in the field: effectiveness and complications. *J Trauma* 1998;44:98.
14. Martin RR, Bickell W, Mattox KL, et al. Prospective evaluation of preoperative volume resuscitation in hypotensive patients with penetrating truncal injuries. *J Trauma* 1991;31:1033.
15. Baxt WG, Berry CC, Epperson MD, et al. The failure of prehospital trauma prediction rules to classify trauma patients accurately. *Ann Emerg Med* 1989;18:1.

2. INITIAL EVALUATION AND MANAGEMENT OF SEVERELY INJURED PATIENTS(1)

AXIOM The priorities of care at the scene of an accident include establishment of the airway, maintenance of adequate ventilation, and control of external bleeding.

EMERGENCY DEPARTMENT MANAGEMENT

The trauma team should be activated before critically injured patients arrive in the ED. Petrie et al. (2) noted that trauma patients with an injury severity score (ISS) greater than 12 did significantly better if a trauma team was activated and handled the initial resuscitation (vs. management on an individual service-by-service basis). A team captain also should be designated before trauma resuscitations. This individual should resolve any questions regarding the ranking of trauma therapy implemented on a patient at a particular time. Traditionally, this team captain is a surgeon with a special interest in trauma.

The revised trauma score (RTS) and ISS for evaluation of results can help to indicate the efficacy of the trauma program. Osler et al. (3) recently showed that the New Injury Severity Score (NISS) significantly outperforms the ISS as a predictor of mortality. The NISS is defined as the sum of the squares of the Abbreviated Injury Scale scores of each of the patient's three most severe Abbreviated Injury Scale injuries, regardless of the body region in which they occur. Thus three critical injuries, all within the abdomen, could provide an NISS of 75 and an ISS of 25.

Forcing an unwilling patient to lie supine can lead to a sequence of combativeness, restraints, medications for sedation, and endotracheal intubation, all of which can be very traumatic. This sequence can sometimes be circumvented by simply talking to the patient and understanding the patient's desire to control his or her own airway.

AXIOM An uncooperative or restless patient should be assumed to be hypoxic until proven otherwise.

Restless patients not responding to oxygen require early endotracheal intubation to correct hypoxia and provide adequate ventilation.

Pneumatic Antishock Garment

Although pneumatic antishock garments (PASGs) can help to immobilize pelvic and lower-extremity fractures and reduce associated blood loss, this device has relatively little value in hypotensive patients in urban trauma centers. If one uses a PASG, one also should recognize that it can cause compartment syndromes, particularly if applied with high pressures for prolonged periods (4).

Prehospital Intravenous Lines

Starting intravenous fluids at the scene is counterproductive if the transit time to the hospital is less than 15 minutes. Indeed, excess fluids could restart bleeding that has temporarily ceased.

Establishing Intravenous Lines

If the patient has severe hypovolemic shock, causing venous collapse, or if there is a history of previous intravenous narcotic use, it may be difficult to establish rapid venous access in peripheral veins. In such patients, subclavian veins are often the quickest sites for establishing intravenous access.

Subclavian vein catheters should generally be inserted by making the percutaneous puncture at the junction of the middle and medial thirds of the clavicle while advancing the needle perpendicular to the median plane and parallel to the floor toward the suprasternal notch. This technique is best performed with the patient in the Trendelenburg position. The incidence of successful insertion of these catheters is extremely high. The incidence of complications, such as pneumothorax, has been less than 1.5% at the Detroit Receiving Hospital for many years. In patients with chest wounds, subclavian vein catheterization should be performed on the side of the injury to reduce the chances of also collapsing or damaging the uninjured lung.

Percutaneous catheterization of the internal jugular vein is also excellent for rapid large-bore catheter venous access, particularly in patients who require immediate operative intervention. The skin-puncture site is about 0.5 cm to 1.0 cm above the top of the triangle formed by the sternal and clavicular heads of the sternocleidomastoid muscle. The needle is directed caudally at the ipsilateral nipple. Medial deviation of the needle may lead to inadvertent puncture of the carotid artery.

Injuries sustained to the neck or upper chest require at least one venous access to be inserted in a lower extremity. If the injury is in the abdomen, one or two intravenous lines should be inserted into a tributary of the superior vena cava.

Cardiopulmonary Resuscitation

Open thoracotomy can be performed as part of the emergency room resuscitation with reasonable expectation for success in patients who have a stab wound of the chest and have had a cardiac arrest just before or soon after arrival in the ED. However, open cardiac massage in the ED is rarely successful in patients with cardiac arrest due to gunshot wounds, penetrating intraabdominal injuries, or severe blunt trauma to the head or trunk.

Control of External Bleeding

External bleeding in most patients is best controlled by direct digital pressure. This is particularly true in patients with small deep wounds adjacent to vessels and in patients with neck wounds. Control of major bleeding in an extremity should not be attempted by blindly clamping in the depths of the wound.

Tourniquets are rarely needed, but if used, the pressure should be applied over the most proximal portion of the extremity wound, and the cuff pressure should be well above the systolic pressure. If the tourniquet pressure is slightly below the systolic pressure, it will allow arterial blood to enter the extremity, and this will cause increased venous bleeding.

Shock

AXIOM Continued shock after trauma is usually due to continued bleeding or inadequate resuscitation.

Hemorrhage is the most common cause of shock in critically injured patients. Patients arriving at the hospital in shock after blunt trauma are likely to be bleeding from intraperitoneal injuries, pelvic or long-bone fractures, or intrathoracic wounds. Hypovolemic shock after trauma also may occur from translocation of fluids into burned, contused, or contaminated tissues.

Hypovolemic shock with consequent cerebral hypoxia is a major factor leading to death in patients with head injury. Damaged brain tissue is particularly sensitive to a decrease in cerebral perfusion or oxygenation.

Hypotension to systolic pressures below 90 mm Hg in patients with spinal cord injuries is primarily caused by dilatation of superficial capacitance and resistance vessels. Intoxication with alcohol or other drugs may accentuate this phenomenon. Other sites of injury also must be anticipated, particularly if the systolic pressure is below 80 mm Hg, if the patient is tachycardic, or if the skin is cool and clammy.

During resuscitation with balanced electrolyte solutions (BESs), one should avoid glucose infusions to counter the tendency toward stress-induced hyperglycemia.

Even if no glucose is given, hyperglycemia tends to occur after trauma because of an increase in catecholamine, glucagon, cortisol, and growth hormone release.

The Three Phases of Shock

The body's physiological responses to hypovolemic shock may be divided into three phases (5).

1. Phase 1 is the period of shock and active hemorrhage. This phase extends from the time of the injury to the completion of the resuscitation and surgery for control of bleeding.
2. Phase 2, which is the period of extravascular fluid sequestration, begins after the bleeding is controlled and resuscitation is completed, and extends until the time of maximal weight gain. This fluid-sequestration phase averages 24 to 36 hours in patients receiving 15 or more units of blood during phase 1.
3. Phase 3, which is the mobilization and diuretic period, extends from the time of maximal weight gain to the end of diuresis, as reflected by maximal weight loss.

The expansion of the extravascular space after shock and trauma appears to include both the interstitial and intracellular compartments. The obligatory nature of this third-space expansion is somewhat similar to that seen in burn patients. Studies indicate that during phase 2, the volume of the interstitial space may increase by more than 10 L, and the total extravascular fluid increase may exceed 20 L in some patients (5).

Grading Hemorrhage

A grade 1 hemorrhage is an acute loss of 10% to 15% of the circulating blood volume. This is about 750 to 1,000 mL blood in an average 70-kg adult and is usually associated with some tachycardia and oliguria, but there is usually no decrease in blood pressure (BP) or organ function.

A moderate, or grade 2, blood loss is defined as an acute loss of 20% to 25% of the blood volume or approximately 1,250 mL to 1,750 mL of blood in a 70-kg adult. Such blood loss will usually cause some tachycardia (100 to 120 beats/min), a reduced pulse pressure, and more severe oliguria (due to renal vasoconstriction, causing decreased renal blood flow and glomerular filtration). Patients who are seen in the ED with a grade 1 or 2 hemorrhage can usually have their circulatory volume fully restored by the administration of 2 to 3 L of a BES.

Changes in pulse pressure often correlate with changes in stroke volume and can be used as an index of the adequacy of fluid resuscitation. During hemorrhage, any reduction in cardiac output causes an even greater reduction in renal blood flow (because of renal artery vasoconstriction). There will also be increased renal absorption of sodium and water, resulting in a decreased urine output (6).

AXIOM Urine output can be an important guide to the adequacy of fluid resuscitation in injured and burned patients.

A grade 3 hemorrhage represents a severe acute loss of 30% to 35% of the blood volume or approximately 2,100 mL to 2,450 mL in a 70-kg adult. It is usually associated with hypotension, severe tachycardia (120 to 140 beats/min), oliguria, and cold clammy skin. Complete restoration of the circulating blood volume can usually be achieved by the prompt infusion of 4 to 5 L of BES along with 1 or 2 units of blood. Patients who receive multiple blood transfusions of packed red cells require approximately 1.6 L of a BES for each transfusion by the time the operative intervention is completed (6).

Grade 4 hemorrhage represents catastrophic hemorrhage with severe shock. It occurs with an acute loss of at least 40% to 45% of the circulating blood volume or about 3 L of whole blood loss in a standard 70-kg man. This usually causes a precipitate decrease in BP, which may not be obtainable by the cuff technique. There is also a marked catecholamine release, causing the skin to be cold and clammy.

The response to a fluid challenge of 20 mL/kg of a BES over 5 minutes also provides some information about the amount of blood loss. A rapid and sustained improvement in the BP and patient's condition implies a blood loss of less than 10% to 20%. An improvement that is only transient tends to indicate a 20% to 40% blood loss or continuing hemorrhage or both. If there is little or no response to the fluid bolus, the blood loss usually exceeds 40% of the estimated blood volume.

Colloids

Use of colloids (especially albumin) to treat hypovolemic hypotension is very controversial, but may be of some value in patients who are severely hypoproteinemic. Albumin is expensive, and it may also impair production of immunoglobulins (7) and coagulation factors (8). Hetastarch or dextran, especially in doses exceeding 1,500 mL in the first 24 hours, may increase the tendency to bleeding.

Blood

Failure to respond to 40 mL/kg of a BES given over 10 minutes should make one consider prompt movement to the operating room (OR) to control bleeding and to start type-specific blood.

The transfusion of multiple units of packed red blood cells may lead to a coagulation-protein deficiency (6). In patients requiring fewer than 10 transfusions of bank blood or 5 to 6 units of cell-saver blood, there is no clinical or laboratory evidence to support the prophylactic use of fresh frozen plasma (FFP) or platelets. However, FFP and platelet supplementation should be administered if there is excessive oozing (microvascular bleeding) or if the platelet count is less than 50,000/mm^3 or both.

Hemodynamic Effects of the Trendelenburg (Head-Down) Position

In anesthetized patients with coronary artery disease, Reich et al. (9) found that a 20° Trendelenburg head-down position caused a slight (10%) increase in systemic BP, cardiac index, and filling pressures. However, this position decreases cerebral blood flow by increasing the jugular venous pressure and impeding cerebral venous drainage. The head-down position also may cause respiratory distress because of cephalad displacement of intraabdominal contents and the resultant elevation of the diaphragm. The hemodynamic effects of passive leg raising are similar to those of the Trendelenburg position and do not have as many adverse effects.

Hemodynamic Monitoring

Patients with grade 1 or grade 2 hemorrhage can usually be monitored adequately with observation of the skin, urine output, cuff BP, and heart rate. These patients usually stabilize rapidly with crystalloid resuscitation.

AXIOM Large variations in systolic BP during the ventilatory cycle may be an early sign of hypovolemia or pericardial tamponade (10).

During the initial resuscitative and operative procedure(s), the relative amounts of blood and BES needed for patients with a class 3 hemorrhage can be partially guided by serial hemoglobin or hematocrit measurements, in addition to careful observation of any changes in systemic and central venous pressures and urine output. Patients with class 4 hemorrhage should have invasive monitoring of arterial BP, arterial blood gases, and central venous pressure (CVP). If the patient is still hemodynamically unstable, especially in an intensive care unit (ICU), monitoring of pulmonary artery wedge pressure and pulmonary artery oxygen saturation (S_vO_2) also should be considered.

Airway Control

AXIOM The combination of shock and acute respiratory distress is highly lethal unless corrected rapidly.

When a patient is in acute respiratory distress after a penetrating chest wound, one must immediately rule out pericardial tamponade, tension pneumothorax, or a massive hemothorax. If pericardial tamponade is suspected, rapid beneficial results can often be obtained by a pericardiocentesis. This is usually performed by inserting an 18-gauge spinal needle just to the left of the xiphoid, with the tip of the aspirating needle directed superiorly and to the right.

If the patient is in severe respiratory distress and if the trachea is shifted away from a tympanotic hemithorax with no breath sounds, rapid aspiration with a large needle inserted into the second intercostal space at the midclavicular space can temporarily relieve a tension pneumothorax while preparations are made to insert a chest tube.

AXIOM Open chest wounds should not be covered or closed until a chest tube is in place.

If a chest tube evacuates 1,500 mL to 2,000 mL of blood and the patient is still bleeding rapidly out the chest tube or is hemodynamically unstable, a thoracotomy is indicated.

Intraabdominal Bleeding

AXIOM The most urgent threat to life in patients with abdominal injury is severe intraperitoneal hemorrhage from injuries to the liver, spleen, or major vessels. If a diagnostic peritoneal lavage (DPL) is negative, hypotension is almost always a result of other causes.

The definition of a positive DPL after penetrating abdominal injury is variable. The red cell count for a positive DPL is much lower with penetrating injury than with blunt trauma and is probably in the range of 10,000/mm^3. The most common cause for a false-negative DPL after blunt trauma is a ruptured diaphragm. The most common cause for a false-positive DPL is a pelvic fracture.

With bowel injury, a DPL may show an increased white cell count, amylase, or alkaline phosphatase in the aspirate. In selected patients, abdominal computed tomography (CT) scans with oral and intravenous contrast may be helpful if the diagnosis of an injury with less sophisticated techniques has been inconclusive. Flat and upright films of the abdomen after blunt trauma may demonstrate retroperitoneal air along the lateral border of the right psoas muscle and around the right kidney due to blunt rupture of the retroperitoneal duodenum.

A persistent increase in serum amylase levels at 6 hours or 12 hours, coinciding with increasing abdominal pain and tenderness, is suggestive of pancreatic injury. If a diagnosis of pancreatic injury is being considered and an intraperitoneal injury has been ruled out, an abdominal CT scan may demonstrate edema around the pancreas in the lesser sac, and sometimes actual division of the midportion of the pancreas may be seen on fine cuts.

Genitourinary Tract Injuries

If the genitourinary evaluation is performed in conjunction with assessment for other organ injuries in a stable patient, the renal evaluation can be performed more accurately on an abdominal CT scan with oral and intravenous contrast rather than an intravenous pyelogram.

Extremity Injuries

Early complete evaluation of neurovascular function is an important part of the initial examination of extremity injuries before radiographs or any attempts at reduction are performed.

⊘ FREQUENT ERRORS

1. **Not following the priorities *of correction of airway, ventilation, and circulation problems in multiply injured patients.***
2. **Not having a designated team captain *to oversee management of severely injured patients.***
3. **Forcing all trauma patients to lie flat *on a cart even when they are hemodynamically stable and are not a spine injury risk and can obviously breathe better sitting up.***
4. ***Starting an* emergency subclavian line on the uninjured side *of a patient with chest trauma.***
5. ***Assuming that* continued hypotension *in a trauma patient is due to factors other than persistent severe bleeding or inadequate fluid resuscitation.***
6. **Using diuretics *rather than fluids to increase urine output during the fluid-sequestration phase.***

SUMMARY POINTS

1. When the transit time from the site of injury to the closest skilled emergency center is less than 15 to 20 minutes, time spent starting intravenous fluids at the scene is usually counterproductive.

2. Once a team captain is identified, all participants of the trauma care team must respect his or her position as the final decision maker.

3. One should assume that an uncooperative or restless patient is hypoxic until proven otherwise.

4. Subclavian catheterization should be performed on the side of injury in patients with chest wounds to reduce the chances of collapsing an uninjured lung.

5. With injuries in the neck or upper chest, at least one venous access should be inserted in a lower extremity. If the injury is in the abdomen, at least one intravenous route should be placed in a tributary of the superior vena cava.

6. If a patient has had a cardiac arrest of less than 5 minutes duration due to a stab of the chest, an open thoracotomy with internal cardiac massage is indicated in an appropriate ED setting.

7. If tourniquets are not applied properly, they can increase bleeding and tissue loss.

8. Continued shock after trauma is usually due to continued bleeding or inadequate resuscitation.

9. Shock or hypoxia in a patient with a head injury can rapidly make the brain injury much worse.

10. Resuscitation from shock in adults and older children should not be done with glucose-containing solutions.

11. Significant fluid shifts out of the vascular space continue for 24 to 48 hours or longer after bleeding has been controlled.

12. Whenever an acute mild-to-moderate blood volume loss occurs, early administration of 3 times that amount of a BES will usually restore the blood volume to normal.

13. In young and previously healthy individuals, loss of 20% to 25% of the blood volume may be associated with minimal or no arterial hypotension.

14. Even if the arterial BP in a trauma patient is normal, it may be associated with a significant reduction in cardiac output, and urine output, and stroke volume.
15. In most hypovolemic patients, urine output is an important guide to the adequacy of fluid resuscitation.
16. Severe oliguria during and immediately after traumatic shock should not be treated with diuretics, except after aggressive fluid loading and as a very last resort to help prevent oliguric renal failure.
17. The CVP can be useful in monitoring trauma patients who are not responding hemodynamically as expected.
18. Large respirophasic variations in systolic BP may be an early sign of hypovolemia or pericardial tamponade.
19. The combination of shock and acute respiratory distress is rapidly lethal unless corrected promptly.
20. Open chest wounds with an underlying lung injury should not be covered or closed until a chest tube is in place.
21. The most urgent threat to life in patients with abdominal injury is severe intraperitoneal hemorrhage from injuries to the liver, spleen, or major vessels.
22. The most common cause for a false-negative DPL after blunt trauma is a ruptured diaphragm, and the most common cause for a false-positive DPL is a pelvic fracture.
23. If a patient has a gunshot wound that may have entered the peritoneal cavity, a laparotomy should generally be performed.
24. It may take 6 to 12 hours or more for bowel leakage to produce signs and symptoms of peritonitis.
25. Patients with severe blunt abdominal trauma should have radiographs of the abdomen to help identify the retroperitoneal air that may be present in patients with duodenal rupture.
26. Obtaining serial serum amylase measurements after blunt abdominal trauma can facilitate the diagnosis of pancreatic injury by demonstrating an increase in serum amylase levels at 6 hours or 12 hours, especially if it coincides with increased abdominal pain and tenderness.
27. Early complete evaluation of neurovascular function is an important part of the initial examination of extremity injuries, especially before any attempts at reduction are performed.

REFERENCES

1. Lucas CE, Ledgerwood AM. Initial evaluation and management of severely injured patients. In: Wilson RF, Walt AJ, eds. *Management of trauma: pitfalls and practice*. Philadelphia: Williams & Wilkins, 1996:13–27.
2. Petrie D, Lane P, Stewart TC, et al. An evaluation of patient outcomes comparing trauma team activated versus trauma team not activated using TRISS analysis. *J Trauma* 1996;41:870.
3. Osler T, Baker SP, Long W. A modification of the injury severity score that both improves accuracy and simplified scoring. *J Trauma* 1997;43:922.
4. Aprahamian C, Gessert G, Banoyk DF, et al. MAST-associated compartment syndromes (MACS): a review. *J Trauma* 1989;29:549.
5. Lucas CE. Resuscitation of the injured patient: the three phases of treatment. *Surg Clin North Am* 1977;57:3.
6. Lucas CE, Ledgerwood AM. Hemodynamic management of the injured. In: Capan LM, Miller SM, Turndorf H, eds. *Trauma anesthesia and intensive care.* Philadelphia: JB Lippincott, 1991:83.
7. Faillace DF, Ledgerwood AM, Lucas CE, et al. Immunoglobulin changes after varied resuscitation regimens. *J Trauma* 1982;22:1.
8. Lucas CE, Ledgerwood AM, Mammen EF. Altered coagulation protein content after albumin resuscitation. *Ann Surg* 1982;196:198.
9. Reich DL, Konstadt SN, Raissi S, et al. Trendelenburg position and passive leg raising do not significantly improve cardiopulmonary performance in the anesthetized patient with coronary artery disease. *Crit Care Med* 1989;17:313.
10. Coyle JP, Teplick RS, Long MC, et al. Respiratory variations in systemic arterial pressure as an indicator of volume status. *Anesthesiology* 1983;59:A53.

3. CARDIOPULMONARY RESUSCITATION AFTER TRAUMA(1)

Cardiac arrest can be defined as a sudden cessation of effective cardiac output (CO). It may be due to asystole, ventricular fibrillation (V-fib), or any condition that reduces CO to a negligible level.

> ⊘ **PITFALL**
>
> ***If a physician, confronted by a patient with a possible cardiac arrest, delays resuscitation because of uncertainty about the diagnosis, the chances for survival with intact neurologic function decrease precipitately.***

Trauma can precipitate acute myocardial ischemia or infarction (MI) because of the related hemorrhage, hypoxia, anxiety, or pain. If the myocardial ischemia is severe enough, it can progress to cardiac arrest with or without an antecedent period of shock. In young healthy individuals, cardiac arrest usually results from exsanguination from major blood vessels or asphyxia caused by damage to the airway, lungs, chest wall, or diaphragm.

A patient with hypovolemic cardiac arrest rarely survives if external cardiac massage and nonintubated ventilation are performed for more than 5 minutes before arrival at the hospital; however, at least one other center recommends that, with penetrating wounds of the chest, resuscitative efforts may be applied even if prehospital cardiopulmonary resuscitation (CPR) has been performed for up to 15 minutes (2).

Prehospital cardiac arrest management should include immediate establishment of an airway and ventilation with 100% oxygen, preferably by an endotracheal tube. External cardiac massage in the presence of truncal trauma is apt to cause more harm than good.

DIAGNOSIS

The cardinal signs of cardiac arrest include

- Lack of a palpable pulse;
- Absence of an audible heart beat; and
- Loss of cerebral or brainstem function (such as unresponsiveness and apnea).

If there is loss of pulses during a trauma resuscitation, but the cardioscope reveals a fairly normal rhythm, a true cardiac arrest probably has not occurred.

Attempts to breathe or gasp do not always stop immediately after a cardiac arrest. The patient may continue to have some respiratory effort for 20 to 30 seconds after the heart has stopped. If the end-tidal CO_2 ($P_{ET}CO_2$) is monitored on a capnograph, a sudden decrease to levels near zero is diagnostic of either a cardiac arrest, accidental disconnection of the ventilatory tubing, or movement of the endotracheal tube out of the trachea.

> ⊘ **PITFALL**
>
> ***If the diagnosis of cardiac arrest is made after the patient has had a convulsion, brain damage has generally already occurred.***

AXIOM Although regurgitation of gastric contents can be the cause of a cardiac arrest, the regurgitation is usually due to relaxation of sphincters after the cardiac arrest.

INITIAL EMERGENCY DEPARTMENT MANAGEMENT

Defibrillation

AXIOM Early defibrillation is the most important determinant of survival from sudden cardiac arrest. If there is any delay in defibrillating the heart, the chances of successful resuscitation are reduced.

The Advanced Cardiac Life Support (ACLS) starting dose for external defibrillation is 200 joules. If the V-fib is not terminated by the first attempt, a second shock should be given immediately at 300 joules, followed by a third defibrillation at 360 joules if the second shock also was unsuccessful.

⊘ PITFALL

If severe metabolic acidosis or hypoxemia is allowed to persist, it may be impossible to defibrillate the patient.

Endotracheal Intubation

Cardiac arrest in critically injured patients in the Emergency Department (ED) typically occurs during or shortly after endotracheal intubation. This can occur as a result of any one of at least seven reasons:

1. **Inadequate preintubation oxygenation**: Two to three minutes of effective ventilation with 100% O_2 increases the arterial Po_2 of most patients to 300 mm Hg or more. This is usually enough oxygen to prevent hypoxemia even if the patient is then apneic for 2 to 3 minutes.

AXIOM Pulse oximetry with occasional arterial blood gas analysis should be used in all patients with severe trauma, especially during and after emergency intubation.

2. **Esophageal intubation**: Some ways to ensure that the endotracheal tube is placed properly in the trachea include the following:

   Visualize the tube going between the vocal cords;
   Note the compliance of the pilot balloon: when the cuff is being inflated, the pressure in the pilot balloon is less if the tube is in the esophagus;
   Note the compliance of the ventilating bag: it is initially easier to ventilate the stomach than the lungs;
   Look for anterior and lateral chest-wall motion as the ambu bag is squeezed;
   Auscultate both axillas and the epigastrium: if the breath sounds in the epigastrium are better than those in the lateral chest, the tube is in the esophagus; and
   Measure the end-tidal carbon dioxide with a capnograph or disposable $ETCO_2$ detector; the $ETCO_2$ in the esophagus is close to 0.

AXIOM If there is any suspicion that the "endotracheal" tube is in the esophagus, it should be kept in place while another endotracheal tube is inserted.

3. **Intubation of a main-stem bronchus**: Poor breath sounds on one side, usually the left, in an intubated patient with chest trauma are frequently due to an endotracheal tube being inserted in too far rather than a left hemopneumothorax.
4. **Excess ventilatory pressures**: If the patient is hypovolemic, excessive positive-pressure ventilation will further reduce venous return. This can make the hypotension worse and cause a cardiac arrest. Hypovolemic patients should be ventilated cautiously until the hypovolemia is at least partially corrected and venous return is improved. If the lung has blebs or a penetrating injury, bagging the patient vigorously can cause a tension pneumothorax. Even with normal lungs, ventilatory pressures exceeding 60 to 80 cm H_2O can cause interstitial emphysema or a pneumothorax.
5. **Systemic air embolism**: Any patient with a lung injury and hemoptysis should be considered at risk for developing a systemic air embolus, especially if positive-pressure ventilation is used. In addition, patients with hemoptysis are at risk for flooding normal alveoli with blood, which can cause severe hypoxemia (3).

AXIOM Any cardiovascular or neurologic deterioration occurring during or just after endotracheal intubation and positive-pressure ventilation should be considered a result of systemic air emboli until proven otherwise.

6. **Vasovagal responses**: Vasovagal responses are rare after trauma, but they occur with increased frequency in patients with abnormally slow pulse rates during insertion of endotracheal, nasogastric, or chest tubes.
7. **Development of severe alkalosis**: Patients who have emergency intubation are often vigorously hyperventilated; this can decrease the P_{CO_2} to less than 20 mm Hg. If the plasma bicarbonate level is normal (24 mEq/L), this degree of hypocarbia will increase the arterial pH to 7.70.

AXIOM Sudden severe alkalosis with a pH of 7.70 can reduce ionized calcium and magnesium levels by 12% to 24% (4% to 8% decrease for each 0.1 pH increase), and this can cause severe arrhythmias.

Thoracotomy

Most surgeons agree that with the proper personnel and facilities, resuscitative thoracotomy should be performed on patients who have a cardiac arrest (resulting from a penetrating wound, particularly a stab wound, of the chest or extremities) within 5 minutes of arrival in the ED. The objectives of an ED resuscitative thoracotomy are to

1. Release cardiac tamponade;
2. Control intrathoracic bleeding;
3. Treat or prevent air embolism;
4. Redistribute the available blood flow to vital organs (brain and heart) by cross-clamping the descending thoracic aorta; and
5. Optimize CO by performing open cardiac massage (4).

Release of Pericardial Tamponade

Pericardial tamponade is said to be characterized by Beck's triad, which includes hypotension, distended neck veins, and muffled heart tones. In the hypovolemic patient, distended neck veins may not appear until fluid resuscitation has begun, and even then, Beck's triad is often falsely positive or falsely negative (5).

AXIOM The quickest way—before pericardiocentesis or thoracotomy—to increase the blood pressure (BP) in a patient with pericardial tamponade is to administer intravenous fluids.

Control of Intrathoracic Hemorrhage

Life-threatening intrathoracic hemorrhage requiring a thoracotomy occurs in fewer than 10% of patients after penetrating trauma and is most frequently the result of bleeding from lung injuries (6). If a major systemic vessel is involved, bleeding should be controlled with proximal and distal clamping. If the aorta is involved, side clamping, digital pressure, or a rapid running suture under a finger is used to control the bleeding until an adequate heartbeat is obtained.

Providing an Airway

If an endotracheal tube cannot be inserted in less than 30 seconds, that attempt at intubation should stop, and the patient should be ventilated by a mask with 100% oxygen for 2 to 3 minutes before attempting intubation again. If an adequate airway cannot be established rapidly with an oral airway or endotracheal tube in an apneic patient, an emergency coniotomy (cricothyroidotomy) should be performed.

Optimizing Oxygen Delivery

If spontaneous cardiac function resumes, an attempt should be made to optimize tissue oxygen delivery (DO_2) to make up for the oxygen deficit that accumulated during the cardiac arrest. If a pulmonary artery (PA) catheter is in place, one can increase the circulating blood volume until the cardiac index (CI) is 4.0 to 4.5 L/min/m^2 or until the CO will not increase with further increase of the central venous pressure (CVP) and pulmonary artery wedge pressure (PAWP) by using fluid or blood. Inotropes also may be used to increase CI. Oxygen-carrying capacity can be maximized by increasing hematocrit levels to 35% to 40% or higher. If these measures fail to increase the oxygen consumption (VO_2) in a previously normal individual to 150 mL/min/m^2 or higher within 12 hours of injury, there is an increased incidence of multiple organ failure (7).

External Cardiac Massage

External CPR increases cerebral venous and intracranial pressures, which can reduce cerebral perfusion pressures (CPPs) and oxygenation. In contrast, direct or open massage of the heart does not occlude the veins in the chest and therefore can provide perfusion pressures much closer to normal.

Experimental and clinical data suggest that, for a successful outcome, CPR should produce at least 20% of the normal CO and a coronary perfusion pressure (which is equal to the aortic diastolic pressure minus right atrial diastolic pressure) of at least 20 to 30 mm Hg (8). These pressures are more likely to be approached during external CPR if high-dose epinephrine (0.1 to 0.2 mg/kg) is administered.

Other Considerations. The ideal rate for cardiac massage in adults is about 80 compressions per minute. Inexperienced personnel tend to massage the heart too rapidly, thereby reducing filling time between compressions. The addition of interposed abdominal compressions (IACs) to standard CPR may improve survival after in-hospital cardiac arrest (9).

AXIOM After 20 minutes of unsuccessful resuscitation, further interventions are likely to be futile, except when cardiac arrest occurs during hypothermia.

The incidence of iatrogenic injuries from external CPR range from 10% to 40%, with about 30% of the victims having iatrogenic rib fractures and almost 20% having sternal fractures (10). Less frequent, but potentially lethal, complications include lacerations to the heart, large vessels, liver, spleen, or gastroesophageal area.

Evaluating CPR Effectiveness. Blood pressure, skin color, state of consciousness, and electrocardiographic changes should be closely monitored to evaluate the effectiveness of the resuscitative efforts during CPR. Direct intraarterial pressure monitoring may also be helpful, but the aortic pressures generated during precordial compression have been found to correlate poorly with CO.

AXIOM Acid–base monitoring during cardiac resuscitation should include arterial and mixed venous blood gases, lactate levels, and end-tidal CO_2 (11).

Studies in animals and humans during CPR have demonstrated increased systemic venoarterial P_{CO_2} differences directly proportional to the reduced pulmonary blood flow. Normally, arterial blood has a pH that is 0.05 to 0.06 higher, a bicarbonate that is 1.1 mEq/L lower, and P_{CO_2} that is 6 to 8 mm Hg lower than central venous or mixed venous blood. In patients with a low CO, the P_{CO_2} differences may be increased two- to fourfold.

With external CPR, the increase in $P_{ET}CO_2$ directly correlates with pulmonary blood flow, coronary perfusion pressure (CPP), and CO (12). If the $P_{ET}CO_2$ stays less than 10 mm Hg during CPR, the successful resuscitation is extremely unlikely. If spontaneous circulation is restored, an abrupt further increase in $P_{ET}CO_2$ occurs to levels that transiently exceed prearrest values. This is the result of the washout of the increased venous CO_2.

Open-Chest (Direct) Cardiac Massage

In normovolemic cardiac arrest, open cardiac massage has been shown to generate aortic pressures that are about 60% of prearrest values (4). External chest compressions, in contrast, provide only 3% to 10% of the normal coronary and cerebral perfusion.

If a cardiac arrest within the past 5 minutes is the result of a penetrating chest wound, the physician should not hesitate to perform open cardiac massage. Prerequisites for performing open cardiac massage should include a physician experienced in performing thoracotomies and direct cardiac massage, and an ED/OR system that can rapidly provide the needed surgical support.

Thoracotomy Techniques

The initial incision of choice for ED thoracotomy for open CPR is an anterolateral thoracotomy on the side of the thoracic injury. Extension of the incision across the sternum and into the other hemithorax can be accomplished quickly with a Lebsche knife or rib shears. If better exposure of the superior mediastinum is needed, the superior sternum can be split in the midline. This incision can also be extended into the right or left neck or supraclavicular fossa as needed for control of more distal injuries to arch vessels.

The pericardial sac is opened for optimal internal cardiac massage, relief of any suspected tamponade, and operative control of any heart wounds. Resuscitation after opening the pericardial sac can be discontinued if

- There is no cardiac activity;
- The heart is completely empty; and
- The patient has had no signs of life for more than 5 minutes.

If the heart is beating, the bleeding is controlled with a fingertip and efforts at cardiorrhaphy are delayed until the initial resuscitative measures have been completed. In the nonbeating heart, suturing should be done rapidly before defibrillation. Ventricular wounds are often closed with 2-0 nonabsorbable horizontal mattress sutures tied over Teflon pledgets. Lacerations of the atria or large veins can often be repaired with simple running 3-0 nonabsorbable sutures.

For massive wounds of the ventricle or inaccessible posterior wounds, the patient should be placed on cardiopulmonary bypass, if rapidly available, to accomplish a proper unhurried closure. If bypass is not rapidly available, a saline slush may be applied over the heart, and the superior and inferior vena cava can be occluded temporarily to facilitate myocardial repairs.

If the heart is completely empty or internal defibrillation does not rapidly result in vigorous return of cardiac activity or both, the descending thoracic aorta should be occluded to maximize coronary and cerebral perfusion. However, if the heart begins to beat and if the systolic BP in the proximal aorta is allowed to exceed 160 to 180 mm Hg, the resultant strain on the left ventricle can cause acute distention with resultant failure and pulmonary edema.

Clinical Results of Emergency Department Thoracotomy

In a review of 11 reports by Moore et al. (4), the survival rate with an ED thoracotomy for trauma was 27% (81 of 296) for patients in shock, 13% (65 of 511) for patients with no vital signs, and 2.3% (15 of 651) for patients with no signs of life. The overall survival rate was 11% (161 of 1,458). Our overall survival rate with ED thoracotomy at Detroit Receiving Hospital (DRH) was 10% (26 of 272). The survival rate with stab wounds (20%; 14 of 69) was much better than for gunshot wounds (6%; 12 of 203). If the DRH patients with no signs of life at the scene are excluded, the survival rates were 25% and 8%, respectively.

Monitoring Preload

After a cardiac arrest, there may be persistent severe left ventricular failure allowing the left atrial pressure to increase rapidly and pulmonary edema to develop in spite of a low CVP (13). Under such circumstances, PAWPs may reflect left heart filling pressures better than the CVP.

Drug Therapy

If there is essentially no tissue perfusion, it is not unusual for the central venous or pulmonary arterial pH to decrease below 7.0 within 4 to 5 minutes of cardiac arrest. If V-fib is terminated by an electric shock but quickly recurs, various drugs may be used to attempt to reduce the irritability of the heart. However, before giving drugs, one should ascertain that the patient is not severely acidotic, alkalotic, hypoxic, or hypothermic.

α-Adrenergic Agents

With asystole, **epinephrine** is the best drug available for stimulating the heart. α-adrenergic agents, such as epinephrine, can increase successful return of spontaneous circulation with CPR by increasing diastolic aortic pressure and CPP. The usual initial intravenous or intracardiac dose of epinephrine is 0.01 to 0.02 mg/kg or 0.5 to 1.0 mg (10 mL of a 1:10,000 solution) in an average-sized adult. This may be repeated every 3 to 5 minutes. The various other doses of epinephrine that may be tried include

1. Intermediate: 1 to 5 mg every 3 to 5 minutes;
2. Escalating: 1 mg, then 3 mg, and then 5 mg, 3 minutes apart; and
3. High dose: 0.1 mg/kg every 3 to 5 minutes.

Epinephrine may be especially important if a cardiac arrest occurs during a high spinal anesthetic (14); however, although high-dose epinephrine may improve the initial CPR success rate, it probably does not increase the number of central nervous system (CNS)-intact patients leaving the hospital alive.

AXIOM If the physician is unable to start an intravenous line promptly in a patient with a cardiac arrest, epinephrine can be given through the endotracheal tube.

Some of the drugs that may be used to treat hypotension after resuscitation include **dopamine**, **epinephrine**, and **norepinephrine**. The ACLS guidelines suggest the use of low-dose norepinephrine for a systolic BP less than 70 mm Hg because high doses of dopamine tend to have a greater dysrhythmogenic effect (15).

The only indication for **isoproterenol** in acute cardiac care is for temporary control of hemodynamically significant atropine-resistant bradyarrhythmias and refractory torsades de pointes (15). Under such circumstances, isoproterenol can be infused at 1 to 2 μg/min. This may produce a significant increase in cardiac output; however, higher doses increase cardiac irritability.

Dopamine is a naturally occurring catecholamine that has various dose-dependent effects. At 1 to 3 μg/kg/min, dopamine is predominantly a splanchnic vasodilator (causing increased blood flow to the kidneys and other viscera). Dopamine, in doses of 5 to 15 μg/kg/min, acts primarily as a positive inotropic agent and increases CO and BP (16). Larger doses of dopamine tend to have an increasing alpha effect so that, with doses above 30 to 40 μg/kg/min, its effects tend to be primarily those of a vasoconstrictor.

Dobutamine is a synthetic adrenergic-like drug with inotropic and vasodilator effects. At doses of 5 to 15 μg/kg/min, it increases cardiac output and slightly reduces systemic vascular resistance. Blood pressure tends to remain constant. Dobutamine tends to cause less of an increase in pulmonary artery pressure and heart rate than dopamine.

Bicarbonate

AXIOM Bicarbonate should be withheld or given with extreme caution during cardiac arrests or shock.

The arterial P_{CO_2} ($P_{a}CO_2$) should be lower than [(1.5)(HCO_3) + 12]. In other words, if the arterial bicarbonate is 12.0 mEq/L and the $P_{a}CO_2$ is 40 mm Hg, the patient is said to have an "excess $P_{a}CO_2$" of 10.0 mm Hg. If an excess P_{CO_2} is present, bicarbonate administration can cause a paradoxic intracellular acidosis. Alkalemia from increased plasma bicarbonate levels also shifts the oxyhemoglobin dissociation curve to the left, thereby decreasing oxygen release at the tissue level. Alkalosis also reduces cerebral blood flow.

Calcium Salts

During a cardiac arrest, plasma ionized calcium levels may decrease abruptly (17); however, there is no evidence that suggests that administration of calcium salts improves outcome during CPR. Nevertheless, calcium may be helpful in patients with severe hyperkalemia, severe ionic hypocalcemia from multiple blood transfusions, or calcium channel–blocker overdoses.

AXIOM Administration of calcium is not advised during CPR except when cardiac arrest is associated with hyperkalemia, hypocalcemia, or calcium channel–blocking drugs.

Atropine

Atropine administration is indicated in cases of severe bradycardia with associated hypotension. The usual dose is 0.5 to 1.0 mg intravenously with a maximal dose of 0.04 mg/kg (3 mg in a 70-kg person). When adequate ventilation, effective cardiac massage, and the various drugs are unsuccessful in correcting symptomatic bradycardia, an external (transcutaneous) cardiac pacemaker may be considered.

Antiarrhythmic Agents

Ventricular tachycardia (V-tach) and unifocal or multifocal premature ventricular contractions may respond dramatically to **lidocaine**. The usual dose for dangerous premonitory arrhythmias is 1.0 to 1.5 mg/kg bolus with 0.5 to 0.75 mg/kg repeated in

5 to 10 minutes as needed. Once an adequate response has been obtained, lidocaine levels may be maintained by an intravenous infusion of 1 to 4 mg/min.

Bretylium is a potent alternative for treating recurrent V-fib/tach that is refractory to lidocaine. It initially releases norepinephrine at adrenergic nerve endings, and the resultant sympathomimetic effects (which may cause severe hypertension) last for about 20 to 30 minutes (18). Bretylium then prevents synaptic norepinephrine release, causing a decrease in systemic vascular resistance. Although bretylium, like lidocaine, raises the threshold for V-fib to occur, it differs from lidocaine in that the energy requirements for defibrillation are not increased.

Procainamide has a mechanism of action similar to that of lidocaine. However, it is generally reserved for treating multiple premature ventricular contractions (PVCs), V-tach, and wide complex tachyarrhythmias that are resistant to lidocaine (11). It is a second-line agent because it has a greater myocardial depressant effect than lidocaine, and it is more likely to cause severe hypotension. The usual dose of procainamide is 20 to 30 mg/min i.v. until either the arrhythmia is suppressed, the QRS is lengthened by 50%, hypotension occurs, or the patient receives a maximum of 17 mg/kg. If the arrhythmia is suppressed, a drip can then be started at 1 to 4 mg/min.

Adenosine is a purine nucleotide that suppresses SA and AV nodal function and is effective in terminating reentrant supraventricular tachycardias (11). Adenosine's short half-life (less than 10 seconds) and high efficacy (90% to 95%) make it an attractive drug to use during emergencies. Adverse effects are usually transient because of the kinetics of the agent and its rapid rate of elimination. The usual dose of adenosine is 6 mg over 1 to 3 minutes, followed by 12 mg if no response is seen in another 1 to 2 minutes.

Magnesium administration has been shown to suppress refractory V-tach, V-fib, and multifocal atrial tachycardia (MAT). It also reduces the incidence of post-MI arrhythmias in some patients (19). Magnesium should be administered in 1- to 2-g i.v. infusions over 5 to 60 minutes, depending on the urgency of the situation. It can then be continued as a maintenance i.v. drip at 0.5 to 1.0 g/h for 12 to 24 hours.

Quinidine is a potent antiarrhythmic drug that is used primarily to treat atrial tachyarrhythmias after the patient has been digitalized. The usual dose is 200 mg every 4 to 8 hours.

Digoxin may be used to treat rapid atrial fibrillation or flutter after cardiac resuscitation. The total intravenous dose is 1.0 to 1.5 mg administered over 12 to 18 hours in divided doses. In more urgent situations, 1 mg can be given in divided doses over 1 hour.

Arrhythmias during digitalis therapy are fairly frequent, particularly in patients with hypokalemia or hypercalcemia. **Dilantin**, **Digibind** (an antibody to digoxin), and **magnesium** may be useful in managing such arrhythmias.

EFFORTS TO IMPROVE CEREBRAL PERFUSION

After CPR, there is often prolonged impairment of cerebral blood flow. Six types of treatment have been used to try to reduce the amount of brain damage developing during or after experimental circulatory arrest.

1. **Brain-oriented life support**: Protocols designed to reduce postischemic brain damage by maintaining normal BP, blood gas values, and blood composition after restoration of spontaneous cardiac activity seem to improve overall cerebral function in both animal models and patients.
2. **Blood-flow promotion**: Hemodilution and moderate hypertension have improved outcome after 12 minutes of cardiac arrest in dogs (20).
3. **Barbiturates**: Barbiturates reduce cerebral oxygen consumption during postarrest hypoperfusion and have other beneficial effects, such as free-radical scavenging (21); however, no clinical benefits have been noted.
4. **Calcium entry blockers**: Long-term outcome studies with nimodipine after global brain ischemia in monkeys (22) showed beneficial results. However, the Brain Resuscitation Clinical Trial II using lidoflazine after arrest did not show any improvement in outcome when compared with controls (23).

5. **Free-radical scavengers**: The use of a cocktail of various free-radical scavengers has produced a modest, but significant improvement in outcome after asphyxial cardiac arrest in dogs; however, superoxide dismutase (SOD) or deferoxamine or both administered after global brain ischemia in humans showed no effect on survival or neurologic deficit scoring (24).
6. **Insulin-like growth factors**: White et al. (25) pointed out that these substances have the potential to reverse phosphorylation of elf-2 alpha, promote effective translation of the messenger RNA (mRNA) transcripts generated in response to ischemia and reperfusion, enhance neuronal defenses against free radicals, and stimulate lipid synthesis and membrane repair.

Fogel et al. (26) found that, after cardiac arrest, serum neurospecific enolase levels exceeding 33 mg/mL predicted persistent coma with a high specificity (100%) and a positive predictive value of 100%.

WHEN TO STOP ATTEMPTS AT CARDIAC RESUSCITATION

The only definite contraindication to cardiac resuscitation is an obvious normothermic death or a terminal disease in which the patient's suffering would only be prolonged. In addition, cardiac resuscitation should not be continued if there are unreconstructible injuries, uncontrollable bleeding, or apparent brain death demonstrated by fixed dilated pupils and absence of all reflexes for more than 20 to 30 minutes without hypothermia. Even without these injuries or signs, if adequate myocardial function cannot be restored after 30 minutes of effective massage, further attempts at resuscitation are generally futile.

⊘ FREQUENT ERRORS

1. ***Any delay in beginning CPR in a patient who apparently has no effective cardiac output.***
2. ***Failure to look for and rapidly correct the initial cause of a cardiac arrest.***
3. ***Failure to attempt preoxygenation of a "live" patient before attempting endotracheal intubation.***
4. ***Failure to use pulse oximetry to monitor critically injured patients in the ED.***
5. ***Failure to promptly check the position of the endotracheal tube after it is inserted.***
6. ***Failure to recognize a cardiac arrest until the patient has had a seizure or has regurgitated gastric contents.***
7. ***Failure to recognize that any new cardiovascular or neurologic symptoms developing soon after beginning positive-pressure ventilation may be caused by air emboli.***
8. ***Administration of bicarbonate for severe acidosis without checking for excess "P_{CO_2}" or decreased end-tidal CO_2 levels.***
9. ***Delay in cardioverting cardiac arrhythmias if the patient is hypotensive.***
10. ***Use of external cardiac massage in a patient with severe truncal trauma.***
11. ***Failure to immediately defibrillate electrically a patient who has just had a cardiac arrest.***

SUMMARY POINTS

1. Prehospital cardiac arrest is almost uniformly lethal if it persists for more than 5 minutes or results from problems that cannot be rapidly corrected.

2. Preintubation oxygenation can be extremely important in patients in acute respiratory failure after trauma.

3. Pulse oximetry should be used in all patients with severe trauma, especially during and after emergency intubation.

4. If there is any suspicion that the "endotracheal" tube is in the esophagus, it should be kept in place while another endotracheal tube is inserted.
5. Even if the endotracheal tube is correctly placed initially, it is easy for it to move down into a main-stem bronchus, especially on the right, particularly if the patient is small and agitated.
6. Severe hemoptysis after trauma is an indication for an emergency thoracotomy, especially if there is evidence of air embolism.
7. Any new cardiovascular or neurologic changes occurring during or just after endotracheal intubation and positive-pressure ventilation should be considered due to systemic air emboli until proven otherwise.
8. Sudden severe alkalosis (pH 7.70) can reduce ionized calcium and magnesium levels by 12% to 24% (4% to 8% decrease for each 0.1 pH increase), which may cause severe arrhythmias.
9. Ventricular tachycardia without hypotension can often be treated with medications alone, but immediate cardioversion is indicated if there is associated hypotension, chest pain, congestive heart failure (CHF), or signs of end-organ hypoperfusion.
10. If an adequate airway cannot be rapidly established with an oral airway or endotracheal tube in an apneic patient, an emergency coniotomy (cricothyroidotomy) should be performed.
11. Although patients with severe trauma require a minute ventilation that is at least twice normal, excessive ventilatory pressures can reduce venous return, and this can cause a cardiac arrest if the patient is severely hypovolemic.
12. Vigorous external cardiac massage can cause severe thoracoabdominal organ damage, especially in patients with recent truncal surgery or trauma.
13. If patients with an otherwise good prognosis have a cardiac arrest due to a mechanical problem (such as pericardial tamponade) and do not respond rapidly to closed cardiac massage, open cardiac massage may substantially improve their chances of survival.
14. Because many patients who have had cardiac arrest have a tendency to develop CHF, a large fluid bolus should not be given unless there is evidence of hypovolemia.
15. If a patient remains hypotensive after an otherwise successful cardiac resuscitation, insertion of a pulmonary artery catheter should be considered.
16. Acid–base monitoring during cardiac resuscitation should include arterial and mixed venous blood, lactate levels, and expired CO_2.
17. The $P_{ET}CO_2$ is a relatively good indicator of the quantity of pulmonary blood flow, especially during closed-chest CPR. During surgery, a $P_{(a\text{-}ET)}CO_2$ exceeding 10 mm Hg usually indicates inadequate pulmonary blood flow.
18. Early defibrillation is the most important determinant of survival from sudden cardiac arrest.
19. Persistent hypotension in trauma patients is usually caused by hypovolemia from continued bleeding.
20. α-adrenergic agents, such as epinephrine, increase the likelihood of a successful return of spontaneous circulation with CPR by increasing diastolic aortic pressure and CPP; but CNS-intact survival may not be increased.
21. Epinephrine should be administered in increasing doses if there is no satisfactory response to CPR within 2 to 3 minutes.
22. Isoproterenol should not be given if the patient has a tachycardia.
23. The administration of calcium is not advised during CPR except when cardiac arrest is associated with hyperkalemia, hypocalcemia, or calcium channel–blocking drugs.
24. Atropine may be used to help prevent asystole in high-degree A-V blocks, but it is usually indicated only during symptomatic bradycardia, endomyocardial disease (EMD), or asystole.
25. Lidocaine may be of benefit for preventing V-fib, but once V-fib occurs, lidocaine may make it more difficult to cardiovert it to a sinus rhythm.
26. Bretylium may be a potent alternative for recurrent V-fib/tach that is refractory to lidocaine.
27. If an intravenous line cannot be started promptly in a patient with a cardiac arrest, epinephrine can be given via the endotracheal tube.

28. Open cardiac massage is much more effective than closed-chest compression in patients with chest or abdominal trauma.
29. Resuscitative thoracotomy and open cardiac message will only on rare occasion successfully resuscitate a patient who has a cardiac arrest secondary to blunt trauma.
30. The quickest way (before pericardiocentesis or thoracotomy) to increase the BP in a patient with pericardial tamponade is to rapidly give intravenous fluids.
31. At the time of ED thoracotomy, further attempts at resuscitation should cease if there is no cardiac activity, the heart is completely empty, and the patient has had no signs of life for more than 5 minutes.
32. Thoracic aortic cross-clamping can greatly improve coronary and cerebral blood flow and reduce intraabdominal bleeding, but the systolic BP should not be allowed to exceed 160 mm Hg.
33. After cardiac resuscitation, one should increase oxygen delivery (D_{O_2}) until oxygen consumption (V_{O_2}) is above normal or will not increase any further as the D_{O_2} is increased.

REFERENCES

1. O'Neil BJ, Wilson RF. Cardiopulmonary resuscitation after trauma. In: Wilson RF, Walt AJ, eds. *Management of trauma: pitfalls and practice.* 2nd ed. Philadelphia: Williams & Wilkins, 1996:28–50.
2. Pasquale MD, Rhodes M, Cipolle MD, et al. Defining "Dead on Arrival": impact on a level one trauma center. *J Trauma* 1996;41:726.
3. Wilson RF, Soullier GW, Wienck RG. Hemoptysis in trauma. *J Trauma* 1987;27:1123–1126.
4. Moore JB, Moore EE, Harken AH. Emergency department thoracotomy. In: Moore EE, Mattox KL, Feliciano DV, eds. *Trauma.* 2nd ed. Norwalk, CT: Appleton & Lange, 1991:181–193.
5. Wilson RF, Bassett JS. Penetrating wounds of the pericardium or its contents. *JAMA* 1966;195:513–518.
6. Washington B, Wilson RF, Steiger Z. Emergency thoracotomy: a four-year review. *Ann Thorac Surg* 1985;40:188.
7. Moore FA, Haenel JB, Moore EE, et al. Incommensurate oxygen consumption in response to maximal oxygen availability predicts post-injury multiple organ failure. *J Trauma* 1992;33:58.
8. Paradis NA, Martin GB, Bovell D, et al. Coronary perfusion pressures during CPR are higher in patients with eventual return of spontaneous circulation. *Ann Emerg Med* 1989;18:478.
9. Halperin HR, Chandra NC, Levin HR. Newer methods of improving blood flow during CPR. *Ann Emerg Med* 1996;27:553.
10. Krischer JP, Fine EG, Davis JH, et al. Complications of cardiac resuscitation. *Chest* 1987;92:287–291.
11. Weil MH, Gazmuri RJ, Rackow EC. The clinical rationale of cardiac resuscitation. *Dis Month* 1990;36:431.
12. Sanders AB, Kern KB, Otto CW, et al. End-tidal carbon dioxide monitoring during cardiopulmonary resuscitation: a prognostic indicator of survival. *JAMA* 1989;262:1347–1351.
13. Wilson RF, Sarver E, Birks R. Central venous pressure and blood volume determinations in clinical shock. *Surg Gynecol Obstet* 1971;132:631.
14. Rosenberg JM, Wortsman J, Wahr JA, et al. Impaired neuroendocrine response mediates refractoriness to cardiopulmonary resuscitation in spinal anesthesia. *Crit Care Med* 1998;26:533.
15. Guidelines for cardiopulmonary resuscitation and emergency cardiac care. *JAMA* 1992;268:2201.
16. Wilson RF, Sibbald WJ, Jaanimagi JL. Hemodynamic effects of dopamine in critically ill septic patients. *J Surg Res* 1976;20:163–172.
17. Urban P, Scheidegger D, Buchmann B, et al. Cardiac arrest and blood ionized calcium levels. *Ann Intern Med* 1988;109:110–113.
18. Hanyok JJ, Chow MS, Kluger J, et al. Antifibrillatory effects of high dose

bretylium and a lidocaine-bretylium combination during cardiopulmonary resuscitation. *Crit Care Med* 1988;16:691–694.
19. Ceremuzynski L, Jurgizil R, Kulakowski P, et al. Threatening arrhythmia and acute myocardial infarction are prevented by IV $MgSO_4$. *Am Heart J* 1989;118: 1333.
20. Safar P, Stezoski SW, Nemoto EM. Amelioration of brain damage after 12 minutes cardiac arrest in dogs. *Arch Neurol* 1976;33:91.
21. Siesjo BK. Cell damage in the brain: a speculative synthesis. *J Cereb Blood Flow Metab* 1981;1:155.
22. Steen PA, Gisvold SE, Milde JH, et al. Nimodipine improves outcome when given after complete cerebral ischemia in primates. *Anesthesiology* 1985;62:406.
23. Robers MC, Nugent SK, Stidham GL. Effects of closed-chest cardiac massage on intracranial pressure. *Crit Care Med* 1979;7:454.
24. Krause GS, White BC, Aust SD, et al. Brain cell death following ischemia and reperfusion: a proposed biochemical sequence. *Crit Care Med* 1988;16:714.
25. White BC, Grossman LI, O'Neil BJ, et al. Global brain ischemia and reperfusion. *Ann Emerg Med* 1996;27:588.
26. Fogel W, Krieger D, Veith M, et al. Serum neuron-specific enolase as early predictor of outcome after cardiac arrest. *Crit Care Med* 1997;25:1133.

4. BLOOD REPLACEMENT[1]

AXIOM Prompt correction of severe blood-volume deficits in the critically injured patient may be lifesaving; however, inappropriate use of blood and fluids can cause severe complications.

CRYSTALLOIDS

The terms "crystalloid" and "colloid" refer to solute particles that will or will not pass through a semipermeable membrane. Isotonic fluids, such as Ringer's lactate and normal saline, distribute evenly throughout the extracellular space. In healthy adults, equilibration of these balanced electrolyte solutions (BESs) with the extracellular space occurs within 20 to 30 minutes after infusion. After 1 hour, about one third of the volume infused remains in the intravascular space. In contrast, glucose in water equilibrates with the entire body water so that only about one fifteenth (60 to 70 mL of 1 L) will remain in the vascular space.

⊘ PITFALL

The major pitfall to avoid during fluid resuscitation is inadequate or slow administration. One usually needs 3 to 4 L of crystalloid to replace a 1,000-mL blood loss.

The adequacy of intravascular volume repletion is indicated by

- Stable mean arterial pressure of at least 70 to 80 mm Hg;
- Heart rate decreasing to less than 100 to 110 beats/min;
- Warm extremities with good capillary refill;
- Adequate central nervous system function;
- Urine volume of at least 0.5 to 1.0 mL/kg/h;
- Absence of lactic acidosis; and
- Core temperature above 35°C.

Recently some studies supported the use of gastric mucosal pH (pH_i) as a guide to the adequacy of resuscitation (2). In general, a pH_i below 7.30 indicates inadequate splanchnic perfusion. Wilson et al. (3) also found that a low end-tidal P_{CO_2} (<22 mm Hg) or arterial to end-tidal P_{CO_2} differences of 10 to 13 mm Hg or more after resuscitation were associated with an increased mortality rate (50% to 53% vs. 18% to 23%).

In older patients with underlying cardiopulmonary problems, monitoring of pulmonary artery wedge pressure, cardiac output, mixed venous oxygen saturation, and serum lactate levels also should be used to guide fluid administration (4).

Normal (0.9%) saline and Ringer's lactate are the most frequently used crystalloids for resuscitation and, generally, can be given interchangeably. The theoretic concern that large volumes of normal saline produce a "dilution acidosis" or hyperchloremic acidosis is seldom a problem clinically. The excess circulating chloride ions are normally excreted by the kidney quite readily.

AXIOM Administration of large quantities of saline solution in patients with continued inadequate tissue perfusion or ketoacidosis can contribute to the development of a hyperchloremic (nonanion gap) metabolic acidosis.

Although crystalloids can expand the intravascular volume, they dilute the remaining red cells and protein, reducing the oxygen-carrying capacity, buffering ability, and colloid osmotic pressure of the blood. "Edema safety factors," which limit the tendency for reduced colloid oncotic pressure to increase extravascular lung water (EVLW) include increased lymphatic flow, diminished pulmonary interstitial oncotic pressure, and increased interstitial hydrostatic pressure (3). When the total crystalloid volume administered is controlled to prevent volume overload, there is usually no difference in lung function in patients with shock resuscitated with crystalloids or colloid solutions.

AXIOM Crystalloid resuscitation of the critically injured patient usually does not impair pulmonary function unless there is lung damage or the patient develops right-sided heart failure.

Acute loss of up to 30% of the blood volume may be adequately replaced with crystalloid alone if given rapidly in quantities equal to three to four times the blood lost. Nevertheless, in critically injured patients who have been hypotensive, it is my practice to maintain the hemoglobin concentration above 10.0 g/dL, without giving large amounts of albumin.

⊘ PITFALL

Large quantities of Ringer's lactate given to patients with severe liver disease may precipitate a severe lactic acidosis.

Lactate may be metabolized very slowly when liver function or perfusion is impaired. In patients with advanced cirrhosis, normal or half-normal saline with an ampule of sodium bicarbonate (44.6 mEq) in each liter of fluid is preferable to Ringer's lactate. Normal (0.9%) saline contains 154 mEq/L each of sodium and chloride, and Ringer's lactate contains 130 mEq/L sodium, 109 mEq/L chloride, 28 mEq/L lactate, 4 mEq/L potassium, and 3 mEq/L calcium. Half (14 mEq) of the lactate is *l*-lactate, which can undergo hepatic metabolism and is converted to bicarbonate to release 14 mEq of free base per liter of solution. The other 14 mEq/L of lactate is *r*-lactate, which can be excreted unchanged in the urine. In patients with renal failure, the 4 mEq/L of potassium may contribute to a hyperkalemic state, in which case, normal saline should be substituted. Similarly, normal saline is preferred to Ringer's lactate in hypercalcemic, hyperkalemic, or hyponatremic states. In the presence of established hyperchloremic metabolic acidosis, Ringer's lactate is preferred because it provides a bicarbonate source and reduces the administered chloride load.

AXIOM Because of the calcium present in Ringer's lactate, it should not be infused with or in the same intravenous (i.v.) tubing as bank blood.

COLLOIDS

The normal plasma colloid oncotic pressure (COP) of 28 mm Hg is an important factor in determining the distribution of fluid across capillary membranes. A high COP will "pull" fluid into the capillaries, which tends to restore intravascular volume and reduce interstitial edema.

A profound reduction in COP may reduce left ventricular compliance, increase pulmonary extravascular water, decrease tissue oxygen delivery, and impair wound healing (4).

Albumin

AXIOM Albumin may be of value for expanding blood volume, especially in severely hypoproteinemic patients, but it is expensive, and excessive amounts can cause cardiac, pulmonary, and renal problems.

The average molecular weight (MW) of endogenous albumin is 65,000. About 12 to 14 g is synthesized daily by the liver, and it accounts for about 80% of the plasma COP (5). A normal adult has 4 to 5 g of albumin per kilogram body weight in the extracellular space, but only about 30% to 40% of this is present in the intravascular compartment, resulting in a normal serum level of about 3.5 to 5.0 g/dL. Much of the endogenous albumin in the interstitial space is tissue bound and unavailable to the circulation. Unbound or "free" interstitial-space albumin returns to the vascular compartment through lymphatic drainage. The half-life of albumin in the body is about 20 to 22 days (5).

AXIOM In severe injury or stress, hepatic albumin synthesis decreases, and the production of acute-phase reactants such as fibrinogen and C-reactive protein increase significantly.

Administered albumin distributes itself throughout the extracellular space. The plasma half-life of exogenous albumin is usually about 12 to 16 hours. In severe shock or sepsis, the hourly disappearance rate of exogenous albumin increases from a normal 7% to 8% per hour to more than 30% per hour (6).

Albumin is available as a 5% or 25% solution in isotonic saline. It is prepared by fractionating blood from healthy donors and heating it to 60°C for 10 hours, which inactivates the hepatitis viruses and the human immunodeficiency virus (HIV). Plasma volume expansion resulting from infusion of 500 mL of 5% albumin ranges from 250 to 750 mL (6). The 25% albumin solution contains 12.5 g of albumin in 50 mL of buffered solution containing approximately 130 to 160 mEq/L sodium. The infusion of 100 mL of 25% albumin solution (25 g albumin) increases the intravascular volume about 300 to 600 mL (average, 450 mL) over 30 to 60 minutes (7).

In addition to its plasma volume-expansion effects, albumin may have other clinically useful properties including binding and inactivation of proteolytic enzymes, maintenance of microvascular permeability to protein, and scavenging of free radicals (8).

⊘ **PITFALL**

Infusion of albumin, especially to hypotensive patients, may rapidly reduce ionized calcium levels and contribute to myocardial failure or shock.

Each gram of albumin binds about 0.8 mg of calcium and may temporarily reduce ionized calcium levels, producing a negative inotropic effect on the myocardium.

Dextran

AXIOM Low molecular weight dextran (Dextran 40) can be an effective colloid, but it may cause increased bleeding from open wounds, difficulty with typing and cross-matching of blood, and occasional anaphylactoid reactions.

Dextran is a glucose polymer formed from sucrose by the bacterium *Leuconostoc mesenteroides*. D-40 and D-70 contain particles with molecular weights ranging from 10,000 to 80,000 and 40,000 to 100,000, respectively (7). Particles less than 15,000 MW are rapidly filtered by the kidney, and 50% to 75% of these are lost in the urine in 15 to 30 minutes; however, while in the circulation, they exert osmotic activity. Larger particles (MW of 15,000 to 50,000) are lost more slowly in the urine, but approximately 40% of the Dextran with a molecular weight less than 50,000 is excreted in the urine within 24 hours. After 24 hours, the particles remaining in the circulation have an average MW of more than 80,000. These particles are taken up by the reticuloendothelial system and enzymatically degraded to glucose at a rate of 70 to 90 mg/kg/day and metabolized to carbon dioxide and water.

Dextran has at least two properties of an ideal plasma volume expander: a relatively long dwell time in the circulation and ultimate biodegradability (9). A 500-mL bolus of D-40 produces an intravascular volume expansion of 750 mL within the first hour and 1,050 mL within 2 hours. This volume expansion may persist for up to 8 hours in hypovolemic patients.

In addition to improving the overall cardiac output, dextran also improves blood flow in the microvasculature by coating endothelial and blood cell surfaces, decreasing viscosity, and preventing red blood cell (RBC) sludging.

⊘ PITFALL

If dextran is given with multiple blood transfusions, it may be difficult to determine the cause of reactions or increased hemorrhage.

Anaphylactoid reactions to dextran can be clinically identical to anaphylactic reactions; however, anaphylactoid reactions occur with synthetic compounds and do not involve reagin (immunoglobulin E; IgE). In contrast, anaphylactic reactions involve naturally occurring compounds and involve reagin (IgE). The incidence of anaphylactoid reactions to dextran is probably less than 0.1%. If there is an allergic reaction, it usually occurs within half an hour after the infusion is begun and is usually manifested only by urticaria, rash, nausea, and bronchospasm.

⊘ PITFALL

If the blood bank is not informed of the recent administration of dextran to a patient who requires blood transfusions, it may fail to obtain a proper type and cross-match.

Dextran can interfere with the cross-matching of blood by inhibiting RBC aggregation. This is handled best by drawing blood before dextran infusions. If dextran was started before the blood sample was obtained, the blood bank should be notified so that the dextran can be washed off the RBCs before the cross-matching.

⊘ PITFALL

If dextran is given to patients with large open wounds, excessive blood loss may occur.

Dextran decreases platelet adhesiveness and can precipitate fibrinogen, factor VIII fibrin monomers, and von Willebrand factor. This can result in prolonged bleeding times and increased incisional bleeding; however, at doses less than 20 mL/kg/day (1.5 g/kg/day), clinical bleeding is usually not encountered (10).

Because dextran particles with MWs less than 50,000 are rapidly filtered through the glomerulus, an osmotic diuresis can occur almost immediately. This may result in a diuresis that may make hypovolemia and oliguria worse. In oliguric patients, the dextran may precipitate within the renal tubules and can cause acute renal failure.

Hydroxyethyl Starch

AXIOM Hydroxyethyl starch (Hetastarch, HES) is an effective colloid for expanding blood volume, but excessive use can cause increased bleeding.

Hydroxyethyl starch (hetastarch, HES) is a synthetic starch molecule derived almost entirely from amylopectin (7). HES is available for clinical use as a 6% solution in normal saline. Plasma volume expansion after infusion of HES is approximately 100% to 170%. This is equal to or slightly greater than the volume expansion produced by D-70 or 5% albumin. HES also has a plasma retention time of 12 to 48 hours, which is slightly longer than that with D-70 or albumin.

Administering HES to subjects who are bleeding, especially in doses exceeding 20 mL/kg/day, can cause a number of coagulation and bleeding changes including

1. Reduction in fibrinogen levels because of hemodilution;
2. Prolongation of partial thromboplastin and bleeding times;
3. Shortening of thrombin, reptilase, and urokinase-activated clot lysis times; and
4. Reduction in factor VIII complex concentration to a greater degree than accounted for by hemodilution (11).

These findings are suggestive of enhanced fibrinolysis and a direct interaction of HES with factor VIII.

Serum amylase levels may double after HES administration. This occurs because plasma amylase forms complexes with HES molecules, creating large macroamylase particles, which are excreted in the urine at a much slower rate than the usual amylase molecules.

Pentastarch

Pentastarch is a low-molecular-weight form of HES with a lower MW of 63,000 (7). Pentastarch is more rapidly and completely degraded by circulating amylase than is HES and, therefore, it is more rapidly and effectively eliminated directly in the urine. The potential advantages of pentastarch include a greater degree of plasma volume expansion per volume infused, faster onset, and more rapid elimination from the blood. The effects of pentastarch on coagulation appear to be proportional to its degree of hemodilution only.

Pentastarch has been used successfully as an adjunct to leukopheresis, but clinical trials showed that it may also be a useful colloid in fluid resuscitation. Doses of pentastarch up to 2,000 mL/day appear to be well tolerated, and its volume-expanding capability is slightly greater than that of 5% albumin.

Fresh Frozen Plasma

AXIOM Fresh frozen plasma (FFP) can correct deficiencies in clotting factors (not platelets) and antithrombin, but it can also transmit blood-borne diseases.

The main indication for use of FFP is the presence of multiple coagulation-factor deficiencies. It takes 20 to 40 minutes to thaw and must be given through a filter. If used within 2 hours of thawing, it contains normal levels of coagulation factors. Delays decrease the coagulation-factor activity, especially for factor VII.

AXIOM Compatibility testing for FFP is not required, but it should be ABO compatible.

Crystalloids Versus Colloids

AXIOM Successful resuscitation is primarily dependent on the adequacy of fluid replacement and not on the composition of fluid itself.

Controversies over the type of fluid used for resuscitation ("colloid vs. crystalloid") centers mainly on issues relating to philosophy, side effects, and economics (12; Table 4-1).

HYPERTONIC SALINE SOLUTIONS

AXIOM Hypertonic saline can rapidly expand blood volume, but it can cause excess vasodilation and serum sodium levels greater than 160 to 165 mEq/L.

Hypertonic saline solution (HSS; 1,200 to 2,500 mOsm/L) has been shown to resuscitate patients effectively with less edema formation and better tissue perfusion than normal saline solution (NSS; 13). In addition to pulling intracellular fluid into the

Table 4-1. ***Crystalloids versus colloids***

Colloid proponents argue	Crystalloid proponents argue
The key problem in shock is a loss of circulating blood volume, thus making replacement with colloid appropriate	The key problem in shock is shrinkage of the ECF; therefore, replacement with crystalloids is more appropriate
Crystalloids, because of the prompt equilibration with extracellular fluid (ECF), must be infused in amounts exceeding estimated losses by at least three to four times	Fluid overload causing congestive heart failure and/or pulmonary edema is less likely to occur with crystalloids because of their rapid equilibration with ECF
Crystalloids reduce the colloid osmotic pressure, thus favoring the development of pulmonary edema (17)	Administered colloids may cross the pulmonary capillary membrane in patients with increased microvascular permeability, pulling water along with them
	Crystalloids are free from the risk of occasional (less than 0.05%) anaphylactoid reactions, which can occur with any colloid solution, especially synthetic colloids
	Colloids, except possibly for FFP (18), have adverse effects on coagulation either by dilution of the factors or by actually interfering with their production or function
	Fluid resuscitation with colloids is 10 to 100 times more expensive than equivalent blood volume expansion with crystalloid infusions

extracellular space, hypertonic saline also is reported to exert direct inotropic actions on the myocardium, cause vasodilation, decrease intracranial pressure (ICP), and enhance vagally mediated reflex venoconstriction (14). In a study of 34 patients with moderate to severe head injuries, Shackford et al. (15) found that hypertonic saline tended to cause a decrease in ICP, whereas (isotonic) Ringer's lactate tended to increase it. In uncontrolled hemorrhage experiments, small-volume hypertonic resuscitation (vs. no resuscitation) can improve arterial blood pressure and survival (16).

AUTOLOGOUS TRANSFUSION (AUTOTRANSFUSION)

AXIOM Autotransfusion can reduce blood-bank needs and reduce the risk of blood-borne diseases, but if used in excess, especially in patients in shock, it can cause coagulopathies.

The advantage of autotransfusion is that blood can be available for administration without delays or a need for a cross-match. Of greater importance to many individuals has been the concern over transmission of disease with bank blood. With autotransfusion, the risk of transmitted disease such as hepatitis, acquired immunodeficiency syndrome (AIDS), malaria, and syphilis is eliminated. Furthermore, no hemolytic, febrile, or allergic reactions have been reported during autotransfusion.

AXIOM Autotransfusion with blood contaminated with intestinal contents is not absolutely contraindicated, especially if no other blood is available, if the autotransfused red cells are washed well, and if antibiotics are given in full dose.

Blood collected during operations may or may not be washed, but it must be filtered before reinfusion. Although washing the collected RBCs takes some time, it is advantageous because it removes fibrin, cellular debris, free hemoglobin, potassium, and various procoagulants, and anticoagulants. Extensive autotransfusion of blood washed with normal saline can cause a hyperchloremic metabolic acidosis plus significant decreases in protein, calcium, and magnesium levels (17).

AXIOM Autotransfusions are safest if used in moderation and if the RBCs are carefully washed before infusion.

The administration of large volumes of autotransfused blood may also cause thrombocytopenia and decreased levels of coagulation factors. In patients with extensive tissue damage or prolonged shock, this may increase the incidence of disseminated intravascular coagulation (DIC) and activation of fibrinolytic mechanisms. Increased bleeding due to heparinization also may occur as a result of residual heparin that is reinfused despite washing of the autotransfused RBCs.

In general, the amount of autotransfused blood should be limited to 3,000 mL or less (18). If autotransfusion is used in a trauma victim, it should be considered an adjunct to the use of cross-matched blood available from the blood bank. Patients who are autotransfused should have serial coagulation studies, which include platelet count, platelet function, prothrombin time (PT), partial thromboplastin time (PTT), and fibrinolytic activity. Coagulation abnormalities should be treated as needed.

BLOOD TRANSFUSIONS

AXIOM Young, healthy individuals can do well with a hemoglobin of 7.0 g/dL if they are hemodynamically stable and their bleeding is controlled.

As a general rule, a hematocrit of 20% to 25% provides adequate oxygen delivery if blood volume and cardiac output are normal or increased and the hemoglobin is at least 90% saturated with oxygen. In most critically ill or injured patients, a hematocrit of at least 30% to 35% is preferable. In patients with severe sepsis or cardiopulmonary dysfunction, a hematocrit of 35% to 40% is preferred.

Almost all blood transfusions today are packed RBCs. An average unit of packed RBCs is approximately 250 to 350 cc, with an average hematocrit between 60% and 80%.

Frozen Red Blood Cells

After mixing with glycerol solutions, RBCs can be frozen at –80°C (–176°F), at which temperature they can be maintained indefinitely (19). When needed, the RBCs are thawed by direct immersion into a stirring bath at 37°C (98.6°F). The thawed cells are washed, centrifuged to remove the glycerol solution, and resuspended in a saline–glucose solution, producing a final hematocrit of 35% to 55%. The advantages of frozen cells are

1. No citrate or other additives are required;
2. There are no incompatible antibodies;
3. The risk of hepatitis is reduced;
4. There is less chance of sensitization by plasma proteins, white cells, or platelets; and
5. Blood can be stored indefinitely.

Because of the time required to prepare and thaw them, however, frozen RBCs are of little benefit for acute resuscitation.

Blood Types

The "safest" type of blood to administer is that which has been fully cross-matched, because of a decreased risk of hemolytic reactions. Unfortunately, full cross-matching of blood may take 30 to 45 minutes or even longer if delays of transportation to and from the blood bank are incurred. Thus fully cross-matched blood is not rapidly available for emergency resuscitation.

O-Negative Blood

⊘ PITFALL

If physicians give type O un–cross-matched blood when it might be possible to delay infusion for 5 to 10 minutes by using other fluids or colloids, they greatly increase the risk of complications.

Because type O blood contains no cellular antigens, it is theoretically safer to give to patients regardless of their blood type with minimal risk of a donor antigen versus recipient antibody hemolytic reaction. The major benefit of O-negative blood is that it is available for transfusion without a cross-match. However, because the plasma of O-negative blood does contain anti-A and anti-B antibodies, significant minor transfusion reactions can occur if large volumes are infused. If more than 4 units of O-negative blood is administered to a patient with a different blood type, "admixture" situations may complicate subsequent cross-matching of blood (20).

Type-Specific Blood

Blood of the recipient's type (i.e., type-specific blood) that has not been cross-matched can generally be administered quite safely and can usually be released for transfusion within 10 to 15 minutes of arrival. This is generally thought to be preferable to giving O-negative un–cross-matched blood.

Problems with Massive Transfusions

Patients who require massive transfusions of 10 or more units of blood within 24 hours have a mortality rate that averages about 50%. In a series of 339 of our trauma patients receiving massive transfusions, the mortality rate averaged 47%. In those receiving 10 to 19 units of blood, the mortality rate was 28% (51 of 182); in those receiving 20 to 39 units, the mortality rate increased to 65% (78 of 121); and in those receiving 40 or more units, the mortality rate was 83% (30 of 36). The presence of a systolic blood pressure less than 80 mm Hg for 30 minutes or more and the presence of preexisting disease also were important. In 146 patients who received 10 or more units of blood but had no preexisting disease, were younger than 65 years, and had shock for less than 30 minutes, the mortality rate was only 17% (25 of 146). In contrast, massively transfused patients who had any of these problems had a mortality rate of 69% (134 of 193; $p < 0.0001$).

In examining acid–base balance during and after massive transfusions, it was noted that the patients who died had a lower mean (±SD) pH (7.08 ± 0.15 vs. 7.21 ± 0.15; $p < 0.001$), and a higher mean P_{CO_2} (47 ± 16 mm Hg vs. 43 ± 9 mm Hg; $p < 0.01$). Even more interesting was the progression of these acid–base changes in the 28 trauma patients with the most severe acidosis. During the first 2 hours in the operating room (OR), the mean pH in those who survived in the OR actually tended to be lower than that of those who died in the OR (6.92 ± 0.12 vs. 7.03 ± 0.22; $p = 0.11$). Over the next 2 hours, however, the patients who survived developed a higher pH (7.22 ± 0.09 vs. 7.08 ± 0.14; $p < 0.005$) and lower P_{CO_2} (39 ± 9 mm Hg vs. 54 ± 10 mm Hg; $p < 0.0001$). Indeed, no massively transfused patients with a persistent metabolic and respiratory acidosis survived.

Reactions

The administration of blood products may produce hemolytic or nonhemolytic reactions. Although the signs and symptoms of a major transfusion reaction are readily discernible in most patients, they may be extremely difficult to identify in a patient who is anesthetized, especially if he or she is in shock. Under these conditions, the first sign of a major transfusion reaction may be the sudden onset of urticaria, increased bleeding from open wounds, or hypotension.

⊘ PITFALL

If the usual signs of incompatibility are watched only during the first few minutes of a transfusion, recognition of significant reactions may be missed entirely.

Nonhemolytic Reactions

The most frequent types of reactions are nonhemolytic and involve the development of fever, urticaria, hives, or asthma after the administration of blood. The incidence of these reactions is approximately 2% to 10% (20). They may be related to leukocytes or proteins, and the incidence of these reactions may be reduced by the use of packed RBCs, washed RBCs, or special filters for the removal of leukocytes.

Hemolytic Reactions

AXIOM The most severe hemolytic transfusion reactions are generally caused by simple clerical errors.

Major hemolytic transfusion reactions occur from the interaction of antibodies in the plasma of the recipient with antigens in the RBCs of the donor. The majority of these cases (45%) are the result of clerical errors in which mistakes were made in the identification of blood samples or in the administration of blood to the wrong patient.

With O-negative blood, half of the fatal hemolytic reactions resulted from previously unidentified antibodies. In the remaining half, continued administration of type O blood caused non-O patients to develop "admixture" blood types with difficulty in subsequent cross-matching.

Major hemolytic transfusion reactions generally declare themselves clinically before 50 to 100 mL of blood has been infused. Nonhemolytic febrile or allergic reactions may not occur until all units of blood have been administered. Most febrile or allergic reactions occur in spite of a satisfactory type and cross-match. In a series of 624 transfusion reactions studied at Detroit Receiving Hospital, only 35 were found to involve a factor that might have been predicted by cross-matching or prevented with more care. These included transfusion of blood to the wrong patients in five instances.

If a major transfusion reaction is suspected, the transfusion should be stopped immediately and the remainder of the stored blood, plus a sample of the patient's blood, should be sent to the blood bank for repeated cross-match and analysis. Diphenhydramine (Benadryl; 50 mg) is given intramuscularly or intravenously immediately and every 6 hours as needed for urticaria, itching, or other allergic phenomena. If the patient is not in danger of overload, i.v. fluids should be administered rapidly with 12.5 to 25.0 g of mannitol to ensure a copious urine output of 100 to 200 mL/h. One to two ampules of sodium bicarbonate may be added to each liter of i.v. fluid to alkalinize the urine to a pH of at least 6.5. If shock occurs, adrenaline, hydrocortisone, and additional fluids also should be administered.

Changes in Blood During Storage

Although transfused blood is essential for its oxygen-carrying capacity in hypovolemic patients, its use in large quantities may cause significant problems. The effects of the anticoagulant preservative solution and refrigeration include reduced RBC viability, increased plasma hemoglobin, abnormal potassium concentrations, and reduced RBC concentrations of adenosine triphosphate (ATP) and 2,3-diphosphoglycerate (2,3-DPG; 21). The ATP content of the RBCs is maintained at normal levels for about 3 weeks in the blood bank, but at 35 days, it is only 50% of normal (22). Lower levels of ATP result in decreased deformability of red cells, thereby interfering with blood flow through capillaries.

AXIOM Blood that has been recently transfused can carry oxygen to the tissues but may not release it properly for several hours.

Levels of 2,3-DPG, although now better maintained than in previously used preservatives, are still only 70% of normal in bank blood at 14 days, 30% at 21 days, and 5% at 35 days. These low levels of 2,3-DPG greatly reduce oxygen availability to the tissues and may be a critical factor if cardiac output or the arterial P_{O_2} or both are low. Regeneration of 2,3-DPG in the patient without shock is rapid after transfusion, and levels usually increase to more than 50% of normal within 4 to 12 hours.

AXIOM The two most common causes of increased postoperative bleeding in a patient who has received massive transfusions are inadequate surgical hemostasis and thrombocytopenia.

After 24 to 48 hours of storage, there are virtually no functioning platelets in bank blood. Trauma patients with massive fluid and transfusion requirements frequently have platelet counts that are significantly decreased and continue to decline for 2 to 3 days. Although it is generally agreed that thrombocytopenia is the most important defect causing diffuse microvascular bleeding after massive blood transfusions (23), one must look for surgical causes of bleeding that may have been overlooked while the patient was hypotensive.

Table 4-2. ***Change in platelet count, prothrombin time (PT), and accelerated partial thromboplastin times (aPTT) with the number of units of blood (X ± SD)***

	10–19 Units	20–39 Units	40+ Units
Platelets*	72 ± 50 (89)	52 ± 38 (90)	41 ± 70 (27)
PT**	18 ± 10 (89)	21 ± 11 (82)	27 ± 20 (25)
aPTT**	62 ± 47 (89)	89 ± 68 (92)	132 ± 13 (26)

( ) = Number of patients; * × 10^3; ** seconds

In a recent study, platelet counts averaged 50,000/mm^3 after 20 or more blood transfusions (24). The mean platelet count decreased with the units of blood given from 72,000 to 52,000 to 41,000/mm^3 after 10 to 19, 20 to 39, and 40 or more units of transfused blood (Table 4-2). Any patient who is receiving massive blood transfusions and develops diffuse microvascular bleeding should be considered for platelet transfusions to increase the platelet count to at least 50,000/mm^3 and preferably to 80,000 to 100,000/mm^3.

During storage of whole blood, a marked decrease in coagulation factors occurs. By day 14, approximately 25% of factor VIII and 60% of factor V are lost (25). In a recent review, we found that the mean activated PTT (aPTT) increased from 62 to 89 to 132 seconds as the units of blood given increased from 10 to 19, to 20 to 39, to 40 or more within 24 hours (Table 4-2). Hypothermia and increased duration of shock increased the aPTT. The mean PT increased from 18 to 21 to 27 seconds as the number of blood transfusions in 24 hours increased from 10 to 19, to 20 to 39, to 40 or more, respectively.

In patients with unresponsive life-threatening hemorrhage, the use of unrefrigerated fresh whole blood may substantially reduce the need for FFP, cryoprecipitate, and platelets often needed in the treatment of posttransfusion coagulopathies (26).

⊘ PITFALL

If excessive operative bleeding in a critically injured patient is assumed to be due to a coagulopathy, the surgeon may not spend the time and effort needed to obtain proper hemostasis.

By far, the most frequent cause of excessive bleeding at the time of surgery is an inadequate effort by the surgeon in tying, suturing, or coagulating open vessels. Indeed, during a difficult operation in a poor-risk patient, the surgeon may, in frustration, attribute continued, excessive bleeding to a platelet or clotting defect. As a result, he or she may attempt to terminate the anesthetic as soon as possible, hoping that the hemostatic agents or packs or both will control the bleeding.

If a coagulation problem does develop or is suspected, the initial coagulation tests should include a platelet count, PT, and aPTT. More sophisticated tests include bleeding time, thrombin times, euglobulin lysis time, and direct measurement of fibrinogen and other individual clotting factors.

AXIOM If sophisticated clotting studies are not available in a patient who may have a coagulopathy, observation of 2 to 3 mL of blood placed in a clear stoppered test tube, and inverted once a minute, may provide valuable information on the blood's ability to clot.

If 2 to 3 mL of blood in a clean test tube clots within 5 to 10 minutes, it is unlikely that there is a significant deficit of platelets or other clotting factors. If the clot involves all the blood that was present, the fibrinogen level is probably greater than 100 mg/dL. If the clot begins to retract within an hour, at least 75,000 platelets/mm^3 are present.

AXIOM Blood for clotting studies should not be drawn from an indwelling catheter.

If blood drawn directly from a vein does not clot properly in the test tube, the patient probably has a deficit of platelets or other clotting factors. Blood drawn from a venous or arterial line may have heparin present from various flushing solutions, and this can prevent blood drawn from such catheters to clot properly.

Meticulous hemostasis, rapid complete correction of hypovolemia, and keeping the core temperature at 35°C or higher are the best prophylaxis and treatment for coagulation abnormalities during an operation. Hypothermic patients are particularly apt to develop a prolonged PTT (Table 4-3).

If large quantities of packed RBCs are administered, FF plasma and packed platelets may be needed, as indicated by clinical or laboratory abnormalities. Fresh frozen plasma contains normal levels of coagulation factors if administered within 2 hours of thawing.

Electrolyte Problems

During the storage of whole blood, plasma levels of potassium, ammonia, lactate, and hemoglobin increase, whereas bicarbonate and pH levels decrease. Potassium levels in the plasma may increase by up to 1 mEq/day, and the actual amount of potassium administered may exceed 6.6 mEq per unit of packed RBCs (18).

Table 4-3. ***Changes in accelerated partial thromboplastin times (aPTT) correlated with core temperature in patients receiving massive transfusions****

Core temperature	Number of patients	aPTT (sec) X ± SD
35°C or more	18	48 ± 41
34.0–34.9°C	24	66 ± 54
32.0–33.9°C	43	87 ± 63
Less than 32°C	25	120 ± 79

*≥10 units of blood in 24 hours

AXIOM Patients who have had recent massive transfusions can be hyperkalemic or hypokalemic.

In spite of the increased potassium levels in transfused blood, hypokalemia is encountered almost as frequently as hyperkalemia in patients who are given massive blood transfusions. Of a series of 409 patients receiving 10 or more units of blood, 130 (32%) developed serum potassium levels greater than 5.0 mEq/L, and 19% developed hypokalemia (27). If the serum potassium levels were corrected for the arterial pH (i.e., reduced 0.5 mEq/L for each 0.10 the pH was less than 7.40), only 5% had hyperkalemia and 47% had hypokalemia.

AXIOM Administration of large quantities of bank blood infused at a rate faster than 1 unit every 5 minutes in patients with shock, cirrhosis, or hypothermia can cause severe cardiovascular dysfunction due to citrate toxicity or ionic hypocalcemia or both.

A healthy, well-perfused adult with adequate hepatic function can tolerate the amount of citrate in 1 unit of blood every 3 to 5 minutes without requiring supplementation with calcium; however, patients who are hypothermic or are in shock while receiving massive transfusions may develop plasma citrate levels as high as 60 to 100 mg/dL. As these levels are approached, plasma levels of ionized calcium may decrease significantly. This may produce muscle tremors and changes in the electrocardiogram (ECG), such as prolongation of the QT interval and depression of the P and T waves. Irreversible ventricular fibrillation may follow, particularly if citrate levels of greater than 60 mg/dL are achieved. Excess citrate also may have a direct depressant effect on the myocardium separate from its effect on ionized calcium.

AXIOM Calcium does not usually have to be given with blood transfusions unless large amounts (greater than 6 to 10 units) are given rapidly (more than 1 unit every 5 minutes) and the patient is in heart failure or shock.

Plasma ionized calcium levels less than 0.85 m*M* may interfere with cardiovascular function, and infusion of calcium may be of some benefit in patients who are hemodynamically unstable (28). Ionized calcium levels of 0.7 or less have been associated with a significant increase in mortality.

In a recent series of 116 critically ill or injured patients who had 10 to 19 units of blood within 24 hours, 37 (32%) had very low ionized calcium levels (0.69 m*M* or less; 27). In 118 patients receiving 20 or more units, 71 (60%) had severe hypocalcemia. Of the patients who were given too much calcium and developed an ionic hypercalcemia, none survived.

Hypothermia

AXIOM Coagulation defects, arrhythmias, and impaired cardiovascular function in patients receiving massive transfusions are frequently the result of associated hypothermia (less than 32°C to 33°C).

Hypothermia (core body temperature less than 35.0°C) is often seen during massive blood transfusions in the OR, no matter how much effort is made to prevent it by warming i.v. fluids or using heating blankets and heated ventilator gases. Because myocardial contractility becomes impaired below temperatures of 32°C to 34°C, a vicious cycle of hypothermia and progressively deteriorating cardiovascular function can develop. The hypothermia also may interfere with coagulation mechanisms. Patients maintaining a core temperature below 32°C during massive transfusions have a mortality rate exceeding 85% (24).

AXIOM Once bleeding is controlled, every effort should be made to warm the patient to at least 34°C to 35°C as soon as possible.

Pulmonary Dysfunction

McNamara (29) noted that when more than 5 units of blood was infused through a standard blood filter, there was a decrease in P_{aO_2} within 48 hours, and the decrease in P_{aO_2} was proportional to the amount of blood transfused (29). Another study, however, noted that when multiple transfusions were the only risk factor for adult respiratory distress syndrome (ARDS), the problem developed only in patients receiving 23 or more units of blood within 12 hours (30).

AXIOM One should assume that there will be some degree of pulmonary dysfunction if a patient receives more than 20 units of blood and has been in shock more than 30 minutes.

Infectious Complications

AXIOM Non-A, non-B hepatitis is one of the biggest threats to life in patients surviving more than a month after massive blood transfusions.

Approximately 85% to 98% of posttransfusion hepatitis is of the non-A, non-B type, and most of the remainder is hepatitis B (31). Non-A, Non-B hepatitis has an incubation period of 8 weeks (compared with 11 weeks for hepatitis B); however, clinical signs and symptoms may appear in 10% of patients as early as 2 weeks after transfusion. Seventy-five percent of the infected patients are anicteric and relatively asymptomatic and have only mild increased levels of liver enzymes [aspartate aminotransferase (AST) and alanine aminotransferase (ALT)]. Nevertheless, 40% to 50% of all cases of fulminant viral hepatitis are caused by the non-A, non-B type, and the mortality rate in fulminant hepatitis may approach 87% to 100%. Non-A, non-B hepatitis also has a higher rate of chronicity (up to 36%) compared with the 5% to 10% risk associated with hepatitis B.

About 1% to 2% of all AIDS cases result from blood transfusions (32). In 1995, Klein (33) estimated the risk of various infections per unit of blood transfused in the United States as 1:5,000 for viral hepatitis, 1:200,000 for human T-cell leukemia–lymphoma virus (HTLV), and 1:420,000 for HIV infection.

Bacterial Infections

As many as 2.3% of all blood units prepared may be contaminated with bacteria that are capable of using citrate as a carbon source and of growing at low temperatures. The septic reaction to contaminated blood may produce a picture similar to that of a hemolytic transfusion reaction; however, hemolysis does not commonly occur with septic reactions. These reactions can usually be differentiated by microscopic examination of the blood product given, by determining the presence or absence of hemoglobin in the urine, and by a review of the transfusion cross-match by the blood bank.

Other diseases that may be transmitted through blood transfusions include malaria, syphilis, brucellosis, cytomegalovirus (CMV), trypanosomiasis, babesiosis, Chagas' disease, toxoplasmosis, leishmaniasis, and infectious mononucleosis.

Sepsis is a major problem in patients with massive transfusions who survive at least 48 hours. All of the survivors in one series of patients requiring 20 or more units of blood developed some type of infection (27). The increased tendency to develop sepsis after massive blood transfusions increasingly appears to be the result of impaired host defenses. Moore et al. (34) also showed that blood transfusion is an early and consistent risk factor for postinjury multiple organ failure and infection, independent of other variables.

Stroma-free Hemoglobin

AXIOM Encapsulated "stroma-free" hemoglobin (SFH) can carry oxygen, but it is inefficient in releasing its oxygen to tissues. It also can cause cardiovascular and renal problems.

As purer hemoglobin preparations have been developed, the major remaining problem with SFH has been its very high oxygen affinity, which limits its ability to release oxygen to tissues. Recently developed products, including polymerized pyridoxalated hemoglobin (SFH-PLP) with a P_{50} of 20 mm Hg, appear to have overcome this problem partially (35). Experimental data also suggested that lysosome-encapsulated human hemoglobin can readily substitute for circulating red cells and can maintain aerobic metabolism in hypotensive animals (36).

Perfluorocarbons

AXIOM Currently available fluorocarbons can carry oxygen, but they can be very toxic and are probably of little value except with severe anemia (Hb less than 5 g/dL) in patients who will not accept blood transfusions.

Short half-life, prolonged tissue retention, and potential toxicities place significant limitations on the use of perfluorocarbons as a blood substitute (37). Nevertheless, intraoperative infusion of these agents, as an adjunct to normovolemic hemodilution, can provide additional oxygen and a margin of safety not obtainable from standard crystalloid and colloid solutions. This type of application could reduce the allogeneic use of blood and thereby reduce the incidence and severity of complications due to blood transfusions.

⊘ FREQUENT ERRORS

1. ***Delayed or inadequate replacement (or both) of extracellular fluid deficits.***
2. ***Using fresh frozen plasma to correct volume deficiencies in a patient with normal coagulation.***
3. ***Excessive autotransfusion (more than 6 units) to patients who are likely to develop a coagulation abnormality.***
4. ***Giving un–cross-matched type O, Rh-negative blood to a patient who could be treated with crystalloids or colloids for another 5 to 10 minutes so that type-specific blood could be given.***
5. ***Assuming that excessive bleeding during surgery is the result of a coagulopathy, without carefully looking for open vessels that can be controlled surgically.***
6. ***Failure to give calcium to a patient who is in persistent shock and has been given 6 or more units of blood faster than 1 unit every 5 minutes.***
7. ***Assuming a patient is hyperkalemic because he or she has received massive blood transfusions.***
8. ***Giving bicarbonate to a patient who has received massive transfusions and has a combined metabolic and respiratory acidosis.***
9. ***Giving blood products when not really necessary.***
10. ***Failure to look closely for nosocomial infections in patients who have received massive transfusions.***

SUMMARY POINTS

1. Prompt correction of severe blood-volume deficits in the critically injured patient may be lifesaving; however, inappropriate use of blood and fluids can cause significant complications.

2. Administration of large quantities of saline solution in patients with continuing inadequate tissue perfusion or ketoacidosis can contribute to the development of a hyperchloremic (nonanion gap) metabolic acidosis.

3. Crystalloid resuscitation of critically injured patients does not usually impair pulmonary function unless there is concomitant lung damage.

4. Because of the calcium present in Ringer's lactate, it should not be infused with or in the same i.v. tubing as bank blood.

5. Albumin may be of value for expanding a reduced blood volume, especially in severely hypoproteinemic patients, but it is very expensive, and excessive amounts can cause cardiac, pulmonary, and renal problems.

6. Dextran 40 can be an effective colloid, but it may cause increased bleeding from open wounds, difficulty with type and cross-matching of blood, and occasional anaphylactoid reactions.
7. Hydroxyethyl starch (HES) is an effective colloid for expanding blood volume, but excessive use can cause increased bleeding.
8. The increased plasma amylase levels after HES administration are caused by formation of macroamylase molecules and do not reflect pancreatic problems.
9. Fresh frozen plasma (FFP) can correct deficiencies in clotting factors (not platelets) and antithrombin, but it also can transmit blood-borne diseases (hepatitis).
10. Compatibility testing for FFP is not required, but it should be ABO compatible.
11. Successful resuscitation is primarily dependent on the adequacy of fluid replacement not on the composition of the fluid itself.
12. Hypertonic saline can rapidly expand blood volume, but it can cause excess vasodilation, and serum sodium levels greater than 160 to 165 mEq/L may cause reactions.
13. Autotransfusion can reduce blood-bank needs and reduce the risk of blood-borne diseases, but if used in excess, especially in patients in shock, it can cause coagulopathies.
14. Autotransfusion of blood contaminated with intestinal contents is not absolutely contraindicated, especially if no other blood is available, the autotransfused red cells are washed well, and antibiotics are given in full dose.
15. Autotransfusions are safest if used in moderation and if the red cells are carefully washed before infusion.
16. Young, healthy individuals can do well with a hemoglobin of 7.0 g/dL if they are hemodynamically stable and the bleeding is controlled.
17. The most severe hemolytic transfusion reactions are generally caused by simple clerical errors so that bank blood is given to the wrong patient.
18. Blood that has been recently transfused can carry oxygen to the tissues, but it may not release it properly for several hours.
19. The two most common causes of increased postoperative bleeding in a patient who has received massive transfusions are inadequate surgical hemostasis and thrombocytopenia.
20. If laboratory clotting studies are not available in a patient who may have a coagulopathy, observation of 2 to 3 mL of blood placed in a clear stoppered test tube and inverted once a minute may be used to evaluate clotting.
21. Blood for clotting studies should not be drawn from an indwelling vascular catheter.
22. Patients who have had recent massive transfusions can be hyperkalemic or hypokalemic.
23. Administration of large quantities of bank blood infused at a rate faster than 1 unit every 5 minutes in patients with shock, cirrhosis, or hypothermia, can cause severe cardiovascular dysfunction because of citrate toxicity or ionic hypocalcemia or both.
24. Calcium does not usually have to be given with blood transfusions unless large amounts (more than 6 to 10 units) are given rapidly (more than 1 unit every 5 minutes) and the patient is in heart failure or shock.
25. Coagulation defects, arrhythmias, and impaired cardiovascular function in patients receiving massive transfusions are frequently the result of an associated hypothermia.
26. Once bleeding is controlled, every effort should be made to warm the patient to 35°C as rapidly as possible.
27. One should assume that there will be some degree of pulmonary dysfunction if a patient receives more than 20 units of blood and has been in shock more than 30 minutes.
28. Non-A, non-B hepatitis is often the biggest threat to life in patients surviving more than a month after massive blood transfusions.
29. The majority of trauma patients requiring massive blood transfusions will develop a nosocomial infection postoperatively.

30. Encapsulated SFH can carry oxygen, but it is relatively inefficient in releasing its oxygen to tissues. It can also cause cardiovascular and renal problems.
31. Currently available fluorocarbons can carry oxygen, but they can be very toxic and are of little value except with very severe anemia (Hb less than 5 g/dL) in patients who will not accept blood transfusions.

REFERENCES

1. Wilson RF. Blood replacement. In: Wilson RF, Walt AJ, eds. *Management of trauma: pitfalls and practice.* 2nd ed. Philadelphia: Williams & Wilkins, 1996:51.
2. Guzman JA, Lacoma FJ, Kruse JA. Relationship between systemic oxygen supply dependency and gastric intramucosal PCO_2 during progressive hemorrhage. *J Trauma* 1998;44:696.
3. Wilson RF, Tyburski JG, Kubinec SM, et al. Intraoperative end-tidal carbon dioxide levels and derived calculations correlated with outcome in trauma patients. *J Trauma* 1996;41:606.
4. Mikulaschek A, Henry SM, Donovan R, Scalea TM. Serum lactate is not predicted by anion gap or base excess after trauma resuscitation. *J Trauma* 1996;40:218.
5. Chan STF, Kapadia CR, Johnson AW, Radcliffe AG, Dudley HAF. Extracellular fluid volume expansion and third space sequestration at the site of small bowel anastomoses. *Br J Surg* 1983;70:36–39.
6. Wilson RF, Sarver E, Birks R. Central venous pressure and blood volume determinations in clinical shock. *Surg Gynecol Obstet* 1971;132:631.
7. Nearman HS, Herman ML. Toxic effects of colloids in the intensive care unit. *Crit Care Clin* 1991;7:713.
8. Emerson TE. Unique features of albumin: a brief review. *Crit Care Med* 1989;17:690.
9. Shoemaker WC, Schluchter M, Hopkins JA. Fluid therapy in emergency resuscitation: clinical evaluation of colloid and crystalloid regimens. *Crit Care Med* 1981;9:367.
10. Alexander B, Odake K, Lawlor J, et al. Coagulation, hemostasis and plasma expanders: a quarter-century enigma. *Fed Proc* 1975;34:1429.
11. Stump DC, Strauss RG, Heinriksen RA, et al. Effects of hydroxyethyl starch on blood coagulation, particularly factor VIII. *Transfusion* 1985;25:349.
12. Ledingham IM, Ramsey G. Hypovolemic shock. *Br J Anesth* 1986;8:169.
13. Shackford SR, Fortlage DA, Peters RM, et al. Serum osmolar and electrolyte changes associated with large infusions of hypertonic sodium lactate for intravenous volume expansion of patients undergoing aortic reconstruction. *Surg Gynecol Obstet* 1987;164:127.
14. Dubick MA, Wade CE. A review of the efficacy and safety of 7.5% NaCL/6% dextran 70 in experimental animals and in humans. *J Trauma* 1994;36:323.
15. Shackford SR, Mackersie RC, Holbrook TL, et al. The epidemiology of traumatic death: a population-based analysis. *Arch Surg* 1993;128:571.
16. Matsuoka T, Hildreth J, Wisner DH. Uncontrolled hemorrhage from parenchymal injury: is resuscitation helpful? *J Trauma* 1996;40:915.
17. Halpern NA, Alicea M, Seabrook B, et al. Cell saver autologous transfusion: metabolic consequences of washing blood with normal saline. *J Trauma* 1996;41:407.
18. Gervin AS. Transfusion, autotransfusion, and blood substitutes. In: Mattox KL, Moore EE, Feliciano DV, eds. *Trauma.* Norwalk, CT: Appleton & Lange, 1988:159.
19. Meryman HT, Hornblower M. A method for freezing and washing red cells using high glycerol concentration. *Transfusion* 1972;12:145.
20. Barnes A. Transfusions of universal donor and uncross-matched blood. *Bibl Haematol* 1980;46:132.
21. Baker RJ, Moinichen BS, Nyhus LM. Transfusion reaction. *Ann Surg* 1969;169:684.
22. Sohmer PR, Scott RL. Metabolic burden of massive transfusion. In: *Massive transfusion in surgery and trauma.* Alan R. Liss, 1982:272.
23. Hewson OR, Neale PB, Kumar N, et al. Coagulopathy related to dilution and hypotension during massive transfusion. *Crit Care Med* 1985;13:387.

24. Wilson RF, Dulchavsky SA, Soullier G, et al. Problems with 20 or more blood transfusions in 24 hours. *Am Surg* 1987;53:410.
25. Latham JT, Bove JR, Weirich L. Chemical and hematologic changes in stored CPDA-1 blood. *Transfusion* 1982;22:158.
26. Erber WN, Tan J, Grey D, Lown JAG. Use of unrefrigerated fresh whole blood in massive transfusion. *Med J Aust* 1996;165:11.
27. Wilson RF, Binkley LE, Sabo FM, et al. Electrolyte and acid-base changes with massive transfusions. *Am Surg* 1992;58:535.
28. Bashour TT. Hypocalcemic acute myocardial failure secondary to rapid transfusion of citrated blood. *Am Heart J* 1984;108:146.
29. McNamara, JJ. Microaggregates in stored blood: physiologic significance. In: Chaplin H, Jaffee ER, Lenfort C, Valeri CR, eds. *Preservation of red blood cells.* Washington: National Academy of Science, 1972:315.
30. Pepi PE, Potkin RT, Rheu RH, et al. Clinical predictors of the adult respiratory distress syndrome. *Am J Surg* 1982;144:124.
31. Blum HE, Vyas GN. Non-A, non-B hepatitis: a contemporary assessment. *Haematologia* 1982;15:162.
32. Hardy AM, Allen JR, Morgan M, et al. Incidence rate of acquired immunodeficiency syndrome in selected populations. *JAMA* 1985;253:215.
33. Klein HG. Allogenic transfusion risks in the surgical patient. *Am J Surg* 1995; 170:21.
34. Moore FA, Moore EE, Sauaia A. Blood transfusions: an independent risk factor for postinjury multiple organ failure. *Arch Surg* 1997;132:620.
35. Leppaniemi A, Soltero R, Burris D, et al. Early resuscitation with low-volume polyDCLHb is effective in the treatment of shock induced by penetrating vascular injury. *J Trauma* 1996;40:242.
36. Takaori M, Fukui A. Treatment of massive hemorrhage with liposome encapsulated human hemoglobin (NRC) and hydroxyethyl starch (HES) in beagles. *Artif Cells Blood Substitut Immobil Biotechnol* 1996;24:643.
37. Spence RK. Perfluorocarbons in the twenty-first century: clinical applications as transfusion alternatives. *Artif Cells Blood Substitut Immobil Biotechnol* 1995;23: 367.

5. GENERAL PRINCIPLES OF WOUND CARE[1]

STAGES OF WOUND HEALING

Healing begins from the moment of injury. In open wounds, the stages of healing are usually referred to as inflammation, proliferation, maturation, and remodeling. In wounds that are closed promptly, epithelialization begins before there is proliferation of collagen (Figure 1;2,3).

Inflammation

Celsus (30 B.C. to 45 A.D.) characterized the signs of inflammation as heat (calor), redness (rubor), swelling (tumor), and tenderness or pain (dolor). This inflammatory response, which usually lasts 2 to 5 days, is important for the phagocytosis of foreign materials and dead tissue. The inflammatory phase also generates a variety of soluble mediators, which help regulate the subsequent stages of wound healing.

The polymorphonuclear leukocytes are important for controlling any bacterial contamination that is present at the time of wounding. The mononuclear cells come into the wound later and become increasingly abundant after 24 to 72 hours. In addition to aiding in bacterial phagocytosis and tissue debridement, the macrophages influence the subsequent course of wound healing by stimulating the proliferation of fibroblasts and endothelial cells.

Fibrin, which is produced in the wound by conversion of circulating plasma fibrinogen, promotes hemostasis, and provides a scaffolding for the ingrowth of cells. Fibronectins are high-molecular-weight glycoproteins that facilitate the attachment of migrating fibroblasts to the fibrin latticework within the wound. Various growth factors also can have a profound effect on wound healing (4).

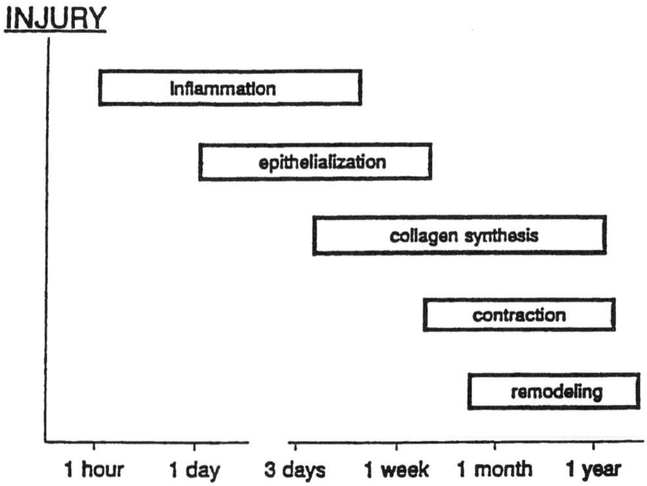

FIG. 5-1. The sequence of events in wound healing. Note the amount of overlap of the various stages (Peacock JL et al., Wound healing in the physiologic basis of surgery, ed. by O'Leary JP; Williams & Wilkins, Philadelphia 1993:p100).

AXIOM In the presence of extensive tissue injury or heavy bacterial contamination, the inflammatory phase will be prolonged, and wound healing may be greatly delayed.

Epithelialization

The process of epithelialization includes detachment, migration, proliferation, and differentiation (2,3). Within 24 hours after injury, cells at the base of the epidermis along the wound margins increase their rate of mitosis, detach themselves from the underlying dermis, and migrate across the wound to cover any exposed dermis.

AXIOM Open wounds that are allowed to dry out will epithelialize slowly.

Proliferative Phase

The proliferative phase, also known as the cellular phase or phase of fibroplasia, is characterized by the deposition of collagen by fibroblasts in the wound. It begins on the third to fifth day and usually lasts at least 21 to 28 days. The time required for mesenchymal cells to differentiate into fibroblasts and form collagen is known as the "lag phase" of wound healing.

AXIOM Collagen is the most important component supporting the healed wound.

Collagen can be synthesized by fibroblasts, osteoblasts, smooth-muscle cells, chondrocytes, epithelial cells, and endothelial cells. In the cell, the appropriate sequences of amino acids are synthesized into polypeptide chains at ribosomes.

After hydroxylation with proline and lysine, the polypeptide chains fold into a helical formation that is then excreted from the cell as a procollagen. Procollagen peptidase, which is on or near the cell surface, then converts the procollagen into tropocollagen. Tropocollagen then undergoes assembly into collagen filaments, which combine to form collagen fibers. As the collagen matures, the polypeptide chains composing each tropocollagen unit form strong intramolecular bonds mediated by lysyl amine oxidase. Intermolecular cross-linking between tropocollagen molecules also occurs and further strengthens the collagen complex.

Maturation

The process of maturation (remodeling of collagen and extracellular matrix) continues for months after reepithelialization has occurred and is responsible for the changes in the physical properties of the scar. Type III collagen, which is abundant in the early scar, is gradually replaced by type I collagen. The immature scar is often raised, erythematous, and pruritic; however, as maturation progresses, the water content of the scar decreases, thereby allowing the collagen fibers to lie closer together, and the ideal scar becomes flat, white, soft, and nonirritating (2,3).

AXIOM Maturation of a wound involves a continuous process of collagen lysis and collagen synthesis and usually persists for at least 6 to 12 months.

The breakdown of collagen (collagenolysis) in maturing wounds and in stable scars is caused by collagenase, which is secreted by polymorphonuclear leukocytes, macrophages, and epithelial cells. This degradation of collagen is as important as collagen production in wound remodeling. Loss of the proper equilibrium between collagen production and degradation can lead to excessive deposition of collagen, as in hypertrophic scars or keloids.

By the end of 2 weeks, most skin wounds have gained only about 12% of their preinjury tensile strength, and by 4 to 6 weeks, only 50% of the preinjury tensile strength has returned. After 6 to 12 months, it is still usually only 90% of normal (2,3).

AXIOM Scars are usually not considered fully mature and generally should not be revised until at least 1 year after the initial repair.

Defective deposition of wound collagen can be a serious problem in some patients. DaCosta et al. (5) found, in a study of wound-healing in a rat model, that diphenylhydantoin significantly increased wound tensile strength compared with controls and may be of benefit in clinical situations in which there is defective wound collagen deposition.

HEALING OF OPEN WOUNDS

The typical sequence of biologic events involved in the healing of open wounds includes control of infection, resolution of inflammation, angiogenesis, regeneration of a functional connective tissue matrix, contraction, resurfacing, and remodeling.

Healing of open wounds progresses through stages similar to those seen in closed wounds, but wound contraction assumes a much more important role. Wound contraction is maximal between 5 and 15 days after wounding and is mediated to a great extent by the myofibroblasts and their specialized connections with the surrounding extracellular matrix.

AXIOM Wound contraction is decreased by skin grafting, and full-thickness grafts impede wound contraction more than split-thickness grafts.

Factors Affecting Wound Healing

The presence of bacteria in a wound (contamination) does not necessarily imply that infection (with invasion of the tissues) is present; however, if β-hemolytic streptococci are present or if the bacterial count exceeds 10^5/per gram of tissue, infection is likely to be present. Local infection retards wound healing, but systemic sepsis decreases wound healing even further by causing reduced macrophage chemotaxis and phagocytosis.

AXIOM One of the best ways to prevent wound infection in a contaminated case is to leave the skin and subcutaneous tissue open.

Protein depletion is particularly apt to impair healing if it results in edema in the wound or if it is associated with a deficiency of critical amino acids, such as cystine, which is essential for collagen synthesis (3).

AXIOM Malnutrition resulting in an acute decrease in lean body mass of 15% has been shown to result in decreased strength of healed skin wounds and colon anastomoses (6).

Corticosteroids inhibit inflammation, fibroplasia, collagen synthesis, and neovascularization, and thereby greatly reduce the rate of healing of wounds. They also increase susceptibility to infection because of their immunosuppressive effects; however, retinoic acid (vitamin A) in high doses (25,000 IU per day) may reverse the healing retardation caused by cortisone (7).

Diabetes mellitus can cause a wide variety of problems, including vascular disease, which may delay wound healing. Severe hyperglycemia, especially if associated with ketoacidosis, causes a delayed response to injury and impairs the function of white blood cells. Endothelial cells in diabetics show decreased adhesion and cell growth on nonenzymatically glycosylated laminin (8).

AXIOM Even if distal pulses feel normal, wound healing in patients with diabetes mellitus tends to be impaired, particularly if blood glucose levels are not under good control.

Vitamin C (ascorbic acid) is required as a cofactor in the hydroxylation of proline and, consequently, is essential for collagen synthesis. Indeed, chronic severe lack of vitamin C can even cause previously well-healed wounds to break down.

Zinc is necessary for the activity of DNA and RNA polymerases and transferases that are needed for proper epithelialization and fibroblast proliferation. Ferrous iron and copper also are necessary for normal collagen synthesis.

Significant blood loss causing hypovolemia has a detrimental effect on wound healing in animals because of decreased tissue oxygenation; however, healing is generally unaffected if normal blood volume is maintained and hematocrit levels do not decrease below 15%.

Oxygen is necessary for cell migration and proliferation and for protein and collagen synthesis. Increasing tissue oxygen tension with hyperbaric oxygen may further enhance wound healing. Although oxygen tension is relatively low in healing wounds, anything that interferes with the delivery of oxygen to the wound (e.g., anemia, cardiovascular disease, diabetes, radiation) will have a detrimental effect on wound healing.

Evaluation of the Wound

A good history should elicit the mechanism of injury and indicate the depth and probable amount of contamination of the wound and the possibility of foreign bodies, thereby stimulating efforts to locate and remove them.

An examination of facial lacerations should include evaluation of the underlying sensory and motor nerves and their function. The depths of the wounds should be carefully visualized and not just palpated to determine whether there has been extension into the oral cavity. Lid lacerations also must be carefully examined to determine whether the eye is involved. Any wound in the area of the parotid gland or duct should be carefully examined, by using ductograms as needed, to rule out salivary gland involvement. Examination of extremity wounds should include distal testing for sensation, motor function, capillary refill, and joint mobility.

Many foreign bodies can be seen on plain radiographs; however, about 10% of glass and other foreign bodies in tissue are not radiopaque. In such cases, a xeroradiograph can help to determine whether foreign bodies are present in the depths of the wound.

MANAGEMENT OF THE WOUND

Hemostasis

Clamps or suture ligatures used in blind attempts to obtain hemostasis in the depths of a wound can damage important vessels or nerves. Direct local pressure with gloved fingers or compression with sterile dressings is much safer.

Tourniquets are seldom needed except above major amputations and, if used incorrectly, can increase bleeding and cause much harm. A tourniquet should ideally be at least 2 to 3 inches wide so that the pressure is evenly distributed (a blood pressure cuff makes an excellent tourniquet). The pressure applied must also be high enough to prevent arterial inflow. If the tourniquet is applied for too long, it can cause irreversible distal ischemic damage.

Hematomas

A hematoma, especially because of the iron present in blood, is an ideal culture medium for bacteria and, acting as a foreign body, it also prevents or inhibits the delivery of phagocytic cells to the area. Therefore, one should attempt to obtain meticulous hemostasis before closing any deep wound. If all of the oozing cannot be stopped, hematoma formation should be prevented with a pressure dressing, closed suction, or both.

WOUND CLEANSING

In the emergency department, all wounds should immediately be covered with sterile dressings until they can be properly treated. Before examination or repair, the surrounding skin should be carefully scrubbed with a contact antimicrobial agent (preferably povidone–iodine). The povidone–iodine solution, which is bactericidal, should not be applied to the wound itself because it is cytotoxic. Full-strength hydrogen peroxide and Dakin's solution also are injurious to tissue cells.

AXIOM One should not irrigate a wound with anything that would not be used to irrigate eyes.

After adequate debridement, the wound can be cleansed by irrigating it with a pulsating jet lavage. Pulsating pressure irrigation systems generally produce much better cleansing of contaminated wounds than do other techniques. Indeed, irrigation with pressures as high as 70 pounds per square inch may be needed to remove adequately bacteria and certain types of debris. A 35-mL syringe with a 19-gauge plastic needle attached also can provide high-pressure irrigation (9). If the wound is to be closed, fresh drapes and gloves should be used before placing the closing sutures.

Local Anesthesia

Local anesthesia should be injected slowly by using a very small needle (25- to 30-gauge) to minimize the pressure–pain effect during the injection. Buffering the local anesthesia with bicarbonate solution (1:10) also reduces the pain caused by the local anesthetic. The addition of epinephrine can improve hemostasis during the procedure; however, epinephrine is usually contraindicated in digits and the penis because the vasoconstriction may cause ischemia and further tissue loss. If injected into small fascial compartments, local anesthetics also can cause local ischemia or impair venous return or both.

If a digital block is performed, care must be taken to prevent digital artery obstruction from the pressure of the injected anesthetic. One also should avoid injecting the local anesthetic into blood vessels because of the rapid systemic toxicity it can produce.

Debridement

Meticulous removal of nonviable tissue is essential for optimal wound healing. Use of magnification when treating soft-tissue facial wounds may provide improved debridement and less irregular wound edges. If a wound is contaminated excessively or is more than 8 to 12 hours old, it can be converted to a relatively clean, fresh wound by excising the entire wound.

Foreign Bodies

Prosthetic grafts or other foreign materials should not be placed in grossly contaminated wounds. Nonabsorbable sutures such as silk and cotton also should be used as little as possible because they may act as foreign bodies and perpetuate infection with resultant chronic draining sinuses. If absorbable sutures are used for tying off small vessels, slowly absorbable varieties are usually preferable to catgut because they cause less local inflammatory response while being absorbed.

WOUND CLOSURE

Severely contaminated wounds should not be closed. If there is any question regarding the number of bacteria in the wound, a biopsy can be performed on the tissue. A small portion of viable tissue (250 mg) can be removed and processed by a rapid slide technique to determine the level of bacterial contamination. If there are more than 100,000 (10^5) organisms per gram of tissue, bacterial contamination is often too great to allow normal wound healing without infection (10).

Occasionally, wounds of the face with tissue of questionable viability may be closed because of the excellent blood supply in the face and the better cosmetic result that can be obtained by performing a primary repair. Although skin and subcutaneous tissues can be left open, tissue such as bowel, cartilage, tendons, vessels, and bones should be covered with at least one layer of tissue such as peritoneum, fascia, or muscle.

Animal and human bite wounds should not be closed. Cat saliva contains 10^8 organisms per milliliter of fluid, and animals that eat meat tend to cause more heavily contaminated wounds than non–meat eaters. Human saliva contains at least 10^6 to 10^8 organisms/mL. People with poor dentition may have bacterial counts exceeding 10^{10} to 10^{12}/mL.

AXIOM Contaminated wounds that are closed by secondary intention will generally provide much better cosmetic results than primary closures that become infected.

Quirinia and Viidik (11) found that delayed primary closure (at 3 days) of ischemic wounds in rats resulted in wounds that were as strong as wounds closed primarily (when tested 10 days after wounding). Thus it appears that ischemic or contaminated wounds may safely be left open for a few days before suturing.

Wound Configuration

A jagged, irregular wound running perpendicular to the "wrinkle lines" is likely to have retarded healing with a poor cosmetic result. Wherever possible, wound edges should be straight, sharp, and parallel to the wrinkle lines. If the wound must be debrided or lengthened to achieve this, it should be done without hesitation.

Whenever possible, the skin edges should be slightly everted to compensate for the tendency for the scar to sink in slightly as it heals. Such eversion can usually be achieved with fine vertical mattress sutures.

Wound Tension

Wound edges should come together with little or no tension. Relaxing incisions or freeing more tissue at the level of the superficial or deep fascia may help to bring wound edges together with less tension.

Suture Materials

Foreign bodies, including sutures, greatly increase the risk of infection in wounds (12). Nonabsorbable monofilament sutures generally cause much less tissue reaction than absorbable and braided sutures and are less apt to promote development of infections. Braided sutures leave more interstices for bacterial adherence and proliferation and tend to result in a higher incidence of wound infections.

Areas such as the face, which has a high density of dermal appendages, should have the epidermal sutures placed only through the depth of the epidermis. If the dermis is included in the sutures, suture tracks can occur if these stitches are left in place for as short a period as 4 days.

Full-Thickness Skin Loss

If the tissue loss in a fresh clean wound is too extensive to allow a direct closure, a partial-thickness skin graft can be used as either a temporary or permanent surface repair. The donor site should match the wound area as closely as possible for color and amount of hair. Supraclavicular and postauricular skin are good color matches for the face. For most other parts of the body, the anterior thigh is quite satisfactory.

AXIOM Avulsed or surgically removed skin can be an important source of split-thickness grafts in trauma patients.

During the first 24 hours (before the establishment of new vascular and lymphatic channels in the graft), skin grafts are nourished by fluid from the host tissue by a process referred to as imbibition.

In wounds with questionable devitalized tissue or contamination, one can use autograft, homograft, or heterograft as temporary biologic dressings. Such grafts are often far superior to the usual dressings applied to these wounds.

Full-thickness skin grafts should seldom be used to treat fresh wounds (except for clean wounds of the head and neck by experienced surgeons). Full-thickness grafts vascularize very slowly and require optimal conditions and postoperative care; however, when they do take, the color and function of the graft are usually better than those achieved with split-thickness grafts. Full-thickness grafts are particularly good in children because the growth potential of split-thickness grafts is limited.

The graft should be pressed down firmly to provide uniform complete tissue contact. In concave defects, the fine sutures used to tack the graft in place should be left long enough to be tied over a stent as a pressure dressing. If the wound is on an extremity, a splint should be applied to prevent undue motion at the wound site.

AXIOM Full-thickness skin grafts do not take as easily as partial-thickness skin grafts, but the cosmetic result and function of full-thickness grafts are usually much better.

Completely avulsed extremity tissue, except for fingertips, is usually contaminated and too thick to allow adequate revascularization. Partial avulsions on extremities, especially if long and narrow or if pedicled distally, are apt to die; therefore, if the tissue is clean, it should be converted to a fat-free partial-thickness graft. Amputated portions of a composite structure such as the eyelid, nose, or ear can sometimes be sutured back in place with success. Partial or complete avulsions on the face and neck usually heal well if sutured promptly and if the surrounding tissue is healthy.

Ohtsuka et al. (13) were the first to report on the use of a free omental graft for soft-tissue reconstruction of the lower extremity. Free vascularized omental flaps may be used to cover deep defects in the lower leg, and pedicled flaps may be used to cover proximal groin, thigh, or hip defects extending into the hip joint.

A properly applied sterile dressing can protect the wound from additional bacterial contamination and further injury. A dressing of absorptive gauze also helps to move exudate away from the skin. Clinical studies have shown that wounds treated with occlusive dressings have less pain, swelling, and tenderness, and the cosmetic results of the scars are often superior.

A wound that is likely to become very edematous, due to either a dependent position or tissue damage from the injury, can be gently compressed with gauze wrappings to minimize the edema formation and the pain.

Some wounds, especially over joints or in highly mobile areas, may benefit from a period of immobilization by a stiff dressing or even a splint or cast. Limiting mobility tends to reduce pain and edema formation and increase the coaptation of wounded structures during the healing period; however, in elderly patients, joint stiffness may develop very rapidly.

Bacterial Prophylaxis

Patients with deep penetrating wounds, which should all be considered contaminated, may benefit from at least 1 to 2 days of prophylactic antibiotics. Patients with penetrating injuries who have not had a tetanus booster inoculation in the last 10 years also are more vulnerable to tetanus infection, especially if there is any ischemic or necrotic tissue, which facilitates proliferation of anaerobic organisms. Treatment of these tetanus-prone wounds should include a tetanus toxoid booster plus tetanus immunoglobulin (Hypertet).

AXIOM The immunization status of all patients with open wounds should be carefully ascertained. If the history is in doubt, one should assume that the patient is inadequately immunized against tetanus.

Patients whose wounds were inflicted by animals that are prone to rabies infection must be closely questioned. If suspicion is sufficiently high, a prophylactic course of rabies immunization should be undertaken.

Removal of Sutures

If the underlying tissues are closed properly, sutures on the face should be removed in 3 to 4 days to reduce the chances of permanent stitch marks. Sutures in the skin of the abdomen or chest can usually be removed in 7 days, whereas sutures on the hands, feet, or legs should often be left in place for 10 to 14 days. If the wound is in an area that is subject to much movement or if the patient is apt to heal poorly, Steri-strips may have to be left in place for an additional 1 to 2 weeks.

Wound Infection

The likelihood of an infection depends on the interaction between the patient's host defenses and the dose and virulence of the microorganisms. A susceptible wound is one that contains devitalized tissue or is inadequately perfused or both. Foreign bodies and hematomas retained in a wound also promote bacterial growth.

Radiation changes or ischemia due to vascular disease are local factors that reduce resistance to infection. Certain systemic conditions (e.g., diabetes mellitus, corticosteroids, shock, burns, renal disease, cancer, and immunosuppressive agents) also impair host resistance.

When viewed in the clinical or operating room setting, a wound can be classified as clean, clean–contaminated, contaminated, or infected. A clean wound is nontraumatic and free of inflammation; it is created in the operating room; no break in surgical technique has occurred; and the respiratory, alimentary, and genitourinary tracts have not been violated. A clean–contaminated wound also is nontraumatic, but it is characterized by a minor break in surgical technique or the involvement of the gastrointestinal, genitourinary, or respiratory tracts without significant spillage of contents. Contaminated wounds include all traumatic wounds and all wounds caused by a dirty source, contaminated with feces, containing a foreign body, or containing devitalized tissue. Wounds receiving delayed treatment also are considered to be contaminated.

AXIOM Biopsies of infected tissue usually provide better cultures than the pus present in the center of the abscess.

The treatment of a wound infection should include prompt and appropriate drainage. A sample of any wound discharge is submitted for Gram staining, aerobic and anaerobic culture, and determination of bacterial sensitivity. Antibiotics to cover the microorganisms most likely to be present are initiated before obtaining the culture results.

AXIOM The most important aspect of the early management of any infected wound is adequate drainage; antibiotics often are not needed.

Hypertrophic Scars and Keloids

The hypertrophic scar is characterized by the deposition of excess collagen that remains within the borders of the scar bed. Keloids extend beyond the boundaries of the original wound and have continued growth. Wounds that are perpendicular to the lines of facial expression are more likely to become hypertrophic than are those that lie parallel to the wrinkle lines (14).

Wounds that heal over a very thin layer of remaining dermis, such as a burn, have an increased chance of developing excessive scarring. Hypertrophic scars and keloids are more commonly found in regions of tension (deltoid, parasternal, back), in wounds with retained foreign bodies (ear lobes), in wounds complicated by inflammation or infection, and in families with a history of excessive scarring.

When wounds on the hands or face or above the clavicles are sufficiently healed in a patient with a history of abnormal wound healing, external compression can be applied. This may take the form of a compression elastic garment, such as Jobst garment, or an external plastic mold, such as the clear plastic Uvex.

CHRONIC WOUNDS

The initial treatment of chronic wounds is removal of all necrotic debris. The bacterial count should then be assessed by both qualitative and quantitative analyses. If the bacterial count is greater than 100,000 organisms per gram of tissue or if any β-hemolytic *Streptococcus* are present, the wound should be treated with topical antimicrobials, such as silver sulfadiazine or mafenide acetate. Because the scar tissue around chronic wounds makes these areas relatively ischemic and decreases the ability of systemic antibiotics to penetrate into the edges of the open wound, it should be excised as completely as possible.

AXIOM Systemic antibiotics do not penetrate chronic scarred wounds well, but they are indicated if there is surrounding cellulitis or evidence of sepsis.

The underlying cause of the chronic wound should be removed if at all possible. If the wound is a pressure sore, the patient should be placed on a mattress that will reduce exposure to excessive pressure and ischemia.

⊘ FREQUENT ERRORS

1. ***Inadequate attention to blood flow to wounds in older individuals and those with diabetes mellitus.***
2. ***Inadequate attention to replenishment of vitamin C and zinc in malnourished individuals who have large or difficult wounds.***
3. ***Assumption that a foreign body is not present in a wound because it does not show on radiograph.***
4. ***Use of a tourniquet or hemostats to control bleeding from a deep wound on an extremity when direct local pressure might be adequate.***
5. ***Inadequate irrigation of contaminated wounds.***
6. ***Irrigation of wounds with solutions that may be irritating to the tissue.***
7. ***Not switching to dry drapes around a clean wound after the drapes have become saturated with fluid.***
8. ***Use of multiple subcutaneous sutures to eliminate dead space.***
9. ***Assumption that skin sutures will provide adequate hemostasis for deep bleeding wounds.***
10. ***Failure to use closed drainage in a wound if there is residual dead space, oozing, or both.***
11. ***Reliance on antibiotics rather than adequate incision and drainage to treat a wound infection.***

SUMMARY POINTS

1. The five stages of wound healing (which tend to overlap) include inflammation, epithelialization, collagen synthesis, contraction, and remodeling.
2. In the presence of extensive injury or heavy contamination, inflammation can be greatly prolonged, and wound healing may be greatly delayed.
3. Open desiccated wounds epithelialize more slowly than wounds with appropriate dressings.
4. Collagen is the most important component in the strength of a healed wound.
5. Scars are usually not considered fully mature and generally should not be revised until at least 1 year after the initial repair.
6. Wound contraction is decreased by skin grafting, and full-thickness grafts impede wound contraction more than split-thickness grafts.
7. Open wounds containing any β-hemolytic streptococci or more than 10^5 other bacteria per gram of tissue should not be closed, even if they look good clinically.
8. One of the best ways to prevent wound infection in a contaminated case is to leave the skin and subcutaneous tissue open.
9. One should be prepared for delayed healing in patients receiving corticosteroids.
10. Even if distal pulses feel normal, wound healing in patients with diabetes mellitus tends to be impaired, particularly if blood glucose levels are not under good control.
11. Prolonged severe lack of vitamin C can cause previously well-healed wounds to break down.
12. Anything reducing oxygen tension below normal in a wound can retard its healing.
13. Hemostasis is generally best obtained initially by accurately applying direct external pressure.
14. Use of a tourniquet, especially outside the operating room, can be extremely dangerous because it can rapidly cause irreversible distal ischemia.
15. All traumatic wounds are contaminated.
16. If there is any chance that a local anesthetic may interfere with perfusion of a digit or some other anatomic structure, one should not combine it with epinephrine (adrenaline).
17. If a wound is contaminated excessively or is more than 8 to 12 hours old, it can be converted to a relatively clean, fresh wound by excising the entire wound.
18. The number of bacteria in a wound, not its age, determines if it is safe to close at a particular time.
19. Contaminated wounds that close by secondary intention will generally provide much better cosmetic results than primary closures that become infected.
20. Whenever possible, wounds should be closed parallel to tension and wrinkle lines and should be slightly everted.
21. A large number of sutures placed in subcutaneous tissue to reduce dead space increases the risk of infection.
22. If all dead space in a wound cannot be obliterated, the wound should be left open or kept evacuated with a closed drainage system.
23. Wounds closed with nonabsorbable monofilament sutures generally heal better and have fewer infections than those closed with absorbable and braided sutures.
24. Foreign bodies, including sutures, increase the risk of infection in wounds.
25. Use of braided sutures leaves more interstices for bacterial adherence and proliferation and tends to result in a higher incidence of wound infections.
26. Skin sutures in the face should incorporate as little dermis as possible and should be removed early, often within 3 to 4 days.
27. Whenever possible, fresh traumatic wounds should be closed primarily, without use of complicated reconstruction techniques.
28. Avulsed or surgically removed skin can be an important source of split-thickness grafts.

29. In large open wounds, partial-thickness autografts or allografts may be the ideal temporary biologic dressing.
30. Full-thickness skin grafts do not take as easily as partial-thickness skin grafts, but the cosmetic result and function of full-thickness grafts are usually much better.
31. Drains should be used only for specific definable reasons: the obliteration of dead space, continued oozing, or provision of egress for bile, pancreatic juice, or intestinal contents.
32. Excessive edema in wounds can be painful, and it can slow the healing of the wound and increase the chance of infection.
33. The tetanus-immunization status of all patients with an open wound should be carefully ascertained. If the history is in doubt, one should assume that the patient is inadequately immunized against tetanus.
34. Biopsies of infected tissue usually provide better cultures than the pus that is present in the center of an abscess.
35. The most important aspect of the early management of any infected wound is adequate drainage; antibiotics often are not needed.
36. Wounds that are perpendicular to the lines of facial expression are more likely to become hypertrophic than those that lie parallel to the wrinkle lines.

REFERENCES

1. Wilson RF, Balakrishnan C. General principles of wound care. In: Wilson RF, Walt AJ, eds. *Management of trauma: pitfalls and practice.* Philadelphia: Williams & Wilkins, 1996:70–84.
2. Cohen IK, Diegelmann RF. Wound healing. In: Greenfield LJ, ed. *Surgery: scientific principles and practice.* Philadelphia: JB Lippincott, 1993:86–102.
3. Peacock JL, Lawrence WT, Peacock EE Jr. Wound healing. In: O'Leary JP, ed. *The physiologic basis of surgery.* Baltimore: Williams & Wilkins, 1993:95–111.
4. Greenhalgh DG. The role of growth factors in wound healing. *J Trauma* 1996;41: 159.
5. DaCosta ML, Regan MC, Sader MA, et al. Diphenylhydantoin sodium promotes early and marked angiogenesis and results in increased collagen deposition and tensile strength in healing wounds. *Surgery* 1998;123:287.
6. Ward MW, Danzi M, Lewin MR, et al. The effects of subclinical malnutrition and refeeding on the healing of experimental colonic anastomosis. *Br J Surg* 1982;69: 308.
7. Ulland NE, Gartner MH, Richards JR, et al. Retinoic acid restores transforming growth factor $beta_1$ concentrates in a steroid-impaired wound healing model. *Surg Forum* 1994;45:714.
8. Subin B, Tuan TL, Cheung D, et al. Cellular and molecular pathogenesis of defective healing in diabetes mellitus. *Surg Forum* 1994;45:707.
9. Edlich RF, London SD. Wound repair: from ritual practice to scientific discipline. *J Trauma* 1996;40:326.
10. Krizek TJ, Robson MC, Kho E. Bacterial growth and skin graft survival. *Surg Forum* 1967;18:518.
11. Quirinia A, Viidik A. Effect of delayed primary closure on the healing of ischemic wounds. *J Trauma* 1996;41:1018.
12. Mehta PH, Dunn KA, Bradfield JF, Austin PE. Contaminated wounds: infection rates with subcutaneous sutures. *Ann Emerg Med* 1996;27:43.
13. Ohtsuka H, Toriga K, Itoh W. Free omental transfer to lower limbs. *Ann Plast Surg* 1980;4:70.
14. Robson MC, Raine TR, Smith DJ, et al. Principles of wound healing and repair. In: James EC, Corry RJ, Perry JF, eds. *Basic surgical practice.* Philadelphia: Hanley & Belfus, 1987:69.

6. ANESTHESIA FOR THE TRAUMA PATIENT[1]

PREOPERATIVE MANAGEMENT

Preanesthetic Assessment

AXIOM Although there is such a thing as "minor surgery," there is no such thing as a "minor general anesthetic."

Rapid movement of a severely traumatized patient from the emergency center to the operating room (OR) provides little opportunity for a careful preanesthetic evaluation. Nevertheless, one should try to get as much detail as possible about the mechanism of injury, physical status of the patient at the scene, and prehospital therapy.

In the preanesthetic evaluation of a trauma patient, the anesthesiologist benefits from knowing

1. Past or intercurrent cardiovascular, respiratory, renal, or endocrine disease;
2. Current medications;
3. Allergies or untoward reactions to previous medications;
4. Previous use of drugs such as cocaine, opiates, or steroids; and
5. Time of the patient's last food or drink in relation to the injuries.

The lack of an optimal preanesthetic assessment, when combined with surgical uncertainty about the extent of a patient's injuries, leads the trauma-oriented anesthesiologist to be liberal in the use of invasive monitoring and to be extremely careful with the administration of drugs that may depress the circulation (2).

Specific laboratory investigations, such as a complete blood count (CBC), urinalysis, blood urea nitrogen (BUN), serum creatinine, and electrolytes, should be performed as rapidly as possible, even if the results are not available at the beginning of anesthesia. Blood should also be drawn for typing and cross-matching, and the status of blood availability (cross-matched, type-specific, or type O Rh-negative) should be known as rapidly as possible.

⊘ **PITFALL**

Assuming that normal hemoglobin and hematocrit levels in a trauma patient indicate that the blood volume also is normal.

The hemoglobin concentration (Hgb) or hematocrit (Hct) needed in a trauma patient for safe anesthesia is a matter of considerable meta-analytic opinion. The efficiency of oxygen transport and uptake in the tissues does not seem to deteriorate until the Hct is below 30%, unless the patient has severe cardiac or pulmonary disease. However, survival in postoperative critically ill patients may decrease when the hematocrit is below 32%.

AXIOM Hypoglycemia may occur in some patients with severe alcoholism or cirrhosis, but the great majority of acute trauma patients are hyperglycemic and should not be given glucose with the resuscitation fluids.

Preanesthetic coagulation workups are not routinely indicated, unless major blood loss is anticipated. In such instances, serial platelet counts, prothrombin times (PTs), and accelerated partial thromboplastin times (aPTTs) may provide useful information. If a coagulopathy is suspected, additional tests should include bleeding time, thrombin time, and fibrinogen levels.

Trauma Protocols

AXIOM Well-designed trauma protocols should provide the level of care to injured patients at 2:00 a.m. that is available when the most experienced members of the team are present at 2:00 p.m.

Even when resuscitators are of equivalent training, those who follow a scientifically developed algorithm have less morbidity and mortality than those who function in a less structured fashion.

The surgeon and anesthesiologist should apprise each other of their plans, needs, and concerns. The "fix everything now" approach makes good communication a key to successful outcome. Immediately on transporting an unstable patient to the OR for emergency surgery, the surgeon and anesthesiologist should discuss the patient's condition, the nature and severity of the injuries, and the planned operative procedures. Available historic information, positioning, and difficulties with the airway or vascular access also should be discussed at this time.

Intraoperatively, the surgeon and anesthesiologist should communicate continuously about any significant changes in vital signs, laboratory determinations, and ongoing therapy with blood, fluid, and drugs. Surgical interference with ventilation or circulation, such as by compression of the lung or vena cava, should be announced in advance. Clamping or unclamping of the aorta or anticipated maneuvers associated with major blood loss also should be announced well ahead of time. Conversely, the anesthesiologist should notify the surgeon of changes in any physiologic parameters so that the surgeon can help determine whether these changes are related to the surgical activity or the condition of the patient.

AXIOM Operative procedures should be ranked in the event that the patient's condition deteriorates so badly that surgery must be discontinued.

Control of the Airway

All severely injured patients should be breathing 90% to 100% oxygen soon after entering the emergency system. Adequate preoxygenation and denitrogenation can prevent hypoxemia for up to 2 to 3 minutes after the patient stops breathing effectively during endotracheal intubation.

AXIOM Critically injured patients with impending ventilatory failure should be intubated immediately by the most experienced individual present.

The initial major decision of the anesthesiologist is whether to keep the patient awake (breathing on his own) until the endotracheal tube is passed and then induce anesthesia, or to administer anesthesia or a muscle relaxant or both before intubation. Although the latter option may provide better conditions for intubation, if immediate intubation is not possible, an emergency airway must be provided almost immediately.

AXIOM Aspiration of vomitus or blood into the lungs can occur suddenly at any time before surgery, but it is most apt to occur when inducing anesthesia and instrumenting the upper airway.

Most general anesthetics and paralytic agents relax the esophagogastric and pharyngoesophageal sphincters. Alcohol and nicotine also reduce the tone of these sphincters, and there is the additional danger that intragastric pressure may be increased from air swallowing, particularly if mask-to-face artificial ventilation has been used.

The preanesthetic evaluation of trauma patients, no matter how abbreviated, includes an examination of the airway. Some questions that should be answered during this evaluation include

- Is it safe and possible to extend the head and neck?
- Does the patient's mouth open widely? and
- Is the submandibular space large enough and the tissues filling it pliable enough to permit displacement of the base of the tongue during direct laryngoscopy?

If the answers to these questions are all affirmative and there are no associated airway, craniofacial, or cervical injuries, intubation during rapid-sequence induction is the preferred technique.

The decision to use direct laryngoscopy on the awake patient is often aided by a quick "look–see" with a warm laryngoscope blade during the preanesthetic assessment. It is wise to have a suitable endotracheal tube ready because sometimes the tube can be readily passed at this point.

Controlled (Rapid) Sequence Induction

Most anesthesiologists choose a "rapid-sequence" induction technique for trauma patients requiring emergency surgery. This helps to prevent regurgitation and aspiration of gastric contents, but it requires preoxygenation and denitrogenation by mask to prevent severe hypoxia during the intubation. Anesthesia is induced with an appropriate intravenous agent, and succinylcholine is given to relax the patient's musculature to facilitate intubation. Alternatively, large doses of nondepolarizing neuromuscular blocking agents may be substituted for succinylcholine. The trachea is rapidly intubated, and the cuff is inflated to protect the airway. Proper tube placement is confirmed by auscultation and appropriate levels of exhaled carbon dioxide.

During the induction, a skilled assistant stabilizes the head (to prevent aggravation of any cervical spine injuries) while a second assistant presses backward on the cricoid cartilage to prevent the passage of gastric or esophageal contents in the laryngopharynx. The cricoid pressure is maintained until the cuff on the endotracheal tube has been inflated and proper placement of the tube has been confirmed.

AXIOM Rapid-sequence induction has the potential of producing either an easy intubation or a catastrophe.

The main disadvantage of rapid-sequence induction is that, when anesthesia has been induced, there is no turning back. The patient is rendered apneic at a time when oxygenation is difficult to assure without an endotracheal tube. In addition, if facial injuries do not allow the close application of a face mask, preoxygenation may be impossible or inadequate. Copious foreign material or blood may obscure the view even if the patient has not vomited.

Succinylcholine is usually avoided in patients who have sustained a severe eye injury with an "open globe." In such circumstances, paralysis for intubation is provided by a large dose of a nondepolarizing relaxant with or without the use of a small initial "priming" dose (4).

The induction of general anesthesia is frequently accompanied by respiratory standstill, and bag–mask ventilation may be inadequate because of the mechanical airway obstruction that caused the respiratory distress in the first place. This combination of a technically difficult intubation and airway distress often dictates the need for an emergency cricothyroidotomy. A catheter cricothyroidotomy with jet ventilation can generally provide sufficient oxygenation to permit controlled creation of a surgical airway.

Anatomically difficult intubations in patients who are ventilating adequately can sometimes be performed over a catheter or wire. A large needle is introduced into the trachea or the cricothyroid membrane, and a long, large-bore vascular catheter or a long "j-wire" is advanced retrograde through the larynx and then into the pharynx (3). The end of the catheter or wire is grasped, and an endotracheal tube is advanced over the guide and through the larynx. Alternatively, the guide wire may be passed through the working channel of a fiberoptic bronchoscope. Intubation then proceeds antegrade over the wire, under direct vision. The catheter is then withdrawn from the trachea, and the endotracheal tube is advanced further down, to a position 3 to 4 cm above the carina.

Intubation of Patients with Head Injury

AXIOM Whenever possible, head-injured patients should be examined by the neurosurgeon before an analgesic or sedative is given.

Endotracheal intubation of a patient with a severe closed-head injury is a major concern because intracranial pressure (ICP) can increase precipitately during the procedure (4). Even mild drug-induced respiratory depression with its associated hypercapnia can result in a rapid increase in ICP.

AXIOM One should not attempt to correct hypertension due to a head injury until the cause of the increased ICP has been corrected surgically or by other means.

If a head-injured patient is severely hypertensive, cautious use of β-blockers has been recommended to control ICP. Systemic vasodilators, such as sodium nitroprusside, nitroglycerin, and hydralazine, can reduce the systemic blood pressure (BP), but they also tend to increase cerebral blood flow and ICP.

Failed Intubation

AXIOM Before one attempts endotracheal intubation, particularly in an unstable trauma patient, an alternate technique for rapidly providing an airway should be immediately available.

Failure of endotracheal intubation in a critically injured patient who has been rendered apneic can be terrifying, but a cricothyroidotomy can usually be performed within a few seconds, provided the anterior neck anatomy is normal. If this is not possible, a 14-gauge intravenous cannula can be passed through the cricothyroid membrane or anterior upper trachea, attached to wall or tank oxygen (50 psi), and flushed about 20 times a minute. Great care should be taken to ensure that the cannula is in the trachea, as mediastinal insufflation of large quantities of oxygen under pressure can be catastrophic. Although a properly placed catheter intermittently flushed with wall O_2 can usually keep the patient oxygenated for at least 20 to 30 minutes, CO_2 retention can be a problem, especially if the catheter technique is continued for longer periods.

Sedating the Intubated Patient

Once an endotracheal tube has been passed, the awake patient should be made comfortable with small doses of intravenous anesthetics or narcotics, unless full anesthesia is to be induced for surgery. The experience of being paralyzed and awake is very distressing.

LOCATIONS FOR VENOUS CATHETERS

At least two large-bore (16-gauge or larger) cannulas should be placed, preferably in veins not apt to have injuries proximally. For wounds of abdomen or lower extremities, upper extremity venous catheters are preferred. If a superior vena cava tributary in the chest may be injured, at least one large intravenous catheter should be inserted in a vein leading to the inferior cava.

Venous Catheter Monitors

Most trauma patients are relatively young and without previous cardiovascular disease, and there is usually little need for central venous or pulmonary artery monitoring catheters. However, radial artery cannulation can be very useful for BP measurement and for obtaining repeated blood samples for analysis.

Central venous pressure catheters can be particularly helpful for evaluating preload when there are questions about the patient's fluid status. They also can help in the diagnosis of pericardial tamponade and detection of changes in the circulation from clamping the aorta. In addition, central venous oxygen saturations can be reflective of the overall adequacy of tissue oxygenation (5). If there is severe underlying cardiac or pulmonary disease, a pulmonary artery wedge pressure (PAWP) catheter can be very helpful.

Analgesia and Sedation

AXIOM Premedication designed to reduce patient anxiety is contraindicated if the patient is hemodynamically unstable.

Anxiety may be an early manifestation of circulatory inadequacy or hypoxemia, and attempts at controlling it pharmacologically may result in cardiovascular or respiratory collapse. Nevertheless, if a stable patient is extremely frightened, intravenous agents such as the short-acting narcotic, fentanyl, or the short-acting benzodiazepine, midazolam, may be cautiously titrated to effect.

AXIOM Titrated small doses of intravenous narcotics are generally the safest premedication for anesthesia.

Judicious intravenous administration of narcotics to an injured patient can make the transfer from a stretcher to an x-ray or OR table much more tolerable. Because inadvertent narcotic overdose resulting in hypotension, respiratory depression, or excessive somnolence can be easily antagonized with intravenous naloxone, intravenous narcotics are the first choice for premedication.

The peripheral, splanchnic, and renal vasoconstriction caused by pain and hypovolemia not only reduce the size of the faster compartments of the volume of distribution, but they also decrease the rate of drug elimination by the liver and kidneys. If hypothermia is present, drug elimination will be further retarded. The patient may also have recently taken other drugs that may have an additive effect. For example, at least 50% of trauma patients are intoxicated to some degree with alcohol.

Intravenous Administration of Medications

Peripheral vasoconstriction prevents the subcutaneous and intramuscular routes of administration from working reliably. Poor perfusion of muscle and fat also allows a reservoir of the drug to lie in the tissues from which it can be mobilized when the integrity of the circulation is restored, producing a possible overdose in the patient.

The safest method for providing analgesia after severe trauma is to give small frequent intravenous doses until the patient is no longer severely distressed by the pain. The intermittent doses should be spaced far enough apart to allow time for each dose to exert its effect. This is about 5 to 7 minutes in the case of morphine, and 2 to 3 minutes with fentanyl.

Uncooperative Patients

Sedation, other than that produced by analgesics for severe pain, is seldom indicated preoperatively unless the patient is unruly and physically resisting attempts to provide treatment. Sometimes such restlessness may be due to hypoxia, but if such behavior is sufficiently self-destructive to endanger the patient's life, the use of sedation and muscle relaxants along with mechanical ventilation and oxygen is justified to bring an impossible situation under control.

INTRAOPERATIVE MANAGEMENT

AXIOM Every effort should be made to prevent or rapidly correct hypothermia in patients with severe trauma.

A heated, humidified, breathing circuit and warming blankets should be set up to prevent hypothermia and help warm the patient. Rapid-infusion devices that can warm fluids to 40°C to 42°C should be primed, and the intravenous fluids should be prewarmed. Until the patient is anesthetized and draped, the OR temperature should be kept at 75°F (23°C). After the patient is draped, if blood loss is controlled and the core temperature is above 35°C, it is safe to cool the room to normal levels.

During general anesthesia, the monitoring of trauma victims should minimally include an electrocardiogram, urine output via an indwelling Foley catheter, BP (arterial line or cuff), core temperature probe, and oxygen saturation (pulse oximeter). One should also have the endotracheal tube connected to a capnography machine to monitor exhaled CO_2 concentrations.

If the patient is hypovolemic, depression of sympathetic tone by a normal dose of anesthetic may cause sudden severe cardiovascular collapse. Consequently, general anesthesia for trauma victims should be induced with the minimal amount of agent that will obtund consciousness and provide needed relaxation.

⊘ PITFALL

If the depth of anesthesia is reduced to maintain an adequate BP, patients may have severe pain and anxiety without being able to show it.

Hypotensive, unintubated patients require rapid induction and endotracheal intubation. Reduced doses of ketamine, etomidate, thiopental, or other induction agents are supplemented with large doses of muscle relaxants to allow rapid intubation.

Currently the induction agent of choice for unstable hypovolemic patients is very small doses of ketamine or etomidate; however, ketamine has the theoretic disadvantage of being a sympathetic stimulant, which could cause vasoconstriction and further reduce cardiac output, even though the BP may increase. It is also a direct myocardial depressant, and it may decrease myocardial contractility in a patient who already has a low ejection fraction (6).

General Anesthesia

Maintenance of general anesthesia is usually safest with low concentrations of a volatile inhalation anesthetic carried in 100% oxygen. Until the patient is fully resuscitated and stable, it is probably wise to avoid nitrous oxide, which does not allow the use of high oxygen concentrations. Nitrous oxide also has the potential to greatly increase the size of a pneumothorax, bowel gas, and air bubbles in the circulation.

Local Anesthesia

In the trauma setting, local anesthesia is rarely chosen, except for the repair of superficial lacerations, the insertion of thoracostomy tubes, or the placement of catheters for vascular access. Because of the tissue acidosis that may occur in trauma patients, local anesthetics can be less effective, and the likelihood of systemic toxicity is increased.

Regional Anesthesia

Regional anesthetic techniques can be useful for single-limb injuries, and they will usually not interfere with systemic sympathetic tone. Regional techniques also allow one to closely monitor the patient's level of consciousness after head injury.

Intravenous perfusion (Bier) blocks require little patient cooperation and can be performed on upper or lower extremities with equal success; however, care must be taken to choose a correctly sized tourniquet, and the tourniquet must remain inflated during the entire procedure.

Formal nerve blocks in an upper or lower extremity require more cooperation from the patient than local anesthesia because the elicitation of paresthesias is required; however, extended analgesia for the extremity can be attained. In the upper extremity, placing a catheter in the axillary sheath usually provides excellent anesthesia for limb or digit replantations.

AXIOM The main disadvantage of regional anesthesia is that the amount of anesthetic required usually limits the anesthetic technique to only one extremity.

Spinal or Epidural Anesthesia

The use of spinal or epidural anesthesia in acute trauma patients is debatable. For cooperative, stable patients, they can provide a safe, comfortable method for performing surgical procedures on the lower limbs. In addition, epidural techniques can also provide superb analgesia postoperatively.

One should take every precaution not to allow an epidural or low spinal anesthetic to become a total spinal anesthetic with resultant inadequate spontaneous ventilation. Under such circumstances, emergency endotracheal intubation can be extremely difficult.

Another problem is the sympathetic block, which correlates with the extent of sensory anesthesia, so that a patient who is anesthetized enough to permit a thorough intraabdominal examination will generally also have an extensive sympathetic block.

AXIOM Spinal or epidural techniques should be avoided if there may be preexisting hypovolemia or if there is any expectation of significant intraoperative bleeding.

Monitoring

As soon as the airway is secured and the patient is well oxygenated and anesthetized, consideration should be given to inserting catheters as needed for further resuscitation and monitoring. If not already in use, electrocardiogram (ECG) leads, pulse oximeter, and an esophageal temperature probe can be placed.

AXIOM A single large intravenous cannula with a fast-infusion device is safer and easier to control than two to three smaller intravenous lines.

An arterial catheter for BP monitoring and for frequent blood sampling can be very helpful in patients who may become unstable. If the patient is still hypotensive after what seems to be a reasonable amount of fluid, a central venous or pulmonary artery catheter or both should be inserted.

AXIOM Continued hypotension, even in the face of massive fluid resuscitation, generally is a result of continued bleeding, but one should also look for cardiac tamponade and tension pneumothorax.

Urine output can be a useful measurement of circulatory function, provided the patient does not have to excrete an osmotic load (e.g., radiographic contrast media, mannitol, or glucose) or has not received diuretics. After severe trauma, there may be a lag of up to 2 hours after adequate crystalloid resuscitation before antidiuretic hormone levels are low enough to allow the kidneys to open up and produce an adequate urine output of at least 0.5 to 1.0 mL/kg/h.

Fluid Management

The initial approach to fluid resuscitation during anesthesia is to give enough warmed crystalloid, colloid, blood or a combination of these to maintain a mean BP of at least 60 to 70 mm Hg (to maintain normal cerebral perfusion) and a urine output greater than 0.5 mL/kg/h. At the same time, the hematocrit should be kept above 20% to 25% in the previously fit patient, and 27% to 32% in patients with preexisting cardiopulmonary disease.

Adjuncture Maneuvers

In persistently hypotensive patients with adequate fluid loading, infusions of dopamine, with or without dobutamine, or both in doses of 5 to 20 μg/kg/min may be helpful. However, if the patient is acidotic, epinephrine may be more effective (2). Care must be exercised when administering these agents to patients who are cold and acidotic, as the likelihood of producing a serious dysrhythmia is increased.

Sodium bicarbonate may be required for the treatment of persistent severe metabolic acidosis (pH below 7.10) not responsive to other therapy. However, one must carefully monitor arterial and venous pH and P_{CO_2} and not allow the P_{CO_2} to increase above a level equal to $[(HCO_3)\ (1.5) + 12]$. In other words, a patient with an arterial bicarbonate of 10 mEq/L should not have a P_{CO_2} above 25 mm Hg.

POSTOPERATIVE MANAGEMENT

Transfer from the Operating Room

Transfer to the postanesthetic care unit (PACU) or surgery intensive care unit (SICU) can be as demanding of attention by the anesthesiologist as the period of intraoperative resuscitation. Respiratory support with controlled ventilation, positive end-expiratory pressure (PEEP), and high concentrations of oxygen should be maintained at the same level as provided intraoperatively. A battery-powered pulse oximeter allows continuous measurement of arterial oxygen saturation during transport. The ECG and intraarterial pressure also should be monitored electronically en route to the recovery room or ICU. Small, lightweight, battery-powered infusion devices make continuous drug infusions during transport quite safe and convenient. Finally, adequate personnel to move the patient's bed, ventilator, and other equipment should be available so that the anesthesiologist can concentrate on monitoring and ventilation.

ICU/PACU Care

The patient waking from a general anesthetic will often have a period of severe sympathetic overactivity. The BP can usually be brought under control with a short-acting β-blocker (e.g., esmolol). Sodium nitroprusside infusions are rarely needed.

The patient, in the absence of painful surgical stimuli, may "renarcotize" himself or herself when the blood levels of opiate medications mobilized from extravascular tissue become higher than needed. If there have been acid–base and electrolyte abnormalities, the reversal of muscle relaxants also may have been inadequate during the surgery.

The monitoring and vigilance of the OR must be continued into the postoperative period, preferably in a critical care area. The handing-over process should be standardized, so that the patient does not get into difficulties through a lack of continuity of care.

Postoperative Pain Relief

For most postoperative and posttraumatic pain involving the lower chest, abdomen, pelvis, or lower extremities, epidural analgesia provides the best pain relief. Short et al. (7) found that intrapleural analgesia (for the management of blunt traumatic chest-wall pain) was no more effective than opioid analgesics.

CHRONIC PAIN

The major problems seen with chronic pain include causalgia or reflex sympathetic dystrophy or both. Disorders previously considered to be classic reflex sympathetic dystrophy and causalgia have recently been classified as chronic regional pain syndrome (CRPS; 8). CRPS type I (i.e., classic reflex sympathetic dystrophy) and type II (i.e., causalgia) are poorly understood conditions that may occur after trauma to the extremities. The main symptoms include chronic severe pain, swelling, skin discoloration, and contracture.

If untreated, symptoms of CRPS may continue for months or even years. The exact cause is uncertain, but it is considered to involve sympathetic nervous system dysfunction. Various treatment modalities have been tried, including physiotherapy, sympathetic blockade, and steroid administration. Muramatsu et al. (9) recently described successful treatment of 17 consecutive patients with chronic regional pain syndrome by using manipulation therapy and regional anesthesia.

⊘ FREQUENT ERRORS

1. ***Delay of surgery for diagnostic studies that are not immediately necessary for providing a safe, effective anesthetic.***
2. ***Failure to have an emergency drug and equipment setup ready on a 24-hour basis.***
3. ***Allowing oneself to be rushed into a method of anesthetic management that, on reflection, one would not ordinarily choose.***
4. ***Failure to anesthetize the patient adequately before starting endotracheal intubation.***
5. ***Beginning a general anesthetic without adequate routes of intravenous administration and without adequate blood products or substitutes immediately available.***
6. ***Failure to anticipate and be prepared for the possibility of regurgitation and resultant aspiration during attempts at endotracheal intubation.***
7. ***Failure to have an adequate plan and necessary equipment to manage a failed intubation.***
8. ***Failure to communicate with others involved in the anesthetic–surgical management of the patient.***
9. ***Failure to maintain continued vigilance immediately after surgery and during transfer to the recovery room or ICU.***

SUMMARY POINTS

1. Although there is such a thing as “minor surgery,” there is no such thing as a “minor general anesthetic.”

2. Well-designed trauma protocols should provide the level of care to injured patients at 2:00 a.m. that is available when the most experienced members of the team are present at 2:00 p.m.

3. A failure to discuss surgical and anesthetic strategies preoperatively can lead to major intraoperative difficulties for the entire patient-care team.
4. Operative procedures should be ranked in the event that the patient's condition deteriorates so badly that surgery must be discontinued.
5. Critically injured patients with impending ventilatory failure should be intubated immediately by the most experienced individual present.
6. Before one attempts endotracheal intubation, particularly in an unstable trauma patient, an alternate technique for rapidly providing an airway should be immediately available.
7. Aspiration of vomitus or blood into the lungs can occur suddenly at any time before surgery, but it is most likely to occur when inducing anesthesia and instrumenting the upper airway.
8. "Rapid-sequence induction" has the potential of producing either an easy intubation or a catastrophe.
9. Whenever possible, head-injured patients should be examined by the neurosurgeon before an analgesic or sedative is given.
10. One should not attempt to correct hypertension due to a head injury until the increased ICP has been corrected surgically or by other means.
11. Being awake and paralyzed can be a very terrifying experience for the patient.
12. Failure of the patient to respond appropriately to what should be adequate resuscitative fluid is an indication for CVP or PAWP monitoring.
13. Titrated small doses of intravenous narcotics are generally the safest premedication for anesthesia.
14. Although pain from trauma may be of a magnitude demanding larger than normal amounts of narcotic analgesics, the sensitivity of these patients to these agents may be considerably increased.
15. Every effort should be made to prevent or rapidly to correct hypothermia in patients with severe trauma undergoing major surgery.
16. Nitrous oxide should generally be avoided in patients with severe chest or abdominal trauma.
17. The main disadvantage of regional anesthesia is that the amount of anesthetic required usually limits the anesthetic technique to only one extremity.
18. One should take every precaution to avoid having an epidural or low spinal anesthetic become a total spinal anesthetic with resultant inadequate spontaneous ventilation.
19. Spinal or epidural techniques should be avoided if there may be preexisting hypovolemia or if there is any expectation of significant intraoperative bleeding.
20. A single large intravenous cannula with a fast-infusion device is safer and easier to control than two to three smaller intravenous lines.
21. Lack of adequate communication between anesthesia and ICU or other postanesthesia personnel is one of the major causes of suboptimal care immediately after surgery.

REFERENCES

1. Abrams KJ, Bryan-Brown CW. Anesthesia for the trauma patient. In: Wilson RF, Walt AJ, eds. *Management of trauma: pitfalls and practice.* 2nd ed. Philadelphia: Williams & Wilkins, 1996:85.
2. Coveler LA. Anesthesia. In: Moore EE, Mattox KL, Feliciano DV, eds. *Trauma.* 2nd ed. Norwalk, CT: Appleton & Lange, 1991:219–229.
3. King HR, Wang LF, Khan AK, Wooton OJ. Translaryngeal guided intubation for difficult intubation. *Crit Care Med* 1987;15:869.
4. Orshaker JS, Whye DW. Head trauma. *Emerg Med Clin North Am* 1993;11:165.
5. Scalea TM, Houman M, Fuortes M, et al. Central venous blood oxygen saturation: an early accurate measurement of volume during hemorrhage. *J Trauma* 1988;28: 725.
6. Lippman M, Appel PL, Mok MS, et al. Sequential cardiorespiratory patterns of anesthetic induction with ketamine in critically ill patients. *Crit Care Med* 1983; 11:730.
7. Short K, Scheeres D, Mlakar J, et al. Evaluation of intrapleural analgesia in the

management of blunt traumatic chest wall pain: a clinical trial. *Am Surg* 1996; 62:488.

8. Janig W. The puzzle of "reflex sympathetic dystrophy": mechanism, hypotheses, open questions. In: *Reflex sympathetic dystrophy: a reappraisal: progress in pain research and management.* Seattle, WA: IASP Press, 1996:1–24.
9. Muramatsu K, Kawai S, Akino T, et al. Treatment of chronic regional pain syndrome using manipulation therapy and regional anesthesia. *J Trauma* 1998;44: 189.

7. DIAGNOSTIC AND INTERVENTIONAL RADIOLOGY IN TRAUMA[1]

RADIOLOGIC DIAGNOSTIC MODALITIES IN ACUTE TRAUMA

Plain Film

Plain film radiography is the best way to visualize the skeleton during the initial examination; however, it has only modest value in the assessment of anatomically complex regions, such as the pelvis, face, and the base of the skull, where it has been replaced or greatly supplemented by computed tomography (CT).

Contrast Studies

Contrast studies and fluoroscopy may be of value in esophagography, cystourethrography, sinography, and intravenous pyelography (IVP). When done properly, a normal IVP can be accepted with only a slight risk of missing a major injury. When an IVP is done as a rapid preoperative test, its usefulness is generally limited to the determination of presence or absence of renal function in both kidneys. CT scanning provides much better detail, and it also provides information on other injuries that may be present.

Radionuclide Imaging

Radionuclide imaging (RN) has had extensive use in pediatric abdominal trauma; however, it now has only limited application compared with CT scans.

Liver Scans

Liver scans are seldom indicated in the initial study of hepatic injury, but they can be helpful later when evaluating the patient for a possible hepatic hematoma or abscess or subphrenic collections. Scanning of the lungs also can be helpful in the diagnosis of pulmonary embolism or other causes of reduced circulation to the lungs.

Ultrasound

Ultrasound may be of value for detecting collections of fluid, particularly in the pericardium, but also in the abdomen and retroperitoneum. Even in skilled hands, however, ultrasound is not reliable for the diagnosis of solid-organ injury, and it cannot differentiate intraperitoneal hemorrhage from other causes of intraperitoneal fluid, such as ascites. Recently sonography also has been used in the detection, preoperative localization, and confirmation of surgical retrieval of foreign bodies in the distal extremities.

Computerized Tomography

Computerized tomography is becoming increasingly valuable to traumatologists because it

- Combines high image resolution with the capacity to demonstrate soft-tissue and skeletal injuries simultaneously;
- Differentiates between normal and abnormal soft tissue;
- Delineates the extent of hematomas;
- Detects intraperitoneal blood; and
- Differentiates blood from ascitic and diagnostic peritoneal lavage (DPL) fluid.

In addition, CT is unsurpassed in assessment and follow-up of head injuries, and it is being used increasingly for the diagnosis of penetrating abdominal trauma and vascular injuries. The newer spiral CT scanners add even greater resolution to these studies and may even be accurate enough to rule out traumatic rupture of the aorta (TRA).

Magnetic Resonance Imaging

Magnetic resonance imaging (MRI) is particularly helpful for detecting soft-tissue abnormalities. A major limitation of MRI is the length of time necessary to complete studies. In addition, life-support equipment containing ferromagnetic alloys cannot be allowed near the magnet.

Angiography

Angiography continues to be the most reliable diagnostic procedure for detection of vascular injury. Angiography should be performed whenever vascular injury is suspected and immediate surgery is not required. Examination of the abdominal and pelvic arteries requires insertion of an intraarterial catheter, fluoroscopic control, and serial filming.

Therapeutic Angiography

Therapeutic angiography is indicated in certain cases of arterial injury when hemostasis can be attained by the angiographer. This is especially rewarding if the surgical approach is extremely hazardous (e.g., pelvic ring disruption) or technically difficult (e.g., the vertebral artery; 2).

Single-Stick Arteriograms

If there is inadequate time to obtain a formal arteriogram, a "single-stick" arteriogram can sometimes be very helpful. The procedure involves insertion of a needle into the femoral or axillary artery, hand injection of radiopaque contrast, and plain film radiography. Compression of the proximal vessel and rapid injection of 50 mL or more contrast through a relatively large (16- to 18-gauge) needle help to improve the quality of the studies.

Digital Subtraction Angiography

Digital subtraction angiography (DSA), by virtue of computerized subtraction and enhancement of the image, creates high-quality images with less contrast medium. Real-time projection of the study on the screen at the time of injection allows immediate diagnosis of major injuries without waiting for film processing. Intravenous DSA (IV-DSA) is not recommended unless an arterial approach is impossible. The amount of contrast used for IV-DSA is greater than for intraarterial DSA (IA-DSA), and the images are often of inferior quality.

Carbon Dioxide Angiography

In patients who require angiography but cannot take iodine contrast solutions, carbon dioxide may be used. Although the images are not as definitive as routine contrast studies, they are satisfactory for most cases and extremely safe.

Contrast-Induced Nephropathy

Contrast-induced nephropathy is the third leading cause of hospital-acquired acute renal failure (3). Predisposing factors include preexisting renal insufficiency, dehydration, diabetes mellitus, advanced age, and increased volumes of contrast media. Renal vasoconstriction induced by contrast media appears to be an important etiologic factor.

Hans et al. (4) prospectively studied 55 patients with chronic renal insufficiency (serum creatinine of 1.4 to 3.5 mg/dL) who underwent abdominal aortography and arteriography of the lower extremities. Group 1 (28 patients) received dopamine, 2.5 μg/kg/min, beginning 1 hour before arteriography and continuing for 12 hours. Group 2 received an equal volume of saline for the same period. Creatinine clearance did not change significantly from baseline after arteriography in the dopamine group; however, the control group showed a significant linear decrease in creatinine clearance.

MEDICOLEGAL ASPECTS OF RADIOLOGY

In the current litigious atmosphere, it is often considered negligent not to have radiographs made of all injured areas, even if the physician believes such examinations are unnecessary. Careful clinical notes, with appropriate instructions given to the patient to return if symptoms persist, should eliminate a large percentage of unnecessary radiographic examinations without prejudicing the patient's well-being or jeopardizing the physician.

AXIOM If treatment is the same and outcome identical regardless of the radiographic results, the radiologic examination is not needed.

PREREQUISITES FOR EFFECTIVE EXAMINATIONS

AXIOM In most instances, the amount of information that a radiologist can provide from reading radiographs is directly proportional to the information supplied to him by the clinician.

In dealing with possible fractures, it is particularly helpful to know the exact site of tenderness when trying to evaluate a shadow that could be a normal variant or the result of an old injury. Statements such as "bruised left shoulder with crepitus," "marked swelling of face and left eyelid," or "board-like abdomen with no bowel sounds" can be very helpful to the radiologist.

Children, combative individuals, and patients with multiple injuries may require sedation or anesthesia before or during angiography or CT, or both. The duration of most examinations can be shortened and their quality dramatically improved if the patient is able to cooperate with the x-ray technician.

Radiographic Reports

Films should be processed and interpreted rapidly so that repeated examinations, when needed, can be obtained without moving the patient unnecessarily. Ideally, all films also should be reviewed by the clinicians so that discrepancies between the clinical picture and the radiologic interpretation can be discussed with the radiologist.

AXIOM Radiographs should always be cross-checked with the patient's identification and clinical features. In a busy emergency department (ED), it is easy to attach incorrect identification to radiographs.

Negative or Normal Radiographs

AXIOM Negative or normal radiographs do not mean that a fracture or injury is not present. Some fractures are not visible on the initial radiographs even with examinations of the highest quality. Patients with suspected fractures of non–weight-bearing bones but negative radiographs can be given a splint or sling and instructions to return if symptoms persist.

Fractures of the carpal navicular are frequently not seen on the original radiographs. If such a fracture is suspected, but the original films are negative, a cast or splint should be applied to the forearm and hand and the radiographs repeated in 1 or 2 weeks. A radionuclide bone scan can reliably detect many of these fractures 24 hours after the injury if a definitive diagnosis is necessary.

When clinical evidence suggests the possibility of a fracture of the femoral neck, the patient should be kept at bed rest until the question is resolved. Occasionally, as little as 1 day can be sufficient time to permit visualization of a fracture line on radiograph. Plain film tomography and CT scans are usually diagnostic. Cases that are still equivocal may need a nuclear bone scan or MRI.

Children younger than 12 years often require radiographs of both the injured and normal extremities. Sometimes this is the only way that normal anatomic variations of the growing skeleton can be differentiated from changes due to trauma. In addition, because the ends of the long bones in children are partially uncalcified cartilage, severe disruptions at the epiphyses can occur with relatively little radiologic change.

AXIOM Pathologic fractures should be suspected whenever a fracture occurs after relatively mild trauma.

RADIOLOGIC EXAMINATION OF SPECIFIC AREAS

Skull

Patients with a skull fracture have a greatly increased chance of developing a lesion that needs neurosurgical intervention (5); however, a significant number of patients who do not have a skull fracture and are initially clinically alert, later deteriorate and need neurosurgical intervention.

If skull radiographs are obtained, it is an error to assume that no skull fracture is present (especially in the basilar area) because no fracture line is readily visible on a skull radiograph or on CT scans of the head; thin-section CT of the skull base is needed reliably to exclude this diagnosis.

Brain

The best procedure for evaluating a patient with a possible significant intracranial injury is a nonenhanced CT scan of the brain. Hematomas, pneumocephalus, tissue loss, contusion, the exact location of foreign bodies and bone fragments, and remote intracranial effects of the injury can all be visualized.

AXIOM Plain films of the skull should be discouraged if a CT scan will be performed because plain films generally cannot show the presence of injury to the brain.

Face

Preliminary plain films are not very helpful in assessment of facial injuries. Fractures of the paranasal sinuses and orbits are frequently difficult to recognize on plain films, but the presence of an air—-fluid level in a sinus after injury may be a clue to recognition of an otherwise inapparent fracture. If one maxillary sinus seems more opaque than the other, this can be caused by overlying soft-tissue swelling or fluid or blood within the sinus or a combination of these. One should also look for a depressed fracture of the orbital floor.

CT scans can be used to confirm the findings seen on plain films, and they will also often identify other fractures. If a facial fracture is suspected, but no definite bone fragments are identified on plain radiographs because the area in question is obscured by overlying structures, CT scans in both the axial and coronal planes are usually definitive.

Spine

Many patients with blunt trauma are brought to the ED with a cervical collar in place. With the collar left in place, a cross-table lateral view of the cervical spine is obtained as soon as possible. If this film is normal and the patient cooperates, one can also obtain open mouth (OM) and anteroposterior (AP) views. If these views are also negative and the patient has a normal neurologic examination, the collar is removed, and oblique views can be obtained.

Four radiologic signs that can occur with unstable spinal fractures include displacement of vertebrae, widened interspinous spaces, widened apophyseal joints, and widened vertebral canal (4). In addition, many significant cervical spine injuries are accompanied by abnormal prevertebral soft-tissue shadows.

The C-7 to T-1 interspace is injured in 3% to 9% of patients with cervical spine injuries, but not uncommonly, several radiographs of this area must be taken, including swimmer's views, before the seventh cervical and the top of the first thoracic vertebra can be seen clearly.

AXIOM When considering vertebral alignment, the posterior borders of the vertebral bodies are more reliable guidelines than the anterior borders.

With any type of spinal trauma, CT or MRI is the best way to assess the integrity of the spinal canal, its possible compromise by bone fragments, and the craniovertebral junction. With penetrating wounds of the spine, CT also can localize foreign bodies and bone fragments.

Assessment of any compression on the spinal cord is aided significantly by intrathecal contrast media or MRI. Multiplanar reconstruction of the CT images also allows intensive study of the spine and soft tissues without unnecessary manipulation of the patient.

Neck

With penetrating wounds of the neck, laceration of the upper airway or esophagus may be suspected radiologically by the presence of air in the soft tissues of the neck and mediastinum and particularly in the retropharyngeal space. If the space between the pharynx and cervical spine on lateral view of the neck is more than 4 mm from C-1 to C-4, an abnormal fluid collection should be suspected. At C-5, the prevertebral soft tissue may normally be as thick as the body of the vertebra. Abnormal collections of air or fluid in the mediastinum or pleural spaces also should make one suspect a pharyngeal or esophageal injury.

Angiography is of particular value in assessing penetrating injuries high in the neck between the angle of the mandible and the base of the skull, especially if the vertebral arteries may be involved (6). Vascular injuries accompanying an unstable cervical spine fracture in neurologically intact patients should be managed by angiography to eliminate the risk of iatrogenic quadriplegia (2).

Chest

In patients with severe hypotension, plain films to rule out a hemothorax or pneumothorax are extremely important. Subtle signs of a ruptured hemidiaphragm may also be seen and targeted for further assessment. The mediastinum also should be evaluated to rule out possible injury to the aorta or its major branches.

Injuries to the anterior noncalcified cartilaginous ends of the ribs are seldom detectable. In addition, almost half of all fractures of the lateral and posterior osseous portions of the rib are invisible on the initial radiologic examinations of the chest, even in retrospect.

A pneumothorax can often be detected best by looking for a "thin white line." When air is in the pleural space, the visceral pleura seen tangentially is outlined by air within the lung on one side and pneumothorax air on the other side, producing a thin white line, which is about 1.0 mm thick and should be seen in two dimensions.

A skin fold overlying the chest may mimic a pneumothorax, especially when the radiograph is taken with the patient in a supine position. However, the only dimension that a skin-fold line has is length, and it is not a white line.

AXIOM More than 1,000 mL of pleural fluid may not be apparent on routine radiographs of the chest in supine patients.

Pleural fluid is not seen well when radiographs are taken of supine patients. Although large amounts of pleural fluid on one side can be suspected on recumbent films because of the increased density of the hemithorax, upright and decubitus views are often necessary to see smaller collections. If even slight blunting of the costophrenic angle is seen on an upright film, it can usually be assumed that at least 200 to 300 mL of fluid are present. A subpulmonic pleural effusion should be suspected on an upright chest radiograph if the top of the dome of the diaphragm is shifted laterally rather than located in the middle of the hemithorax.

It may occasionally be difficult to differentiate between a large pleural effusion and atelectasis with a mass producing a whited-out hemithorax. As a general rule, the heart or mediastinum is usually shifted toward the side of a major atelectasis. In contrast, a large pleural effusion will tend to shift the mediastinum away from the area of opacification.

If the medial border of the alleged effusion has a meniscus sign, but the lateral border of the alleged pleural effusion does not also have a meniscus sign, the opacification may be due to atelectasis. Contusion of the lung produces transudation of fluid and blood into and around the bronchioles and alveoli, increasing the density of the involved area.

Although minimal amounts of thoracic subcutaneous emphysema can be expected with any penetrating injury, large amounts, particularly if they occur after blunt trauma, suggest damage to the trachea or large bronchi.

Heart

If the normal pericardial cavity rapidly fills with more than 200 mL of blood or fluid, tamponade usually occurs, but the enlargement of the heart shadow may be so slight that it can be easily overlooked on chest radiograph. Echocardiography has been increasingly suggested for the workup of precordial penetrating or blunt trauma, but 5% to 10% false negatives have been reported. Computed tomography also may be used to screen stable patients at risk for penetrating cardiac injury (7).

Mediastinum

Large mediastinal hematomas (especially from a traumatic rupture of the aorta) are readily recognized on plain chest films if they widen the superior mediastinum, displace midline structures (trachea and nasogastric tube) to the left, depress the left main bronchus, and obliterate normal tissue interfaces. Mediastinal width, whether absolute or as a percentage of thoracic diameter, is only moderately sensitive and poorly specific for traumatic rupture of the aorta. Smaller hematomas may not be recognized at all if the chest radiograph is not subjected to meticulous inspection by an experienced radiologist.

On the CT scan, the presence of soft-tissue-density material around the aorta or one of its branches may represent hematoma or mediastinal fat. If the normal dark mediastinal fat is displaced or infiltrated, it is possible that a hematoma is adjacent to a major vessel, and an arteriogram is needed. Rapid spiral CT techniques have significantly improved CT evaluation of vascular structures and may be almost as good as aortography.

AXIOM Most mediastinal hematomas are produced by injury to venous or small arterial structures. Nevertheless, if the CT demonstrates mediastinal hemorrhage adjacent to the aorta, aortography is warranted.

Miller et al. (8), in a series of 104 patients who had a CT scan of the chest and an aortogram, had five patients with TRA. Only three were interpreted as having a mediastinal hematoma on CT scan, but one was apparently performed without intravenous contrast and one was misread by a radiology resident. Three aortic branch injuries were also missed.

In another study, Durham et al. (9) reported that six aortic injuries were detected by aortography, but only four had positive CT scans, for a sensitivity of only 67%.

There was some interreader variation, and the quality of the CT scans is not really known.

In contrast, in a recent review, Raptopoulos (10) indicated that normal findings on chest CT scans exclude aortic injury rather well. Indeed, Fisher et al. (11) found that CT was at least as good as aortography for excluding aortic injury. Raptopoulos (10) believed that overwhelming evidence suggests that CT can be used for screening patients with suspected aortic transection, especially those who are hemodynamically stable and are undergoing CT for other injuries.

AXIOM Aortograms to rule out TRA should visualize the entire thoracic aorta and its major branches.

Diaphragm

On the initial plain films of the chest or abdomen, diaphragmatic injuries should always be suspected when the diaphragm is elevated, when it moves abnormally, or if unusual gas shadows are seen above the diaphragm, especially on the left, or with a combination of these.

The diagnosis of diaphragmatic injury is sometimes first made when the end of a nasogastric tube is noted to pass from the abdomen into the left chest. Occasionally, insufflation of 200 to 300 mL of air into the stomach through a nasogastric tube may outline the stomach or intestine in the chest.

Herniation of the bowel into the chest is often better seen with the patient supine, because intrathoracic abdominal contents may slide back below the diaphragm when the patient is upright.

Abdomen

AXIOM Hemodynamically unstable patients should not be sent to the radiology department for CT scans, except for a very rapid CT scan of the brain in an individual strongly suspected of having a life-threatening intracranial hematoma that must be drained immediately.

The most reliable radiologic study for assessment of blunt abdominal trauma is a CT scan of the abdomen and pelvis. At the time of abdominal imaging, a limited screening examination of the chest also can be performed within minutes to identify or rule out mediastinal hematomas. However, one also must be aware that seat-belt injuries of the lumbar spine may be subtle and may require additional studies (12). The injuries most likely to be missed on CT scan are those involving the intestine (13). Other injuries likely to be missed are those of the mesentery, diaphragm, and pancreas.

The oral contrast consists of a 2% water-soluble iodinated material diluted in water. Ideally, 300 to 600 mL of this oral contrast solution are administered via nasogastric tube within 30 minutes of the onset of the study, and the nasogastric tube is withdrawn into the esophagus to decrease streak artifact. The intravenous contrast consists of 100 mL of a 60% iodinated substance, given after an initial scan is performed.

In general, the better the intravenous and oral contrast administration, the more likely it is that any pathology will be seen on CT; however, Kinnunen et al. (13) noted that omission of the oral contrast medium does not jeopardize the essential diagnoses, and it saves time.

Penetrating abdominal trauma is frequently evaluated by plain film radiography. Such films can be helpful for documentation of entrance and exit wounds and foreign body location. The presence of a small pneumoperitoneum may be seen only on upright or left lateral decubitus views.

On supine abdominal films, a "double wall" sign can help make a diagnosis of intraperitoneal air. On a standard supine film of the abdomen, air located within the bowel lumen outlines only the intraluminal side of the bowel. In patients with a ruptured viscus, air may outline both the mucosal and serosal sides of the bowel wall, producing a positive double-wall sign.

Although a preoperative CT is rarely necessary with penetrating abdominal trauma, a CT scan with colon contrast can help determine the need for laparotomy in patients who have been stabbed in the flank or back.

Duodenum

Rupture of the duodenum after blunt trauma is characterized by obliteration of the right psoas shadow and the presence of bubbles of air in the right perinephric space or along the borders of the psoas muscle or both.

A large intramural hematoma involving the retroperitoneal portion of the duodenum can produce a picture of a high small-bowel obstruction. A duodenal mass on CT after trauma has also proved effective in making the diagnosis of intramural duodenal hematoma.

Liver and Spleen

Although arteriography and CT scans are more precise methods for evaluating liver and spleen injuries, a number of indirect signs seen on plain films can help make the diagnosis. For example, fractures of the lower ribs associated with a mass in the region of the liver or spleen is suggestive of blood or hematoma. With some splenic injuries, the gastric air bubble may be displaced to the right, or the splenic flexure may be depressed.

Pelvis

Accurate diagnosis of the bone and ligament injuries in a fractured pelvis is best made with CT scans with multiplanar and three-dimensional reconstruction (14). Venous and osseous pelvic bleeding can generally be controlled by external fixation of the pelvic fracture. Continued arterial pelvic hemorrhage, often from posterior branches of the internal iliac artery, can usually be controlled by angiographic embolization (15).

Urinary Tract

An excretory urogram (IVP) can be performed without prior preparation, by bolus administration of 60% contrast medium in a dose of 1.0 mL/lb, up to 150 mL. Damage to a renal artery is suggested when a kidney is not visualized. Renal vein injuries can produce a swollen nonvisualized kidney. Parenchymal injuries can be manifested by distortion of the collecting system or extravasated contrast material. Injuries of the renal pelvis, parenchyma, and ureters are best evaluated by dynamic CT studies. Injuries to the urinary bladder are best evaluated by retrograde cystography.

Extremities

The forearm and lower leg both have two bones. If either one of the two bones is fractured, the transmitted force frequently fractures or dislocates the other bone, often at the end remote from the injury.

AXIOM With any suspected fracture, the radiologic examination should include the proximal and distal joints of the suspected bones.

After a fall on an outstretched hand, persistent localized wrist pain with no fracture showing on radiographs of the hand, wrist, and forearm indicates a possible fracture of the navicular. If findings are suggestive of navicular fracture, tailored navicular views may increase diagnostic accuracy.

Undisplaced fractures of the femoral neck can be very difficult to diagnose radiologically at times. The difficulty is even greater when the patient has demineralized bones. Conventional plain film tomography, CT, radionuclide bone scans, and MRI are useful for definitive diagnosis, but at progressively increased cost.

Fractures of the knee are frequently associated with an accumulation of fat and blood in the knee joint. This lipohemarthrosis can easily be detected on a cross-table lateral view of the knee.

Frequently patients will come to the ED with ankle pain after a misstep off a curb. If only ankle radiographs are ordered, one can miss a fracture of the base of the fifth metatarsal.

Vascular injuries in extremities occur with varying frequency in association with fractures and dislocations. Angiography is recommended whenever the probability of vascular injury is relatively high. For example, injury to the popliteal artery is common with dislocations of the knee.

When an injured extremity is pulseless in spite of appropriate traction, angiography is important. It is advisable to do the angiogram before any orthopedic surgery to avoid lengthy delays in diagnosis of vascular injuries.

RADIOLOGY DURING RECOVERY FROM TRAUMA

Postoperative abdominal complications are often best diagnosed by CT. CT is especially important in diagnosing and localizing intraabdominal abscesses, which may be multiple in up to 45% of infected patients (16).

RECOGNIZING CHILD ABUSE

The problem of unexplained fractures in infancy has received widespread attention, but difficulties remain when guardians vehemently deny injuring their child. Fractures that suggest abuse include scapular fractures, fractures involving the small bones of the hands and feet, lateral clavicular fractures, and sternal and spinal fractures. It also should be remembered that lesions that have a low specificity for abuse (e.g., long-bone fractures) achieve a higher specificity when a history of trauma is absent or inconsistent with the injuries (17).

⊘ FREQUENT ERRORS

1. ***Failure to provide the appropriate clinical information to the radiologist and x-ray technicians.***
2. ***Being satisfied with (and not repeating) inferior radiologic examinations.***
3. ***Forgetting that many injuries cannot be recognized radiologically, particularly at the time of the initial examination.***
4. ***Sending an uncooperative patient to the radiologist for CT scans of the head, chest, or abdomen.***
5. ***Failure to compare current films with old radiographs if they are available.***
6. ***Failure to obtain radiographs of the joints proximal and distal to a suspected fracture.***
7. ***Failure to obtain radiographs of the uninjured arm or leg in a child if the bones and growth centers in the injured side are confusing.***

SUMMARY POINTS

1. If treatment is the same and outcome identical regardless of the radiograph, the radiologic examination is unnecessary.

2. In most instances, the amount of information that a radiologist can provide from reading radiographs is directly proportional to the information supplied by the clinician.

3. Radiographs should always be cross-checked with the patient's identification and clinical features. In a busy ED, it is easy to attach incorrect identification to a radiograph.

4. Negative or normal radiographs do not mean that a fracture or injury is not present. Some fractures are not visible on the initial radiographs, even with examinations of the highest quality.

5. Pathologic fractures should be suspected whenever a fracture occurs after relatively mild trauma.
6. Plain films of the skull should be discouraged if a CT scan of the head will be performed.
7. Proper immobilization is essential to ensure that a patient's injury is not aggravated by motion during radiologic studies.
8. When considering spinal alignment, the posterior borders of the vertebral bodies are more reliable guidelines than the anterior borders.
9. If a recent fracture has occurred, cortical bone should be interrupted.
10. The "thin white line" sign is valid only for small to medium-sized pneumothoraces.
11. Large quantities of pleural fluid may not be easily visible on routine radiographs of the chest in a supine patient.
12. When a small pleural effusion is suspected but is difficult to see on routine chest radiographs, decubitus views can be very helpful.
13. Any true finding on CT scan will be present on adjacent cuts or more than one view. Artifacts are not usually consistent from film to film.
14. Most mediastinal hematomas are produced by injury to venous or small arterial structures; nevertheless, if the CT demonstrates mediastinal hemorrhage adjacent to the aorta, aortography is warranted.
15. Aortograms to rule out TRA should visualize the entire thoracic aorta and its major branches.
16. In general, hemodynamically unstable patients should not be sent to the radiology department for CT scans, except for a very rapid CT scan of the brain in an individual strongly suspected of having a life-threatening intracranial hematoma that must be drained immediately.
17. In general, the better the intravenous and oral contrast administration, the more likely it is that abdominal pathology can be seen on CT.
18. When checking for the double-wall sign of free intraperitoneal air on a supine film, one should find an isolated portion of bowel that has no overlapping loops.
19. With any suspected fracture, the radiologic examination should include the joints proximal and distal to the area of concern.

REFERENCES

1. Guyot DR, McCarroll KA, Wilson RF. Diagnostic and interventional radiology in trauma. In: Wilson RF, Walt AJ, eds. *Management of trauma: pitfalls and practice.* 2nd ed. Philadelphia: Williams & Wilkins, 1996:105.
2. Ben-Menachem Y, Handel SF, Thaggard A III, et al. Therapeutic arterial embolization in trauma. *J Trauma* 1979;19:944.
3. D'Elia JA, Gleason RE, Aldey M, et al. Nephrotoxicity from angiographic contrast material: a prospective study. *Am J Med* 1982;72:719.
4. Hans SS, Hans BA, Dhillon R, et al. Effect of dopamine on renal function after arteriography in patients with pre-existing renal insufficiency. *Am Surg* 1998;64:432.
5. Feuerman T, Wackym PA, Gade GF, et al. Value of skull radiography, head computed tomographic scanning, and admission for observation in cases of minor head injury. *Neurosurgery* 1988;22:449.
6. Sclafani SJA, Panetta T, Goldstein AS, et al. The management of arterial injuries caused by penetration of zone III of the neck. *J Trauma* 1985;25:871.
7. Nagy KK, Gilkey SH, Roberts RR, et al. Computed tomography screens stable patients at risk for penetrating cardiac injury. *Acad Emerg Med* 1996;3:1024.
8. Miller FB, Richardson JD, Thomas HA, et al. Role of CT in diagnosis of major arterial injury after blunt thoracic trauma. *Surgery* 1989;106:596.
9. Durham RM, Zuckerman D, Wolverson M, et al. Computed tomography as a screening exam in patients with suspected blunt aortic injury. *J Trauma* 1993;35:161.
10. Raptopoulos V. Chest CT for aortic injury: maybe not for everyone. *Am J Roentgenol* 1994;162:1053.

11. Fisher RG, Chasen MH, Lamki N. Diagnosis of injuries of the aorta and brachiocephalic arteries caused by blunt chest trauma: CT versus aortography. *Am J Roentgenol* 1994;162:1047–1052.
12. Taylor GA, Eggli KD. Lap-belt injuries of the lumbar spine in children: a pitfall in CT diagnosis. *Am J Roentgenol* 1988;150:1355.
13. Kinnunen J, Kivioja A, Poussa K, et al. Emergency CT in blunt abdominal trauma of multiple injury patients. *Acta Radiol* 1994;35:319–322.
14. Noh HM, Scott WW, Fishman EK. Imaging of pelvic trauma: the role of CT with multiplanar and three-dimensional reconstruction. *J South Orthop Assoc* 1996;5:111.
15. Ben-Menachem Y, Handel SF, Ray RD, et al. Embolization procedures in trauma: the pelvis. *Semin Intervent Radiol* 1985;2:158.
16. Sclafani SJA. Radiologic intervention for post-traumatic abscesses. *Semin Intervent Radiol* 1985;2:182.
17. Chapman S. Radiological aspects of non-accidental injury. *J R Soc Med* 1990;83:67.

8. TRAUMA IN INFANTS AND CHILDREN[1]

STATISTICS

Trauma is the leading cause of death for young children older than 1 year, with nearly 15,000 children dying of trauma annually. Indeed, in young children, trauma accounts for more deaths than all other causes combined and results in more than two thirds of the deaths in young boys. For each death, there are another 40 to 50 nonlethal injuries requiring hospital admission (2).

⊘ PITFALL

The most common pitfall in the management of injured children is to assume that they are small adults and treat them accordingly.

Children tend to sustain characteristic injuries at different levels of growth and development. During the first 6 years of life, falls are the predominant form of injury. In the elementary school years, bicycle accidents and automobile–pedestrian injuries predominate. As children enter the midadolescent years, high-speed motor vehicle accidents and wounds associated with violent crime become the primary sources of trauma, much as in adults.

Children have a higher incidence of head trauma, partly because the head represents a larger proportion of a child's surface area than it does in adults. Isolated head injury accounts for 19% of pediatric trauma deaths, and head injury combined with another body part injury accounts for about 70% of mortalities.

AXIOM A child's relatively compliant body may have little external evidence of serious internal damage.

Pediatric Trauma Score

The pediatric trauma score (PTS) was devised and tested as a triage tool to identify children who might require care in a pediatric trauma center (3). The PTS has six components, which can be scored as +2 (least severe problem), +1 (moderate problem), or −1 (most severe problem). The components include size of the child (more than 20 kg, 10 to 20 kg, less than 10 kg), airway (normal, maintainable, unmaintainable), central nervous system (CNS; awake, obtunded, comatose), systolic blood pressure (BP; more than 90, 50 to 90, less than 50 mm Hg), open wounds (none, minor, major), and fractures (none, one closed, open, or multiple). Children with a PTS more than 8 rarely die, whereas those with a PTS of 0 or less have a mortality approaching 100%. With scores between 0 and 8, a linear relation is found between decreasing PTS and increasing potential for death. Thus any injured child whose PTS in the field is 8 or less should be transported to the highest level trauma care facility in the area.

Resuscitation

Although the incidence of cervical spine injuries is lower in children than in adults, neck immobilization with sand bags with proper taping is important until appropriate radiologic studies have ruled out this injury.

Children can lose heat quickly. Their surface area is large compared with both their mass and blood volume. In addition, they have less insulating fat and thinner skin than adults. A trauma room for children should be equipped with both a room thermostat and overhead warmers. All blood and other intravenous fluid infused should be warmed to 40°C to 42°C.

⊘ PITFALL

A child should not be allowed to lose heat by exposure to room-temperature air and unwarmed intravenous solutions.

Ileus is more common in children than in adults, and early gastric intubation to prevent severe gastric distention with vomiting and aspiration is important. If there is any midfacial or anterior head trauma in infants or trauma leading to suspicion of a cribriform plate injury, the gastric tube should be placed through the mouth and not the nose.

AXIOM Because infants are obligatory nasal breathers, occlusion of the nose by injuries or foreign bodies, such as nasogastric tubes, may severely impair ventilation.

Establishment of an airway by pulling the mandible and tongue forward in a child is most easily done with a chin-lift maneuver, which avoids neck extension. Most children can be adequately ventilated with a bag and mask, but intubation is required for severe head or thoracic trauma. In the acute situation, oral intubation is recommended over nasal. Tracheostomy is rarely indicated and can be difficult to perform in a child. If the airway is unstable and the patient cannot be intubated, a temporary needle catheter cricothyroidotomy can be performed.

AXIOM Restlessness or any change in mental status in an injured child should be attributed to hypoxia until proven otherwise.

If the nasal passages cannot be cleared in an infant with respiratory distress, an oral airway or endotracheal tube should be inserted. The proper size endotracheal tube to use in a child may be estimated from the size of the child's external nares or little finger. The endotracheal tubes used in children should be uncuffed and allow some leakage of air to prevent laryngotracheal trauma, which can cause subglottic edema, ulceration, and eventual stenosis.

A child's tongue is much larger in relation to the oral cavity than that in an adult, and the infant's larynx and glottis are also more cephalad, making endotracheal intubation more difficult. In addition, because of the infant's large occiput, the neck is already flexed and the head slightly extended when the child is lying in a supine position.

AXIOM There is little distance in an infant between the position of an endotracheal tube that is inserted too far and one that is not in far enough.

Care must be taken to pass the endotracheal tube only 2 to 3 cm below the vocal cords, and the tube should be marked at this point. Palpation of the tip of the tube in the trachea at the point between the clavicular heads is a reliable method of positioning the tube in the midtrachea of infants; however, the position of the tube should also be checked by listening for breath sounds over both lung fields before securing the tube. Failure to secure the tube properly in the infant and to prevent excessive movement of the neck also can result in bronchial intubation or accidental extubation.

AXIOM Because of the inaccuracy of checking endotracheal tube position by physical examination in infants or young children, a chest radiograph is always obtained to ascertain endotracheal tube position as soon as it has been secured.

In a child with acute obstruction of the upper airway who cannot be intubated immediately, a large-bore needle (14- to 18-gauge) may be placed through the cricothyroid membrane. As in adults, wall oxygen can be attached to the needle and a hole cut in the tubing can be occluded intermittently to ventilate the child as a temporizing maneuver. Surgical cricothyroidotomy is rarely, if ever, indicated in infants or children because it can cause severe upper airway problems and has been associated with the later subglottic stenosis.

AXIOM Infants ventilate primarily with their diaphragms; therefore, anything pressing on or irritating the diaphragm can greatly reduce the ability of a child to breathe properly.

AXIOM The mediastinum shifts easily in infants and young children; consequently, any problem in one hemithorax, such as a flail chest, can severely impair ventilation and venous return.

Although the newborn has much smaller lungs than an adult in terms of total lung capacity (63 vs. 86 mL/kg) and vital capacity (35 vs. 70 mL/kg), the minute ventilation (210 vs. 90 mL/min/kg) and oxygen consumption (6.4 vs. 3.5 mL/min/kg) are much greater (4).

Shock and Vascular Access

Pediatric patients in shock can have a normal systolic BP because of their ability to increase heart rate and to vasoconstrict while in the supine position as compensation for blood losses in excess of 15% to 20%. Inadequate tissue perfusion in young children should be diagnosed primarily by tachycardia, tachypnea, decreased responsiveness, and decreased urine output.

In the noncrying child, the systolic BP should generally be at least 80 plus twice the age in years, and the diastolic pressure should be two thirds of the calculated systolic pressure. The normal heart rate is 120 beats/min at 0 to 1 years, 100 beats/min at 1 to 5 years, and 80 beats/min after age 5 years. Because infants have a relatively fixed stroke volume, any pathologic process or drug that decreases heart rate also will decrease cardiac output, and this must be avoided in infants with significant blood loss.

In children, hypovolemia is best treated by keeping the patient warm and rapidly administering 20 mL/kg lactated Ringer's solution as a bolus in 5 to 10 minutes. If there is no response, a second bolus is administered rapidly. If there is still no response, type-specific or O-negative blood (10 mL/kg) is rapidly given, along with further crystalloid. One should also consider prompt operative control of the bleeding sites.

Whenever time permits, compatibility testing should be performed before beginning blood transfusions. Maternal serum can be used for cross-matching infants younger than 1 week, because immunoglobulin G (IgG) blood group antibodies are passively transferred from the mother to the infant during gestation (5). For older infants and children, samples for compatibility testing are obtained from the patient. However, infants younger than 4 months rarely produce antibodies against blood group antigens. Therefore, patients in this age group do not require repeated compatibility testing, even if different donors are used, unless plasma-containing components, such as whole blood, have been transfused.

AXIOM Whenever possible, blood less than 5 days old should be selected for transfusion to young children.

Young children do not increase the 2,3-diphosphoglycerate (2,3-DPG) in transfused red blood cells as rapidly as do adults. Although the 2,3-DPG levels in transfused red cells may return to normal within a few hours in adults, there is often a much longer delay in young children.

The "three-for-one" rule used for estimating crystalloid replacement for blood loss applies in children as it does in adults. During operative intervention, third-space requirements of lactated Ringer's are similar to those in adults at about 3 to 10 mL/kg/h depending on the operative site. If the hematocrit is 40% or more in the newborn or more than 30% in the older infant or child, colloid may be given for intravascular volume replacement in lieu of blood. This can be given as 5% albumin in lactated Ringer's in doses of 10 to 20 mL/kg over a 2- to 3-hour period in addition to maintenance fluid.

Although the ideal vascular access in severely injured children, as in adults, is one or two large-bore upper extremity lines, this may not always be possible. A saphenous vein cutdown at the ankle is safe and efficient. Internal jugular vein and subclavian vein catheterization are possible even in the smallest child by trained and experienced personnel; however, the anatomy in children is somewhat different from that in adults. In addition, inserting these catheters in a struggling, awake child is associated with a higher incidence of pneumothorax and arterial puncture than in adults.

AXIOM If no vascular access is available in an emergency, nearly all resuscitation drugs, except $NaHCO_3$, can be given to children via an endotracheal tube.

Intraosseous Infusions

AXIOM If adequate vascular access cannot be obtained in a reasonable period for resuscitation of a hemodynamically unstable child, the intraosseous route should be considered until other venous access is obtained.

An intraosseous needle or spinal needle can be placed relatively easily into the marrow cavity of the proximal tibial plateau. The distal femur, distal tibia, sternum, clavicle, and humerus also may be used. For tibial infusions, the needle should be placed 2 or 3 cm distal to the tibial tuberosity on the anterior medial surface of the proximal tibia. The needle is inserted perpendicular to the bone or pointing 60° inferiorly, with the bevel directed up. Pressure and a rotary motion are used until a decrease in resistance is noted, indicating that the medullary cavity has been entered. It is not always possible to aspirate marrow, but the fluid should run easily without a pump.

Intraosseous infusions have included saline, glucose, blood, sodium bicarbonate, atropine, dopamine, epinephrine, diazepam, antibiotics, phenytoin, and succinylcholine (6). Reported complications with intraosseous infusions, such as cellulitis, osteomyelitis, extravasation, and hematoma, are relatively uncommon.

Maintenance fluid is administered on a milligram per kilogram body weight basis as 5% dextrose solution in 0.2% normal saline (NS) plus 2 mEq potassium chloride (KCl) per 100 mL of intravenous fluid. Because premature infants and stressed full-term infants may have a depletion of liver glycogen, they should be maintained on a 10% dextrose solution in 0.2% NS, and the serum glucose levels should be monitored at regular intervals at the bedside.

Maintenance fluid needs per day are 100 mL/kg for the first 10 kg, 50 mL/kg for the next 10 kg, and then 20 mL/kg for each kilogram over 20 kg of body weight. Thus a 30-kg child requires (10 × 100) + (10 × 50) + (10 × 20), or 1,700 mL maintenance fluid per day.

Urine Output

A full-term infant, in response to water deprivation, can increase urine osmolality to only 500 to 600 mOsm/kg (7). Consequently the needed urine output for a low-birth-weight infant to excrete its solute load may be as high as 4 mL/kg/h. For a normal newborn, it is 1.5 to 2.0 mL/kg/h, and for a child, 0.5 to 1.0 mL/kg/h is usually adequate. In situations in which there is an increase in protein catabolism, such as after trauma, the solute load may be significantly greater, and a higher urine output is required.

AXIOM A urine osmolality of 600 mOsm/kg in a newborn usually indicates hypovolemia.

Hypothermia

Hypothermia has been shown to stimulate the secretion of catecholamines and muscle shivering, and this can cause severe metabolic acidosis, especially if tissue perfusion is impaired. The infant who is hypothermic may be refractory to therapy for shock, may develop bleeding disorders, and may have a prolonged effect from any anesthetic agents given.

The high ratio of body surface area (BSA) to body mass, the small glycogen stores in the liver, and a thin skin with minimal subcutaneous tissue (allowing increased conductive heat loss) all greatly affect a child's ability to maintain its core temperature. The temperature at which the metabolic activity keeps caloric production at a basal level is also much higher for the newborn and infant than for an adult.

AXIOM To help prevent hypothermia, injured infants should be treated in a warm environment maintained between 24°C and 27°C (75°F to 80°F).

In the neonatal nursery, babies are kept warm with radiant warmers, cellophane wraps to decrease convection losses, and warming of inspired gases. The temperature of a pediatric operating room should be kept at 24°C to 27°C.

Fluids for preparation of the skin and irrigation of body cavities should be warm and should not be allowed to soak the infant's skin and back, resulting in evaporative heat loss. Placement of eviscerated intestine in a plastic bag or maintaining it within the abdominal cavity is also helpful for decreasing the amount of evaporative heat loss during celiotomy. When the baby is covered by the sterile sheets, a heating blanket and extremity wraps must be used.

CARDIAC ARREST AND DRUGS

AXIOM Children who experience a cardiac arrest after trauma need oxygen, fluid, and blood rather than multiple drugs or electric shocks.

Attempts to defibrillate hypoxemic and hypovolemic children are generally futile (8). Nevertheless, if cardiac arrest or hypotension persists after adequate oxygen has been provided and blood volume has been restored, cardiopulmonary resuscitation (CPR) drugs in pediatric doses may be helpful (Table 8-1).

If ventricular fibrillation occurs, children can usually be defibrillated promptly with only a 2- to 4 watt-second (joules)/kg shock.

Monitoring

All members of the team caring for seriously injured children should know the range of normal values for the vital signs in infants and young children. Thus a systolic BP

Table 8-1. ***Pediatric doses of resuscitation drugs***

Drugs	Dose	Purpose
$NaHCO_3$	1 mEq/kg (1 mL/kg of an 8.4% solution 0.5 mEq/kg in neonates (also in neonates dilute in an equal volume of D5W)	Correction of metabolic acidosis
Atropine	0.02 mg/kg up to 1 mg	Increased heart rate (in children cardiac output is often rate dependent)
Epinephrine	0.01 mg/kg 0.1 mL/kg of a 1:10,000 solution	Chronotropic and inotropic
Isoproterenol	0.1 to 1.0 μg/kg/min 0.6 × kg = mg to add to 100 mL; then 1 mL/hr delivers 0.1 μg/kg/min	Continuing chronotropic and inotropic Bradycardia
Dopamine	5–20 μg/kg/min 6 × kg = mg to add to 100 mL; then 1 mL/hr delivers 1 μg/kg/min	Low dose increases renal perfusion Higher doses are pressor
Dobutamine	5–15 μg/kg/min 6 × kg = mg to add to 100 mL; then 1 mL/hr delivers 1 μg/kg/min	Inotropic and pressor
Lidocaine	1 mg/kg; then 20–50 μg/kg/min	Treatment of ventricular tachyarrhythmias
Bretylium	5 mg/kg	Treatment of ventricular tachyarrhythmias

of 80, heart rate of 120 beats/min, and respiratory rate of 40 breaths/min might be normal in an infant but would be evidence of shock or acute respiratory distress or both in an older child. Bradycardia in an injured child is an ominous sign of impending cardiovascular collapse.

AXIOM The most valuable noninvasive monitor in injured children is serial physical examinations by a well-trained physician. The most helpful blood tests are serial hematocrits.

For children with evidence of a severe head injury who are younger than 6 years, the children's coma score (CCS), which has a maximum score of 11, should be used rather than the Glasgow Coma Scale (9; Table 8-2).

Patients with severe head trauma or multisystem injury should have arterial and central venous lines. Swan–Ganz catheters are seldom used in children and should

Table 8-2. ***Children Coma Scale (CCS)***

Ocular response	4 Pursuit of object with eyes 3 Pupils nonreactive *or* EOM paralyzed 2 Fixed pupils *and* EOM paralyzed
Verbal response	3 Cries 2 Spontaneous breathing 1 Apneic
Motor response	4 Flexes and extends 3 Withdraws from painful stimuli 2 Flaccid

EOM = extraocular muscles

be limited to patients who are older than 2 years or weigh more than 8 kg and who have cardiac or pulmonary disease that might limit the value of central venous pressure (CVP) monitoring.

DIAGNOSTIC STUDIES

Blood Tests

As soon as an intravenous route is established, blood should be drawn for a type and cross-match and for measuring hemoglobin and hematocrit. Other useful blood tests may include liver enzymes, amylase, and blood gases (10). If the patient can void, the urine can be evaluated with a dipstick. Recent studies indicated that gross hematuria, microscopic hematuria with 50 or more red blood cells/high power field (RBC/HPF), or any microscopic hematuria persisting beyond 24 hours indicates a need for an intravenous pyelogram (IVP) or computed tomography (CT) scan with intravenous contrast (11). Microscopic hematuria less than 50 RBC/HPF does not usually demand urgent study. Most urine dipsticks are positive for blood at 10 RBC/HPF or more.

Roentgenograms

Plain films of the neck, chest, and pelvis are usually done as part of the resuscitation protocol for children with severe blunt trauma. Radiographic evaluation for possible extremity fractures, however, can usually wait until resuscitation is completed, unless there is a peripheral neurovascular problem.

When a CT scan is done for abdominal trauma, both oral and intravenous contrast should generally be used. The intravenous contrast may demonstrate bleeding sites and distinguish between hematomas and blood vessels. They generally also provide a much better evaluation of both kidneys than does a standard IVP. If the duodenum is obstructed by an intramural hematoma or laceration, the oral contrast study will usually be diagnostic.

Children with a history of loss of consciousness, but improving levels of consciousness, are admitted for observation and do not routinely have a CT scan of the head. Head CT scans are, however, obtained on children with any persistent alteration in the level of consciousness, any focal neurologic signs, or any acute CNS deterioration.

Abdominal CT scans should be performed on all patients with an equivocal abdominal examination, abnormal vital signs, or abnormal laboratory evaluation. In addition, if the trauma includes a pelvic or femoral fracture, an abdominal CT scan can help differentiate blood loss into the abdomen from that occurring into and around the fracture sites.

Arteriography should be performed on any extremity with a fracture or dislocation associated with abnormal pulses. The presence of an audible Doppler pulse does not rule out vascular injury in a child. Even though biphasic pulses can sometimes be heard distal to a completely obstructed artery, it is unlikely that triphasic sounds will be found under such circumstances.

TREATMENT

The free-water clearance of children is less efficient than that in adults, so they tend to develop more edema with resuscitation fluids, and the diuretic phase usually occurs later than in adults. Consequently, the presence of peripheral edema should not be a reason to withhold fluid that may be necessary to maintain adequate tissue perfusion.

AXIOM Injured children can develop peripheral edema even when they are still hypovolemic.

Head Injuries

AXIOM Scalp injuries in children may bleed excessively and should be sutured promptly to control hemorrhage.

After an adequate resuscitation, volume restriction or the judicious use of mannitol or both (while still maintaining an adequate cerebral perfusion) may help control increased intracranial pressure. If there is intracranial hypertension, monitoring of CVP and arterial blood gases (ABGs) is indicated.

During recovery from severe head trauma, many children will often regress to an earlier stage of development (12). Children who are walking may no longer be able to do so after the injury. Those who were toilet trained may need diapers again.

AXIOM It is becoming increasingly clear that defects in intelligence, cognitive abilities, psychosocial behavior, and motor, speech, and language recovery may not be fully apparent until 2 to 3 or more years after severe head injury (12).

Chest Injuries

Penetrating injuries to the chest are rare in young children. When they do occur, they are more frequently the result of fractured ribs or clavicles rather than of external missiles.

The bony and cartilaginous structures of young children are extremely flexible. Whereas fractured ribs are often seen in teenagers and adults who have severe blunt chest trauma, simple fractures and flail chest are uncommon in younger children; however, because of the elasticity of the chest wall, the force of the trauma can be transferred directly to the underlying pulmonary parenchyma, resulting in a pulmonary contusion in nearly 60% of children with severe thoracic injuries.

Because the mediastinum of the child is very mobile, a pneumothorax can easily cause angulation of the great vessels (reducing venous return) and compression of the lung and trachea (reducing minute ventilation). Consequently, early chest-tube decompression is important. Chest tubes are not inserted low in the chest because, in a child, the diaphragm may be quite high because of intraabdominal injury, gastric distention, or respiratory effort. Chest tubes also must be inserted with great caution in children because the greater chest-wall compliance increases the chance of iatrogenic injury to underlying structures.

Abdominal Injuries

Before 1960, optimal management of significant abdominal trauma was routine laparotomy. Prompted by the report of Lowe et al. (13) of 1.6% mortality, 19% morbidity, and 3% readmission rates for adhesive bowel obstruction after negative laparotomies, a selective nonoperative approach was developed. The increased incidence of postsplenectomy sepsis also provided impetus for selective nonoperative management of splenic and liver trauma.

AXIOM Whenever possible, injuries to the liver or spleen, especially in children, should be treated nonoperatively.

Any child with abdominal trauma who fails to stabilize with resuscitation with blood equal to half of the calculated blood volume requires laparotomy. A CT scan with intravenous and oral contrast can be helpful in the evaluation of abdominal trauma in children. Some of the indications for CT scanning in injured children with stable vital signs include suspected intraabdominal injury, slowly declining hematocrit or requirement for persistent fluid resuscitation, head injuries with altered consciousness, other injuries requiring general anesthesia, and urine with more than 50 RBC/HPF.

Diagnostic peritoneal lavage (DPL) can be used to exclude abdominal injury in children with life-threatening extraabdominal injury who require operations for those problems. It also may be useful to evaluate peritoneal injury in selected patients with abdominal stab wounds or children with persistent shock of unknown origin.

Although DPL is a highly sensitive test for peritoneal injury, presence of intraperitoneal blood is not generally considered an indication for laparotomy in a child.

Powell et al. (14) found that nearly a third of children operated on just because of increased red cells on DPL had injuries that did not require surgical intervention.

Splenic Injuries

The spleen is the most commonly injured intraabdominal organ in children, but surgery is not usually needed. Considerations that have led to a more conservative, nonoperative approach to splenic injuries during childhood include the realization that the incidence of overwhelming postsplenectomy infection (OPSI) for trauma in children is more than 85 times higher than that in the normal population. Furthermore, the mortality rate in those developing this syndrome is close to 50% (15). Although sepsis may occur any time after splenectomy, the risk is greatest during the first 2 years after splenectomy and occurs most frequently in children younger than 5 years.

The spleen is particularly important in the defense against infection in children because it produces several substances, such as immunoglobulins and tuftsin, that are important in phagocytosis of encapsulated organisms such as the pneumococcus, *Haemophilus influenzae*, and meningococcus (15).

AXIOM The great majority of children with splenic injuries can be safely treated nonoperatively.

In general, children who require replacement of more than half their blood volume (i.e., more than 40 mL/kg of blood replacement) within the first 24 hours after injury require operative intervention. Those with less bleeding can usually be treated nonoperatively.

Even if surgery is required because of continued bleeding, at least part of the spleen can often be salvaged. Ligation of hilar vessels, repair of lacerations with absorbable sutures, wrapping with polyglactin 910 (Vicryl) mesh, or application of hemostatic agents [such as absorbable gelatin sponge (Gelfoam), absorbable cellulose fabric (Surgicel), microfibrillar collagen (Avitene), or fibrin glue] or a combination of these to torn parenchyma can control most splenic hemorrhages.

Liver Injuries

The liver is the second most frequently injured intraabdominal organ during childhood. An isolated injury of the liver without involvement of its associated large vessels (portal vein, hepatic veins, or suprarenal inferior vena cava) can usually be treated nonoperatively.

Duodenal Injuries

AXIOM A child with pain from midabdominal trauma, plus persistent nausea and vomiting and no peritoneal signs, should be suspected of having duodenal obstruction by an intramural hematoma.

Duodenal hematomas are relatively common in children. They frequently occur after falling on the handlebars of a bicycle. Vomiting or high nasogastric-tube output 24 hours after injury should arouse suspicion of this problem and is an indication for an upper gastrointestinal series, which typically shows a "coiled-spring sign" or a cutoff in the duodenum or both, usually in the second portion.

Treatment includes decompression of the child's stomach with a nasogastric tube plus total parenteral nutrition. Whereas the majority of duodenal hematomas will resolve within 10 days of injury, complete resolution of the obstruction may take up to 3 weeks. Large hematomas discovered at operations done for other reasons, or those not resolving by 14 days, should be treated by surgical evacuation of the hematoma via a serosal incision, which is then closed.

Small Intestinal Injuries

Children after direct blows to the abdomen can develop mesenteric hematomas plus antimesenteric perforations and have acute abdominal pain; however, the diagnosis of small bowel perforation is often delayed in children because the peritoneal signs tend to develop slowly.

With small bowel injuries in children, peritoneal signs may not develop until more than 24 hours after the injury. Furthermore, because of a rapid development of ileus, there may also be minimal free intraperitoneal air (16). Signs of peritoneal irritation are the most consistent evidence of traumatic hollow viscus perforations in children and are a strong indication for peritoneal lavage (17).

Colon and Rectal Injuries

Because rectal injuries may be very painful and because the children often cannot cooperate, proper examination may not be possible except under general anesthesia.

AXIOM Except for straddle injuries, most isolated rectal injuries in children are caused by child abuse or deviant sexual activity (18).

Mucosal or superficial anal injuries usually resolve with conservative treatment. Full-thickness injuries above the level of the internal sphincter should be protected by a sigmoid colostomy and presacral drainage.

Pancreatic Injuries

Of particular concern in children is a complete pancreatic transection because a distal pancreatic resection frequently requires a concomitant splenectomy. Consequently, the distal pancreas is generally preserved by anastomosing the injured end of the distal pancreas to a Roux-en-Y loop of jejunum. The injured portion of the proximal pancreas can then be stapled or oversewn and drained.

Urinary Tract Injuries

AXIOM With any perineal trauma, sexual abuse must be suspected, and cultures and specimens for examination should be obtained from the vagina, rectum, and mouth.

Whenever possible, a spontaneously voided urine specimen should be obtained and analyzed on all severely injured children, particularly for red blood cells. After the child has voided, a urethral catheter may be placed to monitor urine output; however, any suspicion of a urethral injury, especially in boys, warrants a retrograde urethrogram before insertion of a Foley catheter. If a bladder injury is suspected, cystography, with oblique views and postevacuation films, is obtained. Intraperitoneal injuries must be repaired at surgery, but small extraperitoneal bladder ruptures can often be managed with catheter drainage alone.

Renal injuries with a mild extravasation of urine on CT or IVP may be observed after careful evaluation; however, delayed operative intervention may be required for large or progressively enlarging retroperitoneal hematomas or fluid collections (19).

Musculoskeletal Injuries

Most fractures in children can be treated with closed reduction, but internal fixation may be indicated for specific fractures, particularly those involving joint surfaces, if the fracture fragments are not aligned well by closed reduction.

Spinal injuries are infrequent in children and may be difficult to diagnose because of the differences in the radiographic appearance compared with adults. Children can also have spinal cord injury without radiologic abnormality (SCIWORA) and, therefore, thorough physical examination supplemented with CT scan is necessary in suspected cases (20).

Vascular Injuries

The most common cause of damage to blood vessels in children is iatrogenic from needles used for therapeutic or diagnostic purposes; nevertheless, vascular injuries in children require early diagnosis and aggressive operative management to prevent ischemia, which could cause growth retardation of that limb.

AXIOM The presence of distal pulses in a child does not rule out a significant proximal arterial injury.

If vascular injury is suspected in a child, objective studies such as Doppler pressure measurements or flow-wave analysis or arteriography or a combination of these may be required. Unfortunately, arteriography has its own inherent risks in small children and infants and should be done by someone experienced in the technique and only if the vessel would be repaired if an injury were found.

The most important differential diagnosis is between partial occlusion and spasm of an injured vessel. Vascular spasm is often due to damage to adjacent soft tissue, hemorrhage into surrounding tissue, or trauma to the vessel wall, but it will usually disappear within 3 hours. If impaired perfusion of the extremity persists beyond 3 hours, vascular damage is likely; if there is poor perfusion or absent pulses longer than 6 hours, thrombosis or transection of the vessel is almost certain.

Burns

Children are particularly susceptible to accidental burns, most of which cover less than 20% of the total BSA and are generally a result of hot water. The burns are generally partial-thickness injuries that can be adequately treated by initial debridement of large blisters and topical closed antibiotic dressings with silver sulfadiazine or mafenide. Most face burns are treated open with bacitracin ointment.

Children with any size burn to the hands, face, feet, or genitalia, as well as any partial-thickness injury more than 8% BSA or full-thickness injury more than 3% BSA are admitted to the Burn Unit. For children younger than 1 year, these criteria are halved. If the burns appear deep, early excision and grafting are carried out, keeping in mind that skin grafts add to the total percentage of the BSA that has a partial-thickness injury.

When calculating the surface area of a burn in children, one must consider the age differences in body proportions, particularly the larger surface area of the head and smaller surface area of the lower extremities in infants. For example, in a 1-year-old child, the head may be 17% of the BSA, whereas each lower extremity is only 11.5% (Fig. 8-1).

Children with 10% or more BSA burn will usually require intravenous support. If the burn is 20% or more, or if the genitalia are involved, a urethral catheter is necessary. Nasogastric tubes are used frequently for prevention of ileus and vomiting and later for enteral feedings. Providing adequate intravenous fluids to severely burned children for the initial 24 to 48 hours is extremely important. Many burn fluid formulas are available for guiding such fluid therapy. The projected fluid requirement (mL) for the burn itself for the first 24 hours is

$$\%\ \text{BSA} \times \text{weight (kg)} \times 2 \qquad (1)$$

Maintenance fluids also must be given to children.

CHILD ABUSE AND NEGLECT

AXIOM A history of repeated "minor traumas" resulting in significant injuries should make one suspicious of child abuse or an underlying congenital anomaly.

Approximately 1,000,000 children are abused in the United States every year, and it is estimated that between 2,000 and 5,000 children die annually as a result of this abuse, usually from major head and abdominal injuries.

Children's Hospital of Michigan
DETROIT MICHIGAN

BURN SHEET

BURN RECORD. AGES—BIRTH - 7½

DATE OF OBSERVATION ________________________

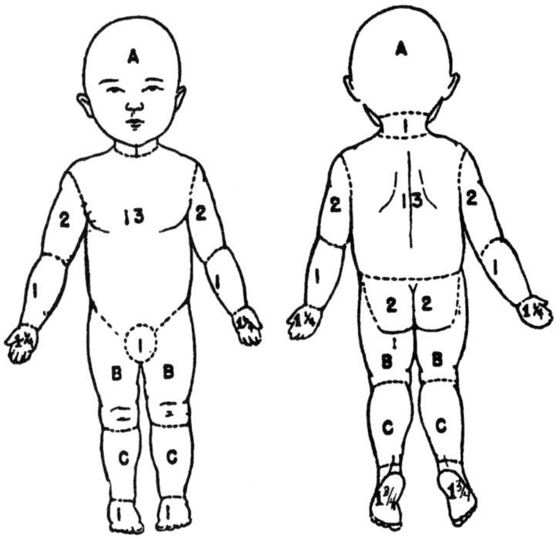

% BURN BY AREAS

AREA	% 2°	% 3°
HEAD		
NECK		
UPPER ARM		
FOREARM		
ANTERIOR TRUNK		
POSTERIOR TRUNK		
GENITALS		
BUTTOCKS		
THIGHS		
LEGS		
FEET		
HANDS		
TOTAL		

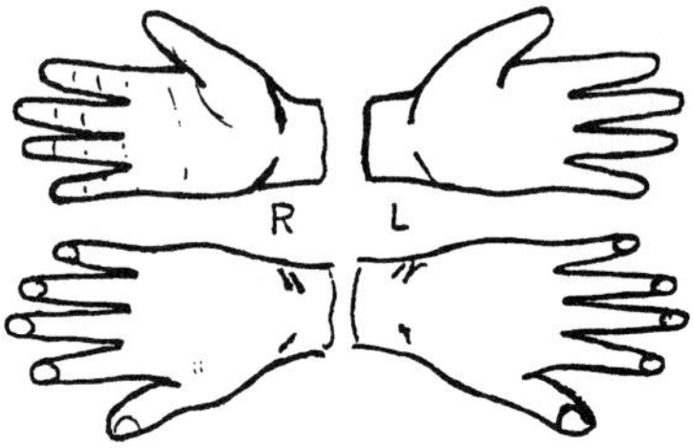

RELATIVE PERCENTAGES OF AREAS AFFECTED BY GROWTH

AREA	AGE 0	1	5
A = 1/2 of Head	9 1/2	8 1/2	6 1/2
B = 1/2 of One Thigh	2 3/4	3 1/4	4
C = 1/2 of One Leg	2 1/2	2 1/2	2 3/4

WEIGHT ________________ HEIGHT ________________

SURFACE AREA ________________________

TYPE OF BURN ________________________

COMMENT ____

____

________________________ M.D.

FIG. 8-1. Burn sheet: ages birth through 7.5 years.

Locking a child in a car on a hot summer day, or in a room with poisons and matches, may be more neglect than abuse, but can lead to just as severe an injury. Lack of immunizations, unusual prior hospitalizations, and a mechanism of injury inconsistent with the examination should also raise suspicion.

⊘ FREQUENT ERRORS

1. ***Treating injured children, especially infants, as if they were small adults.***
2. ***Failure to recognize that severe internal injuries may be present in children with little external evidence of trauma.***
3. ***Inadequate concern about the patency of the nasal passages in young infants.***
4. ***Delay in decompressing the stomach in infants with major trauma.***
5. ***Interpreting and treating agitation as anxiety when it is actually due to hypoxia.***
6. ***Failure to give glucose during fluid resuscitation of infants and small children.***
7. ***Inadequate efforts to prevent and correct hypothermia.***
8. ***Assuming that vital signs in children are the same as those in adults.***
9. ***Failure to consider abuse or neglect in the etiology of a child's injury.***
10. ***Assuming that an edematous injured child cannot be hypovolemic.***
11. ***Operating for isolated liver or spleen injuries if the child can be hemodynamically stabilized with transfusions of less than half of blood volume.***
12. ***Lack of effort to preserve at least part of a badly injured spleen.***

SUMMARY POINTS

1. Injury is the most frequent health problem affecting children and adolescents in the United States.

2. When trauma occurs, the child's relatively compliant body may have little external evidence of serious internal damage.

3. Early decompression of the stomach is extremely important in severely injured children.

4. Restlessness or any change in mental status in an injured child should be attributed to hypoxia until proven otherwise.

5. Because infants are obligatory nasal breathers, occlusion of the nose by injuries or foreign bodies, such as nasogastric tubes, may severely impair ventilation.

6. There is little distance in an infant between the position of an endotracheal tube that is inserted too far and one that is not inserted far enough.

7. Because of the inaccuracy of checking endotracheal tube position by physical examination, a chest radiograph should be obtained to ascertain endotracheal tube position as soon as it has been secured.

8. If ventilation of an infant or child cannot be promptly provided with an endotracheal tube, a large needle inserted into the trachea and attached to intermittent wall oxygen can be lifesaving.

9. Infants ventilate primarily with their diaphragms; therefore, anything pressing on or irritating the diaphragm can greatly reduce the ability of a child to breathe properly.

10. Gastric dilatation can seriously interfere with ventilation and with the abdominal evaluation of critically injured children.

11. The mediastinum shifts easily in children; consequently, any problem in one hemithorax can severely impair ventilation and venous return.

12. Inadequate tissue perfusion in young children should be diagnosed primarily by tachycardia, tachypnea, decreased responsiveness, and decreased urine output; hypotension tends to occur relatively late.

13. Whenever possible, blood less than 5 days old should be selected for transfusion to young children.

14. One should not use a scalp vein for intravenous access when rapid fluid administration may required.

15. If no vascular access is available, nearly all resuscitation drugs, except $NaHCO_3$, can be given to children via an endotracheal tube.

16. If adequate vascular access cannot be obtained in a reasonable period for resuscitation of a hemodynamically unstable child, the intraosseous route should be considered until other venous access is obtained.

17. Severe hypoglycemia can develop rapidly in infants unless some glucose is given in their intravenous maintenance fluids.
18. A urine osmolality of 600 mOsm/kg in a newborn usually indicates hypovolemia.
19. To help prevent hypothermia, injured infants should be treated in an environment maintained between 24°C to 27°C (75°F to 80°F).
20. All intravenous solutions, including blood, given to an injured child should be warmed to 40°C to 42°C.
21. Children who experience a cardiac arrest after trauma need oxygen, fluid, and blood rather than multiple drugs or electric shocks.
22. Bradycardia in an injured child is an ominous sign of impending cardiovascular collapse.
23. Oxygen desaturation usually occurs before bradycardia develops, allowing time to correct the developing pulmonary or cardiovascular problem before it becomes serious and difficult to reverse.
24. Bowel perforation is less frequent with blunt trauma to the liver or spleen in children than in adults.
25. Whenever possible, injuries to the liver or spleen, especially in children, should be treated nonoperatively.
26. Peritoneal lavage is indicated in injured children who require immediate surgical intervention for extraabdominal injuries or who have suspected abdominal injuries causing hemodynamic instability.
27. The great majority of children with splenic injuries can be safely treated nonoperatively.
28. Children who have isolated liver or spleen injuries generally do not require operative intervention unless they require replacement of more than half their blood volume (i.e., more than 40 mL/kg of blood replacement) within the first 24 hours.
29. A child with pain from midabdominal trauma, nausea, vomiting, and no peritoneal signs should be suspected of having duodenal obstruction by an intramural hematoma.
30. The diagnosis of small bowel perforation is often delayed in children because the peritoneal signs tend to develop slowly.
31. With a torn pancreas in a child, the distal pancreas is preserved if at all possible so that a splenectomy can be avoided.
32. With any perineal trauma, sexual abuse also must be considered, and cultures and specimens for examination should be obtained from the vagina, rectum, and mouth.
33. Children with fractures through growth centers must be monitored carefully because of the serious effects such injuries can have on long-term growth and function.
34. The presence of distal pulses in a child does not rule out a significant proximal arterial injury.
35. With major arterial trauma, blood flow to an extremity may be adequate to maintain viability of the limb but still be inadequate for normal growth.
36. Burns in children are considered to be a result of abuse or neglect until proven otherwise.
37. A history of repeated "minor trauma" resulting in significant injuries should make one suspicious of child abuse or an underlying congenital anomaly.

REFERENCES

1. Long JA, Klein MD. Trauma in infants and children. In: Wilson RF, Walt AJ, eds. *Management of trauma: pitfalls and practice.* 2nd ed. Philadelphia: Williams & Wilkins, 1996:128.
2. Rouse TM, Eichelberger MR. Trends in pediatric trauma management. *Surg Clin North Am* 1992;72:1347.
3. Ramenofsky ML, Ramenofsky MB, Jurkovich GJ, et al. The predictive validity of the pediatric trauma score. *J Trauma* 1988;28:1038–1042.
4. Searpelle EM, ed. *Pulmonary physiology in the fetus, newborn and child.* Philadelphia: Lea & Febiger, 1975:168.

5. Pediatric transfusions practice. In: Snyder EL, ed. *Blood transfusion therapy.* Arlington, VA: American Association of Blood Banks, 1983:49.
6. Guy J, Haley K, Zuspan SJ. Use of intraosseous infusion in the pediatric trauma patient. *J Pediatr Surg* 1993;28:158.
7. Aperia A, Broberger O, Thodenius K, et al. Renal control of sodium and fluid balance in newborn infants during maintenance therapy. *Acta Pediatr Scand* 1975;64:725.
8. Hazinski MF, Chahine AA, Holcomb GW III, et al. Outcome of cardiovascular collapse in pediatric blunt trauma. *Ann Emerg Med* 1994;23:1229.
9. Raimondi AS, Hirschauer J. Head injury in the infant and toddler: coma scoring and outcome scale. *Child's Brain* 1984;11:12–35.
10. Isaacman DJ, Scarfone RJ, Kost SI, et al. Utility of routine laboratory testing for detecting intra-abdominal injury in the pediatric trauma patient. *Pediatrics* 1993;92:692.
11. Lieu TA, Fleisher GR, Mahboubi S, et al. Hematuria and clinical findings as indications for intravenous pyelography in pediatric blunt renal trauma. *Pediatrics* 1988;82:216–222.
12. Greenspan AI. Functional recovery following head injury among children. *Curr Probl Pediatr* 1996;26:170.
13. Lowe RJ, Boyd DR, Folk FA, et al. The negative laparotomy for abdominal trauma. *J Trauma* 1972;12:853–861.
14. Powell RW, Green JB, Ochsner MG, et al. Peritoneal lavage in pediatric patients sustaining blunt abdominal trauma: a reappraisal. *J Trauma* 1987;27:6.
15. Francke EL, Neu HC. Postsplenectomy infection. *Surg Clin North Am* 1981;61: 135.
16. Ford EG, Senac MO Jr. Clinical presentation and radiographic identification of small bowel rupture following blunt trauma in children. *Pediatr Emerg Care* 1993;9:139–142.
17. Ulman I, Avanoglu A, Ozcan C, et al. Gastrointestinal perforations in children: a continuing challenge to nonoperative treatment of blunt abdominal trauma. *J Trauma* 1996;41:110.
18. Black CT, Pokorny WJ, McGill CW, et al. Anorectal trauma in children. *J Pediatr Surg* 1982;17:501.
19. Levy JB, Baskin LS, Ewalt DH, et al. Nonoperative management of blunt pediatric major renal trauma. *Urology* 1993;42:418.
20. Pang D, Pollack IF. Spinal cord injury without radiographic abnormality in children: the SCIWORA syndrome. *J Trauma* 1989;29:654.

9A. SPECIAL PROBLEMS OF TRAUMA: THE AGED[1]

Trauma can be especially devastating to the aged. The elderly tend to have different types of injuries, and their responses and ultimate outcome reflect the effects of underlying diseases and the changes that occur in organ function with time.

AXIOM The relation between the condition of a car (or patient) and its age is not as important as how well it was made (genetics), the miles that it has been driven (wear and tear), and the care and maintenance (general health habits) that it has received.

In 1984, unintentional injury accounted for almost 24,500 deaths of persons age 65 and older. This death rate of 86 per 100,000 population was more than twice the accidental death rate of those age 25 to 44 years (35 of 100,000; 2). Elderly trauma patients also have a poor long-term prognosis, with up to 88% of survivors requiring nursing home placement or full-time in-home assistance. Indeed, of elderly patients who have a fall requiring care in a hospital, about half will die within 1 year (3).

⊘ PITFALL

One should not treat elderly patients less vigorously just because of a theoretically shorter life expectancy.

In 1989, the average 65-year-old could expect 17 additional years of life. The average life expectancy for a 75-year-old was 11 years, and for the average 85-year-old, it was 6 years (4). Nevertheless, Kilaru et al. (5) found that, of patients older than 65 years admitted with a diagnosis of closed head injury and an admission Glasgow Coma Scale (GSC) score of 7 or less, 74% were dead at the end of a 38 ± 3-month follow-up, and all of the survivors were in persistent vegetative or dependent functional states. In like manner, Battistella et al. (6) found that 12% of trauma patients who were 75 years and older died within 6 months of being discharged from the hospital.

CAUSES OF TRAUMA IN THE ELDERLY

Falls

Falls are the leading cause of injury in the elderly and are the second most frequent cause of elderly trauma deaths. They cause about 7 million injuries and 10,000 deaths per year and are usually the result of accumulated defects and diseases (3).

Older people are less coordinated and have less stable gaits. Impaired vision, hearing, and memory make any environment dangerous. Medical problems, such as vertigo, cardiac dysrhythmias, anemia, transient ischemic attacks, unstable joints, spontaneous fractures, epilepsy, and electrolyte imbalances, also contribute to an increased tendency to fall. Drugs, especially sedatives, antihypertensives, diuretics, hypoglycemic agents, and alcohol, also are contributing factors.

Gubler et al. (7) found that injured patients older than 65 years had a more than twofold increased risk for subsequent trauma admissions (when compared with otherwise similar uninjured individuals). The risk of subsequent admissions for new trauma among the injured group (compared with the uninjured group) increased with age, injury-severity scores, and the presence of preexisting comorbid conditions.

Motor Vehicle Accidents

In 1989 in the United States, approximately 5,170 elderly individuals were killed as drivers or passengers in motor vehicle accidents, and an additional 7,200 were killed as pedestrians (8).

Elderly pedestrian trauma victims have an extremely high mortality rate. Champion et al. (9) found that the death rate for pedestrian accidents in the elderly (32.6%) was about 2.5 times that of younger individuals (13.5%)

Burns

In some burn units, the elderly constitute as many as 20% of the admissions; the mortality rate for elderly patients with larger than 15% burns is 80% or more (10). Pneumonia in elderly burn victims is almost uniformly fatal regardless of the organism involved.

IMPAIRED ORGAN FUNCTION IN THE ELDERLY

Much of the "fragility" of elderly patients who are injured is related to a loss of "physiological reserve" in multiple organ systems. In a study of patients from Detroit Receiving Hospital (DRH), the incidence of hypertension and cardiac disease increased significantly in trauma patients who were age 50 years or older. The mortality rate for admitted trauma patients was 1.8% for those age 14 to 49 years and reached a maximum of 12.9% in those who were age 70 to 79 years.

MacKenzie et al. (11) showed that the incidence of preexisting medical problems in individuals older than 65 years was 36% to 40%. In individuals with no preexisting medical conditions, the mortality rate averaged about 3%, but if more than two medical problems were present, the mortality rate may exceed 25% (12).

⊘ PITFALL

Assumption that confusion in an elderly patient is due to senility rather than to problems that are correctable by improving cerebral oxygenation.

Tranquilizers and barbiturates should be used with special care in elderly patients, because they can cause or potentiate confusion.

Cardiac Mechanisms

Cardiac output, stroke volume, and maximal heart rate decrease about 0.5% to 1.0% per year after age 20 years (13). Myocardial conduction is slowed, and contraction times are prolonged. This predisposes the heart to reentry dysrhythmias and limits the heart's ability to increase its rate in response to added stress. Because systemic vascular resistance also tends to increase in elderly patients, the cardiovascular system is particularly susceptible to pump failure in response to trauma.

Because older patients frequently have significant narrowing of important vessels, arterial flow to vital organs may be very pressure dependent. Consequently, the likelihood of cerebral or myocardial infarction increases markedly if significant hypotension occurs.

⊘ PITFALL

If serial electrocardiograms (ECGs) and enzyme studies are not obtained in elderly patients who have been hypotensive, many silent myocardial infarctions will be missed.

Patients with chronic cardiac failure have usually been treated with a low-salt diet and diuretics for some time, and they can have severe deficiencies in sodium, potassium, chloride, magnesium, and calcium. These electrolyte abnormalities may be manifested clinically by weakness, decreased tolerance of blood loss, lethargy, hypotension, and abnormal responses to many drugs, especially anesthetics.

The excitability of the myocardium and its conducting system, along with the patient's responses to many drugs, are altered by massive blood transfusions, persistent hypotension, impaired ventilation, and acidosis. If hypothermia develops, it further impairs cardiac performance and increases the tendency to arrhythmias.

Elderly patients with cardiovascular disease should, whenever possible, have their pulmonary arterial wedge pressure (PAWP), cardiac output, oxygen delivery, and oxygen consumption optimized preoperatively, intraoperatively, and postoperatively, for at least 24 to 48 hours (14). Even in stable, normovolemic patients, general anesthesia often reduces cardiac output by more than 20% to 30%.

Pulmonary Mechanisms

The aging lung progressively loses its elasticity. Even though total lung capacity (TLC) tends to remain constant with age, residual volume tends to increase from a normal of 20% to 25% in young adults to 35% to 45% of the TLC in the elderly, with a corresponding decrease in expiratory and inspiratory reserve volumes and vital capacity (15). Aging also causes alveolar ducts to dilate and many interalveolar septa to disappear, thereby further reducing functional alveolar volume.

Because of a reduced stability of the pulmonary "skeleton," the terminal bronchioles collapse earlier in expiration, increasing the "closing volume" of the lungs (15), predisposing the patient to the development of atelectasis.

Because of all these changes and a decreased diffusion capacity, there is an almost linear decline in the arterial PO_2 of 3 to 4 mm Hg per decade after age 20 years; however, there is little change in the P_aCO_2 in normal subjects. Nevertheless, if the patient has severe chronic obstructive pulmonary disease (COPD), the P_aCO_2 may increase to levels exceeding 55 to 60 mm Hg. At these P_aCO_2 levels, hypoxia is the main drive to ventilation.

⊘ PITFALL

The use of oxygen on an emphysematous patient with chronic severe hypercarbia can lead to severe respiratory acidosis or respiratory arrest or both.

Because bicarbonate levels change much more slowly than PCO_2, the PCO_2 can be rapidly reduced by putting a patient on a ventilator. Because the patient with a chronic respiratory acidosis has increased bicarbonate levels to partially compensate for the increased P_aCO_2, sudden hyperventilation can produce a severe combined alkalosis, which in turn reduces potassium and ionized magnesium and calcium levels and can cause dangerous arrhythmias.

⊘ PITFALL

In patients with chronic hypercarbia, the P_aCO_2 should not be reduced by more than 5.0 mm Hg per hour.

The efficacy of protective airway reflexes decreases in the elderly, increasing the likelihood of aspiration of oropharyngeal secretions during trauma or surgery. Increased disorders of swallowing and of the upper and lower esophageal sphincter in the elderly also predispose them to aspiration of oral or gastric secretions. All this, together with preexisting emphysema or bronchitis, increases the chances of elderly patients developing postoperative atelectasis and pneumonia.

AXIOM At least 50% of elderly patients undergoing major thoracic or upper abdominal surgery develop postoperative complications, and of these, two thirds are pulmonary (16).

Renal Mechanisms

After age 30 years, there is an average 1.5% reduction per year in renal mass, the number of glomeruli, and the filtration rates, and this occurs with increasing rapidity after age 50 years (17). Effective renal blood flow and glomerular filtration rate decrease by almost 50% between the third and tenth decades.

In healthy, young individuals, the kidneys can concentrate to a specific gravity of 1.035 and a maximal osmolality of about 1,400 mOsm/kg; however, specific gravities greater than 1.024 and urine osmolalities greater than 750 mOsm/kg are rarely achieved after age 70 years. As a result, older individuals usually need a larger urine volume to maintain adequate excretion of nonvolatile acid and metabolites.

As the muscle mass decreases, creatinine production also decreases, and thin elderly individuals involved in little physical activity normally have serum creatinine levels of 0.6 to 0.8 mg/dL. Decreased protein intake also tends to reduce blood urea nitrogen (BUN) levels. Consequently, creatinine clearance is a far more reliable index of renal function in the elderly than are the BUN and serum creatinine levels. Indeed, even with normal serum creatinine levels, creatinine clearance may be as low as 33% of normal by age 70 years.

A gradual decline in hepatic function occurs after age 50 years, particularly regarding its capacity to conjugate lipid-soluble drugs (18). This results in prolonged high serum concentrations and reduced dosage requirements for such drugs.

Musculoskeletal Mechanisms

Osteoporosis, characterized by a decrease in the mass of histologically normal bone and consequent loss of strength and resistance to fractures, causes clinical problems in almost half of all elderly people. Causes of osteoporosis include reduced secretion of estrogen, decreased physical activity, inadequate consumption of calcium, or a combination of these. Osteoporosis also contributes to the high incidence of hip fractures in the elderly.

AXIOM The osteoporosis and reduced activity of advanced age combine to increase bone fragility and the incidence and severity of fractures.

Nutritional Mechanisms

An abnormal glucose tolerance develops in 50% of patients older than 70 years (12,13), and this can occasionally cause severe problems, especially during intravenous hyperalimentation after trauma.

AXIOM Many elderly individuals, even those who are obese, have subclinical malnutrition.

As a result of inefficient utilization, protein requirements tend to increase in the elderly so that the current recommended daily allowance for protein of 0.8 g/kg/day is probably inadequate for older patients who are traumatized (19).

AXIOM Close attention to drug dosing is extremely important in the elderly because of a wide variety of physiologic changes including decreased protein binding and reduced hepatic metabolism and renal excretion (Table 9A-1;20).

Table 9A-1. ***Geriatric physiologic changes that contribute to adverse drug reactions***

Physiologic changes	Adverse drug reactions
Decrease in total body water by 10%–15%	Reduced half-life and distribution of water-soluble drugs
Increased body fat 18%–30% in men 30%–45% in women	Increased half-life and distribution of fat-soluble drugs
Decrease in lean body mass by 20%–30%	Higher weight-corrected dosage
Reduction in functional glomeruli by 30%	Reduced renal excretion
Decrease in hepatic blood flow by 40%–45%	Decrease in metabolic excretion and oxidation
Decrease in cardiac output	

Immune Mechanisms

Because of decreased cell-mediated and humoral immune responses, the incidence and mortality rate of infections increases in the elderly; however, the signs, symptoms, and laboratory changes with sepsis may be greatly decreased, and early diagnosis may be extremely difficult.

INITIAL EVALUATION AND MANAGEMENT

AXIOM Elderly patients should be examined as if some degree of trauma or dysfunction is present in all organ systems.

Hypotension and impaired tissue perfusion in the elderly should be corrected rapidly by aggressive fluid therapy; however, such patients are also easy to overload with fluids. If the patient is bleeding, one should try to control the hemorrhage before large amounts of fluids, blood, or both are given.

AXIOM The best guide to continued fluid therapy is the hemodynamic response to the previous fluid bolus.

If the patient responds only transiently to aggressive fluid resuscitation, the cause of the hypotension must be rapidly determined. Although hypotension after trauma is usually due to continued bleeding or inadequate resuscitation or both, one also must look for tension pneumothorax, pericardial tamponade, myocardial contusion, or cardiac disease.

SPECIFIC INJURIES IN THE ELDERLY

Head Injuries

With increasing age, the dura becomes more tightly adherent to the skull, making the development of epidural hematomas (EDHs) less common. The progressive loss of brain volume with age helps to protect it from contusion, but it also makes subdural hematomas (SDHs) more likely to occur (21). Indeed, SDHs are three times more common in the elderly than in younger patients, and because there is an increased subdural space, a relatively large SDH may cause only a gradual neurologic decline. Lucid intervals in the elderly are usually also caused by SDHs, whereas in younger patients, they are characteristically caused by EDHs.

Chest Trauma

AXIOM It is probably wise to consider all elderly patients with localized chest pain and tenderness after trauma to have rib fractures, even if the fractures are not apparent on the initial radiographs.

Because of the rigid chest wall and osteoporosis, blunt chest trauma to the elderly frequently results in rib fractures. Even a relatively mild injury with a few fractured ribs requires careful pulmonary monitoring and may make it necessary for an elderly patient to receive ventilatory support for several days.

Even in patients with severe chronic hypercarbia who depend on hypoxia to sustain their respiratory drive, administration of some oxygen to improve the Po_2 is usually very beneficial. Although some believe that endotracheal intubation can be hazardous for the elderly and may increase the risk of pneumonia, it should be performed promptly if there is inadequate ventilation that cannot be rapidly improved by other techniques, such as an epidural block for reducing the pain from fractured ribs.

Abdominal Trauma

Elderly patients may not tolerate an unnecessary laparotomy very well, but any delay in treating bleeding or a bowel leak in the abdomen is apt to be lethal.

AXIOM The diagnostic approach to abdominal trauma in the elderly is similar to that used in younger patients; however, there is a greater need for an early accurate diagnosis.

Musculoskeletal Injuries

Osteoporosis in the elderly predisposes them to fractures from relatively mild trauma. Consequently, elderly injured patients should have a very careful physical examination, and radiographs should be obtained on any bone that may be fractured. Fractures that are particularly likely to occur in the elderly include Colles' fractures, hip fractures, and fractures of the head of the humerus.

Abuse of the Elderly

The incidence of abuse to elderly individuals is estimated to be at least 10%, with 40% of these defined as victims of moderate to severe abuse (22). In 1980, the United States Senate Special Committee on Elder Abuse reported that there were up to 2,500,000 cases of geriatric abuse, neglect, or mistreatment each year in the United States. It is estimated that only one in six cases of geriatric abuse comes to the attention of authorities (22).

SPECIAL CONSIDERATION FOR TRAUMA SURGERY IN THE ELDERLY

Preoperative Considerations

With trauma care in the elderly, often less than optimal results must be acceptable to keep morbidity or mortality or both to a minimum. One example is accepting the deformity of a Colles' fracture to provide early mobilization to maintain wrist and hand function. Another example might be leaving a colostomy in place in high-risk elderly patients who are bedridden rather than risk reoperative bowel surgery.

AXIOM The preoperative workup of elderly trauma patients should be designed to discover the presence and severity of all major organ dysfunctions.

In a survey of elderly women with hip fractures, significant dysfunction of at least one organ was found in 92% (23). This included cardiovascular disease in 78%, mental abnormalities in 39%, pulmonary diseases in 14%, endocrinopathies in 12%, and neurologic disturbances in 10%.

Many elderly patients are taking multiple medications. In one series, 87% of the patients were receiving medications for a variety of problems before their hip fracture. Digitalis preparations, β-blockers, calcium channel blockers, and antihypertensives are among the most common medications used by the elderly.

A suggested preoperative approach to severely injured elderly patients involves transfer to a special-care unit where a pulmonary artery catheter can be introduced to allow cautious optimization of cardiac function and oxygen delivery (24). Surgery is performed as soon as cardiopulmonary function has been optimized. The physiologic surveillance of the patient is continued for at least 24 and preferably 72 hours postoperatively. With this approach, the mortality rate in a monitored group of elderly patients was 3%, as opposed to 29% in a similar but unmonitored group.

Choice of Anesthesia

Many surgeons and anesthesiologists believe that surgery in the elderly should be performed under regional, rather than general, anesthesia whenever possible, because it may have a less suppressive effect on most organ systems, especially the heart and the lungs.

AXIOM Preoperative, intraoperative, and postoperative optimization of cardiac and pulmonary function is more important than the type of anesthetic used for a surgical procedure.

Fluid Requirements During Surgery

Fluid requirements in elderly trauma patients, if corrected for the smaller amount of lean body mass that is present with aging, are similar to those of younger patients; however, hypertensive patients, particularly those receiving prolonged diuretic therapy, often have a chronically contracted blood volume, total body potassium and magnesium deficits, and a reduced ability to concentrate urine.

In addition, the optimal hematocrit in elderly trauma patients is probably higher than that in younger individuals, and this is best determined by attempts to optimize oxygen delivery and consumption. Experience at Detroit Receiving Hospital agrees with that of Horst et al. (25), who found that elderly trauma survivors tended to have higher hemoglobins than did nonsurvivors (12.1 g/dL vs. 10.5 g/dL). The survivors also had a higher O_2 delivery (608 ± 168 mL/min/m^2 vs. 483 ± 210 mL/min/m^2).

Preventing Hypothermia

Some of the factors reducing the ability of elderly patients to maintain an adequate core temperature include slowed basal metabolism, reduced ability to shiver under anesthesia, and reduced delivery of oxygen and glucose to the tissues.

A decrease in rectal or esophageal temperature to less than 34°C to 35°C can rapidly lead to coagulopathies and organ dysfunction. Use of heating pads, coverage of unused body parts with "space blankets," warm intravenous fluids, room temperatures of 75°F to 80°F or more, and incandescent heating lamps also can be helpful.

Shivering postoperatively in hypothermic patients can increase oxygen consumption by more than 400%. If pulmonary and myocardial reserves are limited, it can cause myocardial ischemia, hypoxemia, increased systemic vascular resistance, anaerobic metabolism, and lactic acidosis (26).

Length of Operation

AXIOM Operations in the elderly should be as short as possible, but one should try to prevent the need for additional procedures.

Morbidity and mortality in trauma surgery are often related to the duration of the surgical procedure; nevertheless, one longer operation is generally safer than two shorter operations of the same total duration. Although it is generally believed that splenorrhaphy is preferable to splenectomy, it is probably safer to perform a rapid splenectomy in an elderly person with a badly injured, salvageable spleen to prevent the possibility of later hypotension or need for a second operation or both.

Postoperative Management

Scalea et al. (27), prospectively evaluating multiply injured geriatric patients in an intensive care unit (ICU), showed that survival was increased from 7% to 53% by early admission to the ICU and placement of a Swan–Ganz catheter to optimize cardiovascular function.

Early mobilization of patients after trauma is important for reducing the risk of atelectasis, pneumonia, pulmonary embolus, and decubiti; however, the greatest benefit of early mobilization is probably the psychologic lift it provides.

Complications

Pulmonary complications are the most common posttraumatic problems experienced by geriatric patients, and the incidence is particularly higher in individuals with preexisting chronic bronchitis or emphysema and heavy tobacco use. The incidence and severity of such complications can be reduced by early mobilization, chest physiotherapy, encouraged coughing and deep breathing, and incentive spirometry. Judicious use of narcotics and maintenance of effective nasogastric decompression also can help reduce pulmonary complications.

AXIOM Myocardial ischemia is best prevented by keeping the heart rate and blood pressure (BP) within normal limits.

Patients with preexisting coronary artery disease are particularly prone to develop myocardial ischemia if hypotension develops or if stress causes a combination of hypertension and tachycardia. Changes in the pulse–pressure product (PPP; heart rate × systolic BP) correlate with changes in myocardial oxygen demand. Dahn et al. (28) found that verapamil could reduce systolic BP and heart rate after aortic surgery, thereby reducing the PPP and myocardial oxygen demand.

Factors predisposing elderly trauma patients to the development of venous thrombosis include reduction of venous flow rate (as a result of bed rest, congestive heart failure, hypovolemia, or venous congestion) and hypercoagulable states.

Deep venous thrombosis is classically prevented by early mobilization, elevation of the lower extremities, and active and passive leg exercises. External pneumatic compression stockings, by providing rhythmic compression of the legs, also reduce the risk of deep venous thrombosis. Even if the pneumatic stockings are applied only to the arms, they can provide some protection by increasing plasma levels of fibrinolysins.

AXIOM Acute oliguric renal failure is probably best prevented by maintaining as high a urine output as possible (without using diuretics) and by avoiding nephrotoxic drugs.

Elderly patients are not only more likely to develop infections, but they are also less likely to show the typical fever, leukocytosis, and local signs and symptoms that can help provide an early diagnosis. In elderly patients who are not improving as fast as they should, the empiric removal and culture of indwelling intravenous catheters is often helpful. In patients who are deteriorating after abdominal surgery or trauma and have no evidence of infection clinically or radiologically, a "blind laparotomy" may be indicated; however, for eradication of pus to improve survival rate, it must be done before multiple organ failure develops.

Factors that contribute to the development of postoperative restlessness or delirium in elderly patients include hypoxemia, hypotension, fluid and electrolyte abnormalities, various medications, unfamiliar environments, sleep deprivation, excessive stress responses, and sepsis. In general, with recovery from the acute stress and transfer from an intensive care environment, the majority of elderly patients will recover their preinjury mental status.

Surgical Outcomes

In a series by Oreskovich et al. (16), the overall mortality rate in elderly trauma patients admitted to a hospital was 15%. This was quite similar to the results of a study by Champion et al. (29), in which the mortality rate of injured patients older than 65 years was 19.0%, which was almost twice as high as the mortality rate of 9.8% in similarly injured individuals younger than 65 years.

Rehabilitation After Surgery

AXIOM Optimal rehabilitation begins when the trauma patient is first seen.

Rehabilitation of the elderly can be a long and tedious process, but the sooner it is started, the shorter and more effective it will be. DeMaria et al. (30) found that with aggressive treatment, 89% of elderly survivors of trauma returned home, and 57% returned to living independently.

AXIOM Home care should be provided as soon as services that can be provided only in a hospital are no longer necessary.

⊘ FREQUENT ERRORS

1. ***Delay or avoidance of necessary surgery in elderly patients because of their increased risk.***
2. ***Use of tranquilizers and barbiturates to control restlessness in elderly patients.***
3. ***Failure to optimize PAWP and O_2 delivery in elderly, high-risk patients who need a general anesthetic.***
4. ***Reliance on certain levels of central venous pressure (CVP) or PAWP or both to determine the amount of fluid loading an elderly patient will receive (rather than reliance on the response to a fluid challenge).***
5. ***Rapid correction of chronic acid–base and fluid and electrolyte problems.***
6. ***Delay or reluctance or both to provide nasotracheal suction or bronchoscopy for pulmonary toilet in elderly patients who will not breathe and cough adequately.***
7. ***Assumption that renal function in an elderly patient is normal because the urine output is good and the BUN and serum creatinine are "within normal limits."***
8. ***Assumption that an elderly patient who is still awake after head trauma cannot have a large subdural hematoma.***
9. ***Attempts to obtain optimal reduction of fracture fragments, especially in the upper extremities, at the expense of mobility.***
10. ***Reliance on a relatively low hematocrit to maintain an adequate O_2 delivery in patients who have cardiac or pulmonary dysfunction or both.***
11. ***Use of multiple operations to correct a problem in the elderly rather than relying on one larger operation to correct all the problems.***

SUMMARY POINTS

1. The relation between the condition of a car (or patient) and its age is not so important as how well it was made (genetics), the miles that it has been driven (wear and tear), and the care and maintenance that it has received (general health status).
2. Most falls in the elderly are the result of their accumulated defects and diseases.
3. Elderly pedestrians struck by motor vehicles have the highest mortality rate of all injury victims.
4. Tranquilizers and barbiturates should be used sparingly in elderly patients, because they can cause or potentiate confusion.
5. Elderly patients with cardiac disease tend to have a small margin of safety between a preload that prevents hypotension and one that causes overt heart failure.
6. Elderly patients with cardiovascular disease should have their PAWP, cardiac output, oxygen delivery, and oxygen consumption optimized preoperatively, intraoperatively, and postoperatively, for at least 24, and preferably, 72 hours.
7. Significant renal impairment may exist in elderly patients in spite of "normal" serum creatinine and BUN levels.
8. The osteoporosis and reduced activity of advanced age combine to increase bone fragility and the incidence and severity of fractures.
9. Many elderly individuals, even those who are obese, have subclinical malnutrition.
10. Elderly patients should be examined as if some degree of trauma or dysfunction were present in all organ systems.
11. Resuscitation of elderly trauma victims should generally be more aggressive than that in younger individuals.
12. The best guide to continued fluid therapy is the response to the previous fluid bolus.
13. One must have a high index of suspicion for subdural hematomas in elderly patients with head trauma.
14. It is probably wise to consider all elderly patients with localized chest pain and tenderness after trauma to have rib fractures, even if they are not apparent on the initial radiographs.
15. Elderly patients tolerate continued intraabdominal bleeding or peritoneal contamination very poorly.
16. If one does not look for abuse in elderly trauma victims, it will generally not be detected or prevented (or both) from recurring.
17. The preoperative workup of elderly trauma patients should be designed to discover the presence and severity of all major organ dysfunctions.
18. Urgent surgery on elderly trauma patients should be performed as soon as their organ function can be made optimal.
19. Preoperative, intraoperative, and postoperative optimization of cardiac and pulmonary function is more important than the type of anesthetic used for procedures.
20. The optimal hematocrit in elderly trauma patients is probably higher than that in younger individuals, and this is best determined by attempts to optimize oxygen delivery and consumption.
21. Elderly, high-risk patients should have their preload optimized preoperatively, and the optimal preload should be maintained intraoperatively and for at least 48 hours postoperatively.
22. Hypothermia can occur quickly and easily in the elderly, and the hypermetabolism to correct it can put great stress on the cardiovascular system.
23. Operations in the elderly should be as short as possible, but one should try to prevent the need for additional operations.
24. Myocardial ischemia is best prevented by keeping hypotension, hypertension, and tachycardia to a minimum.
25. Acute oliguric renal failure is probably best prevented by maintaining as high a urine output as possible (without using diuretics) and by avoiding nephrotoxic drugs.

26. Frequently sepsis is not recognized in the elderly until multiple organ failure begins to develop, and then it is often too late to save the patient.
27. Restlessness is due to hypoxemia until proven otherwise.
28. Optimal rehabilitation begins when the patient is first seen.

REFERENCES

1. Wilson RF, Bender JS, Gass J. Special problems of trauma in the aged. In: Wilson RF, Walt AJ, eds. *Management of trauma: pitfalls and practice.* 2nd ed. Philadelphia: Williams & Wilkins, 1996:146.
2. National Safety Council. *Accident facts.* Chicago: National Safety Council, 1986.
3. Rubenstein LZ. Falls in the elderly: a clinical approach. *Top Primary Care Med* 1983;138:273.
4. U.S. National Center for Health Statistics. *Vital statistics of the United States.* U.S. National Center for Health Statistics, Hyattsville, MD,1989:74.
5. Kilaru S, Garb J, Emhoff T, et al. Long-term functional status and mortality of elderly patients with severe closed head injuries. *J Trauma* 1996;41:957.
6. Battistella FD, Din AM, Perez L. Trauma patients 75 years and older: long-term follow-up results justify aggressive management. *J Trauma* 1998;44:618.
7. Gubler KD, Maier RV, Davis RD, et al. Trauma recidivism in the elderly. *J Trauma* 1996;41:952.
8. Fife DD, Barancik JI, Chatterjee MS. Northeastern Ohio trauma study: injury rates by age, sex, and cause. *Am J Public Health* 1984;74:473.
9. Champion HR, Copes WS, Buyer D, et al. Major trauma in geriatric patients. *Am J Public Health* 1989;79:1278.
10. Anous MM, Heimbach DM. Causes of death and predictors in burned patients more than 60 years of age. *J Trauma* 1986;26:135.
11. MacKenzie EJ, Morris JA, Edelstein SL. Effect of preexisting disease on length of hospital stay in trauma patients. *J Trauma* 1989;29:757.
12. Milzman DP, Boulanger BR, Rodriguez A, et al. Preexisting disease in trauma patients: a predictor of fate independent of age and injury severity score. *J Trauma* 1992;32:236.
13. Fairman R, Rombeau JL. Physiologic problems in the elderly surgical patient. In: Miller A, ed. Rowlands J, contrib ed. *Physiologic basis of modern surgical care.* Washington, DC: Mosby, 1988:1108.
14. Rao TLK, Jacobs KH, El-Etr AA. Reinfarction following anesthesia in patients with myocardial infarction. *Anesthesiology* 1983;59:499.
15. Brandstetter RD, Kazemi H. Aging and the respiratory system. *Med Clin North Am* 1983;67:419.
16. Oreskovich MR, Howard JD, Copass MK, et al. Geriatric trauma: injury patterns and outcome. *J Trauma* 1984;24:565.
17. Miller JH, McDonald RU, Shock NW. Age changes in maximum rate of renal tubular resorption of glucose. *J Gerontol* 1952;7:196.
18. McLeskey CH. Anesthesia for the geriatric patient. *Adv Anesth* 1985;2:32.
19. Young EA. Nutrition, aging, and the aged. *Med Clin North Am* 1983;67:295.
20. Hartford CE, Kealey GP, Wilmore DW, et al. Pharmacokinetics in surgical practice. In: *American College of Surgeons: care of the surgical patient.* Vol. 1. New York: Scientific American, 1988:11.
21. Kirkpatrick JB, Pearson J. Fatal cerebral injury in the elderly. *J Am Geriatr Soc* 1978;27:489.
22. Rathbone-McCuan E, Voyles B. Case detection of abused elderly patients. *Am J Psychiatry* 1982;139:189.
23. Haljamae H, Stefansson T, Wickstrom I. Preanesthetic evaluation of the female geriatric patient with hip fracture. *Acta Anesth Scand* 1982;26:393.
24. Schultz RJ, Whitfield GF, LaMura JJ, et al. The role of physiologic monitoring in patients with fractures of the hip. *J Trauma* 1985;25:309.
25. Horst HM, Obeid FN, Sorensen VJ, et al. Factors influencing survival of elderly trauma patients. *Crit Care Med* 1986;14:681.
26. MacIntyre PE, Pavilion EG, Dwersteg JR. Effect of meperidine on oxygen con-

sumption, carbon dioxide production, and respiratory gas exchange in postanesthesia shivering. *Anesth Analg* 1987;66:751.
27. Scalea TM, Simeon HM, Duncan AO. Geriatric blunt trauma: improved survival with early invasive monitoring. *J Trauma* 1990;30:129.
28. Dahn MS, Wilson RF, Lange MP, et al. Hemodynamic benefits of verapamil after aortic reconstruction. *J Vasc Surg* 1989;9:806–811.
29. Champion EW, Mulley AG, Goldstin RL, et al. Medical intensive care for the elderly. *JAMA* 1981;246:2052.
30. DeMaria EJ, Kenney PR, Merriam MA, et al. Aggressive trauma care benefits the elderly. *J Trauma* 1987;27:1200.

9B. SPECIAL PROBLEMS OF TRAUMA: DRUG-ADDICTED PATIENTS(1)

Illicit use of drugs is a major problem in trauma, with studies showing evidence of cocaine in up to 54% of trauma victims (2). In addition, more than 80% of violent crime may be associated with the use of illegal drugs.

AXIOM Failure to manage trauma patients' addictions as well as their injuries can greatly increase morbidity and mortality.

Illicit drug use can produce difficulties from either "too little," which can produce severe withdrawal symptoms, and "too much," which can cause severe physiologic changes because of the side effects of the drug. Indeed, many of the signs and symptoms produced by addiction or withdrawal can be confused with those resulting from various injuries.

HISTORY

Failure to elicit a history of drug use or to obtain laboratory evidence confirming such use can lead to disastrous results. It also is important to interview any friends or family who accompany the patient to the emergency department; however, they also may be reluctant to provide accurate information.

DIAGNOSIS

⊘ PITFALL

If the diagnosis of drug use is overlooked preoperatively, withdrawal may occur under anesthesia when it is much more dangerous and difficult to treat.

Respiratory Problems

Unexplained respiratory difficulty after trauma should make the physician suspicious of a narcotic or barbiturate overdose (3). Although a rapid pulse rate after trauma is usually indicative of hypovolemia, tachycardia associated with a normal or increased blood pressure may be an early clue to the presence of cocaine, amphetamines, or hallucinogens. In contrast, patients with bradycardia and hypotension may have taken large doses of depressants, such as narcotics, barbiturates, or tranquilizers. Patients with sluggish but widely dilated pupils and with no evidence of head injury should be suspected of having taken excessive doses of barbiturates or tranquilizers.

Mental Status

Changes in the mental status of a trauma patient should not be considered drug related until all other causes (brain injury, hypoxia, hypoglycemia, etc.) have been excluded and the diagnosis of drug use is established.

Although vague neurologic signs or symptoms are often caused by drugs, unconsciousness associated with localizing signs is more apt to be a result of head injury. Radiographs and blood glucose, barbiturate, salicylate, and alcohol levels should be obtained to aid in the differentiation of traumatic and drug-induced coma.

TYPES OF DRUG ADDICTION

For practical purposes, the various narcotic drugs, including heroin, morphine, meperidine, and codeine, can be considered one group. Other categories include barbiturates and tranquilizers, hallucinogens [lysergic acid diethylamide (LSD), mescaline, and peyote], and adulterants (agents such as strychnine, atropine, belladonna, talcum powder, and quinine that are frequently mixed with "street drugs").

Narcotics

Cocaine

Cocaine is a naturally occurring alkaloid derived from the South American shrub *Erythroxylon coca*. It is usually sniffed or inhaled, but it can also be injected. "Crack" cocaine is a neutral form of the drug, like freebase, that is made without solvent extraction.

AXIOM The intense "high" of cocaine plus the central stimulatory properties can lead to rapid addiction, even with only one or two uses.

Physiologic Effects

Cocaine has both local anesthetic and sympathomimetic actions on multiple organs. It blocks presynaptic reuptake of the neurotransmitters norepinephrine and dopamine, thereby potentiating the effects of both circulating catecholamines and direct sympathetic stimulation. The cardiovascular effects of cocaine include dose-dependent increases of mean arterial pressure (MAP), heart rate, myocardial oxygen consumption ($M\text{V}O_2$), and coronary vasospasm, leading to acute myocardial ischemia or arrhythmias or both. Prolonged cocaine use also may lead to myocardial lesions similar to those seen after chronic sympathetic stimulation from a pheochromocytoma.

AXIOM Excessive stimulation of the cardiovascular system is the most frequent manifestation of severe cocaine toxicity.

Anesthetic Interactions

Cocaine can interact adversely with a number of anesthetic agents, such as halothane, so that the myocardium is greatly sensitized to the effects of catecholamines (4). Development of sudden cardiac arrhythmias or unexplained myocardial decompensation in the midst of massive blood and fluid replacement after severe injury is more frequent in patients taking cocaine.

AXIOM Strokes and acute myocardial infarctions in young drug users are often caused by cocaine.

The sudden, severe increase of blood pressure caused by an acute ingestion of cocaine can result in a hypertensive crisis, and cocaine is the primary cause of stroke in young patients (5). Cocaine also may induce acute aortic dissection. Patients with brain trauma may be at a much greater risk for intracranial hemorrhage if they are taking cocaine. The pulmonary effects of cocaine include pulmonary edema, bronchospasm, and transient pulmonary infiltrates accompanied by fever. These changes may be difficult to differentiate from direct trauma or the pulmonary response to hypovolemic shock and massive blood replacement.

Cocaine also may cause rhabdomyolysis and acute myoglobinuric renal failure. A great increase in motor activity probably also contributes to the myonecrosis and acute renal failure (6). Gastrointestinal ischemic syndromes, including perforation, have been noted in conjunction with cocaine use (7). The acute abdominal pain caused by cocaine-induced vascular spasm can interfere greatly with accurate assessment of patients with possible abdominal injuries.

Signs and Symptoms of Cocaine Use

AXIOM Acute psychotic behavior may be a result of cocaine, but central nervous system (CNS) injury or hypoxia must be ruled out first.

High doses of cocaine, as with other stimulants, can cause impaired judgment, disinhibition, impulsiveness, compulsively repeated actions, paranoia, and extreme psychomotor agitation (8). Panic attacks, paranoid ideation, and psychotic behavior may be associated with violence and sometimes with homicidal intent; indeed, drug-related injuries are frequent during this phase.

Treatment

Treatment of patients with cocaine overdose is primarily supportive. The cardiovascular and pulmonary problems are probably best handled by providing ventilatory support and optimizing hemodynamic function with a Swan–Ganz catheter.

Heroin

Heroin is derived from morphine, the principal product of the poppy *Papaver somniferum* (8). Its effects are mediated by endogenous opiate receptors that function as neurotransmitters, neurohormones, and modulators of neurotransmission throughout the CNS. Drug-related injuries from heroin include overdose, mycotic aneurysms, and myriad infectious complications.

One of the main problems with heroin is the unpredictable quantity of active drug, toxic additives, and contamination in each dose. The additives used to dilute heroin typically include quinine, strychnine, lidocaine, sugar, talcum, and starch. Because the dilution is uncontrolled, there is frequent bacterial contamination.

Signs and Symptoms

The patient with a heroin overdose will usually be somnolent, stuporous, or in a profound coma (8). The breathing pattern tends to be slow and shallow, resulting in a significantly reduced minute ventilation.

AXIOM Narcotic overdose should be part of the differential diagnosis in somnolent patients with depressed ventilation, pulmonary congestion, vasodilation, hypotension, or a combination of these.

Heroin causes a decrease in systemic vascular resistance (SVR) that is augmented by a concomitant release of histamine (8). Therefore opiate-intoxicated patients can have severe hypotension with relatively mild hypovolemia.

Occasionally young heroin addicts exhibit mental confusion with progressive cardiac failure that is resistant to the usual forms of therapy. Patients with this difficulty should be given ventilatory and cardiovascular support as needed plus narcotic antagonists.

Treatment

Naloxone, given in intravenous doses of 0.4 mg, repeated every few minutes as necessary, can cause a dramatic reversal of the respiratory depression and peripheral vasodilation resulting from opiate toxicity. Excessive naloxone, however, can precipitate opiate withdrawal, thereby greatly complicating therapy. Because the effective half-life of naloxone is shorter than that of most opiates, redosing of naloxone every few hours may be necessary until the circulating opiate is excreted.

Other Narcotic Problems

Withdrawal

Withdrawal from narcotic addiction can be dangerous, especially if it occurs during an anesthetic or in the immediate postoperative period. The associated rhinorrhea, lacrimation, confusion, sweating, cramping, and diarrhea can cause severe fluid and electrolyte problems. The resulting clinical picture can be extremely confusing and very difficult to treat.

With methadone, signs and symptoms of withdrawal may not occur until 24 hours after the last dose (2). The physiologic changes can be especially dangerous in hypovolemic patients under general anesthesia.

AXIOM The addicted trauma patient who is in shock and is immediately taken to the operating room will often not manifest withdrawal symptoms until under anesthesia or postoperatively.

Ongoing Narcotic Use

Sudden deterioration of an addict's condition in the hospital without explanation, just when it seems that the patient is improving, should alert the physician to the possibility that narcotics have been given to the patient by friends or family. On several occasions, visitors have injected heroin into the intravenous lines of critically ill patients, causing sudden unexplained deaths.

Barbiturates and Tranquilizers

Overdoses

Overdoses of barbiturates and tranquilizers tend to produce lethargy, slurred speech, inability to solve simple mental problems, and confusion. Severe overdoses also may cause bradycardia and hypotension. Treatment of barbiturate or tranquilizer intoxication varies with the severity of the symptoms and CNS depression. Gastric lavage, if feasible, should be carried out as soon as possible with a large 40 to 50F Ewald tube to remove any drug still retained in the stomach.

After the stomach is emptied, administration of activated charcoal should reduce the absorption of any residual agent that may have reached the intestines. If there is severe respiratory depression, a ventilator is used to maintain adequate blood gases. If the patient becomes hypotensive, large volumes of fluid may be needed to fill the dilated vascular space. Occasionally, inotropic drugs or vasoconstrictors or both also may be needed to maintain a satisfactory blood pressure and tissue perfusion.

AXIOM Treatment of barbiturate overdoses involves emptying the stomach and decreasing drug absorption with charcoal plus support of pulmonary, cardiac, and renal function.

Excretion

Short-acting barbiturates, such as pentobarbital (Nembutal) and thiopental (Pentothal), are metabolized primarily by the liver. Long-acting barbiturates, such as phenobarbital, are excreted by the kidneys (2). The excretion of both types of barbiturates is increased by alkalinizing the serum and urine and maintaining a urine output of at least 100 to 200 mL/h.

Postoperative Withdrawal

Postoperative barbiturate withdrawal may cause seizures, delirium, hyperpyrexia, tachycardia, coma, and death. If thiopental is used to induce anesthesia, the barbiturate addict may have a repeated respiratory crisis. Then when the anesthetic wears off, the patient may develop withdrawal. Barbiturate withdrawal in the postoperative period may require intramuscular injections of short-acting barbiturates in doses exceeding 100 mg/h. This dose is then gradually reduced at a rate of about 100 mg/day.

AXIOM Of the various drugs that may be abused, barbiturates are the most likely to cause death as a result of acute withdrawal.

Hallucinogens

AXIOM Bizarre suicide attempts should make one suspect hallucinogen intoxication.

Signs and Symptoms of Hallucinogen Use

Patients under the influence of hallucinogens often have wild visual images, which may precipitate self-inflicted wounds and suicidal gestures. This type of addiction should be suspected when the physician is confronted with a bizarre suicide attempt. A "good trip" can cause euphoria and tranquility. A "bad trip" can cause excitability, disorientation, inappropriate verbiage, and occasional fits of rage. Overdoses can produce death, seizures, or unconsciousness. Physical findings can include mydriasis, hyperthermia, piloerection, hyperglycemia, and bradycardia.

Medication Interactions

Preoperative medications for patients suspected of taking hallucinogens should not include atropine-like drugs because these may potentiate the anticholinergic effects of hallucinogens. Generally, the safest drug for control of hallucinogenic effects is intramuscular diazepam (Valium) in doses of 5 to 10 mg every 2 to 4 hours as needed.

Adulterants

The most important adulterants mixed with street drugs include lidocaine, atropine, strychnine, and quinine (2). Any of these agents may cause lethal and incapacitating effects. Local anesthetic adulterants, such as lidocaine or tetracaine, can cause CNS stimulation with tremors, agitation, or seizures, especially after prolonged exposure.

Classic signs of **atropine** toxicity include tachycardia, fever, cutaneous flushing, dilated pupils, and extreme dryness of the skin and mucous membranes. Severe overdoses should be managed with short-acting barbiturates, hypothermia as needed, and intravenous fluids. Eye patches should be applied to prevent blinding from the excessive light that might otherwise reach the retina through dilated pupils. Methacholine may be useful in substantiating the diagnosis of atropine toxicity (2). Lack of rhinorrhea, lacrimation, salivation, sweating, and cramps after 10 to 20 mg of methacholine subcutaneously is virtually diagnostic of atropine toxicity.

Symptoms of **quinine** toxicity can include tinnitus, headache, nausea, and blurred vision. Chronic poisoning can produce photophobia, dyslogia (impairment of reasoning), blindness, cramps, vomiting, and a characteristic papular scarlatina-like rash. A clue to identifying a chronic user of quinine is the presence of an unexplained hemolytic anemia. Treatment is primarily symptomatic.

Strychnine, which is a competitive antagonist of the CNS inhibitory neurotransmitter glycine, tends to cause apprehension, nausea, abdominal cramps, and constricted facial muscles followed by spasms of extensor muscles, opisthotonos, and frank seizures. Strychnine also may cause rhabdomyolysis and myoglobinuric acute renal failure. Treatment includes short-acting barbiturates to control seizures plus ventilatory support as needed.

VIRAL DISEASES ASSOCIATED WITH ADDICTION

Hepatitis

Estroff et al. (9) noted 85% seropositivity for hepatitis B in intravenous heroin and cocaine addicts. Approximately 25% of practicing surgeons in this country carry antibody to hepatitis antigens (10). Two to three hundred health care personnel die each year of occupationally acquired hepatitis, many more than those of acquired immunodeficiency syndrome (AIDS). These deaths could have been prevented by the prophylactic use of hepatitis B vaccine.

AIDS

At least 4% of the injured patients treated at the Detroit Receiving Hospital are human immunodeficiency virus (HIV) positive (8).

AXIOM All urban patients with penetrating injuries should be considered to be hepatitis and HIV positive until proven otherwise.

Sloan et al. (11) found that young urban trauma patients were 15.3 to 17.6 times more likely to be HIV positive than the trauma population overall. Other demographic factors associated with an increased risk of HIV infection in urban trauma patients included penetrating trauma, nonwhite race, male gender, positive drug or positive alcohol screens (or both), and city residence (12). For example, 10% of the trauma patients seen at Johns Hopkins Hospital, Baltimore, Maryland, have tested positive for HIV. The percentage increases to 19% for male victims of penetrating trauma between the ages of 25 and 34 years.

Gerberding et al. (13) at San Francisco General Hospital observed 130 consecutive surgical procedures to determine the risk of accidental exposure to blood. Parenteral exposure to blood occurred in 1.7% of the cases, whereas cutaneous exposure occurred in an additional 4.7%. Most of the cutaneous exposures could have been prevented by appropriate techniques such as double gloving and wearing impermeable garments.

Diagnosis

Standard tests for HIV are too time consuming to be of use in the emergency setting; however, several findings should alert the surgeon that the patient may be infected. Preoperatively, an abnormally low white count should serve as a clue. Intraoperatively, splenomegaly and retroperitoneal lymph node enlargement are common findings. Enlarged lymph nodes should be sampled and sent for culture as well as histologic analysis. The presence of cytomegalovirus or an atypical mycobacterium is virtually diagnostic of AIDS.

AXIOM Very low white blood count (WBC), weight loss, and multiple enlarged lymph nodes should make one very suspicious of an underlying HIV infection.

⊘ FREQUENT ERRORS

1. ***Not paying adequate attention to a patient's drug addiction and considering only the problems caused by the trauma.***
2. ***Failure to consider drug withdrawal as a cause of unusual behavior during or after a general anesthetic.***
3. ***Assuming that unusual behavior in an injured drug addict is due to the illicit drug and not the trauma or a correctable metabolic problem.***
4. ***Forgetting that hypertension in a cocaine overdose may hide an underlying hypovolemia.***

5. ***Forgetting that cocaine can cause acute cerebrovascular accidents and myocardial infarctions in young individuals.***
6. ***Failure to follow universal precautions when treating a patient who may be a drug addict.***

SUMMARY POINTS

1. Failure to manage patients' addictions as well as their injuries can greatly increase mortality and morbidity.

2. The intense "high" of cocaine plus the central stimulatory properties can lead to rapid addiction, even with only one or two uses.

3. Excessive stimulation of the cardiovascular system is the most frequent manifestation of severe cocaine toxicity.

4. Strokes and acute myocardial infarctions in young drug users are often due to cocaine.

5. Acute psychotic behavior may be a result of cocaine, but CNS injury and hypoxia must be ruled out.

6. Heroin-related problems may be caused by infection, various additives, its inherent pharmacologic toxicity, or direct injury to the lungs.

7. Narcotic overdose should be part of the differential diagnosis in somnolent patients with depressed ventilation, pulmonary congestion, vasodilation, hypotension, or a combination of these.

8. The addicted trauma patient who is in shock and is immediately taken to the operating room often does not manifest narcotic withdrawal symptoms until under anesthesia or postoperatively.

9. Treatment of barbiturate overdoses involves decreasing drug absorption with charcoal and support of pulmonary, cardiac, and renal function.

10. Of all the drugs that may be abused, barbiturates are the most likely to cause death as a result of acute withdrawal.

11. Bizarre suicide attempts should make one suspect hallucinogen intoxication.

12. One cannot rely on an addicted patient's history on time and doses of any drug.

13. All urban patients with penetrating trauma should be considered hepatitis and HIV positive until proven otherwise.

14. Very low WBC, weight loss, and multiple enlarged lymph nodes should make one very suspicious of an underlying HIV infection.

REFERENCES

1. Wilson RF, Bender JS, Gass J. Special problems of trauma in addicted patients. In Wilson RF, Walt AJ, eds. *Management of trauma: pitfalls and practice.* 2nd ed. Philadelphia: Williams & Wilkins, 1996:160.
2. Parran TV, Weber E, Tasse J, et al. Mandatory toxicology testing and chemical dependence consultation follow-up in a level one trauma center. *J Trauma* 1995; 38:278.
3. Soderstrom CA, Dailey JT, Kerns TJ. Alcohol and other drugs: an assessment of testing and clinical practices in U.S. trauma centers. *J Trauma* 1994;36:68.
4. Barash PG, Koprieva CJ, Langou R, et al. Is cocaine a sympathetic stimulant during general anaesthesia? *JAMA* 1980;243:1437.
5. Levine SR, Brust JCM, Futrill N, et al. Cerebral vascular complications of the use of the "crack" form of alkaloidal cocaine. *N Engl J Med* 1990;323:699.
6. Herzlich BC, Arsura EL, Pagala M, et al. Rhabdomyolysis related to cocaine abuse. *Ann Intern Med* 1988;109:335.
7. Lee HS, LaMaute HR, Pizzi WF, et al. Acute gastroduodenal perforations associated with use of crack. *Ann Surg* 1990;211:15.
8. Lucas CE, Joseph AJ, Ledgerwood AM. Alcohol and drugs. In: Moore EE, Mattox

KL, Feliciano DV, eds. *Trauma.* 2nd ed. Norwalk, CT: Appleton & Lange, 1991: 677–687.
9. Estroff TW, Extein IL, Malaspina R, et al. Hepatitis in 101 consecutive suburban cocaine and opiate users. *Int J Psychiatr Med* 1986;16:237.
10. West DJ. The risk of hepatitis B infection among health professionals in the United States: a review. *Am J Med Sci* 1984;287:26.
11. Sloan EP, McGill BA, Zalenski R, et al. Human immunodeficiency virus and hepatitis B virus seroprevalence in an urban trauma population. *J Trauma* 1995; 38:736.
12. Kelen GR, Fritz S, Qaguish B, et al. Substantial increase in human immunodeficiency virus infection in critically ill emergency patients: 1986 and 1987 compared. *Ann Emerg Med* 1989;18:378.
13. Gerberding JL, Littell C, Tarkington A, et al. Risk of exposure of surgical personnel to patients' blood during survey at San Francisco General Hospital. *N Engl J Med* 1990;322:1788.

9C. SPECIAL PROBLEMS OF TRAUMA: ALCOHOLIC PATIENTS(1)

An estimated 76,000,000 people in the United States are affected by alcohol abuse at some time, and motor vehicle accidents are the leading cause of death in these individuals. Of the 50,000 deaths due to motor vehicle accidents annually, more than 50% are alcohol related (2). Indeed, two of every five Americans will be in an alcohol-related motor vehicle accident (MVA) sometime during their lives (3). In addition, alcohol is a factor in up to 67% of home injuries, drownings, fire fatalities, and job injuries.

ACUTE ALCOHOLISM

AXIOM The main problem in treating acutely intoxicated trauma victims is the increased incidence of diagnostic errors.

Many injured patients who are intoxicated are uncooperative, and some are extremely loud and belligerent. Not infrequently, those with minimal injuries will insist loudly on immediate intensive care, whereas those with the most severe trauma often cannot be made to appreciate fully the seriousness of their injuries. The physical examination is often incomplete because of poor patient cooperation, so that mistaken or delayed diagnoses in acutely intoxicated patients are not infrequent.

⊘ PITFALL

If it is not appreciated that acute alcoholic intoxication can seriously impair a patient's judgment, some badly injured intoxicated patients may be allowed to leave the hospital without adequate care.

Although the desire to "treat and street" disruptive alcoholic patients is very high, especially if they are "repeaters," such an attitude should be avoided until it is quite certain that no serious problem exists and that a responsible and sober individual will watch over them.

⊘ PITFALL

If alcoholics are not roused and checked frequently after they have fallen asleep, serious neurologic lesions may not be detected until too late.

Basic rules to be followed with all acutely intoxicated patients who have had head trauma include

1. Complete vital signs should be taken at least every 30 minutes;
2. "Sleeping" patients should be aroused at least every 30 minutes for a neurologic examination, which includes pupillary size and reaction and deep tendon reflexes;
3. Computed tomography (CT) scans of the brain should be obtained on all alcoholics with head trauma who have any lateralizing signs or do not "wake up" within 4 to 6 hours; and
4. Alcoholism should not be accepted as a cause of unconsciousness if the blood level of alcohol is less than 150 mg/dL.

Respiratory Complications

Almost all severely intoxicated patients who are supine tend to "snore" because of a partial upper airway obstruction caused by a flaccid tongue falling back into the pharynx. If the cervical spine radiographs are negative and if it does not appear that turning the patient on his or her side will aggravate any other injuries, moving the patient into this position can readily solve this problem.

Alcoholics are also prone to aspirate their oral or gastric secretions, and this can cause severe acute respiratory infections, including lung abscesses. If there is any evidence of aspiration, it should be treated vigorously with prompt bronchoscopy and ventilatory assistance as needed.

Hemodynamic Effects of Alcohol

AXIOM Alcohol blunts the ability of the body to compensate for acute hemorrhage.

Gettler and Allbritten (4) noted that intoxicated dogs were more likely to have a decreased compensatory response to hemorrhage resulting in a lower mean arterial pressure (MAP), increased tendency to metabolic acidosis, and an increased mortality rate (30% vs. 0 in the controls).

AXIOM Alcohol tends to blunt the ventilatory and vasoconstrictor response to hemorrhagic shock.

Alcohol increases the incidence of arrhythmias in humans and may be part of the cause of the increased mortality rate from hemorrhagic shock in inebriated patients (5). In addition, chronic alcoholics often have evidence of cardiomyopathy.

With severe intoxication, the negative inotropic effect of alcohol combined with a decreased systemic vascular resistance (SVR) can cause a reduction in MAP far out of proportion to the actual amount of blood loss. Consequently, many injured, intoxicated patients have severe hypotension even though the blood volume loss is relatively small.

AXIOM Ethanol tends to cause vasodilation and a negative inotropic effect, and this can increase the amount of hypotension that occurs with blood loss.

Acute Withdrawal (Delirium Tremens)

One of the most common severe alcohol-related metabolic problems after operation is delirium tremens (DTs). The full-blown syndrome in the trauma patient usually does not manifest for at least 24 to 48 hours, and in some instances, it may be delayed for 4 to 5 days or longer. Patients with confusion but without hallucinations are classified as having mild or class I DTs. Class II includes auditory hallucinations, and class III includes visual hallucinations. Class IV patients also have total body tremulousness or generalized convulsions or both.

AXIOM Acute restlessness in alcoholics should not be considered a result of alcohol withdrawal or DTs until hypoxia, head trauma, sepsis, hypoglycemia, and electrolyte abnormalities have been ruled out.

Signs and Symptoms

The first indications of an impending attack of DTs are restlessness and mental irritability. In severe untreated forms, DTs are characterized by a disoriented, disheveled patient who is constantly moving, rearranging bedclothes, tugging at his restraints, and often incontinent. The obvious tremor is so grossly disorganized that even simple chores become impossible. Patients may actively hallucinate and engage in imagined conversations. They may shout or scream in anguish to ward off imaginary people or animals who threaten them. Vomiting, dehydration, hyperthermia, hypovolemia, severe electrolyte imbalances, and aspiration pneumonitis occur frequently and can progress rapidly to death unless treated aggressively.

⊘ PITFALL

Confusing the early manifestations of hypoxia or sepsis with DTs.

Approximately 10% of patients with symptoms of severe acute alcohol withdrawal experience seizures. Ninety percent of these seizures occur between 7 and 48 hours after cessation of drinking, with a peak incidence between 12 and 24 hours. Withdrawal seizures have an abrupt onset, tend to be generalized tonicoclonic in nature, and are usually associated with a loss of consciousness. In contrast, focal seizures imply focal cerebral disease, and craniocerebral trauma must be suspected.

AXIOM Focal seizures during alcohol withdrawal are a result of head trauma until proven otherwise.

Physiologic Effects

The most frequent cause of death after operation in injured patients with DTs is an arrhythmia that is often related to hypokalemia or hypomagnesemia. Serum potassium levels often decline below 3.0 mEq/L during alcohol withdrawal and remain low despite intravenous replacement. Hyponatremia, hypophosphatemia, and hypomagnesemia are also frequently encountered during alcohol withdrawal and must be addressed. Chronic alcoholics can have very low serum magnesium levels, but even if the serum magnesium levels are normal, the total body content is often severely reduced. If the patient develops full-blown DTs, 12 g i.v. or more of $MgSO_4$ may be required daily. In addition, the patient may need 6 to 8 L or more of balanced electrolyte solution per day to reverse the tendency to dehydration. If vomiting occurs, nasogastric suction should be begun.

AXIOM Serum levels of potassium, magnesium, phosphorus, and sodium should be watched carefully in patients who may develop DTs or other alcohol-withdrawal symptoms.

Medications

Trace elements and vitamins, especially potassium, magnesium, calcium, thiamine, and nicotinic acid, should be routinely added to the intravenous solutions of patients likely to go into alcohol withdrawal. Isolation or restraint of the patient should be avoided if possible at this point, as these measures only increase anxiety and metabolic demands.

Diazepam (Valium) is generally a safe drug in alcoholics, and it can be given orally, intramuscularly, or intravenously with a fairly wide margin of safety. Large quantities of sedatives or tranquilizers, in addition to restraints and a reasonably quiet environment, are often required to control agitation. Such sedation, however, may be a great problem in patients being observed for a head injury and may also increase the incidence of aspiration pneumonia.

Convulsions should be controlled or prevented with intravenous or intramuscular diazepam or dihydrohydantoin (Dilantin), but hypoglycemia should be eliminated as a possible etiologic factor. When boluses of glucose are given, they should be preceded by 100 mg of thiamine every 12 hours to help prevent Wernicke's encephalopathy (6).

CHRONIC ALCOHOLISM

Chronic alcoholism is the most frequent cause of cirrhosis in the United States. In addition, chronic alcoholism can cause damage to a wide variety of other organ systems.

AXIOM One should never rely completely on a history provided by a chronic alcoholic patient.

Physiologic Effects

The neurologic changes of chronic alcoholism can make it extremely difficult to obtain a reliable history and to determine whether significant head trauma has occurred. Korsakoff's syndrome or similar problems can result in medical histories that are extremely misleading. Wernicke's syndrome, characterized by ophthalmoplegia, nystagmus, pupillary alterations, and ataxia with tremors, can cause severe central neurologic changes that are not usually localized. The peripheral neuropathy of chronic alcoholism may also cause the patient to lose peripheral sensation, coordination, and strength.

The cardiovascular changes of advanced cirrhosis include a reduced ability to tolerate hypotension and an increased tendency to congestive heart failure. These patients rely on hepatic artery blood flow to nourish the liver, and hypotension in these patients is associated with an extremely high incidence of liver failure and death. Cardiomyopathies also are common, so there may be minimal tolerance between hypovolemic hypotension and fluid overloading.

AXIOM Cardiac filling pressures must be monitored closely in chronic alcoholics because of the small margin that they may have between hypovolemic hypotension and overt cardiac failure.

In the past, it was thought that most cardiac problems in chronic alcoholics resulted from a thiamine deficiency, as in beriberi heart disease; however, many of these patients respond only partially to large doses of thiamine. Furthermore, these patients are overly sensitive to digitalis, especially if acidosis and hypotension are present. Consequently, extra care must be taken to avoid fluid overload. Conversely, even though severe ascites may produce some respiratory distress, complete removal of the fluid can cause hypovolemia and hypotension to develop rapidly, unless adequate fluids and protein are administered as the ascitic fluid reaccumulates at the expense of the functional extracellular fluid (ECF).

AXIOM Reaccumulation of ascitic fluid after laparotomy in a cirrhotic patient can rapidly cause severe hypovolemia.

Gastrointestinal Bleeding

Gastrointestinal bleeding in chronic alcoholics can be due to esophageal varices, gastric erosions, or peptic ulcers. Bleeding from esophageal varices can have a high mortality, regardless of the mode of therapy. Diagnosis is generally made endoscopically, and any varices found can be sclerosed during the endoscopy. Vasopressin (pitressin) at 0.2 to 0.4 U/min or more i.v. or into the superior mesenteric artery is often effective. Nitroglycerin is often given intravenously or as a skin patch with the vasopressin to prevent excessive hypertension. Recently intravenous somatostatin analogues have been found to be more effective than vasopressin (7).

Coagulation Problems

Severe coagulation problems, especially prothrombin deficiencies, can be encountered in chronic alcoholics. Vitamin K may not restore the prothrombin time to normal if the liver disease is severe, and if emergency surgery is required, 6 to 12 units of fresh frozen plasma may be required to correct the coagulopathies rapidly.

AXIOM If at all possible, surgery should be delayed until the prothrombin time is within 3 to 5 seconds of normal (control) values.

Hepatic Injuries in Cirrhotics

Patients with alcoholic cirrhosis and either blunt or penetrating hepatic injuries can be very difficult to treat. One should avoid anesthetics such as fluothane that require detoxification by the liver. Because of the portal hypertension, minor liver lacerations may bleed profusely, and obtaining exposure to posterior wounds can be very difficult. In such cases, one should consider early placement of intraabdominal packs and reexploration of the patient in 48 to 72 hours. Packing with omentum and use of fibrin glue also may be helpful.

Postoperative Resuscitation

Some general rules in the postoperative management of the chronic alcoholic include

1. Liberal use of glucose, trace elements, and vitamins;
2. Avoidance of excess water and salt;
3. Early cleansing of blood from the gastrointestinal tract; and
4. Administration of intestinal neomycin in selected cases.

AXIOM Continued or recurrent postoperative bleeding in cirrhotics in spite of a reasonable correction of the prothrombin time and platelet count should be controlled surgically as soon as possible.

General debility, poor resistance to infection, and elevation of the diaphragm by ascites all increase the chances of postoperative pneumonitis and respiratory failure (6). Complete gastrointestinal decompression, vigorous bronchial toilet, and early ventilatory assistance, as needed, are mandatory. Tamura et al. (8) recently found that acute ETOH intoxication inhibits several arms of immune defense, causing attenuation of T-cell function, decreased bacterial clearance from the lungs, and impaired macrophage bactericidal activity.

ETOH dose-dependently attenuated superoxide production by polymorphonuclear lymphocytes (PMNs) with significance at 0.3% ETOH. Elastase release was attenuated starting at 0.2% ETOH, and CD11b expression was reduced starting at 0.4% ETOH. Thus clinically relevant concentrations of ETOH can attenuate PMN functions that are critical in host defense against invading pathogens.

Impaired liver function coupled with an increased protein load to the liver from blood transfusions and absorption of blood from injured tissue, sets the stage for hepatic encephalopathy. Cleansing of the gastrointestinal tract of blood with enemas and cathartics as soon as possible and the use of parenteral and intestinal antibiotics may help reduce the formation of ammonia by intestinal bacteria. Histamine (H_2) blockers or antacids or both should be begun immediately postoperatively to decrease the chances of stress gastric bleeding.

OUTCOMES OF TRAUMA

AXIOM Overall, intoxicated drivers in MVAs tend to have higher morbidity and mortality rates than do sober drivers.

Luna et al. (9) noted that mortality rates in intoxicated patients are almost double those of nonintoxicated patients with comparable injuries. By using data collected over 5 years on more than a million drivers, Waller et al. (10) found that alcohol-involved drivers had serious and fatal injuries 1.7 to 2.1 times as often as their sober counterparts with matched collisions.

Tinkoff et al. (11) found a mortality rate of 30% in 40 cirrhotic trauma victims admitted to two Pennsylvania hospitals. This was significantly higher than the 7% mortality rate predicted by TRISS methods. Most of the deaths were due to sepsis and multisystem organ failure. Predictors of poor outcome on admission included ascites, increased prothrombin time, hyperbilirubinemia, and the need for a laparotomy.

⊘ FREQUENT ERRORS

1. ***Failure to look carefully for alcoholic intoxication in MVA victims, especially those with an altered state of consciousness.***
2. ***Attributing a tendency to be uncooperative and sleepy only to alcohol.***
3. ***Considering central nervous system (CNS) changes a result of acute alcoholic intoxication, even after 4 to 6 hours of observation.***
4. ***Failure to look for other drugs in patients who are obviously intoxicated.***
5. ***Assuming that focal seizures in an alcoholic are a result of alcohol withdrawal.***
6. ***Failure to monitor serum electrolytes, especially potassium and magnesium, closely enough in alcoholic patients.***
7. ***Assuming that total body magnesium levels are normal if serum levels are normal, and thereby failing to provide adequate magnesium to chronic alcoholic patients.***
8. ***Failure to provide adequate fluid to cirrhotic patients who have had a laparotomy and may rapidly reaccumulate ascitic fluid.***
9. ***Failure promptly to correct the prothrombin time and platelet count in cirrhotic who are bleeding postoperatively and thereby continuing to assume that the excess bleeding does not require surgical control.***

SUMMARY POINTS

1. There is a high incidence of diagnostic errors in acutely intoxicated trauma victims.

2. Acutely intoxicated patients are prone to aspirate or to develop severe pulmonary infections or both.

3. Alcohol blunts the hemodynamic and ventilatory response to acute hemorrhage.

4. Ethanol tends to cause vasodilation and a negative inotropic effect, and this can increase the amount of hypotension that occurs with blood loss.

5. Severe metabolic acidosis in a chronic alcoholic without evidence of shock or tissue ischemia may be a result of methanol ingestion.

6. Acute restlessness in alcoholics should not be considered a result of alcohol withdrawal until hypoxia, head trauma, sepsis, hypoglycemia, and electrolyte abnormalities have been ruled out.

7. Focal seizures during alcohol withdrawal are a result of head trauma until proven otherwise.
8. Serum levels of potassium, magnesium, phosphorus, and sodium should be watched carefully in patients who may develop DTs or other alcohol-withdrawal symptoms.
9. Chronic alcoholics can have rather severe total body magnesium deficits, even though serum magnesium levels are normal.
10. Cardiac filling pressures must be monitored closely in chronic alcoholics because of the small margin of safety between hypovolemic hypotension and overt cardiac failure.
11. Reaccumulation of ascitic fluid after laparotomy in cirrhotic patients can rapidly cause severe hypovolemia.
12. If at all possible, surgery should be delayed until the prothrombin time is within 3 to 5 seconds of the normal (control) values.
13. Continued postoperative bleeding in cirrhotics, in spite of correction of the prothrombin time and platelet count, should be controlled surgically as soon as possible.

REFERENCES

1. Wilson RF, Bender JS, Gass J. Special problems of trauma in alcoholics. In: Wilson BF, Walt AJ, eds. *Management of trauma: pitfalls and practice.* Philadelphia: Williams & Wilkins, 1996:167–172.
2. Maull KI. Alcohol abuse: its implications in trauma care. *South Med J* 1982; 75:794.
3. Lucas CE, Joseph AJ, Ledgerwood AM. Alcohol and drugs. In: Moore EE, Mattox KL, Feliciano DV, eds. *Trauma.* 2nd ed. Norwalk, CT: Appleton & Lange, 1991: 677–687.
4. Gettler DT, Allbritten FF. Effect of alcohol intoxication and the respiratory exchange and mortality rate associated with acute hemorrhage in anesthetized dogs. *Ann Surg* 1963;158:151.
5. Gleenspon AJ, Schaal SF. The "holiday heart": electrophysiologic studies of alcohol effects in alcoholics. *Ann Intern Med* 1983;98:135.
6. Goulinger RC. Delirium in the surgical patient. *Am Surg* 1989;55:549.
7. Imperiale TF, Teran JC, McCullough AJ. A meta-analysis of somatostatin versus vasopressin in the management of acute esophageal variceal hemorrhage. *Gastroenterology* 1995;109:1289.
8. Tamura DY, Moore EE, Patrick DA, et al. Clinically relevant concentrations of ethanol attenuate primed neutrophil bactericidal activity. *J Trauma* 1998;44: 320.
9. Luna GK, Maier RV, Sowder L, et al. The influence of ethanol intoxication on outcome of injured motorcyclists. *J Trauma* 1984;24:695.
10. Waller PF, Stewart JR, Hansen AR, et al. The potentiating effects of alcohol on driver injury. *JAMA* 1986;256:1461.
11. Tinkoff G, Rhodes M, Diamond D, et al. Cirrhosis in the trauma victim. *Ann Surg* 1990;211:172.

10. HEAD INJURIES[1]

INCIDENCE

AXIOM Head injury is the leading cause of mortality and morbidity after trauma.

Each year in the United States, 350,000 to 500,000 patients have a head injury severe enough to be hospitalized (2). At least 50,000 of these patients die because of their head traumas, and another 50,000 to 60,000 are severely disabled.

In an average year, the neurosurgical department of Detroit Receiving Hospital (DRH) sees more than 1,000 adult patients with head injuries. During a 2-year period (1992 through 1993), 1,050 patients with head injuries were admitted to DRH. Of these, 69% were mild [Glasgow Coma Scale (GCS) score of 13 to 15], 10% were moderate (GCS of 9 to 12), and 21% were severe (GCS score of 3 to 8). The in-hospital mortality rates with these three groups were 2%, 7%, and 46%, respectively.

TYPES OF BRAIN INJURY

Primary

Primary brain injury is the damage produced directly by the original mechanical forces. Abrupt deceleration with a rapidly moving head brought to a sudden halt causes the brain to collide with the inner surface of the skull. Shearing forces result from the differential acceleration and rebound, and contusions or lacerations may occur as the brain comes up against the more irregular contours of the skull (such as the lesser sphenoid wing) or the edges of the dura (such as the undersurface of the falx cerebri). As the brain moves away from the cranial vault on the side opposite the area of impact, tearing of bridging veins may occur, resulting in a subdural hematoma (SDH). The rebound of the brain also may result in contusion or hematoma in the area of brain striking the inner surface of the skull opposite the site of impact. This is referred to as a contrecoup injury.

Rotational acceleration is the most important factor in causing axonal disruption, hemorrhage, and brain edema. This shear–strain damage tends to be most disruptive to axons at the interface of gray and white matter, primarily in the frontal and temporal lobes and in the corpus callosum.

Mass lesions, such as hematomas or severe localized cerebral edema can cause an abrupt increase in intracranial pressure (ICP) with resultant cerebral ischemia. If subarachnoid hemorrhage also is present, this can cause increased vasospasm, causing even more ischemia.

Secondary

Secondary injury occurs after the initial trauma and is usually caused by ischemia or hypoxia or both. Injuries occurring to the brain after the primary injury lead to further damage of neurons. Hypotension and hypoxia are particularly important and, even if they are present only briefly, can double the mortality rate after head trauma (2).

AXIOM Hypoxemia and hypotension, which are the most frequent systemic insults causing severe secondary brain injury, should be prevented or corrected very rapidly.

Arterial hypoxemia is commonly seen when patients with severe head injuries arrive in the emergency department (ED) and is usually due to hypoventilation. Brainstem movement at the moment of impact can cause loss of consciousness and, because the brainstem controls respiration, hypoventilation is also likely to occur. Other causes of hypoxemia, especially in patients with multiple injuries, may include upper-airway obstruction, flail chest, hemothorax, pneumothorax, pulmonary contusion, or a combination of these.

Hypotension [systolic blood pressure (BP) less than 90 mm Hg] accompanies head trauma in about 35% of severely injured patients and increases mortality from 27% to 50% (3). Stochetti et al. (4) noted that of 49 patients with traumatic brain injury (TBI) evaluated at the accident scene, 27 (55%) had an arterial saturation less than 90%, and 12 (25%) had a systolic BP less than 100 mm Hg.

Because cerebral autoregulation is often greatly impaired by trauma, cerebral blood flow (CBF) changes directly with the systemic arterial pressure; consequently, even mild hypotension can greatly increase the brain ischemia caused by the injury itself.

A hematocrit of less than 30% leads to reduced blood oxygen-carrying capacity, and this can also make cerebral ischemia worse. Miller and Becker (3) found a mortality rate of 52% when anemia accompanied head injury. Other important systemic causes of secondary brain injury include hyperglycemia and hyperthermia.

Mechanisms of Trauma Damage

AXIOM Increased intracellular calcium can cause a number of reactions that can increase secondary brain damage.

The molecular events leading to further vascular and neuronal damage after TBI include formation of free radicals and lipid peroxidation. The appearance of microhemorrhages 12 to 18 hours after brain injury has been linked to postischemic reperfusion with iron-dependent oxygen radical–mediated peroxidation of polyunsaturated fatty acids in the cell membrane (5) and is found in more than 50% of patients dying of severe head trauma.

AXIOM Excessive release of excitatory amino acids after head trauma can greatly aggravate secondary brain injury.

The excitatory amino acid neurotransmitters glutamate (Glu) and aspartate (Asp), which are released in increased quantities after trauma, can produce cell swelling, vacuolization, and eventual cell death when applied directly to neurons (6). They also can cause seizures and general central nervous system (CNS) neuronal destruction when administered *in vivo.*

AXIOM Magnesium deficiencies contribute to the severity of secondary brain injury.

In vivo nuclear magnetic resonance studies after TBI demonstrated significant declines in intracellular free Mg^{2+} concentrations, which can cause secondary injury by disruption of membrane integrity plus the reductions in high-energy phosphate metabolism and resultant tissue acidosis (7).

Skull Fractures

Most skull fractures are linear; however, severe impact can produce subsidiary fracturing, resulting in a stellate pattern. Linear fractures that cross the middle meningeal artery or a dural sinus can be particularly dangerous because they may be associated with development of an epidural hematoma. Depressed skull fractures are usually more serious than linear fractures because of the increased incidence of injury to underlying dural sinuses and brain tissue. Depressed fractures are particularly important if the depression is greater than the thickness of the skull. Emergency surgical intervention may be necessary if the fracture is compound, if the dura is torn, or if intracranial vessels are ruptured.

AXIOM Patients with skull fractures are much more likely to have severe underlying brain injuries.

As a general rule, patients with skull fractures are about 50 times more likely to have an intracranial lesion requiring surgery. In addition, basilar skull fractures can injure cranial nerves and blood vessels traversing the foramina at the skull base. If a fracture extends into the paranasal sinuses or mastoid air cells, it can cause a cerebrospinal fluid (CSF) leak and subsequent infection.

Concussions and Contusions

Concussion refers to a transient loss of consciousness that may result from temporary dysfunction of either cortical hemispheric neurons bilaterally or the reticular activating system (RAS). There is little or no apparent tissue damage with concussions on computed tomography (CT) scans; however, positron emission tomography (PET) scans may show rather extensive metabolic lesions, and there is often some amnesia for events occurring just before and during the injury.

AXIOM Although cerebral concussions are generally considered mild head injuries, extensive subclinical damage may be present.

Cerebral contusions, as contrasted with concussions, imply tissue injury with capillary damage and interstitial hemorrhage. Although contusions can produce some neurologic deficit, they usually exert their major effect as a nidus for hemorrhage, swelling, or posttraumatic epilepsy.

Diffuse axonal injury (DAI) characteristically involves the corpus callosum, the dorsal lateral quadrant of the midbrain, and subcortical white matter (8). Initially it was thought that the tearing of axons that is often seen occurs at the moment of injury, causing the severed axon to extrude a ball of axoplasm called a "retraction ball." Increasing numbers of investigators now believe the axons are not torn at the moment of injury but rather are "perturbed," setting the stage for progressive intraaxonal changes, eventually leading to axonal disconnection.

Intracranial Hematomas

AXIOM The most frequent indication for a craniotomy after head injury is the need to evacuate an intracranial hematoma.

Intracerebral hematomas may occur in up to 23% of patients with severe head injuries. Small intracerebral hematomas are best treated nonsurgically by improving cerebral oxygen delivery and by keeping the ICP at normal levels; however, accessible hematomas larger than 30 cc or causing a midline shift greater than 5 mm in severely impaired or deteriorating patients should have prompt surgical evacuation.

Subdural Hematomas

AXIOM Much of the relatively poor prognosis associated with acute SDHs is due to the underlying brain damage.

Subdural hematomas (SDHs) may be acute (seen within 24 hours of injury), subacute (seen between 24 hours and 10 days), or chronic (seen after 10 days). They are most commonly the result of rupture of veins that bridge the space between the brain and the dura. On CT scan, they often appear as a whitened thick "smudge" next to the skull, often with a shift of the midline and hemorrhage in the subjacent white matter (Fig. 10-1).

Acute subdural hematomas, except for small asymptomatic collections, are best treated by prompt craniotomy and evacuation. Because of the underlying brain damage, the preoperative increased ICP and midline shift may persist after evacuation of the hematoma. Chronic subdural hematomas and subacute hematomas that have liquified can often be treated with evacuation and continuing drainage through burr holes rather than through the large bone flap often required for drainage of acute collections (9).

Epidural Hematomas

AXIOM Epidural hematomas are uncommon, but with prompt surgical evacuation, they usually have a good prognosis.

Epidural hematomas (EDHs) occur in only about 3% of patients with severe head trauma (9). The hematoma collects where dura has been stripped from the skull, and they are usually associated with temporal bone fractures with resultant laceration of the middle meningeal artery. On CT, the EDH characteristically shows a sharp biconvex white density adjacent to the skull (Fig. 10-2).

Expansion of the hematoma causes further dural separation. The classic clinical course includes an initial period of unconsciousness from the primary insult (con-

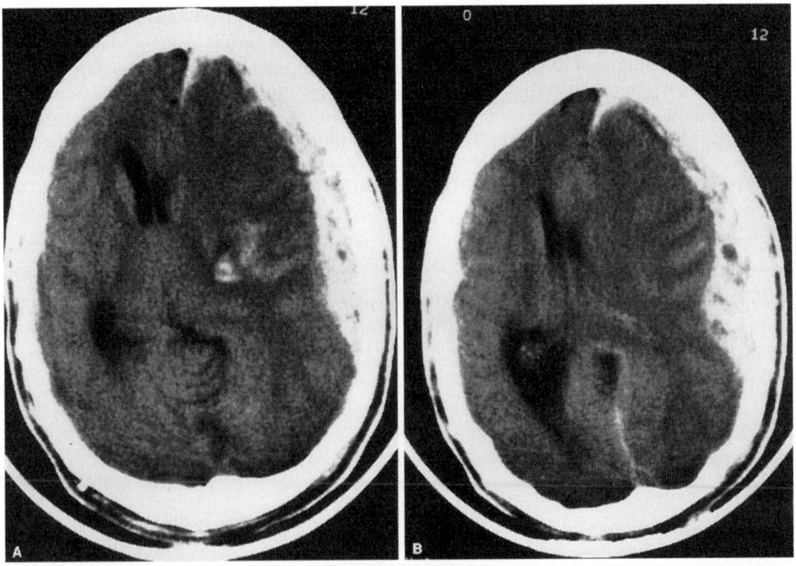

FIG. 10-1. (A,B) Acute subdural hematoma. The CT slices demonstrate the crescentic smudge of a large acute subdural hematoma. Massive shift of the midline structures and hemorrhage in the subjacent white matter also is present.

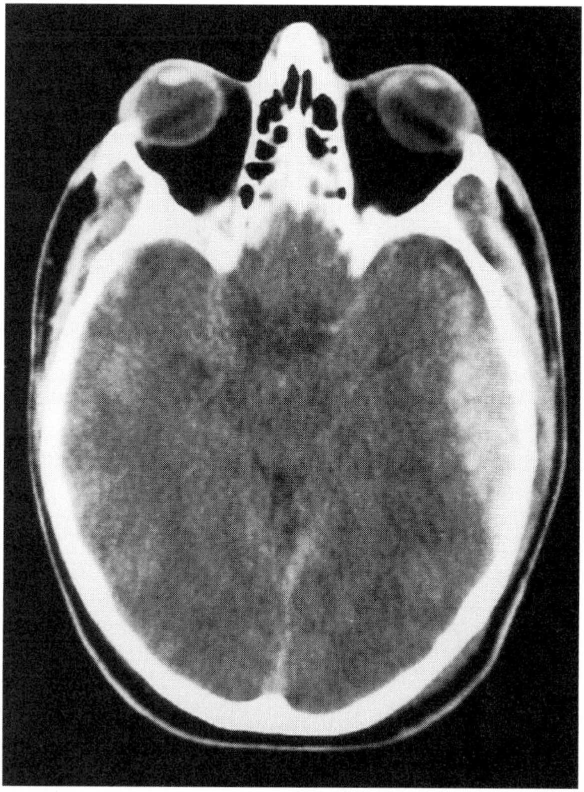

FIG. 10-2. Epidural hematoma. CT shows a sharp biconvex density.

cussion) and then neurologic recovery ("lucid interval"), followed over several hours by headache, loss of consciousness, and progressive neurologic deterioration.

AXIOM A lucid interval in a young patient with head trauma should warrant special efforts to rule out an acute EDH.

A lucid interval occurs in only a minority of patients with EDHs and may also occur in alcoholic patients who have a chronically shrunken brain and an acute SDH. About one third of the patients with EDHs never regain consciousness, and about one third never lose it. When a patient with an EDH loses consciousness again, neurologic deterioration may progress very rapidly. As with other symptomatic intracranial hematomas, treatment is prompt surgical evacuation. If symptoms are progressing rapidly, a bolus of intravenous mannitol (50 to 100 g) and hyperventilation to a P_{CO_2} of 25 to 30 mm Hg may gain some time while the patient is being rushed to the operating room (OR).

Subarachnoid Hemorrhage

Greene et al. (10) found that patients with a nonpenetrating head injury who also had a traumatic subarachnoid hemorrhage (tSAH) on the admission head CT scan had a much higher incidence of increased ICP at the time of ventriculostomy placement (versus those without tSAH). These patients also had a higher incidence of hypoxia and hypotension and spent more days in intensive care units (ICUs), had more total hospital days, and had worse Glasgow Outcome Scale scores at the time of hospital discharge.

Brain Herniation

As a result of supratentorial swelling or hematoma or both, the brain may herniate through the dural hiatuses or the foramen magnum. Herniation of the medial portion of the temporal lobe through the tentorial hiatus causes midbrain compression, which can result in loss of consciousness and decerebrate rigidity. Compression of the oculomotor nerve against the tentorium results in dilatation of the ipsilateral pupil. At the same time, there is often a herniation of the cingulate gyrus under the falx cerebri (pericallosal herniation). This may be severe enough to compress the anterior cerebral artery and produce weakness of the contralateral lower extremity.

Hemorrhagic necrosis of the medial temporal lobes and brainstem tegmentum (Duret's hemorrhages), as well as infarctions in the distribution of the posterior cerebral artery, also may be caused by transtentorial herniation.

AXIOM If, after head trauma, a decompressive craniotomy is not performed before herniation occurs, a successful outcome is very unlikely.

CEREBRAL BLOOD FLOW

Normal CBF is approximately 55 mL/100 g/min. Changes in the electroencephalogram (EEG) usually occur if the blood flow is less than 25 mL/100 g/min, and the threshold for infarction is about 18 mL/100 g/min.

Local CBF is regulated by several factors, including P_aCO_2, P_aO_2, blood pressure, and cerebrovascular resistance (CVR). For every 1 mm Hg decrease in P_aCO_2 (between 20 and 60 mm Hg), cerebral blood flow decreases 2% to 3% (15). Thus a P_aCO_2 less than 20 to 25 mm Hg may cause CBF to be less than half normal. Hypoxia has little effect on CBF until the PO_2 is less than 50 mm Hg (Fig. 10-3).

Cerebral perfusion pressure (CPP), defined as the difference between mean systemic arterial pressure and the ICP, is the pressure gradient across the brain that drives CBF. Normally, CBF varies directly with the metabolic needs of the brain over a wide range of CPP. This autoregulation is often lost with severe brain trauma or if the CPP decreases to less than 50 mm Hg (12).

If CBF is reduced, the brain may extract up to 67% of the oxygen from the blood to maintain cerebral metabolism. If jugular bulb oxygen saturation decreases to less than 55%, severe cerebral ischemia is present.

AXIOM A jugular bulb oxygen saturation less than 55% after severe head injury is an indication of cerebral ischemia (13).

An increasing number of studies show that injured brain tissue has a reduced blood flow. Yoshino et al. (14) performed dynamic CT scanning on 42 patients within 6 to 12 hours of severe head injury and found that 17 (68%) of 25 fatally injured patients had severe brain ischemia. By using xenon (Xe 133) to measure CBF, Muizelaar (15) found that of 186 patients with head trauma and a GCS of 8 or less, 24 (13%) had severe global cerebral ischemia (CBF of 18 mL/100 g/min or less). Of the 24 patients with cerebral ischemia, 15 (63%) continued to be vegetative or died. Of the other 160 patients with severe cerebral injury who were not ischemic, only 59 (37%) had a similar poor outcome.

Increased Intracranial Pressure

Most traumatic cerebral edema is vasogenic, resulting from increased leakage of plasma ultrafiltrate through hyperpermeable capillary membranes into the extra-

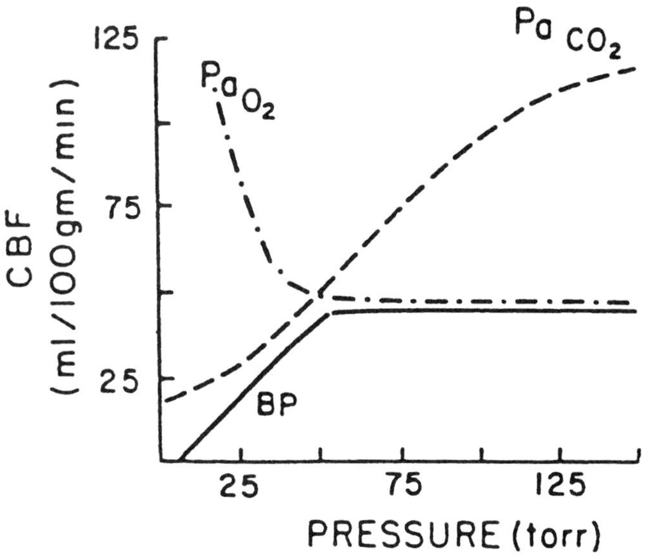

FIG. 10-3. Cerebral blood flow. Response to changes in P_aO_2, P_aCO_2, and mean arterial blood pressure (11).

cellular space. However, there is also some cytotoxic edema as a result of cellular injury from the trauma itself and from hypoxic or ischemic insults. The cytotoxic edema from hypoxia or ischemia primarily affects astrocytes in the gray matter.

AXIOM According to the Monro–Kellie hypothesis, any increase in the intracranial volume of blood, brain, or CSF causes a reciprocal change in the others, so that the intracranial volume remains constant; otherwise, the ICP increases.

The intracranial volume in adult humans is about 1,600 to 1,800 mL. Of this, about 80% to 90% is brain, 5% to 10% is blood, and 5% to 10% is CSF. If the brain swells or there is an intracranial hematoma, the CSF is displaced into the spinal subarachnoid space, and blood is displaced into extracranial veins. As long as there is displaceable blood or CSF, an increase in intracranial volume causes only a small increase in ICP. Once there is no more blood or CSF to displace, the ICP increases rapidly with any further increase in intracranial volume.

AXIOM After head injury, the ability of the brain to reduce CSF in response to an increasing ICP can be severely limited.

A normal ICP is 5 to 10 mm Hg or less. An ICP of 10 to 20 mm Hg requires careful observation, and any ICP above 20 to 25 mm Hg after an acute brain injury should be treated urgently. Indeed, the prognosis of patients with persistent or irreversible high ICP (more than 30 to 50 mm Hg) is very poor.

AXIOM Regardless of the cause of an increased ICP in head trauma, inability to reduce it promptly to less than 20 mm Hg is generally indicative of a poor prognosis.

Intracranial Pressure Monitoring

Several fundamental points about ICP monitoring should be emphasized. First, the information obtained is only as reliable as the system providing the information. If the monitor is not properly inserted or if the system is not properly calibrated, the information may be meaningless. Second, ICP monitoring provides information about only one aspect of the patient's condition. The ICP is of little value without knowledge of the disease being treated, the overall clinical condition of the patient, and the ICP dynamics.

The main indications for ICP monitoring in trauma are

1. If there is a reasonable chance that the ICP is significantly increased;
2. When treatment is to be undertaken for an increased ICP; and
3. When frequent, accurate assessment of neurologic status is not possible.

Several methods of ICP measurement are available (16). A catheter placed into a lateral cerebral ventricle and connected to a standard strain-gauge transducer allows not only continuous ICP monitoring, but also permits withdrawal of CSF as needed or desired to control an increased ICP. However, it may be difficult to insert such a catheter when hematoma or diffuse brain swelling distorts or decreases the size of the lateral ventricles or both.

Although a subarachnoid bolt is easily inserted under almost any circumstances, it may provide erroneous readings, depending on its placement relative to the site of injury (16). Epidural bolts have the lowest risk of complications, but they are less accurate than ventricular catheters or subarachnoid bolts and do not permit withdrawal of CSF. Many centers now monitor the ICP by using an intracerebral fiberoptic sensor that is easy to place and can provide accurate information.

AXIOM If facilities for ICP monitoring are not available, one should assume that the ICP is increased if the GCS is 7 or less and begin appropriate therapy.

At any given mean BP, an increase in ICP will reduce the CPP, which should be maintained above 70 mm Hg to ensure adequate blood supply to the brain. As part of the Cushing response to an increased ICP, about 20% of patients admitted with head injury develop significant systemic hypertension. Although some increase in BP may produce a beneficial increase in CPP, severe systemic hypertension, by increasing capillary filtration pressures and transcapillary fluid movement into damaged areas, may increase brain swelling and cause further increase of ICP and ischemia (17).

AXIOM Hypertension after a head injury should be treated by removing the underlying cause of the increased ICP; if this is not possible, β-blockers may be given cautiously; vasodilators tend to increase ICP (15).

Because there is only one (occasionally incompetent) valve in each internal jugular vein (18) and no valve in the vertebral veins, the ICP will vary somewhat with the cerebral venous pressure (CVP) and the degree of head elevation. Thus increased intrathoracic pressure, as from hypervolemia or a head-down position, can increase CVP and ICP.

DIAGNOSIS OF HEAD INJURIES

Physical Examination

Level of Consciousness

It is particularly important to obtain information about any changes in the level of consciousness or other neurologic function occurring before the initial examination in the hospital. In patients in whom it is difficult to differentiate between a dazed state and true unconsciousness, the presence and duration of any posttraumatic amnesia can be very helpful.

If the period of unconsciousness is short (i.e., less than 5 minutes), patients with a completely normal neurologic examination should still be carefully observed for at least 6 to 12 hours. Patients with periods of unconsciousness lasting more than 5 minutes, or prolonged retrograde amnesia, even with no neurologic changes, should be observed closely for at least 24 hours.

Associated Injuries

⊘ PITFALL

Failure to look carefully beyond the obvious head injury in patients with blunt trauma may cause neglect of important associated injuries.

An important complicating factor in patients with head injuries is the high incidence of associated injuries. At least one in four patients with blunt head injury has associated injuries of other parts of the body. Up to 6% of head-injured patients have coincident cervical spine injuries, and up to 26% of patients with cervical spine injuries have head injuries (19). Kaups and Davis (20), however, in a study of 202 patients with gunshot wound (GSW) of the head, obtained cervical spine clearance either clinically, radiographically, or by review of postmortems and found that indirect spinal injury occurred in none of their patients.

The patient's head is examined carefully for injury, particularly signs of basilar skull fracture. These include periorbital ecchymoses (raccoon's eyes), subscleral hemorrhage, telocanthus (widening of the distance between the inner canthi), retroauricular hematoma (Battle's sign), hemotympanum, and CSF rhinorrhea or otorrhea. The carotid arteries in the neck are palpated and auscultated, and the presence of ecchymosis or hematomas overlying them is noted.

AXIOM All patients with major trauma should be assumed to have a head injury and cervical spine fracture until proven otherwise.

Neurologic Evaluation

As soon as possible, a complete neurologic evaluation should be performed on all seriously injured patients. This may not be possible initially in unstable patients; however, as part of a cursory neurologic examination, one should evaluate and record the level of consciousness and pupillary and motor responses.

AXIOM The *sine qua non* of head-injury management is repetitive careful neurologic examinations and timely intervention.

Glasgow Coma Score

The mental status and state of consciousness usually provide the most sensitive indication of the amount of brain injury and any tendency to deterioration. Patients who are unable to speak or follow commands have a much greater incidence of serious brain injury and a much poorer prognosis. The GCS score should be determined at least every 30 minutes during the early stages of injury. Because one third of the GCS score is based on verbal response, allowance must be made for this in patients who are intubated. For example, an intubated patient who opens his eyes to pain and withdraws an extremity from pain has a GCS score of 6/10 (Table 10-1).

Meredith et al. (21) found that the eye and motor scores can be used to accurately predict the total GCS-derived verbal score equal to -0.3756 + motor score $\times$ 0.5713 + eye score $\times$ 0.4233. Thus if the eye score is 4 and the motor score is 6, the estimated

Table 10-1. ***Glasgow Coma Scale***

1. Eye opening	
Spontaneous	4
To voice	3
To pain	2
None	1
2. Verbal response	
Oriented	5
Confused	4
Inappropriate words	3
Incomprehensible words	2
None	1
3. Motor response	
Obeys command	6
Purposeful movement (pain)	5
Withdraw (pain)	4
Flexion (pain)	3
Extension (pain)	2
None	1
Total GCS Points (1 + 2 + 3)	3–16

verbal score is $-0.38 + 6(0.57) + 4(0.42) = -0.38 + 3.42 + 1.68 = -0.38 + 5.10 = 4.72 = 5$. If the eye score is 3 and the motor score is 4, the verbal score is $-0.38 + 4(0.57) + 3(0.42) = -0.38 + 2.28 + 1.26 = 3.16 = 3$.

Examination of Pupils

AXIOM One cannot rely on neurologic assessments until adequate perfusion and oxygenation have been obtained.

Severe hypotension, even without a brain injury, can cause a patient to be comatose. For example, pupils that are fixed and dilated during a cardiac arrest often become small and reactive if cerebral perfusion is reestablished promptly.

The size, shape, and reactivity of the pupils to light allow evaluation of the integrity of the second and third cranial nerves and the midbrain. The reaction of the pupils to light, the extraocular movements, and the visual fields also should be carefully checked, if possible.

AXIOM Not infrequently, a unilateral dilating pupil that is still reactive to light is the first sign of an expanding mass in the temporal lobe or an epidural hematoma in the middle fossa.

Caloric Testing

With caloric testing, the patient lies supine with the head elevated 30 degrees (9). The integrity of the tympanic membrane should be ascertained by direct inspection before irrigating the ear. By using a tuberculin syringe, 0.2 mL of ice water is instilled deep into the external ear canal. The nystagmus (fast component) is normally toward the opposite ear in an awake patient and to the same side in a comatose patient. These responses test the third, sixth, and eighth cranial nerves and nuclei as well as the ascending brainstem pathways from the pontomedullary junction to the mesencephalon. Obviously, injury to the vestibular apparatus or its nerve also can impair these reflexes.

AXIOM The mnemonic for a normal oculovestibular (caloric) response is "COWS" (cold, opposite; warm, same); that is, normally the fast nystagmus is toward the opposite side if the ear is irrigated with cold water.

Motor and Sensory Testing

Purposeful movement indicates intact motor pathways from the cortex on down, whereas abnormal flexor and extensor posturing are generally signs of severe neurologic impairment (9). Deep tendon reflexes and passive muscle tone in the extremities should be assessed for symmetry. Sensory examinations in serious head injury are usually limited to the response to painful stimuli.

The first cranial nerve can be tested with simple solutions with a distinctive odor (methylsalicylate, rose water, tincture of benzoin, etc.). The sensory function of the fifth cranial nerve and the motor function of the seventh cranial nerve can be checked by examination of the corneal reflexes (1).

Gross examination of hearing should be carried out, and the external ear canals should be examined for CSF drainage and for bleeding through or behind the tympanic membranes. The functions of the lower cranial nerves X and XII may be evaluated by observing the patient's ability to swallow and the function of the palate and tongue during that process.

Ventilatory Patterns

AXIOM A significant deterioration in the state of consciousness is almost invariably associated with development of an abnormal ventilatory pattern (22).

Many patients exhibit some degree of respiratory depression after head injury. Consequently, the airway should be cleared and intubation performed at the first suspicion of inadequate ventilatory effort or of depressed gag or cough reflexes or a GCS of 8 or less.

There are three types of phasic respiration seen with CNS problems (22):

1. Some patients exhibit a **Cheyne–Stokes variant**, which is a regular, cyclic variation in respiratory depth from hyperventilation to hypoventilation without apneic periods. This pattern is generally associated with a mild degree of coma.
2. **True Cheyne–Stokes** respiration consists of regular cycles of hyperventilation followed by apnea due to an exaggerated ventilatory response to increasing P_aCO_2. This hyperpnea then reduces the P_aCO_2 to the point at which the respiratory drive is abolished until reaccumulation of CO_2 again stimulates hyperventilation. True Cheyne–Stokes respiration is usually associated with severe brain injury.
3. **Ataxic ventilation** is characterized by inspiratory and expiratory phases that are irregular in both rate and amplitude, with intervening periods of apnea. This pattern is also described as gasping or cluster breathing with expiratory pauses. The respiratory rate is usually slow, and the minute ventilation is significantly decreased. This is generally an indicator of very severe brainstem damage and is almost always a terminal sign.

Laboratory Assessment

Victims of severe brain injury should have arterial blood gas determinations, and venous blood should be sent for complete blood count (CBC), platelet count, coagulation profile, electrolytes, blood alcohol levels, and type and cross-match. Urine should be sent for standard chemical and microscopic analysis and for toxicologic screening. In addition to arterial blood gas analyses, it is wise to monitor the patient's tissue oxygenation constantly with a pulse oximeter.

AXIOM The presence of alcohol or illicit drugs should be checked in all patients with a head injury.

Severe head injuries are frequently complicated by coagulation abnormalities, which cannot only increase bleeding into the brain and from associated injuries but also delay needed neurosurgical procedures.

Radiologic Studies

Skull radiographs are generally indicated if

1. There has been a loss of consciousness for more than a few seconds;
2. There is a scalp laceration that may be associated with a fractured skull; or
3. The patient has clinical evidence of a basilar skull fracture.

Occasionally, an air–fluid level in the sphenoid sinus is the only evidence of a basilar skull fracture. Linear skull fractures are often best delineated and the margins of a depressed fracture most clearly defined on plain skull radiographs.

Early and appropriate use of CT scanning without intravenous contrast can help detect significant intracranial lesions before there is severe clinical deterioration. Altered mental status and focal hemispheric deficits are the best clinical predictors of the presence of hematoma that requires emergency surgery and indicate a need for CT scanning regardless of the GCS score.

AXIOM Computed tomography scanning is the most accurate method to localize and quantify intracranial mass lesions.

A minimum of four axial cuts demonstrating the parasagittal sulci, lateral ventricles, middle fossae, and posterior fossa are usually obtained with CT scans of brain-injured patients. If a patient is deteriorating rapidly, a single CT axial cut at the level of the lateral ventricles will detect the majority of surgical mass lesions requiring immediate craniotomy.

Angiography

Cerebral angiography is done rarely for head injuries now, but it can play an important role in the detection of traumatic aneurysms, arteriovenous fistulas, and carotid or vertebral arterial injuries (9). In addition, isodense subdural collections can at times be difficult to define by CT, but they are generally delineated quite well by cerebral angiography.

AXIOM Cerebral angiography may be the only readily available means of diagnosing traumatic intracranial mass lesions if CT scanning is unavailable.

Electrophysiologic Monitoring

Judson et al. (23) showed that absence of the somatosensory-evoked cortical potentials (SSEPs) within the first 24 hours is an important negative prognostic sign. In 100 intubated patients with closed-head injury with an initial GCS of 9 or less, absence of SSEPs on one or both sides during the first day after injury predicted death or major disability with a specificity of 95%. Prolonged cortical conduction time did not predict a poor outcome if SSEPs were present bilaterally.

TREATMENT OF HEAD INJURIES

Initial Management

The first objective in the treatment of patients with head injuries is prevention of conditions known to cause secondary brain injury. Ideally, efforts to maintain adequate ventilation, oxygenation, and tissue perfusion should be initiated at the scene of the accident.

AXIOM Although not all patients with head injury require neurosurgical consultation, they all require prompt resuscitation and frequent careful neurologic assessment.

Criteria often used for ventilatory assistance in patients with head injury include

1. Clinical respiratory distress, a rate above 30/min or below 10/min, or an abnormal ventilatory pattern;
2. Motor posturing or absence of a motor response to pain;
3. Abnormal or deteriorating arterial blood gases;
4. Repeated convulsions;
5. Increasing or high ICP;
6. Signs of aspiration or pulmonary edema; and
7. Concurrent severe pulmonary or cardiac injury.

The arterial Po_2 in patients with acute severe head injury should be maintained at 80 mm Hg or higher (95% oxyhemoglobin saturation), and the minute volume should be adjusted to provide arterial Pco_2 levels between 35 and 40 mm Hg. Positive end-expiratory pressures (PEEPs) less than 10 cm H_2O do not appear to increase ICP if the head is elevated 30 degrees.

Administration of Drugs

Rapid-sequence intubation with succinylcholine or vecuronium is preferable to awake, blind nasotracheal intubation in head-injured patients. Administration of a single bolus dose of esmolol (a very short-acting β-adrenergic blocker) has been shown to effectively blunt the increase in heart rate and mean arterial BP that often occurs in response to intubation. Fentanyl, intravenously in a dose of 3 to 5 μg/kg about 1 to 3 minutes before intubation, also is effective in blunting the increase in heart rate and mean arterial BP often seen with intubation (24). Intravenous lidocaine (1.5 mg/kg), given 2 to 3 minutes before intubation, can often prevent an increase in ICP during intubation and may have a directly beneficial effect on the injured brain (25).

AXIOM Although emergency intubation of head-injured patients without appropriate premedication can cause an abrupt increase in ICP, there is not always time for such medications.

Barbiturates have also been shown to attenuate the increase in ICP often seen with intubation, and they also decrease the cerebral demand for oxygen (26). Thiopental is an ultrashort-acting barbiturate that has extremely rapid onset and a duration of action similar to that of succinylcholine; however, in induction doses (3 to 5 mg/kg), it can be a potent cardiovascular depressant. Therefore, in hemodynamically compromised patients, one should either reduce the dose to 0.5 to 1.0 mg/kg or use another agent, such as fentanyl or etomidate.

Administration of Fluids

AXIOM Even if the ICP is increased, hypotension in head-injured patients is still usually best treated by administering fluids.

It may seem a paradox to give fluids to correct hypotension in a patient receiving diuretics to reduce the ICP, but the purpose of mannitol therapy is to dehydrate the brain, not to reduce the blood volume. A normal blood volume with slightly hyperosmolar plasma (300 to 320 mOsm/L) is the desired therapeutic aim. Thus fluid losses should be monitored and the fluid carefully replaced. If a vasopressor is needed, 5 to 10 μg/kg/min of dopamine, with its inotropic action and tendency to increase the systemic BP, is often the best choice.

Quereshi et al. (27) found that hypertonic (3%) saline or acetate infusions tended to decrease ICP and lateral displacement of the brain in patients with cerebral edema after trauma or brain surgery. It also improved the mean GCS score.

Controlling the Intracranial Pressure

AXIOM In addition to keeping the CVP as low as possible and mild hyperventilation to an arterial P_{CO_2} of 35 mm Hg, one can use head elevation, mannitol, and furosemide to keep the ICP less than 20 mm Hg.

Head-of-bed elevation has been used for many years to decrease ICP. Indeed, Feldman et al. (28) showed that head-of-bed elevation from 0 to 30 degrees results in a decreased ICP without a statistically significant decrease in CPP, CBF, cerebral metabolic rate, or CVR.

Use of the loop diuretics furosemide and ethacrynic acid to treat an increased ICP is somewhat controversial. Although they do not reliably reduce ICP, they can help reduce the extent of secondary brain injury by decreasing glial swelling. Administering loop diuretics before beginning mannitol therapy may help prevent the initial hypervolemia and pulmonary congestion that may be seen when mannitol therapy is begun. They may also potentiate the rate and duration of the ICP reduction produced by mannitol.

In areas with intact autoregulation, mannitol tends to cause cerebral vasoconstriction. This causes an immediate decline in ICP by much as 27% with a corresponding improvement in CPP (29). In patients with large areas of impaired autoregulation, mannitol infusion will decrease ICP by only about 5%, but CBF may increase by as much as 17%.

Mannitol also improves microcirculatory blood flow by decreasing blood viscosity and by decreasing red blood cell aggregation at the capillary level. However, mannitol, if given very rapidly in large doses, can cause a transient hypotension by dilating skeletal muscle vessels (30).

AXIOM Patients with signs of cerebral herniation or rapid CNS deterioration should receive mannitol (1.0 to 1.5 g/kg) by rapid intravenous infusion while at least a limited CT scan through the cerebral hemispheres is attempted before surgery.

Hyperventilation reduces ICP by constricting pial and cerebral arterioles. This vasoconstriction, however, is relatively transient because of rapid return of the brain interstitial pH to normal levels (31). Hyperventilation can also further reduce blood flow to damaged ischemic brain tissue. The general tendency is now to try to improve CBF after head trauma and keep the P_{CO_2} at about 35 mm Hg.

AXIOM Hyperventilation and hypocapnia are most effectively used for early, temporary control of ICP.

Some neurosurgeons believe that all patients with moderate to severe head injuries should receive prophylactic diphenylhydantoin at a loading dose of 18 mg/kg intravenously in normal saline over a 30-minute period while BP and the electrocardiogram (ECG) are monitored (9). Other neurosurgeons believe that one should not give diphenylhydantoin (Dilantin) until at least one or two early seizures have occurred. Seizures occurring after 24 to 48 hours are always treated. For control of ongoing seizures (with or without prophylactic diphenylhydantoin), 5 to 10 mg of diazepam can be given intravenously. This may be repeated as needed at 10- to 15-minute intervals to a maximum dose of 30 mg.

Operative Management

Patients with open depressed skull fractures or penetrating brain injuries should be given a first-generation cephalosporin in full dosage. For GSWs, gram-negative aerobes and anaerobes also should be covered. Tetanus prophylaxis should be provided as indicated.

Scalp lacerations should be carefully explored for possible fractures or skull penetration. If the galea is lacerated or if the scalp injury is extensive or complex, it should be explored and closed in the OR. Lacerations of the galea should be closed as a separate layer.

Skull Fractures

Undisplaced linear fractures of the cranial vault without associated scalp lacerations do not require specific treatment. Open linear fractures, however, have a small but definite risk of osteomyelitis. The overlying laceration must be carefully cleaned, debrided, and closed, preferably in the OR. One dose of an antistaphylococcal antibiotic may be of benefit, but longer courses of prophylactic antibiotics are not usually recommended.

A closed, depressed skull fracture does not usually have any effect on neurologic deficits that may be present. Some neurosurgeons believe that a depressed skull fracture, particularly over the motor strip of the cerebral cortex, increases the tendency to posttraumatic epilepsy and should be elevated.

The treatment of basilar skull fractures is largely concerned with the recognition and care of any associated cranial nerve or vascular injuries and prevention of CSF fistulas. Surgical decompression has been advocated in injuries to the optic or facial nerves if there is evidence of deteriorating function (32).

Because most traumatic CSF rhinorrhea and almost all CSF otorrhea resolve spontaneously, a trial of conservative therapy with bed rest and head positioning to minimize CSF drainage is warranted. If the CSF leakage does not slow after 3 to 4 days, one may try repeated lumbar punctures or a lumbar drain. Prophylactic antibiotics are usually not recommended because they do not reduce the incidence of infection, and if infection does occur, it is more likely to be caused by antibiotic-resistant organisms (33). If the fistula persists for more than 7 to 10 days, repair via an intradural approach is indicated.

AXIOM Early surgical closure of CSF leaks should be undertaken for widely diastatic fractures, bone fragments displaced into brain, copious CSF flow, or increasing pneumocephalus.

Intracranial Hematomas

Operative intracranial decompression is required in about 12% of patients with an acute head injury causing unconsciousness (9). Such decompression should be performed before the patient shows clinical evidence of tentorial herniation. Progressively diminishing responsiveness, development of unilateral pupillary dilatation, abnormal flexor or extensor posturing, and increasing arterial hypertension and bradycardia associated with periodic breathing are signs that third nerve and brainstem compression have already occurred from tentorial herniation.

AXIOM An intracranial hematoma that causes increasing neurologic dysfunction, an ICP persistently greater than 25 mm Hg, or more than 5 mm midline displacement should be evacuated as soon as possible.

Head-injured patients with a GCS score of 9 or less who are found to have an intracranial mass lesion causing a midventricular shift of more than 5 mm, an ICP greater than 25 mm Hg, or neurologic deterioration should have the lesion evacuated immediately (9). If the midline shift is less than 5 mm, the clinical status is stable, and the ICP is controllable, one can continue to observe the patient carefully and repeat the CT scan in 24 hours.

AXIOM Mass lesions should be evacuated quickly in patients with a GCS score of 8 or less if further brain damage is to be prevented.

If no mass lesion is seen in a patient with a GCS score of 13 or less, the most likely explanation is brain swelling, which does not benefit from operative decompression (9); however, if the ICP is persistently greater than 25 mm Hg or if there is neurologic deterioration, the patient should have a repeated CT scan and operative decompression as indicated.

AXIOM In general, the sooner an intracranial mass lesion is drained, the better the results.

Of patients who come to the hospital in an awake, alert state and then deteriorate, at least 70% to 80% have a mass lesion, such as a SDH or EDH, which needs to be drained as soon as possible. In patients with acute SDHs, Seelig et al. (34) found a 90% mortality rate when the operation occurred more than 4 hours after injury, compared with a mortality rate of only 30% in patients with similar lesions who had surgery within 4 hours of injury.

AXIOM Very rarely, a rapidly expanding intracranial hematoma must be evacuated without preoperative localization.

Suggested locations for the initial trephine openings for nonlocalized hematomas are

1. Frontocoronal: 3 cm lateral to the midline at the coronal suture (on a line about 2 cm anterior to the ear);
2. Temporal: 2 cm anterior to the ear and 2 cm superior to the zygoma; and
3. Parietal: 2 cm above and 2 cm posterior to the top of the ear (Fig. 10-4).

For nonlocalized hematomas, burr holes should be made bilaterally. The use of bilateral frontal, temporal, and parietal burr holes, particularly when supplemented by ultrasound evaluation during surgery, can accurately identify extradural and intracerebral hematomas in more than 90% of patients.

AXIOM Although the intracranial space can be decompressed to some extent through burr holes, adequate evacuation of the majority of intracranial hematomas requires a bone flap.

Irreparably damaged areas of brain contusion can act as a nidus for edema or hemorrhage and may be resected if larger than 1 to 2 cm (9). Over the frontal or temporal areas, one may be relatively aggressive with such debridement. In more functionally vital areas, resections must be done very judiciously to avoid adding to the neurologic deficit.

Intracerebral hematomas larger than 3 to 4 cm diameter (30 mL volume) near the surface may be evacuated. More deeply placed clots require evacuation if they are

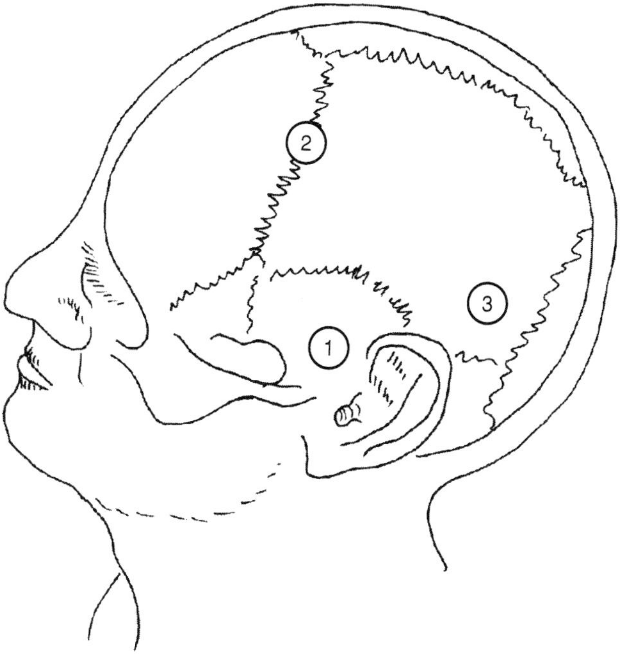

FIG. 10-4. Suggested sites for emergency trephine openings if the intracranial hematoma has not been localized preoperatively. **1:** Temporal: 2 cm anterior to the ear and 2 cm superior to the zygoma. **2:** Frontocoronal: 3 cm lateral to the midline at the coronal suture. **3:** Parietal: 2 cm above and 2 cm posterior to the ear.

large enough to produce significant shift, but such aggressiveness should be tempered by the risk of increasing the neurologic deficit.

Occasionally sudden massive brain swelling will develop during the operation (9). This is usually due to hyperemia from defective cerebrovascular autoregulation but may also be caused by hypoventilation. Consequently, the endotracheal tube position and bilateral breath sounds should be promptly checked. Additional mannitol boluses and increased ventilation will often reverse such acute swelling, but this therapy may need to be repeated several times. Swelling unrelieved by such means may respond to 500-mg boluses of thiopental, up to a total dose of 1 to 2 g. If all of these measures fail, decompression via frontal or temporal lobectomy has been occasionally performed.

Penetrating Injuries

The management of penetrating stab wounds of the head is analogous to that of compound depressed fractures (9). In cases in which the penetrating object is still in place, no attempt should be made to extract it until the patient is in the OR with a craniotomy flap turned to expose the wound tract. If it is likely that a major vessel is involved, the preliminary evaluation should include angiography.

Patients with penetrating brain injuries resulting from GSWs and any reasonable chance for survival should be given mannitol and broad-spectrum antibiotics as soon as they are seen. The scalp, cranial, and dural entrance wounds are thoroughly debrided. Irreparably damaged cerebral cortex is removed, and the debridement is extended as far as is safely possible along the wound tract to remove all devitalized tissues, bone, missile fragments, hematoma, and foreign bodies. Intraoperative ultrasound may be a useful adjunct for removing foreign bodies safely. A watertight dural closure at the end of the case is critical, and the wound should be covered by full-thickness scalp, which is closed without tension. This may require extensive undermining of the scalp or even rotation flaps.

Postoperative Management

Intracranial pressure is monitored until it stabilizes, we hope at a normal level, for at least 24 hours. This usually means that the ICP catheter and transducer will be in place for 3 to 8 days. If an intraventricular catheter is used, it should probably be removed after 8 days because the incidence of complications, especially infection, greatly increases after that time (35).

Sudden discontinuance of osmotic therapy may be associated with a significant increase in ICP "rebound," as water is shifted from the vascular space into brain tissue. This effect is more pronounced if the serum osmolarity is more than 320 mOsm/kg (11). The rebound can be moderated by limitation of fluid intake or by furosemide therapy, but one must be careful not to allow hypotension to develop.

Barbiturates

Barbiturates can be effective in reducing an increased ICP in patients who are unresponsive to standard therapy. The therapeutic effects of barbiturates may due to

1. Reduction of ICP by cerebral vasoconstriction (probably the major effect);
2. Reduction of cerebral metabolism and oxygen requirements (36); or
3. Reduction of free-radical damage to brain cells (37).

Although good results have been reported with barbiturates, especially in patients refractory to aggressive therapy that includes CSF drainage, hyperventilation, and mannitol, serious questions remain about their influence on survival and long-term morbidity (38).

AXIOM Barbiturates are probably of greatest value in reducing brain damage in patients who have persistently high ICPs in spite of all other therapy.

Before barbiturate therapy is begun, the patient should be normotensive [mean arterial pressure (MAP) above 70] and normovolemic [pulmonary artery wedge pressure (PAWP) of about 8 to 12 mm Hg]. Thus a pulmonary artery (PA) catheter, arterial line, and ICP monitor are often needed to accurately assess both the cardiovascular and cerebral effects of the barbiturates. The rectal temperature also should be monitored closely and not allowed to decrease below 32°C because the combination of barbiturates and hypothermia can cause severe cardiac arrhythmias, particularly in younger patients.

The barbiturates are usually administered as intravenous pentobarbital in an initial dose of 5 to 10 mg/kg and continued as a 1.5 mg/kg/h drip until the ICP decreases below 15 to 20 mm Hg or until serum barbiturate levels are 3 to 5 mg/dl (36). Levels above 5 mg/dl do not seem to increase the therapeutic effects of barbiturates but can cause the EEG to become isoelectric.

AXIOM The only way to monitor the neurologic status of a patient in barbiturate coma reliably is with evoked potentials and, if these deteriorate, one should promptly obtain a repeated CT scan.

Barbiturate levels are maintained at 3 to 5 mg/dl by continuous intravenous infusion until the ICP remains normal for at least 24 to 48 hours (9). The dosage is then tapered gradually over 4 days to avoid the sudden deterioration that may follow abrupt discontinuation. If the ICP increases during the tapering, the barbiturate therapy should be resumed.

Ventilatory Support

Mechanical ventilation should be continued postoperatively until the patient becomes alert enough to follow two-stage commands or until the ICP remains normal for several days. This usually takes a week or less, but in some cases, more than 2 to 3 weeks of ventilatory support may be necessary.

AXIOM In adults, continuous ventilatory support may not only help to control the ICP, but it may also prevent the hypoxic brain damage that might be caused by unexpected respiratory insufficiency.

Sedation or neuromuscular blockade or both may help the patient to breathe synchronously with the ventilator. Repeated small doses (1 to 3 mg) of intravenous morphine will usually allow proper ventilatory support without unduly masking the neurologic status. In the presence of severe central hyperventilation, intravenous muscle relaxants, such as pancuronium or vecuronium, may be needed.

AXIOM Hypercarbia, struggling, or coughing during pulmonary physiotherapy, tracheal suctioning, or therapeutic bronchoscopy, even in the presence of coma, can cause severe increases in ICP.

Optimizing Oxygen Delivery

AXIOM In patients with severe head injury, a PA catheter should be inserted and efforts made to optimize oxygen delivery to the brain.

If possible, one should attempt to optimize DO_2 to the brain by ensuring that the total DO_2 is at least 600 mL/min/m^2 and that it is increased until the VO_2 will no longer increase or it is at least 150 mL/min/m^2. This is best done by achieving a cardiac index of at least 4.0 to 4.5 L/min/m^2 with a hemoglobin level of 12 gm/dl and an S_aO_2 of 95% to 98%.

Catheterization of the jugular bulb with a cannula passed retrograde up the internal jugular vein permits sampling of cerebral venous damage and has been used increasingly in some centers in attempts to optimize CBF (39). An arterial–jugular bulb oxygen content difference [$C_{(a\text{-}jb)}O_2$] greater than 8.0 vol% or a jugular bulb oxygen saturation [$S_{jb}O_2$] less than 55% to 60% generally indicates cerebral ischemia and should be corrected promptly. A $C_{(a\text{-}jb)}O_2$ greater than 6.0 vol% in a head-injured patient with an increased ICP is borderline and should be treated, because any further reduction in CBF may lead to severe cerebral ischemia. In such circumstances, the indicated therapy might include mannitol, which reduces ICP while increasing CBF.

AXIOM If a jugular bulb catheter is in place, one should try to keep the $C_{(a\text{-}jb)}O_2$ differences less than 6 vol% and the $S_{jb}O_2$ above 55% to 60%.

Fluid and Electrolyte Management

Diabetes insipidus (DI) may be seen after basilar skull fractures causing injury to the pituitary stalk or hypothalamus (40). The decreased antidiuretic hormone (ADH) secretion can result in severe polyuria and progressive dehydration. In the absence of excess fluid, diuretics, or hyperglycemia, DI should be suspected if the urine output exceeds 200 to 300 mL/h. The increased free-water loss of DI should be replaced with hypotonic saline and appropriate potassium at a rate that includes the previous hour's urine output. Serum sodium and potassium levels should be checked frequently until the DI is controlled. Aqueous vasopressin can be given intermittently, at a dosage adjusted to the urinary output. Prolonged DI may be treated with longer-lasting vasopressin tannate in oil. Desmopressin acetate (DDAVP), a synthetic analogue of arginine vasopressin, can be administered intravenously or intranasally.

Head injury will occasionally cause the syndrome of inappropriate ADH secretion (SIADH), which should be suspected if hyponatremia is associated with high urine osmolarity and urine sodium concentrations greater than 20 mEq/L. The SIADH may be made much worse by overadministration of free water, which cannot be excreted because of the increased ADH. Excess release of atrial natriuretic peptide (ANP) by the atria in response to stress may mimic SIADH because it can cause increased urinary sodium loss and hyponatremia. SIADH is best treated by dehydration, but hypertonic saline solutions may be required if the patient has CNS irritability or the serum sodium is less than 120 mEq/L or both. Rapid correction (faster than 0.5 mEq/L per hour) of chronic hyponatremia may cause central pontine myelinolysis.

Nutrition

Patients with severe cerebral trauma tend to develop a severe hypermetabolic state that peaks around the third day and lasts about 1 week (41). In some patients with isolated head injury, the negative nitrogen balance may exceed 30 g/day. Such patients require a high caloric and protein intake to avoid nitrogen wasting with its attendant possibilities of impaired host defenses, decubitus ulcers, and infections. Bruder et al. (42) found that sedation of head-injured patients (to avoid coughing and straining against the ventilator and to decrease restlessness to control ICP) reduced energy expenditure from about 60% over calculated basal energy expenditure (BEE) to levels only about 22% above the BEE.

AXIOM Patients with severe head injury should be started on nutritional support as soon as possible.

Enteral feeding, preferably into the jejunum, should be started as soon as possible if there are no gastrointestinal problems to preclude its use. If there will be any delay in getting enteral nutrition rapidly up to a goal of 30 to 35 nonprotein kcal/kg/day and 1.5 to 2.0 g amino acids or protein/kg/day, one should start total parenteral nutrition (TPN). Because patients with severe head injuries have an increased tendency to gastroesophageal reflux (43), there may be an advantage to providing early gastric decompression with a gastrostomy tube. Use of gastrostomy and jejunostomy tubes inserted at laparotomy plus an early tracheostomy help to reduce the incidence and severity of sinus infections resulting from indwelling nasal catheters.

Blood glucose levels, nitrogen balance, and respiratory quotient should be monitored carefully. Experimental evidence indicates that hyperglycemia above 200 mg/dl tends to cause harmful lactic acidosis in the injured brain (44). Although high blood glucose levels in adults seem to correlate with poorer survival, it is not known whether these results can be altered by treatment.

General Management

Head Elevation

Once patients with head injuries have been adequately resuscitated, they should generally be kept in semi-Fowler's position, with 20 to 30 degrees of head elevation, to decrease jugular venous pressure (45). Even if the cervical spine is uninjured, the head should be maintained in a neutral position, by padding if necessary, because rotation, flexion, or extension of the neck may partially block the jugular veins and increase ICP.

Preventing Hyperthermia

Body temperature should be kept within normal limits. Hyperpyrexia unrelated to infection is seen in about 15% of brain injuries as a result of blood in the ventricles or damage to the hypothalamus or brainstem (12). If fever develops, antipyretics plus cooling blankets, as needed, should be instituted promptly.

AXIOM It is generally accepted that hypothermia can protect the injured brain, but hyperthermia damages it (46).

Recent studies consistently showed that in brain-injured patients, the brain temperature tends to be significantly higher than the core body temperature. Indeed, Rumana et al. (47) found that brain temperatures exceed systemic core temperatures in head-injured patients by an average of 2.0°F (1.1°C).

Neurogenic Pulmonary Edema

Neurogenic pulmonary edema (NPE) can be defined as a state of increased lung water occurring in association with acute diseases of the nervous system, in the absence of cardiac or pulmonary disorders or hypervolemia (48). It is characterized by a fulminant onset of pulmonary vascular congestion and exudation of protein-rich edema fluid, often in patients with subarachnoid or intracerebral hemorrhage.

The most popular theory concerning the mechanism of NPE is that a massive sympathetic discharge produces a dramatic increase in peripheral vascular resistance, causing a shift of blood into the pulmonary vasculature. The increased pulmonary arterial and venous pressures can cause structural capillary damage with increased capillary permeability (49).

AXIOM Fluid overload greatly increases the tendency to neurogenic pulmonary edema.

Treatment of NPE involves keeping cardiac filling pressures as low as possible while maximizing CBF. Increasing the FiO_2 is important, but an FiO_2 greater than 0.60 may eventually cause oxygen toxicity. Adding PEEP can often produce a dramatic improvement in oxygenation, but excess PEEP can decrease cardiac output and may also increase ICP; however, McGuire et al. (50) found that, in patients with increased ICP, increasing PEEP levels to 15 cm H_2O did not increase the ICP or decrease the CPP.

Acute Respiratory Distress Syndrome

It can be difficult to distinguish between neurogenic pulmonary edema and acute respiratory distress syndrome (ARDS) in head-injured patients; however, they are treated in the same way except for the increased efforts to keep ICP low in NPE. If ARDS does develop, one should look very carefully for uncontrolled sepsis.

Fat Embolism

Fat embolism can be an important cause of hypoxemia and CNS changes in patients who have multiple extremity fractures (51). The pulmonary or CNS changes or both usually become evident 12 to 36 hours after the trauma, and fat embolism syndrome should be strongly suspected if the platelet count is lower than expected.

Gastrointestinal Bleeding

AXIOM Gastric pH must be monitored carefully in all head-injured patients and kept above 4.5 to 5.5 with appropriate medications.

Gastrointestinal (GI) bleeding is common after severe head injury, and up to 30% of comatose patients treated in an ICU will show clinical evidence of blood loss from the GI tract (52). The probable cause of ulcers associated with head trauma is increased gastric acidity resulting from hypothalamic stimulation of vagal activity or mucosal ischemia or both. Perforation of a Cushing's ulcer should be suspected in any head-injured patient who develops abdominal distention and ileus with increased fever or leukocytosis.

Coagulation Problems

AXIOM Damaged brain tissue is a powerful procoagulant and can cause a severe consumptive coagulopathy.

Clotting disorders, particularly disseminated intravascular coagulation (DIC), are quite common after severe brain trauma and may represent a significant contributing factor in patients dying as a result of hemorrhage or intractable cerebral edema or both (53). Appropriate therapy involves improving CBF, restoring blood volume, and administering clotting factors (such as cryoprecipitate and fresh frozen plasma) and platelets as needed.

TREATMENT OUTCOMES

The Glasgow Outcome Scale for patients with head injury provides a basis for comparing the results of treatment in different centers and for evaluating new therapeutic measures as they are introduced. The categories include

1. Good recovery: complete neurologic recovery or only minor deficits that do not prevent the patient from returning to his or her former level of function;
2. Moderately disabled: deficits that prevent normal function but allow self-care;
3. Severely disabled: marked deficits that prevent self-care;
4. Vegetative: no evidence of higher mental function; and
5. Dead.

As age increases, the chances of a good recovery after severe head trauma decrease significantly. Quigley et al. (54) noted that of their patients with a GCS score of 5 or less, abnormal pupils, and age of 50 years or older, none were functional survivors. Compared with adults, children have an improved survival and rate of recovery. Nevertheless, even in children, a low GCS score and absent pupillary reaction and brainstem reflexes after an adequate resuscitation correlate highly with a poor outcome.

Even patients with "minor" head injuries can have significant cognitive defects for at least 3 to 6 months (55). Another problem is the failure by many investigators to differentiate between the cognitive consequence of TBI and postconcussion symptoms (56). In young children, the cognitive defects may not be fully appreciated until months or years after hospital discharge (57).

⊘ FREQUENT ERRORS

1. ***Inadequate attention to other, less obvious injuries.***
2. ***Any delay in restoring an adequate blood pressure and correcting hypoxemia.***
3. ***Delay in intubating patients with severe head injury.***
4. ***Assuming that there is little or no neurologic defect in patients with "mild head injuries."***
5. ***Efforts to reduce an increased ICP without attention to maintaining a more than adequate CPP.***
6. ***Delay in obtaining a CT scan in patients with moderate to severe head injury.***
7. ***Delay in measuring ICP in patients who may require a craniotomy to evacuate an intracranial hematoma.***

8. ***Inadequate frequency of careful neurologic examinations, especially in intoxicated individuals.***
9. ***Failure to act promptly on any change in pupil size or reactivity or other CNS deterioration.***
10. ***Failure to take strong steps to rule out and prevent spinal cord injury.***
11. ***Failure to have prompt repeated CT scans of the head in patients who deteriorate neurologically.***
12. ***Correcting hypertension in a patient with a head injury without first giving attention to its cause.***
13. ***Failure to monitor urine output and osmolarity closely in head-injured patients.***

SUMMARY POINTS

1. Head injury is the leading cause of mortality and morbidity after trauma.

2. If subarachnoid hemorrhage is seen on the CT scan, there is an increased likelihood of the patient developing cerebral vasospasm.

3. Hypoxemia and hypotension, which are the most frequent systemic insults causing secondary brain injury, should be prevented or corrected rapidly.

4. When cerebral autoregulation is impaired by trauma, CBF changes directly with the systemic arterial pressure.

5. Increased intracellular calcium or excessive release of excitatory amino acids after head trauma can greatly aggravate secondary brain injury.

6. Magnesium deficiencies contribute to the severity of secondary brain injury and may be present even with normal serum levels.

7. Patients with skull fractures are much more likely to have severe underlying brain injuries.

8. Although cerebral concussions are generally considered mild head injuries, extensive subclinical damage may be noted on PET scans.

9. Much of the relatively poor prognosis associated with acute SDHs is due to the underlying brain damage and any delay in evacuating the SDH.

10. Epidural hematomas are uncommon but usually have a good prognosis if they are promptly evacuated.

11. A lucid interval should warrant special efforts to rule out an acute EDH.

12. An arteriovenous oxygen difference of 8 mL/dL or more or a jugular bulb oxygen saturation less than 55% to 60% is an indication of cerebral ischemia indicating a need to decrease ICP and increase CPP and Do_2.

13. Endotracheal intubation of patients with severe head injury (GCS score, 3 to 8) is generally indicated for prevention of secondary hypoxic brain damage.

14. According to the Monro–Kellie hypothesis, any increase in the intracranial volumes of blood, brain, or CSF causes a reciprocal change in the others, so that the intracranial volume remains constant; otherwise, the ICP can increase abruptly.

15. Regardless of the cause of an increased ICP in head trauma, inability to promptly reduce it to less than 20 mm Hg is generally indicative of a poor prognosis.

16. If facilities for ICP monitoring are not available, one should assume that the ICP is increased and should begin appropriate therapy if the GCS score is 7 or less.

17. Hypertension after a head injury should be treated by removing the cause of the underlying increased ICP, not by giving vasodilators; if a drug must be given, β-blockers are preferred.

18. The *sine qua non* of head-injury management is repetitive careful neurologic examinations and timely intervention.

19. If, after head trauma, a decompressive craniotomy is not performed before cerebral herniation occurs, death or severe disability is almost certain.

20. One cannot rely on neurologic assessments in a patient who is in shock or severely hypoxic or hypercarbic.

21. Not infrequently, a unilateral dilating pupil that is still reactive to light is the first sign of an expanding mass in the temporal lobe or an epidural hematoma in the middle cranial fossa.
22. The mnemonic for a normal oculovestibular (caloric) response is "COWS" (Cold, Opposite; Warm, Same); that is, normally the fast nystagmus is toward the opposite side if the ear is irrigated with cold water.
23. A new focal motor deficit is an important sign that the patient with head injury needs immediate, aggressive care.
24. The presence of alcohol or illicit drugs should be checked in all patients with a head injury.
25. Although skull fractures do not generally require treatment, they indicate a much greater likelihood of severe underlying brain damage.
26. One should assume that all patients with blunt head injuries have associated cervical spine fractures until ruled out by complete clinical and radiologic examinations.
27. CT scanning is the most accurate and expeditious method to localize and quantify intracranial mass lesions.
28. Although not all patients with head injury require neurosurgical consultation, they all require prompt resuscitation and frequent, careful neurologic assessment.
29. Although emergency intubation of head-injured patients without appropriate premedication can cause an abrupt increase in ICP, there is not always time for such medications.
30. Even if the ICP is increased, hypotension in head-injured patients is still usually best treated initially by administering fluids.
31. In addition to keeping the CVP as low as possible and hyperventilating the patient to an arterial P_{CO_2} of 35 to 40 mm Hg, one can use head elevation, mannitol, and furosemide to keep the ICP less than 20 mm Hg.
32. Patients with signs of cerebral herniation or rapid CNS deterioration should be hyperventilated and given mannitol (1.0 to 1.5 g/kg) by rapid intravenous bolus while attempting to obtain at least a limited CT scan through the cerebral hemispheres before surgery.
33. Early closure of CSF leaks should be undertaken for widely diastatic fractures, bone fragments displaced into brain, extremely copious CSF flow, or increasing pneumocephalus.
34. An intracranial hematoma that causes increasing neurologic dysfunction, an ICP persistent greater than 25 mm Hg, or more than 5 mm midline displacement should be evacuated as soon as possible.
35. Mass lesions should be evacuated quickly in patients with a GCS score of 8 or less if further brain damage is to be prevented.
36. Barbiturates are probably of greatest value in reducing brain damage in patients who have persistently high ICPs in spite of all other therapy.
37. The only way to monitor the neurologic status of a patient in barbiturate coma reliably is with evoked potentials and, if these deteriorate, one should obtain a repeated CT scan.
38. Hypercarbia, struggling, or coughing during tracheal suctioning, or therapeutic bronchoscopy, even in the presence of coma, can cause severe increases in ICP and should be prevented with muscle relaxants as needed.
39. If a jugular bulb catheter is in place, one should try to keep $C_{(a-jb)}O_2$ differences less than 6 vol% and the $S_{jb}O_2$ above 55% to 60%.
40. Patients with severe head injury should be provided with complete nutritional support as soon as possible, preferably enterally, but glucose levels should be kept below 200 mg/dl.
41. Gastric pH should be monitored carefully in all head-injured patients and kept above 4.5 to 5.5 with appropriate medications.
42. Damaged brain tissue is a powerful procoagulant and can cause a severe consumptive coagulopathy.

REFERENCES

1. Michael DB, Wilson RF. Head injuries. In: Wilson RF, Walt AJ, eds. *Management of trauma: pitfalls and practice.* 2nd ed. Philadelphia: Williams & Wilkins, 1996:173.

2. Shackford SR, Mackersie RC, Davis JW, et al. Epidemiology and pathology of traumatic deaths occurring at a level I trauma center in a regional system: the importance of secondary brain injury. *J Trauma* 1989;29:1392.
3. Miller JD, Becker DB. Secondary insults to the injured brain. *J R Coll Surg Edinb* 1982;27:292.
4. Stocchetti N, Furlan A, Volta F. Hypoxemia and arterial hypotension at the accident scene in head injury. *J Trauma* 1996;40:764.
5. Muizelaar JP. Cerebral ischemia-reperfusion injury after severe head injury and its possible treatment with polyethyleneglycol-superoxide dismutase. *Ann Emerg Med* 1993;22:1014.
6. Siesjo BK. Basic mechanisms of traumatic brain damage. *Ann Emerg Med* 1993; 22:959.
7. Vink R, McIntosh TK, Demuduk P, et al. Decline in intracellular free Mg^{2+} is associated with irreversible tissue injury after brain trauma. *J Biol Chem* 1968; 263:757.
8. Povlishock JT. Pathobiology of traumatically induced axonal injury in animals and man. *Ann Emerg Med* 1993;22:980.
9. Lahaye PA, Gade GF, Becker DP. Injury to the cranium. In: Moore EE, Mattox KL, Feliciano DV, eds. *Trauma.* 2nd ed. Norwalk, CT: Appleton & Lange, 1991: 247.
10. Greene KA, Jacobowitz R, Marciano FF, et al. Impact of traumatic subarachnoid hemorrhage on outcome in nonpenetrating head injury. Part II: relationship to clinical course and outcome variables during acute hospitalization. *J Trauma* 1996;41:964.
11. Shapiro HM. Intracranial hypertension: therapeutic and anesthetic considerations. *Anesthesiology* 1975;43:445.
12. Miller JD, Bell BA. Cerebral blood flow variations with perfusion pressure and metabolism. In: Wood JH, ed. *Cerebral blood flow: physiologic and clinical aspects.* New York: McGraw-Hill, 1987:119–130.
13. Bouma GJ, Muizelaar JP, Choi SC, et al. Central circulation and metabolism after traumatic brain injury: the elusive role of ischemia. *J Neurosurg* 1991;75:685.
14. Yoshino E, Yamaki T, Higuchi T, et al. Acute brain edema in fatal head injury: analysis by dynamic CT scanning. *J Neurosurg* 1985;63:830.
15. Muizelaar JP. Cerebral ischemia-reperfusion injury after severe head injury and its possible treatment with polyethyleneglycol-superoxide dismutase. *Ann Emerg Med* 1993;22:1014.
16. Ward JD. Intracranial pressure monitoring. In: Champion HR, Robbs JV, Trunkey DD, eds. *Rob and Smiths' operative surgery: trauma surgery, part I.* 4th ed. London: Butterworths, 1989:217–223.
17. Durward QJ, Del Maestro RF, Amacher A, et al. The influence of systemic arterial pressure and intracranial pressure on the development of cerebral vasogenic edema. *J Neurosurg* 1983;59:803.
18. Dresser LP, McKinney WM. Anatomic and pathophysiologic studies of the human internal jugular valve. *Am J Surg* 1987;154:220.
19. Michael BD, Guyot DR, Darmody WR. Coincidence of head and cervical spine injury. *J Neurotrauma* 1989;6:177.
20. Kaups KL, Davis JW. Patients with gunshot wounds to the head do not require cervical spine immobilization and evaluation. *J Trauma* 1998;44:865.
21. Meredith W, Rutledge R, Fakhry SM, et al. The conundrum of the Glasgow Coma Scale in intubated patients: a linear regression prediction of the Glasgow verbal score from the Glasgow eye and motor scores. *J Trauma* 1998;44:839.
22. Shogan SH, Kindt GW. Injuries of the head and spinal cord. In: Zuidema GD, Rutherford RB, Ballinger WF, eds. *The management of trauma.* Philadelphia: WB Saunders, 1985:207.
23. Judson JA, Cant BR, Shaw NA. Early prediction of outcome from cerebral trauma by somatosensory evoked potentials. *Crit Care Med* 1990;18:363.
24. Helfman SM, Gold MI, DeLisser EA, et al. Which drug prevents tachycardia and hypertension associated with tracheal intubation: lidocaine, fentanyl, or esmolol? *Anesth Analg* 1991;72:482.

25. Nagao S, Murota T, Momma F, et al. The effect of intravenous lidocaine on experimental brain edema and neural activities. *J Trauma* 1988;12:1650.
26. Eisenberg HM, Frankowski RF, Constant CF, et al. High-dose barbiturate control of elevated intracranial pressure in patients with severe head injury. *J Neurosurg* 1988;69:15.
27. Quereshi AI, Suarez JI, Bhardwaj A, et al. Use of hypertonic (3L) saline/acetate infusion in the treatment of cerebral edema: effect on intracranial pressure and lateral displacement of the brain. *Crit Care Med* 1998;26:440.
28. Feldman Z, Kanter MJ, Robertson CS, et al. Effect of head elevation on intracranial pressure, cerebral perfusion pressure, and cerebral blood flow in head-injured patients. *J Neurosurg* 1992;76:207.
29. Rosner MJ, Coley I. Cerebral perfusion pressure: a hemodynamic mechanism of mannitol and the postmannitol hemogram. *Neurosurgery* 1987;21:147.
30. Bouma GJ, Muizelaar JP, Bandoh K, et al. Blood pressure and intracranial pressure-volume dynamics in severe head injury: relationship with cerebral blood flow. *J Neurosurg* 1992;77:15.
31. Muizelaar JP, van der Poel HG. Cerebral vasoconstriction is not maintained with prolonged hyperventilation. In: Hoff JT, Bertz AL, eds. *Intracranial pressure VII.* Berlin: Springer Verlag, 1989:899.
32. Guyer DR, Miller MR, Long DM, et al. Visual function following optic canal decompression via craniotomy. *J Neurosurg* 1985;62:631.
33. Choi D, Spann R. Traumatic cerebrospinal fluid leakage: risk factors and the use of prophylactic antibiotics. *Br J Neurosurg* 1996;10:571.
34. Seelig JM, Becker DP, Miller JD, et al. Traumatic acute subdural hematoma: major mortality reduction in comatose patients treated under 4 hours. *N Engl J Med* 1981;304:1511.
35. Narayan RK, Kishore DRS, Becker DP, et al. Intracranial pressure: to monitor or not to monitor? *J Neurosurg* 1982;56:650.
36. Kassell NF, Hitchon PW, Gerk MK, et al. Alterations in cerebral blood flow, oxygen metabolism, and electrical activity produced by high dose sodium thiopental. *Neurosurgery* 1980;7:598.
37. Godin DV, Mitchell MJ, Saunders BA. Studies on the interaction of barbiturates with reactive oxygen radicals: implications regarding barbiturate protection against cerebral ischemia. *Can Anaesth Soc J* 1982;29:203.
38. Schwartz ML, Tator CH, Rowed DW, et al. The University of Toronto Head Injury Treatment Study: a prospective, randomized comparison of pentobarbital and mannitol. *Can J Neurol Sci* 1984;11:434.
39. Sari A, Matayoshi Y, Yonei A, et al. Cerebral arteriovenous oxygen content difference during barbiturate therapy in patients with acute brain damage. *Anesth Analg* 1986;65:1196.
40. Griffin JM, Hartley JH, Crow RW, et al. Diabetes insipidus caused by craniofacial trauma. *J Trauma* 1976;16:979.
41. Wilson RF, Tyburski JG. Metabolic response and nutritional therapy in patients with severe head injuries. *J Head Trauma Rehabil* 1998;13:11.
42. Bruder N, Raynal M, Pellissier D, et al. Influence of body temperature, with or without sedation, on energy expenditure in severe head-injured patients. *Crit Care Med* 1998;26:568.
43. Saxe JM, Ledgerwood AM, Lucas CE, et al. Lower esophageal dysfunction precludes safe gastric feeding after head injury. *J Trauma* 1993;35:170.
44. Prough DS, Coker LH, Lee S, et al. Hyperglycemia and neurologic outcome in patients with closed-head injury. *Anesthesiology* 1988;69:A584.
45. Durward QJ, Amacher AL, Del Maestro RF, et al. Cerebral and cardiovascular responses to changes in head elevation in patients with intracranial hypertension. *J Neurosurg* 1983;59:938.
46. Marion DW, Penrod LE, Kelsey SF, et al. Treatment of traumatic brain injury with moderate hypothermia. *N Engl J Med* 1997;336:540.
47. Rumana CS, Gopinath SP, Uzura M, et al. Brain temperature exceeds systemic temperature in head-injured patients. *Crit Care Med* 1998;26:562.

48. Theodore J, Robin ED. Pathogenesis of neurogenic pulmonary oedema. *Lancet* 1975;2:749.
49. Rosner MJ, Newsome HH, Becker DP. Mechanical brain injury: the sympathoadrenal response. *J Neurosurg* 1984;61:76.
50. McGuire G, Crossley D, Richards J, et al. Effects of varying levels of positive end-expiratory pressure on intracranial pressure and cerebral perfusion pressure. *Crit Care Med* 1997;25:1059.
51. Shier MR, Wilson RF. Fat embolism syndromes: traumatic coagulopathy with respiratory distress. *Surg Ann* 1980;12:139.
52. Larson GM, Koch S, O'Dorisio TM, et al. Gastric response to severe head injury. *Am J Surg* 1984;147:97.
53. Clark JA, Finelli RE, Netsky MG. Disseminated intravascular coagulation following cranial trauma. *J Neurosurg* 1980;52:266.
54. Quigley MR, Vidovich D, Cantella D, et al. Defining the limits of survivorship after very severe head injury. *J Trauma* 1997;42:7.
55. Kibby MY, Long CJ. Minor head injury: attempts at clarifying the confusion [Review]. *Brain Injury* 1996;10:159.
56. Powell TJ, Collin C, Sutton K. A follow-up study of patients hospitalized after minor head injury. *Disabil Rehabil* 1996;18:232.
57. Greenspan AI. Functional recovery following head injury among children. *Curr Probl Pediatr* 1996;26:170.

11. SPINAL CORD INJURIES(1)

INCIDENCE

Between 8,000 and 10,000 spinal cord injuries (SCIs) occur in the United States annually. The most common causes of SCIs are motor vehicle accidents (48%), falls (21%), assaults (15%), and sports-related accidents (14%; 2). Most sports-related injuries result from diving into shallow water. Indeed, Tyroch et al. (3) found that spinal cord damage was potentially preventable in 74% of blunt injuries and 66% of the penetrating injuries.

Almost 50% of these injuries involve the cervical spinal cord, particularly the C-5 to C-6 area, and lead to tetraplegia in 32% to 45%. Of injuries below the cervical spinal cord, 54% result in complete paraplegia. Thoracolumbar and lumbar spine fractures account for 20% to 30% of all spine fractures, and the neurologic injury usually involves the conus medullaris or cauda equina.

In patients with multiple injuries, the spine may not be given adequate attention. In one study of patients with cervical SCIs, 67% had associated limb fractures, 53% had intrathoracic injuries, and 33% had an associated head injury (4). Approximately 70% of patients with thoracic SCI had pneumothorax, hemothorax, or other associated intrathoracic injuries.

ANATOMY, BIOMECHANICS, AND PHYSIOLOGY

Trauma severe enough to injure the spinal cord almost always disrupts the ligaments or joints that maintain the stability of one vertebra on another, thereby increasing the risk of further spinal cord damage from any inadvertent movement. The cervical spinal cord is most vulnerable to injury because there is more motion in this region, and there is relatively little mechanical support for the vertebrae (5).

The upper cervical spine is particularly vulnerable to axial loading if force is applied to the top of the skull. This tends to cause burst fractures through the lateral masses of C-1 (Jefferson fractures). Hyperextension of the neck due to force applied to the forehead can cause fractures through the odontoid, usually at its base. More severe hyperextension can cause fractures of the pedicles of C-2 (hangman's fracture).

In the lower cervical spine (C-5 to C-7), the most common types of fractures and dislocations are hyperflexion injuries, which are likely to cause unstable fractures involving the C-5 or C-6 vertebra. These fractures also tend to be associated with significant neurologic injury.

Rotation combined with flexion injuries can cause unilateral locked facets with about 25% subluxation of one vertebral body relative to an adjacent vertebral body. If the injury is more severe, it can cause bilateral facet dislocation with a greater than 50% anteroposterior (AP) vertebral body length displacement. These injuries are usually stable and not associated with significant ligamentous disruption, abnormal mobility, or neurologic injury (5).

In the thoracic spine, fractures usually result from direct blows or extreme hyperflexion injuries. Compression or burst fractures from motorcycle or bicycle accidents are generally the result of axial loading to the upper thoracic spine. The thoracolumbar junction is particularly vulnerable to hyperflexion injuries, especially because much of the normal lower-back flexion and extension occurs at this level. Extreme hyperflexion with axial loading tends to cause compression fractures of the T-12 or L-1 vertebrae, often with severe ligamentous injury and retropulsion of bone fragments into the spinal canal.

Lumbar spine injuries are most commonly the result of hyperflexion, and this tends to cause compression or burst fractures.

AXIOM All spinal fractures should be treated as if they are very unstable.

PATHOPHYSIOLOGY OF SPINAL CORD INJURY

Actual mechanical transection of the spinal cord is rare, even in patients with severe neurologic disability; however, neural action potentials will not cross the injured area. Almost immediately after injury to the spinal cord, there is disruption of vascular structures in that area (6). This causes a dramatic local decrease in spinal cord blood flow, followed by development of punctate areas of hemorrhagic necrosis in the central gray matter of the cord. Within minutes, these small areas of hemorrhagic necrosis tend to coalesce into larger lesions, which then extend outward toward the peripheral white matter of the cord. These histologic changes with SCIs reach a maximum approximately 72 hours after trauma and may extend for two segments proximally and distally.

Most of the changes seen are caused by secondary neurochemical phenomena occurring at a cellular level, starting immediately after the injury (7). The early biochemical events can be characterized as an uncoupling of oxidative phosphorylation and a shift to anaerobic glycolysis. The resultant depletion of adenosine triphosphate (ATP) leads to inactivation of calcium-dependent ATPase. As a consequence, there is a sharp increase in intracellular calcium, which activates calcium-dependent phospholipase A2. This, in turn, acts on membrane phospholipids and liberates arachidonic acid. Ultimately, lipid peroxides and various free radicals accumulate and disrupt the protein and phospholipid bilayer of cell membranes.

Although gray matter is usually ischemic after SCI, white matter tends to be hyperemic after injuries that are incomplete, and ischemic if there is a complete SCI (8). Vascular autoregulation is lost in the injured area, so that its blood flow varies with systemic arterial blood pressure (BP).

Swelling of spinal cord tissue in and around the area of injury tends to occur rapidly after local trauma (9). Initially this appears to be a vasogenic phenomenon, and intravascular fluids rapidly escape into the extravascular space because of increased capillary permeability. During the second 24 hours after trauma, the fluid shifts continue, but they become increasingly cytotoxic in nature. The resultant intracellular swelling not only can deform the neural elements but can also occlude local capillaries.

EMERGENCY MANAGEMENT OF SPINAL CORD INJURIES

Spine Immobilization

AXIOM During the extrication from vehicles, prehospital transport, and the initial resuscitation of any patient with a possible SCI, one should take all necessary precautions for immobilizing the potentially injured spine.

The simplest and perhaps the most effective method of immobilizing the cervical spine is use of a long spinal board plus application of sandbags to both sides of the head and neck with adhesive tape applied across the forehead. Hard cervical collars, such as the "Philadelphia collar," can provide similar immobilization if adhesive tape is applied across the collar and across the forehead to a long spinal board to secure that portion of the head. The thoracolumbar spine can be effectively immobilized by keeping the patient strapped to a backboard with bedrolls placed on either side of the body to minimize movement.

Initial Resuscitation

AXIOM Patients with high SCIs tend to have a relative hypovolemia and some impairment of cardiac function.

Because of the systemic vasodilation seen with high SCIs, there is a relative hypovolemia, and large amounts of fluids may have to be administered rapidly to maintain adequate spinal cord perfusion. In the patient who does not respond to 2 to 3 L of fluid resuscitation, a vasopressor may be required, and the possibility of significant associated injuries should be considered.

DIAGNOSIS

Patient History

Special attention should be paid to the mechanism of injury. Hyperflexion injuries or flexion with rotation are more common with motor vehicle accidents. Falls typically cause hyperextension injuries, and axial loading is often the result of diving into shallow water.

AXIOM A head injury accompanied by loss of consciousness is associated with an injury to the cervical spine in 6% to 15% of patients (11).

If the patient is conscious, one should try to determine whether the patient has any pain along the spine or any abnormality of strength or sensation. Radicular pain, numbness, or paresthesias also are important and may indicate transient damage to the spinal cord or cauda equina.

AXIOM If an adult with blunt trauma is alert, is not intoxicated, has no distracting injuries, and has no neck or back symptoms, the patient does not have a significant spine injury and requires no spine radiographs or precautions (12).

Kaups and Davis (13), in a study of 202 patients with gunshot wound (GSW) of the head, found no evidence of indirect spinal injury.

Physical Examination

In patients with severe blunt trauma, the entire spine must be palpated very carefully, looking for any deformity, tenderness, or hematomas. A high index of suspicion must be maintained whenever tenderness is encountered anywhere along the spine, even in the absence of any neurologic deficit. Such patients should be regarded as having a spine injury until proven otherwise.

The initial neurologic evaluation must be thorough and should include an accurate description of the level of any sensory and motor dysfunction. Sensory testing should include touch and pain sensation, including sharp/dull discrimination. Joint-position sense should be determined carefully because posterior column pathways are likely to remain intact after incomplete cord injuries.

Sacral function is tested by evaluating perianal sensation, rectal sphincter tone, and the bulbocavernosus reflex. When this reflex is present, the bulbocavernosus muscle and anal sphincter contract when the glans penis is squeezed or the dorsum of the penis is tapped.

The bladder should be catheterized to detect residual urine as an indication of bladder denervation. The hourly urine output also may be an excellent indicator of the adequacy of fluid resuscitation and BP.

If spotty sensory or motor abnormalities are found, an incomplete cord lesion or peripheral nerve damage is present. If no sensory perception or muscle power is present distal to the level of injury, a complete cord lesion is present.

AXIOM The clinical level of a complete spinal cord lesion is the lowest nerve root providing good sensation and active muscle control.

The usual markers for evaluating cervical spinal nerve root function include

C-4: Sensation over the shoulders and down over the chest, almost to the nipple line; voluntary control of the diaphragm, trapezius, and sternocleidomastoid muscles;
C-5: Sensation over the lateral arm; voluntary control of deltoid and biceps muscles (can abduct the arm at the shoulder);
C-6: Sensation over the thumb and index finger; voluntary control of radial wrist extensors (can flex at the elbow and extend at the wrist);
C-7: Sensation over the long and ring fingers; voluntary control of wrist flexors, pronator teres, triceps, and finger extensors (can flex at the wrist and extend at the elbow);
C-8: Sensation over the little finger; voluntary control of finger flexors; and
T-1: Sensation over the medial arm; voluntary control of intrinsic hand muscles.

The dermatomes for sensory function of the lumbosacral nerve roots include

L-1: Pubis and lower abdomen;
L-2: Anterior thigh;
L-3/4: Knee;
L-4: Medial lower leg;
L-5: Lateral lower leg and big toe;
S-1: Fifth toe and heel;
S-2: Back of thigh;
S-3: Buttocks;
S-4: Perineum; and
S-5: Perianal skin.

Although some overlap occurs, the motor functions of the nerve roots to the lower extremities include

L-2: Flexion at the hip;
L-3/4: Extension at the knee [knee deep tendon reflex (DTR)];
L-4: Dorsiflexion at the ankle;
L-5: Dorsiflexion at the toes;
S-1: Plantar flexion at the toes (ankle DTR); and
S-2/3: Anal sphincter contraction

Incomplete Spinal Cord Injuries

The central cord syndrome is characterized by more neurologic impairment in the upper extremities than in the lower extremities, and greater neurologic loss in the distal portions of the limbs than proximally (Fig. 11-1). Although bowel and bladder control may be lost in the more severe cases, pain perception (sharp/dull) is usually maintained around the anus and in the perineum. These lesions are more likely to occur in older traumatized patients who have a hyperextension injury and an underlying cervical spondylosis with spinal canal narrowing. Usually some clinical improvement occurs after this injury, but up to 50% of patients will have permanent motor deficits, particularly in their hands (14).

Anterior spinal cord syndrome is the result of trauma or ischemia to the anterior portion of the spinal cord, usually due to clamping of the descending thoracic aorta. It is characterized by complete loss of motor function and pain (including sharp/dull discrimination) and temperature sensation below the injured segment. Because preservation of the dorsal columns occurs, joint position (proprioception) and

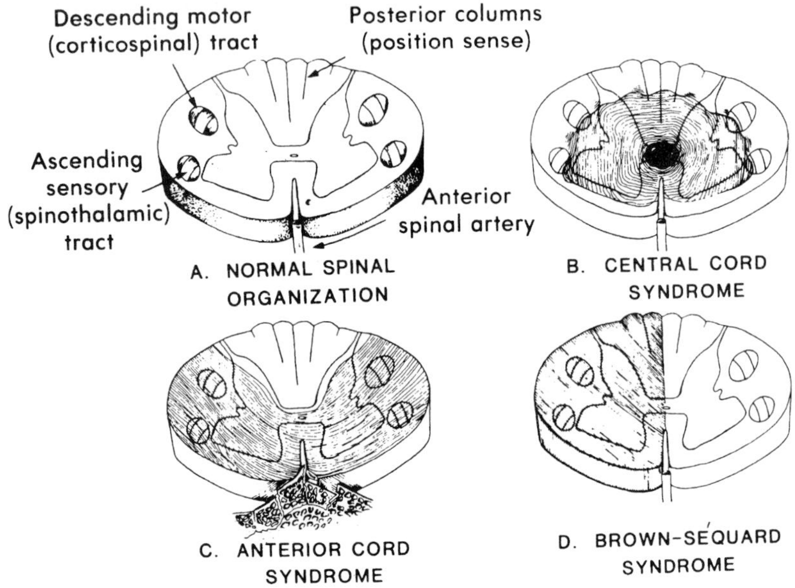

FIG. 11-1. The neurologic deficits after an incomplete spinal cord injury reflect the neurologic function of the portions of the spinal cord involved in the injury. **A:** Normal spinal cord organization. **B:** Central cord syndrome. The motor deficit affects the upper limbs more than the lower limbs. The extent of the damage in the central spinal cord determines the extent of the neurologic dysfunction. **C:** Anterior cord syndrome. Motor function and pain sensation are lost below the level of spinal cord injury. Position sense, which is carried by the intact posterior columns, is relatively well preserved. **D:** Brown–Sequard syndrome. This syndrome is characterized by loss of motor function on the side ipsilateral to the spinal cord lesion and loss of pain and temperature sensation on the contralateral side (9).

deep-pressure sensation remain intact. The prognosis for recovery from this type of injury is poor, and fewer than 10% of patients regain functional motor control (15).

The **Brown–Sequard syndrome** is the result of injury to half of the spinal cord. This causes interruption of motor function, position, and vibratory sensation on the same side as the injury and interruption of pain and temperature on the contralateral side. This rare syndrome most often occurs with penetrating injuries of the spine, such as with knife or GSWs. Clinically, some gross sensory and motor sparing usually is evident, and most patients make a fairly good recovery (15).

Lesions involving the **conus medullaris** (the lowest portion of the spinal cord) can cause bilateral symmetric lower extremity deficits and disturbances of bowel and bladder function (9). In contrast to cauda equina lesions, there is little or no radicular pain. Early decompression of a traumatic injury to the conus medullaris is important and may improve the chances of recovery. Although the motor deficit usually resolves completely, there is generally some permanent sensory impairment.

Lesions of the **cauda equina** tend to cause asymmetric lower extremity deficits (9). Radicular pain or dysesthesia in the legs is often a major complaint, but sensation around the anus (S-2, S-3, S-4) and bowel and bladder control are usually retained. Timing of surgery to decompress cauda equina lesions is not so critical in determining outcome as with conus medullaris deficits.

Spinal cord concussion is a rare, temporary injury to the spinal cord that is usually caused by deceleration trauma to the neck (16). Neurologic function below the level of the injury is lost instantaneously, but returns spontaneously within 24 to 48 hours. This lesion occurs in 3% to 4% of all patients with SCIs and is most common when preexisting degenerative disease has narrowed the spinal canal. Because this lesion may be present, caution is advised in predicting neurologic recovery on the basis of the acute presentation.

⊘ **PITFALL**

It is unwise to predict neurologic outcome within 48 hours of an apparently complete SCI.

Spinal cord injury without radiographic abnormalities usually occurs in children and has been called the **SCIWORA syndrome** (17). The elasticity of the anterior and posterior longitudinal ligaments in children, as well as the immaturity of the osseous elements of the developing vertebrae, can allow rather extensive momentary subluxation of vertebrae in response to deforming forces, without radiographic evidence of injury.

Radiologic Examination

AXIOM The extent of bony deformation seen on radiography after trauma does not represent the full bony excursion and damage occurring at the time of injury.

All severely injured patients must be presumed to have sustained unstable spinal injuries, and the assessment of the cervical spine is begun with a cross-table lateral, on which one should demonstrate all seven cervical vertebrae plus the top portion of the body of T-1. On this film, one should carefully check

1. Alignment of the anterior line of the vertebral bodies;
2. Posterior line of the vertebral bodies;
3. Junction of the laminae with the spinous processes;
4. Tips of the spinous processes; and
5. Thickness of the soft-tissue shadows anterior to the vertebral bodies.

It is frequently not possible to determine directly the integrity of the spinal ligaments and stability of the spine on the basis of radiologic evaluations; however, the presence of ligamentous injury and instability can usually be inferred from certain radiographic characteristics, which include (Fig. 11-2; 18):

1. Greater than 5 mm of subluxation;
2. Bilateral jumped facets;
3. Burst fractures with bone fragments in the canal;
4. Widening of the interspinous space; and
5. Fractures of the posterior elements and the vertebral body.

AXIOM Absence of the typical signs of spinal fractures does not guarantee stability.

Spinal stability after traumatic fractures is frequently assessed according to the "three-column theory" (19). The three columns evaluated by such analysis include

1. Anterior half of the vertebral body and the anterior longitudinal ligament;
2. Posterior half of the vertebral body, the facets, facet capsules, and posterior longitudinal ligament; and
3. Spinous process, lamina, and interspinous ligament.

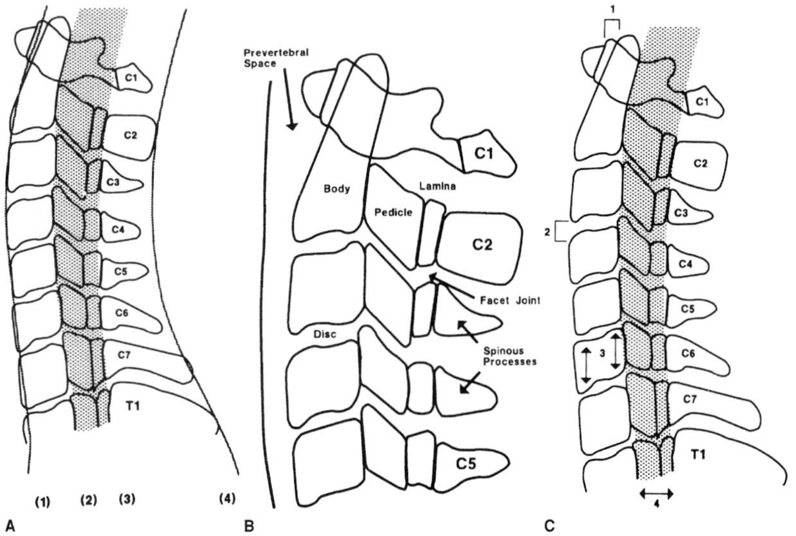

FIG. 11-2. A: In evaluating the cervical spine on a lateral radiography, one should see all seven cervical vertebrae plus the top portion of the body of T-1. The alignment of the anterior portions of the vertebral bodies, the posterior vertebral bodies, the junction of the laminae with the spinous processes and the tops of the spinous processes, and the tips of the spinous processes should all be checked carefully. **B:** When reviewing radiographs of the cervical spine, one should look closely at various components of the prevertebral space, the alignment of the vertebral bodies, the disc spaces, the pedicles, the laminae, the facet joints, and the spinous processes. **C:** Measurements that may be helpful in evaluating a lateral radiograph of the cervical spine for injuries include (a) atlantodental interval (normal, 2.5 to 3.0 mm), (b) superior vertebral body inferior vertebral alignment (should be <2.7 mm difference), (c) anterior to posterior bone height in a vertebrae body (should be <3 mm difference), (d) spinal canal width (should be ≥13 mm), and (e) <5 mm prevertebral space (18).

When two of the three spinal columns are damaged, the spine is considered to be unstable.

After the patient has been adequately resuscitated, more complete evaluation of the spine can be obtained with additional plain films, tomography, computed tomography (CT) scans, or magnetic resonance imaging (MRI). In spinal trauma, CT is useful to assess the integrity of the spinal canal, to detect its possible compromise by bone fragments, and to investigate the craniovertebral junction. MRI can be especially helpful for evaluating soft-tissue changes, such as ligament rupture, herniated disc, and spinal cord abnormalities.

AXIOM In patients without SCI and without spinal fracture on the initial plain radiographs, flexion/extension views or CT scan may be useful to determine stability of the spinal column.

AXIOM If the radiologic examination is negative or equivocal in patients with suggestive signs or symptoms, one can obtain an MRI scan or myelography followed by a CT scan of suggestive areas.

TREATMENT

Drug Administration

Because it is believed that SCI is at least partially the result of local ischemia and resultant toxic free radicals, many compounds have been tested in an effort to improve neurologic outcome.

Corticosteroids

Massive doses of corticosteroids can have a wide variety of effects on tissues, including decreased lipid peroxidation and free radical production in injured tissue. Patients taking part in a national drug trial (20), who received methylprednisolone within 8 hours of injury, showed slight but significant improvement in motor function and sensation at 6 months. As a result of these data, it has generally been believed that one should give massive steroids (30 mg/kg methylprednisolone by intravenous push, followed by 5.4 mg/kg/hr for 24 hours) to patients as soon as possible after SCI.

In another National Acute Spinal Cord Injury Study, the results of a randomized, controlled trial in patients with acute SCI were reported (21). Efficacy was evaluated for methylprednisolone administered for 24 versus 48 hours and for tirilazad mesylate [a potent inhibitor of lipid peroxidation developed to treat central nervous system (CNS) trauma] administered for 48 hours. All patients received a bolus of 30 mg/kg methylprednisolone before being randomized to receive 24 hours of methylprednisolone at 5.4 mg/kg (n = 166), 48 hours of methylprednisolone (n = 167), or a 2.5-mg/kg bolus infusion of tirilazad every 6 hours for 48 hours (n = 166). Patients receiving 48 hours of steroids had improved functional outcome relative to those receiving 24 hours of treatment, when treatment was initiated at 3 to 8 hours after injury; however, this improved outcome was at the cost of a higher incidence of severe sepsis and pneumonia. All other complications and mortality occurred with equal frequency. Patients who received tirilazad for 48 hours recovered at rates similar to those receiving 24 hours of steroids.

Prendergast et al. (22) questioned the value of steroids in SCIs caused by penetrating trauma (22).

GM-1 Ganglioside

Gangliosides, which are complex acidic glycolipids present in high concentrations in CNS cells, form a major component of the cell membrane and are located predominantly in the outer portion of the cell membrane bilayer (23). Experimental evidence suggests that these substances augment neurite outgrowth, induce regeneration and sprouting of neurons, and restore neuronal function after injury.

In a drug trial (24), the patients treated with GM-1 ganglioside had a significantly greater improvement in neurologic function at 1 year than did patients treated with a placebo. The increased recovery in the GM-1 group was attributable to initially paralyzed muscles that regained useful motor strength rather than to strengthening of weak muscles.

General Management

Cervical Spine Fractures

For cervical spine fractures associated with subluxation or angulation, axial traction is generally applied to the skull (5). Because overdistraction may damage the brainstem or upper cervical spinal cord, it is important to monitor the patient's neurologic status closely and to check lateral cervical spine radiographs as each increment of weight is added. Widening of the disc space or interspinous distance is a sign that further distraction may be hazardous.

AXIOM Closed manipulation of the cervical spine to reduce fractures is not recommended.

The only braces that immobilize the cervical spine enough to allow proper healing of unstable cervical spine fractures are the halo brace and the Minerva jacket. Stable

CSIs, such as unilateral locked facets, can be treated adequately in a sternal occipital mandibular immobilization (SOMI), four-poster, or Yale brace (5).

Types of Cervical Spine Fractures

Rotatory subluxation of C-1 is rare, but it can cause a very painful torticollis. After reduction with traction, continued treatment of this injury is based on the degree of subluxation. Complete subluxation should be treated for 3 months in a halo brace. Less severe subluxations, commonly seen in children, may be treated for a shorter time with a collar.

Jefferson fractures (involving the lateral masses of C-1) are usually stable and can be treated with a Philadelphia collar. If there are associated ligamentous injuries, a halo brace is recommended for 3 months (5).

Odontoid fractures are the most common upper cervical spine fractures. Avulsion of the tip of the odontoid (type I fracture) is a stable injury and can usually be treated adequately with a Philadelphia collar for 6 weeks (5). Type III odontoid fractures extend into the body of the C-2 vertebra and usually heal well when immobilized with a halo brace for at least 3 months. Treatment of type II odontoid fractures, which occur at the base of the odontoid, is somewhat controversial. Young patients with nondisplaced type II odontoid fractures generally heal with only halo-brace immobilization. However, internal fixation is often necessary for patients 60 years or older if the odontoid is displaced more than 4 mm.

Hangman's fractures (fractures through the pedicles of C-2) result from hyperextension of the cervical spine. They usually are treated with halo-brace immobilization for at least 3 months.

Fracture dislocations of the lower cervical vertebrae, which are often associated with severe ligamentous and bony disruption, usually cannot be treated adequately with external braces alone (25). After the subluxation is reduced, the involved vertebrae are fused intraoperatively. A posterior approach to fuse the laminae and spinous processes is used most often. Patients are usually then kept in a rigid neck support for 6 weeks to 3 months, depending on the stability of the fixation.

For **compression or burst fractures**, an anterior approach may be necessary to remove retropulsed bone fragments and replace them with a fibular or iliac crest strut–graft. This can be supplemented with internal fixation. Otherwise, external support with a halo brace is recommended.

Thoracic Spine

Simple compression fractures of the thoracic spine without subluxation are usually stable, and surgery is not necessary (5). A rigid external brace for 3 months may help to reduce pain. Severe compression (comminuted or burst) fractures or subluxed vertebrae require operative stabilization. When fragments of bone have been retropulsed into the spinal canal, causing neurologic injury, surgical decompression is required; however, the role of surgical treatment in patients with fragments in the canal and no neurologic injury is still debated.

Thoracolumbar Spine (T-12 to L-1)

Mild compression fractures of the thoracolumbar spine are usually stable and are best managed with a rigid "tortoise shell" thoracolumbar brace to hasten healing and diminish pain. If a neurologic deficit is present, one has to search for a herniated disc, epidural hematoma, or bone fragments in the spinal canal. These are best detected with MRI or myelography and CT scan.

If a burst fracture, retropulsed fragments, or subluxation is present with a neurologic deficit, surgical decompression of the spinal cord and stabilization is required. Rigid external thoracolumbar braces are generally used for at least 3 months after such surgery.

Lumbosacral Spine

Mild compression fractions can be treated conservatively, but severe fractures and subluxations should be treated surgically.

Penetrating Spine Injuries

AXIOM Because of the risk of meningitis, anyone with a cerebrospinal fluid (CSF) leak from the spine for more than 24 to 48 hours should have primary closure of the dura.

Patients who sustain GSWs or stab wounds to the spine occasionally require surgery to repair the dura if there is a persistent CSF leak (5). In patients with GSWs that pierce the small bowel or colon and then penetrate the vertebral column, the need for surgical exploration and debridement of the spine is controversial.

Surgical Management

Timing of Surgery

The role of early surgery in the management of acute SCI is controversial. Arguments used to support early surgical intervention in SCI include

1. It may provide better restoration of bone alignment;
2. Earlier decompression of neural tissue may improve ultimate neural function;
3. Early stabilization reduces the risk of secondary spinal cord damage; and
4. Early mobilization of the patient reduces the incidence of pulmonary and other complications.

Counterarguments to early surgical intervention in SCI include

1. Adequate alignment can usually be obtained by skeletal traction and closed manipulation;
2. Early removal of bone fragments from the spinal canal usually does not improve neurologic recovery;
3. The benefits of early mobilization can also be obtained by a program of active physiotherapy (9); and
4. The SCI is often made worse.

AXIOM Indications for early surgery on SCIs include (a) a progressively worsening neurologic deficit; (b) persistent leaking of CSF from a spine wound; and (c) failure to achieve spinal alignment by closed methods (9).

Rehabilitation

AXIOM An effective rehabilitation program begins immediately after admission to the hospital.

The initial objective in spinal cord rehabilitative programs is to maintain a full range of motion in all joints (9). This requires early attention to proper positioning of all portions of the body and to passive and active range-of-motion exercises. As soon as practical, self-range techniques should be taught, and the importance of a daily routine to maintain maximal motion should be emphasized. The use of orthotics to maintain joint motion and to assist in stretching contractures also is important for maintaining a functional range of motion. Muscle strengthening should be started simultaneous with the range-of-motion programs to retard atrophy in normal muscle and to assist in regaining strength in neurologically compromised areas. Electrical stimulation may be of some assistance in maintaining strength in marginally functioning muscles until reinnervation occurs.

COMPLICATIONS OF SPINAL CORD INJURIES

Cardiovascular Problems

Spinal cord injury above T-1 or T-2 with disruption of the descending sympathetic fibers from the hypothalamus and midbrain results in loss of sympathetic vasomotor tone throughout the body. The resultant vasodilation not only reduces systemic vascular resistance but also increases vascular capacity (26). There may also be some myocardial dysfunction. The decreases in afterload, preload, and contractility can cause significant hypotension, or "neurogenic shock." Consequently, a systolic BP of 80 mm Hg or less is not unusual immediately after SCI, but the heart rate is generally only 70 to 80 beats/min, and the skin is usually warm and dry.

AXIOM If a patient with a high SCI has a systolic BP <80 mm Hg, rapid heart rate (>90 to 100 beats/min), or cool, clammy skin (or a combination of these), one should suspect other injuries causing hypovolemia.

Although a systolic BP of 80 mm Hg in a vasodilated patient may not interfere with tissue perfusion, it is certainly not optimal for the injured spinal cord tissue. If possible, without giving excessive amounts of fluid or vasoactive agents, one should attempt to keep systolic BP at 100 to 110 mm Hg or higher (27).

AXIOM If central venous pressure (CVP) and BP continue to be low after aggressive fluid resuscitation in a patient with a high SCI, one should suspect an associated injury causing continued blood loss.

Electrocardiogram Findings

Changes in the ECG after cervical SCI consistent with subendocardial ischemia have been described clinically and experimentally. Other ECG changes that may be seen include ST-segment and T-wave abnormalities, sinus pauses, shifting sinus pacemaker, nodal escape beats, runs of atrial fibrillation, multifocal premature ventricular contractions, ventricular tachycardia, or a combination of these.

Sinus Bradycardia

Sinus bradycardia after SCI is caused by loss of sympathetic input to the heart, with unopposed parasympathetic stimulation through intact vagus nerves (9). Increased parasympathetic stimulation by tracheal suctioning can make this bradycardia worse and may even cause asystole. In patients who are extremely sensitive to parasympathetic stimulation, intermittent use of atropine (0.5 to 1.0 mg) may be necessary. In rare cases, a pacemaker may be required.

AXIOM Patients with high SCIs need careful cardiac monitoring during tracheal suctioning.

Preoperative Monitoring

When early surgery is contemplated for a patient with a high SCI, the preoperative placement of a pulmonary artery catheter to determine the optimal cardiac filling pressure is increasingly recommended. The optimal pulmonary arterial wedge pressure (PAWP) should then be maintained intraoperatively and for at least 48 hours after surgery. If there is intraoperative hypotension in spite of optimal filling pressures, vasoconstrictors, such as phenylephrine, are generally preferable to inotropic agents.

Hyperkalemic Crises

Denervated muscles tend to have greatly increased sensitivity to succinylcholine, manifested as sustained contractions and a massive release of potassium.

Consequently, succinylcholine can precipitate a hyperkalemic crisis and should be avoided during the first 6 months after a high SCI.

AXIOM Use of succinylcholine is contraindicated for at least 6 months after SCIs.

Postural Hypotension

Postural hypotension may be a big problem in patients with complete or nearly complete high spinal cord lesions. Syncopal episodes in these patients may be minimized by using elastic stockings and an abdominal binder, both of which may aid venous return to the heart.

Venous Thromboembolism

Venous thromboembolism is a major risk in patients with SCIs. Eventually almost all paralyzed patients will develop deep-vein thrombosis (DVT) of the lower extremities, and up to 10% will develop significant pulmonary emboli (28). The use of low-dose heparin to minimize these complications has been advocated by some; however, other clinicians found more value in instituting a routine of leg elevation (while the patient is confined to bed), thigh-high elastic stockings, pneumatic compression stockings, and frequent passive range-of-motion exercises (12).

Autonomic Hyperreflexia

Immediately after SCI, there is a period of "spinal shock," which refers to the hyporeflexia and absent reflexes that may persist for several days. Some time after 48 to 96 hours, spinal reflexes tend to return to the distal portion of the spinal cord, and the patient may develop intermittent episodes of hypertension, diaphoresis, and diffuse pallor, which are often referred to as autonomic hyperreflexia (29). These episodes usually occur with injuries above T-6 and involve up to 50% of patients with complete cervical SCIs.

Autonomic hyperreflexia results when a sensory stimulus enters an isolated segment of the spinal cord below the injury level, initiating a "mass reflex" of excessive sympathetic and somatic activity. Common stimuli initiating this response include an overdistended bladder or gut, irritation of cutaneous pressure sores, or sudden decreases in arterial BP, such as during the induction of anesthesia.

AXIOM After spinal shock has resolved, an overdistended bladder, pressure sores, or hypotension can initiate a phenomenon known as autonomic hyperreflexia, which can cause severe hypertension, diaphoresis, and diffuse pallor.

Because autonomic hyperreflexia can be extremely painful and can cause severe damage to the patient, preventive measures should be taken as soon as there is any suggestion that this problem is developing. If an improvement is not noted soon after removing the apparent stimulus, diazoxide or hydralazine (Apresoline) can be given to control the BP. In chronic or recurrent cases, phenoxybenzamine hydrochloride (Dibenzyline) has helped to prevent further episodes.

Pulmonary Problems

Pathophysiology

Atelectasis and pneumonia are common in patients with high spinal cord lesions and are the leading cause of death. In one series, a 40% mortality rate in tetraplegic patients was largely attributed to pulmonary complications (29).

AXIOM Need for prolonged ventilatory assistance in tetraplegic patients can often be prevented by aggressive, sterile pulmonary toilet and toilet position changes.

Adequate spontaneous ventilation may be impossible with very high cervical spine injuries because the diaphragm, the most important muscle for ventilation, is innervated by the C-3 to C-5 segments. In addition, if the diaphragm is weak, the abdominal contents may push toward the head while the patient is supine, thereby restricting pulmonary capacity.

The upper accessory muscles of respiration, such as the trapezius, scalenus, and sternocleidomastoid muscles, are innervated by C-1 to C-3 and usually are spared, but the tidal volume they produce by increasing the AP diameter of the upper chest is not enough for adequate ventilation (5).

Injuries to cervical cord segments C-3 through C-5 may be associated with sleep apnea, sometimes referred to as "Ondine's curse" (9). Patients with this problem ventilate adequately while awake but lose their central respiratory drive while asleep. This syndrome is more likely to occur if the patient is given CNS depressants.

Management of Pulmonary Problems

A rigorous program of postural drainage on a regular basis can be assisted by devices such as Roto beds. The "quad" cough, or rapid application of upper abdominal pressure every 2 to 3 hours, also may be helpful in mobilizing secretions. Removal of all catheters from the pharynx helps to reduce upper airway secretions and will decrease the danger of aspiration of oral contents. Gastric feedings increase the risk of aspiration into the lungs, and gastric decompression should be maintained until it is evident that the stomach is emptying properly. Jejunostomy feedings provide less risk of aspiration, unless there is distal obstruction.

AXIOM In patients with excess secretions requiring prolonged ventilatory support, a tracheostomy may greatly increase patient comfort and improve pulmonary toilet, but it often reduces the patient's ability to cough.

During the first 2 weeks after a high SCI, in addition to continuous monitoring of pulse oximetry and forced vital capacity (FVC), arterial blood gases (ABGs) should be measured at least once daily. A FVC less than 10 mL/kg or a Pco_2 greater than 45 mm Hg with an arterial pH less than 7.40 is usually an indication for ventilatory assistance.

Gastrointestinal Complications

⊘ PITFALL

Failure to initiate early gastric suction in patients with SCI.

A severe adynamic ileus usually develops promptly after SCI (9). In uncomplicated cases, without associated injuries to the abdomen or retroperitoneum, peristalsis gradually returns over the next 3 to 5 days. Failure to prevent gastrointestinal dilation prolongs the ileus and greatly increases the risk of aspiration and atelectasis.

In patients with high SCIs, the unopposed parasympathetic stimulation can greatly increase gastric secretions and contribute to the development of stress gastritis or ulcers, particularly while high-dose corticosteroids are being given. Consequently, a combination of intravenous histamine (H_2) blockers and frequent instillations antacids (Maalox) into the nasogastric tube is often required to keep the gastric pH greater than 4.5 to 5.5.

Peritonitis

Because quadriplegic patients cannot feel abdominal pain, progressive bowel distention resulting in necrosis and perforation can go unrecognized (5). One should also be suspicious of the presence of peritonitis if there is an unexplained fever, increase of the white blood cell count or amylase, increasing abdominal distention, or a combination of these.

AXIOM One should obtain abdominal and pelvic CT scans if there is any suspicion of an intraabdominal problem in a patient with SCI.

Malnutrition

Patients with SCIs can rapidly develop severe negative nitrogen balance (exceeding 20 to 25 g/day) as a result of the trauma and the muscle "denervation." To deliver adequate calories and protein, intravenous nutrition is usually required initially. If the patient cannot take an adequate oral diet by 5 days after trauma, insertion of a percutaneous endoscopic gastrostomy (PEG) or a feeding jejunostomy may be beneficial.

Genitourinary Complications

The sympathetic component innervation of the bladder is derived from T-11 to L-2, and the parasympathetic innervation from S-2 to S-4. During the period of spinal shock, the contractile ability of the bladder is lost, resulting in an areflexic bladder that tends to distend and develop overflow incontinence (9). After resolution of the spinal shock, reflex bladder activity returns because the spinal micturitional reflex arc is usually intact in the spinal cord below the lesion. This results in an "automatic bladder," which has spastic bladder muscles that tend to cause urinary frequency.

The initial management of patients with SCI usually requires an indwelling bladder catheter to help monitor fluid intake and output accurately. Later, the bladder is catheterized only intermittently to decrease the risk of urinary tract infection, which has a high frequency in both tetraplegic and paraplegic patients (31).

Heterotopic Ossification

Heterotopic ossification (myositis ossificans) is an inflammatory process of unclear origin involving voluntary muscles below the level of the SCI, primarily around major joints, such as the hips, knees, and elbows. It is characterized by calcium deposits within the muscle tissue and decreased range of motion. This process, which occurs in approximately 30% of all patients with SCIs and in up to 70% of tetraplegics, results in a significant limitation of motion in at least half of those affected (32). Therapy includes attempts to reduce the inflammation accompanying the bone formation and to maintain a normal range of motion until maturation of the process is complete.

Muscle Spasticity

AXIOM Muscle spasticity can often be controlled by early muscle stretching, which helps to maintain a full range of motion and decreased muscle tone.

If noninvasive techniques fail to control muscle spasticity adequately, baclofen, beginning at 20 mg/day in divided doses and increasing until maximal benefit is achieved, may be effective. The addition of diazepam in small doses also may help. In cases that are refractory to these medications, clonidine in doses of 0.2 to 0.4 mg/day has been used with some success (33).

Skin Complications

AXIOM Skin breakdown resulting in decubiti is the most common avoidable complication of SCI.

Pressure sores developing over bony prominences are the single most frequent cause of prolonged hospitalization and increased medical costs with SCI. Decubitus ulcers develop in at least 32% of tetraplegic and paraplegic patients, most frequently over the bony prominences of the sacrum (39%), heels (14%), and ischium (9%; 5). Loss of sensation to the skin keeps patients from shifting and turning as they normally would. The prolonged pressure causes local ischemia, which leads to necrosis and ulcer formation.

These ulcers are best prevented by minimizing the pressure against any body surface and by frequent redistribution of pressure over the body, such as by "log-rolling" the patient side-to-side every 2 hours (9).

Psychiatric Issues

Spinal cord injury almost always causes severe emotional distress, which manifests as overt anger or indifferent withdrawal behavior (or both) that can last up to 2 years. In addition, at least 5% to 10% of quadriplegic patients attempt suicide at some point. Overt or covert self-neglect is a common sign of this adjustment problem (34).

PROGNOSIS

The prognosis for victims of SCI depends primarily on the severity and location of the injury and the age of the patient; however, early use of comprehensive spinal cord rehabilitation facilities is an important factor in a successful rehabilitation. Patients with tetraplegia have the highest mortality rate, and 15% to 37% of these patients die during the first year after their injuries (35). The early mortality rate for all patients with SCIs is about 11%, but for those aged 50 years or older, it increases to 39%.

The most common causes of death for patients with SCIs are respiratory problems (21%), cardiovascular problems (15%), accidents, poisonings, or violence (10%), and infections (9%). Up to 20% of those who require ventilator assistance die in the first 3 months (36).

Unfortunately, up to 7% of patients with SCIs have a progressive decrease in neurologic function or develop painful dysesthesias months to years after injury (37). A common cause of this is posttraumatic spinal cord syrinx that develops when hemorrhagic or necrotic lesions cavitate, leaving a space that can take on fluid and thereby compress surrounding spinal cord tissue. Such patients may have substantial neurologic improvement and pain relief after surgical drainage of the cyst.

Posttraumatic back and radicular pain of unclear origin (not caused by a syrinx) are not uncommon after SCI. These conditions may respond to appropriate physical therapy and intrathecal baclofen injections.

⊘ FREQUENT ERRORS

1. ***Failure to assume that all unconscious patients and patients with severe blunt injuries have spine injuries until proven otherwise.***
2. ***Forgetting that the amount of spinal deformity that occurred at the time of injury may be much greater than the extent of the injury seen on plain radiographs later.***
3. ***Reliance on fluids alone to correct hypotension in patients with high SCIs.***
4. ***Failure to consider associated injuries as a possible cause of continued hypotension after high SCI, especially if tachycardia is present.***
5. ***Predicting neurologic outcome within 48 hours of injury.***
6. ***Failure to look for evidence of increasing spinal cord compression as a possible cause of deteriorating neurologic dysfunction.***
7. ***Failure to ensure early, complete gastric decompression with a nasogastric tube.***
8. ***Failure to keep the gastric pH greater than 4.5 to 5.5.***
9. ***Delaying passive and active range-of-motion exercises.***
10. ***Failure to take special efforts to prevent decubiti.***

SUMMARY POINTS

1. All spinal fractures should be treated as if they were very unstable.
2. During the extrication from vehicles, prehospital transport, and the initial resuscitation of any patient with a possible SCI, one should take all necessary precautions for immobilizing the potentially injured spine.
3. Patients with high SCIs tend to have a relative hypovolemia and some impairment of cardiac function.
4. If an adult with blunt trauma is alert, is not intoxicated, has no distracting injuries, and has no neck or back symptoms, the patient does not have a significant spine injury and requires no spine radiographs or precautions.
5. All unconscious trauma victims should be assumed to have an SCI until proven otherwise.
6. The clinical level of a complete spinal cord lesion is the lowest nerve root providing good sensation and active muscle control.
7. In patients without SCI and without spinal fracture on the initial plain radiographs, flexion/extension views may be useful to determine the stability of the spinal column.
8. If the radiologic examination is negative or equivocal in patients with suggestive signs or symptoms, one can obtain an MRI scan or myelography followed by a CT scan of suggestive areas.
9. Because of the risk of meningitis, anyone with a spinal CSF leak for more than 24 to 48 hours should have primary closure of the dura.
10. Removing a bullet from the spinal canal is generally not recommended unless there is an incomplete neurologic injury.
11. Indications for early surgery of SCIs include (a) a progressively worsening neurologic deficit; (b) persistent leaking of CSF from a spine wound; and (c) failure to achieve spinal alignment by closed methods.
12. An effective rehabilitation program begins immediately after admission to the hospital.
13. If possible, without giving excessive amounts of either fluid or vasoactive agents, one should attempt to keep systolic BP at 100 to 110 mm Hg or higher.
14. If the CVP and BP continue to be low after aggressive fluid resuscitation, one should suspect an associated injury causing continued blood loss.
15. Patients with high SCIs need cardiac monitoring during tracheal suctioning.
16. Use of succinylcholine is contraindicated for at least 6 months after SCIs.
17. After spinal shock has resolved, an overdistended bladder, pressure sores, or hypotension can initiate a phenomenon known as autonomic hyperreflexia, which can cause severe hypertension, diaphoresis, and diffuse pallor.
18. In patients with excess secretions requiring prolonged ventilatory support, a tracheostomy may greatly increase patient comfort and improve pulmonary toilet, but it often reduces the patient's ability to cough.
19. A continuous intravenous drip of an H_2 blocker or frequent instillation of antacids or both should be used for patients with SCIs to keep the gastric pH greater than 4.5.
20. One should obtain abdominal and pelvic CT scans if there is any suspicion of an initial or later intraabdominal problem in a patient with SCI.
21. Gentle passive and active exercises to maintain the range of motion of all joints should be started as soon as possible after SCI.
22. Muscle spasticity can often be controlled by early muscle stretching, which helps to maintain a full range of motion and also decreases muscle tone.
23. Skin breakdown resulting in decubiti is the most common, avoidable complication of SCI; decubitus ulcers can develop in as short a time as one-half hour.

REFERENCES

1. Highland T, Salciccioli G, Wilson R. Spinal cord injuries. In: Wilson RF, Walt AJ, eds. *Management of trauma: pitfalls and practice.* 2nd ed. Philadelphia: Williams & Wilkins, 1996:203.

2. Kennedy EJ, ed. *Spinal cord injury: the facts and figures.* Birmingham: University of Alabama, 1986:1.
3. Tyroch AH, Davis JW, Jaups KL, et al. Spinal cord injury: a preventable public burden. *Arch Surg* 1997;132:778.
4. Mackersie RC, Shackford SR, Garfin SR, et al. Major skeletal injuries in the obtunded blunt trauma patient: a case for routine radiologic survey. *J Trauma* 1988;28:1450.
5. Marian D, Clifton G. Injury to the vertebrae and spinal cord. In: Moore EE, Mattox KL, Feliciano DV, eds. *Trauma.* 2nd ed. Norwalk: Appleton & Lange, 1991:261–275.
6. Sasaki S. Vascular change in the spinal cord after impact injury in the rat. *Neurosurgery* 1982;10:360.
7. Tator CH. Update on the pathophysiology and pathology of acute spinal cord injury. *Brain Pathol* 1995;5:407.
8. Fehlings MG, Tator CH, Linden RD. The relationships among the severity of spinal cord injury, motor and somatosensory evoked potentials and spinal cord blood flow. *Electroencephalogr Clin Neurophysiol* 1989;74:241.
9. Kopaniky DR. Pathophysiology of spinal cord disruption and injury. In: Miller TA, ed. *Physiologic basis of modern surgical care.* St. Louis: CV Mosby, 1988:789.
10. DeLorenzo RA. A review of spinal immobilization techniques. *J Emerg Med* 1996; 14:603.
11. Micheal DB, Guyot DR, Darmody WR. Coincidence of head and cervical spine injury. *J Neurotrauma* 1989;6:177.
12. Velmahos GC, Theodorou D, Tatevossian R, et al. Radiographic cervical spine evaluation in the alert asymptomatic blunt trauma victim: much ado about nothing. *J Trauma* 1996;40:768.
13. Kaups KL, Davis JW. Patients with gunshot wounds to the head do not require cervical spine immobilization and evaluation. *J Trauma* 1998;44:865.
14. Stauffer ES. Rehabilitation of posttraumatic cervical spinal cord quadriplegic and pentaplegia. In: Sherk HH, et al., eds. *The cervical spine.* Philadelphia: Lippincott, 1989:521.
15. Stauffer ES. Diagnosis and prognosis of acute cervical spinal cord injury. *Clin Orthop* 1975;112:9.
16. Del Bigio MR, Johnson GE. Clinical presentation of spinal cord concussion. *Spine* 1989;14:37.
17. Kriss VM, Kriss TC. SCIWORA (Spinal cord injury without radiographic abnormality) in infants and children. *Clin Pediatr* 1996;35:119.
18. Rozycki GS, Champion HR. Radiology of the cervical spine. In: Maull KI, ed. *Advances in trauma.* Vol. 5. St. Louis: Mosby Year Book, 1990:37–47.
19. Harris JH Jr, Harris WH, Navelline RA. *The radiology of emergency medicine.* 3rd ed. Baltimore: Williams & Wilkins, 1993:152.
20. Bracken MB, Shepard MJ, Collins WF, et al. A randomized, controlled trial of methylprednisolone or naloxone in the treatment of acute spinal cord injury: results of the Second National Acute Spinal Cord Injury Study. *N Engl J Med* 1990;322:1405.
21. Bracken MB, Shepard MJ, Holford TR, et al. Administrations of methylprednisolone for 24 or 48 hours or tirilazad mesylate for 48 hours in the treatment of acute spinal cord injury: results of the Third National Acute Spinal Cord Injury randomized controlled trial. *JAMA* 1997;277:1597.
22. Prendergast MR, Saxe JM, Ledgerwood AM, et al. Massive steroids do not reduce zone of injury after spinal cord injury (SCI) [Abstract]. *J Trauma* 1993;35:168.
23. Ledeen RW. Ganglioside structures and distribution: are they localized in the nerve endings? *J Supramol Struct* 1978;8:1.
24. Geisler FH, Dorsey FC, Coleman WP. Recovery of motor function after spinal-cord injury—a randomized, placebo-controlled trial with GM-1 ganglioside. *N Engl J Med* 1991;324(26):1829.
25. Bucholz RD, Cheung KC. Halo vest versus spinal fusion for cervical injury: evidence from an outcome study. *J Neurosurg* 1989;70:884.

26. Lehmann KG, Lane JG, Piepmeier JM, Batsford WP. Cardiovascular abnormalities accompanying acute spinal injury in humans. *J Am Coll Cardiol* 1987;10:46.
27. Silver JR. Immediate management of spinal injury. *Br J Hosp Med* 1983;29:412.
28. Myllynen P, Kammonen M, Rokkanen P. Deep venous thrombosis and pulmonary embolism in patients with acute spinal cord injury: a comparison with nonparalyzed patients immobilized due to spinal fractures. *J Trauma* 1985;25:541.
29. Erickson RP. Autonomic hyperreflexia: pathophysiology and medical management. *Arch Phys Med Rehabil* 1980;61:431.
30. Ballamy R, Pitts FW, Stauffer ES. Respiratory complication in traumatic quadriplegia. *J Neurosurg* 1973;39:596.
31. Erickson RP, Merritt JL, Opitz JI. Bacteriuria during follow up in patients with spinal cord injury: I. rate of bacteriuria in various bladder emptying methods. *Arch Phys Med Rehabil* 1982;63:409.
32. Finerman GAM, Stover SL. Heterotopic ossification following hip replacement or spinal cord injury: two clinical studies with EHDP. *Metab Bone Dis Relat Res* 1981;45:337.
33. Morris JA Jr., Limbird TJ, MacKensie E. Rehabilitation of the trauma patient. In: Moore EE, Mattox KL, Feliciano DV, eds. *Trauma*. 2nd ed. Norwalk, CT: Appleton & Lange, 1991:820.
34. MacLeod AD. Self-neglect of spinal injured patients. *Paraplegia* 1988;26:340.
35. Janssen L, Hansebout RR. Pathogenesis of spinal cord injury and newer treatments: a review. *Spine* 1989;14:23.
36. Daverat P, Gagnon M, Dartigues JF, et al. Initial factors predicting survival in patients with spinal cord injury. *J Neurol Neurosurg Psychiatry* 1989;52:403.
37. Piepmeier JM, Jenkins NR. Late neurological changes following traumatic spinal cord injury. *J Neurosurg* 1988;69:399.

12. OCULAR TRAUMA[1]

Approximately 500,000 individuals sustain eye injuries every year (2). Of the more than 60,000 patients who sustain ocular injuries serious enough to require hospitalization, about 20,000 have open wounds of the eyeball or ocular adnexa. Recently there also has been increased recognition of airbag-induced eye injuries (3).

EYE AND FACIAL TRAUMA PROGNOSIS

Penetrating ocular injuries generally have the worst prognosis with up to 40% resulting in blindness; however, up to 70% of eyes with penetrating injuries treated promptly with modern microsurgical techniques can regain functional vision (4).

AXIOM Patients with severe facial injuries should be suspected of also having significant eye injuries.

In one series, 67% of patients with blunt maxillofacial trauma had associated ocular injuries of which 18% were serious and 3% resulted in blindness (5). In other series, ocular injuries have been present in 10% to 40% of orbital and periorbital fractures (6) and in up to 8% of head-injured patients (6).

Pelletier et al. (7) recently reported on 127 patients with head and neck injuries at a regional trauma center. Ophthalmology initially assessed 41 patients, whereas 86 were seen by another specialty. These specialties referred 23 of their patients with ocular signs and symptoms to ophthalmology. In the remaining 63 patients, signs and symptoms indicative of potentially more serious ocular problems (subconjunctival hemorrhage, lid laceration, diplopia, infraorbital anesthesia, ptosis, periorbital ecchymosis) were recorded in the charts of 39 (61.9%) patients, yet no ophthalmologic assessment was performed.

EYE ANATOMY

From a functional standpoint, the eye can be divided into two parts: an anterior chamber with a radius of about 8 mm containing the cornea and lens, and a posterior chamber with a radius of about 12 mm containing the retina and optic nerve.

The eyeball is flattened vertically and has a diameter of about 24 mm in the anteroposterior (AP) axis. The cornea and lens act to refract incident rays of light so that they focus a sharp image on the fovea. The fovea is a special area of the macula, which in turn is a specialized portion of the retina positioned about 3.5 mm lateral (temporal) to the optic disc.

A progressive decrease occurs in the number of rods, and a progressive increase occurs in the number of cones as one moves from the periphery of the macula toward the central fovea. No rods exist in the fovea itself. It has only cones, with each cone connected to only one ganglion cell instead of many; thus the impulse at the fovea is much purer and the resultant image received by the brain much sharper than those originating from elsewhere in the retina. Because of this, the fovea is the only part of the retina capable of having 20/20 vision. Visual acuity decreases as the image is focused outside to the fovea, decreasing to 20/200 at the edge of the macula and over the rest of the retina. When vision cannot be corrected to at least 20/200, the individual is said to be legally blind.

AXIOM Because visual pathways cross at the optic chiasm, injury anterior to the chiasm can cause unilateral visual dysfunction, whereas injury at or posterior to the chiasm can cause bilateral visual dysfunction.

Mechanisms of Visual Dysfunction

If incident light, after being refracted by the cornea and lens, is not focused on the fovea, a refractive error exists. If the focal point is anterior to the fovea because the eye is too long or has a cornea that has too much converging power, myopia (nearsightedness) is present. Conversely, if the focal point is posterior to the fovea because the eye is too short or has a cornea that is too flat, hyperopia (farsightedness) results.

In the normal eye, a clear path exists between the front of the cornea and the fovea. Any opacity between the two may cause visual disturbances. The opacities may take the form of corneal scars, blood in the anterior chamber (hyphema), cataracts, or vitreous hemorrhage.

SPECIFIC EYE TRAUMA: MECHANISMS OF INJURY

Corneal Abrasions

The cornea is covered with a layer of epithelium overlying a basement membrane (Bowman's membrane; 4). This epithelium protects the corneal stroma against infection and is necessary for the cornea to remain in its normal, relatively dehydrated, clear state. The corneal sensory nerves lie just beneath the corneal epithelium. If the corneal epithelium is removed or damaged, the nerve endings become exposed, causing severe pain.

Corneal abrasions are most commonly caused by minor trauma, such as a fingernail or particulate matter striking the eye (4). Multiple extremely fine linear abrasions of the superior third of the cornea (the "ice rink sign") suggest the presence of a foreign body under the upper lid. Overuse of contact lenses, particularly the hard variety, also can cause corneal abrasions.

Chemical Injuries

AXIOM Alkali injuries of the eye are much more severe than those caused by acid.

The most severe ocular damage is caused by highly alkaline compounds. Strong alkali can cause complete liquefaction necrosis of the cornea and severe intraocular inflammation, resulting in dense, permanent corneal scarring, cataracts, glaucoma, ocular ischemia, and necrosis of intraocular contents. Acids do not cause as much ocular damage because they tend to coagulate protein, which then acts as a barrier to further penetration. Although concentrated acids may render the corneal epithelium white and opaque, with time, the opaque epithelium sloughs, and it is usually replaced by normal epithelium so that permanent damage to vision is rare.

Blunt Ocular Trauma

Severe concussive injury to the eye may cause damage to the soft tissues of the globe, including the choroid, iris, ciliary body, or retina, or a combination of these. A severe orbital or retroorbital hematoma can cause marked proptosis and increase the intraorbital pressure sufficiently to occlude the central retinal artery, producing pain and an abrupt loss of vision.

Fracture of the floor of the orbit may be accompanied by herniation of orbital tissue into the maxillary antrum, producing enophthalmos and double vision. There also will be limitation of upward gaze if the inferior rectus muscle is trapped. Fracture of the roof or medial wall of the orbit can cause orbital emphysema (air in the orbit), which may be followed by orbital cellulitis. Bony fractures at the apex of the orbit may cause damage to the optic nerve by direct contusion, pressure from adjacent hematomas, or lacerations by bony fragments.

Penetrating Ocular Trauma

The prognosis of penetrating eye trauma is related primarily to its location and the extent of damage. In general, the more posterior and larger the laceration, the worse the prognosis (8). Through-and-through injuries have a particularly dismal prognosis. Penetrations or lacerations of the cornea, anterior chamber, lens, or a combination of these can generally be treated with meticulous microsurgical closure, contact lens, intraocular lens, optical corrections, or even corneal transplantation with a high rate of visual rehabilitation (4).

AXIOM Early microsurgery to correct penetrating eye injuries can save much vision that would otherwise be lost.

Posterior penetrating eye injuries, in addition to damaging the retina directly, may result in foreign material in the vitreous, and this creates a nidus for growth of scar tissue throughout the vitreous cavity. This scar tissue, derived in part from metaplastic fibroblasts and retinal pigment epithelial cells, also contains contractile proteins that have the potential to contract and induce retinal tears. Despite successful initial reattachment of the retina, the scar contracture may cause recurrent retinal detachment.

AXIOM Parenterally administered antibiotics penetrate the eye poorly, making it particularly important to reduce the risk of endophthalmitis by prompt surgical repair of open eye injuries whenever possible.

Sympathetic Ophthalmia

Sympathetic ophthalmia is a bilateral inflammation of the uveal tract (iris, ciliary body, and choroid) associated with penetrating injury to one eye (4). Untreated, this inflammation may result in loss of the uninjured eye. Evidence suggests that the risk of sympathetic ophthalmia may be reduced if the injured eye is enucleated within 2 weeks of the injury. This has prompted some physicians to recommend prompt removal of an injured eye when it has very poor visual potential; however, the development of the sympathetic ophthalmia is very unlikely with improved vitreous microsurgery. Furthermore, early enucleation does not guarantee protection for the other eye, and early use of corticosteroids or cytotoxic agents can allow retention of good vision in the majority of patients who develop sympathetic ophthalmia.

AXIOM The risk of sympathetic ophthalmia does not justify the primary removal of a severely traumatized eye unless the vision of that eye is completely lost.

DIAGNOSIS

History

An accurate history can provide valuable clues for early diagnosis and optimal treatment of eye injuries. Several historical items that are particularly important include (4):

1. How well can the patient see now?
2. Are one or both eyes affected?
3. Are there any other symptoms besides decreased vision?
4. What was the vision in the affected eye(s) before injury? Was that with or without corrective lenses?
5. Is there a history of eye disease, injury, or surgery?

With chemical injuries, it must be determined immediately exactly what the agent is, and copious irrigation should be begun immediately.

With foreign-body or pellet injuries, the probable size, velocity, and chemical constituents of the pellet should be obtained. The toxicity and management of intraocular pellets vary significantly depending on whether they are lead, steel, or copper.

Physical Examination

⊘ PITFALL

If visual acuity and visual fields are not checked during the initial physical examination, the diagnosis of important eye injuries may be delayed.

A check of visual acuity can usually determine how well the eyes and visual pathways are functioning and alert the examiner to the possible existence of subtle eye injuries. If the patient has poor vision, even in otherwise normal-appearing eyes, one should suspect a significant injury and ensure that an emergency complete ophthalmic examination is performed.

Visual acuity should be tested with the examiner making sure that the other eye is properly covered. With a Rosenbaum near 2d-vision card, one can easily check visual acuity at the bedside or in the emergency department. A standard eye chart or near–vision card is preferable so that one can assign a numeric value to the patient's visual acuity; however, when one is not available, a newspaper, magazine, or even package label may be used.

AXIOM In checking near visual acuity, especially in patients older than 40 years, it is imperative that the patients wear their reading glasses if they normally use them.

If the patient cannot read even large print, it is important to determine whether the patient can at least count fingers, see gross movements of the examiner's hands, or perceive light (4). As long as the patient has any vision, there is some potential for successful repair of the eye, no matter how severely damaged it appears.

AXIOM Pain from a corneal abrasion or chemical injury may result in the vision being assessed as poorer than it really is.

Topical anesthesia (0.5% proparacaine) can relieve much of the pain and tearing that can occur with mild eye injuries and allow patients to keep their eyes open for examination; however, use of any medication that may affect pupil size and reactions in patients with head injury should first be discussed with the physicians evaluating the patient's central nervous system (CNS) status.

In an alert, cooperative patient, visual fields can be easily determined. As with visual-acuity testing, each eye is evaluated individually after covering the other eye. The eye being tested fixates on the examiner's nose, and the patient is asked what part of the face is missing. Visual-field defects and central scotomas may be detected in this manner. To detect hemianopsias and quandrantanopsias, the patient is asked to stare at the examiner's nose while fingers are presented in the periphery. The patient is asked how many fingers are being presented while fixating on the examiner's nose.

AXIOM If the patient has normal visual acuity and visual fields, the chance of serious injury to the eye or visual pathways is unlikely; however, if subnormal results are obtained, a vigorous investigation is needed.

During external examination of the globe itself, the primary question to be answered is, "Is the globe ruptured?" Clues to rupture or perforation of the globe include

1. Presence of brown tissue (the iris or ciliary body) protruding through a laceration;
2. Obviously soft, shrunken eye;
3. Teardrop-shaped or eccentric pupil;
4. Sticky, clear material (vitreous) on the surface of the globe;
5. Hyphema blood in the anterior chamber; and
6. History of a high-velocity foreign-body injury.

AXIOM On discovery that an eye globe is ruptured, further examination is unnecessary. The eye should be covered with a protective shield until it can be examined by an ophthalmologist in an appropriate environment.

When a lid laceration is present, one should determine whether the margin or the nasal aspect of the lid has been violated. Although simple lid lacerations may be repaired by nonophthalmologists, those involving the lid margin or lacrimal system are best repaired by an ophthalmologist who is prepared to cannulate the lacrimal drainage system and deal with the problem of sutures passing through the posterior aspects of the lid and lid margin.

Orbital floor fractures can often be diagnosed by palpation of a step-off in the orbital margin. Orbital fractures also should be suspected when the patient has hypesthesia involving the cheek or upper lip, as a result of injury to the infraorbital nerves (4).

The Marcus–Gunn pupil indicates an abnormality in afferent pupillary function and should be considered when unexplained vision loss occurs in one eye. To perform this test, the reaction of each pupil to light is observed. A bright light shining into the normal eye will cause both pupils to constrict; however, the same light shining into the abnormal eye will cause the pupils to dilate for a short period. Situations in which this may be encountered after trauma include contusion of the optic nerve, retinal detachment, or vitreous hemorrhage.

Eversion of the upper lid is often necessary to detect and remove conjunctival foreign bodies. Foreign bodies have a tendency to embed themselves in the conjunctiva on the inner surface of the upper lid. Then, as the eye blinks, these foreign bodies rub against the cornea, causing areas of corneal abrasion.

Corneal abrasions may be invisible to the observer without the use of fluorescein, which stains areas of the cornea that have been denuded of epithelium because of abrasions, chemical injury, or a foreign body (4). The tip of a fluorescein strip should be wet, preferably with a commercial irrigating solution, and then touched to the conjunctiva. By blinking, the patient disperses the fluorescein in the preocular tear film. Then by using a penlight with a blue filter or a Wood's light, areas of fluorescence corresponding to areas of injury can be seen quite easily.

Laboratory Evaluation

Radiography

Any patient with severe blunt trauma to the midface or a suspected penetrating eye injury should have a complete set of orbital radiographs. Orbital floor fractures are most easily visualized by using a Water's view. Sometimes the fracture itself cannot be visualized but should be suspected if there is clouding of the maxillary sinus (due to herniation of blood or tissue into it through the orbital floor defect). Metallic fragments and foreign bodies made of leaded glass can often also be detected on plain AP and lateral orbital films (5).

Precise localization of intraocular foreign bodies requires the use of computed tomography (CT) or echographic (ultrasonographic) techniques or both. CT scans also may occasionally diagnose a suspected orbital floor fracture not visualized on plain films.

AXIOM Magnetic resonance imaging (MRI) can help evaluate soft-tissue injuries; however, the use of very high magnetic fields is contraindicated in patients who may have a metallic intraocular foreign body, which might be magnetically pulled through delicate intraocular tissues (4).

Echography

Echographic (ultrasonographic) examination of the globe and orbit can be useful for detecting and localizing foreign bodies and for determining the gross anatomy of the eye (8). When the fundus cannot be visualized because of hemorrhage or cataract, B-scan echography is the only nonsurgical technique for determining whether vitreous or choroidal hemorrhage is present and whether the retina is detached.

TREATMENT

Chemical Injuries

AXIOM Chemical burns of the eyes are best treated by early, copious irrigation.

The treatment of chemical injuries to the eyes is immediate with on-site copious irrigation with any solution that is nontoxic to the eye. There is often severe pain with alkali eye injuries, and topical anesthesia may be needed to allow adequate irrigation. During the irrigation, the lids should be held open and the stream of irrigating fluid should be directed into the superior and inferior fornices to wash away any particulate matter that may have lodged there (4). Additional irrigation should be performed in the emergency department. The fornices also should be cleaned with moistened swabs to remove any possible retained particulate matter. If, after 30 minutes of irrigation, the pH in the cul-de-sac normalizes, it is safe to discontinue irrigation. Topical antibiotics and cycloplegia are started once the pH normalizes.

Orbital Hypertension

Bleeding within the orbit or swelling of retrobulbar tissues can occasionally increase the pressure within the orbit to more than 20 to 30 mm Hg. At such pressure, blood flow to the optic nerve and posterior eye may be so impaired that blindness can result. When orbital hypertension is suspected because of evidence of local trauma, severe proptosis, eye pain, decreasing vision, or a combination of these, a lateral canthotomy may be required on an emergency basis.

The lateral canthus, after being anesthetized with lidocaine, is grasped with toothed forceps, and a hemostat is angled laterally and slight inferiorly, with the lateral lower eyelid margin contained within the jaws. The hemostat is advanced with open jaws into the fornix, and then closed, crushing the tissue. Scissors are then introduced along the same path, and the lateral canthal tendon is divided. If additional relaxation is required, the inferior crus to the lateral canthal tendon can be completely separated.

Eyelid Injury

AXIOM The three essential requirements for successful eyelid surgery under local anesthesia include adequate sedation, complete anesthesia, and an immobile eye.

Complete anesthesia refers to the use of local, regional, or general anesthesia so that there is no pain that might cause the patient to move the eye or eyelids during the procedure. Local or regional anesthesia can often be used for surgical management of closed-eye injuries and injuries to the ocular adnexa in cooperative adults (2). Children and uncooperative adults rarely tolerate eye surgery while conscious.

Although infiltration of individual eyelid nerves can produce satisfactory analgesia, infiltration of local anesthetic agents through the lacerated wound edges is much simpler and usually equally effective. When this approach is used, the anesthetic should be injected into the neurovascular plane of the eyelid, which lies between the firm tarsal plate and the orbicularis oculi muscle (Fig. 12-1; 2).

Topical anesthesia also is usually needed to manipulate the conjunctiva during repair of lid lacerations. Local anesthesia for the lids can be provided by injection of a few milliliters of 1% lidocaine or 0.5% bupivacaine with or without epinephrine (1:200,000). Topical anesthesia of the cornea and conjunctiva can be provided by two to three drops of 1% tetracaine. This treatment also allows the measurement of the intraocular pressure (IOP) and removal of foreign bodies lodged on the eye surface.

A crucial part of eyelid repair is the meticulous reapproximation of the lacerated eyelid margins and tarsal plates (Fig. 12-2). Failure to reapproximate the lacerated borders accurately may result in lid notching, which can lead to severe eye damage over time. Eyelid margins can be repaired with 6-0 sutures reapproximating first the meibomian gland orifices, and then the anterior lash line, and finally the gray line. Several 5-0 absorbable sutures can be used to repair the torn tarsus, taking care not to enter the posterior boundary of the lid, where it can cause corneal irritation and abrasion.

AXIOM With any lid laceration near the medial canthus, a canalicular laceration should be suspected.

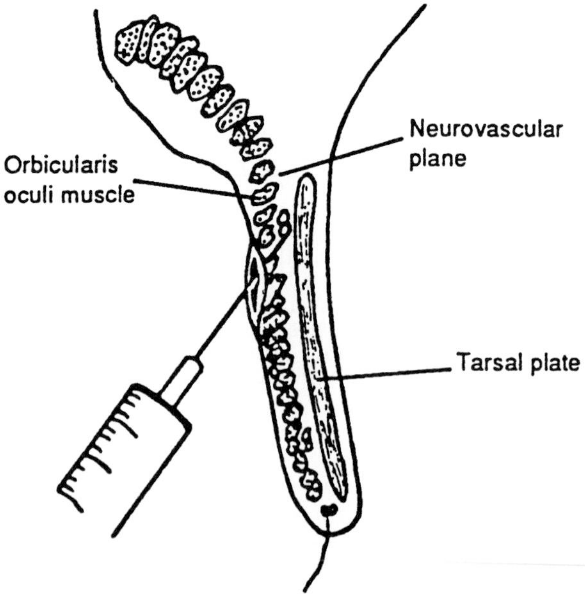

FIG. 12-1. Sagittal section of the eyelid showing orbicularis oculi muscle anteriorly, tarsal plate posteriorly, and neurovascular plane in the middle. Satisfactory analgesia can be obtained by injection of local anesthetic agent within the neurovascular plane. From ref. 2, with permission.

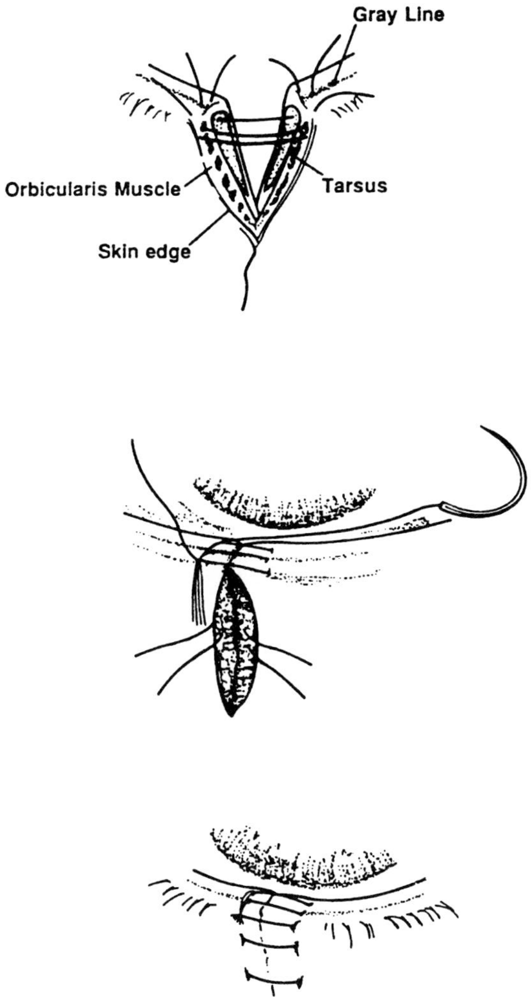

FIG. 12-2. Three-suture technique to repair eyelid-margin laceration with minimal loss of tissue. From ref. 13, with permission.

When the medial portion of an upper or lower eyelid has been lacerated, thorough examination of the extent of the laceration should be performed to determine the integrity of the lacrimal drainage system. If there is any possibility that a canaliculus has been injured, it should be probed and irrigated with a fluorescein solution.

AXIOM If a laceration involving a canaliculus of the eye is not repaired properly, persistent tearing can result.

Corneal Abrasions

Patients with a corneal abrasion typically are seen with a red eye, severe pain, tearing, and photophobia. If the corneal abrasion is not obvious, the instillation of a topical anesthetic will bring immediate relief of pain. After the symptoms are relieved, fluorescein should be instilled in the eye. With fluorescein staining, denuded corneal epithelium appears green under white light and fluoresces as bright green under cobalt blue light. Normal cornea with intact epithelium does not stain.

Corneal abrasions caused by vegetable matter may require intensive treatment to prevent or treat fungal keratitis, but corneal abrasions caused by clean objects, such as a sheet of paper, require only an eye patch and observation.

Treatment of corneal abrasions is best achieved by instilling an antibiotic ointment (e.g., gentamicin) in the eye and applying a pressure patch to prevent the patient from opening the eye. This relieves pain and helps to prevent infection. In addition, the patch immobilizes the eyelids, thereby allowing uninterrupted ingrowth of corneal epithelium.

To place a pressure patch on the eye, two eye pads are placed across the patient's closed lids (4). The patches are then taped in place firmly with multiple strips of adhesive paper or plastic tape. Before the patching, the examiner should instill a topical cycloplegic agent, either 1/4% scopolamine or 1% cyclopentolate, in the affected eye. This will partially relieve patient discomfort. Uncomplicated corneal epithelial defects often heal within 24 to 48 hours, depending on the size of the defect.

⊘ PITFALL

Steroids should never be used in the presence of a corneal epithelial defect because they can rapidly make an undetected herpes simplex or bacterial keratitis much worse.

Inability to Close Eyes

AXIOM If, because of severe brain, eyelid, or facial nerve injury, patients cannot completely close their eyes, exposure damage to the cornea can occur rapidly despite intensive medical and nursing care.

Taping the eyelids shut, placing plastic wrap over the orbital areas in unconscious patients, and instilling eye ointment such as Lacri-lube can help to prevent the eyes from drying and developing corneal ulcers.

Corneal Foreign Bodies

The majority of corneal foreign bodies are superficially embedded, and although they can cause severe pain, they do not usually cause serious injury (4). After a careful examination of the eye to eliminate a penetrating injury, the examiner may attempt removal of the foreign body by gently rolling a moistened cotton swab across the cornea. If this is unsuccessful, ophthalmologic consultation should be obtained.

Corneal Ulcers

If, during the treatment of a corneal abrasion, the surrounding cornea develops an infiltrate (which makes it hazy), a corneal ulcer is probably present. An immediate ophthalmic consult should be obtained and the patient admitted to the hospital.

Corneal Lacerations

Corneal lacerations may range from small, subtle, self-sealing lacerations to large gashes with prolapse of intraocular contents. Because the cornea contains 70% of the eye's refractive power, an injury to the cornea may have profound effects on vision;

however, with small, self-sealing corneal lacerations, normal vision and appearance are usually retained.

AXIOM The optimal treatment of full-thickness corneal lacerations is expeditious surgical repair to restore the eye's integrity and to prevent intraocular infection and complications.

Because corneal lacerations heal with scar formation, vision may be compromised; however, early meticulous microsurgical repair plus careful attention to the placement of the sutures should minimize the scarring.

Penetrating Ocular Injuries

⊘ PITFALL

Any eye suspected of perforation should be protected from further damage by a metal shield until it is formally repaired.

As soon as the diagnosis of an open eye wound is made, broad-spectrum antibiotics are given intravenously to achieve high bacteriocidal levels in the eyes. These are continued for only 48 to 72 hours if no growth is evident on intraoperative culture of the wound. When there is concern regarding vegetable matter contamination of the eye, antibiotics such as clindamycin, which are active against *Bacillus* species, are added to provide broad-spectrum coverage. Tetanus prophylaxis is administered to all patients with an open eye wound or eyelid lacerations.

A preoperative CT scan of the orbits aids in eliminating retained intraocular foreign bodies and in delineating any unsuspected concomitant intracranial injuries. The metallic eye shield does not interfere with high-resolution CT.

Before the repair, magnetic intraocular foreign bodies, if present, may be removed with a giant magnet. Some magnetic fragments and all nonmagnetic fragments are removed from the posterior segment of the eye by using vitrectomy and vitreous microsurgery.

Although an open eye should be considered an emergency and should generally be repaired within the first 24 hours, there is little difference in the eventual visual outcome in eyes immediately repaired versus those whose repair is delayed by 24 to 36 hours. Untrained operating room personnel, inadequate anesthesia, a tired surgeon, and unavailable surgical equipment all serve to make a repair suboptimal.

⊘ PITFALL

A ruptured globe should not be repaired immediately if the circumstances for repair are unfavorable.

Most penetrating ocular injuries are complicated by some degree of intraocular injury, such as lens damage, vitreous hemorrhage, vitreous loss, retinal incarceration in the wound, retinal detachment, or significant choroidal hemorrhage. Many ocular trauma surgeons believe that these cases are managed more effectively by primary wound closure and delayed definitive management rather than by a single, comprehensive surgical procedure.

Delaying definitive intraocular repairs for 5 to 10 days allows a decrease in orbital congestion and periocular tissue swelling, partial or complete resolution of choroidal hemorrhage, and spontaneous separation of the vitreous from the underlying retina. This also allows a more complete preoperative evaluation, including echography.

Delayed surgical intervention on the eye should be coordinated with repair of other facial fractures that will require placement of external hardware (4). Such hardware may render introduction of microinstruments into the eye physically impossible. Additionally, when the eye is filled with gas after intraocular repair to tamponade the retina, it may be necessary to keep the patient in a prone position for several days.

Hyphema

Hyphemas (blood in the anterior chamber) usually result from contusive injuries to the eye that traumatize the vasculature of the iris. Because normal vision depends on a clear path from the cornea to the macula, a large hyphema can interfere with vision.

The initial collection of blood in the anterior chamber usually resolves spontaneously without complications; however, in 9% to 32%, rebleeding will occur, usually between the second and fifth day (9). When permanent visual loss is caused by hyphema, it is almost always the result of rebleeding, which causes corneal staining or hemorrhagic glaucoma with subsequent optic atrophy. Because of this, the two basic principles of the treatment of traumatic hyphema include prevention of rebleeding and control of IOP.

AXIOM All patients with hyphemas, even if very small, are admitted and placed on strict bed rest with head elevation plus sedation to prevent anterior chamber hypertension and rebleeding.

Daily ophthalmic evaluations are performed on patients with traumatic hyphema with specific attention to IOP and the condition of the corneal endothelium. It is important to control IOP in these patients by using osmotic agents, carbonic anhydrase inhibitors, topical β-blockers, or a combination of these. If early corneal blood staining or persistently increased IOP occurs due to hyphema, the blood should be removed surgically from the anterior chamber. Carbonic anhydrase inhibitors should not be used in patients with sickle cell anemia because this agent slows the clearance of sickled red cells from the anterior chamber.

AXIOM All black patients with hyphemas should be checked for the presence of sickle hemoglobin.

Rebleeding recurs in approximately 10% to 30% of hyphema patients, generally within the first 5 days (10). Aspirin and nonsteroidal antiinflammatory drugs are avoided because they increase the risk of rebleeding. Many medical regimens have been advocated to minimize the risk of rebleeding, but only Amicar (epsilon aminocaproic acid), an antifibrinolytic agent, has proved effective in randomized, double-blind trials; however, the side effects (hypotension, dizziness, nausea, and vomiting) have limited its widespread use.

Lens Injuries

Severe contusive or penetrating trauma causing violation of the lens capsule causes the lens fibers to imbibe aqueous humor, lose their clarity, and opacify. A traumatic cataract that is visually significant obscures the fundus and is usually easy to detect with a penlight examination or with an ophthalmoscope. Definitive treatment involves the removal of the cataract and subsequent visual rehabilitation with an intraocular or contact lens.

Vitreous Hemorrhage

Vitreous hemorrhages are commonly seen in penetrating or severe contusive eye injuries. Normally, the vitreous is a clear hydrogel that permits the uninterrupted passage of light from the posterior aspect of the lens to the macula. Any collection of blood in the vitreous will decrease visual acuity and limit retinal evaluation.

Because retinal detachments and retinal holes are frequently associated with vitreous hemorrhages, nonvisual means of detection, such as ocular ultrasonography, are needed. The treatment of unresorbing blood from the vitreous cavity is the surgical removal of the blood and the associated vitreous. If a retinal detachment also is present, it can be repaired at the same time.

Retinal Injuries

Retinal detachments may be caused by penetrating or contusive eye injuries and must be detected and repaired surgically as soon as possible. Patients will usually complain of flashing lights and "floaters" or loss of visual field as the retina detaches, but they may remain asymptomatic until the macula detaches, at which time visual acuity is severely diminished.

⊘ PITFALL

All patients with ocular or periocular trauma need complete fundus examinations, including visualization of the retinal periphery with indirect ophthalmoscopy, to detect retinal holes, tears, or detachments.

Optic Nerve Damage

Visual loss may occur after blunt trauma because of optic nerve avulsion or infarction or because of compression by a nerve sheath hematoma, edema, or bone fragments. The history is vital in diagnosing the nature of the optic nerve injury. If the patient noticed immediate total loss of vision at injury, it is likely that the patient has optic nerve avulsion or infarction, for which there is no successful therapy. Conversely, a history of slowly progressive visual loss after blunt craniofacial trauma suggests the presence of increasing compression of the optic nerve, and prompt neuroradiologic evaluation of the optic canal for fracture is mandatory.

When neuroradiologic evaluation with CT scans demonstrates fractures in the optic canal, visual loss may be due to compression of the optic nerve, and prompt transcranial or transethmoidal decompression of the optic canal may provide dramatic restoration of vision.

When blunt orbital or cranial trauma causes vision loss in the presence of an afferent pupillary defect, traumatic optic neuropathy exists. Treatment includes large doses of intravenous corticosteroids given as a 30 mg/kg loading dose of methylprednisolone sodium succinate (Solu-Medrol) followed 2 hours later by 15 mg/kg and then 15 mg/kg every 6 hours (11). If visual acuity improves, the steroids should be continued as long as vision is improving for up to 72 hours. In the unconscious patient, grading of the afferent pupillary defect is the only indicator of progression. Although the prognosis for regaining useful vision is guarded, excellent results have been reported.

Orbital Fractures

The orbital contents are protected by a thick, bony ring consisting of the supraorbital ridge, the glabella, and the infraorbital and lateral orbital rims. The bones of the medial wall, floor, and roof are almost eggshell thin.

AXIOM Computed tomography is the best method for evaluating the extent of orbital fractures.

Evaluation of orbital-floor and medial-wall fractures is incomplete without high-resolution CT scanning of the orbits. Orbital fractures can usually be localized well by axial views, but additional helpful information can often be obtained with the aid of oblique and coronal reconstructions. These can help to evaluate the size and extent of any orbital fractures and any involvement of the inferior rectus muscle or the optic nerve.

⊘ PITFALL

With fractures extending into the orbital apex or orbital canal, surgery in or around the orbit can cause traumatic optic neuropathy with marked loss of vision.

Most authorities believe that significant residual diplopia, entrapment of orbital contents, or large fractures with significant enophthalmos are indications for surgical repair of orbital fractures. Repair of orbital-floor fractures is often delayed 7 to 14 days, so that orbital swelling and hemorrhage can subside. Surgical repair of the orbit also should be delayed until hyphema or other ocular injuries (e.g., ruptured globe) have resolved or have been repaired.

⊘ PITFALL

Surgical repair of a blow-out fracture may be contraindicated if it is on the side of the only eye with vision.

The medial wall (lamina papyracea) is the thinnest portion of the orbit and is easily fractured. These fractures are easily missed, and CT scans may show only a subtle step-off of medial wall bone or blood in the ethmoid sinus. These fractures are particularly easy to miss if the patient is asymptomatic. The presence of orbital emphysema on radiograph or CT should make one very suspicious of a medial wall fracture; however, surgical repair of medial-wall orbital fractures is needed only rarely, and then only if medial rectus entrapment or damage to the lacrimal system is present.

Orbital-roof fractures can involve the frontal sinus and anterior cranial fossa and can be associated with significant intracranial injury. Cerebrospinal fluid leaks and carotid cavernous fistulas can occur if the fracture extends along the base of the skull. Ptosis with upward-gaze palsy can occur as a result of injuries to the superior division of the oculomotor nerve.

Anterior Ischemic Optic Neuropathy

Shaked et al. (12) noted that anterior ischemic optic neuropathy (AION) can be a complication of hemorrhagic shock. This is a devastating disorder characterized by a sudden blindness that may be unilateral or bilateral. This loss of vision is painless and may be complete or partial. Sometimes the condition is reversible and temporary, but in other cases, the loss of vision is permanent. AION is associated with systemic disorders such as chronic hypertension, diabetes mellitus, chronic renal failure, atherosclerosis, vasculitis, or cardiac disease. Many cases of AION occur spontaneously; however, acute hypotension and anemia are the most significant causative factors. In the trauma patient, this pathology may not be discovered until late because the patient may be unconscious for a prolonged period.

⊘ FREQUENT ERRORS

1. ***Failure to promptly check visual activity and visual fields in patients with possible eye trauma.***
2. ***Failure to check visual acuity with the patient wearing his or her usual glasses.***
3. ***Failure to promptly and adequately irrigate the eyes after possible chemical injury.***

4. ***Failure to promptly consult an ophthalmologist when the patient has a potentially serious eye injury.***
5. ***Missing corneal lesions because of failure to use fluorescein staining.***
6. ***Failure to completely examine the globe in patients with penetrating eyelid injuries.***
7. ***Improper closure of lacerations involving the free margin of the eyelids.***
8. ***Using corticosteroids on a corneal lesion that could be caused by a viral or bacterial infection.***
9. ***Failure to promptly and adequately protect a ruptured or lacerated eye globe.***
10. ***Failure to admit and aggressively treat patients with a "minor" hyphema.***
11. ***Failure to carefully evaluate the eyes in patients with midface fractures, especially when a "tripod" fracture is present.***
12. ***Failure to promptly use CT to evaluate the orbit further in patients with suspected but unproven fractures on plain radiography.***
13. ***Failure to adequately protect the corneas when the eyelids cannot cover them properly.***

SUMMARY POINTS

1. Patients with severe facial injuries should be suspected of also having significant eye injuries.

2. Because visual pathways cross at the optic chiasm, injury anterior to the chiasm can cause unilateral visual dysfunction, whereas injury at or posterior to the chiasm can cause bilateral visual dysfunction.

3. Alkali injuries of the eye are generally much more severe than those caused by acid, and copious irrigation should be begun immediately.

4. Posttraumatic posterior intraocular hypertension can rapidly occlude the retinal artery and cause blindness.

5. Parenterally administered antibiotics penetrate the eye poorly, making it particularly important to reduce the risk of endophthalmitis by prompt surgical repair of open eye injuries whenever possible.

6. Although a penetrating injury to one eye can cause the development of sympathetic ophthalmia, with resultant blindness in the other eye, this possibility is very unlikely with improved vitreous microsurgery.

7. In checking visual acuity in patients older than 40 years, it is imperative that patients wear their reading glasses if they normally use them.

8. Pain from a corneal abrasion or chemical injury may result in the vision being assessed as poorer than it really is.

9. If the patient has normal visual acuity and visual fields, the chance of serious injury to the eye or visual pathways is unlikely; however, if subnormal results are obtained, a vigorous investigation is needed.

10. Once it is discovered that an eye globe is ruptured, further examination is unnecessary. The eye should be covered with a protective shield until it can be examined by an ophthalmologist in an appropriate environment.

11. Superficial corneal injuries are diagnosed most readily by fluorescein staining.

12. Magnetic resonance imaging (MRI) can help to evaluate soft-tissue injuries; however, the use of very high magnetic fields is contraindicated in patients who may have a metallic intraocular foreign body, which might be magnetically pulled through delicate intraocular tissues.

13. Any trauma that injured an eyelid also may have injured the eye.

14. The three essential requirements for successful eye surgery under local or regional anesthesia include adequate sedation, complete anesthesia, and an immobile eye.

15. With any lid laceration near the medial canthus, a canalicular laceration should be suspected.

16. If a laceration involving the canaliculus of the eye is not repaired properly, persistent tearing can result.

17. A delay of 12 to 24 hours, until optimal patient and operative conditions can be obtained, will not compromise the outcome of most eyelid lacerations.
18. If because of severe brain, eyelid, or facial nerve injury, patients cannot completely close their eyes, exposure damage to the cornea can occur rapidly despite intensive medical and nursing care.
19. The optimal treatment of full-thickness corneal lacerations is expeditious surgical repair to restore the eye's integrity and to prevent intraocular infection and complications.
20. All patients with hyphemas, even if the hyphemas are very small, are admitted and placed on strict bed rest with head elevation plus sedation to prevent anterior chamber hypertension and rebleeding.
21. All black patients with hyphemas should be checked for the presence of sickle hemoglobin.
22. If early corneal blood staining or persistently increased intraocular pressure occurs because of hyphema, the blood should be removed surgically from the anterior chamber.
23. When hyphema is present, it is important to rule out injury to other portions of the eye and optic nerve.
24. A traumatic cataract in a child with a vague or inconsistent history of trauma should alert the examiner to the possibility of child abuse, and the appropriate agencies should be notified.
25. Progressive loss of vision after blunt eye or face trauma requires emergency ophthalmologic evaluation and treatment to save as much vision as possible.
26. About 60% of patients with midface fractures have injuries to the eyes that should be evaluated by an ophthalmologist.

REFERENCES

1. Spoor TC, Ramocki JM, Kwitro GM. Ocular trauma. In: Wilson RF, Walt AJ, eds. *Management of trauma: pitfalls and practice*. 2nd ed. Philadelphia: Williams & Wilkins, 1996:225.
2. Capan LM, Mankikar D, Eisenberg WM. Anesthetic management of ocular injuries. In: *Trauma: anesthesia and intensive care.* Philadelphia: JB Lippincott, 1991:357–384.
3. Duma SM, Kress TA, Porta DJ, et al. Airbag-induced eye injuries: a report of 25 cases. *J Trauma* 1996;41:114.
4. Bracker G, Parke DW II, Hamill MB. Injury to the eye. In: Moore EE, Mattox KL, Feliciano DV, eds. *Trauma*. 3rd ed. Norwalk: Appleton & Lange, 1995:279–290.
5. Holt JE, Hot GR, Blodgett JM. Ocular injuries sustained during blunt facial trauma. *Ophthalmology* 1983;90:14.
6. Hardy RA. Ocular trauma. *Mil Med* 1996;161:465.
7. Pelletier CR, Jordan DR, Braga R, et al. Assessment of ocular trauma associated with head and neck injuries. *J Trauma* 1998;44:350.
8. Kramer M, Hart L, Miller JW. Ultrasonography in the management of penetrating ocular trauma. *Int Ophthalmol Clin* 1995;35:181.
9. Spoor TC, Hammer M, Belloso H. Traumatic hyphema: failure of steroids to alter its course: a double-blind prospective study. *Arch Ophthalmol* 1980;98:116.
10. Thomas MA, Parrish RK II, Fener WJ. Rebleeding after traumatic hyphema. *Arch Ophthalmol* 1986;104:206.
11. Anderson RI, Panse WP, Gross CE. Optic nerve blindness following blunt forehead trauma. *Ophthalmology* 1982;89:445.
12. Shaked G, Gavriel A, Roy-Shapira A. Anterior ischemic optic neuropathy after hemorrhagic shock. *J Trauma* 1998;44:923.
13. Catalano RA. *Ocular emergencies.* Philadelphia: WB Saunders, 1992:118.

13. TRAUMA TO THE FACE[1]

Except for airway problems, massive bleeding, or aspiration of blood into the lungs, patients seldom die of facial injuries (2); however, one should always consider the possibility of brain or cervical spine injuries in patients with severe maxillofacial trauma. Up to 4% of patients with facial fractures have associated cervical spine injuries (3).

MECHANISM OF FACIAL INJURY

Knives usually injure only soft tissue, but intracranial and orbital penetration also can occur. With gunshot wounds of the face, the tongue, floor of the mouth, and deeper structures are frequently injured. Close-range shotguns, rifles, and high-velocity military missiles can produce massive destruction and loss of tissue.

The nasal bones, the zygoma, the mandibular ramus, and the frontal sinus are less tolerant to blunt impact than are other facial bones. For instance, a 30-mile/hour collision can easily result in 80 *g* forces, which is sufficient to cause fractures of these facial bones, while sparing others (4); however, even minor impacts in elderly people with osteoporotic facial bones may produce severe complex fractures.

TYPES OF FACIAL INJURY

Soft-tissue injuries of the face can bleed severely; however, because of the rich vascularity of the face, primary closure, after proper irrigation and debridement, is possible even with wounds for which treatment has been delayed for as long as 36 hours. Hematomas of the nasal septum or auricular cartilages, conversely, require urgent surgery. If hematomas in these structures are not drained promptly, they can cause pressure necrosis of the cartilage and secondary septal defects or external ear deformities.

Mandibular Fractures

After the nose and the zygoma, the mandible is the third most frequently fractured facial bone (5). Mandible fractures tend to occur in weaker areas of the bone, such as the condyles, the subcondylar area, the angle, or the body in the area of the second bicuspid (6). In elderly edentulous persons with thin cortical bone, the mandible is often broken in the symphyseal and parasymphyseal areas.

AXIOM If a mandible has one fracture line, one must look very carefully for other fracture lines that may not be readily apparent on standard radiography because more than 50% of mandibular fractures occur in more than one site.

The inferior neurovascular dental bundle is at risk in fractures occurring between the mental foramen anteriorly and the mandibular foramen posteriorly in the ramus; however, the fibrous sheath surrounding the bundle provides considerable support and explains the low incidence of permanent nerve damage.

Lower-lip numbness caused by damage to the inferior alveolar nerve or its branches is generally transient, and hemorrhage from a transected inferior alveolar artery often ceases spontaneously.

Mandibular muscles are divided into four functional categories that include

1. Elevators (masseter, anterior temporalis, medial pterygoid);
2. Depressor–retractors (anterior digastric, geniohyoid, mylohyoid);

3. Retractors (posterior temporalis); and
4. Protrusors (lateral pterygoid).

Of the three mandible-elevator muscles (which close the mouth), the masseter is the strongest. The depressor–retractor muscles opening the mouth include the anterior belly of the digastric, the geniohyoid, and the mylohyoid, all of which originate from the hyoid bone (Fig. 13-1).

In bilateral parasymphyseal fractures, the fractured segment of the mandible is pulled downward and backward by the digastric, mylohyoid, and geniohyoid muscles. Such a pull may retract the tongue and intraoral soft tissues into the pharynx, causing airway obstruction.

Temporomandibular Joint Dislocation

Considerable pain and muscle spasm are present in almost all patients with TMJ dislocations; however, injection of a few milliliters of local anesthetic into the connective tissue of the TMJ capsule can relieve the pain and muscle spasm and sometimes results in spontaneous reduction of the dislocation (7). If this measure is ineffective, one can often reduce the dislocation by depressing the mandible with the thumbs pushing down on the back teeth and simultaneously providing gentle elevation with the fingers from outside the mouth. Rarely, with severe force against the point of the open jaw, a condyle may actually be pushed back into the middle cranial fossa.

Central Midface Fractures

Rene LeFort in 1901 noted three relatively constant patterns with facial fractures.

1. In LeFort I or Guerin's fractures, a horizontal fracture line separates the maxillary alveolar process from the rest of the maxilla.
2. The LeFort II fracture is pyramidal and begins in the midline at the thick portion of the nasal bone, extends laterally through the lacrimal bones and inferior rim of the orbit, and then continues downward near the zygomaticomaxillary sutures.
3. In LeFort III injuries, a combination of frontal and maxillary fractures cause separation of the midface and the anterior base of the skull from the main body of the cranium, resulting in dysjunction of parts of the frontal bone, orbital roof, or sphenoid bone (or a combination of these; Fig. 13-2).

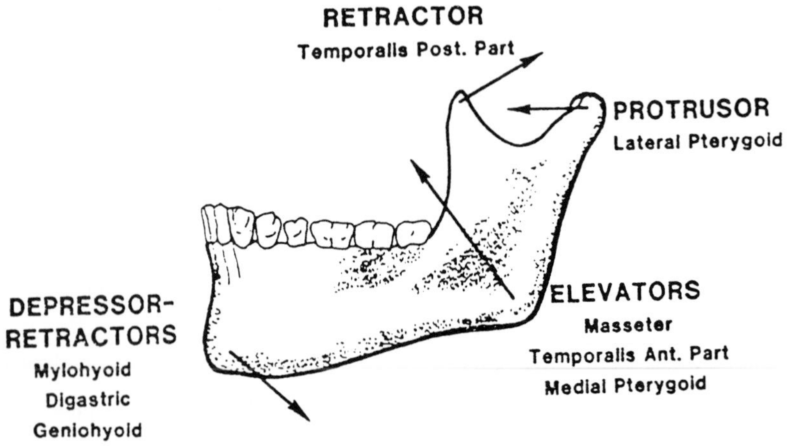

FIG. 13-1. The elevator, depressor–retractor, retractor, and protrusor muscles of the mandible and the direction of fragment displacement produced by them (arrows). From ref. 2, with permission.

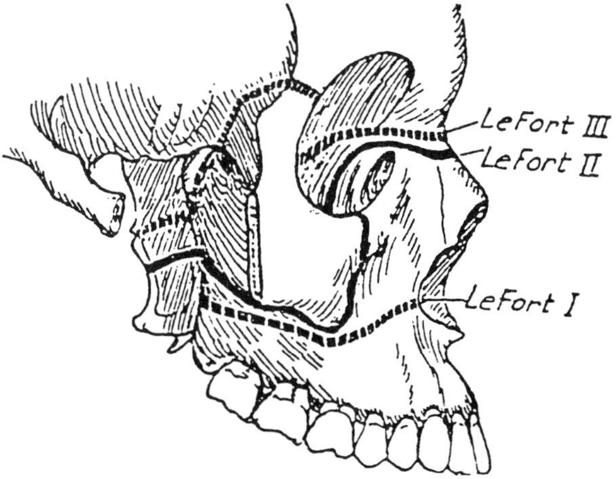

FIG. 13-2. LeFort's lines of fracture on lateral view. From ref. 19, with permission.

When a LeFort III fracture occurs, the entire midface tends to move backward and downward, parallel to the base of the cranium, causing the face to be elongated and flattened (2). The posteriorly displaced midface can impinge on the oropharynx and nasopharynx, potentially causing airway obstruction (Fig. 13-3).

AXIOM One should look carefully for cerebrospinal fluid (CSF) rhinorrhea or airway obstruction or both in patients with LeFort III fractures.

Nasal Fractures

The projection of the nose beyond the rest of the face and the delicate structure of its bones make nasal fractures the most commonly encountered bony injury of the face. With such fractures, one should look for a nasal septal hematoma that should be drained promptly. Radiographic studies typically add little to the clinical diagnosis; however, computed tomography (CT) scans may be required to differentiate simple nasal fractures from complex nasoethmoid fractures that require early surgical intervention to prevent infection.

Nasoethmoid Fractures

Nasoethmoid fractures should be suspected when severe trauma to the central face causes epistaxis, depression of the nasal dorsum, severe pain and tenderness over the upper nose, bilateral "black eyes" (spectacle hematomas), inferomedial orbital rim fractures, or a combination of these (2). The bony injuries can easily be missed because of the severe soft-tissue swelling.

AXIOM A nasoethmoid fracture should be suspected in patients with bilateral periorbital ecchymosis (spectacle hematomas or "raccoon eyes").

Bilateral black eyes suggest the possibility of fractures in the base of the skull anteriorly. Severe ocular injury with initial or subsequent loss of sight may be present in up to 30% of patients with nasoethmoid fractures. Telecanthus, which is an increased distance between the medial canthal ligaments, also may be observed

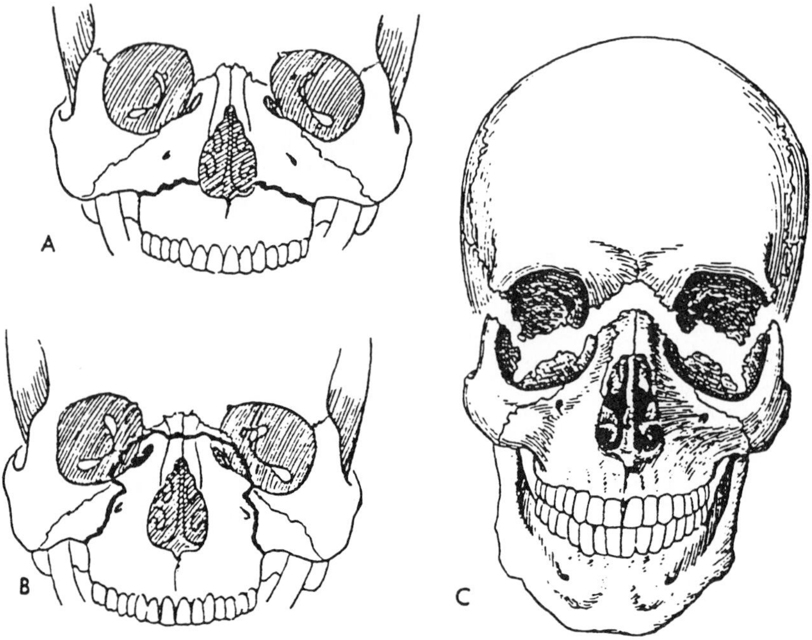

FIG. 13-3. LeFort's classification of midfacial fractures. **A:** LeFort I, horizontal fracture of the maxilla, also known as Guerin's fracture. **B:** LeFort II, pyramidal fracture of the maxilla. **C:** LeFort III, craniofacial disjunction. From ref. 19, with permission.

either immediately after injury or a few days later as the swelling disappears (8). Telecanthus suggests the presence of an unstable, complex, maxillofacial injury that often requires aggressive management by using a combined craniofacial approach (9).

Lateral Midface Fractures

Lateral midface fractures primarily involve the zygomatic arch, but they also may involve the malar bone and the orbit (2). The displaced zygomatic fragment may impinge on the mandibular coronoid process and produce limited mouth opening, which must be differentiated from trismus resulting from pain and temporalis muscle spasm. The displaced zygomatic fragment also may intrude on the lateral wall of the maxilla and produce infraorbital nerve damage. Orbital fractures can affect eye movement if the external ocular muscles are entrapped by fracture fragments or if the globe prolapses into the maxillary sinus.

Upper Facial Fractures

Upper facial fractures also are called "frontobasilar fractures" and tend to involve the frontal bone, frontal sinus, and anterior cranial fossa (2). Concomitant nasoethmoid, supraorbital, zygomatic, and cranial-base fractures are common associated injuries. Frequent complications of these fractures include frontal lobe contusions or lacerations, CSF rhinorrhea, pneumocephalus, and periorbital emphysema.

EMERGENCY MANAGEMENT

AXIOM Facial fractures generally do not pose an immediate threat to life unless they compromise the airway or are associated with extensive bleeding; however, associated injuries of the cervical spine and brain must be suspected when attempting airway-management techniques (2).

Airway Problems

Causes

Up to 6% of patients seen in the emergency department with serious maxillofacial injuries require emergency tracheal intubation to relieve airway obstruction or improve oxygenation (2). Respiratory distress in a patient with acute maxillofacial injury is most commonly caused by an upper airway obstruction, but other problems, such as a pneumothorax, pulmonary contusion, pulmonary aspiration, or combination of these factors, also must be considered. If consciousness is impaired because of associated craniocerebral trauma, the tongue can fall back against the posterior wall of the pharynx and occlude the airway. Blood, tooth fragments, dentures, and foreign bodies in the pharynx also may occlude the upper airway or may be aspirated into the tracheobronchial tree.

Signs and Symptoms

In conscious patients with marginal breathing difficulty, a fairly reliable way to establish the need for immediate airway management is to ask them if they are getting enough air. If these patients cannot answer or cannot stick out their tongues fairly easily, they should be intubated.

Breathing is characteristically noisy in a patient with partial airway obstruction, although the respiratory efforts of a totally obstructed patient are silent. When inspiratory stridor occurs, it is assumed that the upper airway is at least 70% occluded. Intercostal retraction, paradoxic movement of the lower neck and chest, flaring of alae nasi, and stridor are also important signs of upper airway obstruction.

Relief of Obstruction

Many conscious patients with maxillofacial injury breathe more comfortably if they are leaning forward in a sitting position. In this position, the intraoral soft tissues tend to move forward, and may relieve some upper airway obstruction.

AXIOM Patients with severe facial injuries who are hemodynamically stable and have their spine cleared or immobilized should be allowed to sit up if they can breathe more effectively and comfortably in that position.

If airway occlusion after a maxillofacial injury is caused by simple loss of soft-tissue tone, anterior traction on the jaw or tongue or proper placement of an oral or nasal airway usually relieves the problem (2). A nasal airway is less likely to cause gagging than is an oral airway, but it should not be used if a fracture of the central midface is suspected.

AXIOM All patients with facial trauma should have the mouth carefully examined for blood clots, foreign bodies, vomitus, and loose teeth or dentures.

Airway obstruction is occasionally caused by posterior displacement of the entire midface after fracture of the pterygoid plates. Insertion of the fingers into the mouth and palpation of the pterygoid plates immediately posterior and medial to the last upper molar teeth can confirm this diagnosis. If the palate can be pulled anteriorly with the fingers, this can reposition the entire maxilla and relieve any airway obstruction that is present, but it must be done carefully and expeditiously, because the fingers in the mouth can cause severe gagging or vomiting.

AXIOM Paralyzing a patient to insert an endotracheal tube may be fatal if intubation or provision of a surgical airway cannot be accomplished promptly.

In LeFort II and especially LeFort III fractures, which may involve the base of the skull, nasal endotracheal intubation is generally contraindicated unless done over a thin fiberoptic scope to ensure accurate placement in the airway. Nasally introduced gastric tubes carry similar risks.

Cricothyroidotomy (Coniotomy)

AXIOM One should always be prepared to perform an emergency cricothyroidotomy in adults with severe facial injuries and respiratory distress because attempts at endotracheal intubation may fail or cause complete airway obstruction (2).

A cricothyroidotomy is generally preferred to a tracheostomy for emergency airway control because it is easier and faster to perform; however, it is contraindicated if a laryngeal injury, particularly a cricotracheal separation, is suspected. One of the other major problems with cricothyroidotomy is the ease with which the relatively small tube (usually 6 mm or less) that is generally used can be occluded by blood or secretions.

In performing a cricothyroidotomy, the cricothyroid membrane is usually incised 1.5 to 2.0 cm transversely with a pointed scalpel blade, and the opening is widened with a medium or large hemostat. A 6-mm tracheostomy tube is then inserted.

In children with respiratory difficulty who cannot be intubated, a 14-gauge intravenous catheter may be inserted percutaneously through the cricothyroid membrane in the midline and directed caudally. Ventilation through the catheter is accomplished by connecting it to a high-pressure (50 psi) oxygen source with a hole in the tubing that allows intermittent insufflation of oxygen.

Tracheostomy

An emergency tracheostomy is required only rarely during management of maxillofacial injuries, but it is the procedure of choice when evidence of a serious laryngeal injury exists. Whenever possible, the airway should be controlled initially by endotracheal intubation performed over a flexible thin endoscope.

Cervical Spine Injuries

AXIOM All patients with maxillofacial trauma (especially those with neck pain, tenderness, muscle spasm, or any neurologic deficits) should be assumed to have cervical spine injury until proven otherwise.

Cervical spine injury is reported in up to 6% of patients with maxillofacial trauma (2). Injuries associated with mandibular fractures typically involve the first or second cervical vertebra, whereas middle or upper facial trauma is typically associated with injuries of the lower cervical spine (10).

AXIOM During endotracheal intubation, the head must be stabilized by another individual to reduce motion of the neck to a minimum.

Hemorrhage

Severe bleeding from facial lacerations can usually be controlled with digital pressure until the lacerated vessel is identified. Blind probing of facial wounds with surgical clamps should be discouraged because of the potential for damage to important nerves or ducts.

Bleeding into the walls of fractured sinuses may often be stopped by simple manual repositioning of the bone fragments or by intermaxillary fixation. Anterior packing of the nose with one-half-inch wide adaptic gauze moistened with a petroleum jelly–based ointment often stops mild-to-moderate bleeding from the nose or sinuses. Combined anterior and posterior nasal packing is occasionally necessary to control more severe or persistent (or both) posterior epistaxis.

Posterior packing can be performed by inserting a 16F or 18F Foley catheter with a 30-mL balloon passed through a nostril until its tip is seen in the pharynx. The balloon then is filled with air or water and pulled up gently against the choana. The balloon should be inflated only after the tip is seen in the pharynx because if it entered the cranial vault via a fracture of the cranial base and the balloon was then inflated, it could cause severe damage. Alternatively, a 4 × 4-inch antibiotic-impregnated gauze pad may be tied into a roll with heavy sutures; this pad is then tied to the tip of a nasally inserted Foley catheter that is withdrawn until the gauze is snugly secured against the posterior nasal opening into the pharynx. Anterior gauze is then packed up against the posterior pack.

If bleeding from an identified vessel is profuse, and radiologic intervention is not available or is not successful, surgical ligation of the feeding vessel is the treatment of choice. External carotid artery ligation alone is seldom effective because of the rich collateral circulation between the facial, maxillary, and lingual arteries. Ligation of the external carotid artery plus clipping of the anterior and posterior ethmoid arteries along the medial orbital wall is more likely to be successful (11).

AXIOM Angiography and embolization with absorbable gelatin sponge (Gelfoam) or other substances is the treatment of choice for nasal bleeding that persists in spite of repositioning of facial fractures and insertion of a posterior nasal pack.

Komiyama et al. (12) showed that intractable oronasal bleeding resulting from severe craniofacial injuries can be successfully treated with transarterial embolization by using Gelfoam pledgets, polyvinyl alcohol particles, or platinum coils.

ASSOCIATED INJURIES

The incidence of brain injury in patients with maxillofacial trauma after motor vehicle accidents (MVAs) varies from 15% to 48% (5). The risk of serious brain injury is particularly high in upper facial injuries.

The incidence of associated eye injuries in patients with maxillofacial fractures is extremely varied and ranges from 3% to 67% in large series; however, only 18% of these injuries are serious, and only 3% cause blindness (13).

Associated thoracoabdominal injuries, which are seen in 5% to 15% of patients seen in the emergency department with maxillofacial injuries (2,5), may increase the need for early endotracheal intubation.

DIAGNOSIS OF MAXILLOFACIAL INJURIES

History

The time and mechanism of the injury should be sought from the patient, emergency medical service (EMS), police, or any witnesses. The type and direction of the injuring forces frequently determines the pattern of facial bone injury. Symptoms, such as localized pain, tenderness, or crepitation, should make one suspect an underlying fracture even when no palpable deformity exists. Numbness or paralysis in the distribution of a specific nerve, facial asymmetry or deformity, or visual disturbance, should also suggest fracture.

AXIOM Malocclusion almost always indicates a fracture of the jaws or teeth.

Any history of drug use, excess alcohol ingestion, or loss of consciousness should be noted with respect to the diagnosis of occult central nervous system injury. The patient's dental history and any prior radiographs are important not only to document missing teeth and dentures but also as a guide for later reconstruction.

Physical Examination

Examination of the face during the secondary survey begins by checking all lacerations for foreign bodies. Lacerations of the scalp and face also should be carefully palpated and examined for any evidence of underlying fractures. All lacerations near an eye should be carefully screened for associated penetrating trauma to the globe.

The approximate position of Stensen's duct from the parotid gland is on a line drawn from the tragus to the middle upper lip. Where this line crosses the anterior border of the masseter is the position of its entrance into the oral cavity and also marks the location of the buccal branches of the facial nerve. Any lacerations in this area should lead to suspicion of a parotid duct laceration.

AXIOM Deep lacerations of the cheek, especially posteriorly, should be suspected of involving the parotid duct or branches of the facial nerve or both.

The major motor nerves of the face are the facial nerve, which supplies the facial muscles, and the motor branch of the trigeminal nerve, which supplies many of the muscles of mastication (masseter, temporalis, and the medial and lateral pterygoids). Injury to the motor branch of the trigeminal is rare, but facial nerve injuries are not uncommon and are easily missed.

The patient is inspected for facial asymmetry. Does the oral commissure droop on one side, indicating injury to the buccal branch of the facial nerve? Are the forehead wrinkles absent on one side, indicating injury to the temporal branch of the facial nerve? Patients are then asked to smile, show the teeth, wrinkle the forehead, and close the eyes. Inability to perform these maneuvers or asymmetry is strongly suggestive of facial nerve injury.

AXIOM Because most of the major sensory nerves of the face traverse facial bones, any area of hypesthesia or anesthesia should make one suspect an underlying fracture.

Although the mental nerve may be injured by deep chin lacerations, numbness of the lip or gum should make one suspect a mandibular fracture until proven otherwise. Similarly, the infraorbital nerve exits the maxilla after traversing the orbital floor and supplies the side of the nose, cheek, and upper lip. Numbness in those areas, although occasionally a result of a direct blow to the cheek, is frequently evidence of an orbital floor or maxillary fracture.

Examination of the Facial Bones

The bones of the face should be examined by very careful palpation for any step-offs, irregularities, or asymmetry. Facial edema can develop so rapidly that a severely depressed zygoma fracture may be quickly obscured; however, careful palpation generally reveals the asymmetry.

⊘ PITFALL

Reliance on radiographic evidence alone to diagnose facial fractures will lead to missed fractures that would have been easily detectable by physical examination.

By standing above the patient and looking down the facial axis, the examiner's index fingers can be stabilized on the supraorbital margin and then the middle fingers used to assess zygomatic depression on either side (2). Particularly noticeable are step-offs at fracture sites. With "tripod" fractures at the zygomaticofrontal, zygomaticomaxillary, and zygomaticotemporal sutures, step-offs usually are palpable at the upper lateral and lower orbital margins, and the zygomatic arch is depressed. The supraorbital margin and glabellar regions are palpated for frontal bone fractures. Point tenderness is usually present at fracture sites, but it is not always diagnostic. The nose is examined for asymmetry, and the nasal bones are palpated for depression.

⊘ PITFALL

Failure to ask and look for dental malocclusion can easily lead to missed maxillary or mandible fractures.

Additional testing involves grasping and pulling on the maxillary alveolus in several areas to determine whether the underlying bone moves. If an isolated segment of the maxilla can be moved from its position with the other bones, an alveolar fracture is present.

Nasoethmoid or nasoorbital fractures usually are seen as a depressed nasal dorsum, and if mistaken for a simple nasal fracture, the consequences could be disastrous. With nasoethmoid or nasoorbital fractures, the lacrimal bones also are usually fractured, and the medial canthi are displaced laterally, causing telecanthus.

Examination of the Ears

The ears are inspected for hematomas, which may need to be drained before they cause pressure necrosis of the adjacent ear cartilage, which can result in a "cauliflower ear." Blood in the middle ear cavity often indicates a basal skull fracture (2); however, bleeding also may occur from small wounds in the external auditory canal, which may occasionally be caused by condylar fractures and dislocations. One must also look carefully for a CSF leak (otorrhea).

AXIOM Bleeding from an ear after trauma should be considered the result of a basilar skull fracture until proven otherwise.

Examination of the Nose

The nasal bones are carefully palpated to assess for deformities. An endonasal examination also should be conducted to assess septal deviation and to detect the presence of a septal hematoma. If a septal hematoma is found, it should be drained promptly to prevent pressure necrosis of underlying cartilage.

With severe nasoethmoid fractures, a CSF leak is detected in approximately one third of patients within the first 24 hours of the injury. By 48 hours, a CSF leak is evident in more than half of patients (14). If a commercial paper reagent test identifies glucose in fluid draining from the nose, it is probably CSF.

AXIOM When bloody CSF is placed on filter paper, there will generally be a "bull's eye sign" with an outer clear ring caused by the CSF and an inner ring of blood with or without nasal fluid.

Examination of the Mouth

In the oral cavity, the locations of loose or missing teeth are documented (2). Lacerations of the tongue and floor of the mouth that have stopped bleeding can be easily overlooked and are often best palpated. Mandibular fractures are often compound into the mouth, either directly or via a tooth socket, where a small amount of bleeding may herald the presence of the fracture.

Radiologic Examinations

Plain Film Radiography

Equipment for airway management and other types of resuscitation should be provided during transport to radiology. Frequent monitoring of the level of consciousness and vital signs should be continued during the radiographic examinations. If available, a pulse oximeter should be used continuously to monitor arterial oxygen saturation.

A facial series includes views of the maxilla, zygoma, orbits, and frontal bone. The Water's view is usually included and is particularly useful for evaluating the zygoma, maxilla, and orbits. The symmetry of the zygomatic arches can often be best examined in a submentovertex view. For the mandible, a panorex, which shows the lower maxilla and mandible from condyle to condyle on one film, is most useful.

AXIOM Condyle fractures are missed easily and can cause considerable functional disability and deformity.

Computed Tomography

Computed tomography has replaced plain radiography for evaluating facial fractures in many centers, not only because it eliminates the problems of positioning, but also because of its ability to provide more detailed information. With sophisticated computer software, two-dimensional CT data can also be reformatted to create three-dimensional CT images (3-D CT).

TREATMENT

Soft-Tissue Facial Injuries

With proper use of ice-cold compresses, most contusions resolve within 24 to 72 hours. Small hematomas may be treated expectantly; however, large clots should be evacuated through incisions made along lines of relaxed skin tension (i.e., wrinkle lines).

AXIOM If a large hematoma is neglected, the surrounding tissue may form a thick capsule, while the center liquifies. Once this occurs, such a collection may require repeated aspirations, and contraction of the hematoma capsule can result in an unsightly depressed scar.

It is generally best to repair facial lacerations as soon as they are seen; however, the patient's condition may not allow this. When repair is delayed, an effort should be made to irrigate and cleanse the wound and cover it with a sterile dressing as soon as possible. Fortunately, because of the luxuriant blood flow to the face, most facial wounds, with the possible exception of human bites, may be safely closed up to 24 to 36 hours after injury.

For most injuries involving the skin and subcutaneous tissues, local anesthesia is the method of choice; however, general anesthesia in an operating room is preferred for very extensive injuries, uncooperative patients, or possible injuries of special structures, such as the facial nerve or parotid duct.

For local anesthesia on the face, 0.5% lidocaine (Xylocaine) with epinephrine is generally used. It has been suggested that epinephrine should not be used in the ear or the tip of the nose because of the possible detrimental effects of the excessive vasoconstriction that it can cause.

Wound Debridement

The skin around any open wound should be thoroughly cleaned and then the wound irrigated with copious amounts of sterile saline. Particularly dirty wounds should be irrigated with several liters of saline and scrubbed with moistened gauze. Pulsatile jet lavage can be very effective for removing hair, dirt, clothing, and other foreign matter from wounds. A mild cleaning agent, such as chlorohexidine (Hibaclens) or hexachlorophene (pHisoHex), is recommended for especially dirty wounds.

With severe injuries, some tissue may look marginally viable; however, the blood supply to the face is so good that it will usually survive. If excess tissue is debrided, a good cosmetic repair may be extremely difficult to achieve.

Most dog bites of the face can be closed after they are thoroughly cleaned and debrided. Human bites are almost never closed primarily. These should be cleansed, debrided, and dressed. After proper wound care and antibiotics for 3 to 4 days, they can usually be closed secondarily.

"Road burns" with traumatic tattooing caused by asphalt, tar, or dirt embedded in the abrasions can cause permanent pigmentation of the skin. Removing debris embedded in the skin requires adequate local or general anesthesia. A sterile scrub brush can be very helpful for removing these particles. If the particles are deeply imbedded, they may be picked out with a No. 11 blade.

Repair of Lacerations

Ideally, the edges of lacerations should be debrided of injured tissue until the wound edge is perpendicular to the skin surface. In most cases, this means an elliptical excision of the wound.

AXIOM Skin closures should be parallel to the natural skin creases (relaxed skin tension lines) whenever possible.

Absorbable subcutaneous and dermal sutures are initially placed to line up the edges on the skin closure. These sutures should be placed in a buried, simple fashion so that the knots will not be close to the epidermis. The skin is then closed with a fine, nonabsorbable, nonreactive suture.

Skin wounds should be repaired with a slight eversion whenever possible because a perfectly flat repair will become depressed when the inevitable scar contraction occurs. Depressed scars look worse because the irregularity causes harsh shadows to appear, making the scar more noticeable.

Special Areas

Lips

With lacerations through the cutaneous vermilion border of the lips, the first suture should be placed at this boundary precisely to line up the skin and vermilion so that there is a smooth, continuous line throughout the border (Fig. 13-4). After this key suture is placed, the deeper sutures can be placed. It is especially important that the orbicularis oris muscle continuity be restored with deep sutures. For nasal-rim lacerations, the key suture is placed at the lower border of the alar rim to ensure a continuous, smooth line without notching.

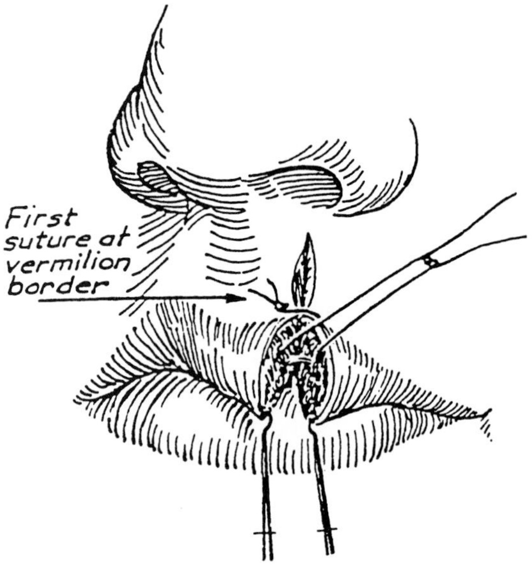

FIG. 13-4. Repair of vertical lacerations of the vermilion–cutaneous margin. The suture should be used to approximate the vermilion–cutaneous border. This will avoid conspicuous irregularity of this portion of the lip after healing. From ref. 19, with permission.

External Ear

The key suture for repair of the helix of the external ear is placed at the outer rim to prevent notching. The underlying cartilage must also be carefully approximated for optimal results.

Eyelid

A full-thickness laceration through an eyelid requires meticulous technique. The key suture is placed through the ciliary margin at the "gray line," which is the border of the tarsus and orbicularis. Two additional sutures are then placed, first through the tarsus and then through the orbicularis muscle at the ciliary margin. Once the lid margin is repaired, the orbicularis muscle and skin are closed in layers. No conjunctival repair is necessary.

AXIOM Lacerations at the medial lid margin should be inspected very carefully for a canalicular injury.

Parotid Duct

A transected parotid duct should be repaired in the operating room. The buccal branches of the facial nerve also are often involved and should be explored and repaired as necessary. The duct is repaired over a stent that is brought out through the buccal opening.

Facial Nerve

It is easiest to repair facial nerve lacerations at the time of injury in the operating room by using a microscope and microsurgical monofilament suture; however, if microsurgical expertise is not available, the wound should be closed and the patient referred to a plastic surgeon. Nerve repairs done within 2 to 3 weeks of injury generally provide the same results as early repair.

Facial Fractures

There has been a virtual revolution in the treatment of facial fractures after the introduction and application of craniofacial surgery begun by Paul Tessier more than 20 years ago. Within the past decade, techniques using wide, direct exposure of fracture sites combined with rigid miniplate fixation and immediate cranial bone grafting have made the most complex facial fractures amenable to primary repair. This obviates the need for extremely difficult secondary reconstruction with its usual inferior results.

Contemporary facial fracture repair (1,5) is characterized by

1. Precise preoperative imaging of fractures;
2. Precise preoperative plans of bony reconstruction;
3. Early one-stage repair whenever possible;
4. Adequate exposure of all fractures, by using "degloving" of the entire facial skeleton as necessary;
5. Precise reduction of all fractures in three dimensions by using immediate bone grafts as needed; and
6. Rigid interosseous fixation, particularly with self-tapping miniplates.

These advances, however, have not supplanted two basic principles of facial bone repair.

1. Teeth must be returned to their normal occlusal relation; and
2. The repair proceeds from an unbroken or a stabilized segment to an adjacent fracture fragment, which is reduced and then rigidly fixed to the adjacent stable bone.

In this way, multiple fractures are repaired in a stepwise fashion, each fixed segment being used to align and stabilize the next.

AXIOM If a plastic surgeon with craniofacial capabilities is not present, one has 7 to 10 days to transfer the patient with severe facial fractures for proper primary treatment.

Mandible Fractures

⊘ PITFALL

Failure to reduce a mandible to a proper occlusal relation can cause severe functional problems with the jaws.

A stable mandible fracture may be managed in a closed fashion by bringing the teeth into centric occlusion and then holding the mandible in place with arch bars or interdental wiring.

Unstable mandible fractures that must be opened are approached through lower labial buccal sulcus incisions for fractures of the symphysis and body. Oral or cutaneous incisions are used for fractures of the angle and ramus. If an external incision is used, care should be taken to avoid injuring the marginal mandibular branch of the facial nerve. An intraoral approach avoids this risk, but reducing the fragments with this approach can be very difficult without special maxillofacial instruments. Fixation of these fractures classically consists of simple wiring of the fragments together, combined with intermaxillary fixation.

Mandible fractures also can be treated by fixation with special miniplates and screws (15). This can provide rigid, stable fixation, and intermaxillary fixation can be avoided. It is critically important that the patient's pretraumatic dental occlusion be reestablished first with interdental fixation.

PITFALL

Failure to obtain centric occlusion with intermaxillary fixation before fixation of the remaining fragments can result in severe malocclusion.

The depressor group of muscles tends to cause lingual displacement of parasymphyseal fracture fragments, even in the presence of intermaxillary fixation. A simple approach is rigid-plate fixation through a lower labial–buccal sulcus incision. After proper plate fixation, arch bars can be applied.

Proper occlusion of a fractured edentulous mandible is reestablished by using intermaxillary fixation to maintain the position of the patient's dentures, when they are available. When dentures are not available, appropriate splints are fabricated and secured to the maxilla and mandible by using wires. Centric occlusion is then established, and intermaxillary fixation is achieved. Another approach places the maxilla and mandible into approximate occlusion, reduces the fracture fragments, and then fixates them with rigid miniplates.

In instances of gunshot or shotgun wounds with severe soft-tissue damage or deficiencies, in which infection is much more likely, the use of an external fixation device can be extremely helpful. Centric occlusion is reestablished first, and then soft-tissue and oral-lining deficiencies can be addressed with appropriate flaps. Once this is accomplished and the external fixator is applied, mandibular bone grafting and rigid fixation can be undertaken later as needed.

Maxillary Fractures

AXIOM All LeFort fractures should be explored and accurately reduced under direct vision.

For LeFort I fractures, the teeth are placed into centric occlusion, and the fractures are fixed with miniplates across the buttresses. After proper centric occlusion has been established, only the maxillary arch bar is needed to keep the segment in position, and a soft diet is prescribed for 4 weeks. With very unstable alveolar segments or with noncompliant patients, complete intermaxillary fixation is maintained for 4 weeks.

For LeFort II and III fractures, incisions are made in the lower lids to explore the zygomatic–maxillary sutures, orbital floor, and medial orbital wall. In LeFort III fractures, an additional coronal incision is made in the anterior scalp, and the upper face is degloved to expose the nasofrontal region and the zygomatic arch. In this way, the displaced segments can be reduced into exact anatomic position and secured with miniplates under direct vision.

PITFALL

Failure to recognize and properly treat a comminuted maxillary fracture may lead to a shortened face, which can be extremely difficult to correct secondarily.

Zygomatic Fractures

The zygomatic arch usually fractures in at least two locations and becomes depressed. Unlike most facial fractures, the arch can simply be elevated into position, and it generally does not need internal fixation. With tripod fractures, however, the fragments require fixation. Because tripod fractures also include an orbital floor fracture, the floor of the orbit is routinely explored through the lower lid incision while the zygoma is being reduced.

Orbital Floor Fractures

Enophthalmos or impaired eye motion is a clear indication for operative reduction of orbital fractures. Small floor fractures without limitation of upward gaze, enophthalmos, or inferior displacement of the globe or herniation on CT can be treated without surgery; however, the patient should be monitored closely to detect any delayed enophthalmos or eye-muscle trapping.

Nasal Fractures

Reduction of displaced nasal bones is done by using Ashe forceps under local anesthesia. Unfortunately, the edema that usually develops very rapidly can make judging the adequacy of the reduction extremely difficult, and a secondary reduction is not infrequently necessary for residual deformity. A plaster or preformed splint is then applied for 1 week.

AXIOM Careful follow-up of patients with closed reduction of nasal fractures is important to detect significant residual bony or septal deformities.

Frontonasoethmoid Fractures

Significant sequelae of frontonasoethmoid fractures include

1. Traumatic telecanthus;
2. Ocular injuries;
3. CSF rhinorrhea;
4. Injury to the nasolacrimal apparatus; and
5. Depressed nasal dorsum with inward telescoping of the nose.

Disruption of the nasolacrimal apparatus may occur from direct injury or from impingement by fracture fragments. A "saddle nose" may result from comminution of the nasal dorsum or the loss of dorsal support plus elevation of the nasal tip. CSF rhinorrhea may result from fractures extending into the base of the skull at the cribriform plate.

Nasoethmoid fractures should be accurately reduced under direct vision, preferably through a coronal-degloving scalp and face incision. Bone grafts are then used to restore dorsal projection and nasal length. After this, bilateral medial canthoplasties are performed, and the medial walls of the orbit are bone grafted as needed.

AXIOM A CSF leak is no reason to postpone treatment of facial fractures. In fact, accurate reduction of the fracture fragments may stop the leak.

Surgery for persistent CSF leaks involves patching the fistulous tract with a fascia lata or other material graft (14). This procedure is performed via either a craniotomy or a transethmoid/sphenoid approach.

Frontal Sinus Fractures

Fractures involving only the anterior table are treated if they are displaced. The segments are reduced through a coronal incision or through associated facial lacerations and wired in place.

Fractures involving the anterior and posterior tables of the frontal sinus are explored. Significant posterior table fractures may lead to CSF rhinorrhea because of dural injury, and neurosurgical support should be readily available. If the sinus mucosa is severely injured, it is completely stripped from the sinus cavity, and the sinus is obliterated with outer table cranial grafts.

Panfacial Fractures

A systematic approach to reducing and fixing panfacial fractures is essential. First, the mandibular fractures are reduced and fixed. Next, the maxilla is related to the mandible with intermaxillary fixation. The maxilla is then bone grafted and fixated as necessary. The zygoma is then fixated, paying particular attention to the preservation of facial volume at the zygomatic arches. The orbital floor and walls are then bone grafted, and the nasoethmoid and frontal sinuses are repaired.

POSTOPERATIVE CARE

Airway

The airway is rarely a serious problem after reduction and fixation of facial fractures, particularly with the use of rigid plate fixation, which makes intermaxillary fixation unnecessary. Nevertheless, the endotracheal tube should be left in place at the conclusion of surgery while soft-tissue swelling is evaluated, airway reflexes return, and the patient recovers fully from the anesthetic (2).

AXIOM If intermaxillary fixation is used, a wire cutter should be attached to the patient's wires so that the wires can be rapidly cut if an airway obstruction develops because of blood clots, vomitus, laryngeal spasm, or soft-tissue intrusion.

Infections

Fractures of the mandibular angle, body, or parasymphyseal region appear to have a higher infection rate than zygomatic and maxillary fractures, especially when they are open fractures and involve the teeth (2,16). Prophylactic use of cefazolin, 1 g i.v., 1 hour before surgery, and a similar dose 8 hours later, has been shown to diminish the incidence of postoperative infections in facial fractures during elective definitive surgery (16).

Wound infections with collections of pus are drained as needed. Osteomyelitis is uncommon but, when present, usually involves mandibular fractures. This may require debridement of involved bone, removal of hardware, and the application of an external-fixation device.

Extension of infection into the fascial planes of the head and neck a few days after a facial fracture may jeopardize the airway and are characteristically caused by combinations of aerobic and anaerobic mouth organisms (17). These infections can usually be adequately treated with 400,000 units of aqueous penicillin G every 4 hours for several days plus wide drainage of the abscess. Further antibiotic therapy depends on the condition of the patient and the sensitivities of the specific organisms involved.

Tracheal intubation to secure the airway for abscess drainage is performed under direct vision by using a fiberoptic bronchoscope with the patient sedated and awake (2). Preoperative CT scans of the face and neck can help to determine the degree of airway encroachment.

AXIOM A coniotomy or tracheostomy under local anesthesia without attempts at endotracheal intubation is indicated if the patient's clinical condition or a CT scan reveals severe airway compromise.

The possibility of infective endocarditis after elective dental procedures, in patients with valvular heart disease or prosthetic cardiac valves, has led to the development of an antibiotic prophylaxis protocol by the Committee on Rheumatic Fever and Infective Endocarditis of the American Heart Association (18).

FACIAL FRACTURES IN CHILDREN

AXIOM In pediatric patients, the impact of severe trauma on subsequent facial growth must be carefully monitored, and the patient and the family must be made aware of the possible need for later reconstructive surgery.

Diagnosis and treatment of maxillofacial injuries in children can be extremely difficult (2). The apprehension of the child may make a good physical examination extremely difficult. Complaints, such as pain and malocclusion, also may be difficult for children to express. Obtaining the patient's cooperation for proper radiographic studies also may be a problem. The complex anatomy of the small pediatric mandible, which contains multiple tooth buds and a relatively small amount of cortical bone, also makes interpretation difficult. Thus CT scanning can be invaluable for evaluating both mandibular and maxillary fractures in this age group.

The treatment principles of maxillofacial injury in pediatric patients differ somewhat from those for adults (2). Intermaxillary fixation is maintained for a shorter time than that in adults. The dentition of many pediatric patients also is often not appropriate for application of arch bars and interdental wire fixation. Deciduous teeth, mixed dentition, and small permanent teeth make such treatment difficult. Therefore, open reduction with internal fixation under general anesthesia shortly after injury is considered the treatment of choice by many surgeons.

⊘ FREQUENT ERRORS

1. ***Delay in the treatment of life- or limb-threatening injuries because of distraction by dramatic facial injuries.***
2. ***Blind clamping of bleeding vessels deep in facial lacerations.***
3. ***Missing facial fractures by relying primarily on radiographic examinations.***
4. ***Failure to notice a facial nerve injury because facial edema limits movement on the unaffected side.***
5. ***Failure to look carefully for a parotid duct or facial nerve injury in cheek lacerations.***
6. ***Missing fractures of the maxilla or mandible because of failure to check dental occlusion.***
7. ***Missing an orbital fracture because of failure to look for orbital asymmetry.***
8. ***Missing a condyle fracture of the mandible by relying only on physical examination or inadequate radiographs or both.***
9. ***Failure to slightly evert skin edges during repair of facial lacerations.***
10. ***Failure to obtain centric occlusion before fixating fractures of the maxilla and mandible.***
11. ***Failure to identify and treat the full extent of orbital-floor fractures.***
12. ***Failure to treat complex facial fractures with adequate exposure, primary bone grafts, and rigid fixation.***

SUMMARY POINTS

1. If a mandible has one fracture line, one must look carefully for other fractures that may not be readily apparent on standard radiography.

2. Associated basal skull fractures are not uncommon in LeFort II and III fractures and should be ruled out before embarking on airway manipulation via the nasal route.

3. One should look carefully for CSF rhinorrhea or airway obstruction or both in patients with LeFort III fractures.

4. A nasoethmoid fracture should be suspected in patients with bilateral periorbital ecchymosis (spectacle hematomas or raccoon eyes).

5. With facial fractures, associated injuries of the cervical spine and brain must be suspected when attempting airway management techniques.

6. Patients with severe facial injuries who are hemodynamically stable and who have had their spine cleared or immobilized should be allowed to sit up if they can breathe more effectively and comfortably in that position.

7. All patients with facial trauma should have the mouth carefully examined for blood clots, foreign bodies, vomitus, and loose teeth or dentures.
8. Paralyzing a patient to insert an endotracheal tube may be rapidly fatal if intubation or provision of a surgical airway cannot be accomplished promptly.
9. Nasal tubes are generally contraindicated in patients with midface fractures because they may involve the base of the skull.
10. One should always be prepared to perform an emergency cricothyroidotomy in adults with severe facial injuries because attempts at endotracheal intubation may fail or may completely occlude a partially obstructed airway.
11. All patients with maxillofacial trauma (especially those with neck pain, tenderness, spasm, or any peripheral neurologic deficit) should be assumed to have a cervical spine injury until proven otherwise.
12. Angiography and embolization with Gelfoam or other substances is the treatment of choice for persistent nasal bleeding in spite of repositioning of fractures and insertion of a posterior nasal pack.
13. Malocclusion indicates a fracture of the jaws or teeth until ruled out by careful, complete examination and radiologic studies.
14. Before careful examination of the face, the patient should be positioned so that the light is centered on the midline to avoid visual distortion of facial symmetry.
15. Deep lacerations of the cheek, especially posteriorly, should be suspected of involving the parotid duct or buccal branches of the facial nerve or both.
16. Because most of the major sensory nerves of the face traverse facial bones, any area of hypesthesia or anesthesia should make one suspect an underlying fracture.
17. The most accurate method for determining the presence of facial fractures (except for CT) is careful palpation of bony landmarks (looking for step-offs, irregularities, or asymmetry).
18. Bleeding from an ear after trauma should be considered the result of a basilar skull fracture until proven otherwise.
19. When bloody CSF is placed on filter paper, there will be an outer clear ring caused by the CSF and an inner ring of blood with or without nasal fluid.
20. Condyle fractures are missed easily clinically and on facial films, and they can cause considerable functional disability.
21. CT is now the radiographic method of choice for the diagnosis and operative planning of facial fractures.
22. In all facial soft-tissue injuries, wound debridement should be conservative.
23. Skin closures should be parallel to the natural skin creases (relaxed skin-tension lines) whenever possible.
24. If a plastic surgeon with craniofacial capabilities is not present, one has 7 to 10 days to transfer the patient with severe facial fractures for proper primary treatment.
25. Nasoethmoid fractures should be accurately reduced under direct vision, preferably through a coronal-degloving scalp and face incision.
26. A CSF leak is no reason to postpone treatment of facial fractures. In fact, accurate reduction of facial fractures tends to stop the leak.
27. The best chance of providing an excellent result with facial fractures is during the initial reduction and fixation.
28. In pediatric patients, the impact of severe trauma on subsequent facial growth must be carefully monitored, and the patient and family must be made aware of the possible need for later reconstructive surgery.
29. If intermaxillary fixation is used, a wire cutter should be attached to the patient's wires in case of airway obstruction caused by blood clot or vomitus, laryngeal spasm, or soft-tissue intrusion on the airway.
30. A coniotomy or tracheostomy under local anesthesia without attempts at endotracheal intubation is indicated when the patient's clinical condition or CT scans reveal severe airway compromise.

REFERENCES

1. Sullivan WG. Trauma to the face. In: Wilson RF, Walt AJ, eds. *Management of trauma: pitfalls and practice*. 2nd ed. Philadelphia: Williams & Wilkins, 1996:242.

2. Capan LM, Miller SM, Olickman R. Management of facial injuries. In: Capan LM, Miller SM, Turndorf H, eds. *Trauma: anesthesia and intensive care*. New York: JB Lippincott, 1991:385–408.
3. Bucholz RW, Burkhead WZ, Graham W, Petty C. Occult cervical spine injuries in fatal traffic accidents. *J Trauma* 1979;19:768.
4. Lee KF, Wagner LK, Lee YE, et al. The impact-absorbing effects of facial fractures in closed-head injuries. *J Neurosurg* 1987;66:542.
5. Busuito MJ, Smith DJ, Robson MC. Mandibular fractures in an urban trauma center. *J Trauma* 1986;26:826.
6. Olson RA, Fonseca RJ, Zeitter DL, et al. Fractures of the mandible: a review of 580 cases. *J Oral Maxillofac Surg* 1982;40:23.
7. Edgerton MT, Kenney JG. Emergency care of maxillofacial and otological injuries. In: Zuidema GD, Rutherford RB, Ballinger WF, eds. *The management of trauma*. 4th ed. Philadelphia: WB Saunders, 1985:275.
8. Manson PN. Maxillofacial injuries. In: Siegel JH, ed. *Trauma: emergency and critical care.* New York: Churchill Livingstone, 1987:983.
9. Haug RH, Adams JM, Conforti PJ, Likavec MJ. Cranial fractures associated with facial fractures: a review of mechanism, type, and severity of injury. *J Oral Maxillofac Surg* 1994;52:729.
10. Lewis VL, Manson PN, Morgan RF, et al. Facial injuries associated with cervical fractures: recognition patterns and management. *J Trauma* 1985;25:90.
11. Hassard AD, Kirkpatrick DA, Wong FS. Ligation of the external carotid and anterior ethmoidal arteries for severe or unusual epistaxis resulting from facial fractures. *Can J Surg* 1986;29:447.
12. Komiyama M, Nishikawa M, Kan M, et al. Endovascular treatment of intractable oronasal bleeding associated with severe craniofacial injury. *J Trauma* 1998;44:330.
13. Holt JE, Holt R, Blodgett JM. Ocular injuries sustained during blunt facial trauma. *Ophthalmology* 1983;90:14.
14. Westmore GA, Whittman DE. Cerebrospinal fluid rhinorrhoea and its management. *Br J Surg* 1982;69:489.
15. Touvinen V, Norholt SE, Sindet-Pedersen S, Jensen J. A retrospective analysis of 279 patients with isolated mandibular fractures treated with titanium miniplates. *J Oral Maxillofac Surg* 1994;52:931.
16. Chole RA, Yee J. Antibiotic prophylaxis for facial fractures: a prospective, randomized clinical trial. *Head Neck Surg* 1987;113:1055.
17. Schroeder DC, Sarha ED, Hendricksson DA, Healey KM. Severe infections of the head and neck resulting from gas forming organisms: report of case. *JADA* 1987;114:65.
18. Shulman ST, Amren DP, Bisno AL, et al. Prevention of bacterial endocarditis: a statement for health professionals by the Committee on Rheumatic Fever and Infective Endocarditis of the Council on Cardiovascular Disease in the Young. *Circulation* 1984;70:1123A.
19. Converse JM. *Kazanjian and Converse's surgical treatment of facial injuries.* Baltimore: Williams & Wilkins, 1974:697.

14. INJURIES TO THE NECK[1]

ANATOMY

The sternocleidomastoid (SCM) muscle divides the neck into the anterior and posterior triangles. The anterior triangle of the neck, bounded by the SCM, the midline, and the mandible, contains most of the major vascular and visceral structures, including the airway. It, in turn, is divided into the muscular triangle below the omohyoid, the submaxillary triangle above the digastric muscle, and the carotid triangle between them. The posterior triangle, which is bounded by the SCM, the trapezius, and the clavicle, has relatively few important structures except in the supraclavicular triangle just above the clavicle (Fig. 14-1).

Zone I of the neck, often referred to as the thoracic inlet or outlet, is usually described as the area below the cricoid cartilage. Zone II is the midarea of the neck, and it extends from the cricoid cartilage to the angle of the mandible. This is the most frequent site of penetrating neck trauma, and injuries in this area are relatively easy to expose and repair. Zone III is located above the angle of the mandible. Vascular injuries high in zone III involving the upper portions of the internal carotid or vertebral arteries can be difficult to expose and treat surgically; they should be managed with interventional radiologic techniques whenever possible (Fig. 14-2).

AXIOM In stable patients with penetrating neck injuries, arteriography is important for evaluating injuries in zones I and III.

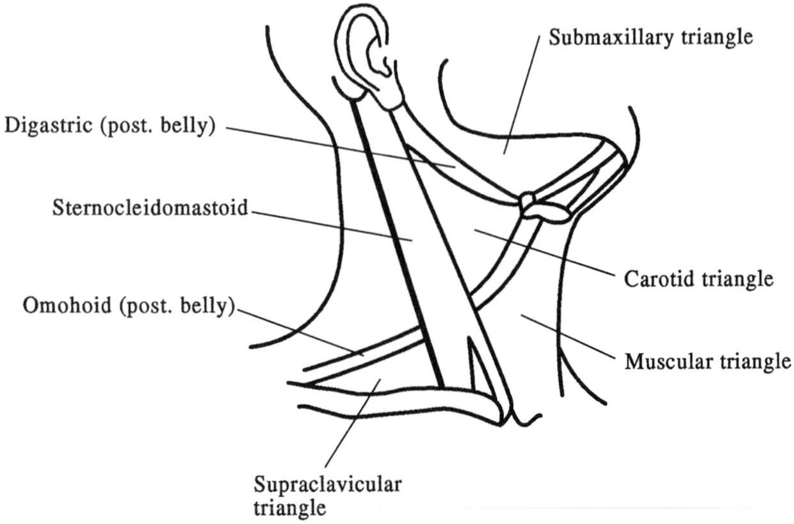

FIG. 14-1. The anterior triangles of the neck lie between the sternocleidomastoid muscles (SCM) and the mandible. It, in turn, is divided into the carotid triangle formed by the SCM, posterior belly of the digastric muscles, and the omohyoid. In the posterior triangle of the neck, most of the important structures lie below the posterior belly of the omohyoid muscle.

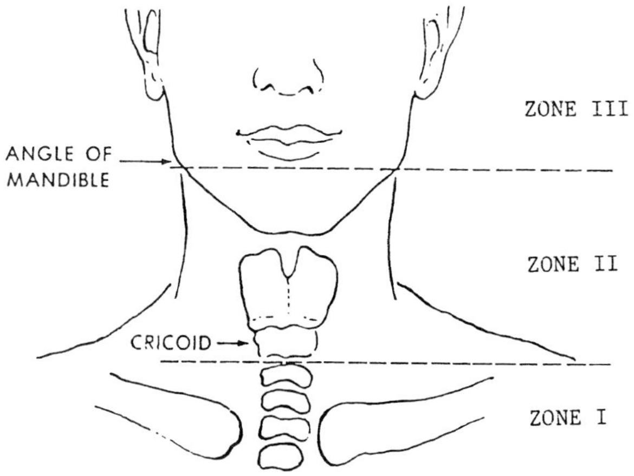

FIG. 14-2. Regions of the neck. (From Roon AJ, Christensen N. Evaluation and treatment of penetrating cervical injuries. *J Trauma* 1979;19:391.)

TYPES OF INJURY

Penetrating Trauma

The approximate incidence of organ injuries with penetrating neck trauma are

Major veins—15% to 25%
Major arteries—10% to 15%
Pharynx or esophagus—5% to 15%
Larynx or trachea—4% to 12%
Major nerves—3% to 8% (2)

Approximately 40% of penetrating neck wounds do not involve an important structure.

Gunshot wounds (GSWs), in addition to directly injuring or tearing structures, may produce shock waves that can devitalize tissue, resulting in later necrosis and leakage. This is especially true with high-velocity missiles (greater than 2,000 to 2,500 feet per second), which are characteristic of military weapons or hunting rifles.

AXIOM All GSWs of the neck should be surgically explored, especially if they cross the midline.

Blunt Trauma

AXIOM Patients with blunt head or neck trauma should have their neck immobilized in the neutral position until radiography or careful examination have eliminated cervical spine fracture or dislocation.

Although neurologic abnormalities seen with cervical spine injuries are usually caused by direct trauma to the spinal cord or brachial plexus, associated vascular injuries with hypotension can make the neurologic picture much worse.

DIAGNOSIS

History

Many significant injuries in the neck are asymptomatic, and diagnosis of an esophageal injury may be particularly difficult. In the series by Weigelt et al., 3 of 10 patients with esophageal trauma had no preoperative signs or symptoms of injury (3). In addition, of 98 other patients with neck trauma without esophageal injury, 25% had symptoms and 26% had signs suggesting such an injury.

AXIOM Esophageal injuries in the neck are particularly difficult to detect or rule out without radiologic and endoscopic support.

With blunt injury to the internal carotid artery (ICA), the time between the injury and appearance of symptoms is variable, occasionally exceeding 2 weeks. Patients with laryngeal trauma frequently complain of neck pain or voice change. Occasionally, they may also have hemoptysis or shortness of breath. Injury to the food passages is suggested by dysphagia or odynophagia.

AXIOM Physical examination of an injured neck is often deceptively negative despite severe underlying injuries to major vessels or the aerodigestive system.

Specific Blunt Trauma Injuries

Cervical Spine

When patients are not completely awake and alert, especially following blunt trauma, one should assume that a cervical spine injury is present until it has been eliminated by appropriate clinical and radiologic examinations.

Vascular Injuries

The patient must be carefully examined for hematomas, a bruit or a thrill, or a peripheral pulse deficit. Other clinical signs suggesting carotid arterial injury include Horner's syndrome, limb paresis or paralysis, or deep coma. These changes may be delayed for up to several days, especially after blunt trauma. Serious vascular injuries in the neck after blunt trauma frequently occur without any overt hematoma formation. Even at exploration, a small subadventitial hematoma may be the only indication of a severe underlying injury.

Hypotensive patients are much more likely to have neurologic symptoms or signs after neck trauma, but these clinical findings may be due largely to impaired central nervous system (CNS) perfusion rather than to direct brain damage.

⊘ PITFALL

Failure to consider an occult, blunt carotid artery injury as a cause of neurologic changes, especially when the brain computed tomography (CT) scan is negative and CNS changes are delayed.

With a possible vascular injury of the neck, one should defer insertion of the nasogastric tube until the patient is anesthetized in surgery; otherwise, a clot at a major vascular injury could be dislodged, and massive bleeding could resume if the patient gags excessively as the tube is being inserted.

Many surgeons have found a poor correlation between clinical signs and symptoms and the presence of an arterial injury. Carducci et al., found that almost one-third of patients with major blood vessel trauma had no signs or symptoms of such injury, particularly when only a major vein was involved (4). Fogelman and Stewart, reporting on 100 consecutive penetrating neck injuries, noted that 43% of patients with vascular injuries were hemodynamically stable, and 70% had no signs of bleeding (5).

Injuries to the Aerodigestive Tract

Injuries to the upper aerodigestive tract may be indicated by subcutaneous emphysema, coughing, or hematemesis. In the series by Weigelt et al., however, 30% of patients with esophageal injury had no clinical signs or symptoms of such a problem (3). Sankaran and Walt emphasized that an important cause of death after penetrating neck wounds is delayed recognition and treatment of esophageal injuries (6).

AXIOM Suspected airway injuries in the neck should be managed emergently in the operating room, especially if there is any evidence that blood is being aspirated into the tracheobronchial tree.

Neurologic Injuries

The neurologic examination for injuries to the neck should include an evaluation of the patient's mental status, cranial nerves, spinal cord, brachial plexus, and sympathetic nerves.

Traumatic Asphyxia

Traumatic asphyxia refers to sudden, severe compression of the chest causing inability to breathe (which is transient in survivors) plus high-grade obstruction of venous return with extravasation of venous and capillary blood into the tissues drained by the superior vena cava. This results in marked violaceous discoloration of the skin of the upper chest, neck, arms, and face, which usually persists for at least several days. Any neurologic changes seen are usually transient.

Laboratory Evaluation

With the exception of a complete blood cell count and type-and-crossmatch, there is usually little need for other routine laboratory tests in previously healthy individuals; however, in patients with liver disease, severe brain injury, or prolonged shock, a prothrombin time, partial thromboplastin time, and platelet count are indicated.

Further Investigation Versus Immediate Surgery

When the patient has been resuscitated and stabilized and the history and physical examination are complete, the surgeon must decide whether to operate promptly, perform more diagnostic tests, or just observe the patient. No disagreement exists about the need for immediate surgery on patients who are hemodynamically unstable or who have had severe hemorrhage or an expanding hematoma. Patients who are hemodynamically stable may undergo further diagnostic evaluations, which may include plain radiographs, contrast swallows, CT scans, arteriography, laryngoscopy, bronchoscopy, or esophagoscopy.

Even when the patient with a zone II injury is stable and there is no apparent vascular or aerodigestive injury, some authors advocate surgical exploration without routine angiography. In contrast, other authors use angiography and other studies routinely to reduce the number of unnecessary surgical explorations (7,8).

⊘ PITFALL

When the need for surgical exploration of a penetrating injury in zone II is obvious, further diagnostic studies tend to delay surgery and increase the chances of severe bleeding, aspiration, or CNS deterioration.

Radiography

AXIOM Lateral radiographs of the neck are indicated in all patients who have had penetrating injuries or severe blunt trauma of the neck.

Lateral radiography of the cervical spine should be obtained in all cases of severe blunt trauma, especially if the head, neck, or upper chest is involved. Anteroposterior and lateral plain films of the neck may reveal subcutaneous emphysema, airway compression, injury to laryngeal structures (especially those that are calcified), tracheal deviation, cervical spine injury, and increased thickness of the anterior paravertebral tissues caused by bleeding or edema. Free air in the neck, particularly in the deep perivisceral spaces, is usually due to an injury to the hypopharynx, but may also be due to an esophageal, laryngeal, or tracheal tear.

AXIOM Increased prevertebral space behind the upper airway is usually due to injuries to the aerodigestive tract.

Increased space between the posterior margin of the upper airway and the anterior border of the vertebral bodies can be helpful. Normally, this distance is less than 4 mm in front of C-3 and C-4 and less than 10 mm in front of C-5, C-6, and C-7. Increased space in this area after trauma is usually due to blood from an adjacent injury, and after 48 to 72 hours, it is often caused by infection.

With blunt trauma to the neck, the first two ribs should be inspected carefully on the radiographs for fracture because such injuries may be associated with an increased incidence of tracheobronchial, myocardial, or vascular injury. Chest radiography is particularly important with penetrating injuries in zone I because of possible associated thoracic injuries, especially hemopneumothorax.

Duplex Scans

Duplex (ultrasonographic) scans can be used to diagnose extracranial carotid arterial disease, including dissections. Color Doppler sonography can be as accurate as angiography in screening clinically stable patients with zone II injuries and no signs of active bleeding (9); however, results are operator dependent.

Arteriography

AXIOM Four-vessel angiography should be performed on all stable patients with suspected penetrating vascular injuries in zones I and III of the neck.

The general indications for angiography in patients with neck trauma are

1. Proximity of injury to the carotid artery, with or without hematoma;
2. Shotgun blasts in which multiple arterial segments may be injured;
3. Precise localization of injury in patients with probable or possible proximal common or high internal carotid injuries to allow planning of appropriate incisions and exposure;
4. Blunt trauma with extensive soft-tissue injury in the neck; and
5. Blunt trauma with neurologic deficits unexplained by CT.

One of the advantages of preoperative angiography is the establishment of a "road map" for the approach to the carotid artery. Angiography also allows one to evaluate the collateral circulation. Although it is widely believed that good crossover circulation exists in most patients through the circle of Willis, only about 20% of individuals actually have complete circles (2,8). Furthermore, many patients have one or more developmental abnormalities that can restrict the effectiveness of the collateral circulation of this vascular ring. In addition, unilateral hypoplastic vertebral arteries are present in approximately 15% of patients (10).

AXIOM Any neck exploration for trauma should include close examination of the vascular and aerodigestive structures, even if preoperative arteriography and other studies do not reveal injuries.

Contrast Swallows

A high index of suspicion for pharyngoesophageal injuries should be maintained in patients with penetrating neck trauma because they are easily missed clinically, radiologically, and endoscopically, and a delay in diagnosis may be associated with a great increase in morbidity and mortality rate (6,8). Extravasation of swallowed contrast material is diagnostic of a pharyngeal or esophageal leak; however, a negative contrast swallow is not reliable, particularly in the neck and especially when done with Gastrografin. Up to 50% of esophageal leaks may be missed on Gastrografin swallows. Even with careful barium studies, up to 25% of esophageal leaks can be missed.

AXIOM If a patient with suspected esophageal injury has a negative Gastrografin swallow, the study should be immediately repeated with barium or an esophagoscopy should be performed.

Some controversy exists as to whether the initial contrast swallow should be done with barium or meglumine diatrizoate (Gastrografin). Gastrografin is used by many physicians because, if a leak is present, the extravasated contrast material is less likely to increase the severity of the inflammatory response and risk of infection; however, if the patient does not have a good cough and gag reflex and Gastrografin is aspirated into the lungs, severe chemical pneumonitis frequently develops. Barium, conversely, is less irritating to the lungs if it is aspirated, and the incidence of false-negative examinations is usually lower.

AXIOM Barium can cause increased inflammation and infection if it enters the mediastinum, but Gastrografin can cause severe pneumonitis if it is aspirated into the lungs.

Computed Tomography Scans

CT scans can clearly demonstrate most laryngeal and associated soft-tissue injuries. This is a particularly important study before surgery on the larynx.

AXIOM Clinically subtle injuries to laryngeal cartilages can usually be demonstrated clearly on CT.

Some patients have peripheral neurologic deficits but no obvious spine injuries. In such patients, CT may demonstrate occult cervical spine fractures, epidural hematomas, or a partially transected spinal cord.

AXIOM Proper CT scanning requires a cooperative patient and should not be attempted in a patient with an unprotected airway injury or unstable vital signs.

Magnetic Resonance Imaging

Magnetic resonance imaging (MRI) can display most of the information provided by CT scans, but with better definition of soft-tissue and vascular injuries; however, the inability of MRI to reliably identify bone injuries and the constraints of its physical setup limit its use in critically injured patients.

Endoscopy

Larynx and Trachea

Endoscopy for a possibly injured larynx should be performed in the operating room as soon as possible after injury. Direct laryngoscopy and bronchoscopy, when done together, are extremely accurate for detecting upper airway injuries (11).

Pharynx and Esophagus

The workup to eliminate pharyngeal or esophageal injuries with penetrating neck trauma often includes a contrast swallow. If an injury to the pharynx or esophagus is suspected and the contrast swallow is negative or equivocal, one should proceed with esophagoscopy. Even if these studies do not reveal injury, the patient should be closely observed in the hospital without oral intake for at least 24 hours.

Although pharyngeal and esophageal injuries can often be seen fairly readily during endoscopy, in some reports, more than half of the perforations have been missed with this procedure (3), particularly when the lesion is small and in the pharynx or cervical esophagus. Esophageal injuries are particularly apt to be missed if the patient is on a ventilator and the esophagus does not expand well during the examination.

TREATMENT

Emergency Management

Patients who are bleeding rapidly or have any suggestion of airway compromise should be brought to the operating room (OR) promptly. In patients with blunt trauma, the neck should be stabilized in a neutral position until injury to the cervical spine can be eliminated.

Nonemergency Management

The management of stable patients with penetrating zone II neck injuries and no evidence of vascular or aerodigestive tract injury remains controversial. The debate centers primarily on whether patients with zone II injuries should have routine surgical neck exploration, or whether the patient should have a complete diagnostic evaluation and have a neck exploration only if the diagnostic studies reveal significant correctable injury.

Mandatory (Routine) Exploration

The primary advantage to performing routine surgical neck exploration is a decreased incidence of missed injuries. Up to 25% of patients undergoing mandatory neck exploration have visceral injuries that are not suspected during the preoperative clinical evaluation (2,8). In addition, negative neck exploration is usually associated with minimal morbidity and no mortality (12). Conversely, missed or delayed recognition of esophageal injuries can be associated with considerable morbidity and mortality (6).

Atta and Walker (13) have emphasized the lethal potential and need for early surgery in patients with gunshot wounds (GSW) or shotgun wounds (SGW) of the neck that cross the midline. In their series, all 11 patients with transcervical GSWs and SGWs sustained vascular or aerodigestive injuries.

Despite its proved efficacy, mandatory exploration does have some disadvantages. The negative exploration rate has been reported to be as high as 67% (2,8). Furthermore, the morbidity of a negative exploration may not be negligible (7).

Selective Conservatism

An alternative method of management is selective conservatism, which has been successful in many centers (14). This technique requires that patients with penetrating neck wounds have angiography, contrast or other radiologic studies, and endoscopy as needed. Surgical neck exploration is undertaken only if these techniques reveal an injury requiring surgical repair.

Using a selective surgical approach, the incidence of negative neck exploration is reduced to approximately 20% and the incidence of missed injuries in many series is negligible (15).

AXIOM Although a policy of selective conservatism reduces the morbidity and mortality rates associated with a negative exploration of the neck, the diagnostic studies done to eliminate significant injuries also have some costs and risks (15).

Maddison noted a 14% incidence of complications with arteriography in patients with penetrating wounds of the neck (16). These may include arterial dissection, occlusion, reactions to intravenous contrast, renal failure, false aneurysms, or hemorrhage. Endoscopy can cause iatrogenic perforation, and contrast swallows may result in aspiration of contrast or gastrointestinal secretions into the lungs.

AXIOM Generally, in patients with penetrating neck wounds in zone II, it may be safer to practice mandatory exploration on GSWs and tend toward selective conservatism with stab wounds.

Technical Considerations

Anesthesia

Whenever possible, neck exploration should be performed under general anesthesia in the operating room; however, one must be very careful when performing endotracheal intubation in anyone with a possible laryngeal or tracheal injury, and one must be prepared to immediately provide a surgical airway. The nasogastric tube can be inserted after the induction of anesthesia so that the patient is less apt to "gag" and so that rapid exploration and treatment could be accomplished if massive bleeding does occur.

AXIOM If the airway occludes suddenly during endotracheal intubation in a patient with a possible laryngeal injury, a large needle or surgical tracheostomy should be rapidly provided.

Positioning and Skin Preparation

Once the airway is assured, appropriate preparations for surgery can be made at a less urgent pace. Under optimal circumstances, the patient should be placed supine with a roll between the scapulae, with the neck in extension, and the head rotated away from the side to be explored. If a cervical spine injury has not been ruled out, the neck should not be extended or turned to the side; but this makes the surgical dissection and exposure more difficult.

Care must be taken during preoperative preparation not to rub the neck vigorously because dislodging a tamponading clot could cause sudden, severe bleeding or embolization.

If time permits, a vascular donor site in one of the thighs should be cleaned and draped if the patient has a potential need for an interposition venous graft or patch.

Incisions

A low, standard "collar" incision 1 to 2 cm above the heads of the clavicles is used in patients whose preoperative evaluation suggests bilateral neck injuries or damage to the lower larynx or trachea. A horizontal incision placed over the midportion of the thyroid cartilage is generally used only if it is fairly certain that the injuries are limited to the larynx.

An anterior sternocleidomastoid incision usually provides ready access to the trachea, thyroid gland, larynx, and carotid artery in a plane anteromedial to the internal jugular vein. Care must be taken to avoid damaging the sympathetic chain, which lies posterior to the carotid sheath on the prevertebral muscles.

If a contralateral injury is suspected intraoperatively, exposure of the other side of the neck may be obtained by extending the lower end of this incision transversely as a "collar" incision or by making a separate oblique incision.

AXIOM Vessels that have any possibility of injury should be thoroughly explored during surgery, because false-negative arteriograms have been reported in up to 10% of patients (17).

With lower neck injuries that may involve great vessels at the thoracic inlet, adequate exposure can usually be obtained through a supraclavicular incision. Exposure of these structures can generally be improved if one also performs a subperiosteal resection of the medial third of the clavicle. If one needs to get to the origins of the innominate, left common carotid, or left subclavian arteries, a median sternotomy incision should be performed.

Management of Specific Injuries

High Internal Carotid Artery Injuries

When a high penetrating ICA lesion is found, adequate exposure of the vessel can be difficult. Access to the vessels and structures close to the base of the skull can be improved by dividing the sternocleidomastoid muscle near its insertion into the mastoid process or dislocating the temporomandibular joint and pulling the mandible forward.

Care must be taken to avoid injury to the hypoglossal nerve (which usually crosses the internal and external carotid arteries about 1.5 to 3.0 cm above their origin) and the spinal accessory nerve (which enters the deep part of the sternocleidomastoid muscle about 3 to 4 cm below the mastoid process).

Bleeding from the distal ICA immediately adjacent to the skull may be controlled best by inserting a Fogarty balloon-tipped catheter into the distal segment and then inflating the balloon. If necessary, the catheter can be left in place for several weeks until the vessel has solidly thrombosed (2).

AXIOM If a carotid artery has an injury that would be difficult or hazardous to repair and the distal stump pressure exceeds 70 mm Hg, the safest treatment is probably ligation of the damaged vessel.

If it is anticipated that the ICA will be clamped for more than 10 to 15 minutes, the patient should be systemically heparinized 2 to 3 minutes before clamping the artery, as long as there are no associated injuries that would preclude such action. Anticoagulation is rarely indicated for patients requiring only a simple rapid repair of the ICA.

Controversy continues as to whether an injured ICA should be repaired if the patient has a major neurologic deficit. In 1964, Wylie et al., showed that ischemic brain tissue caused by an acute stroke can be converted into a hemorrhagic infarct if the responsible occluded vessel is opened and perfusion is reestablished soon after the infarct (18). In 1980, Ledgerwood and colleagues (19) provided direct evidence of the safety of primary repair in five patients who were in coma or with stroke, all of whom underwent primary repair of the injured vessel. Postmortem examination in the patients who died revealed that the deaths were caused by diffuse cerebral edema and not hemorrhagic infarction.

In a literature review, Liekweg and Greenfield studied 233 patients with carotid artery injury and concluded that, in patients with any neurologic deficit short of coma, less morbidity and fewer deaths occurred after repair than after ligation (20).

AXIOM Regardless of the absence or extent of neurologic defects, the ICA should be repaired when prograde flow still is manifest. When no prograde flow exists, the vessel should probably be ligated.

If a subadventitial hematoma is noted at operation, a vertical arteriotomy is made over the area, and the inside of the vessel is inspected for injury.

Internal Carotid Shunts

When bleeding from an ICA injury has been controlled, systemic heparinization is usually recommended (to prevent embolic complications) unless there are concurrent injuries to the eyes, brain, or spinal cord. Following this, it may be advisable to insert a temporary intravascular shunt for added protection to the brain if

1. Backflow from the distal ICA is scant;
2. Stump pressure is less than 40 to 50 mm Hg; and
3. Repair will take more than 5 to 10 minutes because of the extent of the injury or because one must wait while a vein graft or vein patch is being obtained.

Shunts are rarely indicated during repair of common carotid injuries, especially if the distal clamp is applied proximal to its bifurcation into the external carotid artery (ECA) and ICA.

Bypass Grafts

Prosthetic bypass grafts for ICA or common carotid artery (CCA) injuries should be avoided when possible. In one study of six patients with normal preoperative CNS examinations who had bypass grafts for carotid injuries, major strokes developed in two 3 and 7 days postoperatively, presumably from thrombosis of their prosthetic grafts (21).

Extracranial-Intracranial Bypasses

If an injury to the ICA is extensive or if it is necessary to ligate the distal segment, one option available to maintain cerebral blood flow is an extracranial-intracranial (EC-IC) bypass. This is typically accomplished by anastomosing the middle meningeal artery to the middle cerebral artery.

Postrepair Angiography

AXIOM Intraoperative angiography following restoration of blood flow in injured critical vessels is advisable because of the serious consequences of inadequate reconstructions. Approximately 6% of carotid repairs have been shown on postrepair arteriography to require revision (21).

Vertebral Artery Injuries

Injuries to a vertebral artery near its origin from the subclavian artery can be managed by ligation of the proximal segment; however, if any question exists about the blood supply to the posterior brain, an anastomosis of the distal end of the vertebral artery to the side of the CCA can be performed. Higher vertebral artery injuries can usually be controlled by performing proximal and distal ligation.

When the vertebral artery injury is above the sixth cervical vertebra, one can often use interventional radiology to occlude it with autologous clot or other material (22). Vertebral arteriovenous fistulas, which occur in up to 10% to 15% of vertebral arterial injuries, should probably also be treated angiographically whenever possible.

Venous Injuries

The jugular vein is the most frequently injured vessel in the neck, but in many cases, no preoperative evidence of such an injury is manifest. Unless the patient is actively bleeding, isolated jugular vein injuries are seldom important and only rarely require surgical treatment.

Blunt Carotid Injuries

Cogbill and colleagues noted that, although blunt trauma to the carotid artery is rare, it can cause death in up to 40% of patients and permanent neurologic impairment in up to 80% of the survivors (23). With traumatic dissections, a delay of up to 2 to 7 days may occur after the trauma before localizing neurologic findings develop.

AXIOM Blunt carotid artery injuries that cause symptoms usually have a delayed dissection in the media, often with subsequent thrombotic occlusion.

The diagnosis of carotid dissection is usually made with arteriography, which typically shows extensive narrowing of the internal carotid lumen, often extending up to the skull. This "carotid string sign" represents elevation and folding of the intima in the dissected segment. In some instances, carotid arteriography shows a tapered area of narrowing (referred to as a "dunce's cap" deformity) with distal occlusion.

AXIOM When angiography demonstrates blunt carotid injury with dissection of the wall, full anticoagulant therapy should be instituted to prevent thrombus formation.

In the series by Cogbill and colleagues, arterial dissection was managed nonsurgically in 15 (79%) patients, the majority with systemic anticoagulation (23). The mortality rate was 43%; however, most (71%) of their patients had neurologic deficits before or within 12 hours of admission (23). Good neurologic outcomes were achieved in only 22 patients, and these results were largely related to the neurologic status of patients on admission.

Pharynx and Esophagus Injuries

If a pharyngeal or cervical esophageal injury is suspected, it is approached most readily through an incision along the anterior border of the sternocleidomastoid muscle on the side of the injury. If an injury is found, the tear is debrided, as needed, and then closed with two layers of inverting, interrupted, slowly absorbable sutures. If it is difficult to see the mucosa to close the defect properly, a Foley catheter can be inserted through the injury into the pharynx and the inflated balloon can then be pulled back to bring the mucosa up into the operative field. A second layer of sutures is then used to close the muscle layer. Whenever possible, a flap of local muscle, such as the omohyoid, should be used to reinforce or buttress the closure. The area should be drained and a contrast swallow should be performed at 4 to 6 days, before the patient is allowed to eat.

AXIOM With any soft-tissue infection developing in the neck, one should look for missed injuries of the aerodigestive tract or breakdowns of repairs.

In a review by Asensio and colleagues, fistulas developed in 15 of 118 patients with penetrating esophageal injuries (2). All 15 patients recovered fully after wide drainage and intravenous antibiotics were provided.

Occasionally, cervical osteomyelitis may develop following GSWs that have traversed the pharynx or esophagus in the neck before entering the spine. CT scans with contrast are probably the best method for detecting these deep abscesses or collections, but even these studies may be falsely negative in up to 10% to 15% of patients.

Complex Combined Aerodigestive Tract Injuries

AXIOM Patients with combined tracheoesophageal and vascular injuries should be observed particularly carefully for the development of postoperative anastomotic leaks, infections, and fistulas.

Feliciano and colleagues recommend debridement and primary repair of all aerodigestive tract injuries, but with an interposed sternocleidomastoid or strap muscle flap between the suture lines (24). They also recommended avoiding a tracheostomy whenever possible. With extensive esophageal injury and associated laryngotracheal or vascular injuries, they recommended that a cutaneous esophagostomy be created. The authors also recommended that drainage be instituted with closed systems and directed anteriorly, so that the drains do not cross the carotid artery. If a concomitant ipsilateral carotid artery injury has been repaired, the drainage of the neck should be established through the side of the neck opposite the injury.

AXIOM Transcervical neck injuries requiring bilateral neck explorations can cause so much neck edema that one should consider performing a tracheostomy in case there is an inadvertent endotracheal extubation postoperatively.

Neurologic Injuries

Cleanly incised nerves in stable patients should be repaired primarily using magnification lenses as needed to obtain as exact a nerve bundle to nerve bundle repair as possible. With contaminated injuries or with injuries in unstable patients, the ends of the nerve are tagged with nonabsorbable sutures and repaired 1 to 2 weeks later, after skin healing appears to be satisfactory.

⊘ FREQUENT ERRORS

1. ***Delay of needed surgery for a penetrating neck wound in order to perform various diagnostic tests when the neck has to be explored anyway.***
2. ***Failure to obtain preoperative arteriography in stable patients with suspected vascular injuries in zone I or III.***
3. ***Failure to adequately stabilize the neck during surgery in patients with blunt neck injury prior to clearing the cervical spine for injury.***
4. ***Failure to consider a carotid injury in someone with CNS changes but a normal CT scan of the brain after blunt trauma.***
5. ***Reliance on a negative Gastrografin swallow to eliminate esophageal injury.***
6. ***Attempts to follow a policy of selective conservatism on penetrating neck wounds when the needed tests are not readily available.***
7. ***Failure to bring patients with suspected airway injuries to surgery promptly.***
8. ***Failure to repair an injured but patent ICA because a severe neurologic deficit is present.***
9. ***Taking time to repair a complex internal jugular vein injury rather than just ligating it, especially when other severe injuries are present.***
10. ***Failure to look carefully for associated injuries when one finds injury to major vessels or the aerodigestive tract.***
11. ***Failure to adequately buttress and separate repairs of the esophagus and tracheobronchial tree, especially if a vascular repair is also present.***
12. ***Failure to consider that a neck infection after a penetrating neck wound may be due to a missed aerodigestive tract injury or a repair that has leaked.***

SUMMARY POINTS

1. In stable patient with penetrating neck injuries, preoperative arteriography is particularly important for injuries in zones I and III.

2. Penetrating injuries of the neck involve major vessels in 25% to 40% of patients.

3. All GSWs of the neck should be surgically explored, especially if they cross the midline.

4. Patients with blunt head or neck trauma should have their neck immobilized in the neutral position until radiography and careful examination have eliminated cervical spine injury.

5. Neurologic findings after severe blunt head trauma may occasionally be due to carotid or vertebral artery damage in the neck.

6. Many patients with organ damage in the neck requiring an operation have no clinical evidence of such an injury preoperatively.

7. Neurologic signs in patients with penetrating neck injuries may be caused or greatly increased by hypotension.

8. Suspected airway injuries should be managed emergently in the operating room, especially when evidence exists that blood is being aspirated into the tracheobronchial tree.

9. With injuries in the neck, the neurologic examination should include an evaluation of the patient's mental status, cranial nerves, spinal cord, brachial plexus, and sympathetic nerves.

10. The tissue changes of traumatic asphyxia usually resolve spontaneously, but one must look carefully for associated injuries.

11. Lateral radiographs of the neck are indicated in all patients who have had blunt neck injuries.

12. Increased prevertebral space behind the upper airway is usually due to injuries to the adjacent spine or aerodigestive tract.

13. If an alert and oriented patient has full range of nonpainful neck motion, no local tenderness, and no distracting injuries, a significant cervical spine injury is effectively ruled out.

14. Four-vessel angiography should be performed on all stable patients with suspected vascular injuries in zones I and III of the neck.

15. In patients with blunt trauma, presence of focal neurologic changes, despite a normal CT scan of the brain, should make one suspect a carotid injury.

16. Whenever a neck is explored for trauma, the vascular and aerodigestive structures should be examined closely, even if preoperative arteriography and other studies do not reveal injuries.

17. Barium can cause increased inflammation and infection if it enters the mediastinum, but Gastrografin can cause severe pneumonitis if it is aspirated into the lungs.

18. When a patient with suspected esophageal injury has a negative Gastrografin swallow, the study should be repeated with barium or esophagoscopy should be performed.

19. Clinically subtle injuries to laryngeal cartilages can usually be demonstrated clearly on CT.

20. Proper CT scanning requires a cooperative patient and should not be attempted in a patient with an acute, unprotected airway injury or unstable vital signs.

21. When endoscopy is to be performed under topical anesthesia, it is important that the presence of major vascular injuries be eliminated before the procedure because gagging or retching could restart bleeding from injured vessels.

22. If an ecchymosis of the posterior or lateral pharyngeal wall is seen on endoscopy, one should be concerned about a possible underlying vascular injury.

23. When thorough diagnostic studies cannot be performed promptly in patients with penetrating neck injuries, early surgical exploration is generally safer than continued clinical evaluation.

24. A policy of selective conservatism for neck injuries should not be undertaken unless the needed diagnostic tests can be performed promptly and accurately.
25. Although a policy of selective conservatism reduces the morbidity rates associated with a negative exploration of the neck, the diagnostic studies done to eliminate significant injuries also have some costs and risks.
26. With zone II injuries, it is often quicker, safer, and less expensive to explore the neck surgically than it is to get all the studies needed to eliminate significant vascular and aerodigestive tract injuries.
27. Most patients with penetrating neck injuries that also involve the chest do not require chest exploration, unless there is evidence of continued bleeding or an aerodigestive tract injury.
28. When a possibility of vascular injury in the neck exists, a nasogastric tube should not be inserted until the patient is anesthetized because gagging or retching during insertion of the tube could restart bleeding.
29. If the airway occludes suddenly during endotracheal intubation and there is suspicion of a laryngeal injury, a large needle or surgical tracheostomy should be rapidly provided.
30. Unilateral neck explorations are usually best done through an incision along the anterior border of the sternocleidomastoid muscle.
31. During neck exploration, any vessel or aerodigestive structure that is in the path of a knife or anywhere near the presumed tract of a bullet must be examined very carefully.
32. If a carotid artery has an injury that would be difficult or hazardous to repair and the distal stump pressure exceeds 70 mm Hg, the safest treatment is probably ligation of the damaged vessel.
33. Regardless of the absence or extent of neurologic deficits, the ICA should be repaired if prograde flow is still present; if no prograde flow exists, the vessel should be ligated.
34. Prosthetic bypass grafts to restore flow to an injured carotid artery should be avoided if possible because of a possible increased risk of infection and a high rate of later occlusion.
35. Intraoperative angiography following restoration of blood flow in injured critical vessels is advisable because of the serious consequences of inadequate reconstruction, which is present in approximately 6% of such repairs.
36. Interventional radiology should be considered in patients with bleeding or arteriovenous fistulas from high vertebral or very high ICA injuries.
37. Blunt carotid artery injuries that cause symptoms usually have a delayed dissection in the media, often with subsequent thrombotic occlusion, and they should generally be treated with anticoagulants.
38. Blunt carotid injury should be suspected in patients who have severe head trauma and localized neurologic changes but have no lesions on CT scans of the brain to explain the clinical findings.
39. Following repair of penetrating esophageal trauma, the patient should not be allowed to eat until or unless a contrast swallow confirms the clinical impression that no leak is present.
40. Patients with combined tracheoesophageal injuries should be observed carefully postoperatively for the development of anastomotic leaks, infections, and fistulas.
41. Transcervical neck injuries requiring bilateral neck explorations can cause so much neck edema that one should consider performing a tracheostomy in case there is an inadvertent postoperative endotracheal extubation.
42. Injury to the cervical spine by a transpharyngeal GSW, even with the best therapy, greatly increases the risk of later osteomyelitis.

REFERENCES

1. Wilson RF, Diebel L. Injuries to the neck. In: Wilson RF, Walt AJ, eds. *Management of trauma—pitfalls and practice,* 2nd ed. Philadelphia: Williams & Wilkins, 1996:270.

2. Asensio JA, Valenziano CP, Falcone RE, et al. Management of penetrating neck injuries. The controversy surrounding zone II injuries. *Surg Clin North Am* 1991; 71:267.
3. Weigelt JA, Thal ER, Snyder WH, et al. Diagnosis of penetrating cervical esophageal injuries. *Am J Surg* 1987;154:619.
4. Carducci B, Lowe RA, Dalsey W. Penetrating neck trauma: consensus and controversies. *Ann Emerg Med* 1985;15:208–215.
5. Fogelman MJ, Stewart RD. Penetrating wounds of the neck. *Am J Surg* 1956; 91:581.
6. Sankaran S, Walt AJ. Penetrating wounds of the neck: principles and some controversies. *Surg Clin North Am* 1977;57:139.
7. Obeid FN, Hadad GS, Horst HM, et al. A critical reappraisal of a mandatory exploration policy for penetrating wounds of the neck. *Surg Gynecol Obstet* 1985; 160:157.
8. Thal ER. Injury to the neck. EE Moore, KL Mattox, Feliciano DV, eds. *Trauma,* 2nd ed. Norwalk: Appleton & Lange, 1991:305–317.
9. Montalvo BM, LeBlang SD, Nuriez DB, et al. Color Doppler sonography in penetrating injuries of the neck. *AJNR Am J Neuroradiol* 1996;17:943.
10. Mittendorf E, Marks JM, Berk T et al. Anomalous vertebral artery anatomy and the consequences of penetrating vascular injuries. *J Trauma* 1998;44:548.
11. Ford HR, Gardner MJ, Lynch JM. Laryngotracheal disruption from blunt pediatric neck injuries: impact of early recognition and intervention on outcome. *J Pediatr Surg* 1996;30:331.
12. Apffelstaedt JP, Muller R. Results of mandatory exploration for penetrating neck trauma. *World J Surg* 1994;18:917.
13. Atta HM, Walker ML. Penetrating neck trauma: Lack of universal reporting guidelines. *Am Surg* 1998;64:222.
14. Klyachkin ML, Rohmiller M, Charash WE, et al. Penetrating injuries of the neck: selective management evolving. *Am Surg* 1997;63:189.
15. Jurkovich GJ, Zingarelli W, Wallace J, et al. Penetrating neck trauma: studies in the asymptomatic patient. *J Trauma* 1985;25:819.
16. Maddison FE. Patient evaluation and other clinical considerations: basic principles of angiography. Rutherford RB, ed. *Vascular surgery.* Philadelphia: WB Saunders, 1977.
17. Beitsch P, Weigelt JA, Flynn E, Easley S. Physical examination and arteriography in patients with penetrating zone II neck wounds. *Arch Surg* 1994;129:577.
18. Wylie EJ, Hein MF, Adams JE. Intracranial hemorrhage following surgical revascularization for treatment of acute strokes. *J Neurosurg* 1964;21:212.
19. Ledgerwood AM, Mullins RJ, Lucas CE. Primary repair vs ligation for carotid artery injuries. *Arch Surg* 1980;115:488.
20. Liekweg WG Jr, Greenfield LT. Management of penetrating carotid arterial injury. *Ann Surg* 1978;188:587.
21. Fabian TC, George SM, Croce MA, et al. Carotid artery trauma: Management based on mechanism of injury. *J Trauma* 1990;30:953.
22. Sclafani SJA, Scalea TM, Hoffer EK, et al. Interventional radiology in the treatment of internal carotid artery gunshot wounds. *J Vasc Interv Radiol* 1995;6:857.
23. Cogbill TH, Moore EE, Meissnr M, et al. The spectrum of blunt injury to the carotid artery: a multicenter perspective. *J Trauma* 1994;37:473.
24. Feliciano DV, Mattox KL, Graham JM, et al. Five years experience with PTFE grafts in vascular wounds. *J Trauma* 1985;25:71.

15. LARYNGOTRACHEAL TRAUMA[1]

ANATOMY AND PHYSIOLOGY

Larynx

The larynx extends from the epiglottis opposite the third cervical vertebra (C-3) to the cricoid cartilage, which is at the level of C-6 in adults. The skeleton of the larynx has nine cartilages. These include the epiglottis, thyroid, cricoid, two arytenoids, two corniculates, and two cuneiform cartilages. Calcification of the laryngeal cartilages typically begins at 20 to 30 years of age in the thyroid cartilage at its inferior margin and proceeds in a cephalad direction.

Epiglottis

The epiglottis is a leaf-shaped fibroelastic cartilage structure situated at the superior aperture of the larynx. Its pointed lower end (petiole) is attached firmly anteriorly to the posterior surface of the thyroid cartilage in the midline, just below the thyroid notch (Fig. 15-1).

Thyroid Cartilage

The thyroid cartilage is formed from two broad plates that are fused together anteriorly, but which are widely divergent posteriorly. At the top anteriorly, the cartilage has a marked prominence known as the "Adam's apple." The posterior borders of each thyroid cartilage project upward (approximately 2 cm) as a superior horn and downward as a shorter inferior horn on each side. The superior horn of the thyroid cartilage is attached to the greater cornua of the hyoid bone by the lateral thyrohyoid ligament. The inferior thyroid horn articulates with the cricoid cartilage.

Cricoid

The cricoid cartilage is shaped like a signet ring. It is the only completely circumferential structure of the laryngotracheal skeleton. In infants, it represents the narrowest portion of the upper airway (versus the glottis in adults). The posterior portion of the cricoid cartilage is 20 to 30 mm in height, and the smaller anterior portion is only 5 to 7 mm in height in adults.

Arytenoids

The two arytenoid cartilages are small, triangular-shaped cartilages sitting on top of the cricoid posterolaterally. The anterior angle of the base of each arytenoid cartilage projects forward as a vocal process to which the vocal ligament attaches. The lateral (muscular) process serves as a site of attachment for the thyroarytenoid and the lateral and posterior cricoarytenoid muscles.

The two corniculate cartilages (cartilages of Santorini) are small conical structures composed of fibroelastic cartilage; they are attached to the apex of each arytenoid cartilage. The two cuneiform cartilages (cartilages of Wrisberg) are composed of fibroelastic cartilage and lay in the aryepiglottic folds just anterior to the corniculate cartilages.

Glottis

The glottis or vocal apparatus of the larynx includes the two true vocal cords (plica vocalis) and the opening between them (rima glottidis). The supraglottic compartment of the larynx extends from the tip of the epiglottis anterosuperiorly and the apices of the arytenoids posterosuperiorly, to the base of the laryngeal ventricles inferiorly. The vestibule is that portion of the laryngeal cavity extending from its inlet to the vestibular folds (false vocal cords). The laryngeal ventricle is a fusiform fossa

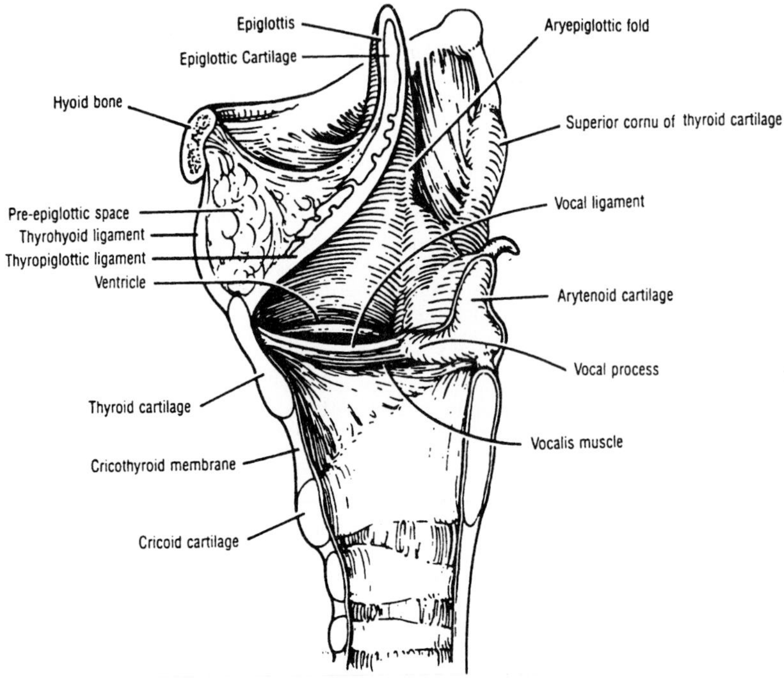

FIG. 15-1. Sagittal view of right hemilarynx highlighting the superior and inferior epiglottic attachments: the hypoepiglottic and thyroepiglottic ligaments, respectively. (From Jeffrey RB, Dillon WP. The larynx. Computed tomography of the head and neck. *Modern Neuro Radiology Series,* 1988:12.4.)

bounded by the crescentic edge of the false cords superiorly and the true cords inferiorly.

The false vocal cords are two folds of mucous membrane enclosing the vestibular ligament on each side. The vestibular ligament extends posteriorly from the angle of the thyroid cartilage to the anterolateral surface of the arytenoid just superior to the attachment of the true cords on the vocal process of the arytenoid.

The true vocal cords extend obliquely from the vocal processes of each arytenoid cartilage and join anteriorly in the midline to form the anterior commissure. The posterior commissure consists of the interarytenoid muscles and overlying mucosa, and it is located between the arytenoid cartilages above the cricoid.

The subglottic region of the larynx extends from the undersurface of the true cords down to the inferior margin of the cricoid cartilage.

AXIOM The only muscle that separates (abducts) the vocal cords is the posterior cricoarytenoid muscle on each side.

Muscles of the Larynx

The extrinsic muscles of the larynx include the infrahyoid or hyoid depressor muscles (omohyoid, sternohyoid, sternothyroid, and thyrohyoid muscles) and the suprahyoid or hyoid levator group (mylohyoid, geniohyoid, digastric, and stylohyoid muscles).

The intrinsic muscles of the larynx act to modify the size of the laryngeal aperture (rima glottidis) between the vocal cords. The cricothyroid muscle is the only "intrinsic" laryngeal muscle that is on the exterior of the larynx, and it is the chief tensor of the vocal cords. The lateral cricoarytenoids are the main adductors of the vocal cords. The deepest fibers of the thyroarytenoid muscle form the vocalis muscle, which is the principal antagonist to the cricothyroid muscle. The vocalis muscle shortens and thickens the vocal cords to enable fine control of the voice. Following contraction of the thyroarytenoid muscle, the vocal cords relax.

Nerves of the Larynx

The superior laryngeal nerve comes off the vagus nerve high in the neck, and it passes posteriorly and medial to the carotid sheath. It subsequently divides into a small, external branch and a thicker, internal one. The external laryngeal nerve passes posterior to the superior thyroid artery and is purely motor to the cricothyroid muscle and some of the inferior pharyngeal constrictor fibers. The internal laryngeal nerve supplies sensation to the larynx above the vocal cords and may contribute some motor or proprioceptive fibers to the interarytenoid muscle.

AXIOM Loss of the superior laryngeal nerve paralyzes the cricothyroid muscle. This reduces the tension of the vocal cord and produces a weak, husky voice.

On the right, the recurrent laryngeal nerve runs up into the neck after crossing the anterior surface of the first part of the subclavian artery to continue medial to the common carotid artery in the right tracheoesophageal groove. On the left, the recurrent laryngeal nerve comes off the vagus nerve on the anterior surface of the aortic arch and continues around the descending thoracic aorta just distal to the ligamentum arteriosum. The left recurrent nerve then runs upward in the neck in the left tracheoesophageal groove.

AXIOM Patients with an aberrant origin of a subclavian artery have a "non-recurrent" recurrent laryngeal nerve, which can easily be injured during thyroid surgery.

Both recurrent laryngeal nerves are closely associated with the branches of the inferior thyroid artery on each side. The nerves enter the larynx under the inferior pharyngeal constrictors, just posterior to the articulation of the inferior horn of the thyroid cartilage with the cricoid cartilage.

The recurrent laryngeal nerves supply sensation to the vocal cords and to the lower portion of the larynx. It is also the motor nerve to all of the intrinsic muscles except the cricothyroid. With unilateral recurrent nerve injury, the airway is typically uncompromised, but the voice is hoarse and breathy, and there is early vocal fatigue. With bilateral recurrent nerve injury, airway obstruction can occur rapidly in some patients because of the bilateral vocal cord abductor paralysis. The paralyzed vocal cords become lax and can approximate or can be up to 3 to 4 mm apart. There is usually no dyspnea at first, but there is immediate loss of voice. Airway obstruction can occur suddenly at almost any time.

Mechanism of Phonation

During quiet respiration, the normal arytenoid cartilages are abducted and in close proximity to the inner margin of the posterior portions of the thyroid cartilages. With phonation, the normal arytenoid cartilages move medially and rotate inward, away from the inner margin of the thyroid cartilage. Adduction, or apposition of the vocal cords, is accomplished through the complex interaction of the intrinsic laryngeal musculature, including the thyroarytenoid, the lateral cricoarytenoid, and the interarytenoid muscles.

Cervical Trachea

The cervical trachea extends from the cricoid cartilage to the thoracic inlet at the level of the sternal manubrium. The trachea varies from 13 to 22 mm in width and is supported anteriorly and laterally by 16 to 20 U-shaped rings of hyaline cartilage, which keep its lumen open. The posterior portion of the trachea is closed by a fibrous membrane on which lies the trachealis muscle and mucous membrane. The entire (cervical and thoracic) trachea is about 9 to 15 cm long, and almost half of it (the cervical trachea) is above the sternum.

TYPES OF TRAUMA

Penetrating Trauma

The most common organs injured by penetrating neck trauma are major veins in 15% to 30%, major arteries in 10% to 20%, digestive tract (pharynx or esophagus) in 5% to 20%, and upper respiratory tract (larynx or cervical trachea) in 5% to 15%. The incidence of upper airway injury is at least doubled when one of the other systems is also injured (2). Of the airway injuries, the larynx is involved in about one-third of patients, and the cervical trachea is damaged in about two-thirds. In 15% to 20% of gunshot wounds, the airway is injured in two or more locations (3).

AXIOM Approximately 25% of patients with penetrating airway trauma also have an esophageal injury; this is the neck injury most likely to be missed until later in the patient's hospital course.

Blunt Trauma

Supraglottic injuries from blunt trauma include fractures of the hyoid bone or thyroid cartilage. With thyroid cartilage fractures, a depression or widening of the thyroid notch with loss of the thyroid prominence is often seen. With disruption of the thyrohyoid membrane or thyroepiglottic ligament, the epiglottis and soft tissues of the larynx tend to be displaced posteriorly and superiorly.

Transglottic injuries often result from direct blows to the thyroid cartilage and are usually divided into anterior and posterior types. The anterior type is characterized by midline vertical fractures of the thyroid cartilage with extension of the laceration into the true and false cords and the aryepiglottic folds. Posterior injuries tend to cause interarytenoid and thyroarytenoid muscle disruptions with dislocation of the arytenoid cartilages.

Subglottic injuries usually occur in conjunction with cricoid cartilage fractures or as part of a laryngotracheal separation pattern. Fractures of the cricoid usually occur anteriorly in the midline or paramedian position. Cricoid damage plus reactive edema and hemorrhage can rapidly occlude the airway.

Laryngotracheal separations typically occur from shearing forces acting on the neck while it is in a hyperextended position. With complete transection, the larynx tends to retract upward, while the trachea retracts downward so that a gap of 6 to 10 cm or more may develop between the cricoid superiorly and the torn trachea distally.

Causes of Blunt Trauma

The most frequent cause of blunt laryngeal injuries is high-speed motor vehicle accidents. The usual scenario involves the hyperextended anterior neck impacting the steering wheel or dashboard. Upon impact of the neck on the dashboard or steering wheel, the larynx can be crushed against the cervical spine. Such trauma may not only produce severe laryngeal fractures, but it may also cause separation of the cricoid cartilage from the upper trachea.

"Clothesline" injuries to the neck by high-speed contact with a horizontally suspended cord are occurring with increasing frequency because of the proliferation of snowmobilers who often run into fences. Such trauma is a frequent cause of cricotracheal disruption.

AXIOM Laryngeal dysfunction can occur following endotracheal intubation and most often results from laryngeal edema, hemorrhage, or mucosal tears.

Even an apparently uncomplicated endotracheal intubation in a normal upper airway can occasionally cause either arytenoid subluxation by direct trauma or recurrent laryngeal nerve paralysis (RLNP). The mechanism of injury of the latter is believed to be a neuropraxic response of the anterior branch of the recurrent laryngeal nerve (RLN), caused by compression of the abducted arytenoid (from endotracheal cuff inflation) against the internal thyroid lamina. Other predisposing factors in endotracheal tube—-associated RLN injury include an overinflated cuff (which may migrate to the cricoid level) and use of high nitrous-oxide mixtures, which can cause expansion of the balloon cuff over time.

AXIOM Differentiating between arytenoid dislocation and RLNP can be difficult; both may show an immobile vocal cord and asymmetrically positioned arytenoid cartilages on laryngoscopy.

Several reports have indicated that vocal cord paralysis found after tracheal intubation (5) was due to damage to the recurrent laryngeal nerves by an overexpanded cuff, toxic neuritis, and various nonspecific causes. It has also been suggested that some of these unexplained vocal cord paralyses with glottic edema at extubation may actually have been caused by arytenoid dislocation. The distinction may be made through videostroboscopy, which can demonstrate preserved mucosal wave movements of the vocal cord if the problem is arytenoid subluxation.

Laryngotracheal Pathology after Blunt Trauma

The subglottic and supraglottic submucosa allows rapid circumferential accumulation of edema fluid following trauma. Air in the submucosal space resulting from mucosal tears also reduces the luminal diameter of the larynx or trachea.

AXIOM Symptoms of airway obstruction are not usually manifest until there is loss of at least 70% of the cross-sectional area of the airway.

The majority of submucosal edema and hematoma formation developing after trauma usually occurs within 6 hours. Consequently, airway obstruction caused by endolaryngeal swelling is likely to occur before that time unless later coughing, straining, or speaking increases the quantity of subcutaneous air or submucosal bleeding.

Both the thyroid and cricoid cartilages are composed of hyaline cartilage and, consequently, are especially prone to fracture. The cuneiform, corniculate, arytenoid, and epiglottic cartilages are made of fibroelastic tissue; consequently, they are more likely to avulse or dislocate (4). The arytenoid cartilages are especially likely to dislocate, and this greatly interferes with the function of the vocal cords. The hyoid bone, although calcified, is rarely injured because it is protected by the overhanging chin and cushioned by its surrounding muscles.

In cricotracheal separations, the soft tissue surrounding the trachea usually remains intact, providing some airway continuity even though a gap of as much as 8 cm may be present between the separated ends of the airway (5). Paralysis produced by muscle relaxants or weakness from sedatives causes these supporting muscles to lose their tone and can result in sudden airway occlusion. Cricotracheal separation is often also accompanied by avulsion of the recurrent laryngeal nerves.

Associated Injuries with Blunt Trauma

AXIOM Cervical spine injury is frequently associated with blunt laryngotracheal trauma and should be considered present until proven otherwise.

The esophagus is most apt to be lacerated when it is crushed between the thyroid or cricoid cartilage and the sharp edge of an osteophyte or a fragment from a fractured cervical vertebra (6). A combined laryngeal and esophageal injury can sometimes be suspected radiographically because of the presence of an air column in the esophagus (which is usually collapsed).

Closed-head injury is frequently seen in patients with blunt laryngotracheal trauma and may give the false impression that the airway obstruction is due to coma, which relaxes the tongue and allows it to fall back into the pharynx. Maxillofacial injuries are also common in patients with laryngeal trauma, and the airway obstruction may initially be blamed on the facial injuries. This assumption may lead to an emergency cricothyroidotomy that may convert a partial laryngeal airway obstruction to one that is complete.

DIAGNOSIS OF LARYNGOTRACHEAL INJURIES

Signs and Symptoms

Although a voice change is the most common presenting symptom with laryngeal injury, and although many of these patients have neck pain and tenderness, there may be minimal initial symptoms or signs; therefore, a high index of suspicion, based on the mechanism of injury, is essential.

In 10 (22%) of 46 patients with upper airway injuries in the series reported by Cicala et al., the diagnosis was not made from the presenting signs and symptoms (3). In some patients, symptoms are delayed for 24 to 48 hours, and in many patients, the airway problem may not become apparent until an attempt at endotracheal intubation is made.

Other symptoms seen with laryngeal trauma include dyspnea, neck pain, sore throat, voice change, dysphagia, and odynophagia. Occasionally, patients with laryngeal trauma may have hemoptysis.

AXIOM A severe sore throat not improving within 48 hours after a transient endotracheal intubation should be investigated for laryngeal injury.

Physical Examination

Penetrating injuries to the larynx and trachea are usually obvious and can be dramatic in their presentations. The most obvious evidence of blunt laryngeal trauma is neck swelling with a partial airway obstruction or voice change.

AXIOM A sucking neck wound and progressive hypoxemia is virtually diagnostic for a major laryngotracheal laceration.

Many patients with stab or gunshot wound injuries to the larynx or cervical trachea experience dyspnea, with an obvious opening into the airway, characterized by air bubbling through the wound and subcutaneous or deep perivisceral emphysema. With lower cervical tracheal wounds, the patient may also have a pneumothorax with decreased breath sounds on one or both sides of the chest. Persistent localized neck pain with coughing also suggests laryngeal or tracheal injury.

AXIOM The most frequent sign of blunt laryngotracheal trauma is subcutaneous emphysema.

The neck must be carefully examined for subcutaneous emphysema, palpable laryngeal fractures, loss of the normal external architecture of the larynx, soft-tissue swelling, and ecchymosis. Even when the larynx is severely fractured, with marked displacement of its component parts, there may be only minimal external evidence of injury (9).

When a cervical immobilization collar has been applied because of the possibility of a cervical spine injury, it is important that the anterior component of the collar be removed (while the head is held in a neutral position) during the examination of the neck for any signs of injury.

Intolerance of the supine position is occasionally seen in patients with upper airway injury and was present in 30% of patients reported by Fuhrman et al. (8). Posttraumatic positional dyspnea (i.e., severe dyspnea on neck extension) may also be a problem in these patients (7,9).

AXIOM When intubating a patient with blunt trauma to the head or neck, one should be prepared to provide a surgical airway rapidly.

When difficulty occurs in advancing an endotracheal tube or ventilating a patient when the endotracheal tube has supposedly "passed between the vocal cords," one should consider the possibility of a cricoid or tracheal injury. If an airway is still present, one can attempt to intubate the patient using a flexible bronchoscope; however, if the airway is lost, immediate emergency tracheostomy or insufflation of oxygen through a large (12 to 14 gauge) needle in the trachea is required.

An injury to the trachea should also be suspected when evidence of overdistension or abnormal migration of the balloon or tip of an endotracheal tube exists. Tobias et al. noted that the inability to seal a properly placed endotracheal tube with a reasonable amount of air is suggestive of airway discontinuity (10). In one series, the endotracheal tube balloon plugged the site of rupture and minimized the air leak. In patients who have had neck injury and had emergency intubation soon after admission, it may be wise to extubate them using a flexible bronchoscope to examine the cervical trachea and larynx as the patient is being extubated.

Radiographic Evaluation

Plain Films

Plain films of the neck may reveal deep, soft-tissue (perivisceral) emphysema, airway compression, displacement or fracture of laryngeal cartilages (best seen in older patients with calcified cartilages), tracheal deviation, cervical spine injury, or increased thickness of paravertebral tissues caused by bleeding or edema. A lateral view of the neck can be particularly helpful for demonstrating displacement of the epiglottis or distortion of the laryngeal air column.

Following penetrating injury, air in the deep tissues of the neck may occasionally be due to air passing down the missile tract, but it is more likely to be due to injury to air-containing structures. In most patients with severe, blunt laryngeal or upper tracheal trauma, deep cervical and mediastinal emphysema can be seen.

Normally, the body of the hyoid bone is situated entirely below a line drawn along the top of the third cervical vertebral body, and the distance between the cornua of the hyoid bone and the angle of the mandible should be at least 2 cm (11). With tracheal or cricotracheal transection, the hyoid bone is elevated.

Angiography

In stable patients with gunshot wounds, especially when the missile has traversed the midline, four-vessel studies including both carotid and both vertebral arteries should be obtained. If an obvious vascular injury is evident in zone II, arteriography is not necessary.

Contrast Swallows

A high index of suspicion for pharyngoesophageal injuries must be maintained in the patient with penetrating airway injury because a delay in diagnosis is associated with a significant increase in morbidity and mortality rate (12). Up to 50% of pharyngeal or esophageal leaks may be missed on Gastrografin swallow (13). If the study is repeated with barium, up to 25% of pharyngoesophageal injuries can still be missed.

Computed Tomography Scans

Detailed, accurate appraisal of laryngeal damage and airway encroachment can be obtained by computed tomography (CT). It is particularly useful in identifying laryngeal cartilage position and structure in patients in whom endoscopic evaluation of the larynx is obscured by edema and hematoma.

Magnetic Resonance Imaging

Magnetic resonance imaging (MRI) can provide more detailed information about soft-tissue injuries than CT, and it provides better definition of vascular injuries; however, its use in severely injured patients is limited.

Endoscopy

Indirect laryngoscopy can be helpful in alert, cooperative patients who do not have respiratory distress or a threatened airway. It can provide information about vocal cord mobility, mucosal integrity, endolaryngeal hematomas, arytenoid dislocation, and the degree of distortion of the laryngeal lumen. Areas poorly visualized on indirect laryngoscopy include the pyriform apex and postcricoid region.

Direct laryngoscopy should be reserved for physicians who are thoroughly familiar with the procedure and are prepared to handle any complications that might develop. The examiner should also be capable of proceeding with immediate, complete surgical reconstruction of the larynx if needed.

AXIOM If a "stable" patient has a suspected laryngeal injury, a cautious endoscopic examination should be performed before attempting airway intervention.

If immediate endoscopic examination is not possible and the patient has an adequate airway, a waiting period of 3 to 4 days is often advised to allow some of the edema and hematoma to subside. Flexible bronchoscopy has come to be generally considered the single most important technique for the overall diagnosis of airway injury (3). In the face of severe edema, however, the paralaryngeal and endolaryngeal recesses, as well as the subglottic larynx, may be inadequately assessed by this technique.

Flexible bronchoscopy not only minimizes movement of the cervical spine in patients with blunt trauma, but it can also be helpful for diagnosis of lesions in the nasopharynx, hypopharynx, larynx, trachea, and bronchi. In addition, it can be used to provide immediate airway control, if needed, with introduction of an endotracheal tube over the instrument (4,14).

AXIOM Bronchoscopy and laryngoscopy, when done together, are virtually 100% accurate for diagnosing upper airway injuries; however, if they are done individually, there is an occasional false-negative result (15).

Specific features that should be sought during laryngotracheal endoscopy include

1. Hemorrhage or hematoma formation;
2. False passages or mucosal tears;
3. Position of the arytenoids;
4. Size and shape of the laryngeal and tracheal lumens;
5. Presence of exposed cartilage; and
6. Vocal cord mobility.

Hematomas are most likely to involve the false cords, true cords, and aryepiglottic folds. False passages in short-necked individuals have a tendency to be infraglottic, but in long-necked patients, they tend to be supraglottic (16).

The mobility of the vocal cords should be noted carefully whenever the larynx is examined. This is one important advantage of performing the examination under topical anesthesia. In the absence of restrictive endolaryngeal edema or hematoma, bilateral cord paresis suggests thyrocricoid disarticulation with either entrapment or avulsion of the recurrent laryngeal nerves (17). Unilateral cord "paralysis" often indicates a cricoid-arytenoid joint dislocation.

Approximately 40% of recurrent laryngeal nerves divide into anterior and posterior branches 0.6 to 4.0 cm from the cricoid cartilage. Damage to an abductor nerve bundle in the presence of an intact external branch of a superior laryngeal nerve can result in a median or paramedian position of the vocal cord, whereas damage to the adductor nerve bundle tends to produce more of an abducted position.

Occasionally during endoscopy, fractured or dislocated cartilages may be displaced, causing complete occlusion of the airway. If one is not prepared for this possibility, the airway may not be reestablished in 3 to 5 minutes, and the patient may suffer irreparable brain damage.

Delayed diagnosis of laryngotracheal injuries is not unusual, especially when emergency intubation is performed soon after the patient's arrival in the emergency department. The diagnosis is made in some patients because they cannot be extubated because of obstruction of the larynx above a tracheostomy. In one series, laryngotracheal injury was not diagnosed in 37% (7 of 19) of patients until airway stenosis presented 8 days to 3 years after the initial trauma (17).

TREATMENT

Laryngotracheal trauma can usually be managed conservatively if:

- A clinically stable airway is present
- Radiologic and flexible endoscopic examinations fail to show displaced cartilages, mucosal disruptions, or progressing edema or hematoma formation

Conservative therapy includes:

- Bed rest in the semi-Fowler position
- Humidification by face mask with supplemental oxygen
- Intravenous access with hydration
- Systemic steroids
- Prophylactic antibiotics
- Early vaponephrine mist nebulizer treatments to help curtail reactive edema

Providing an Emergency Airway

Incidence

Although many blunt injuries to the larynx can be treated conservatively initially, 15% to 50% of patients with penetrating laryngotracheal injuries require immediate airway management (7). Cicala et al. found that the airway could be managed by observation or intubation in three-fourths of their patients (35 of 46) (3). These patients were observed without being intubated (4 patients), intubated through an obvious airway defect (6 patients), or were endotracheally intubated (25 patients). The remaining 11 (24%) patients required an emergent tracheostomy.

Based on the mechanism of injury, the incidence of acute airway problems was 0% (0 of 8) for stabs, 24% (4 of 17) for gunshot wounds, and 40% (8 of 20) for blunt trauma (3). Based on the location of the injury, the incidence of an acute airway problem with blunt trauma was 14% (1 of 7) for laryngeal injuries above the cricoid, 60% (3 of 5) for cricoid injuries, and 44% (4 of 9) for cervical trachea injuries.

Techniques

If an injured patient in the emergency department (ED) has acute, severe respiratory distress and is about to have a cardiac arrest, it is too dangerous to move the patient to the operating room. Such patients generally require prompt orotracheal intubation (with stabilization of the head for possible cervical spine injuries); however, the attempt at intubation can convert a partial airway obstruction into one that is complete, precipitating a need for an emergency tracheostomy or insertion of a large tracheal needle attached to intermittent wall oxygen. If the intubation seems successful initially, but difficulty is experienced in advancing the endotracheal tube, or if a bulging mass appears on the anterior surface of the neck, a subglottic lesion is probably present, and an emergency airway must be provided.

AXIOM Whenever possible, a suspected upper airway injury should be inspected with a flexible bronchoscope and then intubated with a tube previously placed over the flexible bronchoscope.

Cricothyroidotomy can provide an adequate airway if the injury is limited to the upper larynx. However, it can greatly aggravate any subglottic injuries that are present (9). In addition, obliteration of landmarks by edema, blood, or subcutaneous emphysema can result in severe technical difficulties. The most important disadvantage of this procedure is the possibility of acute airway obstruction by insertion of the cannula into a false passage. This is particularly apt to occur if a cricotracheal separation is present.

AXIOM A coniotomy can be extremely dangerous in patients with subglottic laryngeal injuries.

Management in the Operating Room

AXIOM Acute airway problems are best handled in the operating room with the most experienced anesthesiologist and surgeon present.

The anesthesiologist relies on the surgeon to secure the airway if attempts at intubation fail, and the surgeon relies on the anesthesiologist to provide optimal conditions for the performance of a tracheostomy if one is needed.

Tracheostomy

The operating room is the ideal place to perform a tracheostomy; however, if the airway is lost during an attempted endotracheal intubation in the emergency department, one should either perform an immediate tracheostomy via a vertical midline incision or provide transtracheal oxygenation via a large needle attached to wall oxygen (18). Percutaneous tracheostomies are being used more and more (19), but they should probably not be used in emergency situations.

AXIOM All airway manipulations with a suspected laryngotracheal injury should be performed with the patient conscious and breathing spontaneously.

Because severed laryngeal or tracheal tissues may be held together by the tone of the surrounding muscle, muscle relaxation from a general anesthetic can result in sudden airway obstruction. The risk of aspiration is also much greater in the anesthetized patient. If the patient is extremely uncooperative or apprehensive, a general anesthetic may be necessary.

An emergency tracheostomy following blunt trauma should be performed without extending the neck if the possibility of a cervical spine injury has not yet been eliminated. This increases the technical difficulties and is associated with an increased risk of airway obstruction during the procedure.

Elective or semielective tracheotomies are usually performed through a 3- to 4-cm horizontal incision placed midway between the cricoid cartilage and the suprasternal notch of the sternum. In patients whose superficial cervical landmarks are indistinct, or when an emergency tracheostomy is required, a vertical skin incision is preferable.

The opening in the trachea should be below the area of injury, but ideally above rings four or five, to reduce tension on the repair (by fixation of trachea with tube) and to lessen the likelihood of erosion into the innominate artery.

AXIOM After completion of the tracheostomy, it is important to auscultate the lungs and obtain chest radiography because it is not unusual for a pneumothorax to develop during or after this procedure.

Definitive Laryngotracheal Repair

An increasing number of surgeons favor an early operative approach (within 24 hours) to laryngotracheal repairs and have found no advantage in delay (20). Early exploration and repair facilitates healing by reducing the potential for granulation tissue development and allows for the identification of mucosal, muscular, and cartilaginous injuries, which may be approximated primarily in most patients. Delayed intervention generally results in poorer voice and airway results (8). Indeed, if displaced laryngeal fractures are not reduced and stabilized within 7 to 10 days, the resultant scarring may make later correction extremely difficult, and return of normal function is unlikely.

Specific Injuries

Laryngeal Injuries

In general, patients with laryngeal hematomas should receive broad-spectrum antibiotics. The role of steroids is controversial, but if they are given, the dose for an average-sized adult male should be the equivalent of 200 mg of hydrocortisone daily for 4 to 5 days (21).

Midline fractures of the thyroid cartilage are the most common laryngeal fractures. In some series they occur in more than 80% of patients explored for blunt laryngeal trauma. In about 50% of these patients, the epiglottis is displaced posteriorly with herniation of the periepiglottic contents into the larynx (21).

Fine stainless steel sutures (28 or 30 G) can be used to maintain the position of the large cartilage fragments following reduction (21). If comminution of the fractures is present, placement of a soft conforming endolaryngeal stent for at least 4 to 6 weeks is usually recommended. If moderate-to-severe mucosal tears are present or cartilage is exposed, a laryngofissure should be performed to expose and accurately reapproximate the injured respiratory epithelium, usually with 4-0 or 5-0 absorbable suture. Any area in which mucosal continuity is not provided can be a site of excess granulation tissue formation and subsequent scar contracture. Cartilage exposure may also lead to chondritis with secondary resorption and laryngeal stenosis. If the epiglottis is displaced posteriorly and cannot be returned to its normal position, it should be sutured anteriorly to the remnant of stable thyroid cartilage.

Treatment of arytenoid subluxation or dislocation usually consists of surgical reduction by applying gentle pressure with a laryngeal spatula to reposition the arytenoid on the cricoid facet. Early reduction (within 24 hours) must be performed because the cricoarytenoid joint can quickly become fibrosed and the vocal cord fixed in an unfavorable position. In patients with severe disruptive injuries or in those who cannot attain proper repositioning, submucosal resection of the arytenoid should be performed with meticulous mucosal reapproximation.

Treatment of unstable or displaced cricoid cartilage fractures involves open exploration and repair following a tracheostomy. Limited anterior arch fractures should be reduced and stabilized with fine stainless steel wires placed extraluminally. When the arch is too comminuted to lend itself to interfragmentary repair but it still retains perichondrial attachments, manual reduction through the injury site or tracheostomy incision should be accomplished with internal stenting (using a finger cot or Montgomery T-tube) for 2 to 4 weeks.

If a cricotracheal separation is suspected and the patient can tolerate the trip to the operating room, intubation over a flexible bronchoscope can sometimes be accomplished safely. Many authors prefer to manage these by immediate neck exploration with a tracheostomy performed through a vertical midline incision. When intubation over a bronchoscope is chosen, preparations must be made for potential emergency tracheostomy if obstruction of the airway occurs suddenly.

In many patients with blunt laryngotracheal separation, the injured cricoid and uppermost tracheal cartilage are so badly injured that they must be partially or totally resected. If the cricoid is severely damaged and must be removed, the trachea can be anastomosed directly to the thyroid cartilage. Partial cricotracheal disruptions can usually be repaired directly, and smaller lesions may be sealed with laser photocoagulation.

If a primary repair cannot be performed, the distal trachea should be sutured to the skin as a low tracheostomy to provide an airway (22).

AXIOM Complete cricotracheal separations have a high incidence of associated esophageal injuries, particularly in the postcricoid region; therefore, esophagoscopy is essential with these types of injuries.

Laryngeal Injuries in Children

It is particularly important in children to recognize and treat laryngeal injuries promptly and accurately (23). Delayed or inadequate repairs can result in excess scarring, which can prevent normal growth of the larynx and cause severe distortion of the vocal cords and airway.

When it is impossible to perform an immediate laryngeal repair in a child, it is the recommendation of Holinger and Schild that any stenotic areas that develop later be treated by dilatation and conservative treatment (23). Definitive repair should be delayed, if possible, until puberty. This gives the larynx an opportunity to achieve maximal adult growth and maturity. Beyond puberty, the treatment is the same as in adults.

Recurrent Laryngeal Nerve Paralysis

The function of the vocal cords and the recurrent laryngeal nerves should be closely examined both before and after surgery. With injuries to the cricoid cartilage or cervical trachea, direct neural trauma is more likely to occur (particularly with cricotracheal separation) and a high index of suspicion for this injury must exist.

If the recurrent laryngeal nerves are transected, an epineural repair can be attempted using microsurgical technique; however, most surgeons prefer not to search for recurrent nerves during the initial procedure because they are difficult to identify and there is a danger of damaging adjacent structures.

Tracheal Injuries

Minor Injuries

Most cervical tracheal injuries can be adequately treated through a neck incision. If the tracheal injury is small, it can be repaired without a tracheostomy. If the injury is larger and involves the first portion of the trachea, a tracheostomy should be placed through or below the site of the injury.

Major Injuries

If more than 3 cm of damaged trachea need to be resected, the tension on the suture line often exceeds 1000 g and is associated with an unacceptable incidence of short- and long-term sequelae. In these patients, several options can reduce suture tension and permit an end-to-end anastomosis (22).

Mobilization of the cervical trachea typically provides 1 to 2 cm of added length. A laryngeal release, performed by sectioning the suprahyoid or infrahyoid muscle attachments, or both, can provide another 2.5 to 5.0 cm of length. The suprahyoid release is generally preferred because this causes fewer problems with dysphagia. A right thoracotomy can also be performed to divide the inferior pulmonary ligament and mobilize the thoracic trachea and the hilum of the right lung. This may provide another 5.0 cm of tracheal length; however, 7 cm of tracheal loss (about half the tracheal length) is the upper limit of resection that is usually compatible with primary closure, even using all of these release procedures.

A tracheostomy is usually not necessary following tracheal repairs unless the patient requires prolonged intubation for concomitant injuries. Laryngeal fractures, recurrent nerve injuries, high spinal cord lesions, severe chest trauma, and closed-head injury are some of the other indications for tracheostomy.

AXIOM Often, some subglottic or tracheal stenosis develops postoperatively in patients with cervical tracheal injuries because of excess granulation tissue or scar contracture.

Problems Resulting from Prolonged Intubation

AXIOM Although endotracheal tubes may be lifesaving, their prolonged use may damage the larynx and trachea, especially if a high-pressure balloon cuff is used.

Even if the initial intubation was completely atraumatic, prolonged endotracheal intubation can cause severe mucosal and cartilaginous changes with eventual stricture formation in the larynx and trachea. This is especially likely to occur if the endotracheal tube balloon is inflated excessively. Endotracheal tubes, with "soft" compliant balloon cuffs, are much less likely to damage the trachea, especially if they are not completely inflated and a small amount of air is allowed to escape during expiration.

Many surgeons perform a tracheostomy if endotracheal intubation is required for more than 7 to 10 days. The advantages of an early tracheostomy over prolonged endotracheal intubation are being increasingly recognized (24).

Tracheostomy Tubes

The most likely site for development of tracheal stenosis following a tracheostomy is the tracheostomy stoma itself. The next most frequent site is the junction of the superior and middle third of the trachea where the inflated cuff can cause pressure necrosis of the tracheal cartilages.

OUTCOMES

Up to one-third of all patients who survive an upper airway injury and reach a hospital alive suffer some delays in treatment before the diagnosis is made (7). Preventable deaths occur in up to 10% of patients with upper airway trauma, and these are most likely to occur in patients whose airway injuries are not diagnosed in a timely fashion.

Most surviving patients with severe laryngotracheal injuries have some permanent voice and airway impairment, or a tendency to pulmonary aspiration, or both. Granulation tissue, subsequent scar formation, and voice and airway problems are more frequent after blunt than penetrating neck trauma, because the injury is usually more extensive. Delay of treatment for more than 24 hours also appears to be an important contributor to late complications, especially of late airway stenosis (25).

⊘ FREQUENT ERRORS

1. ***Failure to suspect a laryngeal injury in a patient with neck trauma because the voice seems normal.***
2. ***Failure to realize that a little inspiratory stridor actually means an obstruction of at least 70% of the airway lumen.***

3. ***Assuming that an airway problem in an unconscious patient is only due to prolapse of the tongue.***
4. ***Attempting blind endotracheal intubation in a patient with suspected laryngeal lacerations or fractures.***
5. ***Inserting an endotracheal tube with more force than usual if the tip is through the cords but does not seem to want to advance.***
6. ***Failure to immediately protect the lower airway when bleeding occurs in the upper airway.***
7. ***Use of muscle relaxants in a patient with a possible cricotracheal separation.***
8. ***Attempts to perform an emergency tracheostomy in the emergency department on an uncooperative patient with only a partial airway occlusion.***
9. ***Inadequately assessing the esophagus for associated injuries in patients with laryngotracheal trauma.***
10. ***Assuming that vocal cord dysfunction following blunt laryngeal trauma is only the result of reactive edema or hematoma formation.***

SUMMARY POINTS

1. The only muscle that separates (abducts) the vocal cords is the posterior cricoarytenoid.

2. Loss of the superior laryngeal nerve paralyzes the cricothyroid muscle. This reduces the tension of the vocal cord and produces a weak husky voice.

3. Patients with an aberrant origin of a subclavian artery have a "nonrecurrent" recurrent laryngeal nerve, which can easily be injured during thyroid or laryngeal surgery.

4. Laryngeal dysfunction following endotracheal intubation is usually due to laryngeal edema, hemorrhage, or mucosal tears.

5. Differentiating between arytenoid dislocation and RLNP can be difficult; both may show an immobile lateralized vocal cord and asymmetrically positioned arytenoid cartilages on laryngoscopy.

6. Cricotracheal separation is often accompanied by damage to both recurrent laryngeal nerves.

7. Patients with blunt laryngotracheal trauma should be considered to have a cervical spine injury until proven otherwise.

8. Isolated pharyngoesophageal tears often cause deep cervical emphysema, but tears of the laryngotracheal structures tend to cause massive subcutaneous emphysema.

9. Severe laryngeal damage may be initially associated with minimal symptoms or signs; therefore, a high index of suspicion, partially based on the mechanism of injury, is essential.

10. If an endotracheal tube cannot be passed through the larynx of a trauma victim, one should assume that a laryngotracheal injury is present.

11. Attempts to intubate a patient with an unsuspected airway injury can easily result in complete obstruction of the airway.

12. CT scans are best for evaluating the laryngeal cartilages, and laryngoscopy and bronchoscopy are best for evaluating the mucosa and cord motion.

13. Dysphonia is the most common presenting symptom of laryngeal injury, but presence of a normal voice on admission does not eliminate the possibility of a significant laryngeal injury.

14. A sucking neck wound and progressive hypoxemia is virtually pathognomonic for a major laryngotracheal laceration.

15. Continued severe hemoptysis suggests a combined airway and major vascular injury.

16. Difficulty breathing in the supine position may be a sign of upper airway injury.

17. Whenever intubating a patient with blunt trauma to the head or neck, one should be prepared to rapidly provide a surgical airway if needed.

18. If a patient with an anterior neck injury had emergency intubation soon after arrival in the hospital, one should rule out a laryngeal or tracheal injury by flexible endoscopy later when the patient is being extubated.
19. Injuries to the upper respiratory tract, especially by penetrating trauma, are frequently associated with injuries to the pharynx or esophagus.
20. If a "stable" patient has a suspected laryngeal injury, a cautious endoscopic examination should be performed before attempting airway intervention.
21. Bronchoscopy and laryngoscopy, when done together, are virtually 100% accurate for upper airway injuries; however, if they are done individually, there is an occasional false-negative finding.
22. Damage to the recurrent laryngeal nerves results in varying and somewhat unpredictable vocal cord positions; however, bilateral injury can cause sudden complete airway obstruction.
23. While examining the larynx for injury, one must be prepared to handle sudden complete airway obstruction.
24. The faster a patient with a narrow airway breathes, the greater the airway obstruction and stridor produced.
25. Muscle relaxants or sedatives in patients with complete cricotracheal separation can rapidly cause complete airway obstruction.
26. Patients with an acute airway problem that may be due to trauma to the larynx or trachea should generally be brought to the operating room as soon as possible.
27. Nasotracheal intubation should not be attempted in patients with suspected laryngeal or tracheal trauma.
28. Coniotomy can be extremely dangerous in patients with possible lower laryngeal or tracheal injuries.
29. "Rapid sequence" intubation is usually contraindicated in patients with a possible laryngeal injury; all airway manipulations should be performed, if possible, while the patient is conscious and breathing spontaneously.
30. After completion of a tracheostomy, it is important to auscultate the lungs and obtain chest radiography because pneumothorax may develop in approximately 1% to 5% of such patients during or shortly after the procedure.
31. Complete cricotracheal separations have a high incidence of associated esophageal injuries, particularly in the postcricoid region; therefore, esophagoscopy and careful surgical exploration is essential with these injuries.
32. Although endotracheal tubes may be lifesaving, their presence for prolonged periods may damage the larynx and trachea, especially if the cuff is overinflated.
33. Most surviving patients with severe laryngotracheal injuries will have permanent voice damage and airway narrowing plus a tendency to aspirate oral contents.

REFERENCES

1. Wilson RF, Arden RL. Laryngotracheal trauma. In: Wilson RF, Walt AJ, eds. *Management of trauma—pitfalls and practice,* 2nd ed. Philadelphia: Williams & Wilkins, 1996:285.
2. Asensio JA, Valenziano CP, Falcone RE, et al. Management of penetrating neck injuries—the controversy surrounding zone II injuries. *Surg Clin North Am* 1991;71:267–296.
3. Cicala RS, Kudsk KA, Butta A, et al. Initial evaluation and management of upper airway injuries in trauma patients. *J Clin Anesth* 1991;3:91.
4. Cavo J, Leonard G, Tzadik A. Laryngeal trauma. Maull KI, Cleveland HC, Stauch GO, Wolfert CC, eds. *Advances in trauma.* Chicago: Year Book Medical Publishers, 1986:157.
5. Hermon A, Segal K, Har-El G, et al. Complete cricotracheal separation following blunt trauma to the neck. *J Trauma* 1987;27:1365.
6. Reddin A, Stuart ME, Diaconis JN. Rupture of the cervical esophagus and trachea associated with cervical spine fracture. *J Trauma* 1987;27:564–566.
7. Kelly K, Webb WR, Moulder PV, et al. Management of airway trauma. I. Tracheobronchial injuries. *Ann Thorac Surg* 1985;40:551–555.
8. Fuhrman GM, Stieg FH III, Buerk CA. Blunt laryngeal trauma: classification and management protocol. *J Trauma* 1990;30:87–92.

9. Capan LM, Muller S, Turndorf H. Management of neck injuries. Capan LM, Miller S, Turndorf H, eds. *Trauma: anesthesia and intensive care.* Philadelphia: JB Lippincott, 1991:409–446.
10. Tobias ME, Sack AD, Carter G, et al. Cricotracheal separation in blunt neck injury—the sign of hyoid bone elevation. *S Afr J Surg* 1991;27:189.
11. Polansky A, Resnick D, Sofferman RA, et al. Hyoid bone elevation: a sign of tracheal transection. *Radiology* 1984;150:117.
12. Sankaran S, Walt AJ. Penetrating wounds of the neck: principles and some controversies. *Surg Clin North Am* 1977;57:139.
13. Weigelt JA, Thal ER, Snyder WH, et al. Diagnosis of penetrating cervical esophageal injuries. *Am J Surg* 1987;154:619.
14. Ford H, Gardner MJ, Lynch JM. Laryngotracheal disruption from blunt pediatric neck injuries: impact of early recognition and intervention on outcome. *J Pediatr Surg* 1995:30:331.
15. Noyes LD, McSwain NE, Markowitz IP. Panendoscopy with arteriography versus mandatory exploration of penetrating wounds of the neck. *Ann Surg* 1986;204: 21–31.
16. Couraud L, Velly JF, Martignel N'Daiye M. Post-traumatic disruption of the laryngotracheal junction. *Eur J Cardiothorac Surg* 1989;3:441.
17. Ogura JH, Biller HF. Reconstruction of the larynx following blunt trauma. *Ann Otol* 1971;80:492.
18. Alfille PH, Hurford WE. Upper airway injuries [Editorial]. *J Clin Anesth* 1991;3:88.
19. Graham JS, Mulloy RH, Sutherland FR, Rose S. Percutaneous versus open tracheostomy: a retrospective cohort outcome study. *J Trauma* 1996;245–250.
20. Stanley RB. Value of computed tomography in management of laryngeal injury. *J Trauma* 1984;24:359–362.
21. McKenna J, Jacob HJ. Trauma to the larynx. Walt AJ, Wilson RF, eds. *Management of trauma: pitfalls and practice.* Philadelphia: Lea & Febiger, 1975:294.
22. Mathisen DJ, Grillo H. Laryngotracheal trauma. *Ann Thorac Surg* 1987;43: 254–262.
23. Holinger PH, Schild JA. Pharyngeal, laryngeal, and tracheal injuries in the pediatric age group. *Ann Otol* 1972;81:538.
24. Rodriguez JL, Steinberg SM, Luchetti FA, et al. Early tracheostomy for primary airway management in the surgical critical care setting. *Surgery* 1990;108: 655–659.
25. Reece GP, Shatney CH. Blunt injuries of the cervical trachea: review of 51 patients. *South Med J* 1988;81:1542.

16. THORACIC TRAUMA: CHEST WALL AND LUNG[1]

INCIDENCE

AXIOM Chest injuries cause or contribute to 25% to 50% of the deaths attributed to trauma in the United States annually.

At Detroit Receiving Hospital from 1988 through 1994, chest injuries directly caused at least 20% of deaths occurring in patients who arrived at the hospital alive, and they contributed to the in-hospital deaths in another 15%. Some of these deaths might have been prevented by more rapid and adequate ventilation with an endotracheal tube or chest tube or by more rapid correction of hypotension by earlier surgery or more aggressive infusion of fluids and blood. Virtually all of the deaths occurred in patients who were hypotensive on admission or were in respiratory distress and required prompt endotracheal intubation.

EMERGENCY MANAGEMENT

Initial Resuscitation

As with all trauma victims, the initial step in resuscitation of patients with chest trauma is to ensure the patency of the airway and adequacy of ventilation. The minute ventilation (V_E) should be at least 1.5 to 2.0 times normal. Patients with chest trauma in whom acute, severe respiratory distress develops have high mortality rates. In one of our earlier series, 11% of 1,132 patients admitted with chest trauma were in acute respiratory distress and required endotracheal intubation almost immediately upon entrance to the emergency department (2). Of these patients, 58% died. In that same series, the mortality rate was 7% for patients whose admission systolic blood pressure was less than 80 mm Hg (2). When shock was accompanied by acute respiratory distress, the mortality rate increased to 73%. No person older than 43 years of age with chest trauma survived if both shock and acute respiratory distress were present on admission.

AXIOM The combination of shock and acute respiratory distress is highly lethal.

Initial Diagnosis

The main clinical manifestation of penetrating lung wounds is a hemopneumothorax (2). Hemoptysis is occasionally seen, especially with gunshot wounds and, if severe, is an indication for an emergency thoracotomy to prevent continued flooding of dependent alveoli and to prevent possible air embolism.

AXIOM Severe hemoptysis after chest trauma seldom causes hypotension, but it is an indication for an emergency thoracotomy.

Diagnosis of the cause of respiratory distress after trauma must be made promptly. If the patient makes little or no effort to breathe, central nervous system dysfunction caused by head trauma or drugs is the most likely problem. If the patient is attempting to breathe but is moving little or no air, upper airway obstruction should be suspected. If the patient is attempting to breathe and the upper airway appears to be intact but the breath sounds are poor, hemopneumothorax should be considered. If an endotracheal tube is inserted and the breath sounds are poor on one side, one should check the positioning of the endotracheal tube, but if the breath sounds are still poor, one should treat for a presumed hemopneumothorax.

Airway Control

With any airway or ventilatory problem in a severely injured patient, endotracheal intubation is usually preferred over mask ventilation or nasal oxygen administration because it

1. Allows better control of ventilation;
2. Helps to protect against aspiration of gastric contents; and
3. Provides a means for removal of tracheal secretions.

In an awake individual without midfacial injury who is breathing spontaneously, the most comfortable airway is a nasotracheal tube. If it is not possible to rapidly insert such a tube, an orotracheal tube should be inserted carefully while someone stabilizes the patient's head in the midline. In some instances, a fiberoptic laryngoscope or bronchoscope can be used to visualize the glottis, and the endotracheal tube can then be threaded down over the scope.

Tracheal Intubation

AXIOM Cardiac arrests in the emergency department frequently occur during or just after endotracheal intubation.

Although early tracheal intubation and positive-pressure ventilation of critically injured patients can be lifesaving, the most frequent time for a cardiac arrest to occur in trauma patients in the emergency department is just after or during tracheal intubation. Possible causes for cardiac arrest at that time include the following:

1. Inadequate preintubation oxygenation and ventilation;
2. Unrecognized esophageal intubation;
3. Intubation of the right (or left) mainstem bronchus;
4. Excess ventilatory pressures, further reducing venous return;
5. Development of a tension pneumothorax;
6. Systemic air embolism;
7. Vasovagal response (rare); and
8. Development of severe respiratory alkalosis.

Whenever possible, prior to attempts at endotracheal intubation, one should ventilate the patient for at least six to eight breaths with a bag and mask and 100% oxygen. This usually washes out at least 90% of the nitrogen present and elevates the PaO_2 to more than 300 mm Hg, thereby allowing up to 2 to 3 minutes of apnea without great danger.

With emergency endotracheal intubations, it is possible to insert the tube into the esophagus. Ways to ensure that the endotracheal tube is in the trachea include the following:

1. Visualize the tube going between the vocal cords;
2. Note the compliance of the pilot balloon; the pressure in the cuff balloon is less if the tube is in the esophagus;
3. Look for breath condensation in the tube and note the compliance of the ventilation bag; it is easier to ventilate the stomach than the chest;
4. Auscultate the lateral sides of the chest and epigastrium; and
5. Use capnography to confirm an exhaled PCO_2 measurement exceeding 10 to 20 mm Hg.

⊘ PITFALL

One should not assume that the endotracheal tube is properly situated because some breath sounds can be heard bilaterally in the chest.

If breath sounds are heard more clearly in the epigastrium than over the lungs, one should assume that the endotracheal tube is in the esophagus. If any question exists about the location of the endotracheal tube, it should be replaced; however, one should leave the misplaced tube in the esophagus as an anatomic guide while inserting a new endotracheal tube.

Even if the endotracheal tube is correctly placed initially, it is easy for it to move down into the right mainstem bronchus later, especially if the patient is small and uncooperative. Dronen et al. noted that up to 28% of patients who received cardiopulmonary resuscitation had their endotracheal tube in the right mainstem bronchus at the end of resuscitation (3).

AXIOM When breath sounds are poor over the left hemithorax, one should check the position of the endotracheal tube before treating hemopneumothorax.

When the patient has poor venous return because of hypovolemia, excessive ventilatory pressures can further reduce venous return and cause cardiac arrest. If a lung injury or subpleural blebs are present, bagging the patient vigorously can cause a tension pneumothorax to develop rapidly, further reducing venous return.

⊘ PITFALL

Excessive ventilator pressures after intubation can be rapidly fatal.

Any patient with a lung injury, especially with hemoptysis, should be considered at risk for development of systemic air emboli (4). Consequently, the airway pressure should be maintained as low as possible to avoid this complication. Patients with intrabronchial bleeding are also at risk for flooding normal alveoli with blood and rapidly causing severe hypoxemia.

Vasovagal responses are rare in injured patients, but they can occur during insertion of endotracheal, nasogastric, or chest tubes. One should look for this problem to develop during any invasive procedure if the patient has an inappropriately slow pulse rate.

Patients who have an emergency intubation are often hyperventilated aggressively, and this can drive the PCO_2 down to 20 to 30 mm Hg or lower. If plasma bicarbonate levels are normal (24 mEq/L), an arterial PCO_2 of 20 mm Hg increases the pH to 7.70. A pH increase of 0.10 decreases the PCO_2 by about 10%, reduces serum potassium by about 0.5 mEq/L, and reduces ionized calcium and magnesium levels about 4% to 8%. Thus, a sudden, severe alkalosis can cause hypoxemia and can reduce potassium, ionized calcium, and magnesium levels abruptly; this, in turn, can cause serious arrhythmias.

Surgical Airway

If the patient is in severe respiratory distress and an endotracheal tube cannot be inserted promptly, an emergency cricothyroidotomy (coniotomy) should be performed immediately. If the tube inserted is 6 mm or less in diameter, it can easily be occluded by blood or secretions and should be changed to a tracheostomy in the operating room as soon as it is practical.

In children, the cricothyroid space is usually too small for an endotracheal or tracheostomy tube. A 12- to 14-gauge "catheter-over-a-needle" through the cricothyroid membrane and attached to wall oxygen is preferable as the initial effort to prevent severe hypoxemia. The tubing attached to the cricothyroid catheter should have a hole near the attachment, which can be occluded briefly 10 to 30 times a minute to insufflate the lungs with oxygen. This usually provides adequate oxygenation for up to 20 to 30 minutes, but CO_2 retention can be a problem.

Relief of Hemopneumothorax

⊘ PITFALL

Waiting for chest radiography to confirm the presence of a tension pneumothorax before treating it can be rapidly fatal (Fig. 16-1).

If a hemothorax or pneumothorax is suspected in a patient with acute severe respiratory distress, a "blind" chest tube (i.e., a chest tube inserted without waiting for a chest roentgenogram) should be inserted through the fourth or fifth intercostal space in the midaxillary line on the affected side. Digital examination of the pleural

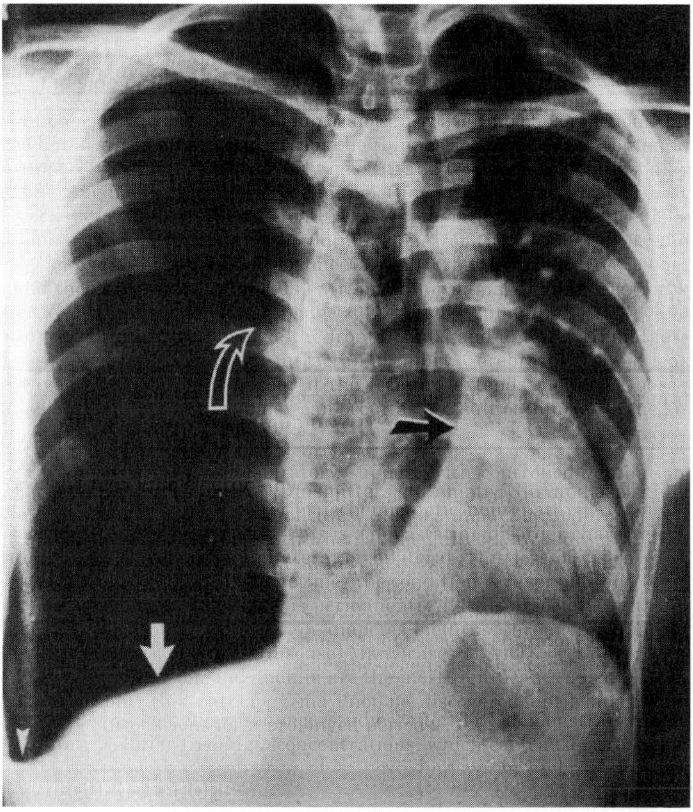

FIG. 16-1. Tension pneumothorax. Signs indicating that the right hemithorax is under tension include depression of the hemidiaphragm (*straight white arrow*), herniation of lung across the midline (*black arrow*), and flattening of the right lung against the mediastinum (*curved open arrow*). Note the small, right hemothorax (*arrowhead*). (From Shulman HS, Samuels TH. The radiology of blunt chest trauma. *J Can Assoc Radiol* 1983;34:204).

cavity before the chest tube is inserted reduces the chances of inserting the chest tube into lung parenchyma (if the lung is stuck to that area by adhesions) or through a high diaphragm.

AXIOM Blind chest tubes should be inserted high and only after finger exploration indicates that it is safe to insert the tube.

If a tension pneumothorax is suspected, a large needle should be immediately inserted into the pleural cavity through the second intercostal space in the midclavicular line to temporarily decompress the pneumothorax while a chest tube is being inserted.

Ventilatory Support

Severe respiratory distress associated with chest trauma and not caused by a pneumothorax or hemothorax is best treated by prompt endotracheal intubation and ventilatory support, particularly if the patient has associated injuries. Ventilatory assistance should also be instituted promptly in patients with a flail chest and marginal ventilation if the patient is in shock, has multiple other injuries, is comatose, requires multiple transfusions, is elderly, or has underlying pulmonary disease. A respiratory rate exceeding 30 to 35 breaths per minute, a vital capacity less than 10 to 15 mL/kg, a negative inspiratory force less than 25 to 30 cm H_2O, and increased ventilatory efforts should also be considered indications for prompt ventilatory support.

A pulse oximeter should be attached to all severely injured patients. Blood gases should also be measured because a pulse oximeter can overestimate arterial oxygen saturation by as much as 2% to 3%. Metabolic acidosis with an arterial P_{CO_2} exceeding 40 to 45 mm Hg is evidence of severe pulmonary dysfunction and also indicates a need for prompt ventilatory support.

An arterial P_{O_2} less than 55 mm Hg while the patient is breathing room air, or less than 80 mm Hg while the patient is breathing supplemental oxygen (equivalent to an FiO_2 of 0.4 or more), is also generally an indication for ventilatory support. Serial arterial blood gas studies indicating increasing pulmonary dysfunction are a strong indication for ventilatory support.

Treatment of Shock

AXIOM Although shock is not usually diagnosed until the systolic blood pressure (BP) is less than 90 mm Hg, a systolic BP of less than 110 in patients with recent severe injuries often indicates inadequate perfusion.

Once adequate ventilation and oxygenation have been ensured, efforts should be directed toward rapidly restoring tissue perfusion, particularly if respiratory distress is also present. In one study, the most frequent causes of shock (systolic BP less than 80 mm Hg) in patients with blunt chest trauma were pelvic or extremity fractures (59%), intraabdominal injuries (41%), and intrathoracic bleeding (26%) (2). In patients with penetrating chest trauma, the most frequent cause of shock, as expected, was intrathoracic injury (74%). The major intrathoracic organ injuries causing the blood loss were the lungs (36%), heart (25%), great vessels (14%), and intercostal or internal mammary arteries (10%).

AXIOM Failure to correct hypotension within 15 to 30 minutes greatly increases mortality rates, especially if the patient requires massive transfusions.

In previously healthy patients who require massive blood transfusions (10 or more units in 24 hours) but have hypotension (systolic BP less than 80 mm Hg) for less than 30 minutes, the mortality rate averages only 9% to 10% (5). If such hypotension is more prolonged (in young, healthy individuals), the mortality rate increases to about 50%. If the massively transfused patients have preexisting disease, or are older than 65 years of age and have shock for more than 30 minutes, the mortality rate exceeds 90%.

When intravenous lines are inserted, a peripheral site is preferred. When peripheral sites are unavailable or monitoring of the central venous pressure or pulmonary arterial wedge pressure is required, a central line should be inserted, usually via a subclavian vein. The catheter is inserted on the side of the injury so that there is less opportunity for a bilateral hemopneumothorax.

⊘ PITFALL

One should not attempt to insert a catheter into a subclavian vein on the side opposite an injured lung because injuries to both lungs can be rapidly fatal.

Some believe that one should use internal jugular veins (rather than subclavian veins) for central lines in patients with chest trauma because attempts at internal jugular vein catheterization are less likely to cause a pneumothorax.

Rarely, the pleural cavity is so full of blood that during an attempt at inserting a subclavian venous catheter, the needle enters the pleural cavity, and then blood is aspirated from the hemothorax, making one believe that the needle and, subsequently the catheter, is in a vein. Obviously, fluid administered through such a line only makes the hemothorax worse and does not improve the patient's vital signs.

Thoracotomy

A large hemothorax or pneumothorax can seriously interfere with ventilation and venous return, and, consequently, it should generally be evacuated as rapidly as possible. If blood is coming out rapidly through the chest tube, vital signs should be followed closely. If the vital signs are improving as the hemothorax is drained and more fluids are given, the pleural cavity should continue to be evacuated. If drainage of a hemothorax causes the patient to become hypotensive, the chest tube should be clamped and an emergency thoracotomy should be performed.

DIAGNOSIS

Signs and Symptoms

The most frequent symptoms of thoracic trauma are chest pain and shortness of breath. The pain is usually well localized to the involved area of the chest wall, but frequently it is referred to the abdomen, neck, shoulders, or arms. Dyspnea and tachypnea are also important symptoms of lung and chest-wall damage, but they are nonspecific and can also be caused by anxiety or pain from other injuries.

⊘ PITFALL

Without careful inspection of the chest wall, one can easily overlook contusions, flail chest, and open or "sucking" chest wounds.

In some patients, a chest wall contusion may be the only external evidence of severe thoracic trauma. Although external bleeding is easily recognized, it may be difficult to determine whether the actual source is intrathoracic or from the chest wall itself. Most chest wounds that communicate with the pleural cavity are readily apparent because of the noise made as air passes through the tissue of the chest wall; however, some of these wounds are open only intermittently and may be discovered only in retrospect.

Segmental fractures (i.e., fractures in two or more locations on the same rib) of three or more adjacent ribs anteriorly or laterally often result in an unstable chest wall. This injury is characterized by a paradoxical inward movement of the involved portion of the chest wall during spontaneous inspiration and outward movement during expiration.

AXIOM Although little or no flail may be apparent initially, as fluid moves into the injured lung and pulmonary compliance decreases, the flail becomes more apparent.

Distended neck veins, especially when the patient is sitting upright, may indicate the presence of pericardial tamponade, tension pneumothorax, air embolism, or cardiac failure. The distended neck veins may not appear until hypovolemia has been at least partially corrected. If the face and neck are cyanotic and swollen, injury to the superior mediastinum with occlusion or compression of the superior vena cava should be suspected. Severe subcutaneous emphysema from a torn bronchus or laceration of the lung can cause massive swelling of the neck and face, quickly obliterating landmarks and, in some instances, completely shutting the eyes.

A scaphoid abdomen may indicate a diaphragmatic injury with herniation of abdominal contents into the chest. A rocking-horse type of breathing may indicate a high spinal cord injury with paralysis of intercostal muscles.

Palpation should begin with determining whether the trachea is in its normal position (in the midline or slightly to the right). Palpation of the chest wall may reveal areas of severe, localized tenderness or crepitation from fractured ribs or subcutaneous emphysema. Because standard radiographs reveal only about 50% of acute rib fractures, areas of severe pain and localized tenderness over injured ribs are often referred to as "clinical" rib fractures.

Dullness to percussion over one side of the chest following trauma may be the first evidence of hemothorax; conversely, hyperresonance tends to indicate the presence of pneumothorax. Pericardial dullness extending more than 1 inch past the point of maximal cardiac impulse may indicate the presence of pericardial tamponade or a large pericardial effusion.

If the breath sounds are equal bilaterally at the bases and apices, the major bronchi are probably intact. Decreased breath sounds on one side usually indicate the presence of hemothorax or pneumothorax, but this may also occur if the endotracheal tube is in too far and is only ventilating one lung. Chen et al. (6) found that 42% (30 of 74) of the pneumothoraces or hemothoraces seen on chest radiograph were missed on auscultation. Although auscultation has a high positive predictive value (98%), "normal breath sounds" do not rule out a hemopneumothorax.

A pneumomediastium should be suspected if a crunching sound (Hamman's sign) is heard over the heart during systole. This finding is present in about 50% of patients with pneumomediastinum, and it is heard best if the patient is in the left lateral decubitus position.

X-Ray Findings

Even with rib detail films, up to 50% of rib fractures are not visible initially. Consequently, with an appropriate history and the finding of localized tenderness over ribs, one can make a diagnosis of clinical rib fractures. Many of these rib fractures can be seen 2 to 4 weeks later when callus or a lytic line develops at the fracture site. Sternal fractures are also easily missed on routine chest films and special lateral views or computed tomography (CT) scans are often required.

Except with direct trauma, such as with a hammer, it usually takes great force to fracture the first and second ribs. In one series, 40% of the patients with fractures of the first and second ribs had severe associated intrathoracic injuries, including myocardial contusion, bronchial tear, or major vascular injury (7). Indeed, first rib fractures are associated with higher mortality rates (15% to 36%) than any other rib fractures because of the frequent association of severe injuries (8).

If a patient with fractured lower ribs, especially ribs 9 through 11, becomes hypotensive and does not have a large hemothorax, tension pneumothorax, or extremity fractures, then intraabdominal bleeding from an injured spleen or liver must be suspected. In one series of 783 patients with rib fractures from blunt chest trauma, 71% of patients admitted in shock had a ruptured intraabdominal viscus (8).

It generally takes great force to cause a scapular fracture. Consequently, when a fracture of the scapula occurs, one should look for underlying damage to ribs, lungs, and great vessels. It is also easy to miss scapula fractures on chest radiographs.

In most patients, radiographic changes of lung contusion appear during the first 4 to 6 hours after injury; in the remaining patients, changes appear within the next 24 hours. These changes are usually a patchy infiltration or consolidation of the lung at the site of injury. The roentgenographic changes frequently appear much worse during the next 24 to 48 hours.

On a good upright chest film, a hemothorax is usually not apparent unless at least 300 mL of blood is present. On a lateral decubitus film, 200 mL may be apparent. If the films are obtained as anteroposterior films with the patient lying prone, a 500- to 1,000-mL hemothorax can easily be missed, especially in obese patients.

AXIOM A moderate hemothorax with up to 500 to 1,000 mL of blood can easily be missed if the chest films are obtained while the patient is lying flat.

If suspicion of pneumothorax exists and it is not seen on the initial chest radiography, the patient should also have expiratory posteroanterior chest films. Generally, a pneumothorax is seen better on expiratory chest films because the pneumothorax space takes up a larger percentage of the involved hemithorax. An apical lordotic view may also show an apical pneumothorax better. A delayed pneumothorax or hemothorax (caused by trauma to the lung parenchyma or intercostal vessels by rib fragments) may occasionally develop more than 12 to 24 hours after the initial injury.

AXIOM Most posttraumatic pneumomediastinums without a pneumothorax are idiopathic, but if their source is not sought aggressively, important aerodigestive injuries may go untreated until too late.

With a pneumomediastinum, one should look closely for an injury to the tracheobronchial tree or esophagus. In most patients, no obvious injury or source can be found. Most "spontaneous" pneumomediastinums are seen in patients with asthma or emphysema.

CT scans of the chest can detect extremely small hemothoraces and pneumothoraces (with volumes less than 50 mL). These "occult" pneumothraces (i.e., seen only on CT scan) do not require a chest tube unless the patient is put on a ventilator (as with general anesthesia).

AXIOM In up to 50% of patients with an occult pneumothorax, a tension pneumothorax develops during ventilatory support.

TREATMENT

Chest Wall Problems

Penetrating Chest Wounds

Probing of penetrating chest wounds to determine their depth or direction can be dangerous because such probing can damage underlying structures or cause severe, recurrent bleeding, pneumothorax, or a sucking chest wound. Bleeding from larger muscles can be profuse and is best controlled initially by local pressure.

AXIOM Occluding a sucking chest wound without simultaneously inserting a chest tube can rapidly cause a tension pneumothorax.

Small, open chest wounds can act as one-way valves, allowing air to enter during inspiration, but allowing none to leave during expiration, thereby causing an increasing pneumothorax, especially if there is an air leak from the lung. With larger chest wall wounds, air may come into the pleural cavity preferentially through the wound in the chest wall rather than through the tracheobronchial tree.

AXIOM If an open chest wound exceeds two-thirds of the cross-sectional area of the trachea in a patient who is breathing spontaneously, effective lung ventilation may cease.

Chest tubes should not be inserted through traumatic holes in the chest wall because they are likely to follow the missile tract into the lung or diaphragm and cause further damage to those organs or restart massive bleeding.

Injuries caused by close-range shotgun blasts or high-powered rifles can destroy such large quantities of tissue that it may be impossible to close the chest wall in the usual manner. Large chest wall defects, after thorough debridement, can be closed with various types of muscle flaps. With large, low chest wounds, the diaphragm may be detached and reimplanted to the chest wall above the wound. The open subdiaphragmatic wound can then be packed with gauze. Thoracostomy tubes are inserted into the involved pleural cavities through separate incisions for pleural drainage.

Subcutaneous Emphysema

Subcutaneous emphysema usually develops because air from damaged lung parenchyma or the tracheobronchial tree has gained access to the chest wall through an opening in the parietal pleura. Although the patient's appearance may be greatly distorted and severe discomfort may be experienced, subcutaneous emphysema by itself does not generally cause any significant ventilatory or hemodynamic problem unless there is an associated pneumothorax.

AXIOM Patients with subcutaneous emphysema after chest trauma should have a chest tube inserted if they are placed on a ventilator, even if a pneumothorax is not seen.

If a pneumothorax is not apparent on chest radiograph, one should be cautious when inserting a chest tube because extensive pleural adhesions may be present. Consequently, if a pleural space cannot be found with a finger inserted through the prospective chest tube site, a catheter should be inserted into the pneumothorax under CT guidance.

Rib Fractures

The pain of rib fractures can greatly interfere with ventilation. Strapping the chest with adhesive tape or a rib belt to relieve the pain may be effective in young, athletic individuals with only a few rib fractures; however, in less vigorous patients, strapping may further reduce ventilation and cause progressive atelectasis.

Probably the best analgesics for mild-to-moderate chest wall pain are acetaminophen with codeine every 4 to 6 hours or ibuprofen 600 to 800 mg every 6 to 8 hours as needed. Meperidine or morphine shots are likely to suppress the cough reflex too much.

An intercostal nerve block is a relatively good way to control severe chest wall pain because it can be accomplished without suppression of the patient's cough and without oversedation. This can usually be accomplished readily by the injection of 2 to 4 mL of a local long-acting anesthetic such as 0.5% to 1% bupivacaine (Marcaine) mixed with 1% lidocaine with epinephrine at the lower edge of each rib to be blocked. Because of the crossover of nerve fibers, it is necessary not only to infiltrate the intercostal nerves of the involved ribs but also to infiltrate two ribs above and two below the fracture sites (Fig. 16-2).

Any portions of the chest wall that are still tender 5 to 10 minutes later should be directly infiltrated. Unless a functioning chest tube is already in place, chest radiographs should be obtained after this procedure to ensure that a pneumothorax has not developed.

AXIOM Thoracic epidural analgesia is usually the best method for controlling chest wall pain.

Periodic injection of morphine-like agents into a spinal epidural catheter can relieve pain more effectively than intercostal blocks (9). The patient should have monitoring in an intensive care unit (ICU) or stepdown-ICU environment because apnea or severe hypoventilation may develop occasionally up to 12 to 16 hours after the last dose. Urinary retention may also occur.

In 1987, Rocco et al. reported significant pain relief and improved minute ventilation by injecting local anesthetics through an intrapleural catheter into the chest in patients with multiple rib fractures (10); however, when Luchette et al. compared the effectiveness of intrapleural analgesia and epidural catheter techniques, epidural analgesic was significantly better (11). It caused less pain at rest, reduced the use of parenteral narcotics, and provided better negative inspiratory pressure and tidal volumes.

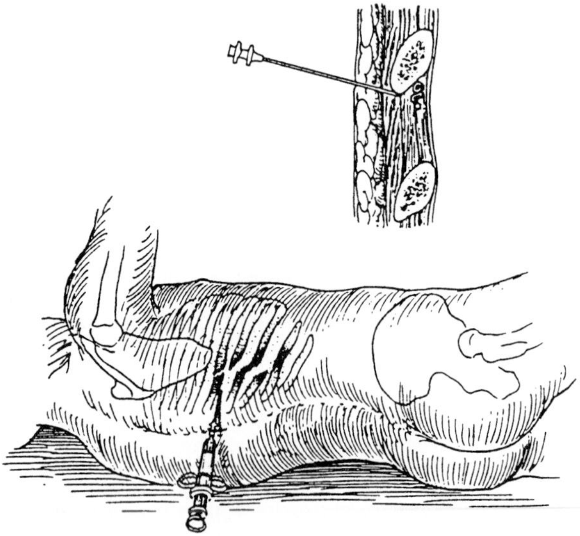

FIG. 16-2. Intercostal nerve block. Inset shows insertion of the needle tip beneath a rib. Ideally, the needle should be angled up a little to get nearer to the intercostal nerve. (From Kirsh MM, Sloan H. *Blunt chest trauma general principles of management.* Boston: Little, Brown 1977:101).

AXIOM If atelectasis or excessive pulmonary secretions develop that cannot be treated adequately with pulmonary physiotherapy and nasotracheal suctioning, bronchoscopy is indicated.

Flail Chest

AXIOM The associated pulmonary contusion is the main cause of the hypoxemia seen with flail chest injuries.

In patients with an unstable chest wall, ventilatory impairment is associated with decreased vital capacity, functional residual capacity, total lung volume, and lung compliance. Patients with a flail chest often are also unable to cough effectively, resulting in a tendency toward accumulation of tracheobronchial secretions, atelectasis, and pneumonitis.

Nonventilator Management

AXIOM Patients with isolated flail chest injuries can often be managed without ventilatory support, especially if the chest pain can be adequately relieved.

Because the magnitude of the flail chest, the underlying pulmonary contusion, and the associated injuries vary from patient to patient, the treatment should be individualized, but it should be provided in an ICU or step-down ICU where the patient can be closely monitored. The treatment is directed primarily toward the relief of pain and prevention of respiratory complications.

Fluid overload can rapidly result in worsening of the pathophysiologic changes of lung contusion (16). Although large volumes of colloid and crystalloids may be required during resuscitation and during the period of obligatory third-spacing of fluid, restriction of fluids thereafter may help reduce the amount of water moving into the contused lung.

Ventilatory Support

In addition to an increasing flail chest as lung compliance decreases with time, the patient may fatigue rapidly because of the decreased efficiency of ventilation and increased muscle effort. Thus, a vicious cycle of decreasing efficiency of ventilation, increasing fatigue, and hypoxemia may progress to a complete respiratory arrest (12).

Indications for early ventilatory support in patients with flail chest include

- Shock
- Three or more associated injuries
- Severe head injury
- Previous severe pulmonary disease
- Fracture of eight or more ribs
- Age greater than 65 years (12)

Although the mortality rate of flail chest injuries is largely related to the numbers and types of associated injuries, early (prophylactic) ventilatory assistance in patients with flail chest and only one or two significant other injuries has been associated with a mortality rate of only 7% (12). This is in sharp contrast to a mortality rate of 69% in similarly injured patients in whom ventilatory assistance was delayed until there was clinical evidence of respiratory failure.

AXIOM If a patient requires ventilatory support, it is much safer to apply it "prophylactically" before actual ventilatory failure develops.

Fixation of Ribs

In patients with a large, unstable chest wall segment who require thoracotomy for other injuries, the flail segment should also be fixed at that time with appropriate devices, for example, intramedullary nails, struts, or wires (13). Some surgeons, especially in European hospitals, greatly prefer treatment with early mechanical fixation of the fractured ribs versus prolonged ventilatory support; however, most U.S. trauma surgeons use rib fixation rarely.

Sternal Fractures

AXIOM Sternal fractures should make one look carefully for an associated myocardial contusion.

In some series reported by radiologists, up to 70% of patients with fractured sternums have had a myocardial contusion (14). Consequently, in patients with fractured sternums from severe trauma, electrocardiograms and creatine phosphokinase (CPK-MB) studies should be done every 8 to 12 hours for the first 24 hours. Echocardiography or radionuclide angiography may also be indicated. However, our experience, and that of other surgeons, suggests that the incidence of a significant myocardial contusion with a fractured sternum is less than 5% (15).

Lung Injuries

Pulmonary Contusions

Treatment of pulmonary contusions primarily involves maintenance of adequate ventilation of the lungs and prevention of pneumonia. Chest physiotherapy, nasotracheal suction, intercostal nerve blocks, and epidural analgesia are used as needed. When ventilatory assistance is required, use of intermittent mechanical ventilation (IMV) and positive end-expiratory pressure (PEEP) usually provides much better ventilation-perfusion matching, better venous return, and quicker weaning than standard assisted or controlled ventilation.

AXIOM If ventilatory pressures are high (plateau or alveolar pressures greater than 30–35 cm H_2O), one should probably use pressure-control ventilation.

Although the type and amount of fluids to be administered to patients with pulmonary contusion are somewhat controversial, the amount of crystalloid solutions given should be just enough to keep the hourly urine output at about 0.5 mL/kg body weight. Patients who have severe unilateral lung injuries and are responding poorly to conventional mechanical ventilation may benefit from synchronous independent lung ventilation provided through a double-lumen endobronchial catheter (16). This technique helps prevent overinflation of the normal lung and underinflation of the damaged lung.

Systemic Air Embolism

If systemic air embolism causes a cardiac arrest, the head should be lowered and an immediate thoracotomy performed to clamp the hilum of the injured lung. Air should then be aspirated from the left heart and aorta. Open cardiac massage with clamping of the ascending aorta may help push air through the coronary arteries. If it is available, cardiopulmonary bypass should be instituted if there is persistent cardiogenic shock.

Intrabronchial Bleeding

Intrabronchial bleeding should be controlled as soon as possible because it can cause death rapidly from severe hypoxemia caused by flooding of dependent alveoli (17). Indeed, relatively small amounts of blood infused into a dog trachea over 30 to 60 minutes can cause severe hypoxemia with minimal changes in $PaCO_2$ or airway resistance. The combination of shock and intrabronchial bleeding is highly lethal and can reduce oxygen transport rapidly to less than 25% of normal. In patients with hemoptysis resulting from trauma, the noninvolved lung must be kept as free of blood as possible, and nasotracheal suction and bronchoscopy should be performed as often as necessary to keep the tracheobronchial tree clear.

If a thoracotomy is necessary, it should be performed with the patient supine (through a midsternotomy or anterior thoracotomy) to prevent the noninvolved lung from being flooded with blood. If the bleeding is severe, a double-lumen endotracheal (Carlens) tube can be used to confine the bleeding to one lung. When a Carlens or similar tube is not available or cannot be inserted, one may insert a smaller (5- to 6-mm diameter) endotracheal tube over a flexible bronchoscope into the left mainstem bronchus. In some instances, bleeding can only be controlled by obstructing the involved bronchus with gauze or the inflated balloon of a Fogarty catheter.

Aspiration

Aspiration of gastric contents is common after severe trauma, especially if the patient is unconscious. After removing as much material as possible from the tracheobronchial tree by endotracheal suction, the patient should have prompt bronchoscopy to remove whatever fluid or food particles remain. Although gastric acid will probably already have caused most of its damage within a few minutes, any remaining food particles should be removed.

AXIOM If aspiration of gastric contents is suspected, bronchoscopy should be performed promptly.

When the patient is lying flat, aspiration pneumonitis tends to involve the posterior portions of the lung, especially the superior segment of the right lower lobe, the posterior segment of the right upper lobe, and the superior segment of the left lower lobe. These pneumonias are often necrotizing and frequently progress to form lung abscesses.

Hemothorax

Hemothorax is caused most frequently by bleeding from lung injuries (18); however, the compressing effect of the shed blood, the large concentration of thromboplastin in the lungs, and low pulmonary arterial pressures combine to help reduce bleeding from torn lung parenchyma. Consequently, most patients with intrathoracic bleeding can be treated adequately by intravenous administration of fluids and evacuation of the hemothorax with a chest tube.

Thoracotomy

If persistent, severe intrathoracic bleeding occurs, it usually arises from large central lung injuries or from damage to systemic arteries.

In a study by Washington et al., only 9% of patients with penetrating chest wounds required a thoracotomy to control continued severe hemorrhage (18). A thoracotomy for intrathoracic bleeding is generally indicated if

1. The patient's vital signs remain or become unstable;
2. More than 1,500 to 2,000 mL of blood is lost from the chest tube in the first 12 to 24 hours, and the patient is still bleeding;
3. Drainage of blood from the chest tubes exceeds 300 mL/h for more than 3-4 hours; and
4. The chest remains more than half full of blood on radiography.

With these last three criteria, emergency thoracotomy is not always necessary if the bleeding slows down to less than 200 mL/h.

If possible, emergency thoracotomies should be performed in the operating room; however, if the patient's condition is considered too precarious to transfer to the operating room, the thoracotomy should be performed in the emergency department.

Thoracentesis

A small, stable hemothorax does not always need to be removed, but it should be carefully observed. If the hemothorax seems large enough to drain, one should avoid needle aspiration and use a chest tube. Needle aspiration of a hemothorax is usually incomplete and may cause a pneumothorax or an infected hemothorax.

Chest Tube (Thoracostomy) Drainage

Blood in the pleural cavity should be removed as completely and rapidly as possible. Blood entering the pleural cavity slowly may not clot because its fibrinogen can quickly layer out on the pleural surface. If hemorrhage is rapid, much of the blood clots before it can defibrinate.

Chest tubes for the treatment of hemothorax should be inserted in the anterior axillary line just behind the lateral edge of the pectoralis major muscle and are directed posteriorly and laterally. A 32- to 40-French chest tube is preferred. The intrathoracic position of the chest tube, its last hole, and the amount of air or fluid remaining in the pleural cavity should be checked with an upright chest film as soon as possible after the chest tube is inserted.

If a significant air leak is present, chest films are best done with portable units at the patient's bedside so as not to risk the development of pulmonary collapse or tension pneumothorax while the patient is without suction en route to the radiology department.

Serial chest auscultation plus daily chest radiography and careful recording of the drainage volume and the severity of any air leak are important guides to the functioning of chest tubes. If a chest tube becomes blocked and a significant pneumothorax or hemothorax is still present, the tube should be replaced. This can often be done easily through the same incision that the previous chest tube occupied.

AXIOM Irrigating an occluded chest tube or passing a Fogarty catheter through an occluded chest tube increases the risk of infection.

If the chest tube is functional and well-placed, but a decubitus film shows a fluid shift, then the hemothorax is partly clotted or loculated and another chest tube may be helpful. If a tube is inserted for bleeding, it should be left in place until the drainage is serous and less than 100 to 150 mL/24 hours; there also should be no air leak for at least 24 hours. While the patient is on a ventilator, many physicians prefer to keep the chest tubes in place to act as a safety valve in case a new pneumothorax suddenly develops.

The patient should be in full inspiration when a chest tube is pulled. Patients have a tendency to gasp with a quick inspiratory effort because of the pleural pain caused as the tube is removed. This sudden gasp can rapidly pull large quantities of air into the pleural cavity just as the tube is being removed.

Following removal of a chest tube, chest radiographs should be obtained to rule out any residual or recurrent pneumothorax. Another chest radiograph should be obtained 12 to 24 hours later to confirm continued, complete expansion of the lungs. If chest radiography after chest tube removal shows a small, stable pneumothorax, it should be observed for another 24 hours. If a residual pneumothorax increases in size or becomes symptomatic, another chest tube should be inserted.

Antibiotics

Much controversy exists concerning the value of prophylactic antibiotics in patients with chest tubes for a traumatic hemothorax or pneumothorax. Nevertheless, if the data from the first six prospective studies on the use of prophylactic antibiotics for chest tubes after trauma are pooled, antibiotics reduced the empyema rate from 9.4% (22 of 234) to 0.8% (2 of 230) and the infection rate from 11.1% to 2.5% ($p<.001$). Total intrathoracic infections were reduced from 17.5% (41 of 234) with placebos to 2.9% (7 of 238) with antibiotics. The validity of those data were confirmed in a metaanalysis by Fallon and Wears (19).

Although antibiotics were given as long as the chest tube was in place in the aforementioned studies, other studies by Cant et al. suggest that antibiotics given for 24 hours are adequate (20); indeed a study by Demetriades et al. suggests that only one dose of antibiotics may need to be given (21).

Autotransfusion

In the patient with massive bleeding into a body cavity, autotransfusion may reduce the need for donor blood and its associated risks. Intrathoracic bleeding is generally ideal for this technique because there is usually no contamination of the blood by bile or intestinal contents. To use the blood for autotransfusion, one needs to add citrate or heparin to the blood as it is being removed.

AXIOM Autotransfusion of more than 6 units of washed red cells can cause a coagulopathy.

Retained Hemothorax

If the chest remains more than one-third to one-half full of blood after 3 to 4 weeks, the retained blood should be removed to prevent delayed empyema or fibrothorax. If the blood is allowed to remain in place for more than 3 to 4 weeks, capillaries grow into the clotted blood from visceral and parietal pleural surfaces. This makes later removal of the blood much more difficult.

If evidence of infection (as reflected by spiking fevers or radiologic studies) develops in a patient with a retained hemothorax, the empyema should be drained promptly. If the empyema is loculated or if it is inadequately controlled with chest tube drainage and antibiotics, a thoracotomy and decortication are usually required. Recently, thoracoscopy has been used successfully to drain and decorticate these empyemas (22).

Pneumothorax

A pneumothorax is not likely to cause significant symptoms unless it

- Is a tension pneumothorax
- Occupies more than 20% to 40% of one hemithorax
- Occurs in a patient with shock or preexisting cardiopulmonary disease

Small, Stable Pneumothorax

A small pneumothorax (less than 1.0 cm wide and confined to the upper one-third of the chest) that is unchanged on two chest roentgenograms obtained 6 hours apart in an otherwise healthy individual can usually be treated by observation alone. In most instances after trauma, however, a chest tube or small catheter should be inserted as a precautionary measure, especially if the patient cannot be observed closely.

AXIOM If a patient is to be put on a ventilator (as with general anesthesia) even the smallest pneumothoraces (even the "occult pneumothoraces" seen only on CT scan) should be treated with a chest tube.

In a study of 4,106 patients with initially asymptomatic stabs of the chest (23), only 12% required a tube thoracostomy for a delayed pneumothorax that did not appear until more than 6 hours after admission. The authors also found that patients with nonprogressive, small (less than 20%) pneumothoraces not requiring chest tubes could be discharged after 48 hours of observation; however, 32% of these patients with "small" pneumothoraces had progression of the pneumothorax and required a chest tube.

Catheter Aspiration

Obeid et al. treated simple, uncomplicated traumatic pneumothorax with catheter aspiration (24). This technique of "catheter aspiration of a simple pneumothorax" (CASP) using a 16-gauge catheter, three-way stopcock, and 50-mL syringe successfully reexpanded the lung in 16 of 17 patients without admission to the hospital. However, the CASP technique was suitable in only 6% of all traumatic pneumothoraces seen.

Chest Tube Drainage

If only a pneumothorax is present, a small- to moderate-sized (24–28 French) chest tube may be inserted anteriorly in the second intercostal space in the midclavicular line; however, a high midaxillary tube is generally preferable. The tube should be directed upward and anteriorly or laterally; it should not be in too far and pressing into the mediastinum. It should also be in far enough so that all of the chest tube holes are inside the pleural cavity. A chest radiograph should be obtained promptly after chest tube insertion to be certain that the tube is properly placed and that the lung is completely expanded.

AXIOM The combination of an air leak plus a persistent pneumothorax space should be eradicated within 24 to 48 hours if possible.

In general, a small- or moderate-sized persistent pneumothorax does not cause complications unless it is associated with a continuing air leak. In like manner, a continuing air leak does not usually cause problems if the lung is completely expanded; however, if a pneumothorax and continued air leak persist for more than 48 hours, the incidence of empyema and bronchopleural fistula is greatly increased. If the pneumothorax space cannot be eradicated with another chest tube, bronchoscopy, and ventilatory support, one should strongly consider a thoracotomy to correct the problem.

Blunt Tracheobronchial Injuries

Blunt tracheobronchial injuries are rare and most patients with such trauma die before they reach the hospital, primarily from severe associated injuries. In a review of 27 patients with tracheobronchial injuries over a 10-year period in Dallas County, only 9 (33%) reached the hospital alive (25).

AXIOM A large air leak, mediastinal air, or persistent pneumothorax following trauma is due to a tracheobronchial injury until proven otherwise.

Shimazu et al. found that endobronchial intubation or a double-lumen endobronchial tube greatly improved ventilation in patients with torn major bronchi (26). Similar benefits were noted by Iwasaki and colleagues who used an Univent tube, which has a movable blocker capable of excluding the injured lung to prevent aspiration of blood into the uninjured lung (27).

SURGICAL APPROACH

In deciding on which side to perform a thoracotomy for exploration and repair of major bronchial injuries, one should be aware that the side of the largest pneumothorax or air leak may not be the side of the injury. Taskinen et al. noted that, of three patients with left-sided injuries, two had massive air leaks to the right side and only one to the left (28). The adventitial tissue surrounding the left main bronchus is so tight that it can often prevent air leakage to the left.

Isolated distal tracheal or proximal right and left mainstem bronchial injuries are best exposed through a right-sided posterolateral thoracotomy. If an associated vascular injury requires the use of a median sternotomy, division of the left innominate vein plus extensive mobilization of the aorta, the arch vessels, and the superior vena cava can provide fairly good exposure of the trachea down to the level of the carina.

Tracheobronchial Repairs

In most patients with tracheal transection, the two segments can be brought together easily without tension, and only rarely should additional length be needed because of loss of tracheal tissue. Up to 5 or even 6 cm of the trachea can be excised, if necessary, and a primary tracheal anastomosis can still be performed (29).

AXIOM Tracheal dissection must be performed carefully to avoid disrupting the tracheal blood supply that comes in laterally or posterolaterally.

Direct cannulation of the distal trachea with a small (7.0 mm), sterile, cuffed tube can provide uninterrupted ventilation while the transected ends of the trachea are mobilized. Most surgeons now use slowly absorbable materials because of the danger of suture granulomas.

Use of a pedicled flap of pericardium, pleura, or intercostal muscle to wrap a tracheal or bronchial anastomosis reduces the risk of air leak and may promote healing. If the tracheal repair is directly adjacent to the repair of a vascular injury, a pedicle flap of pleura or pericardium should be used to separate the suture lines.

Delayed Repairs

Delay in repair of injured bronchi increases the risk of infection and later stenosis. When bronchial stenosis develops and the distal lung is not seriously infected, the stenotic segment can be excised and the bronchus reconstructed after the distal bronchus is thoroughly cleaned (30). If the bronchial injury is extensive, if severe infection is present, or if the rupture is situated in a small bronchus, resection is preferable to reconstruction (31).

Postoperative Management

Postoperative management of the patient with tracheal or bronchial anastomosis requires careful attention to keeping the bronchi clear of secretions, which tend to build up distal to suture lines. Careful endotracheal suctioning is needed so as not to disturb the suture line. Bronchoscopy may be required daily or more frequently if secretions are excessive or if any atelectasis is present (36).

⊘ FREQUENT ERRORS

1. ***Aggressive hyperventilation following emergency endotracheal intubation, especially with penetrating chest trauma.***
2. ***Assuming an endotracheal tube is properly positioned because breath sounds can be heard over both sides of the upper chest anteriorly.***
3. ***Promptly inserting a chest tube (without checking the position of the endotracheal tube) when the breath sounds are reduced on one side after endotracheal intubation.***
4. ***Insistence on chest radiography before insertion of a decompressing needle or a chest tube in a patient with severe respiratory distress or shock that may be due to tension pneumothorax.***
5. ***Failure to provide early monitoring with pulse oximetry or frequent arterial blood gases in patients with chest trauma.***
6. ***Assuming that a hemothorax or a pneumothorax is not present because they were not seen on a supine chest radiograph.***

7. ***Closing or covering a sucking chest wound without prompt insertion of a chest tube on that side.***
8. ***Delay in inserting a chest tube in a trauma patient who has subcutaneous emphysema and will require ventilatory assistance or a general anesthetic.***
9. ***Giving inadequate local pain relief in patients with multiple fractured ribs.***
10. ***Delay in providing ventilatory assistance to a patient who has a flail chest plus two or more other significant injuries.***
11. ***Failure to look carefully for possible associated injuries to the heart or great vessels in patients with fractures of the scapula, sternum, or the first two ribs.***
12. ***Delay in operating on patients with moderate to severe hemoptysis or air embolism after chest trauma.***
13. ***Inadequate or delayed protection of the uninvolved lung in patients with hemoptysis or intrabronchial bleeding.***
14. ***Delayed or inadequate evacuation of a hemothorax after chest trauma.***
15. ***Delayed thoracotomy in patients with thoracic trauma and continued unstable vital signs, a massive hemothorax, or persistent significant bleeding (exceeding 200–300 mL/h).***
16. ***Failure to promptly perform bronchoscopy in a patient with a persistent pneumothorax and large air leak after insertion of one or more chest tubes.***
17. ***Failure to look for tracheobronchial or esophageal injury in patients with a posttraumatic pneumomediastinum.***
18. ***Failure to carefully look for associated vascular or esophageal injuries in patients with penetrating tracheal trauma.***

SUMMARY POINTS

1. Chest injuries cause or contribute to 25% to 50% of the deaths caused by trauma in the United States annually.

2. Shock plus acute respiratory distress requiring prompt endotracheal intubation is a highly lethal combination.

3. Severe hemoptysis after chest trauma seldom causes hypotension, but it is an indication for an emergency thoracotomy.

4. When breath sounds are poor over the right or left hemithorax in a patient with an endotracheal tube, one should check the position of the endotracheal tube before treating a hemopneumothorax.

5. If the patient is in severe respiratory distress and an endotracheal tube cannot be inserted promptly, an emergency cricothyroidotomy (coniotomy) should be performed immediately.

6. If an endotracheal or cricothyroidotomy tube is 6 mm or less in diameter, it can easily be occluded by blood or secretions and should be changed to a tracheostomy in the operating room as soon as it is practical.

7. In patients with chest trauma, persistent impaired ventilation or persistent hypoxemia despite other efforts (i.e., an open airway, relief of chest wall pain, and drainage of any hemopneumothorax) is an indication for ventilatory support.

8. Continuous pulse oximetry should be part of the initial evaluation of anyone with chest trauma.

9. If a patient becomes hypotensive during drainage of a large hemothorax, the chest tube should be clamped and an emergency thoracotomy should be performed.

10. Up to 50% of acute rib fractures are not seen on plain radiographs; therefore, well-localized and persistent tenderness over ribs after chest trauma should be considered to be "clinical" rib fractures if they are not seen on radiography.

11. A moderate hemothorax with up to 500 to 1,000 mL of blood can easily be missed if the chest films are obtained while the patient is lying flat.

12. Occluding a sucking chest wound without simultaneously inserting a chest tube can rapidly cause a tension pneumothorax to develop.

13. If an open chest wound exceeds two-thirds of the cross-sectional area of the trachea in a patient who is breathing spontaneously, effective lung ventilation may cease.
14. Chest tubes should not be inserted through traumatic holes in the chest wall because they are apt to follow the missile tract into the lung or diaphragm and cause further damage to those organs or restart massive bleeding.
15. Patients with subcutaneous emphysema after chest trauma should generally have a chest tube inserted before they are placed on a ventilator.
16. Rib belts and taping of the chest wall to relieve pain from fractured ribs should be avoided except in young, previously healthy individuals.
17. Epidural analgesia is generally the ideal method for controlling chest wall pain so that a patient can cough and breathe deeply.
18. First rib fractures have a higher incidence of associated injuries and death than fractures of any other rib.
19. Although the paradoxical motion of the chest wall in traumatic flail chest injuries can greatly increase the work of breathing, the main cause of the hypoxemia is the underlying lung contusion.
20. Although little or no flail may be apparent initially, as fluid moves into the injured lung and pulmonary compliance decreases, the flail becomes more apparent.
21. If indications for intubating a patient with a flail chest are marginal at the time of admission, the patient should be intubated because the underlying pulmonary contusion and hypoxemia generally get much worse over the next 24 to 48 hours.
22. Prolonged increased work of breathing without relief eventually results in a sudden respiratory arrest.
23. Fluid overloading should be prevented or rapidly corrected in patients with pulmonary contusion.
24. Patients with isolated flail chest injuries can often be managed without ventilatory support, particularly if the chest pain can be adequately relieved.
25. If atelectasis develops or excessive pulmonary secretions cannot be treated adequately with pulmonary physiotherapy and nasotracheal suctioning, bronchoscopy is indicated.
26. If a patient will require ventilatory support, it is much safer to apply it "prophylactically" before actual ventilatory failure develops.
27. Sternal fractures should prompt a search for an associated myocardial contusion.
28. Pulmonary contusions are generally much worse than one would suspect from the initial chest radiographs.
29. In patients with penetrating chest wounds and particularly those with hemoptysis, aggressive positive-pressure ventilation increases the risk of systemic air emboli.
30. Intrabronchial bleeding can rapidly cause flooding of dependent alveoli and severe hypoxemia.
31. If aspiration of gastric contents is suspected, bronchoscopy should be performed promptly.
32. Clots in the pleural cavity release fibrinolysins, and intrapleural clots should be removed as completely and rapidly as possible.
33. Insertion of an exploratory finger before placing a chest tube is important when chest radiographs have not been obtained or when radiography does not clearly show that the lung is away from the chest wall.
34. If the lung has an air leak, the chest tube should not be clamped, even when the patient is being transported.
35. Irrigating an occluded chest tube or passing a Fogarty catheter through it increases the risk of infection.
36. Antibiotics can reduce the incidence of empyema and pneumonia in patients requiring a chest tube for traumatic hemopneumothoraces.
37. Administration of more than 6 units of washed autotransfused red cells can cause a coagulopathy.
38. If chest radiographs performed on admission and 6 hours later in patients with chest trauma are both normal, it is unlikely that additional radiographs are needed except in selected patients.

39. An occult pneumothorax (which is seen only on a CT scan) should be drained with a chest tube or catheter if the patient is to be given ventilator assistance or a general anesthetic.
40. The combination of a persistent pneumothorax space plus a continued air leak frequently results in a pleural infection unless the pneumothorax or air leak can be corrected within 48 hours.
41. Most posttraumatic pneumomediastinums are idiopathic, but if their source is not sought aggressively, important injuries may go untreated until too late.
42. Blunt tracheobronchial injuries usually occur within 2.5 cm of the carina.
43. A large air leak, mediastinal air, or persistent pneumothorax are due to tracheobronchial injury until proven otherwise.
44. A "dropped lung" on an upright chest radiograph is virtually pathognomonic of a complete tear of a major bronchus.
45. Bronchoscopy should be performed in any patient with a suspected airway injury.
46. Bronchial hygiene often with repeat bronchoscopies is especially important after bronchial repairs.
47. Penetrating tracheal trauma often has associated major vascular or esophageal injuries.
48. If a patient is to be put on a ventilator (as with general anesthesia), even the smallest pneumothoraces (even the "occult pneumothoraces" seen only on CT scan) should be treated with a chest tube.

REFERENCES

1. Wilson RF, Steiger Z. Thoracic trauma: chest wall and lung. In: Wilson RF, Walt AJ, eds. *Management of trauma—pitfalls and practice,* 2nd ed. Philadelphia: Williams & Wilkins, 1996:314.
2. Wilson RF, Gibson DEB, Antonenko D. Shock and acute respiratory failure after chest trauma. *J Trauma* 1977;17:697.
3. Dronen S, Chadwick O, Nowak R. Endotracheal tip position in the arrested patient. *Ann Emerg Med* 1982;11:116.
4. Estrera AS, Pass LJ, Platt MR. Systemic arterial air embolism in penetrating lung injury. *Ann Thorac Surg* 1900;50:257.
5. Wilson RF. Complications of massive transfusions. *Surgical Rounds* 1981;4:47.
6. Chen SC, Markmann JF, Kauder DR, Schwab CW. Hemopneumothorax missed by auscultation in penetrating chest injury. *J Trauma* 1997;42:86.
7. Wilson JM, Thomas AN, Goodman PC, et al. Severe chest trauma: morbidity implications of first and second rib fractures in 120 patients. *Arch Surg* 1978;113:846.
8. Bassett JS, Gibson RD, Wilson RF. Blunt injuries to the chest. *J Trauma* 1968;8: 418.
9. Luchette FA, Radfshar MR, Kaiser R, et al. Prospective evaluation of epidural versus intrapleural catheters for analgesia in chest wall trauma. *J Trauma* 1993; 35:165.
10. Rocco A, Reiestad F, Gudman J, et al. Intrapleural administration of local anesthetics for pain relief in patients with multiple rib fractures: preliminary report. *Reg Anesth* 1987;12:10.
11. Luchette FA, Radafshar SM, Kaiser R, et al. Prospective evaluation of epidural versus intrapleural catheter for analgesia in chest wall trauma. *J Trauma* 1994; 36:865.
12. Sankaran S, Wilson RF. Factors affecting prognosis in patients with flail chest. *J Thorac Cardiovasc* Surg 1970;60:402.
13. Borioni R, Ciani R, Guglielmo M, et al. Surgical stabilization of the chest wall. *Ann Thorac Surg* 1992;54:394.
14. Hamilton JR, Dearden C, Rutherford WH. Myocardial contusion associated with fracture of the sternum: important seat belt syndrome. *Injury* 1984;16:155.
15. Shapiro AR, Levi I, Khodann J. Sternal fractures: a red flag or red herring? *J Trauma* 1994;37:59.
16. Adoumie R, Shennib H, Brown R, et al. Differential lung ventilation. Applications beyond the operating room. *J Thorac Cardiovasc Surg* 1993;105:229.

17. Wilson RF, Soullier GW, Wiencek RG. Hemoptysis in trauma. *J Trauma* 1987;27: 1123.
18. Washington B, Wilson RF, Steiger Z, Bassett JS. Emergency thoracotomy: a four-year review. *Ann Thorac Surg* 1985;40:188.
19. Fallon WF, Wears RL. Prophylactic antibiotics for the prevention of infectious complications including empyema following tube thoracostomy for trauma: results of meta-analysis. *J Trauma* 1992;33:110.
20. Cant PJ, Smyth S, Smart DO. Antibiotic prophylaxis is indicated for chest stab wounds requiring closed tube thoracostomy. *Br J Surg* 1993;80:464.
21. Demetriades D, Breckon V, Breckon C, et al. Antibiotic prophylaxis in penetrating injuries of the chest. *Ann R Coll Surg Engl* 1991;73:348.
22. Lang-Lazdunski L, Mouroux J, Pons Francois, et al. Role of videothoracoscopy in chest trauma. *Ann Thorac Surg* 1997;63:327.
23. Ordog GJ, Wasserberger J, Balasubramanian S, et al. Asymptomatic stab wounds of the chest. *Trauma* 1994;36:680.
24. Obeid FN, Shapiro MJ, Richardson HH, et al. Catheter aspiration for simple pneumothorax (CASP) in the outpatient management of simple traumatic pneumothorax. *J Trauma* 1985;25:882.
25. Ecker RR, Libertini RV, Rea WJ, et al. Injuries of the trachea and bronchi. *Ann Thorac Surg* 1971;11:289.
26. Shimazu T, Sugimoto H, Nishide K, et al. Tracheobronchial rupture caused by blunt chest trauma: acute respiratory management. *Am J Emerg Med* 1988;6: 427.
27. Iwasaki M, Kaga K, Ogawa J, et al. Bronchoscopy findings and early treatment of patients with blunt tracheo-bronchial trauma. *J Cardiovasc Surg* (Torino) 1994;35:269.
28. Taskinen SO, Salo JA, Halttunen PEA, Sovijarvi ARA. Tracheobronchial rupture due to blunt chest trauma: a follow-up study. *Ann Thorac Surg* 1989;48:846.
29. Grillo HC. Surgical treatment of postintubation tracheal injuries. *J Thorac Cardiovasc Surg* 1979;78:860.
30. Webb WR. Diagnosis and long-term follow-up of major bronchial disruptions due to nonpenetrating trauma. *Ann Thorac Surg* 1992;33:38.
31. Deslauriers J, Beaulieu M, Archambault G, et al. Diagnosis and long-term follow-up of major bronchial disruptions due to nonpenetrating trauma. *Ann Thorac Surg* 1982;33:32.

17. THORACIC TRAUMA: HEART[1]

PENETRATING INJURY TO THE HEART

Up to 81% of patients with penetrating cardiac wounds die shortly after the injury, either from cardiac tamponade or bleeding (2,3). Bullet wounds are particularly likely to cause death quickly. Of patients lucky enough to reach medical attention, the most important factors for survival are early diagnosis and immediate treatment. Patients with penetrating wounds of the chest, especially from stab wounds, often can be successfully resuscitated from a recent (less than 5 minutes) cardiac arrest by emergency resuscitative thoracotomy.

AXIOM All patients who are in shock and have a penetrating chest injury anywhere near the heart should be considered to have a cardiac injury until proven otherwise (4).

With early, aggressive resuscitation and surgery, up to one-third of patients arriving at a trauma center "in extremis" with cardiac injuries can be saved. For patients who can be brought to the operating room with signs of life and a recordable blood pressure, the survival rates have exceeded 70% for gunshot wounds (GSWs) of the heart and 85% for stab wounds of the heart (5).

Pathophysiology

Patients surviving more than 15 to 30 minutes after a penetrating heart wound usually have relatively small cardiac wounds or pericardial tamponade. In a sense, pericardial tamponade is a two-edged sword: although it may prolong life by reducing the severity of the initial blood loss, it can also be fatal by interfering with venous return and diastolic filling of the heart. Occasionally, a delayed cardiac tamponade can occur days or even weeks after the penetrating chest trauma (6).

AXIOM Pericardial tamponade increases the likelihood of a successful emergency resuscitative thoracotomy for a penetrating injury to the heart.

The normal pericardium cavity cannot easily accommodate rapid accumulation of more than 80 to 100 mL of fluid without increasing the intrapericardial pressure and decreasing cardiac output. At that point, an additional 20 to 40 mL of pericardial fluid can almost double the intrapericardial pressure, thereby greatly restricting cardiac filling and cardiac output. The increased intrapericardial pressure during tamponade decreases diastolic filling of the heart and reduces stroke volume, cardiac output, and arterial blood pressure. The decreased blood pressure causes decreased coronary blood flow, especially to subendocardial tissues; with further increases in pericardial pressure, there is decreased perfusion to both subendocardial and subepicardial tissues (7).

Diagnosis

Physical Examination

AXIOM All patients in shock with penetrating chest wounds between the midclavicular line on the right and anterior axillary line on the left should be considered to have a cardiac injury until proven otherwise.

Beck I Triad

If the only problem with a penetrating heart wound is tamponade and the patient is not hypovolemic, one may find the Beck I triad, which includes

- Distended neck veins
- Hypotension
- Muffled heart tones

The Beck I triad can be deceptive, and may be falsely positive or falsely negative in up to one-third of cases (8).

AXIOM The neck veins in patients with shock from pericardial tamponade do not usually become distended until any coexistent hypovolemia is at least partially corrected.

When fluids are given rapidly to a patient with a cardiac wound that has stopped bleeding and only has pericardial tamponade, the vital signs often improve rapidly after the filling pressures are increased by the fluids.

AXIOM Distended neck veins and hypotension after chest trauma are not always caused by pericardial tamponade.

Breathing abnormally or straining can distend neck veins in the absence of tamponade. A tension pneumothorax, mediastinal hematoma, heart failure, or air emboli can also cause the central venous pressure (CVP) to elevate and blood pressure (BP) to decline.

AXIOM Muffled heart tones are an insensitive and nonspecific sign of pericardial tamponade.

Even with a large, acute pericardial tamponade, which seldom is more than 150 to 200 mL, the heart tones are usually fairly clear, and muffled heart sounds are the least reliable sign in Beck's triad.

Kussmaul Signs

Pericardial tamponade may also cause two Kussmaul signs:

1. Increased distension of neck veins during inspiration; and
2. Pulsus paradoxus.

Paradoxical pulse is characterized by a decrease in systolic blood pressure of greater than 10 to 15 mm Hg during normal inspiration. The "paradoxical" pressure decrease is best determined by listening carefully while taking multiple cuff blood pressures. One notes the highest systolic blood pressure when only one Korotkoff's sound is heard during a ventilatory cycle and then subtracts the highest systolic blood pressure at which all of the Korotkoff's sounds are heard. The difference between these two pressures is the amount of paradox present. The amount of paradox may be increased by hypovolemia or bronchospasm.

AXIOM Bronchospasm is the most frequent cause of pulsus paradoxus in hospitalized patients.

If a CVP catheter is in place and if the venous waves are recorded, various tracings of pericardial tamponade or constrictive pericarditis may be seen. An abrupt decrease in atrial pressures at the beginning of diastole followed by a high, flat-pressure wave has been referred to as the "square-root sign"; however, an acute right ventricular infarction can cause similar changes (9). With constrictive pericarditis, the X descent (after the C wave) may almost disappear and the wave pattern is even flatter (Fig. 17-1).

Diagnostic Tests

Radiographic Studies

If possible, a chest radiograph should be obtained on all trauma victims before they are brought to the operating room. Although chest films are of little help in diagnos-

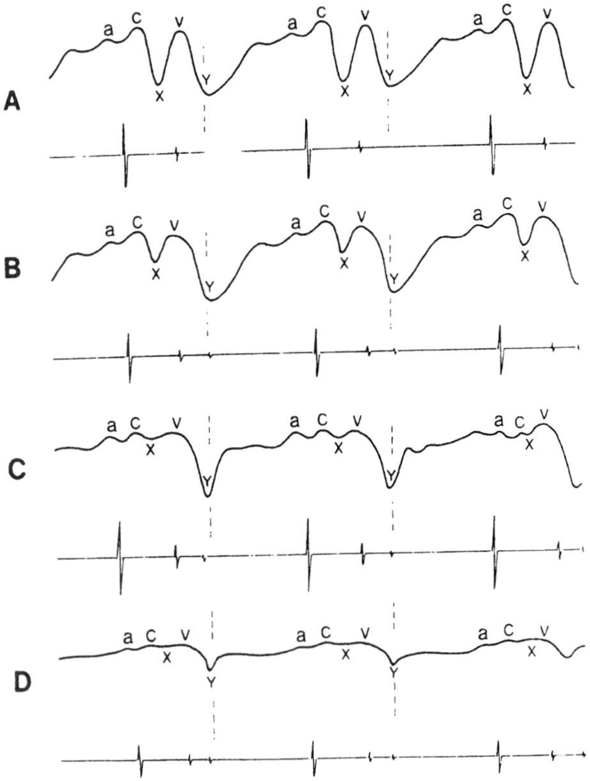

FIG. 17-1. A: Normal right atrial or central venous pressure waves. **B:** A right ventricular infarction or acute right ventricular failure can flatten the atrial waves somewhat and reduce the amount of the X descent. **C:** With constrictive pericarditis, the X descent may almost disappear. **D:** With tamponade, there may be no X descent and the Y descent may become much smaller; the atrial waves also tend to be very flat. With right ventricular infarction, constrictive pericarditis, and pericardial tamponade, the right and left heart diastolic pressures tend to be equal. (From Wilson RF. Injury to the heart and great vessel. In: Henning RJ, Grenvik A, eds. *Critical care cardiology.* New York: Churchill Livingstone, 1989:414.)

ing acute cardiac injury except in unusual cases with intrapericardial air, they may reveal a hemopneumothorax that requires chest tube drainage. If the patient is hemodynamically stable, CT scans can be very accurate (15).

Electrocardiogram

Electrocardiogram (ECG) changes following cardiac injury are usually nonspecific. ST-T-wave changes may indicate pericardial irritation, ischemia, or myocardial damage. New Q waves generally indicate a full thickness myocardial infarction.

Echocardiography

Transthoracic echocardiography (TTE) and epigastric ultrasound can be fairly reliable methods for detecting the presence of increased quantities of intrapericardial fluid (10). TTE, however, is often not immediately available, and up to 5% to 10% false-positive and false-negative results occur.

Pericardiocentesis

AXIOM If blood is obtained on pericardiocentesis and the patient's vital signs improve promptly, a tamponade is almost certainly present.

Pericardiocentesis is not used as a diagnostic procedure very frequently in acutely injured patients with possible tamponade. In at least one series, the incidence of false-negative pericardiocentesis was 80%, and the incidence of false-positive results was 33% (2). In addition to its inaccuracy, pericardiocentesis may injure the heart and cause delays in needed surgery.

Almost all pericardiocenteses are currently done via the paraxiphoid approach (Fig. 17-2). An 18-gauge, 10-cm spinal needle is attached to a stopcock and then to a 20-mL syringe. Pericardiocentesis should be done with continuous ECG monitoring if possible. The needle is passed upward and backward at an angle of 45 degrees for 4 to 5 cm and advanced slowly until the tip seems to enter a cavity. Most authors direct the needle toward the left scapula tip; however, directing the needle toward the right scapula is more likely to parallel the right border of the heart and is less likely to penetrate the right ventricle.

As the needle is advanced, one should aspirate frequently until blood is obtained, cardiac pulsations are felt, or ECG shows an abrupt change, usually premature ventricular contractions (PVCs) or abrupt ST-T wave changes.

AXIOM When a large amount (greater than 20 mL) of blood can be aspirated rapidly and easily during pericardiocentesis, it is likely that one is aspirating blood from the heart rather than the pericardial cavity.

Generally, with penetrating trauma, one-half to two-thirds of the blood in the pericardial cavity is clotted. Consequently, one can usually remove only 4 to 5 mL of blood without manipulating the end of the needle. If 20 mL of blood can be drawn out easily and rapidly, it usually indicates that the blood is being aspirated from the right ventricular cavity.

When immediate thoracotomy is not possible in a patient with positive pericardiocentesis, a plastic catheter inserted over a needle or over a Seldinger wire can be left in place for continued drainage of pericardial blood, as needed, until the cardiac wound can be repaired.

Holes in the right ventricle are frequently found at thoracotomy after attempts at pericardiocentesis. The needle occasionally can cause a fairly large laceration in the right ventricle or a coronary artery and produce tamponade. Other complications, such as arrhythmias, may also occur. A negative pericardiocentesis may also give a false feeling of security that cardiac injury is not present.

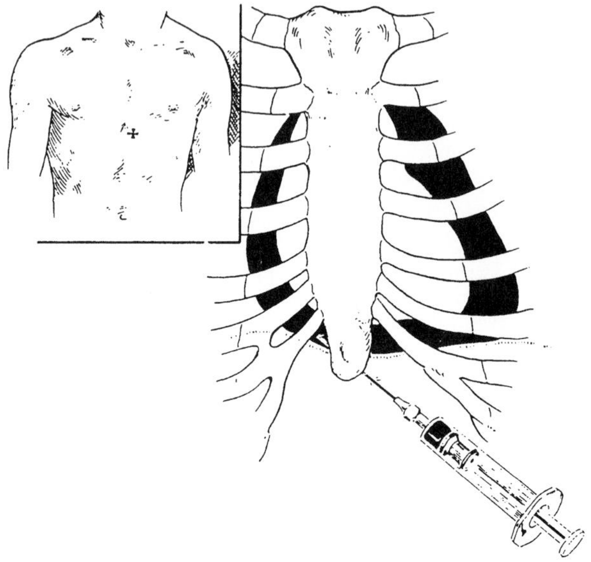

FIG. 17-2. The paraxiphoid technique for pericardiocentesis is usually performed with the needle directed toward the left scapula tip. However, when one aims toward the tip of the right scapula, the needle tends to go parallel to the lateral border of the right heart and is less apt to penetrate the myocardium. (From Wilson RF. Injury to the heart and great vessel. In: Henning RJ, Grenvik A, eds. *Critical care cardiology.* New York: Churchill Livingstone, 1989:415.)

Subxiphoid Pericardiotomy

Another alternative for diagnosing cardiac injury in a patient who is hemodynamically stable is a subxiphoid pericardial window (Fig. 17-3). This can be done under local anesthesia in cooperative individuals, but is generally performed more safely under general anesthesia. If blood is found, as it is in up to 18% of patients (11) and the patient is under general anesthesia, the incision can be extended up as a midsternotomy to repair the cardiac wound. It is not known, however, in how many of these hemodynamically stable patients a problem would have developed if the cardiac wound had not been discovered or treated.

Treatment

Fluid Administration

In patients who are hypotensive and have a low cardiac output, a brief attempt should be made to increase intravascular volume by rapid intravenous infusion of normal (0.9%) saline or Ringer's lactate. If the patient improves and the CVP does not increase as fluid is given rapidly, fluids can be given until the BP and tissue perfusion are adequate. If the CVP increases abruptly with no improvement in tissue perfusion, the patient needs emergency surgery.

AXIOM One of the quickest ways to restore adequate tissue perfusion in a hemodynamically unstable patient with pericardial tamponade is aggressive fluid resuscitation.

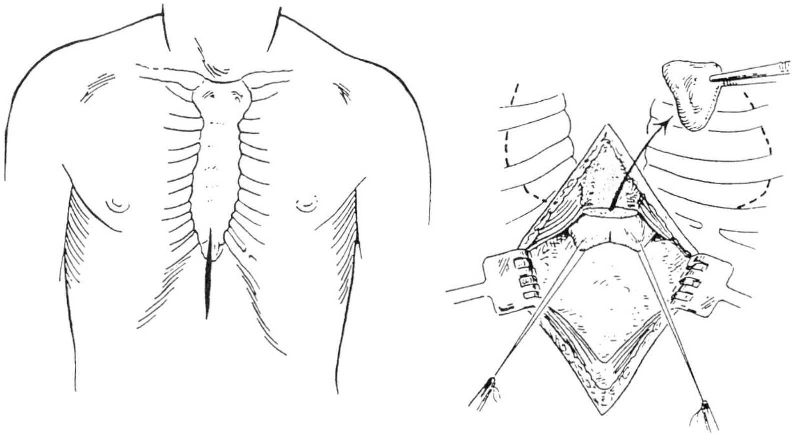

FIG. 17-3. A subxiphoid pericardial window can be performed under local anesthesia in stable patients with suspected paricardial tamponade. The xiphoid process may be removed or split. The diaphragmatic pericardium is pulled inferiorly with traction sutures to facilitate incision of the pericardium. When blood is present in the pericardium, general anesthesia is immediately administered and the incision is extended superiorly into a median sternotomy. (From: Wilson RF. Injury to the heart and great vessel. Henning RJ, Grenvik A, eds. *Critical care cardiology.* New York: Churchill Livingstone, 1989; 416.)

Pericardiocentesis

Pericardiocentesis is primarily a diagnostic procedure, but removal of as little as 5 to 10 mL of blood from the pericardial sac in a hypotensive patient may increase stroke volume by 25% to 50% with dramatic improvement in cardiac output and blood pressure. In selected patients who have small puncture wounds of the heart, pericardiocentesis may be curative, and the patient may not require thoracotomy if the vital signs remain stable.

Emergency Department Thoracotomy

Indications

AXIOM Penetrating wounds of the heart are best treated with emergency thoracotomy and cardiorrhaphy, preferably in the operating room.

In hospitals where adequate facilities, equipment, and trained personnel are present, an emergency department (ED) thoracotomy in patients who arrive with a cardiac arrest from stab of the chest can be lifesaving. Patients who arrive in the ED with no signs of life after a GSW of the chest rarely, if ever, survive. In one study, it was believed that ED thoracotomy for penetrating cardiac injuries is essential for patients who are

1. Clinically dead on arrival in the ED but had some signs of life in transit (survival: 32%); and
2. Deteriorating and have no obtainable blood pressure (survival: 33%).

ED thoracotomies for patients with no signs of life at the scene or within 5 minutes of arrival in the ED are almost invariably futile. Cardiac arrest from blunt trauma or from penetrating brain or abdominal injuries is also almost uniformly fatal (12).

The most frequent time for an injured patient to have cardiac arrest in the ED is during or just after endotracheal intubation. Such cardiac arrests are usually caused by

1. Inadequate preintubation oxygenation;
2. Intubation of the esophagus or right mainstem bronchus; and
3. Excessive ventilatory pressures reducing venous return or causing tension pneumothorax or air embolism.

AXIOM ED thoracotomy for penetrating cardiac injury may be lifesaving for patients deteriorating so rapidly that it is not likely that they will survive movement from the ED to the operating room (4).

Resuscitative ED thoracotomy for trauma should not be performed unless rapid, appropriate backup by the operating room and surgeons is available to properly manage intrathoracic injuries that are likely to be found. The goal of ED thoracotomy is not merely resuscitation of cardiovascular activity, but also salvage of central neurologic function. Patients with isolated stab wounds of the heart and obtainable BP on admission have survival rates often exceeding 90% (13).

AXIOM Whenever the patient can be moved to the operating room with reasonable safety, emergency thoracotomy should be performed there.

Anesthesia

Emergency thoracotomy is often performed with the patient under light general anesthesia administered through an orotracheal tube. If the patient is deeply comatose or in extremis, the operation may be begun without any anesthesia. If some anesthesia is required, drugs such as ketamine, which have little or no cardiodepressant action, cause the least hemodynamic impairment.

Incisions

AXIOM Injuries to the mid or left chest in unstable patients are best explored through the left chest and lesions on the right are best explored through the right chest.

After the patient is intubated, an anterolateral thoracotomy is performed on the side of the injury, one interspace below the male nipple. If the injury is in the midline, a left anterolateral thoracotomy is performed (Fig. 17-4). The incision should be as long as possible, extending from about 1.5 cm lateral to the sternum, to the midaxillary line in the axilla. The incision extends through the intercostal muscles just above the sixth rib into the pleural cavity, being careful not to injure the underlying lung or heart. A rib-spreader is then inserted and opened widely until two hands can fit inside the chest. Cutting the intercostal cartilages above and below the incision may help increase exposure. Frequently, the internal mammary vessels, which lay about 0.5 to 1.0 cm lateral to the sternum, are cut with medial extension of this incision. When this occurs, the vessels must be securely clamped and tied or suture-ligated. One can waste several minutes gaining control of the internal mammary vessels if they are accidentally cut; therefore, one should make an effort to avoid this problem.

If additional exposure is needed, strong consideration should be given to extending the incision across the sternum as bilateral thoracotomy. This allows wide exposure to both sides of the heart and to the proximal great vessels, but it also requires control of both internal mammary arteries.

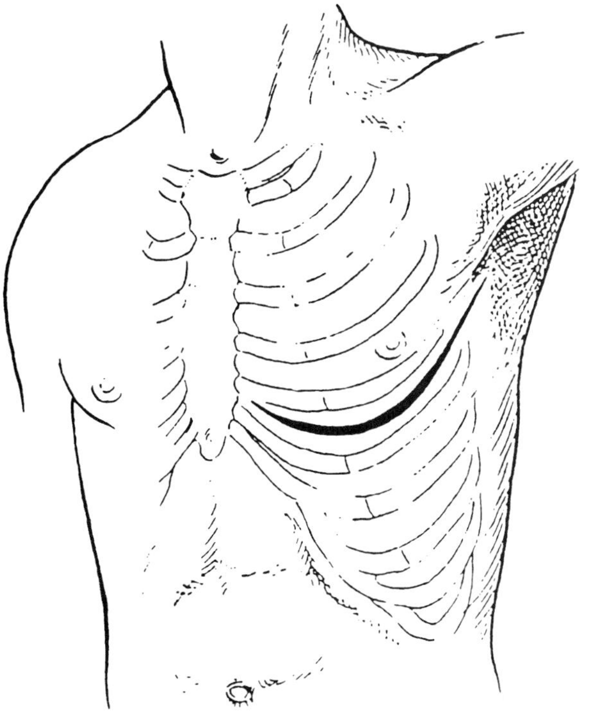

FIG. 17-4. Emergency thoracotomy to treat a stab wound of the heart or to perform open cardiac massage is usually done through an anterolateral thoracotomy incision. The incision extends along the fifth intercostal space with the skin incision placed in the inframammary crease. It extends from just lateral to the sternum to the midaxillary line. (From: Wilson RF. Injury to the heart and great vessel. Henning RJ, Grenvik A, eds. *Critical care cardiology*. New York: Churchill Livingstone, 1989; 418.)

AXIOM If the patient is relatively stable and the cardiac injury is likely to be anterior (as with anterior stab wounds), a median sternotomy can be used to explore the chest.

Even when the pericardial sac is not distended with blood at thoracotomy, it can be difficult to grasp the pericardium with a pickup or forceps. It may be necessary, at times, to "hook" the pericardium with one blade of a scissors and then grab it with a forceps or clamp. Another choice is to make a tiny cut in the pericardium near the diaphram with a scalpel and then elongate the incision with scissors.

The pericardial sac should be opened with scissors in a longitudinal direction 1 to 2 cm anterior (medial) to the left (or right) phrenic nerve. The pericardial incision should extend from the diaphragm below up to the pericardial reflection anteriorly over the ascending aorta. If the pericardial sac is still tight around the heart, a transverse cut of the pericardium inferiorly along the diaphragm may help with exposure. After the pericardium is open, the surgeon should evacuate any liquid blood and clots, begin open cardiac massage if it is needed, and occlude any bleeding cardiac wounds.

Cardiac Wounds

If a cardiac wound is seen, it should quickly be sutured. If it is not convenient to suture the myocardial wound at that time, finger pressure can usually control the bleeding until a repair can be accomplished. A Foley catheter balloon can also be used to occlude the hole while it is being repaired. If a cardiac injury cannot be seen, the heart can be swung out laterally and anteriorly into the left hemithorax to allow better examination. If it is necessary to lift the tip of the heart up, the surgeon should be cautious because this could increase the possibility of air entry into left-sided or posterior cardiac wounds, which could result in sudden, fatal coronary or cerebral air embolism.

Most atrial wounds can be temporarily controlled by the application of a Satinsky vascular clamp and then sewn with a running 3-0 or 4-0 polypropylene suture. Wounds of the ventricles can generally be tamponaded by the surgeon's finger while pledgetted horizontal mattress sutures of 2-0 silk or prolene are passed under the finger and tied by an assistant. When a wound is situated next to a major coronary artery, a pledgetted horizontal mattress suture is placed beneath the artery so as to avoid ligation or compression of the vessel (47). When the left anterior descending coronary artery is involved, use of unnecessarily wide or multiple sutures can cause increased damage to septal perforating branches.

Cardiac Arrest or Hypotension

In patients with severe hypotension or cardiac arrest, one should compress or clamp the descending thoracic aorta to help improve coronary and cerebral blood flow. Because 60% of cardiac output normally goes through the descending thoracic aorta, cross-clamping it can increase blood flow to the coronary and cerebral arteries twofold to threefold.

AXIOM Compressing the descending aorta in a severely hypotensive patient can increase coronary and cerebral blood flow twofold to threefold.

When the cardiorrhaphy has been completed, internal cardiac massage can be performed by compressing the heart between the palms of two hands or between one palm and the sternum. Warm saline poured over the heart may help prevent ventricular fibrillation, which is more likely to occur or recur if the myocardium is hypothermic. If ventricular fibrillation occurs, defibrillation with internal paddles, starting at 20 to 40 watt-seconds and increasing the energy as needed, should be performed. Administration of lidocaine, with or without magnesium, plus correction of severe acidosis or alkalosis may be of benefit for recurrent ventricular fibrillation.

Air Embolism

AXIOM A sudden onset of arrhythmias or hypotension in a patient with open neck veins or a lung injury, especially if hemoptysis is present, should be considered to be the result of air emboli until proven otherwise.

If air embolism is suspected, the head should be lowered and the cardiac chambers and proximal aorta should be aspirated for air immediately. Systemic air embolism is most frequently confirmed by seeing small air bubbles in the coronary arteries. Cardiac massage with full scale cardiopulmonary resuscitation, including clamping of the descending thoracic aorta, is applied vigorously, but is usually unsuccessful.

If a satisfactory rhythm develops, the descending thoracic aorta can be gradually declamped as infusions of fluid and blood are administered, with care being taken to keep the systolic blood pressure greater than 90 to 100 mm Hg. Systolic blood pressures greater than 160 to 180 mm Hg should be avoided when the aorta is clamped because the high pressure may tear open cardiac repairs, excessively dilate the left ventricle (causing irreversible left ventricular failure), or cause intracerebral bleeding.

AXIOM Hypertension and tachycardia greatly increase the workload and oxygen requirements of an injured heart and can cause infarction or overt heart failure.

Special Heart Injuries

Coronary Artery

Laceration of a coronary artery may result in early cardiac tamponade, intrathoracic bleeding, or myocardial infarction. The left anterior descending coronary artery is the most commonly injured vessel. Ligation of the cut ends is the treatment of choice for lacerations of small coronary vessels. Torn proximal coronary arteries may also be ligated if no evidence of cardiovascular dysfunction exists. Such patients must be observed closely. If ligation of a proximal coronary artery results in arrhythmias or impaired hemodynamic function, the vessel should be repaired primarily or, if that is not feasible, it should be bypassed with an internal mammary artery or reversed saphenous vein graft.

Interventricular Defect

An interventricular defect following a penetrating cardiac wound is diagnosed eventually in about 3% to 4% of cases, often late in the postoperative period, but it should be suspected if the patient is in intractable heart failure (14). In most instances, the patient is only mildly to moderately symptomatic, and one can usually wait 2 to 3 months to have the defect repaired.

Cardiac Valve

Most cardiac valve injuries detected postoperatively can be corrected 3 to 6 months later on an elective basis after cardiac catheterization. Occasionally, severe cardiac failure or dysfunction during the initial procedure necessitates an emergency valve repair or replacement.

Ventricular Aneurysms

During a 10-year period at Grady Memorial Hospital, Symbas et al. treated traumatic ventricular aneurysms in five patients, all of which resulted from penetrating trauma (15). The left ventricle is the most common cardiac chamber to develop a traumatic aneurysm, but it may also occur in the right ventricle or in the atria.

AXIOM Pseudoaneurysms of the heart caused by penetrating trauma should be treated surgically because they are basically a contained rupture of the heart.

BLUNT INJURY TO THE HEART

Incidence

Cardiac injury is the most frequent, unsuspected visceral injury responsible for death in fatally injured accident victims, and it accounts for about 25% of deaths at the scene (16). The incidence of cardiac injury after blunt chest trauma in patients who reach the hospital alive probably averages about 15% to 25%, but reports vary from a low of 16% in an autopsy series to a high of 76% in a clinical study (17).

Pathophysiology

AXIOM Myocardial contusion should be suspected in anyone with severe trauma to the anterior chest.

Blunt trauma to the heart can cause a wide spectrum of injuries, including

- Pericardial tears
- Rupture of an outer chamber wall with resulting death from tamponade or bleeding
- Septal rupture
- Valvular injuries, of which the aortic valve is the most frequent
- Direct myocardial injury (contusion)
- Laceration or thrombosis of coronary arteries

Some authors have stressed the differences between myocardial concussion and myocardial contusion (18). With myocardial concussion, no anatomic cellular injury occurs, but some functional damage is demonstrated on two-dimensional echocardiography or other wall-motion studies. With contusion, anatomic injury is demonstrated either by elevated creatinine phosphokinase (CPK-MB) enzymes or by direct visualization at surgery or autopsy.

Emergency Management

Cardiac Rupture

The most severe form of blunt cardiac injury is rupture of the myocardium; this is the heart lesion most frequently found at autopsy in patients dying at the scene of an accident (19). Although some believe that the anterior right ventricle is the most frequent location for blunt cardiac rupture, our experience suggests that tears of the right atrium at its junction with the superior or inferior vena cava are more common in patients reaching the hospital alive.

AXIOM Occasionally, patients with blunt rupture of the right atrium reach the hospital alive, but they usually die rapidly in the ED unless their injuries are recognized and corrected promptly.

Severe cardiac damage should be suspected when shock exists out of proportion to the degree of recognized injury or when shock persists despite rapid fluid resuscitation and control of all other possible sources of hemorrhage. An immediate median sternotomy, preferably with cardiopulmonary bypass, is usually necessary to repair these devastating injuries successfully. If a left anterior thoracotomy incision has been performed and the right heart is injured, the incision needs to be rapidly extended across the midline into the right chest.

Ventricular Septal Defect

In a postmortem examination with 546 victims of blunt cardiac trauma, rupture of the ventricular septum was found in only 30 (5%) and in another study of 152 victims, septal rupture was found in 11 (7%) (19).

Patients with a ventricular septal defect (VSD) from blunt trauma are generally critically ill as a result of the cardiac defect and the associated myocardial and pulmonary contusions. Ventricular septal defect is characterized by a systolic thrill and a harsh, holosystolic murmur that is usually loudest along the left sternal border in the third and fourth intercostal spaces and is transmitted to the right.

AXIOM ECG evidence of cardiac damage plus a new murmur after trauma suggest a valve lesion or VSD.

If severe heart failure develops, prompt cardiac catheterization and rapid surgical repair are required to restore adequate oxygen delivery to the tissues. Although small, traumatic VSDs in the muscular septum may close spontaneously (20), surgical repair, preferably 6 to 8 weeks after trauma, is usually required.

Atrial Septal Defect

Isolated atrial septal defects (ASDs) caused by blunt trauma are extremely rare, and most patients with traumatic ASD die within minutes of injury (21).

Valve Injury

AXIOM The valve injury most likely to be caused by blunt trauma is aortic insufficiency.

Blunt aortic valve injury is usually in the form of rupture of a cusp or at one of the commissural attachments, resulting in acute, severe heart failure. Munshi et al. (22), however, have shown that patients with acute aortic valvular disruption secondary to rapid deceleration trauma can often be managed nonoperatively in the acute setting by carefully titrating the preload and afterload.

Mitral valve rupture is believed to occur when sudden, severe force is applied during the short interval of isovolemic contraction between the closure of the mitral valve and the opening of the aortic valve. Mitral insufficiency may also develop if the valve and adjacent myocardium are sufficiently contused to cause scar formation with later contraction and distortion of the valve apparatus.

Injured valves must usually be replaced, and if the heart failure is not severe, it is preferable to wait 6 to 8 weeks before performing the surgery. Sugita et al. (23) have found that severe posttraumatic tricuspid regurgitation can be corrected by chordal replacement with expanded polytetrafluoroethylene sutures plus a DeVega annuloplasty.

Myocardial Contusion

Incidence

More than 90% of cardiac injuries diagnosed in patients admitted to a hospital after blunt trauma are myocardial contusions (24). The reported average incidence in patients admitted with severe blunt chest trauma is about 5% to 15%. In unstable patients admitted to an intensive care unit (ICU), the incidence, as determined by radionuclide angiography (RNA), may approach 75% (25).

Pathology

The typical pathologic changes seen at autopsy with myocardial contusion include subendocardial and interstitial hemorrhage, large surrounding areas of focal myocardial edema, myofibrillar degeneration, and myocytolysis and infiltration of polymorphonuclear leukocytes (16). This injury may resemble an acute myocardial infarction, but contusions tend to be more patchy. The anterior right ventricular wall is the area most frequently involved, with the anterior interventricular septum and anterior-apical left ventricle being second and third in frequency.

Physiologic Changes

Myocardial contusion can cause rhythm or conduction disturbances, and it impairs myocardial contractility in 10% to 20% of patients studied (26). In patients who have preexisting cardiac disease, multiple other injuries, or prolonged general anesthesia, this impairment can greatly reduce myocardial function and prognosis (24).

AXIOM Myocardial contusions are usually clinically insignificant unless patients have preexisting cardiac disease or other severe injuries or need general anesthesia.

A significant reduction in cardiac output has been found in 65% of patients tested; this is directly related to the amount of contused myocardium. Torres-Mirabal et al. inserted a pulmonary artery catheter into a series of myocardial contusion patients and noted the response to a fluid challenge (27). Of seven patients in whom major complications developed or who died, biventricular failure was demonstrated in three, cardiogenic shock in two, and left ventricular dysfunction in one. It was also found that the cardiac index was only slightly reduced and pulmonary artery wedge pressure (PAWP) only slightly increased in most of these patients; however, when a fluid challenge was administered, the PAWP increased rapidly and little or no increase in cardiac output occurred.

AXIOM The reduced ejection fraction of a contused heart can be compensated for by increased preload and is not usually a problem unless the patient has multiple other injuries or requires general anesthesia.

In another study of blunt chest injury and focal ventricular wall-motion defects as defined by gated cardiac scintigraphy, Sutherland et al. found that the right ventricular ejection fraction (RVEF) was reduced to 29% ± 5% (versus 47% ± 7% in those without wall-motion defects). This was well compensated for by an increased right ventricular end diastolic volume (143 ± 63 versus 93 ± 26 mL/m^2) (28).

Despite these abnormalities, most patients with myocardial contusions have relatively few problems and do not require ICU monitoring unless

1. An arrhythmia, especially PVCs, atrial fibrillation, or a conduction defect is present.
2. Clinical evidence of heart failure exists.
3. Multiple other injuries are present.
4. Preexisting cardiac disease is present.
5. General anesthesia is required, especially if the surgery will be prolonged or is associated with clamping of the aorta or significant blood loss.

AXIOM General anesthesia within 1 month of a diagnosed myocardial contusion can be a significant risk for the development of arrhythmias or hypotension.

In a group of patients studied at the Mayo Clinic by Frazee et al. (18), the incidence of hypotension during general anesthesia was significantly higher in chest trauma patients who had abnormal cardiac wall-motion on two-dimensional echocardiogram than those with normal myocardial motion (23% versus 11%). Furthermore, the incidence of an increased CVP during the hypotension was 50% if the two-dimensional echocardiogram was abnormal.

AXIOM The diagnosis of a myocardial contusion can be made on the basis of new ECG findings, arrhythmias, heart failure, decreased ejection fraction, or increased CPK-MB levels, but evidence of anterior heart wall-motion abnormalities is probably most definitive.

Diagnosis

External evidence of chest injury may not be detectable in up to one-third of patients with blunt cardiac injury. Nevertheless, the majority of patients with myocardial contusion have severe extracardiac injuries, and up to 60% have other thoracic injuries (28).

Signs and Symptoms

AXIOM Any patient involved in a motor vehicle accident at speeds exceeding 35 mph and having an arrhythmia or inappropriate tachycardia should be suspected of having myocardial contusion.

Tachycardia that is out of proportion to the degree of trauma or blood loss may be the first sign of myocardial contusion. Occasionally, an irregular rhythm resulting from atrial fibrillation or premature atrial or ventricular contractions may be noted. Rarely, a patient with myocardial contusion has angina-like pain that is not relieved by nitroglycerin. Differentiation from an acute myocardial infarction may be difficult under such circumstances.

Diagnostic Studies

Radiologic Studies

In some series, the presence of a fractured sternum is the clinical or radiologic finding most significantly associated with myocardial contusion. In one series of 11 patients with sternal fractures studied with RNA, 10 (91%) had functional defects involving the anterior heart (29); however, another series and our own studies suggest that less than 5% of patients with sternal fractures have any evidence of cardiac damage (30).

Electrocardiogram

AXIOM Myocardial contusion seldom causes new arrhythmias more than 24 hours after admission unless significant stress, such as general anesthesia, is added.

An ECG should be obtained initially and at 12 and 24 hours after injury in patients suspected of having a myocardial injury. If no ECG changes are noted by 24 hours, it is unlikely that any will develop later; however, in a series reported by Soliman and Waxman, 23% of the patients with evidence of blunt cardiac injury had initially normal ECGs, but on the second or third hospital day, 12-lead ECG abnormalities developed (31).

AXIOM New atrial fibrillation, multiple PVCs, or conduction disturbances are much more important than ST-T wave changes for diagnosing direct or indirect (ischemic or hypoxic) myocardial injury (31).

Fabian et al. reported that Holter monitoring revealed far more ECG changes than routine or continuous ECG monitoring (32). Of 90 patients monitored for 4 to 5 days for severe anterior chest trauma, 24 had significant arrhythmias (SARR) demonstrated by Holter monitoring. Of these arrhythmias, only 6% were documented by other techniques. The average CPK-MB level in the 24 patients with SARR was 8.3% (versus 2.6% in patients without SARR). The patients with SARR also had lower cardiac indices (2.4 versus 3.2 L/min/m^2); however, it is not clear how many patients with SARR required treatment.

Serum Enzyme Changes

Serum glutamate oxaloacetate transaminase (SGOT), lactate dehydrogenase (LDH), and CPK levels are of relatively little value in diagnosing cardiac injuries. Myocardial (CPK-MB) isoenzyme levels, however, appear to be more accurate (52).

These should be drawn when the patient is first seen in the ED and at 8, 16, 24, and 48 hours after injury. With acute myocardial contusions, the CPK-MB peaks at about 18 to 24 hours.

AXIOM Elevated CPK-MB levels, by themselves, are of relatively little value in predicting the outcome of patients with myocardial contusions.

Most authors consider a ratio of CPK-MB to total CPK of 5% or more to be indicative of myocardial damage (17). Because CPK-MB isoenzyme can also be found in skeletal muscle, pancreas, lung, colon, liver, stomach, and small bowel, CPK-MB fraction may be elevated from a variety of injuries, particularly if the total CPK is very high. Although one series found that no patient whose ECG and CPK-MB results were both negative had a clinical course compatible with important cardiac injury (34), no correlation appeared to exist between the severity of injury and the level of CPK-MB isoenzyme.

Troponin studies have been performed more recently and appear to be more reliable than CPK-MB studies, but their value in diagnosing myocardial contusions is still unclear (35).

Radionuclide Angiography

With first-pass biventricular RNA, the normal LVEF is 62% ± 5% and the normal right ventricular ejection fraction (RVEF) is 50% ± 4% (100). An LVEF less than 50% or an RVEF less than 40% has been interpreted as abnormal. Using this technique, Harley and Mena found that 11 of 12 patients with sternal fractures had abnormalities of ventricular contraction and motion (29); however, only four had ECG changes and none had abnormal CPK-MB levels. Sutherland et al. had similar findings with less than one-third of the patients with abnormal RNA having ECG or CPK-MB abnormalities (25).

AXIOM Gated RNA may be an excessively sensitive technique for detecting clinically significant myocardial contusions.

Single-Photon Emission Computed Tomography

Single-photon emission computed tomography (SPECT) following intravenous injection of thallium can also be used to evaluate for myocardial contusions. This radioactive potassium analogue is extracted from the blood into normally functioning myocardial cells. In a series of 48 patients with blunt chest trauma, 23 had normal SPECT studies and no serious arrhythmias developed in any of these 23; however, in 5 of 25 with abnormal or ambiguous studies, arrhythmias requiring treatment did develop (36).

Two-Dimensional Echocardiography

Two-dimensional echocardiography has many advantages in attempting to make a diagnosis of acute myocardial contusion. The most common abnormality seen with myocardial contusion on two-dimensional echocardiography is right ventricular free-wall dyskinesia, often with some dilation. In addition, some of the patients studied have had mural thrombi attached to the contused myocardium (37).

AXIOM A patient with a normal two-dimensional echocardiogram after blunt trauma is unlikely to have a physiologically significant myocardial contusion.

Transesophageal Echocardiography

Using transesophageal echocardiography (TEE), Shapiro et al. (38) observed regional wall-motion abnormalities consistent with cardiac contusion in 26% of their patients with blunt chest trauma. In their study, performance of the TEE enabled them to make a rapid diagnosis of myocardial contusion and to exclude other causes of circulatory failure, particularly hypovolemia and cardiac tamponade. Pearson et al. (39) found that TEE accurately identified blunt cardiac injury in four patients and aortic injuries in six others. TEE also clearly identified depressed myocardial function in one child.

Pulmonary Artery Catheterization

A pulmonary artery catheter should be inserted to monitor pulmonary artery pressures and cardiac output in anyone with a suspected myocardial contusion and (1) any hemodynamic impairment or (2) need for a major operative procedure under general anesthesia. Although the baseline cardiac output may be relatively normal, a poor response to fluid-loading often occurs.

TREATMENT

AXIOM If possible, patients with myocardial wall-motion abnormalities should not receive general anesthesia for at least 30 days following trauma.

Patients who have no arrhythmias and are hemodynamically stable seldom benefit from continuous cardioscopic monitoring and cardiac precautions. Patients with identifiable CPK-MB changes or wall-motion abnormalities on two-dimensional echocardiography or RNA require careful monitoring if a general anesthetic is given.

Supplemental oxygen should be administered, as needed, to keep the PO_2 greater than 80 mm Hg, and analgesics should be given, as needed, to reduce any tachycardia or increased BP that may be caused by pain. Cardiac dysrhythmias should be diagnosed early and treated with appropriate medication. Low cardiac output or hypotension should be treated with fluids or inotropic agents, guided by the response of the PAWP and cardiac output. In patients with impaired right ventricular function, monitoring of the right ventricular end-diastolic volume index with a special pulmonary artery catheter may be particularly helpful (40).

AXIOM If a patient with a myocardial contusion remains hypotensive despite adequate volume, inotropic support, and correction of any mechanical problems (e.g., tamponade), intraaortic balloon pump (IABP) therapy should be begun.

If intramural thrombus is found on two-dimensional echocardiography in patients with myocardial contusions, it is not clear whether they should have prophylactic anticoagulation (37). Although five of seven patients with chest trauma in one series had echocardiographically proved right ventricular thrombi, none of these patients had subsequent systemic or pulmonary embolization (41). Nevertheless, in patients with proven intramural thrombosis and no contraindication to anticoagulation, one may consider using "mild" to "moderate" heparinization (i.e., 500 to 800 units per hour) (17).

Complications

Posttraumatic Pericarditis

Posttraumatic pericarditis should be suspected in individuals in whom chest pain, fever, and pleural or pericardial effusions develop 2 to 4 weeks after trauma. The blood count often reveals lymphocytosis, and the ECG frequently shows ST-T wave changes consistent with pericarditis. The cause of posttraumatic pericarditis is still largely unknown, but it may be a delayed hypersensitivity reaction to the presence of damaged blood, pericardium, or myocardium in the pericardial cavity (42).

Treatment is primarily symptomatic. Salicylates and rest can often reduce symptoms dramatically within 12 to 24 hours. When no improvement occurs, corticosteroids may be required.

Traumatic Aneurysms

True aneurysms of the heart from blunt trauma are unusual but may occur if a large area of injured muscle undergoes necrosis, stretching, thinning, and eventual dilatation and fibrosis. The patient is usually asymptomatic and is able to perform ordinary activity without discomfort, but an abnormal cardiac silhouette may be discovered during routine chest roentgenography (15). If symptoms develop, they usually are those of congestive heart failure. Occasionally, symptoms of systemic embolization from mural thrombi or dysrhythmias occur. The larger aneurysms should be treated by resection, even in asymptomatic patients (15).

⊘ FREQUENT ERRORS

1. ***Rejecting a diagnosis of pericardial tamponade because the neck veins are not distended.***
2. ***Assuming a pericardial tamponade is not present because an attempted pericardiocentesis was negative.***
3. ***Delaying thoracotomy to perform pericardiocentesis in a patient in severe shock when thoracotomy can be started almost as quickly.***
4. ***Failure to provide adequate fluid resuscitation in an unstable patient with pericardial tamponade because the neck veins are distended.***
5. ***Performing an ED resuscitative thoracotomy on a patient with chest trauma when there is inadequate operating room or surgical backup.***
6. ***Performing a resuscitative thoracotomy when the patient had a GSW or blunt trauma and no signs of life at the scene or for more than 5 minutes before reaching the hospital.***
7. ***Turning a patient who is hemodynamically unstable or has intrabronchial bleeding onto his side to perform a posterolateral thoracotomy.***
8. ***Inadequate or delayed compression of the aorta during thoracotomy or laparotomy in severely hypotensive patients.***
9. ***Allowing the proximal systolic BP to exceed 160 to 180 mm Hg during clamping of the descending thoracic aorta.***
10. ***Inadequate pursuit of a diagnosis of valve injury or septal defect in patients with a murmur after severe chest trauma.***
11. ***Inadequate cardiovascular monitoring of a patient with suspected myocardial contusion before, during, and after general anesthesia.***

SUMMARY POINTS

1. All patients who are in shock and have a penetrating chest injury anywhere near the heart should be considered to have a cardiac injury until proven otherwise.

2. Pericardial tamponade increases the likelihood of successful emergency resuscitative thoracotomy for a penetrating injury to the heart.

3. All patients in shock with penetrating wounds of the chest between the midclavicular line on the right and anterior axillary line on the left should be considered to have a cardiac injury until proven otherwise.

4. The neck veins in patients with shock from pericardial tamponade usually do not become distended until coexistent hypovolemia is at least partly corrected.

5. Distended neck veins and hypotension after chest trauma are not always due to pericardial tamponade.

6. If blood is obtained on pericardiocentesis and the patient's vital signs improve promptly, a tamponade was almost certainly present.

7. When a large amount (greater than 20 mL) of blood can be aspirated rapidly and easily during an attempted pericardiocentesis, it is likely that one is aspirating blood from the right ventricle rather than the pericardial cavity.
8. One of the quickest ways to restore adequate tissue perfusion in a hemodynamically unstable patient with pericardial tamponade is aggressive fluid resuscitation.
9. Penetrating wounds of the heart are best treated with emergency thoracotomy and cardiorrhaphy.
10. ED thoracotomy for penetrating cardiac injury may be lifesaving for patients deteriorating so rapidly that it is not likely that they will survive movement from the ED to the operating room; however, the results are better with OR thoracotomies.
11. Injuries to the mid or left chest in unstable patients are best explored through the left chest, and lesions on the right are best explored through the right chest.
12. If the patient is relatively stable and the cardiac injury is likely to be anterior (as with anterior stab wounds), a median sternotomy can be used to explore the chest.
13. Compression of the descending aorta in a severely hypotensive patient can increase coronary and cerebral blood flow twofold to threefold.
14. Compression of the heart with two hands or between one palm and the sternum reduces the risk of inadvertently entering the heart with a fingertip during open cardiac massage.
15. A sudden onset of arrhythmias or hypotension in a patient with open neck veins or a lung injury, especially if hemoptysis is present, should be considered to be due to air emboli until proved otherwise.
16. Hypertension or tachycardia greatly increase the workload and oxygen requirements of an injured heart and can cause infarction or overt heart failure.
17. Pseudoaneurysms of the heart caused by penetrating trauma should be treated surgically because they are basically a contained rupture of the heart. True aneurysms of the heart are treated surgically if they cause heart failure, arrhythmias, or emboli.
18. Myocardial contusion should be suspected in anyone with severe trauma to the anterior chest.
19. Occasionally, patients with blunt rupture of the right atrium reach the hospital alive, but they usually die rapidly in the ED unless their injuries are recognized and corrected promptly.
20. ECG evidence of cardiac damage plus a new murmur after trauma suggests a valve lesion or VSD.
21. The valve injury most apt to be caused by blunt trauma is aortic insufficiency.
22. Myocardial contusions are usually clinically insignificant unless preexisting cardiac disease, severe injuries, or need for general anesthesia is present.
23. The reduced ejection fraction of a contused heart can be compensated for by increased preload and is not usually a problem unless the patient has multiple other injuries or requires general anesthesia.
24. General anesthesia within a month of a diagnosed myocardial contusion can be a significant risk for the development of arrhythmias or hypotension.
25. The diagnosis of a myocardial contusion can be made on the basis of new ECG findings, arrhythmias, heart failure, decreased ejection fraction, or increased CPK-MB levels, but evidence of anterior heart wall-motion abnormalities may be most definitive.
26. Myocardial contusion seldom causes new arrhythmias more than 24 hours after admission, unless a significant stress, such as general anesthesia is added.
27. New atrial fibrillation, multiple PVCs, or conduction disturbances are much more important than ST-T wave changes for diagnosing direct or indirect (ischemic or hypoxic) myocardial injury.
28. Holter monitoring reveals many more arrhythmias than the usual ECG monitoring systems, but changes seen only on the Holter monitor are less likely to be significant.
29. Elevated CPK-MB levels, by themselves, are of relatively little value in predicting the outcome of patients with myocardial contusion.
30. Gated RNA may be an overly sensitive technique for assessing cardiac function, including left and right ventricular ejection fractions and wall-motion abnormalities.

31. A patient with a normal two-dimensional echocardiogram after blunt trauma is unlikely to have a physiologically significant myocardial contusion.
32. Patients with significant myocardial contusions tend to have relatively flat cardiac function curves in response to fluid-loading, indicating impaired responses to stress.
33. If possible, patients with myocardial contusions and wall-motion abnormalities should not be given general anesthesia for at least 30 days.
34. If a patient with a myocardial contusion remains hypotensive despite adequate volume, inotropic support, and correction of any mechanical problems (e.g., tamponade), IABP therapy should be begun.

REFERENCES

1. Wilson RF, Stephenson LW. Thoracic Trauma. Heart. In: Wilson RF, Walt A, eds. *Management of trauma: pitfalls and practice,* 2nd ed. Philadelphia: Williams & Wilkins, 1996;434.
2. Demetriades D. Cardiac wounds. *Ann Surg* 1985;203:315.
3. Moreno C, Moore EE, Majure JA, Hopeman AR. Pericardial tamponade. A critical determinant for survival following penetrating cardiac wounds. *J Trauma* 1986;26:821.
4. Washington B, Wilson RF, Steiger Z, Bassett JS. Emergency thoracotomy: a four year review. *Ann Thorac Surg* 1985;40:188.
5. Ordog GJ, Wasserberger J, Balasubramanian S, et al. Asymptomatic stab wounds of the chest. *J Trauma* 1994;36:680.
6. Mechem CC, Alam GA. Delayed cardiac tamponade in a patient with penetrating chest trauma. *J Emerg Med* 1997;15:31.
7. Wechsler AS, Auerbach BJ, Graham TC, et al. Distribution of intramyocardial blood flow during pericardial tamponade. *J Thorac Cardiovasc Surg* 1974;68:847.
8. Wilson RF, Basset JS. Penetrating wounds of the pericardium or its contents. *JAMA* 1966;195:513.
9. Lorell B, Leinbach RC, Pohost GM, et al. Right ventricular infarction: clinical diagnosis and differentiation from cardiac tamponade and pericardial constriction. *Am J Cardiol* 1979;43:465.
10. Aaland MO, Bryan FC 3rd, Sherman R. Two-dimensional echocardiogram in hemodynamically stable victims of penetrating precordial trauma. *Am Surg* 1994;60:412.
11. Mayor-Davies JA, Britz RS. Subxiphoid pericardial windows—helpful in selected cases. *J Trauma* 1990;30:1399.
12. Baxter BT, Moore EE, Moore JB, et al. Emergency department thoracotomy following injury: critical determinants for patient salvage. *World J Surg* 1988; 12:671–675.
13. Velmahos GC, Degiannis E, Souter I, et al. Penetrating trauma to the heart: a relatively innocent injury. *Surgery* 1994;115:694.
14. Symbas PN. Traumatic ventricular septal defect. In: Symbas PN, ed. *Cardiothoracic trauma.* Philadelphia: WB Saunders, 1989:95–107.
15. Symbas PN. Traumatic aneurysms of the heart. Symbas PN, ed. *Cardiothoracic trauma.* Philadelphia: WB Saunders, 1989:121–126.
16. Leidtke AJ, DeMuth WE. Nonpenetrating cardiac injuries: a collective review. *Am Heart J* 1973;86:687.
17. Tenzer ML. The spectrum of myocardial contusion: a review. *J Trauma* 1985;25: 620.
18. Frazee RC, Mucha P, Farnell MB, Miller FA. Objective evaluation of blunt cardiac trauma. *J Trauma* 1986;26:510.
19. Parmeley LF, Manion WC, Mattingly TW. Nonpenetrating traumatic injury to the heart. *Circulation* 1958;18:371.
20. Krajcer Z, Cooley DA, Leachman RD. Ventricular septal defect following blunt trauma: spontaneous closure of residual defect after surgical repair. *Cathet Cardiovasc Diagn* 1977;3:409.
21. Rao G, Garvey J, Gupta M. Atrial septal defect due to blunt thoracic trauma. *J Trauma* 1977;17:405.

22. Munshi IA, Barie PS, Hawes AS, et al. Diagnosis and management of acute aortic valvular disruption secondary to rapid-deceleration trauma. *J Trauma* 1996;41:1047.
23. Sugita T, Watarida S, Katsuyama K, et al. Valve repair with chordal replacement for traumatic tricuspid regurgitation. *J Heart Valve Disease* 1997;6:651.
24. Symbas PN. Contusion of the heart. Symbas PN, ed. *Cardiothoracic trauma.* Philadelphia: WB Saunders, 1989:55–76.
25. Sutherland GR, Driedger AA, Holliday RL, et al. Frequency of myocardial injury after blunt chest trauma as evaluated by radionuclide angiography. *Am J Cardiol* 1983;52:1099.
26. McLean RF, Devitt JH, Dubbin J, et al. Incidence of abnormal RNA studies and dysrhythmias in patients with blunt chest trauma. *J Trauma* 1991;31:968.
27. Torres-Mirabal P, Gruenberg JC, Talbert JG, et al. Ventricular function in myocardial contusion—a preliminary study. *Crit Care Med* 1982;10:19.
28. Sutherland GR, Cheung HW, Holliday RL, et al. Hemodynamic adaptation to acute myocardial contusion complicating blunt chest injury. *Am J Cardiol* 1986;57:291.
29. Harley DP, Mena I. Cardiac and vascular sequelae of sternal fractures. *J Trauma* 1986;26:553.
30. Shapira-Roy A, Levi I, Khoda J. Sternal fractures: a red flag or a red herring. *J Trauma* 1994;37:59.
31. Soliman MH, Waxman K. Value of a conventional approach to the diagnosis of traumatic cardiac contusion after chest injury. *Crit Care Med* 1987;15:218.
32. Fabian TC, Cicala RS, Croce MA, et al. A prospective evaluation of myocardial contusion: correlation of significant arrhythmias and cardiac output with CPK-MB measurements. *J Trauma* 1991;31:653.
33. Reynolds M, Jones JM. CPK-MB isoenzyme determinations in blunt chest trauma. *JACEP* 1979;8:304.
34. Miller FB, Richardson JD. Blunt cardiac injury. Common problems in trauma. *Ann Emerg Med* 1982;11:319.
35. Ferjani M, Droc G, Dreux S, et al. Circulating cardiac troponin T in myocardial contusion. *Chest* 1997;111:427.
36. Waxman K, Soliman MH, Braunstein P, et al. Diagnosis of traumatic cardiac contusion. *Arch Surg* 1986;121:689.
37. Timberlake GA, McSwain NE. Thromboembolism as a complication of myocardial contusion: a new capricious syndrome. *J Trauma* 1988;28:535.
38. Shapiro MJ, Yanofsky SD, Trapp J, et al. Cardiovascular evaluation in blunt thoracic trauma using transesophageal echocardiography (TEE). *J Trauma* 1991;31:835.
39. Pearson GD, Karr SS, Trachiotis GD, et al. A retrospective review of the role of transesophageal echocardiography in aortic and cardiac trauma in a level I pediatric trauma center. *J Am Soc Echocardiogr* 1997;10:946.
40. Diebel LN, Wilson RF, Tagett MG, et al. End-diastolic volume: a better indicator of preload in the critically ill. *Arch Surg* 1992;127:817–821.
41. Miller FA, Seward JB, Gersh BJ, et al. Two-dimensional echocardiographic findings in cardiac trauma. *Am J Cardiol* 1982;50:1022.
42. Kirsh MM, McIntosh K, Kahn DR, et al. Postpericardiotomy syndromes. *Ann Thorac Surg* 1970;9:158.

18. TRAUMA TO INTRATHORACIC GREAT VESSELS[1]

ANATOMY OF INTRATHORACIC GREAT VESSELS

The aortic arch begins at the upper border of the second chondrosternal articulation on the right side, and it passes upward and backward and then across and down to the left side of the lower border of the fourth dorsal vertebra. Anomalies or anatomic variants of the aortic arch are present in 25% to 35% of patients. The most frequent variation is a common origin for the right subclavian and right and left common carotid arteries from the innominate artery, which is seen in 10% to 27% of individuals.

The innominate (brachiocephalic) artery is the largest branch off the arch of the aorta. It arises at the level of the border of the second right costal cartilage and ascends obliquely for 1.5 to 2 inches to the upper border of the right sternoclavicular joint where it divides into the right common carotid and right subclavian arteries. It usually has no branches, but in about 10% of patients, a branch, the thyroidea ima, ascends in front of the trachea up to the thyroid isthmus.

The right subclavian artery arises from the innominate artery opposite the right sternoclavicular joint and passes upward and outward behind the scalenus anticus muscle where it ascends slightly above the clavicle. It is covered in front by the right vagus and right recurrent laryngeal nerves. The recurrent nerve then winds around the lower and back part of the vessel to ascend back up to the larynx.

The left subclavian artery typically arises from the left end of the arch of the aorta, opposite the fourth thoracic vertebra. The vagus and phrenic nerves lie anterior and parallel to it. The second portion of the subclavian artery is covered anteriorly by the scalenus anticus muscle. The third portion of the subclavian arteries passes downward and outward from the outer margin of the scalenus anticus to the outer border of the first rib, where it becomes the axillary artery.

PENETRATING TRAUMA

From 1980 to 1990, approximately 30,000 trauma patients were admitted to Detroit Receiving Hospital, only 108 of whom were documented to have great vessel injuries in the chest.

AXIOM Patients with injured thoracic great vessels may suddenly begin to bleed massively again when their blood pressures are restored or when they gag or retch while an esophageal or endotracheal tube is being inserted.

Patients with penetrating injuries of major intrathoracic vessels who survive long enough to reach a hospital generally have their bleeding sites temporarily occluded with blood clot or vessel adventitia. Occasionally, vascular injury results in the formation of a traumatic aneurysm or arteriovenous (AV) fistula, and patients with thoracic vascular trauma are more likely to survive if the injury is within the pericardial cavity where the bleeding may become tamponaded (2).

Types of Vascular Injuries

Symbas and Sehdeva, in a review of 48 patients with successful repairs of penetrating thoracic aortic injuries, noted that 14 had a fistulous communication with a cardiac chamber, nine with an innominate vein, and eight with a pulmonary vessel (3). Most of the 17 patients without fistulas had injuries to the intrapericardial portion of the ascending aorta or had only a small wound to the lower descending thoracic aorta.

AXIOM If more than 25% of the cardiac output goes through an AV fistula, high-output cardiac failure is likely to develop.

A small injury to an artery associated with a contained hematoma often stops bleeding, and the hematoma gradually resolves. In some instances, the opening into the hematoma remains patent, and the hematoma may develop into a false aneurysm with a pseudoendothelial lining. These false aneurysms often enlarge and rupture within a few days, but they occasionally remain relatively stable for many years.

Diagnosis

History and Physical Examination

The size of a knife and its depth and angle of penetration may indicate the vessels or organs most likely to be injured. When two skin wounds are present, it may be helpful to know whether they represent two entrance wounds or single exit and entrance wounds. It is extremely important to know, if possible, the caliber of the bullet and whether it was a high-velocity missile (greater than 2,000 feet per second), which tends to cause far more tissue destruction than knives or low-velocity bullets. High-velocity missile injuries are much more likely to require thoracotomy, even if the bullet did not enter the chest cavity.

The excellent collateral circulation about the shoulder may result in a normal distal pulse even if the innominate or subclavian artery occludes; however, vascular spasm occasionally occurs secondary to adjacent soft-tissue or bony injury and can cause loss of pulses when no demonstrable vessel injury is present at surgery. In a study by Calhoon et al., 64% of 22 patients with proximal thoracic vascular injuries had normal peripheral pulses (4). Nevertheless, if pulse loss is accompanied by another sign of vascular injury, such as bruit or expanding hematoma (present in 68% of the patients reported by Calhoon et al.), arterial injury is present in at least 80% of the patients.

Although probing of penetrating thoracic injuries is not recommended, careful superficial exploration may provide useful information on the direction of the missile tract. One should also auscultate the entire chest and back for bruits. A systolic bruit should lead one to suspect a false aneurysm involving one of the great vessels. A continuous bruit should make one suspect an AV fistula.

A millwheel murmur, believed to be due to air being churned in the heart, may be diagnostic of air embolism. Hamman's sign, which is a crunching sound heard over the precordium during systole, indicates the presence of a pneumomediastinum or pneumopericardium. Occasionally, a large upper mediastinal hematoma can cause an acute superior vena caval syndrome, tracheal compression, or respiratory distress.

Diagnostic Tests

Radiography

AXIOM Virtually all patients with major trauma should have chest radiography as soon as possible after arrival in the ED.

With penetrating injuries of great vessels, a hemothorax is generally apparent on routine radiography of the chest, particularly when an associated pneumothorax provides an air-fluid level. If the patient is lying flat, however, up to 500 to 1,000 mL of blood may cause only a slightly increased haziness over the lung on the involved side. Occasionally, even on an upright chest film, several hundred milliliters of blood may be difficult to identify if it settles under the lung as a subpulmonic collection where it can be mistaken for an elevated diaphragm. Decubitus films, however, generally demonstrate layering of the blood, unless it is loculated or clotted.

Widening of the upper mediastinal silhouette on chest radiography is often present in patients with injury to the aortic arch or its branches. With innominate artery injuries, the widening is usually more superior and to the right than that seen after aortic injury.

When a foreign body pulsates because it lays next to a major vessel, its margins tend to be indistinct on chest films; therefore, a fuzzy foreign body contiguous with mediastinal structures can be an important radiographic clue to vascular injury. Even when angiography is performed and is normal, McFadden et al. believe that a fuzzy foreign body should still be considered an indication for surgery because of the strong likelihood that vascular injury is present (5).

Magnetic Resonance Imaging

Magnetic resonance imaging (MRI) can be as valuable as an arteriogram in most situations, but it should not be attempted in patients with bullets adjacent to great vessels because the MRI could cause the bullet to move, with resultant further tissue damage and bleeding.

Computed Tomography

AXIOM Computed tomography (CT) scans of the chest should not be performed while a patient is hemodynamically unstable.

CT scans can identify many hematomas that may not be apparent on routine radiography. When a persistent extravascular "mass" is adjacent to a great vessel and does not move with position changes by the patient, one should assume a contained hematoma is present. Intravenous contrast is essential for reliably demonstrating false aneurysms on CT. One should also look for irregular vessel contours or intimal flaps.

Arteriography

Arteriography may be particularly helpful for identifying major intrathoracic vascular injuries within contained hematomas, especially those resulting from penetrating wounds of the lower neck. Although valuable information concerning the choice of incision can usually be derived from arteriography, the arteriogram may be falsely negative if the penetration site is temporarily "sealed off" by hematoma or if the radiologic projection is not appropriate.

Venography

Venograms are seldom performed to identify major injuries in the chest. A patient who is actively bleeding from a major venous injury is usually explored emergently because of unstable vital signs or continued blood loss via the chest tubes. After a venous injury stops bleeding, the hemorrhage generally does not recur, and the damaged vessel usually does not require thoracotomy. Nevertheless, we have had at least two isolated innominate vein injuries that bled massively after the patient was hemodynamically stable for more than 24 hours.

Contrast Swallow

A contrast swallow should be performed if the patient is hemodynamically stable and if one suspects an esophageal injury. The patient should be awake and have a good swallowing and cough reflex before attempting a contrast swallow, otherwise there can be aspiration of the contrast material into the lungs. One usually uses Gastrografin first because, if a leak is present, it is believed to be less of an adjuvant to infection and scar formation than barium; however, if the patient aspirates Gastrografin into the lungs, it causes a more severe chemical pneumonitis than barium does.

Bronchoscopy and Esophagoscopy

With penetrating wounds of the central chest or lower neck in hemodynamically stable patients, it is prudent to perform bronchoscopy to eliminate injury to the tracheobronchial tree. Esophagoscopy is done if a contrast swallow is not readily available or does not clearly rule out an esophageal injury.

Treatment

Emergency Thoracotomy

In patients with penetrating chest trauma and severe shock (systolic blood pressure [BP] less than 50 mm Hg), an emergency thoracotomy should be performed. With mild to moderate shock (systolic BP 50 to 89 mm Hg), 2,000 to 3,000 mL of balanced electrolyte solution is infused in 10 to 15 minutes. If shock is persistent or rapidly recurs, or if the patient is actively bleeding, an emergency thoracotomy is indicated.

Occasionally, external hemorrhage from either the suprasternal notch or supraclavicular fossa may be the sole manifestation of a major intrathoracic vascular injury. Insertion of a finger or pack into the stab or gunshot wound site can often reduce the hemorrhage until the vessel can be controlled in the operating room.

AXIOM A moderate or large hemothorax should be promptly evacuated with a chest tube unless the patient requires emergency thoracotomy.

Blood in the pleural cavity should usually be removed as completely and rapidly as possible. If the hemothorax is not removed, it can restrict ventilation and venous return, and the clots present will release fibrinolytic and fibrinogenolytic substances that can act as local anticoagulants and contribute to continued intrathoracic bleeding. If the blood is not removed, it can also form a later fibrothorax or empyema.

AXIOM If a patient needs emergency thoracotomy because of massive bleeding, inserting a chest tube can delay the definitive operative procedure and increase the amount of blood loss.

In patients with massive bleeding into a body cavity, one should consider the use of autotransfusion. Special suction tubes are used and the addition of citrate or heparin to the blood in the suction container prevents it from clotting; however, in emergency situations with continued shock, attempts at autotransfusion can be cumbersome and time-consuming, particularly if adequate type-specific blood is available.

AXIOM Autotransfusion of more than 6 units of blood tends to contribute to development of a coagulopathy.

Although ED thoracotomies can be lifesaving, especially in patients with penetrating wounds of the chest, survival rates are at least twice as good for equivalent injuries if the patient is stable enough to have the emergency thoracotomy done in the operating room.

An antibiotic, such as a first-generation cephalosporin, used primarily to cover staphylococcal or streptococcal contamination, should be given as soon as a chest tube is inserted. Another dose can be given immediately preoperatively if there is more than a 3- or 4-hour delay in performing surgery. If there has been severe hemorrhage, the antibiotics should be given again after the major bleeding has been controlled.

Operating Room Thoracotomy

Indications. Although most cases of intrathoracic bleeding can be treated adequately with intravenous fluids and evacuation of the hemothorax with a chest tube,

9% of our patients with penetrating chest wounds have required a thoracotomy for continuing hemorrhage.

AXIOM If it is obvious that the patient has exsanguinating intrathoracic bleeding, thoracotomy should be performed as quickly as possible and with little or no resuscitation until the bleeding is controlled.

Even if the patient's vital signs are stable, one should perform a thoracotomy for severe, continued bleeding as demonstrated by

1. More than 1,500 to 2,000 mL of blood loss from the chest within the first 12 to 24 hours of injury (with continued bleeding);
2. Blood loss from the chest tubes exceeding 200 to 300 mL/h for 4 to 5 hours or more; and
3. The chest staying more than half full of blood on radiography despite properly positioned chest tubes.

When a chest tube is initially inserted to drain a traumatic hemothorax, blood may come out at an alarmingly rapid rate. If the patient's condition improves as blood is removed and additional intravenous fluids are given, continued drainage of the hemothorax is appropriate; however, if the patient's vital signs deteriorate as blood is removed, the chest tube should be clamped and the patient taken immediately to the operating room.

Incisions. A standard posterolateral thoracotomy provides excellent exposure to almost all parts of the hemithorax including the posterior chest; however, the lateral position of the patient tends to reduce venous return and can cause a precipitous decrease in blood pressure if the patient is hypovolemic. Also, if the patient has blood in the trachea or bronchi, the dependent lung could be flooded, even with a split function endotracheal tube in place.

AXIOM Patients should not be turned onto their side for a posterolateral thoracotomy if there is significant intrabronchial bleeding or if the patient is hypotensive.

A median sternotomy is usually the ideal incision for exploring penetrating wounds of the thoracic inlet or injuries involving the innominate artery or proximal portions of the carotid or right subclavian arteries. Extension of the median sternotomy into the neck along the anterior border of the sternocleidomastoid muscle also provides excellent exposure to the proximal right subclavian and midleft subclavian arteries, as well as the more distal portions of the right common carotid artery (Fig. 18-1).

It can be difficult to approach the origin of the left subclavian artery via a median sternotomy; however, the exposure can be improved by having a vertical sheet roll placed between the shoulder blades so that the shoulders can be pulled back. One could also join the median sternotomy to an anterior second or third intercostal incision.

If a stab wound or gunshot wound has damaged posterior structures, such as the esophagus or azygous or hemizygous veins, it may be difficult to obtain adequate exposure through a median sternotomy without an additional incision along one of the intercostal spaces. Another problem with a median sternotomy is the increased time it can take to perform if a sternal saw is not readily available or if the surgeon does not have a great deal of experience with this approach.

An anterolateral thoracotomy is usually the ideal incision for exploring patients with penetrating chest trauma if they are in severe shock, have moderate to severe hemoptysis, or require internal cardiac massage. The incision is in the fourth or fifth intercostal space. It should start about 2.0 cm lateral to the sternum (to avoid the internal mammary artery) and is continued into the axilla. The ribs are widely sep-

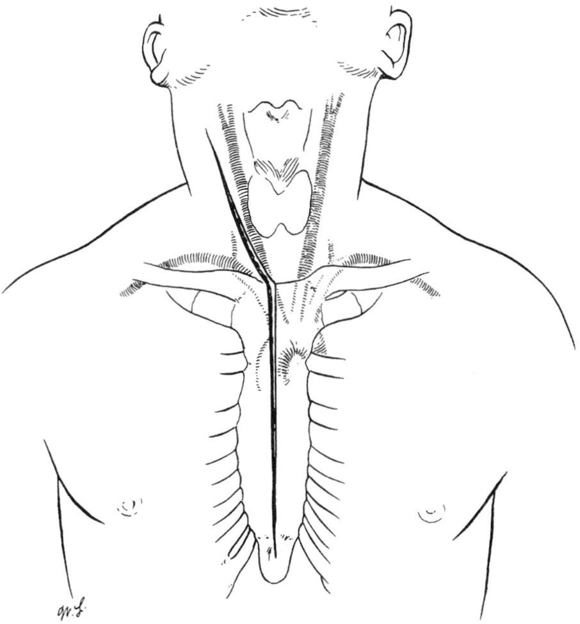

FIG. 18-1. Incision for right brachiocephalic vessels. The innominate artery and the origins of the right common carotid and right subclavian arteries can usually be readily approached through a sternal splitting incision which is extended either into the right neck or along and just above the right clavicle. Resecting the medial portion of the clavicle subperiosteally can further improve exposure to the mid portion of the right subclavian artery. (From Wilson RF. Injury to the heart and great vessels. In: Henning RJ, Grenvik A, eds. *Critical care cardiology.* New York: Churchill Livingstone, 1989:443.)

arated with a rib-spreader. Cutting the costal cartilages of one or two ribs above and below the incision can also help with the exposure.

A bilateral anterior thoracotomy is performed relatively easily by taking a left or right anterolateral thoracotomy, cutting the sternum transversely with rib shears, and connecting that to a contralateral anterolateral incision. Exposure of both pleura cavities and the mediastinum can thus be quickly attained without the need for a sternal saw. If the incisions are extended into both axillae, one usually has excellent exposure to virtually all organs in the chest. An upper median sternotomy and cervical extension can be added if additional exposure in the neck is needed. One must be sure to obtain secure control of the internal mammary vessels, preferably with suture ligatures, when this incision is used.

Intraoperative Resuscitation. Once the bleeding sites are controlled, further dissection should be delayed until the anesthesiologist can administer enough fluid and blood to restore an adequate blood pressure, urine output (at least 1.0 mL/kg/h), and core temperature (≥35°C).

Technical Considerations

AXIOM All hematomas on major vessels should be explored after obtaining proximal and distal control.

We know of at least three patients with aortic injuries from gunshot wounds that were missed at various hospitals and that bled later because the obvious great vessel injuries that were bleeding were repaired, but nonbleeding hematomas outside the presumed trajectory of the bullets were not explored.

During cardiopulmonary resuscitation (CPR) or management of very severe shock, one can clamp the descending thoracic aorta. Cross-clamping of the thoracic aorta should not be done in the ascending aorta or proximal arch without the patient being on cardiopulmonary bypass, but it is usually possible to clamp either the distal arch proximal to the left subclavian artery or the descending aorta safely for at least a few minutes. If proximal aortic pressure increases to over 180 mm Hg, acute left ventricular failure can result.

AXIOM If the systolic BP does not increase to 90 mm Hg within 5 minutes of clamping the descending thoracic aorta, controlling bleeding, and providing aggressive fluid resuscitation, then the patient will almost certainly die intraoperatively.

If an adequate repair of the thoracic aorta cannot be obtained with direct suturing or side-clamping, the aorta should be completely clamped. There are four techniques for handling aortic blood flow with thoracic aortic clamping:

1. Simple cross-clamping of the aorta ("clamp and sew") without shunt or bypass;
2. External heparin-bonded shunts (without systemic heparinization) from the proximal aorta to either the distal thoracic aorta or a femoral artery;
3. Partial or complete cardiopulmonary bypass using an oxygenator and systemic heparinization; and
4. Left atrial or left ventricular bypass via a centrifugal pump to the distal thoracic aorta or femoral artery without an oxygenator and with little or no heparinization.

AXIOM Clamping the upper descending thoracic aorta for more than 30 minutes without providing some blood flow to the distal aorta can result in a high incidence of paraplegia.

The clamp-and-sew technique should be avoided by surgeons who do not have experience with this type of surgery. Clamping of the thoracic aorta in the distal arch or isthmus for more than 30 minutes is associated with a high risk of paraplegia. Monitoring of somatosensory evoked potentials and distal aortic pressure appears to be useful for preventing ischemic spinal cord damage, although their exact role is still unclear (6). A lumbar tap with continuing drainage of cerebrospinal fluid (CSF) may also improve blood flow to the distal spinal cord.

Although it may take more than 30 to 60 minutes to set up cardiopulmonary bypass, especially at night and on weekends, the bleeding sites can generally be controlled by direct pressure during that time. Nevertheless, because patients who sustain intrathoracic vascular injury frequently have associated injuries, the use of cardiopulmonary bypass with systemic heparinization can be hazardous.

Heparin-bonded cannulas and a centrifugal pump (Biomedicus) can be used to pump blood from the left atrium or the apex of the left ventricle into the descending aorta or femoral artery. When no oxygenator is used with this type of pump, little or no heparin is required, and improved results have been obtained (7).

With a contained hematoma, limited dissection is performed to obtain proximal and distal control without disturbing the hematoma. Care must be taken to avoid injury to the left vagus nerve where it crosses over the left subclavian artery and distal aortic arch. If the distal aortic arch is involved, proximal control is generally obtained by cross-clamping the aortic arch between the left common carotid and left subclavian arteries and by clamping the left subclavian artery distal to the hematoma. The distal aorta is cross-clamped below the hematoma. The hematoma can then be opened. Any blood lost should be recovered for autotransfusion.

Aortic Repairs. In most instances, the hole in the aorta is small (or the patient would have rapidly exsanguinated), and lateral aortorrhaphy is often easily accomplished. Mattox noted that the survival rate exceeded 90% for his patients who were normotensive on arrival and had an ascending aortic injury repaired in the operating room (8).

If inspection of the superior mediastinum reveals pulsatile hemorrhage from the transverse aortic arch, a finger (or vascular clamp) can be placed over the hole as the operating surgeon sews under it with a 3-0 or 4-0 polypropylene or polyester suture. An assistant can tie the knots as the surgeon withdraws finger pressure.

When a 2- to 3-inch long aortic tear must be repaired, the best closure technique is a running horizontal mattress suture, which everts about 2 to 3 mm of vessel wall on each side, followed by a simple over-and-over suture across the everted edges. This should be done with the injury isolated by side-clamping or total clamping of the involved aorta.

When possible, sutures in the aorta and large arteries should be tied while the intraluminal pressure is low. If the anesthesiologist cannot decrease the systemic pressure while the aortic sutures are tied, the surgeon can sometimes temporarily apply a side-clamp around the involved aorta while the sutures are being tied.

With all repairs on an opened aorta, the proximal and distal aorta should be flushed before the final sutures are tied. The distal clamp and then the proximal clamp are partly released to evacuate air or clots from the graft and occluded vessels. After the sutures have been tied securely, the distal clamp is removed again to check for any obvious suture line leaks. The proximal clamp is then gradually released so that no abrupt decrease in the patient's blood pressure occurs.

AXIOM When a common carotid artery must be clamped for more than 2 to 5 minutes in a hypotensive patient, one should try to shunt blood flow to the distal vessel.

Repairs of the proximal right (or left) common carotid artery in young patients often do not require internal or external shunting; however, if one of these vessels must be clamped for more than 2 to 5 minutes, one should have some concern about maintaining adequate blood flow to the brain. If the "stump pressure" of the right carotid artery distal to the cross-clamp on the innominate artery is 50 mm Hg or greater, the repair can generally be performed safely without a shunt. If the stump pressure is less than 50 mm Hg or cannot be measured, it may be prudent to insert a temporary external or internal shunt to ensure adequate blood flow to the brain (9). Use of systemic heparinization is not advised by Feliciano and Graham (10) in trauma patients, especially those who have suffered blunt injuries.

Innominate Artery

Innominate (brachiocephalic) artery injuries are rare. Rich and colleagues (11) had only three brachiocephalic artery injuries in their report of 1,000 arterial injuries from the Vietnam War. Of 93 patients with penetrating injuries of the aortic arch reported by Pate et al. (12), only six involved the brachiocephalic artery. Five of these six patients survived operative repair.

Subclavian Artery

Although gangrene of the upper extremity is unusual with ligation of the subclavian artery, especially with penetrating trauma, the injured vessel should be repaired whenever possible. If the subclavian artery is ligated, claudication of the arm may occur, and if the ligation is proximal to the vertebral artery, subclavian steal syndrome may develop. If there is any discrepancy in the length of the vessels, a prosthetic graft should be inserted because the subclavian tears easily, especially if it has been injured by blunt trauma.

Systemic Veins

In most instances, holes in the superior vena cava can be repaired with a lateral venorrhaphy; however, if the inferior or superior vena cava must be completely clamped in the chest, the sudden, severe reduction in venous return can cause cardiac arrest, particularly in hypovolemic patients; however, if the descending thoracic or proximal abdominal aorta is clamped, not as much preload is required, and clamping of an intrathoracic cava is generally tolerated much better.

AXIOM If the inferior or superior vena cava must be occluded in the chest, simultaneous cross-clamping of the descending aorta helps to prevent severe shock or a cardiac arrest.

If the superior vena cava is irreparably damaged, a portion of the internal jugular or left innominate vein is probably the ideal graft; however, one internal jugular vein should be left intact. An injured innominate vein can be ligated; however, if possible, one innominate vein should also be left intact to reduce the likelihood of a superior vena caval syndrome developing postoperatively. Injuries of subclavian veins can be extremely difficult to repair, even with excellent exposure. Ligation proximal and distal to the injury is usually much safer than large or difficult repairs.

Bullets entering large systemic veins or the right heart can embolize to the lungs, whereas bullets entering the pulmonary veins, left heart, or major systemic arteries can embolize to carotid, iliac, femoral, or even popliteal arteries. If a bullet embolus is diagnosed, the entrance wound is controlled and then the bullet is removed from its new position. Fluoroscopy in the operating room can be helpful for tracing these bullets, especially in the central veins or heart, because they can change position rapidly.

The azygous and hemizygous veins run posteriorly in the chest alongside the vertebral bodies and return blood from the posterior chest wall to the superior vena cava. When the patient is cirrhotic, the azygous vein may also return much of the splanchnic blood flow to the heart. Opening the chest and using the rib-spreader to provide better exposure can cause preexisting holes in these veins to enlarge markedly. Under such circumstances, it is better to remove one or two ribs rather than spread them to improve exposure.

Associated Injuries

There is a high incidence of brachial plexus damage if the second or third portion of a subclavian artery has been injured. Delayed neurologic changes after penetrating injury may be due to expanding pseudoaneurysms. Rarely, a phrenic or recurrent laryngeal nerve is injured iatrogenically during surgery. Consequently, the preoperative neurologic status of the patient should be documented as completely as possible.

Concurrent injuries of the tracheobronchial tree or esophagus are not unusual with thoracic vascular injuries. If such injuries are present, the area is contaminated, and one should avoid prosthetic grafts if possible.

Complications of Penetrating Thoracic Vascular Trauma

Atelectasis and pneumonia are best prevented or treated with good pulmonary toilet, deep breaths and coughing after extubation, and nasotracheal suction or bronchoscopy as needed. Epidural analgesia can also be helpful. If the adult respiratory distress syndrome (ARDS) develops, the patient should be given enough positive end-expiratory pressure to decrease the FiO_2 to 0.6 or less as soon as possible. If the ARDS does not respond, one should look for a site of uncontrolled sepsis.

Usually, small residual hemothoraces almost completely resorb spontaneously within 3 to 4 weeks. A retained hemothorax should probably be removed if it

1. Continues to occupy more than one-third of a hemithorax for more than 3 weeks;
2. Causes atelectasis of two or more lung segments; and
3. Is associated with continuing elevated temperature exceeding 101.4°F.

Postoperative Care

Patients with exsanguinating hemorrhage can have postoperative bleeding, hypothermia, coagulopathies, and metabolic acidosis. If the patient is bleeding less than 100 to 200 mL/h, the bleeding usually stops spontaneously, but the chest tubes should be connected to an autotransfusion collection device so that shed blood can be returned to the patient if necessary. Hypothermia is reversed with heating blankets, warmed fluids, and heated ventilator gases. Coagulopathies are corrected by making the patient normothermic and by giving fresh frozen plasma or cryoprecipitate and platelets, as necessary.

AXIOM Excess bleeding following surgery for trauma is often due to inadequate hemostasis by the surgeons.

Follow-up

The most frequent late manifestation of missed major vascular injuries in the chest are arteriovenous fistulas and pseudoaneurysms. Another concern is late infections of vascular grafts, and these may not be apparent until several weeks or months later.

Up to 40% of patients with severe chest trauma or an emergency thoracotomy may have prolonged excess pain, including causalgia. Such patients may respond to repeat stellate ganglion blocks.

BLUNT TRAUMA

Approximately 80% to 90% of patients with blunt trauma to thoracic great vessels, particularly the aorta, die at the scene of the accident or assault, and up to 50% of the remaining patients die within 48 hours if proper treatment is not given (13).

Pathophysiology

Shearing, bending, and torsion stress can combine to produce maximal stress on the inner surface of the aorta just above its point of greatest fixation, the ligamentum arteriosum. The next most common site in survivors is the innominate artery, usually at its origin. Tears in the lower thoracic aorta are uncommon, but tend to occur adjacent to comminuted vertebral fractures. Blunt injuries to the subclavian arteries tend to occur at their origins or where they cross the first rib.

AXIOM Aortography to look for traumatic rupture of the aorta (TRA) should include the entire thoracic aorta and its major branches, including the distal subclavian arteries.

Aortic tears caused by blunt trauma tend to extend obliquely up the isthmus from just above the ligamentum arteriosum toward the inner surface of the arch. If the tear does not involve the adventitia, a false aneurysm may be formed. The false aneurysm tends to expand with time, and if the BP is not adequately controlled, about 50% rupture within 24 hours (13).

Parmley et al. (13) found that, of the patients with traumatic rupture of the thoracic aorta who reach a hospital and survive for 1 hour, if the condition is not diagnosed and treated, 20% to 30% die within 6 hours, 40% to 50% die within 24 hours, and 60% to 80% die within 7 days.

Although the emphasis has generally been to get the patient to the operating room as soon as possible, it is probably much more important to diagnose and treat the patient's other severe injuries first. One should also keep the systolic BP less than 110 to 120 mm Hg and prevent gagging or Valsalva maneuvers. These lesions should be treated like a dissection of the descending thoracic aorta, and surgery should be performed when the conditions for repair are optimal.

Diagnosis

AXIOM The two most important factors in diagnosing TRA are a high index of suspicion because of the mechanism of injury and a widened mediastinum on chest radiograph.

Signs and Symptoms

Even when little or no external evidence of chest injury exists, one should suspect TRA in anyone who has had sudden, severe deceleration, including high-speed "T-bone" motor vehicle accidents. Patients with TRA usually complain primarily of their associated injuries and generally have few or no symptoms related to the aortic injury itself. The most common symptom that may be due to the aortic injury itself is retrosternal or interscapular pain from "stretching" or dissection of the adventitia of the aorta. Less frequent symptoms, resulting from pressure from the hematoma on adjacent structures, include dysphagia, stridor, dyspnea, voice change, or hoarseness.

Only 15 (27%) of 55 patients with TRA in one series sustained identifiable chest wall contusions or rib fractures. Almost all of our patients at Detroit Receiving Hospital with TRA, since our initial report (14), have had some clinical evidence of chest trauma. Physical findings that suggest aortic injury include

1. Upper extremity hypertension;
2. Decreased pulsations or blood pressure in the lower extremities; and
3. Presence of a harsh systolic murmur over the upper chest or posterior interscapular area.

Upper extremity hypertension has been noted in 31% to 43% of patients reported in the literature and has been attributed to compression of the aortic lumen by periaortic hematoma. Hypertension may also be caused by stretching or stimulation of special receptors located in the aortic isthmus (15). This mechanism could account for the upper extremity hypertension that occurs without aortic narrowing and for the slowly resolving postoperative hypertension that is seen in up to one-third of patients successively repaired.

Radiographic Studies

Plain Chest Films

Although the circumstances of the accident and the physical examination may be helpful, the diagnosis of TRA is usually suspected from findings on routine chest radiography. The most frequent radiologic finding is widening of the superior mediastinum, usually to more than 8.0 to 8.5 cm, caused primarily by an associated mediastinal hematoma.

The upper mediastinum appears wider than it really is if chest radiography is obtained

- Anteroposteriorly rather than posteroanteriorly (PA)
- With the patient less than 100 cm from the origin of the x-ray beam
- With the patient lying flat
- With poor inspiration

The optimal chest radiography is obtained with the patient in the so-called Ayella position: an upright PA chest film obtained at a distance of 6 ft (150 cm) from the source of the x-ray beam with the patient leaning forward about 15 degrees (16).

The most accurate chest radiographic sign of TRA is probably deviation of the esophagus or trachea greater than 1 to 2 cm to the right of the spinous process of T-4. In a series by Ayella et al., none of the patients with the esophagus less than 1.0 cm from the midline had TRA (16). In another series of 45 patients, none of the patients with a nasogastric tube in its normal position had TRA (17).

AXIOM A deviation of the esophagus or trachea greater than 2.0 cm to the right in the absence of a left tension pneumothorax after severe chest trauma is usually a result of TRA.

The paratracheal stripe is a linear density on the right side of the tracheal air column (18). It extends from the thoracic inlet to the proximal right bronchus and normally measures less than 5 mm in thickness. When the paratracheal stripe is greater than 5 mm wide or is deviated to the right, this may be another sign of mediastinal hemorrhage (18).

The paraspinal lines lie between the pleura and the lung, projected away from the lateral margin of the thoracic spine. The right paraspinal line is usually not visible on routine chest radiographs, but if it is seen and is displaced to the right in the absence of spinal or sternal fractures, it may be of some diagnostic value. The left paraspinal line may be distinguished from the image of the descending aorta because it is not continuous with the aortic knob. If this line is obviously displaced to the left, it suggests the presence of a mediastinal hematoma (Fig. 18-2) (19).

It often takes great force to fracture the first or second ribs or the sternum, especially in young patients. Consequently, such fractures tend to be associated with an increased incidence of major intrathoracic injuries.

AXIOM One should not assume that a TRA has been eliminated if the initial chest radiograph is "normal."

In up to one-third of patients, widening of the mediastinum and other radiographic changes may not be apparent on the initial chest films (14). Consequently, serial chest films should be obtained in any patient with severe chest trauma at 6- to 8-hour intervals during the first day and then daily for at least the next 2 to 3 days. Up to two-thirds of patients older than 65 years of age with traumatic aortic rupture may not show obvious mediastinal widening (20).

Computed Tomography Scans

The value of CT in screening for TRA is controversial. In 1990, Fenner et al. reported that CT and arteriography had comparable specificity (CT, 96%; arteriography, 92%) and false-positive rates (CT, 3.8%; arteriography, 7.7%) when CT was used as a screening tool for aortic rupture (21). Although some investigators have described cases in which the CT scans did not show a mediastinal hematoma with a TRA, in our experience, this is very rare. Thus, in stable patients with equivocal chest radiographs but with a low clinical suspicion of vascular injury, a CT scan can reliably differentiate mediastinal hematoma from other causes of mediastinal widening (22). The newer spiral CTs tend to be even more accurate.

Magnetic Resonance Imaging

The newer generations of MRI should be ideal for posttraumatic studies of the thoracic vessel if the patient

- Is hemodynamically stable
- Does not require a ventilator
- Can lie still long enough for a proper study
- Does not have a pacemaker or other metallic objects that will be affected by the powerful magnetic field

Aortography

AXIOM If an aortic rupture is suspected because of the mechanism of injury, physical findings, or chest radiographic changes, aortography should be performed promptly.

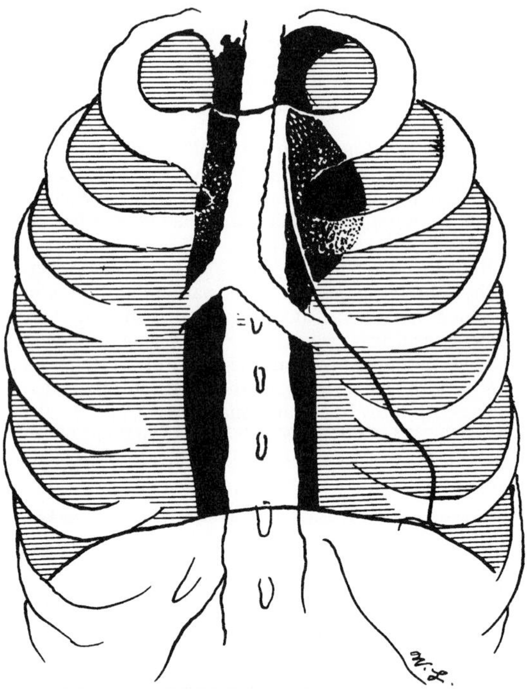

FIG. 18-2. Mediastinal hematomas, indicated by the blackened areas, may thicken and displace the paratracheal stripe laterally by more than 5 mm. Mediastinal hematomas may also displace the right and left paraspinal lines in the lower thorax rather widely from the edge of the thoracic spine. (From Wilson RF. Injury to the heart and great vessels. In: Henning RJ, Grenvik A, eds. *Critical care cardiology.* New York: Churchill Livingstone, 1989:453.)

Thoracic aortography is still considered the "gold standard" for diagnosing TRA, and most trauma surgeons believe that it should be done on all patients who are suspected of having a TRA. While waiting for aortography or surgery, it is important to ensure that the systolic BP does not increase above 110 to 120 mm Hg, using beta-blockers and vasodilators as needed. It is also important to prevent the patient from forcefully gagging or retching, as may occur during insertion of a nasogastric or endotracheal tube.

The most common finding on aortography of a TRA is a pseudoaneurysm of the isthmus of the aorta between the origin of the left subclavian artery and the ligamentum arteriosum. A slight pouching out of the inferior or inner border of isthmus, sometimes referred to as a "ductus bump" is normal, but it is occasionally confused with a traumatic pseudoaneurysm. Ferrera and Ghaemmaghami (23) have noted that a ductus diverticulum may be found in up to 25% of normal aortograms. They also noted that there are angiographic characteristics that are considered typical of this congenital variant, but the incidence of atypical radiologic findings that cannot readily be differentiated from aortic injuries may be as high as 12%.

AXIOM Aortography obtained to eliminate TRA should visualize the entire thoracic aorta and its major branches, out to the first ribs.

Angiographic complications may result from injuring the vessels, passing the catheter through diseased or injured vessels, or injecting contrast material under pressure. In a report by Waugh and Sacharias, it was noted that local complications with conventional angiography occur in 4.1% to 23.2% of patients, and systemic complications occur in 2.2% to 9.4% (24).

Digital Subtraction Angiography

Mirvis et al. studied 61 consecutive patients who had blunt thoracic trauma and obscuration of the aortic knob or mediastinal widening on chest radiography, using intraarterial digital subtraction angiography of the thoracic aorta (25). Digital subtraction aortography was 100% accurate, as indicated by the results of surgery, conventional arteriography, serial chest x-ray studies, and clinical follow-up. The method was 50% faster than conventional aortography and significantly reduced radiographic film costs.

Transesophageal Echocardiography

Shapiro et al. studied 19 patients who had blunt chest trauma with a widened mediastinum with transesophageal echocardiography (TEE). They detected aortic injuries in two patients, and both injuries were confirmed by aortography (26). In one patient, TEE failed to detect an intimal tear that was visualized by aortography. Brooks et al. reported on 450 trauma patients who had TEE (27). Of 21 patients with a wide mediastinum, TEE identified three aortic disruptions, and these were confirmed by aortography. Two patients, however, showed intimal aortic irregularities on TEE just distal to the left subclavian artery which were missed on aortography. In a similar study, Kearney et al. (28) noted that TEE correctly identified five aortic injuries that were confirmed by aortography (four) or thoracotomy (one) for a sensitivity and specificity of 100%. Pearson et al. (29) also found that TEE correctly identified blunt cardiac injury in four patients and aortic injuries in six others.

Treatment

Elective Delays in Surgical Intervention

In a report by Akins et al. in 1981, 14 of 44 patients with TRA had operative therapy delayed for 2 to 79 days with only two (14%) deaths, and five patients did not have operative repairs (i.e., surgery was delayed indefinitely with no deaths) (30). Of 21 patients having "early" operative repair (i.e., within 48 hours), five (24%) died. The 14 patients with elective delays of surgery included 12 patients with severe head injuries, nine patients with extensive pelvic or extremity fractures, three with severe burns, two with large pulmonary contusions, and one with a ruptured colon. A similar experience was reported by Stiles et al. in 1985 (31). Twenty-four patients with thoracic and abdominal aortic injuries became stable after initial fluid replacement. Blood pressures were controlled carefully with vasodilators and beta-blockers while awaiting elective repair of the torn aorta. Only one patient died, and none of the patients bled from the TRA during the elective delay. The mortality rate was much higher in patients who were rushed to surgery at night despite being hemodynamically stable.

Galli et al. (32) recently reported on a series of 42 patients with acute traumatic rupture of the thoracic aorta. Group I (21 patients) underwent immediate repair and, in group II, operation was performed only after intensive medical treatment and management of associated lesions, but with careful monitoring of the aortic tear. The mortality rate in group I patients was 19% and in group II was 0%.

AXIOM When the BP of a patient with proven TRA can be controlled properly, surgery for TRA should be delayed until the best possible circumstances for operative success are available.

Management Priorities with Associated Injuries

AXIOM Unless one is exsanguinating from associated abdominal injuries, TRA should generally be treated before laparotomy for abdominal injuries.

The most life-threatening injury should be corrected first. If all of the injuries are relatively stable, the TRA should be corrected first. If the TRA appears to be stable and the patient is actively bleeding inside the abdomen, laparotomy takes precedence. If the patients' injuries require both a thoracotomy for TRA and a laparotomy for intraabdominal bleeding, the mortality rate may exceed 50%.

Surgical Management

"Clamp and Sew"

AXIOM The clamp/repair technique should not be used if the surgeon is unaccustomed to thoracic aortic surgery or if the repair is likely to require more than 30 minutes of aortic clamp time.

Centers reporting success with the "clamp/repair" technique have had extensive experience with aortic surgery (33). With the clamp/repair technique, the proximal clamp is usually placed on the arch between the left common carotid and left subclavian arteries. A clamp is also placed on the left subclavian artery. The distal clamp is placed as close to the aortic hematoma as possible to avoid interference with the upper intercostal arteries. By avoiding cardiopulmonary bypass and its attendant heparinization, the risk of excessive bleeding is reduced. This may be particularly important in patients with injuries to the brain, eyes, or retroperitoneum.

Critics of the clamp/repair technique have noted that aortic cross-clamping may result in high mortality and morbidity rates, especially if the aorta is clamped for more than 30 minutes (34). In addition, significant hemodynamic and metabolic changes can occur in patients without a shunt or bypass to the distal aorta. Forbes and Ashbaugh noted that simple aortic cross-clamping to repair TRA resulted in a 44% incidence of new neurologic deficits, longer hospitalization, and a higher incidence of pulmonary, gastrointestinal, and septic complications than mechanical circulatory support (35).

External Shunts

Heparin-bonded tubing as a shunt from the ascending aorta or the apex of the left ventricle either to the descending aorta or to a femoral artery can reduce the danger of distal ischemia to the spinal cord and abdominal viscera. It can also prevent proximal hypertension damage to the heart, and the patient does not require systemic heparinization. Verdant et al. reported on use of the shunt in 114 consecutive patients with descending thoracic aortic disease; they found no postoperative paralysis, renal dysfunction, or paraplegia in the survivors (36).

Cardiopulmonary Bypass

Repair of traumatic rupture of the thoracic aorta is often performed under partial cardiopulmonary bypass because it allows increased time for a meticulous repair. A complete cardiopulmonary bypass is seldom used except when repairing tears of the ascending aorta or arch. For lesions involving the aortic isthmus, partial bypass is usually adequate.

Probably the most frequent type of partial cardiopulmonary bypass that has been used has been a femoral vein to femoral artery bypass. This involves use of an oxygenator and requires heparinization of the patient, which can be a significant risk in multiple trauma patients.

If a special vortex (Biomedicus) pump is used with a left atrial-femoral artery bypass, an oxygenator is not needed, and little or no heparinization of the blood is required. In most published series in which this technique was used, few deaths (5%) and no paraplegia have been reported (37). This is increasingly becoming the preferred technique for treating this injury; however, it is important to maintain distal aortic flow at greater than 1.0 L/min to prevent clotting and to maintain an adequate distal BP (Fig. 18-3).

Management of Specific Injuries

Ascending Aorta

Because few patients with rupture of the ascending aorta survive long enough for diagnosis to be established and repair to be carried out, it is encountered clinically in only 2% to 3% of all aortic injuries (38). However, the ascending aorta is the site of rupture in 19% to 25% of patients who die at the scene of the accident.

Most ascending aortic tears occur within the pericardium so that if the tear is complete, there is generally evidence of both shock and pericardial tamponade. Chest x-ray findings typically include a widened superior mediastinum, with or without obscuration of the aortic knob. Aortography usually shows a pseudoaneurysm with an intimal tear seen as an irregular filling defect within the lumen.

Aortic Arch

Operations on the aortic arch involve sophisticated techniques, such as deep hypothermic circulatory arrest and selective cerebral perfusion, to avoid ischemic injury to the brain and viscera when perfusion is interrupted. Howells et al. (39) have pointed out the benefits of hypothermic arrest for surgically correcting blunt injuries of the ascending aorta and aortic arch. Pretre and colleagues (40) described the surgical management of hemorrhage from rupture of the aortic arch in six patients. Bleeding was reduced by keeping the mediastinum under local tension (three

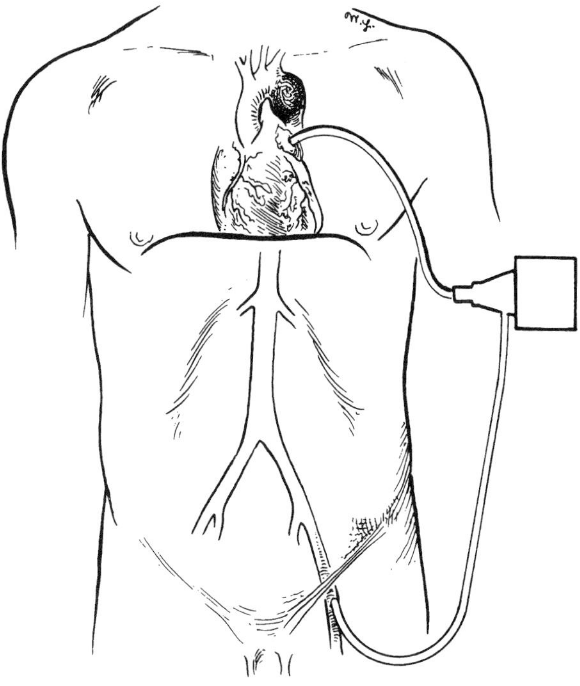

FIG. 18-3. Partial cardiopulmonary bypass with a centrifugal pump. Using this pump to move oxygenated blood from the left atrium directly into the femoral artery allows one to use little or no heparin because an oxygenator is not in the circuit. (From Wilson RF. Injury to the heart and great vessels. In: Henning RJ, Grenvik A, eds. *Critical care cardiology.* New York: Churchill Livingstone, 1989:463.)

patients) or by applying compression on the bleeding site (two patients), or both (one patient) while circulatory support, retransfusion of aspirated blood, and hypothermia were established. The diseased aortic arch was replaced during deep hypothermic (18°C) circulatory arrest for 25 to 40 minutes. In three patients, the brain was further protected by retrograde (two patients) or antegrade (one patient) cerebral perfusion.

Thoracic Aorta Distal to the Isthmus

Thoracic aortic injuries distal to the isthmus should be suspected with severe chest trauma in which a lower thoracic vertebra is crushed. Repair techniques are similar to those used with injuries to the aortic isthmus, but less difficulty should be encountered with clamp/repair technique in this area compared with more proximal aortic injuries.

Innominate Artery

In patients reaching the hospital alive, blunt injuries of the innominate artery are second in frequency only to rupture of the aorta at the isthmus. The diagnosis of blunt injury to the innominate artery may be difficult because no characteristic physical findings are manifest except for some diminution of the right radial or brachial pulse, which occurs in about 50% of patients (2,41). Occasionally, a localized systolic murmur may draw attention to a possible lesion in this area. Chest radiographic findings include widened superior mediastinum; however, the outline of the descending aorta may be preserved, and the trachea and esophagus tend to be deviated to the left.

Weiman et al. (42) recently described five patients with blunt injuries of the brachiocephalic artery seen between 1988 and 1995. All five patients were stabilized preoperatively and underwent repair through a median sternotomy with extension of the incision anterior to the sternocleidomastoid muscle. Restoration of flow to the subclavian and carotid arteries used bypass grafts (four) or primary repair (one). The postoperative neurologic findings were the same as those seen before the operative repair. Cardiopulmonary bypass and heparin or temporary shunts were not used in this series.

Subclavian Artery

Although an occasional subclavian artery is avulsed at its origin because of sudden deceleration, direct trauma to the distal artery with occlusion associated with fractures of the first rib or clavicle is more likely (2,43). The most important sign of a subclavian artery injury is absence of a radial pulse; however, the collateral is so good across the shoulder and upper arm that 15% to 25% of the patients with occlusion of the subclavian, axillary, or high brachial artery have a palpable radial pulse (3). Other physical findings are a pulsatile mass or hematoma or a bruit in the root of the neck. Chest radiography may show a widened superior mediastinum without blurring or obscuration of the aortic knob shadow. Angiography usually shows only an occlusion, but a pseudoaneurysm is occasionally found.

The treatment of acute subclavian artery injury is usually immediate repair; however, in high-risk patients, ligation or angiographic occlusion may be the treatment of choice. When the artery is already occluded, nonoperative care with close observation may be all that is required. When reconstruction of a blunt injury to the distal subclavian artery is required, a graft is usually necessary because the involved vessel may be quite fragile and may not mobilize well. Gore-Tex (PTFE) grafts usually work well in this circumstance.

Babatasi et al. (44) recently reported on endovascular treatment of a traumatic subclavian artery aneurysm.

AXIOM When a subclavian artery is occluded by trauma and no AV fistula, false aneurysm, or distal ischemia is present, there is no critical need to explore the artery, particularly if the patient has severe associated injuries.

Complications of Surgical Treatment

Paraplegia

An anterior spinal cord syndrome resulting in a flaccid paraplegia with varying degrees of sensory loss below T-6 to T-10 is characteristic of the ischemic myelopathy that can occur after prolonged thoracic aortic cross-clamping. Most patients preserve partial function of the posterior columns and have at least some pain and temperature sensation below the level of the spinal injury.

This injury is believed to be due to inadequate anterior spinal artery flow. Collaterals to the anterior spinal artery in the lower chest are inadequate in many patients. Ligation and division of mid and lower thoracic intercostal arteries, particularly the arteria radicularis magna of Adamkiewicz, which is believed to be the major blood supply to the lower spinal cord, can lead to paraplegia, even without prolonged aortic cross-clamping (45).

AXIOM Thoracic aortic cross-clamp times should not exceed 30 minutes unless a bypass or shunt is used to maintain adequate blood flow to the mid and lower thoracic aorta.

The incidence of paraplegia is reduced by maintaining some blood flow to the distal aorta and by draining CSF from a lumbar tap during the case. The physiology of spinal cord perfusion pressure (perfusion pressure = mean aortic pressure − mean CSF pressure) provides the basis for the use of CSF drainage preoperatively, intraoperatively, and postoperatively in patients undergoing thoracic aortic replacement (46). A catheter is introduced by lumbar puncture using local anesthetics at the L3-4 or L4-5 level. It is positioned approximately 10 cm into the intrathecal space, and fluid can be withdrawn via syringe. Recommendations on initial CSF drainage volumes are from 20 to 50 mL. Thereafter, pressure can be continuously monitored and a sterile gravity drainage system can be used to collect fluid, if the CSF pressure becomes greater than 10 mm Hg. The duration of CSF drainage varies between centers; some recommend intraoperative drainage only, whereas others continue it for up to 48 hours until the risk of hemodynamic instability is minimized and the collateral circulation to the spinal cord has stabilized.

Left Heart Failure

Left heart failure after thoracic aortic injury can be due to inadequate coronary blood flow or excessive aortic pressure, such as with thoracic aortic clamping. The pulmonary artery wedge pressure can double after only 2 minutes of thoracic aortic clamping distal to the left subclavian artery (47). Verdant et al. also observed that substantial elevations of left atrial pressure occur when the proximal aortic systolic pressure is maintained above 160 mm Hg (36).

Renal Insufficiency

Although overt renal insufficiency is only rarely described in retrospective studies of patients having the clamp/repair technique, Carlson et al. found some renal dysfunction in all patients studied after that procedure (48).

Pulmonary Problems

Pulmonary problems, particularly atelectasis and pneumonia, are the most frequent postoperative complications after almost all thoracic operations. Careful attention to pulmonary management postoperatively and use of a double-lumen endotracheal tube intraoperatively have decreased the incidence and severity of these problems.

Hypertension

Hypertension in both the upper and lower extremities may persist for several days after repair of TRA, possibly because of stretching or stimulation of baroreceptors located in tissues near the aortic isthmus. If the hypertension is severe, it should be treated with antihypertensive agents.

Vocal Cord Damage
Hoarseness caused by damage to the left recurrent laryngeal nerve as it passes around the aorta just beyond the ligamentum arteriosum may be due to the initial trauma, pressure from an expanding pseudoaneurysm, or iatrogenic injury during dissection and clamping of the aorta. In most instances, the hoarseness is only temporary.

Esophageal Tears
Damage to the esophagus may be caused by the initial trauma, compression by the hematoma, occlusion of its blood supply, or surgical dissection or clamps. Iatrogenic injury, particularly by vascular clamps intended only for the aorta, can occur, especially if a nasogastric tube is not present. If the esophagus has a full thickness injury, the prognosis is poor because, even if the patient survives the surgery, the suture line or prosthetic graft has a greatly increased chance of becoming infected.

Mortality Rates
In most reports, the mortality rates for patients reaching the hospital alive with TRA is 10% to 25%. In those who reach the operating room conscious and with stable vital signs, the mortality rate should be less than 10%. In a review of the literature from 1985 to 1990, the mortality rates with the clamp/repair technique (31.3%) were significantly higher than with techniques that maintained some distal aortic blood flow (7.1% to 11.3%). However, the high mortality rates seen with TRA are often due to the severe associated injuries that frequently accompany this problem. Furthermore, some clamp/repair cases are emergencies when there is no opportunity to use another technique.

⊘ FREQUENT ERRORS

1. ***Failure to obtain arteriography promptly on stable patients who have a penetrating chest wound anywhere near a great vessel or across the mediastinum.***
2. ***Delaying needed surgery to obtain arteriography on unstable patients.***
3. ***Turning a patient with hypotension or significant hemoptysis onto the uninjured side to perform a posterolateral thoracotomy.***
4. ***Taking time to repair a badly injured subclavian artery rather than just ligating it in patients who are hemodynamically unstable.***
5. ***Failing to repair a lacerated but patent carotid artery because a neurologic defect is present.***
6. ***Completely clamping or occluding the superior or inferior vena cava in the chest while the patient is still hypovolemic.***
7. ***Allowing the systolic BP to exceed 120 mm Hg when one suspects a TRA.***
8. ***Assuming that TRA is not present because the initial chest radiograph appears to be normal, despite a suspicious mechanism of trauma.***
9. ***Failing to obtain a CT of the chest when one is already obtaining a CT of the brain after a severe deceleration injury.***
10. ***Assuming that aortography is harmless and is needed on everyone who has even a slight chance of TRA.***
11. ***Assuming radiographically proved TRA must be repaired immediately regardless of the associated injuries, available surgical support, and surgical risk.***
12. ***Using a clamp-repair technique when the surgeon does not have extensive aortic surgery experience or the repair is apt to require more than 30 minutes of aortic cross-clamp time.***
13. ***Repairing other less critical injuries before attempting to repair a TRA.***
14. ***Inadequate warning of the patient and family of the risk of paraplegia when repairing a TRA.***

SUMMARY POINTS

1. Patients with a penetrating thoracic vascular injury may suddenly begin to bleed massively when their BPs are restored or when they gag or retch while an esophageal or tracheal tube is being inserted.
2. If more than 25% of the cardiac output goes through an AV fistula, high-output cardiac failure is likely to develop.
3. A "fuzzy" bullet (due to pulsation of an adjacent vessel) should be considered a radiologic sign of a possible major vascular injury until proven otherwise.
4. CT scans of the chest should not be performed while a patient is hemodynamically unstable.
5. A moderate or large hemothorax should be promptly evacuated with a chest tube unless the patient requires emergency thoracotomy.
6. If a patient needs an emergency thoracotomy because of massive bleeding, inserting a chest tube tends to delay the definitive operative procedure.
7. Autotransfusion of more than 6 units of blood of blood tends to contribute to development of a coagulopathy.
8. If it is obvious that a patient has exsanguinating intrathoracic bleeding, a thoracotomy should be performed as quickly as possible and with little or no resuscitation until the bleeding is controlled.
9. Hypotension that develops or gets worse while a chest tube is draining blood from the chest is an indication for an emergency thoracotomy.
10. Patients should not be turned onto their side for a posterolateral thoracotomy if the patient is hypotensive or has hemoptysis.
11. If the systolic BP does not increase to 90 mm Hg within 5 minutes of clamping the descending thoracic aorta and providing aggressive fluid resuscitation, the patient will almost certainly die intraoperatively.
12. All hematomas on major vessels should be explored after obtaining proximal and distal control.
13. Clamping the upper descending thoracic aorta for more than 30 minutes without providing some blood flow to the distal aorta can result in a high incidence of paraplegia.
14. Probably the safest bypass to the distal aorta is via a centrifugal pump from the left atrium to the distal aorta or femoral artery, and this requires little or no systemic heparinization.
15. When possible, aortic sutures should be pledgetted and then tied while the blood pressure in that area is reduced as much as possible.
16. When a common carotid artery must be clamped for more than 2 to 5 minutes in a hypotensive patient, one should try to shunt some blood flow to the distal vessel.
17. If the inferior or superior vena cava must be occluded in the chest, simultaneous cross-clamping of the descending aorta helps to prevent severe shock or a cardiac arrest
18. When possible, the intrathoracic superior or inferior vena cava should not be cross-clamped while a patient is hypovolemic; if a proximal cava must be clamped, the descending thoracic aorta should also be clamped.
19. If there are concurrent thoracic vascular and aerodigestive injuries, one should avoid prosthetic grafts if possible.
20. Patients reaching the hospital alive with blunt aortic trauma generally have an injury to the isthmus of the aorta.
21. Aortography to look for TRA should include the entire thoracic aorta and its major branches, including the distal subclavian arteries.
22. If a blunt aortic injury is suspected, the systolic BP should be kept below 110 to 120 mm Hg.
23. The two most important factors in diagnosing acute TRA are a high index of suspicion because of the mechanism of injury and a widened mediastinum seen on chest radiograph.

24. One of the main reasons that many unnecessary aortograms are performed for possible TRA is a technically poor initial chest radiograph.
25. A deviation of the esophagus or trachea more than 2.0 cm to the right, in the absence of a left tension pneumothorax, after severe blunt trauma is highly suggestive of a TRA.
26. Fracture of the first or second ribs should make one suspect the presence of severe intrathoracic injuries.
27. If an aortic rupture is suspected because of the mechanism of injury, physical findings, or chest radiographic changes, aortography should be performed promptly.
28. When the BP of a patient with proven TRA can be controlled properly, surgery for TRA should be delayed until the best possible circumstances for operative success are available.
29. Unless the patient is exsanguinating from associated abdominal injuries, TRA should generally be treated before laparotomy for abdominal injuries is undertaken.
30. The clamp/repair technique should not be used if the surgeon is unaccustomed to thoracic aortic surgery or if the repair is likely to require more than 30 minutes of aortic clamp time.
31. A vortex pump with a left atrial-femoral artery bypass requires little or no heparin and is probably the safest technique for preserving distal aortic flow in patients with TRA.
32. When a subclavian artery is occluded by trauma and there is no evidence of an AV fistula, false aneurysm, or distal ischemia, the artery does not have to be explored.
33. Thoracic aortic cross-clamp times should not exceed 30 minutes unless a bypass or shunt maintains an adequate flow to the mid and lower thoracic aorta.
34. A systolic BP above 160 to 180 mm Hg in the aortic arch proximal to an aortic clamp can cause acute left heart failure, especially in patients with recent severe blunt chest trauma.

REFERENCES

1. Wilson RF, Stephenson LW. Trauma to intrathoracic great vessels. In: Wilson RF, Walt AJ, eds. *Management of trauma: pitfalls and practice.* 2nd ed. Philadelphia: Williams & Wilkins, 1996:361.
2. Symbas PN. Trauma to the great vessels. In: *Cardiothoracic trauma.* Philadelphia: WB Saunders, 1989;160–231.
3. Symbas PN, Sehdeva JS. Penetrating wounds of the thoracic aorta. *Ann Surg* 1970;171:441.
4. Calhoon JH, Grover FL, Trinkle JT. Chest trauma—approach and management. *Clin Chest Med* 1992;13:55.
5. McFadden PM, Jones JW, Ochsner JL. The fuzzy foreign body fragment: a subtle roentgenographic clue to mediastinal vascular injury. *Am J Surg* 1985;149:809.
6. Crawford ES, Mizrahi EM, Hess KR, et al. The impact of distal aortic perfusion and somatosensory evoked potential monitoring on prevention of paraplegia after aortic aneurysm operation. *J Thorac Cardiovasc Surg* 1988;95:357.
7. Kim FJ, Moore EE, Moore FA, et al. Trauma surgeons can render operative care for major thoracic injuries. *J Trauma* 1994;36:871.
8. Mattox KL. Symposium: new approaches in vascular trauma. *J Vasc Surg* 1988; 7:725.
9. Marvasti MA, Parker FB Jr, Bredenbery CE. Injuries to arterial branches of the aortic arch. *J Thorac Cardiovasc Surg* 1984;32:293.
10. Feliciano DV, Graham JM. Major thoracic vascular injury. In: Champion HR, Robbs JV, Trunkey DO, eds. *Rob & Smith's operative surgery—trauma surgery.* Part 1, 4th ed. London: Butterworths, 1989;283—-293.
11. Rich NM, Baugh JH, Hughes CW. Acute arterial injuries of Vietnam: 1000 cases. *J Trauma* 1970;10:359.
12. Pate JW, Cole HC, Walker WA, et al. Penetrating injuries of the aortic arch and its branches. *Ann Thorac Surg* 1993;55:586.
13. Parmley LF, Mattingly TW, Manion WC. Nonpenetrating traumatic injury of the aorta. *Circulation* 1958;17:1086.

14. Wilson RF, Arbulu A, Basset J, et al. Acute mediastinal widening following blunt chest trauma: critical decisions. *Arch Surg* 1972; 104:551.
15. Laforet EG. Acute hypertension as a diagnostic clue in traumatic rupture of the thoracic aorta. *Am J Surg* 1965;110:948.
16. Ayella RJ, Hankins JR, Turney SZ, et al. Ruptured thoracic aorta due to blunt trauma. *J Trauma* 1977;17:119.
17. Gerlock AJ, Muhletaler CA, Coulam CM, et al. Traumatic aortic aneurysm: validity of esophageal tube displacement sign. *AJR Am J Roentgenol* 1980;135: 713–718.
18. Woodring JH, Pulmano CM, Stevens RK. The right paratracheal stripe in blunt chest trauma. *Radiology* 1982;143:605.
19. Barcia TC, Livoni JP. Indications for angiography in blunt thoracic trauma. *Radiology* 1983;147:15–19.
20. Gundry SR, Williams S, Burney RE. Indications for aortography in blunt thoracic trauma: a reassessment. *J Trauma* 1982;22:664.
21. Fenner MN, Fisher KS, Sergel NL, et al. Evaluation of possible traumatic thoracic aortic injury using aortography and CT. *Am Surg* 1990;56:497.
22. Creasy JD, Chiles C, Routh WD, et al. Overview of traumatic injury of the thoracic aorta. RadioGraphics 1997;17:27.
23. Ferrera PC, Ghaemmaghami PA. Ductus diverticulum interpreted as traumatic aortic injury. *Am J Emerg Med* 1997;15:371.
24. Waugh JR, Sacharias N. Arteriographic complications in the DSA era. *Radiology* 1992;182:243.
25. Mirvis SE, Pais OS, Gens DR. Thoracic aortic rupture: advantages of intraarterial digital subtraction angiography. *Am J Radiol* 1986;146:987.
26. Shapiro MJ, Yanofsky SD, Trapp J, et al. Cardiovascular evaluation in blunt thoracic trauma using transesophageal echocardiography (TEE). *J Trauma* 1991;31: 835.
27. Brooks WS, Young JC, Cmolik B, et al. The use of transesophageal echocardiography in the evaluation of chest trauma. *J Trauma* 1991;31:1024.
28. Kearney PA, Smith DW, Johnson SB, et al. The use of transesophageal echocardiography in the evaluation of traumatic aortic injury. *J Trauma* 1992;33:155.
29. Pearson GD, Karr SS, Trachiotis GD, et al. A retrospective review of the role of transesophageal echocardiography in aortic and cardiac trauma in a level I pediatric trauma center. *J Am Soc Echocardiogr* 1997;10:946.
30. Akins CW, Buckley MV, Daggett W, et al. Acute traumatic disruption of the thoracic aorta: a ten-year experience. *Ann Thorac Surg* 1981;31:305.
31. Stiles QR, Cohlmia GS, Smith JH, et al. Management of injuries of the thoracic and abdominal Aorta. *Am J Surg* 1985;150:132.
32. Galli R, Pacini D, DiBartolomeo R, et al. Surgical indications and timing of repair of traumatic ruptures of the thoracic aorta. *Ann Thorac Surg* 1998;65:461.
33. Mattox KL, Holzman M, Pickard LR. Clamp/repair: a safe technique for treatment of blunt injury to the descending thoracic aorta. *Ann Thorac Surg* 1985;40: 456.
34. Hunt JP, Baker CC, Lentz C, et al. Thoracic aorta injuries: management and outcome of 144 patients. *J Trauma* 1996;40:547.
35. Forbes AD, Ashbaugh DG. Mechanical circulatory support during repair of thoracic aortic injuries improves morbidity and prevents spinal cord injury. *Arch Surg* 1994;129:494.
36. Verdant A, Cossette R, Dontigny L, et al. Acute and chronic traumatic aneurysms of the descending thoracic aorta: a 10-year experience with a single method of aortic shunting. *J Trauma* 1985;25:601.
37. McCroskey BL, BL, Moore EE, Moore FA, Abernathy CM. A unified approach to the torn thoracic aorta. *Am J Surg* 1991;162:473.
38. Ono M, Yagyu K, Furuse A, et al. A case of Stanford type A acute aortic dissection caused by blunt chest trauma. *J Trauma* 1998;44:543.
39. Howells GA, Hernandez DA, Olt SL, et al. Blunt injury of the ascending aorta and aortic arch: repair with hypothermic circulatory arrest. *J Trauma* 1998;44: 716.

40. Pretre R, Murith N, Delay D, et al. Surgical management of hemorrhage from rupture of the aortic arch. *Ann Thorac Surg* 1998;65:1291.
41. Wilson RF. Injury to the heart and great vessels. In: Henning RJ, Grenvik A, eds. *Critical care cardiology.* New York: Churchill Livingstone, 1989:411–472.
42. Weiman DS, McCoy DW, Haan CK, et al. Blunt injuries of the brachiocephalic artery. *Am Surg* 1998;64:383.
43. Graham JM, Feliciano DV, Mattox KL, et al. Management of subclavian vascular injuries. *J Trauma* 1980;20:537.
44. Babatasi G, Massetti M, LePage O, et al. Endovascular treatment of a traumatic subclavian artery aneurysm. *J Trauma* 1998;44:545.
45. Lynch C, Weingarden SI. Paraplegia following aortic surgery. *Paraplegia* 1982;20:196.
46. Widmann MD, DeLucia A, Sharp WJ, et al. Reversal of renal failure and paraplegia after thoracoabdominal aneurysm repair. *Ann Thorac Surg* 1998;65:1153.
47. Kouchoukos NT, Lell WA. Hemodynamic effects of aortic clamping and decompression with a temporary shunt for resection of the descending thoracic aorta. *Surgery* 1979;85:25.
48. Carlson DE, Karp RB, Kouchoukos NT. Surgical treatment of aneurysms of the descending thoracic aorta: an analysis of 85 patients. *Ann Thorac Cardiovasc Surg* 1983;35:58.

19A. ESOPHAGEAL INJURIES[1]

INCIDENCE AND MORTALITY RATES

Although most busy centers cite only two to four cases of intrathoracic esophageal trauma per year, these injuries are important because of the high mortality and morbidity rates likely to occur if definitive treatment is not accomplished within 12 to 24 hours.

The mortality rate of esophageal injuries is about 5% to 25% for those treated definitively within 12 hours, 10% to 44% for those treated at 12 to 24 hours, and 25% to 66% or higher for those treated after 24 hours (2). Mortality rates are particularly high with perforations of the thoracic esophagus because of the severe suppurative mediastinitis that can develop within 6 to 12 hours.

ANATOMY

In male adults, the esophagus is 25 to 30 cm in length and in its collapsed state measures about 1.5 cm in diameter. The esophagus begins at the cricopharyngeus muscle opposite the sixth cervical vertebra. The lower thoracic esophagus lies behind the left atrium and slightly to the left of the lowest thoracic vertebra. It then enters the abdomen through the esophageal hiatus of the diaphragm to the left of T-11.

The muscular layers of the esophagus consist of an inner circular layer and an outer longitudinal layer that is striated in its proximal one-third and smooth in the distal two-thirds. The esophagus is devoid of serosa but has a rather filmy adventitia.

AXIOM Lack of a serosal covering for the esophagus increases the likelihood of an anastomotic leak.

The major blood supply of the esophagus is segmental and originates from the inferior thyroid artery, bronchial arteries, esophageal branches of the descending thoracic aorta, and the left gastric artery.

Gastroesophageal competence is maintained by the diaphragmatic crura, the intraabdominal segment of esophagus, and the physiologic internal lower esophageal sphincter (LES), which is about 3 to 5 cm in length.

Pathophysiology

With injuries to the thoracic esophagus, resulting leaks are initially confined within the mediastinum, often producing a small sympathetic pleural effusion. Later, the mediastinal pleura breaks down and the pleural effusion rapidly increases. Most of the toxicity of intrathoracic esophageal ruptures is due to regurgitated acidic gastric secretions rather than swallowed saliva. The resulting chemical mediastinitis causes increasing loss of fluid into the inflamed tissues, and this is further increased when infection develops. Indeed, suppurative mediastinitis is one of the most devastating infections that can occur in trauma patients.

ESOPHAGEAL PERFORATIONS

Etiology

Iatrogenic

Up to two-thirds of esophageal injuries are iatrogenic, and more than one-half of these occur during efforts to dilate a stricture (3). Most of the remainder occur during diagnostic endoscopy, usually in a diseased esophagus. With the advent of flexible endoscopy, the risk of perforation has been greatly reduced; however, deep biopsies, dilatation of strictures, forceful dilatation for achalasia, laser surgery for obstructions, and removal of sharp foreign bodies still cause some esophageal injuries.

The most common sites of iatrogenic perforation are at or just above areas that are narrowed anatomically or because of disease. Normally, the esophageal introitus at the cricopharyngeus is the narrowest portion of the esophagus and is the area most prone to perforate. The other frequent sites of perforation, because of anatomic narrowing, are the diaphragmatic hiatus and the area of slight narrowing produced by the left mainstem bronchus.

Penetrating Trauma

Stabs and gunshot wounds may injure the esophagus anywhere along its course, but patients coming to surgery most frequently have involvement of the cervical esophagus (2–4). Most injuries to the cervical esophagus are caused by stab wounds, whereas most intrathoracic or intraabdominal esophageal injuries result from gunshot wounds.

There are several reasons for the relative infrequency of thoracic esophageal injuries. The thoracic esophagus is too deep for most stab wounds, and penetrating trauma that injures the midthoracic esophagus is also likely to involve the heart or great vessels and be rapidly fatal. In our experience of 200 emergency thoracotomies for penetrating trauma, only three patients (1.5%) had an esophageal injury (5).

Blunt Trauma

Esophageal rupture resulting from blunt trauma is rare. In our studies, we found no esophageal injuries in 340 patients admitted with blunt chest trauma (6). Beal et al. (7), in a review of the world experience from 1900 to 1987, found 96 reported cases of blunt esophageal trauma, of which 70% involved the cervical esophagus. The more recent literature includes two reports with a total of 12 patients with blunt pharyngoesophageal perforation resulting in five (42%) deaths (8,9).

Most instances of blunt rupture are probably a result of a sudden increase in intraesophageal pressure. Intragastric pressure transmitted to the esophagus may also play a role. During injury from blunt trauma, the esophagus also may be compressed against preexisting osteoarthritic prominences (resulting in tearing of the esophageal wall) or be severely contused (which subsequently may result in necrosis and perforation).

Diagnosis

AXIOM An esophageal injury should be suspected in all patients who have a penetrating wound in the thoracic inlet or mediastinum and have a pleural effusion or pneumomediastinum.

AXIOM Any new cervical, thoracic, or abdominal symptoms, signs, or x-ray changes after esophageal instrumentation, especially dilatation of an esophageal stricture, are a result of an esophageal leak until proven otherwise.

Signs and Symptoms

The clinical manifestations of a penetrating wound of the esophagus depend upon the site and size of the wound, trauma to neighboring organs, and the time elapsed since the injury. Cervical perforations may cause upper thoracic pain, whereas diaphragmatic irritation may cause shoulder pain. When chest pain occurs because of an esophageal injury, it is often of acute onset (30%), and it is usually severe and continuous, and may be difficult to differentiate from myocardial ischemia (10). Back pain tends to develop later, and it is usually relatively well localized to the actual area of esophageal injury.

A sore throat and slight pain with swallowing are not uncommon for a day or two after any esophageal instrumentation; however, increasing dysphagia (difficulty swallowing) or odynophagia (painful swallowing) should make one suspect esophageal injury.

Vomiting up blood after trauma should make one suspicious of an upper gastrointestinal injury; however, blood from the nose or mouth is often swallowed and may also be vomited. Traumatic insertion of a nasogastric tube, particularly in an uncooperative patient, is a frequent cause of some bleeding. The swallowed blood brought up in the nasogastric tube may then be interpreted as originating from a lower site.

Physical Examination

Although subcutaneous emphysema over the chest usually results from airway or pulmonary injuries, if it is confined to the neck, it may be the first sign of perforation of the esophagus or pharynx. Decreased breath sounds caused by a hydrothorax or pneumothorax after instrumentation of the esophagus or after swallowing a foreign body is virtually diagnostic of an esophageal injury. Occasionally, Hamman's sign, which is a crunching precordial sound synchronous with cardiac systole, can be heard in patients with mediastinal emphysema. This is often heard better if the patient is in the left lateral decubitus position.

The cause of most instances of mediastinal emphysema is unknown. When a source is found, it is usually interstitial emphysema resulting from asthma or a lung injury. Nevertheless, bronchial or esophageal injury should be ruled out if there is any evidence of a pneumomediastinum after trauma.

Fever may occur rapidly with mediastinitis. In older or debilitated patients with a contained leak, little or no fever may be present until quite late in the process. Some upper abdominal tenderness and guarding can be caused by perforations of the lower thoracic esophagus.

AXIOM Abdominal pain and tenderness may be the first signs and symptoms of perforation of the lower thoracic esophagus.

Radiologic Studies

Plain Films

AXIOM Mediastinal or deep cervical emphysema is a result of an aerodigestive injury until proven otherwise.

Free air in the neck after trauma or any instrumentation, particularly in the deep perivisceral spaces, is usually from an injury to the hypopharynx, but it may also result from a tear of the larynx, trachea, or esophagus.

A lateral view of the neck may be particularly helpful in diagnosing injury to the upper esophagus. An increase in the prevertebral space between the posterior pharynx or larynx and the anterior border of the C2-C4 vertebral bodies greater than 4 mm suggests the presence of retropharyngeal inflammation or hematoma. Below C5, the prevertebral space may normally be 1.0 to 1.5 cm wide (11).

With perforations of the thoracic esophagus, plain films of the chest may reveal mediastinal emphysema or widening by fluid or inflammatory reaction. Air-fluid levels in the mid and upper mediastinum may be a result of fluid and air leaking from the esophagus or abscess formation.

AXIOM Pleural effusions with increased amylase levels after chest trauma are a result of esophageal injury until proven otherwise.

Pleural effusions frequently accompany injuries to the thoracic esophagus. With perforations of the upper two-thirds of the thoracic esophagus, a right pleural effusion often occurs; however, with low thoracic esophageal injuries, the left pleural cavity is more likely to be involved. If a nasogastric tube is passed and it enters a pleural cavity, this is diagnostic of an esophageal tear. Occasionally, an upright chest film may show free air under the diaphragm.

Contrast Swallows

As soon as the patient's condition is stable, esophagography should be performed on all patients suspected of pharyngoesophageal injuries. There is some controversy as to whether the initial contrast swallow for a suspected esophageal leak should be done with barium or meglumine diatrizoate (Gastrografin). Gastrografin is used as the initial contrast by many physicians because, if a leak is present, the extravasated Gastrografin is less likely to aggravate the infection; however, Gastrografin is less likely to reveal the leak and, if aspirated, it is more likely to cause a severe pneumonitis.

If the patient is unconscious or has an absent gag reflex, the contrast can be carefully administered through a Foley catheter placed high in the upper esophagus with the balloon inflated to prevent regurgitation of the material. Gastrografin may fail to demonstrate up to 40% to 50% of proven esophageal leaks. The incidence of false-negative examinations with barium is usually less than 25%.

Computed Tomography Scans

Occasionally, a computed tomography scan of the chest may reveal localized collections of air and fluid or even swallowed contrast material that should make one suspect an esophageal injury.

Esophagoscopy

If esophageal injury is suspected and the esophagogram is negative, one should proceed with esophagoscopy. Flexible esophagoscopy is usually safer and easier to perform, but occasionally rigid esophagoscopy may be preferable, particularly if a foreign body is suspected.

Esophageal injury can often be seen readily on esophagoscopy, but smaller lesions, especially in the cervical esophagus, can easily be missed. Esophageal injuries are especially likely to be missed if the esophagus does not expand during endoscopy. Flowers et al. (12) noted a sensitivity of 100% and specificity of 96% when using a flexible scope for the diagnosis of esophageal trauma in 31 patients.

AXIOM When possible, esophagoscopy should be done without ventilatory assistance so that the spontaneous breaths will dilate the esophagus.

Thoracentesis/Chest Tube

If a patient with blunt chest trauma has a hydropneumothorax and the fluid evacuated resembles swallowed saliva or gastric contents (food particles, high amylase, or a pH below 6.0), the diagnosis of esophageal injury is virtually certain. If the patient is asked to swallow methylene blue or some other dye while a chest tube is in place, almost instantaneous appearance of the dye is virtually diagnostic.

Operative Diagnosis

AXIOM The esophagus should be examined carefully for injury at surgery if an adjacent organ was damaged by blunt or penetrating trauma.

With esophageal injuries resulting from penetrating trauma, one must look carefully for associated injuries, which include injury to the trachea (36%–60%), major vessels (18%–45%), and spinal cord (5%–13%) (2–4).

If a suspected esophageal injury cannot be found at the time of surgery, a nasogastric tube or Foley catheter can be passed into the cervical esophagus, and air can be injected by the anesthetist while the esophagus is occluded distally by the surgeon. These maneuvers should distend the esophagus with air, and escape of any bubbles can assist in locating transmural injuries. If there is still a question, one may perform esophagoscopy while the esophagus is exposed.

AXIOM If a laparotomy has been performed because of abdominal pain and tenderness after blunt truncal trauma but the intraabdominal examination is negative, one should suspect a thoracic injury.

Treatment

Treatment of lacerations or rupture of the esophagus should be individualized according to

1. Amount of time between injury and diagnosis;
2. Amount of local inflammation, necrosis, or infection present;
3. Location of the injury (neck, chest, or abdomen); and
4. Preexisting pathology.

Nonoperative Treatment

As a general rule, a nonoperative approach to the management of pharyngoesophageal injuries can be considered if

1. The injury is small.
2. There is no free flow of contrast material into surrounding tissues.
3. There are no other lesions requiring surgical intervention.
4. Antibiotic treatment is started promptly after the injury.
5. There continue to be minimal or no symptoms.
6. There is no evidence of infection.

AXIOM Small iatrogenic injuries of the cervical esophagus or pharynx with a contained leak can often be managed nonoperatively.

Nonoperative treatment of esophageal injuries includes

1. Nothing by mouth;
2. Nasogastric suction (with lesions in the thoracic or abdominal esophagus) to remove any regurgitated gastric acid;
3. Adequate nutrition (preferably via a jejunostomy tube); and
4. Antibiotic therapy.

Early enteral nutrition, preferably into the small intestine just beyond the ligament of Treitz, may help reduce infection and mortality rates. The antibiotics used should cover organisms likely to be present in the mouth, and these are usually quite sensitive to penicillin. In some instances, particularly in more debilitated patients, one may also wish to cover gram-negative aerobes, such as *Escherichia coli,* particularly if the patient is receiving antacid or H2 blocker therapy. One should also be looking for *Candida* species, particularly in older, immunocompromised patients.

AXIOM Antibiotics for treating esophageal perforations should cover mouth organisms well.

Operative Treatment

Incisions

Cervical esophageal injuries are approached most readily through an incision along the anterior border of the sternocleidomastoid muscle. Injuries of the upper and middle third of the thoracic esophagus are best approached via a right posterolateral thoracotomy. The lower third of the thoracic esophagus is usually best approached via a left posterolateral thoracotomy or an anterolateral thoracotomy connected with a midline abdominal incision. If a nasogastric tube has not been inserted previously, it is then placed under the direct control of the surgeon.

Repairs

AXIOM The mucosal tear in an injured esophagus is often longer than the muscle injury.

Once the esophageal wounds are defined, the edges are debrided back to healthy tissue. It is important to clearly visualize the mucosal injury, even if one has to extend the muscle openings at both ends of the perforation.

Esophageal lacerations are usually closed with an inner layer of interrupted inverted sutures of slowly absorbable material and an outer layer of simple Lembert sutures or with horizontal mattress sutures. Some surgeons believe that particular attention should be directed toward incorporating adequate submucosal tissue (which is the strongest layer) in both the inner and outer layer of sutures.

AXIOM When possible, esophageal repairs, especially in the chest, should be buttressed with adjacent viable tissue.

The tissue used to buttress esophageal repairs in the chest can be pleura or intercostal muscle. The lower esophagus may be buttressed with gastric fundus or omentum. Such flaps can be wrapped around the entire esophagus or sutured in place as onlay flaps.

AXIOM With severe injuries in the upper thoracic esophagus, it is safer to reestablish continuity with a gastric bypass and an anastomosis in the neck rather than attempt a complex repair.

For lower thoracic perforations, a gastric fundic patch is extremely effective for buttressing the closure. If the repair narrows the esophagus significantly, a flap of intact gastric fundus can be sutured over the hole as a patch (Fig. 19A-1).

In some instances, although the initial esophageal injury is only a contusion, it may later necrose and leak. Consequently, any contused area should probably be buttressed or covered with a well-vascularized flap of adjacent muscle or pleura.

Drainage

Regardless of the type of procedure used to repair the lower thoracic esophagus, the mediastinum and pleural cavity must be drained well. The mediastinal pleura is incised from the diaphragm up to the thoracic inlet, and two large-bore (32–36 French) chest tubes are inserted to provide ample drainage of the pleural cavity. In addition, a nasal tube can be inserted into the esophagus just proximal to the repair to reduce the amount of swallowed air and oral secretions coming into contact with the repair.

AXIOM The best method for preventing leakage of gastric acid through an esophageal tear is to keep the stomach decompressed with a gastrostomy tube.

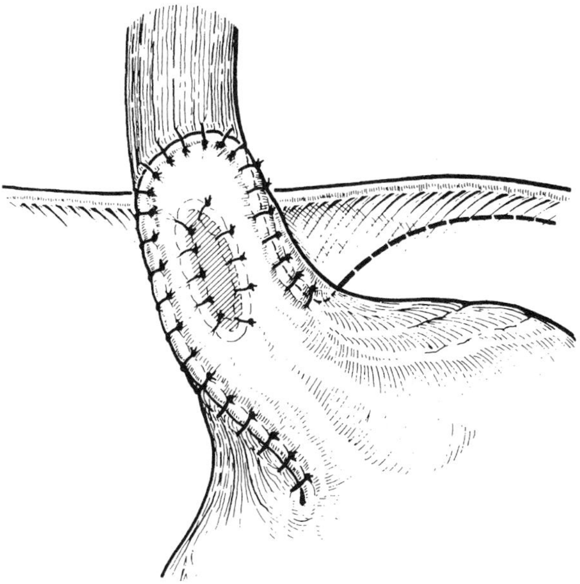

FIG. 19A-1. Gastric fundic patch. For perforations of the lower thoracic esophagus, a gastric fundic patch can be used to close the defect. If closure of the distal esophageal tear or perforation would narrow the esophagus significantly, no attempt should be made to close the lesion primarily. Instead, a flap of intact gastric fundus should be sutured over the hole as a patch. With such flaps, at least half of the esophageal circumference should be covered at least 1 to 2 cm above and below the injury. If the esophageal hole cannot be safely closed directly, one line should be at the edge of the esophageal hole and the other line about 1.0 cm from the hole. Another technique is a complete wrap of the involved lower esophagus with gastric fundus similar to that used for Nissen fundoplication. (From Wilson RF, Steiger Z. Oesophageal injuries. In: Champion HR, Robbs JV, Trunkey DD, eds. *Rob and Smith's operative surgery: trauma, part 1,* 4th ed. London: Butterworths, 1989:334).

The upper esophageal tubes should be left in place for at least 5 to 7 days. At that time, a contrast swallow can be performed around the nasogastric tube. If the repair is intact, oral fluids can be started cautiously. If the repair does not leak and the pleural drainage remains less than 100 mL per day, the chest tubes can be removed.

Enteral Feeding

With injuries to the esophagus, it is prudent to insert a feeding tube into the proximal jejunum about 30 cm distal to the ligament of Treitz whenever possible. Alimentation should be started postoperatively as soon as the patient is hemodynamically stable.

AXIOM Jejunostomy feedings provide the best and safest nutrition for patients with esophageal lacerations.

Treatment after a Delayed Diagnosis

If there has been a delay in diagnosis and if the involved area of the esophagus is necrotic or gross suppuration is present, closure of the esophageal tear should probably not be attempted. After thorough debridement of necrotic or infected tissue, the area is carefully drained to prevent the infection from spreading throughout the neck and down into the mediastinum. Exclusion of the esophagus with a cervical esophagostomy and gastrostomy is also indicated.

AXIOM Whenever possible, severe mediastinitis should be treated by incising the mediastinal pleura over the entire esophagus via a thoracotomy incision and completely debriding and draining the involved tissues.

Esophageal Disruptions

Orringer and Stirling (13) believe that, if esophageal disruption accompanies preexisting esophageal disease or sepsis, esophageal resection often provides the only chance for patient salvage. These authors performed esophagectomy within 12 hours of perforation in ten patients, in 12 to 24 hours in three, and in 3 to 45 days in 11. Gastrointestinal continuity was established with an immediate cervicogastric anastomosis in 11 of 24 patients, and 11 had a cervical or anterior cervical esophagostomy. There were only three hospital deaths (13%), and 19 (90%) of the 21 survivors were eventually able to swallow comfortably. Altorjay et al. (14) also described good results with 27 esophagectomies performed for perforation of the thoracic esophagus. The interval between rupture and esophagectomy was less than 24 hours in only 11 patients (40.7%). Postoperative surgical complications occurred in four patients (14.8%) and nonsurgical complications in seven (25.9%). The hospital mortality rate was 3.7% (1 in 27). In 14 patients, primary reconstruction was performed in the bed of the excised esophagus. There were no anastomotic leaks in this subgroup.

Postoperative Care

Parenteral antibiotics are continued postoperatively for at least 48 hours. The nasogastric tube can be removed as soon as gastrointestinal function returns; however, oral intake is avoided until a contrast esophagogram is obtained 5 to 6 days after surgery. If the repair is intact, clear liquid oral intake can begin. If there is no drainage from the wound after a day or two of oral intake, the drains can be removed.

Complications

Sepsis

The most devastating complication of esophageal perforation is mediastinal infection, and this is usually a result of delayed diagnosis and treatment. Diagnosis of sepsis resulting from an esophageal leak may be difficult, especially in older, malnourished patients who cannot mount a fever or leukocytosis. Computed tomography scans can be helpful for detecting mediastinal abscesses in some patients, but they may be falsely negative in at least 10% to 20% of cases.

AXIOM A “negative” contrast swallow or esophagoscopy does not rule out a mediastinal infection or abscess in a septic patient who has had esophageal surgery or instrumentation.

Suppurative collections above the fourth thoracic vertebra resulting from cervical or high thoracic esophageal injuries can often be drained adequately through a neck incision. Abscesses that are large or located in the lower chest require a thoracotomy to obtain complete drainage of the mediastinum and pleural cavity. Posterior intraabdominal collections can often be drained through the bed of the twelfth rib. In patients in whom severe sepsis develops, esophageal exclusion with a cervical esophagostomy and gastrostomy should be strongly considered.

Although antibiotics are only a second line of defense, they should be given in full dosage for at least 5 to 7 days after esophageal perforation to cover both mouth and gram-negative enteric organisms.

Fistulas

AXIOM Esophageal fistulas in the neck usually heal spontaneously in 2 to 3 weeks; however, fistulas in the chest are much more likely to cause severe sepsis and death.

Treatment of most cervical enterocutaneous fistulas is conservative and is designed to provide adequate drainage of any suppurative collections. One should also look for the factors that tend to keep fistulas open and correct them as soon as possible. These factors include distal obstruction, foreign bodies, malignancy, epithelialization of the tract, and infection. Acute severe malnutrition may also play a role. With thoracic esophagocutaneous fistulas, cervical esophageal exclusion or bypass of the involved esophagus with stomach or colon is frequently necessary.

Tracheoesophageal Fistulas

In most tracheoesophageal fistulas, increased bronchial secretions, pneumonia, or severe coughing develops, particularly when taking liquids. Delayed recognition may occur in individuals with head trauma, particularly if an endotracheal or tracheostomy tube is in place.

Ideally, the diagnosis of tracheoesophageal fistula should be made by esophagoscopy showing tracheobronchial mucosa or an endotracheal or tracheostomy tube. Occasionally, bronchoscopy reveals either the fistula or an indwelling nasogastric tube. If the diagnosis cannot be made in any other manner, small amounts of barium can be given. If cineradiography is available, this may be the best technique for demonstrating the fistula.

When the diagnosis of traumatic tracheoesophageal fistula has been made, an early attempt should be made to exclude, bypass, or close the fistula to prevent continued aspiration pneumonia. If the tracheal and esophageal tissues are not suitable for closure, one can bypass the involved esophagus with stomach or colon brought up substernally to the proximal normal cervical esophagus. The fistula in the esophagus can then be excluded from the bypassed esophagus with staples or sutures. If the involved tissues are not suitable for closure and the patient is too sick for an esophageal bypass, cervical esophageal exclusion and wide drainage of the involved area should be performed. If the tracheal injury can be bypassed with an endotracheal tube, this should also be done.

Strictures

One should suspect an anatomic or functional obstruction of the esophagus if the patient has a great deal of saliva and is drooling excessively. A patient may have no dysphagia until more than 70% to 80% of the normal esophageal lumen is obstructed. Strictures can be confirmed by endoscopy, but contrast swallow is generally preferred because the test is less hazardous and is more apt to show multiple areas of narrowing if they exist.

Short, early strictures can usually be dilated relatively easily to at least 40 to 50 French. Dilatations are safer if performed over a string or flexible wire that has been passed through the stricture into the small bowel or stomach. If a wire or string cannot be passed in the normal direction (prograde), it is often possible to perform a gastrostomy and pass a small semiflexible probe or Jackson dilator up (retrograde) from the stomach into the esophagus and then into the mouth. A string can then be attached to the probe or dilator and pulled out of a gastrostomy. Linked Tucker dilators of gradually increasing size, drawn retrograde through the esophagus via a string through a gastrostomy, are especially useful and safe for esophageal dilatation in children.

Blind dilation without a string or wire to guide the tip of the dilator through the lumen is more likely to result in tears of the esophagus. Mercury-weighted dilators can be used by the patient at home to help maintain the patency of the esophagus once it has been adequately dilated.

If the esophagus of an adult can be dilated to 50 French, swallowing will usually be relatively normal, and repeat dilatations may not be required for at least several weeks. If the esophagus cannot be dilated to at least 40 French in an adult, even after repeated attempts, swallowing will often be impaired and an esophageal resection or bypass should be considered.

Occasionally, a stricture is so severe that it cannot be dilated. In such instances, bypass of the esophagus with stomach or colon (stomach is preferable in adults and colon in children) may be required.

Outcome

The mortality rate of esophageal injuries is still about 5% to 25% for patients receiving definitive treatment within 12 hours, and 25% to 66% or higher for patients receiving treatment after 24 hours (2–4). As a general rule, esophageal injuries in the chest have mortality and morbidity rates more than three times those occurring in the neck.

ESOPHAGEAL FOREIGN BODIES

Etiology

Most foreign bodies are ingested by small children or by adults with psychiatric disease, alcohol abuse, or mental retardation (15). Food impaction in the esophagus typically occurs in patients who are elderly or have a preexisting esophageal stricture, ring, or web. Other predisposing factors include false teeth and poor dentition, resulting in poor chewing of food.

Pathophysiology

About 80% to 90% of ingested foreign bodies pass through the gastrointestinal tract without difficulty, but 10% to 20% lodge in the esophagus at the lower border of the cricopharyngeus muscle, at the level of the aortic arch, or at the LES (15).

Objects that lodge within the esophagus may cause

1. Respiratory compromise resulting from aspiration of secretions or pressure on the trachea;
2. Perforation, causing infection or fistulas; and
3. Pressure necrosis leading to mediastinitis or fistulas.

Although less than 1% of all swallowed objects perforate the gastrointestinal tract, one may see perforation rates as high as 15% to 35% with sharp foreign bodies, such as toothpicks and pins (11,16). Accidentally swallowed sharp foreign bodies may perforate the esophagus at the time they are swallowed or after several hours because of continued local pressure. Foreign bodies may also cause perforation during their removal, particularly if they have sharp hooklike projections.

Diagnosis

Signs and Symptoms

An infant who cannot swallow properly or is salivating excessively should be considered to have an esophageal foreign body until proven otherwise. Most older patients with this problem have additional symptoms, including choking, dysphagia, odynophagia, or sialorrhea (15). The sensation of something sticking in the throat is often also present. With foreign bodies in the esophagus, the sensation of where the object is stuck is usually a few inches above its actual site.

Radiographic Studies

AXIOM On plain x-ray films, coins in the esophagus appear "on face" on a posteroanterior (PA) film and "on edge" in the lateral film (i.e., opposite of a tracheal foreign body).

If the foreign body is radiolucent but holds the esophageal walls apart, air may be seen in that portion of the esophagus. If a swallowed foreign body cannot be located on a lateral neck x-ray film, PA and lateral chest films are obtained. If the foreign body is not seen on those films, an esophagogram may demonstrate it. If a small pledget of cotton saturated with barium sulfate is swallowed, it may hang on a sharp foreign body that might not otherwise be detected.

Esophagoscopy

If the contrast swallow is negative or only a filling defect is seen, esophagoscopy may be diagnostic and therapeutic. It is, however, not unusual for esophagoscopy to miss a foreign body, especially if the lumen is not well distended during the examination.

Treatment

AXIOM Ingestion of a foreign body is an emergency if (1) it causes an acute obstruction, (2) the foreign body is sharp or irregular, or (3) the foreign body is a disk battery (15).

Patients with an esophageal foreign body should be kept in an upright position. Suctioning of oral secretions should be performed as needed, and airway stability should be guaranteed (15). In general, objects that cause complete obstruction or that may cause perforation should be removed as soon as possible.

Esophagoscopic Removal

If the foreign body is seen on endoscopy, it is usually grasped with a forceps appropriate to the object, disengaged from the esophageal wall, and then either removed through a rigid esophagoscope or removed along with the scope as a trailing foreign body.

AXIOM The longer a foreign body remains in the esophagus, the greater the local edema, the greater the difficulty of removal, and the greater the risk of perforation before or during removal.

Catheter Removal

Balloon-tipped catheters (e.g., Foley catheters) have been passed with or without fluoroscopic guidance to help in the removal of some blunt foreign bodies in the proximal esophagus. Typically, a small Foley catheter is inserted past the object, the head and neck are lowered, the balloon is inflated, and the catheter is gently pulled back into the hypopharynx. One should take care to prevent aspiration of the foreign body into the larynx or trachea while it is removed from the esophagus.

Glucagon

If the swallowed object is not sharp and is not causing respiratory symptoms, one can try to have the foreign body pass by itself. Although there have been no controlled studies, glucagon may be helpful because it relaxes smooth muscle and decreases LES tone. A dose of 0.5 mg is injected intravenously and may be repeated once or twice at 10- to 20-minute intervals (15). Aspiration precautions should be used because glucagon may stimulate nausea.

Effervescent Agents

Use of enzymatic digestion of boneless meat with papain is no longer recommended, except when endoscopy is not available, and only if the bolus impaction is of short duration and confirmed by a contrast study. Effervescent agents to distend the esophagus are generally not recommended; however, Karanjia and Rees (17) reported success using cola in six of six food bolus obstructions.

Surgical Removal

If a foreign body cannot be removed in any other manner, surgical removal is required. If the foreign body can be moved at all, it can sometimes be removed endoscopically at surgery without an esophageal incision. If an incision into the esophagus is necessary, it should be in a normal area of the esophagus, proximal to the impacted foreign body.

AXIOM After a foreign body has been removed, radiographic or endoscopic evaluation of the esophagus should be performed to rule out a perforation or underlying esophageal disease.

CHEMICAL INJURIES OF THE ESOPHAGUS

An estimated 26,000 caustic ingestions occur in the United States annually (18). Ingestions in infants and young children are usually accidental and make up approximately 80% of the reported incidents. In teenagers and adults, the majority of caustic ingestions are suicide attempts.

Pathophysiology

The worst caustic injuries are those caused by strong alkali. The damage is due to liquefaction necrosis with dissolution of protein and collagen and rapid penetration of successive tissue layers occurring within seconds of contact. Ingestants with a pH greater than 12 are responsible for the most serious injuries, whereas household bleaches with a pH less than 11 rarely cause serious problems (19). With second- or third-degree burns extending into the muscularis or transmural, there is increased scar tissue and dysmotility by the second to third week (19,20). Strictures form in approximately 20% to 30% of cases of third-degree injuries and are usually evident within 3 to 4 weeks of the ingestion.

Acid causes only about 5% of reported caustic ingestions, and those requiring treatment are usually caused by hydrochloric or sulfuric acid (21). Acids cause damage by coagulation of protein, which retards its continued penetration into the tissues. The most severe damage from acid ingestion tends to occur in the stomach (because of limited contact with the esophagus), predominately along the lesser curvature and in the antrum. Serious esophageal involvement is reported in only 10% to 20% of acid ingestions.

Disk or button batteries used in watches or cameras can cause severe corrosive injury to the gastrointestinal tract when ingested (22). Batteries more than 21 mm in diameter tend to lodge within the esophagus and leak sodium or potassium hydroxide and mercuric oxide.

Pill-induced esophageal injury occurs when the caustic contents of a capsule or tablet remain in the esophagus long enough to produce mucosal damage (23). The agents implicated most frequently are quinidine, doxycycline, tetracycline, emepronium bromide, pirmecillinam, potassium chloride, and aspirin.

Diagnosis

AXIOM Ingested caustic material or a foreign body should be assumed in anyone in whom difficult or painful swallowing suddenly develops, until proven otherwise.

Signs and Symptoms

With accidental caustic ingestions, a history of dysphagia after drinking an unexpectedly bitter or strange-tasting fluid may be the first indication that caustic material might have been ingested. Perioral pain may be the predominant symptom, but dysphagia, odynophagia, chest pain, and sialorrhea suggest substantial esophageal damage. Epigastric pain suggests damage to the stomach or gastroesophageal junction. One should also be alert for delayed chest pain or dyspnea, which may be due to a perforation and may not develop for up to 48 hours.

With an alkali injury of the esophagus, 50% to 90% of patients have a pharyngeal burn, and about 25% to 50% of patients with oral or pharyngeal burns have an esophageal injury (15). Even if there are no obvious burns of the mouth or pharynx, it cannot be assumed that the esophagus is uninjured.

Radiographic Studies

Radiographs of the neck, chest, and abdomen should be obtained after a suspected caustic ingestion to rule out perforation. If there is any suspicion of a perforation, a contrast swallow can also be obtained.

Endoscopy

After appropriate resuscitation, endoscopy should also be performed to guide further therapy and determine prognosis.

AXIOM Because the esophagus is friable and easy to perforate, the scope is not passed beyond the first deep circumferential burn, which indicates a need for full antistricture management.

Treatment

General

If there are extensive burns, much fluid may be lost into the involved tissues. Intravenous catheters should be inserted and the patient given crystalloid to promptly restore adequate hydration and perfusion. Nothing should be administered by mouth until the evaluation is complete.

AXIOM In cases of lye ingestion, the use of emetic agents, charcoal, and nasogastric lavage is contraindicated.

In stable patients who have ingested a small amount of mild alkali (bleaches), one may cautiously give milk, dilute vinegar, or citrus juice (15). In pure acid ingestion, early aspiration of the stomach with a tube, followed by cold fluid lavage, may be of use. Antacids are contraindicated because the heat of neutralization they can produce may cause more damage.

Corticosteroids

The use of corticosteroids for caustic ingestions is controversial. For many years after 1950, when Spain et al. (24) documented that corticosteroids can suppress inflammation, glucocorticoids and antibiotics were used extensively to reduce the risk and severity of stricture formation after caustic ingestions. In 1980, however, Hawkins et al. (25) published a prospective clinical trial that showed no significant advantage to corticosteroids. They also believed that the risks of the corticosteroids outweighed their potential benefits and were probably contraindicated in these injuries. Estrera et al. (20) and Anderson et al. (26) also concluded that there was no benefit from use of steroids.

Although the current tendency seems to be to avoid corticosteroids, an extensive review by Howell et al. (27) of more than 2,000 cases published between 1956 and 1991 suggested that corticosteroids are helpful for second- and third-degree esophageal burns. The steroid treatment group included 283 patients from nine retrospective and two prospective publications. The no-treatment group included 78 patients from three retrospective and three prospective studies. Of the patients with second- and third-degree esophageal burns, the incidence of stricture was 24% (54 of 228) in the corticosteroid treatment group and 52% (13 of 25) in the no-corticosteroid group (27). This difference was significant ($p<.01$). In addition, the steroid-treated patients tended to have a lower mortality rate.

Follow-up

In patients with second- and third-degree burns, barium swallows to assess for stricture formation should be performed at 2, 4, 8, and 12 weeks, even if the patient is swallowing solid food easily (15). Contrast studies are performed sooner if any symptoms develop that suggest the presence of a stricture.

If a stricture appears to be developing clinically or radiologically, the patient should have a string passed as soon as possible for later dilatations. Many physicians believe that the dilatations should be delayed for at least 2 to 3 weeks after the caustic ingestion to reduce the chances of perforating the esophagus, which is still friable. Others have advocated the use of early, frequent dilation of the esophagus beginning 1 week after ingestion to retard stricture formation (25). Nevertheless, patients with severe cicatricial injury should receive early nutrition, either parenterally or preferably via a jejunostomy tube.

If the esophagus cannot be dilated properly, it may be better to excise it early. With severe involvement in children, there is an estimated 1,000-fold increase in the incidence of squamous cell carcinoma in the affected areas of the esophagus (28). Consequently, the development of dysphagia decades after the injury should be anticipated and investigated carefully for a possible malignancy.

⊘ FREQUENT ERRORS

1. ***Delays greater than 6 to 12 hours in repairing esophageal injuries.***
2. ***Failure to understand that an esophageal injury may be present despite normal chest x-ray findings, contrast swallows, and esophagoscopy.***
3. ***Failure to search aggressively for an esophageal rupture or leak if the patient has increased chest pain or fever or a chest radiographic abnormality after an esophagoscopic examination or procedure.***
4. ***Failure to appreciate the severity of the sepsis that can result from minor esophageal leaks into the mediastinum.***
5. ***Failure to adequately examine the patient for an esophageal injury intraoperatively if there is an associated vascular or tracheobronchial injury.***
6. ***Failure to appreciate that fluid leaking via a drain placed near an esophageal repair is indicative of an esophageal leak until proven otherwise.***
7. ***Placing an esophageal anastomosis in the upper chest when it might have been possible to put it in the neck.***
8. ***Failing to buttress an esophageal repair with a flap of viable adjacent tissue.***
9. ***Assuming that insertion of a chest tube without a thoracotomy can completely drain an infected mediastinum.***
10. ***Failure to provide early jejunal enteral feedings and adequate gastric emptying (preferably with a sump-type gastrostomy tube) in patients with a thoracic esophageal leak.***

*11. **Delay in defunctionalizing the esophagus of patients who become septic because of a leaking esophagus.***
*12. **Pulling foreign bodies out of the upper esophagus despite there being a great deal of resistance.***
*13. **Inadequate resuscitation of patients with caustic injuries of the esophagus.***
*14. **Passing an esophagoscope beyond the most proximal site of severe circumferential caustic esophageal injury.***

SUMMARY POINTS

1. Lack of a serosal covering for the esophagus increases the likelihood of anastomotic leaks.
2. Most injuries to the esophagus are iatrogenic and tend to occur at natural or acquired areas of narrowing.
3. If a penetrating wound involves the tracheobronchial tree, one should look carefully for injury to the adjacent esophagus.
4. Tears of the thoracic esophagus can rapidly cause severe mediastinal inflammation and damage from regurgitated gastric secretions or swallowed oral bacteria.
5. An esophageal injury should be suspected in all patients who have a penetrating wound in the thoracic inlet or mediastinum and have a pleural effusion or pneumomediastinum.
6. Any new cervical, thoracic, or abdominal symptoms, signs, or x-ray changes after esophageal instrumentation, especially dilatation of an esophageal stricture, are a result of an esophageal leak until proven otherwise.
7. Abdominal pain and tenderness may be the first sign and symptom of perforation of the lower thoracic esophagus.
8. Increased prevertebral space in the neck may result from a pharyngoesophageal leak.
9. Pleural effusions with increased amylase levels after trauma are a result of esophageal or pancreatic injury until proven otherwise.
10. Gastrografin swallows can miss many esophageal leaks, and, if Gastrografin is aspirated into the lungs, it can cause severe pneumonitis.
11. When possible, esophagoscopy should be done without ventilatory assistance so that the patient's spontaneous breaths will help dilate the esophagus.
12. The esophagus should be examined carefully for injury at surgery if an adjacent organ was damaged by blunt or penetrating trauma.
13. If the patient has a tracheobronchial or vascular injury associated with an esophageal tear, the repairs should be separated by a substantial buttress of viable tissue, preferably muscle.
14. The longer it takes to diagnose and treat an esophageal injury, the greater the tendency toward development of severe sepsis, especially if the mediastinum is involved.
15. If an esophageal injury is more than 24 hours old but there is no evidence of tissue necrosis or infection, one can still attempt to close it, but the repair should be well buttressed with viable adjacent tissue.
16. Small iatrogenic injuries of the cervical esophagus or pharynx with a contained leak can often be managed nonoperatively.
17. Antibiotics for treating esophageal perforations should cover mouth aerobes and anaerobes.
18. The submucosal layer is the strongest layer of the esophagus.
19. Esophageal repairs should be drained by closed catheter systems placed near, but not on, the area of repair.
20. The upper two-thirds of the thoracic esophagus is best approached through a right posterolateral incision; the lowest third is best explored via a left posterolateral incision.
21. The mucosal tear in an injured esophagus is often longer than the muscle injury.

22. With severe injuries in the upper thoracic esophagus, it is safer to reestablish continuity with a gastric bypass and an anastomosis in the neck rather than attempt a complex intrathoracic repair.
23. An esophageal leak in the neck tends to be relatively harmless, whereas esophageal leaks in the chest can rapidly cause severe sepsis.
24. The best method for preventing leakage of gastric acid through an esophageal tear is to keep the stomach decompressed with a sump-type gastrostomy tube.
25. Jejunostomy feedings provide the best and safest nutrition for patients with esophageal lacerations.
26. Severe sepsis resulting from a thoracic esophageal leak is best treated by completely defunctionalizing the esophagus and opening and draining the mediastinum thoroughly.
27. On plain x-ray films, coins in the esophagus appear "on face" on a PA film and "on edge" in the lateral film (i.e., opposite to a tracheal foreign body).
28. Ingestion of a foreign body is an emergency if (1) it causes an acute obstruction, (2) the foreign body is sharp or irregular, or (3) the foreign body is a disk battery.
29. The longer a foreign body remains in the esophagus, the greater the local edema, the greater the difficulty of removal, and the greater the risk of perforation before or during removal.
30. After a foreign body has been removed, radiographic or endoscopic evaluation of the esophagus should be performed to rule out a perforation or underlying esophageal disease.
31. Alkali tends to cause much deeper and more severe esophageal injuries than acid does.
32. Anyone in whom difficult or painful swallowing suddenly develops should be considered to have ingested caustic material or a foreign body until proven otherwise.
33. Although severe symptoms after a possible caustic ingestion indicate an increased likelihood of severe esophageal damage, absence of symptoms cannot be relied upon to rule out significant injury.
34. In cases of lye ingestion, the use of emetic agents, charcoal, and nasogastric lavage is contraindicated.
35. If corticosteroids are used to prevent esophageal strictures after caustic ingestions, care should be taken to prevent the severe complications that they can cause.
36. A "negative" contrast swallow or esophagoscopy does not rule out a mediastinal infection or abscess in a septic patient who has had esophageal surgery or instrumentation.
37. Esophageal fistulas in the neck often heal spontaneously in 2 to 3 weeks; however, fistulas in the chest are much more apt to persist or cause severe sepsis.
38. A "little" dysphagia is often a result of rather severe (greater than 70% to 80%) stenosis.
39. Dilatation of the esophagus is best done over a wire or string to make sure that the dilator does not press excessively against one of the side walls.

REFERENCES

1. Wilson RF, Steiger Z. Esophageal injuries. In: Wilson RF, Walt AJ, eds. *Management of trauma: pitfalls and practice.* Philadelphia: Williams & Wilkins, 1996:388.
2. Wilson RF, Steiger Z. Oesophageal injuries. In: Champion HR, Robbs JV, Trunkey DD, eds. *Trauma surgery,* 4th ed. London: Butterworths, 1989:327–340.
3. Symbas PN. Esophageal injuries. In: *Cardiothoracic trauma.* Philadelphia: WB Saunders, 1989:285–302.
4. Mulder DS, Barkun JS. Injury to the trachea bronchus and esophagus. In: Mattox KL, Moore EE, Feliciano DV, eds. *Trauma II.* Norwalk, CT: Appleton & Lange, 1991:343.
5. Washington B, Wilson RF, Steiger Z, Bassett JS. Emergency thoracotomy: a four-year review. *Ann Thorac Surg* 1985;40:188.
6. Wilson RF, Antonenko D, Gibson DB. Shock and acute respiratory failure after chest trauma. *J Trauma* 1977;17:697.
7. Beal SL, Pottmeyer EW, Spisso JM. Esophageal perforation following external blunt trauma. *J Trauma* 1988;28:1425.

8. Niezgod JA, McMenamin P, Graeber GM. Pharyngoesophageal perforation after blunt neck trauma. *Ann Thorac Surg* 1990;50:615.
9. Chen JY, Chen WJ, Huang TJ, et al. Spinal epidural abscess complicating cervical spine fracture with hypopharyngeal perforation: a case report. *Spine* 1992;17:971.
10. Nevens F, Janssens J, Piessens J, et al. Prospective study on prevalence of esophageal chest pain in patients referred on an elective basis to a cardiac unit for suspected myocardial ischemia. *Dig Dis Sci* 1991;36:229.
11. Sethi DS, Chew CT. Retropharyngeal abscess: the foreign body connection. *Ann Acad Med* 1991;20:581.
12. Flowers JL, Graham SM, Ugarte MA, et al. Flexible endoscopy for the diagnosis of esophageal trauma. *J Trauma* 1996;40:261.
13. Orringer MB, Stirling MC. Esophagectomy for esophageal disruption. *Ann Thorac Surg* 1990;49:35.
14. Altorjay A, Kiss J, Voros A, et al. The role of esophagectomy in the management of esophageal perforations. *Ann Thorac Surg* 1998;65:1433.
15. Shwartz HM, Traube M. Esophageal emergencies. In: Carlson RW, Geheb MA, eds. *Principles and practice of medical intensive care.* Philadelphia: WB Saunders, 1993:1432.
16. Johnson JA, Landreneau RJ. Esophageal obstruction and mediastinitis: a hard pill to swallow for drug smugglers. *Am Surg* 1991;57:723.
17. Karanjia ND, Rees M. The use of Coca-Cola in the management of bolus obstruction in benign esophageal stricture. *Ann R Coll Surg Engl* 1993;75:94.
18. Lovejoy FH. Corrosive injury of the esophagus in children: failure of corticosteroid treatment emphasizes prevention. *N Engl J Med* 1990;323:668.
19. Howell JM. Alkaline ingestions. *Ann Emerg Med* 1986;15:820.
20. Estrera A, Taylor W, Mills LJ, et al. Corrosive burns of the esophagus and stomach: a recommendation for an aggressive surgical approach. *Ann Thorac Surg* 1986;41:276.
21. Zagar SA, Kochhar R, Nagi B, et al. Ingestion of corrosive acids: spectrum of injury to upper gastrointestinal tract and natural history. *Gastroenterology* 1989;97:702.
22. Litovitz TL. Button battery ingestions: a review of 56 cases. *JAMA* 1983;249:2495.
23. Kikendall JW. Pill-induced esophageal injury. *Gastroenterol Clin North Am* 1991;20:835.
24. Spain DM, Molomut N, Haber A. The effect of cortisone on the formation of granulation tissue in mice. *Am J Pathol* 1950;26:710.
25. Hawkins DB, Demeter JM, Barnett TE. Caustic ingestion: controversies in management. A review of 214 cases. *Laryngoscope* 1980;90:98.
26. Anderson KD, Rouse TM, Randolph JG. A controlled trial of corticosteroids in children with corrosive injury of the esophagus. *N Engl J Med* 1990;323:637.
27. Howell JM, Dalsey WC, Hartsell FW, et al. Steroids for the treatment of corrosive esophageal injury: a statistical analysis of past studies. *Am J Emerg Med* 1992;10:421.
28. Appleqvist P. Lye corrosion carcinoma of the esophagus: a review of 63 cases. *Cancer* 1980;45:2655.

19B. THORACIC DUCT INJURIES[1]

ANATOMY

Although there is great anatomic variability in the course of the thoracic duct, it generally starts at the cisterna chyli in the abdominal cavity just anterior to the first or second lumbar vertebra. The thoracic duct continues superiorly, anterior to the vertebral column and the right intercostal vessels, between the azygous vein on the right and the descending aorta on the left. It is posterior to the esophagus until it reaches the level of the fourth to seventh thoracic vertebra. It then curves slightly to the left and occupies a position to the left of the esophagus and just anterior to the vertebral column. The thoracic duct continues into the neck along the left margin of the esophagus up to the level of the transverse process of the seventh cervical vertebra. At this point, it turns laterally behind the carotid sheath and in front of the left vertebral artery. As the duct approaches the medial border of the scalenus anticus muscle, it turns inferiorly in front of the phrenic nerve and the first part of the subclavian artery. It then enters the venous system at the point where the left internal jugular and left subclavian veins meet to form the left innominate vein; however, it may also enter any one of these three veins near that point.

PHYSIOLOGY

Chyle is alkaline and has a specific gravity greater than 1.012 (2). After a meal, chyle usually separates into three layers upon standing: a creamy uppermost layer containing chylomicrons, a milky intermediate layer, and a dependent layer containing cellular elements, mostly small lymphocytes. During fasting, chyle may appear to be only slightly turbid because of its reduced lipid content. Because of its high fatty acid content, chyle is bacteriostatic; however, chyle is nonirritating to the pleura, and it usually does not induce the formation of a pleural peel or fibroelastic membrane if it leaks into the pleural space.

Chyle has a variable protein content (2.2–6.0 g/dL) and a variable fat content (0.4–6.0 g/dL) that includes fat-soluble vitamins (2). Its electrolyte composition is similar to that of serum. Of the cellular elements, lymphocytes of the T-cell type predominate. A few erythrocytes (50–60/mm^3) are also usually present.

Between 1,500 and 2,500 mL of chyle empty into the venous system daily (2). Both the volume and the flow rate of chyle vary considerably, depending on the amount of food and its fat content. The ingestion of fat can increase the flow of lymph in the thoracic duct to two to ten times the resting level of 10 to 15 mL per hour for up to several hours.

AXIOM Prolonged external loss of chyle can result in severe malnutrition, water and electrolyte loss, and lymphopenia with T-cell suppression.

CHYLOTHORAX

Causes

Teba et al. (3), in a special review, indicated that trauma, of either accidental or iatrogenic origin, is the most frequent cause of chylothorax. More chylothoraces result from surgical (iatrogenic) trauma than accidental (nonsurgical) trauma.

AXIOM A chylothorax should be suspected if a delayed pleural effusion develops after severe blunt chest or back trauma, especially if the patient has no rib or spine fractures.

Diagnosis

The symptoms, physical findings, and roentgenologic features of chylothorax are usually those seen with any pleural effusion (2). Occasionally, after trauma, a chylothorax may form at rates exceeding 200 mL per hour, and this can produce respiratory distress within hours.

Latent Period

In traumatic chylothorax, there is usually a latent period of 2 to 10 days between the time of the trauma and the onset of the chylothorax (2). This latent period occurs because the chyle from the ruptured thoracic duct is initially confined to the mediastinum where it forms a chyloma. Eventually, the chyloma ruptures through the mediastinal pleura to produce the chylothorax.

AXIOM Chylothoraces are often delayed in their appearance; therefore, the causal relationship with trauma may be forgotten by the patient.

Diagnostic Tests

In a fasting patient, chyle resembles extracellular fluid with a slightly higher protein content. If almost all of the white blood cells are lymphocytes, one should suspect a chylothorax.

Metabolic and Chemical Changes

The metabolic effects of chylothorax are proportional to the duration and volume of the lymph drainage. The cumulative loss of proteins, fats, electrolytes, bicarbonate, fat-soluble vitamins, and lymphocytes can be substantial and can lead to malnutrition, compromised immunologic status, and metabolic acidosis (4).

If the triglyceride value of the pleural effusion is greater than 110 mg/dL, the patient probably has a chylous effusion, although at times a pseudochylothorax has a triglyceride level exceeding this value. Conversely, an effusion with a high cholesterol level and a triglyceride value below 50 mg/dL has a low probability of being chylous (5).

Radiologic Studies

A detailed magnetic resonance imaging (MRI) examination may diagnose chyle before the effusion is aspirated (6). Because chyle is nonirritating, the pleura adjacent to a chylothorax should be relatively normal. Also, because the chemical composition of chyle can change from that of a thin proteinaceous liquid to that of a lipid emulsion after eating (6), one would also expect the MRI characteristics to change from those of a proteinaceous liquid to those of a lipid after eating.

AXIOM A lymphangiogram to demonstrate the exact site of the leak or obstruction should be considered for every chylothorax that does not respond to nonoperative management and seems appropriate for surgical management (3).

Differential Diagnosis

The differential diagnosis of a chronic milky-white pleural effusion includes a chronic chylothorax, a pseudochylothorax, and empyema (2). Pseudochylothorax (referred to as chyliform pleural effusion) refers to long-standing pleural effusions that have a high concentration of cholesterol or lecithin—-globulin complexes. The milky appearance of an empyema is due to the presence of white blood cells in suspension; with centrifugation, the supernatant usually clears. In both chylothorax and pseudochylothorax, the pleural fluid appears milky or turbid. This characteristic persists after centrifugation and is the result of the high lipid content of the pleural fluid; however, addition of 2 mL of ethyl ether clears the turbidity in chylothorax but not in pseudochylothorax (2).

Treatment

The first principle in the management of a patient with chylothorax is to maintain adequate nutrition and to minimize chyle formation (3). This is necessary to prevent severe nutritional and immunologic derangements from developing because of the removal of large amounts of protein, fat, fat-soluble vitamins, electrolytes, and lymphocytes with repeated thoracenteses or chest tube drainage.

Nonsurgical Treatment

An initial trial of conservative treatment is advocated for traumatic chylothorax because the defect in the thoracic duct frequently closes spontaneously (2,6,7).

Conservative treatment includes complete decompression of the pleural space with tube thoracostomy. The placement of a chest tube also allows apposition of the parietal and visceral pleura and may result in pleurodesis.

If the enteral fat content is reduced to 1.0 g/L, the chest tube drainage may decrease to less than 50 mL/day (3). Because water ingestion may stimulate chyle formation, one may also have to switch to total parenteral nutrition to stop the leak of chyle (8). If the chyle leak can be greatly reduced and the pleural cavity is effectively drained by a chest tube, the leak will stop within 2 to 3 weeks in at least 50% of patients (2).

Lindhorst et al. (8) have recently described the possible role of positive end-expiratory pressure ventilation in the treatment of chylothorax caused by blunt chest trauma. Their treatment of a bilateral chylothorax consisted of high positive end-expiratory pressure ventilation (PEEP), bilateral chest tube thoracostomies, and total parenteral nutrition. The chylothoraces resolved within 4 days of treatment.

Surgical Treatment

Patients with continued high outputs of chyle should be considered for early surgical intervention. Selle and colleagues (9) have suggested the following criteria for surgical therapy:

1. Average daily loss of chyle exceeding 1,500 mL/day in an adult (or 100 mL per year of age in a child) for 5 or more days *or*
2. Persistent drainage of chyle for 14 or more days *or*
3. Development of severe nutritional complications.

AXIOM Large-volume chylous fistulas that do not close after 2 weeks of nonoperative therapy should be closed surgically.

Techniques

If conservative medical therapy has failed, a variety of surgical procedures have been attempted, including pleurodesis with talc, fibrin glue (10), and tetracycline. Successful ligation of a thoracic duct with a thoracoscope has been described by Kent and Pinson (11).

Overall, thoracic duct ligation via a thoracotomy has been the most successful method for treating persistent chylothorax. The surgical exploration is usually performed on the side of the chylothorax. With a bilateral chylothorax, the right side should be explored first (2,7).

At thoracotomy, one attempts to identify the thoracic duct just superior to the diaphragm between the aorta and azygous vein or to locate the site of chyle leakage (2). There are several aids in finding the site of leakage, but probably the best method is to inject 1% Evans blue at a dose of 0.7 to 0.8 mg per kg body weight into the subcutaneous tissue of the leg. Within 5 minutes, the chyle is stained dark blue. One can also give 1 to 2 ounces of cream orally or via a nasogastric tube 30 to 45 minutes before surgery (3). If the leak is identified, the duct is ligated on both sides of the leak. Even with dye injections or enteral fat, however, in most instances, the leak cannot be localized, and one is forced to place mass ligatures incorporating the tissue between the aorta, esophagus, and vertebral bodies.

AXIOM If the origin of a chylous leak in the chest cannot be identified at surgery, the tissue between the aorta, esophagus, and vertebra just above the diaphragm should be ligated in two or three areas 1 to 2 cm apart.

⊘ FREQUENT ERRORS

1. ***Failure to make strong efforts to look for and ligate injured lymphatic ducts during surgical explorations for trauma anywhere near the expected path of the thoracic duct.***
2. ***Failure to adequately monitor and prevent the malnutrition, fluid and electrolyte losses and the lymphopenia that can occur in patients with chylous fistulas.***
3. ***Failure to suspect a thoracic duct injury in a patient in whom a pleural effusion or mediastinal fluid collection develops after neck or chest trauma.***
4. ***Assuming that a nonwhite pleural effusion, even in a patient who is not eating, is not a chylothorax.***
5. ***Assuming that a white pleural effusion after chest or neck surgery or trauma is always a chylothorax.***
6. ***Failure to allow chylous fistulas to close spontaneously by putting the bowel at rest for up to 2 weeks.***

SUMMARY POINTS

1. Because chyle is nonirritating to the pleura and is bacteriostatic, there is generally minimal inflammation and no fibrin peel around a chylothorax.

2. Prolonged external loss of chyle can result in severe malnutrition, water and electrolyte loss, lymphopenia, and T-cell suppression.

3. A chylothorax should be suspected if the patient has a pleural effusion after severe blunt chest or back trauma, particularly if there are no rib or spine fractures.

4. Chylothoraces are often delayed; therefore, the causal relationship with trauma may be forgotten by the patient.

5. During surgery, any injured tissue in the presumed path of the thoracic duct should be securely ligated.

6. Lipoprotein electrophoresis of chyle typically demonstrates triglyceride levels higher than plasma and cholesterol levels lower then plasma.

7. A computed tomography scan of the thorax demonstrating pleural thickening tends to rule out a chylothorax.

8. A lymphangiogram should be considered for every chylothorax that does not respond to nonoperative management and is being considered for surgical management.

9. Most chylous fistulas close spontaneously if the bowel is put at rest.

10. Large-volume chylous fistulas that do not close after 2 weeks of nonoperative therapy should be closed surgically.

11. If the origin of a chylous leak cannot be identified at surgery, the tissue between the aorta, esophagus, and vertebral bodies just above the diaphragm should be ligated.

REFERENCES

1. Wilson, RF. Thoracic duct injuries. In: Wilson RF, Walt, AJ, eds. *Management of trauma: pitfalls and practice,* 2nd ed. Philadelphia: William & Wilkins, 1996:406.
2. Sassoon CS, Light RW. Chylothorax and pseudochylothorax. *Clin Chest Med* 1985;6:163.
3. Teba L, Dedhia HV, Bowel R, Alexander JC. Chylothorax review. *Crit Care Med* 1985;13:49.
4. Siegler RL, Pearce MB. Metabolic acidosis from the loss of thoracic lymph. *J Pediatr* 1978;93:465.
5. Staats BA, Ellefson RD, Budahn LL, et al. The lipoprotein profile of chylous and nonchylous pleural effusions. *Mayo Clin Proc* 1980;55:700.

6. Hom M, Jolles H. Traumatic mediastinal lymphocele mimicking other thoracic injuries: case report. *J Thorac Imaging* 1992;7:78.
7. Dulchavsky SA, Ledgerwood AM, Lucas CE. Management of chylothorax after blunt chest trauma. *J Trauma* 1988;28:1400.
8. Lindhorst E, Miller HAB, Taylor GA, et al. On the possible role of positive end-expiratory pressure ventilation in the treatment of chylothorax caused by blunt chest trauma. *J Trauma* 1998;44:540.
9. Selle JG, Snyder WH, Schrider JT. Chylothorax: indications for surgery. *Ann Surg* 1973;177:244.
10. Akaogi E, Mitsui K, Shoara Y, et al. Treatment of postoperative chylothorax with intrapleural fibrin glue. *Ann Thorac Surg* 1989;48:116.
11. Kent RB, Pinson TW. Thoracoscopic ligation of the thoracic duct. *Surg Endosc* 1993;7:52.

20. GENERAL CONSIDERATIONS IN ABDOMINAL TRAUMA[1]

INITIAL MANAGEMENT

Abdominal injuries account for 13% to 15% of trauma deaths, primarily caused by hemorrhage, but in deaths occurring more than 48 hours after injury, sepsis or its complications are the most frequent cause.

AXIOM The initial resuscitation of patients with severe trauma must promptly ensure an adequate airway and the maintenance of a minute ventilation that is usually at least 1.5 to 2.0 times normal.

Fluid Resuscitation

After adequate ventilation has been ensured, two or more large-gauge intravenous catheters should be inserted, ideally in the upper extremities. Blood is simultaneously drawn for type and cross-matching, hematocrit and hemoglobin measurements, and any other tests suggested by preexisting medical problems.

AXIOM Patients who are bleeding rapidly should have their hemorrhage controlled promptly before aggressive resuscitation with fluids is undertaken.

If the patient is in severe shock on admission and this appears to be related to controllable bleeding, the patient should be rushed to the operating room. If the patient was in relatively mild shock and responds rapidly to the initial resuscitation fluids, one can then perform appropriate diagnostic tests; however, if the patient becomes hypotensive again, indicating that bleeding has recurred, and if the likely source is the abdomen, then the patient should be rushed to the operating room.

AXIOM The failure of 2,000 to 3,000 mL of Ringer's lactate given over 10 to 15 minutes to restore adequate blood pressure and tissue perfusion strongly suggests that the patient is bleeding rapidly and requires urgent control of the bleeding sites.

Gastric Decompression

Early gastric decompression, usually with a nasogastric tube, is particularly important when there is a possibility of intraabdominal visceral damage or when the patient may have eaten or drunk recently. The nasogastric tube also may be a valuable diagnostic tool for revealing injury to the upper gastrointestinal tract.

AXIOM All trauma patients should be assumed to have full stomachs, even if they deny recent ingestion of food or liquids.

Injured patients, particularly anxious adults and crying children, tend to swallow air, especially if they have any respiratory distress. Patients resuscitated with a face mask can also have large amounts of air forced into their stomachs. The resulting distension of the stomach not only increases the chances of vomiting and aspiration, but also raises the diaphragm, increasing the resistance to ventilation.

Fractures involving the midface may involve the cribriform plate. In such circumstances, insertion of a nasal tube can increase the risk of meningeal infection, and there is also a chance that the tube will enter the cranial cavity instead of proceeding down into the pharynx. Consequently, in such patients, tubes to decompress the stomach should be inserted through the mouth.

Urinalysis

A urinalysis should be performed on any patient with suspected abdominal or pelvic damage as a guide both to possible injury of the urinary tract and to the detection of diabetes mellitus or concomitant renal parenchymal disease. If the urine on the dipstick is positive for hemoglobin but has few or no red blood cells (RBCs), one should suspect myoglobinuria. A spontaneously voided specimen is preferable to one obtained with a catheter because the trauma of catheter insertion may in itself cause hematuria.

AXIOM Before inserting a Foley catheter in patients with severe blunt trauma, one should do a rectal examination to check the position of the prostate, look for any rectal blood, and check sphincter tone.

If there is any suspicion of damage to the urethra as a result of (1) blood at the urethral meatus, (2) penile or perineal hematomas, (3) a displaced prostate, or (4) a severe anterior pelvic fracture, a retrograde urethrogram should be performed before a Foley catheter is inserted.

The urinary output monitored via a Foley catheter can be valuable as a guide to the adequacy of vital organ perfusion. A sustained urinary output of 0.5 to 1.0 mL/kg/h in an adult who is not receiving a diuretic and who does not have glycosuria or excess ethanol in the blood is usually reasonable evidence of an adequate tissue perfusion.

Antibiotics

If there is any suspicion of intraabdominal contamination, intravenous antibiotics should be started preoperatively so that adequate blood and tissue levels may be achieved during the operation. If the patient has much blood loss, the antibiotics should be given again as soon as the major hemorrhage has been controlled or if the surgery lasts more than 3 to 4 hours. If no peritoneal soilage is found at celiotomy, no further antibiotics are required for the abdomen. If much peritoneal contamination with distal small bowel or colon contents is found, the antibiotics can be continued for another 24 to 48 hours or longer.

AXIOM Intravenous prophylactic antibiotics that cover enteric gram-negative aerobes and anaerobes are given as soon as possible if intraabdominal contamination is suspected.

A number of different prophylactic antibiotic regimens have been recommended for penetrating abdominal trauma. Most regimens attempt to cover the *Enterobacteriaceae* (gram-negative aerobic enteric bacteria) and *Bacteroides* species (gram-negative anaerobes). A combination of gentamicin and metronidazole should provide adequate coverage for most contamination caused by bowel injuries. If one wishes to use a single antibiotic, cefotetan, Timentin, Unasyn, or Zosyn can be given.

Patients with an uncertain tetanus immunization history and tetanus-prone wounds should also receive tetanus-toxoid and tetanus-immune globulin at different sites.

DIAGNOSIS

In general, the three most common sources of exsanguinating hemorrhage are the abdominal cavity (including the pelvis), the chest, and major vessels in the extremities (3). If a patient is in shock after trauma and if the chest is clear to auscultation or on chest radiograph and there are no major wounds, hematomas, bleeding, or deformities in the extremities, then the abdomen is the most likely source of hemorrhage, and it should be promptly explored.

History

A careful history, when available, may provide valuable clues to the diagnosis of the patient's injuries. Changes in symptoms with time or with posture can be extremely important. A past history, particularly in older individuals, should also be obtained from either the patient or the patient's family. Using the mnemonic "AMPLE" suggested in the Advanced Trauma Life Support courses of the American College of Surgeons, one can inquire about

- *A*llergies
- *M*edications
- *P*ast illnesses
- *L*ast meal
- *E*vents preceding the injury

Any history of diabetes mellitus, coronary artery disease, hypertension, or previous abdominal surgery is also particularly important in patients who may need emergency surgery.

Physical Examination

In many cases of abdominal trauma, the physical examination is the most informative portion of the diagnostic evaluation and should be as complete as the time available and the condition of the patient permit. A systematic approach is highly desirable, leaving the obviously injured areas until last. The more frequently and carefully these examinations are performed, the earlier and more accurately the diagnosis can be made and treatment instituted.

The back of the patient should be examined as carefully as the front. Gunshots or stab wounds can easily be missed in creases of the body, especially if the patient is obese or has large quantities of body hair. If the patient has a possible spine injury, two or preferably three individuals are needed to log-roll the patient carefully so that the back and flanks can be examined.

Physical examination of the penetrated abdomen is conducted in the same manner as that for blunt trauma, with the following exceptions: (1) contamination of open wounds should be avoided, and (2) the entrance wounds of stabs may be cautiously explored, preferably visually, to determine whether there is penetration of the anterior abdominal fascia.

All wounds should be examined and documented. No attempt should be made to label these as exit or entrance wounds in the medical record because this often requires a forensic pathologist. It is prudent to cover each of these wounds with a sterile dressing and a radiopaque marker so that when radiographs are obtained, the location of these wounds can be correlated with the clinical and x-ray findings.

Occasionally, intraabdominal or retroperitoneal blood may cause ecchymosis or purplish discoloration around the umbilicus (Cullen's sign) or in the flanks (Grey-Turner's sign). Such discoloration often requires a few hours to be seen well.

Increasing abdominal distension can be a valuable sign of intraabdominal damage. Measurement of the abdominal girth at the umbilical level soon after the patient's admission can provide a baseline from which subsequent significant changes can be determined early and accurately. For example, if a patient's girth or circumference increases from 34 inches to 35 inches and if one assumes that an enlarging abdomen assumes a somewhat spherical shape, the volume of the abdomen will have increased from 10,876 cm^3 to 11,865 cm^3 (i.e., an increase of 989 mL).

AXIOM If the patient has pronounced involuntary guarding, no other diagnostic studies are indicated, and the patient requires a prompt celiotomy.

Abdominal tenderness is often considered an indication for an exploratory laparotomy after blunt trauma. In a prospective, multiinstitutional study over 22 months at four level I trauma centers reported by Livingston et al. (2), abdominal tenderness in the presence of a negative computed tomography (CT) scan was not predictive of an abdominal injury, and such patients did not benefit from hospital admission and prolonged observation.

AXIOM If the abdomen is much more tender when the abdominal muscles are tensed (as when the patient holds his head up for the pillow), this tends to indicate an injury in the abdominal wall.

Pelvic fractures can be assessed by manual compression on both iliac wings and the pubic symphysis and by motion at the hip joint. Absence of discomfort on performing these three maneuvers usually rules out a significant pelvic fracture. Genital examination should include noting the presence or absence of blood at the urethral meatus or hematomas involving the penis, vagina, or perineum.

On rectal examination, one should check sphincter tone, the integrity of the rectal wall, the presence or absence of blood, and the position of the prostate. If a nonpalpable, dislocated, or high-riding prostate is found, a prostatomembranous disruption of the urethra should be suspected. Vaginal lacerations or disruptions may be caused by pelvic fractures and should be assessed by digital examination; a speculum should also be used if there is a pelvic fracture or other evidence of possible vaginal injury. Both flanks should be carefully examined and palpated.

Gentle percussion of the abdomen can sometimes localize the area of maximal tenderness better than palpation. Percussion can also be used sometimes to determine the location of the top of the liver in the chest to detect hepatomegaly even if the liver is not palpable in the abdomen. Percussion over the spleen may also reveal an enlarged area of dullness that does not move when the patient is turned (Ballance's sign). This suggests the presence of a hematoma around an injured spleen. Free blood or fluid in the peritoneal cavity generally does not cause dullness to percussion over the spleen while the patient is lying on the right side.

AXIOM The presence of bowel sounds is a reassuring indicator of peristalsis, but it is not reliable for ruling out visceral injuries.

Up to 30% of patients have active bowel sounds in the presence of intraperitoneal bleeding or rupture of hollow viscera. Conversely, about 30% of patients who have absolutely no bowel sounds after careful listening for at least 5 minutes have no visceral damage.

Laboratory Studies

Blood Counts

The initial hemoglobin and hematocrit levels do not reflect the amount of recent hemorrhage that has occurred. At least several hours are usually required for hemodilution resulting from transcapillary refill or exogenous fluid to be accurately reflected in the hematocrit. Nevertheless, these values can serve as a baseline and are important if a general anesthetic is necessary. A progressive decrease in hemoglobin and hematocrit levels in the absence of hypotension can also serve as a warning of continuing bleeding, but this tends to be a relatively late finding.

AXIOM A hemoglobin level less than 10.0 g/dL may not provide adequate oxygen transport during anesthesia if the patient is elderly or has cardiac or pulmonary dysfunction.

Serum amylase levels must be interpreted with caution following abdominal trauma. An increasing level of serum amylase or a persistent hyperamylasemia is suggestive, but not pathognomonic, of pancreatic injury.

If there is only minor microscopic hematuria (less than 50 red cells per high power field), a detailed urologic workup is not generally indicated, but a repeat urinalysis is appropriate.

Radiologic Studies

Plain Films

In patients with abdominal trauma, flat and upright films of the abdomen and an upright film of the chest may be helpful. If upright films are not possible because of the poor clinical condition of the patient, a lateral decubitus film of the abdomen may be substituted.

One of the most important initial diagnostic studies in patients with multiple severe trauma is the chest radiograph. This can rapidly indicate whether the pleural cavities are a source of major blood loss or may have damage or disease that can interfere with adequate ventilation and oxygenation. It is also important to examine the lower lung fields and the outlines of the diaphragms carefully to rule out a possible diaphragmatic injury.

Flat films of the abdomen can be of great help in detecting (1) radiopaque foreign bodies such as bullets, (2) separation of loops of intestine by fluid, (3) loss of the psoas shadow, or (4) air around the right kidney or along the right psoas margins. The entrance and exit wounds of any penetrating wound should be covered with a sterile dressing with a radiopaque marker so that the presumed trajectory of the missile or weapon can be determined.

Intraperitoneal blood should be suspected on x-ray if one sees (1) a prominent flank stripe caused by fluid separating the ascending or descending colon from the peritoneal wall; (2) the "hepatic angle sign," which is loss of definition of the usually distinct inferior and right lateral borders of the liver caused by blood accumulation between the hepatic angle and the right lateral peritoneal wall; and (3) the "dog ear sign," which consists of bilateral zones of increased density lying superior to the bladder caused by blood accumulating in the space between the pelvic viscera and its side walls. The presence of one or more of these signs usually indicates the presence of at least 800 mL of intraperitoneal blood.

AXIOM Free air is most reliably seen if the patient is able to remain upright or on his side for at least 10 minutes before the radiologic examination.

Free air on a right or left lateral decubitus abdominal radiograph generally indicates a torn viscus. Air bubbles in or around the right kidney or along the psoas should make one suspect retroperitoneal rupture of the duodenum or right colon. Fractures of lower ribs, spine, or pelvis should direct attention to possible injuries of adjacent organs such as the liver, spleen, or bladder.

If a plain radiograph of the pelvis is negative, it is unlikely that the pelvis is a source of major blood loss, even if further radiographs or a CT scan reveal some fractures. If a severe pelvic fracture is seen on plain film, it could be a source of major hemorrhage.

Contrast Studies

A Gastrografin swallow and upper gastrointestinal series may be helpful for diagnosing injury to the stomach, duodenum, proximal jejunum, or diaphragm. A Gastrografin or barium enema may be helpful for diagnosing rectal or colonic injury.

If injury to the bladder or male urethra is suspected, a retrograde urethrogram and cystogram should be performed.

The role of the intravenous pyelogram (IVP) for diagnosis of renal injury is increasingly questioned because CT scans of the abdomen with intravenous contrast usually provide much clearer delineation of renal anatomy and injuries. If the mechanism of injury, its location, physical examination, or urinalysis suggests a renal injury and the patient is unstable or CT scanning is not rapidly available, one can attempt to get an emergency one-shot IVP in the emergency department or operating room by rapidly infusing 150 to 200 mL of 60% Renografin and obtaining flat films of the abdomen before the infusion and then 1 and 5 minutes later.

Computed Tomography

Intraperitoneal and retroperitoneal blood and most solid organ injuries can be detected in a highly reliable manner with CT scans. Whereas peritoneal lavage often cannot evaluate retroperitoneal injuries accurately, CT scans done with intravenous and oral contrast can provide rather clear images of the duodenum, liver, spleen, and kidneys. CT scans can also be helpful for assessing pelvic and spinal fractures. CT scans are of little help for diagnosing distal small bowel injuries. They are also not very reliable for diagnosing pancreatic or diaphragmatic injuries. Nevertheless, Dowe et al. (3) have noted that a CT finding of mesenteric bleeding or bowel wall thickening *plus* a mesenteric hematoma or infiltration in blunt trauma patients indicated a high likelihood of a mesenteric or bowel injury requiring surgery. However, the finding of a focal mesenteric hematoma or infiltration without adjacent bowel wall thickening was nonspecific and can occur in mesenteric or bowel lesions that do not require surgery.

CT scans are generally not done in hemodynamically unstable patients; however, newer generation CT scanners that can perform these examinations rapidly may obviate this problem to some degree, particularly if the CT scanner is in the emergency department or immediately adjacent to it.

AXIOM The accuracy of abdominal ultrasonography and CT scans is largely determined by the expertise of the individuals performing and interpreting them.

It increasingly appears that the presence of intraperitoneal fluid or an indeterminate RBC count on diagnostic peritoneal lavage (DPL) without evidence of solid organ damage is a strong indication for a laparotomy. Brasel et al. (4) found that the presence of more than trace amounts of free fluid without solid organ injury on CT scan in patients with blunt trauma is a strong indication for exploratory laparotomy, particularly because of the possibility of small bowel injuries.

Cunningham et al. (5) reported on isolated intraperitoneal fluid identified on CT scans in 31 patients with recent blunt trauma. All of these patients underwent laparotomy and 29 (94%) of these procedures were therapeutic. These injuries included bowel (18), mesentery (8), intraperitoneal bladder (5), and undetected solid organ injuries (2). Other organs injured included the stomach, pancreas, ovary, and uterus.

One of the more important criticisms of CT scanning of the abdomen after trauma has been the delay caused by insisting on administration of oral contrast; however, Kinnunen et al. (6) found that omission of the upper gastrointestinal contrast did not jeopardize making the essential diagnoses.

Contrast-enhanced CT enemas (CECTE) using double contrast (intravenous and colonic) or triple contrast (intravenous, oral, and colonic) can also be useful in evaluating penetrating wounds of the flanks or back. In one such series, an injury requiring a celiotomy was successfully ruled out in 92% of the patients on the basis of a CECTE (7).

Ultrasound

There has been increasing interest in the use of ultrasound (US), particularly in emergency departments, to detect collections of fluid in the pericardial, pleural, or peritoneal spaces. Rozycki et al. (8) reported on the use of US in 250 patients with blunt trauma and 55 with penetrating injuries. The time for each US examination averaged 2.5 minutes. There were 41 (13.4%) positive examinations and only two (5%) of these had nontherapeutic laparotomies. There were no false-positive US studies. There were 253 (83%) true-negative and 11 (3.6%) false-negative examinations.

Endoscopy

Injuries that may involve the stomach or duodenum can be investigated with esophagogastroduodenoscopy down to the second or third part of the duodenum. If there is a perforation, however, the air insufflated into the bowel can cause a fairly severe pneumoperitoneum.

With injuries that may involve the rectum or colon, flexible sigmoidoscopy or colonoscopy may be helpful; however, the bowel is usually unprepared. A Fleet's enema may allow examination of the rectum and distal sigmoid colon, but to be able to examine more of the large intestine, a more prolonged cleansing of the colon is usually required.

Local Wound Exploration

One approach to stable patients who have an anterior abdominal stab wound is to perform wound exploration under local anesthesia. If it can be seen that a stab wound does not penetrate the anterior fascia, the patient can be discharged home. If the stab wound does penetrate the fascia, one can elect to perform a laparotomy, perform a DPL, or observe the patient. The incidence of a negative or nontherapeutic celiotomy in patients with evidence of anterior fascial penetration on local wound exploration is about 25% (9). Many surgeons consider this negative exploration rate to be acceptable because the morbidity associated with a negative celiotomy in stab wound victims is only 1.5% to 3.0%; however, the length of stay in hospital after such surgery can be significant.

If a DPL is performed and is negative, a laparotomy is not indicated. If the DPL results are positive only because of increased RBCs, one can elect either to observe the patient carefully or explore the abdomen. If the DPL reveals an elevated white blood cell (WBC) count or that bile, amylase, or food particles are present, the abdomen should be explored.

Diagnostic Peritoneal Lavage

Patients for whom DPL is indicated after blunt abdominal trauma include

1. Patients in whom the physical examination is likely to be falsely negative (e.g., patients with head or spinal cord injuries, severe intoxication, or general anesthesia for another injury);
2. Patients in whom the physical examination is likely to be falsely positive (e.g., lower rib fractures, fractures of lumbar vertebrae, abdominal wall hematomas); and
3. Patients who will not be available for continuous examination (e.g., during angiography, multiple x-ray studies, prolonged neurosurgical or orthopedic operations).

In patients with head injury who require an immediate craniotomy, the DPL can be performed in the operating room. If the lavage is positive, the craniotomy and celiotomy should be performed simultaneously if possible. Positioning of the patient for craniotomies in certain areas of the skull, however, can make a simultaneous celiotomy difficult; nevertheless, if there is significant intraabdominal bleeding, it should be controlled promptly.

Previous abdominal surgery is a relative contraindication to DPL, because adhesions can compartmentalize the peritoneal cavity and predispose the patient to iatrogenic bowel injury. One can make an incision, preferably in the midline, from the previous incisions if possible and do an open DPL.

There are basically three techniques for performing DPL:

1. Open technique;
2. Semiopen technique; and
3. Closed technique.

The open technique is generally safe, but it usually takes more time, and the semiopen technique is almost as safe. In some series, the closed technique has been associated with a high rate of morbidity (6%–8%) (10).

The semiopen technique involves exposure of the midline fascia by sharp dissection followed by a transfascial and transperitoneal puncture using an 18-gauge needle with a stylet. If desired, the fascia can be lifted up on either side of the proposed immature site with stay sutures of clamps to decrease the chances of intraperitoneal or retroperitoneal injury. A guide wire is then threaded through the needle, then a dilator and then the lavage catheter are advanced over the guide wire into the abdomen toward the pelvic cavity.

When the lavage catheter is in place, an attempt is made to aspirate any free intraperitoneal fluid that may be present. If 10 to 20 mL of gross blood is obtained on the initial aspiration, the DPL is considered "positive," and an exploratory celiotomy is usually required. If the initial aspiration recovers no blood, then 15 mL/kg or 1,000 mL, whichever is less, of 0.9% saline solution is allowed to drain by gravity rapidly into the peritoneal cavity. As the fluid is being infused, the patient is turned gently from side to side (except in patients with suspected spinal injury) to ensure good mixing of the infusate fluid with any intraperitoneal fluid. The lavage fluid is then allowed to drain out the same tubing, using gravity, by placing the now empty bottle or container on the floor. At least 200 mL of solution should be recovered, 75 mL of which is sent to the laboratory for analysis.

Inability to read newsprint through the return fluid in the lavage tubing is usually interpreted as "positive." If the fluid is pink, but one can read newsprint through the tubing, the result is interpreted as "indeterminate." Drainage of DPL fluid from a previously placed chest tube signifies a lacerated or ruptured diaphragm. An RBC count of 100,000/mm^3 or more following blunt trauma or a WBC count of 500/mm^3 or more is also considered positive (Table 20-1).

In penetrating trauma, the RBC criterion for a positive finding averages 10,000/mm^3 but varies from 1,000 to 100,000/mm^3. When 10,000 RBC/mm^3 is used as

TABLE 20–1. ***Criteria for Interpretation of Lavage Results in Blunt Abdominal Trauma***

Positive	
	Aspiration >10 mL nonclotting blood
	Lavage fluid comes out Foley catheter or chest tube
	Grossly bloody lavage return
	RBC >100,000/mm^3
	WBC >500/mm^3
	Amylase >175 KU/dL
	Presence of bile, bacteria, and/or particulater matter
Indeterminate	
	Aspiration <10 mL of nonclotting blood
	RBC 50,000 to 100,000/mm^3
	WBC 100 to 500 mm^3
	Amylase 75 to 175 KU/dL
Negative	
	No blood aspirated
	RBC <50,000/mm^3
	WBC <100/mm^3
	Amylase <75 KU/dL

RBC, red blood cell count; WBC, white blood cell count.
From Keating KP, Yeston NS. Diagnostic peritoneal lavage: indications, results, and complications. *Resident and Staff Physician* 1991;37:31.

a criterion for celiotomy, there are about 10% to 15% false-positive findings and a 1.0% false-negative rate. If the major concern is whether a penetrating chest wound injured the diaphragm, as little as 1,000 RBC/mm^3 can be considered positive.

AXIOM If the DPL is "indeterminate" or the number of WBC/mm^3 is suspicious, the DPL can be repeated 3 to 6 hours later.

In many surgeons' hands, DPL has been extremely sensitive (98%–99%) and accurate (97%–98%), and missed injuries are seldom a problem. One of the main problems with DPL is that as many as 20% to 40% of the laparotomies could be avoided, because the increased RBCs result from only minor injuries that could be treated nonoperatively.

The value of DPL in the presence of a pelvic fracture is not clear. There is a fairly high incidence of RBCs passing from the retroperitoneal pelvic hematoma into the peritoneal cavity so that up to 40% of patients with pelvic fractures may have a false-positive DPL by RBC criteria. Indeed, some surgeons believe that, unless more than 10 to 20 mL of gross blood is aspirated at the beginning of the procedure or unless the red cell count in the lavage fluid is 200,000/mm^3 or more, it is unlikely that a laparotomy is required.

AXIOM The clearest indication for DPL is continued hemodynamic instability in a patient with multiple injuries, especially if physical examination of the abdomen cannot be performed reliably.

Laparoscopy

In trauma patients, laparoscopy may be particularly helpful for determining whether a laparotomy is required, and for certain injuries, it can be therapeutic. Ivatury et al. (11) evaluated laparoscopy in 100 patients with penetrating abdominal trauma. The laparoscopy was very accurate for detecting hemoperitoneum, solid organ and diaphragmatic injuries, and retroperitoneal hematomas. For gastrointestinal damage, diagnostic laparoscopy was less accurate, detecting only two of the nine patients with such injuries. The authors concluded that the major role of laparoscopy in penetrating abdominal trauma is in avoiding an unnecessary laparotomy in a patient with only a tangential injury.

There is also some concern that the increased intraabdominal pressure (IAP) might have adverse ventilatory effects. Indeed, if an abdominal vein is injured and venous pressures are very low, in theory, one could quickly cause large amounts of CO_2 to enter the vascular system with resulting CO_2 emboli to the heart and lungs. Another concern is possible creation of a tension pneumothorax in patients with penetrating injuries involving the diaphragm.

Diagnostic laparoscopy may also interfere with intraabdominal blood flow, especially in the presence of hypovolemia. Diebel et al. (12) showed that, with just 10 mm Hg IAP in pigs, hepatic artery flow was reduced by 39%, portal venous blood flow was reduced by 27%, and hepatic microvascular blood flow was reduced by 19%. As IAP was increased, all of these flow parameters decreased even more.

Josephs et al. (13) recently showed that diagnostic laparoscopy with a pneumoperitoneum of 15 mm Hg in normovolemic ventilated pigs increased ICP about 5.3 mm Hg. Thus, diagnostic laparoscopy must be used cautiously in the 30% of patients with blunt abdominal injury trauma who also have an intracranial injury.

If appropriate thoracoscopic skills are available, and if the patient can be intubated with a split function endotracheal tube, one can examine the diaphragm through the chest with a thoracoscope (14). One must be concerned about the pneumothorax produced during thoracoscopy, particularly if the patient has any pulmonary or hemodynamic insufficiency.

Exploratory Laparotomy

In some instances, an exploratory laparotomy may seem to be the best diagnostic test available, even if there are no clear indications for surgery. Although experienced trauma surgeons may have excellent results with this diagnostic technique, the acute morbidity of a nontherapeutic laparotomy may be as high as 19% to 43% (15).

TREATMENT

Nonsurgical Management

With known intraabdominal solid organ injuries in children, there is an increasing tendency for nonoperative management. In a prospective study by Haller et al. (16), all severely injured children with evidence of intraabdominal solid organ injury who remained hemodynamically stable after 40 mL/kg fluid replacement were placed in a prospective nonoperative management protocol. The incidences of eventual operation for each organ injured were

- 28 spleens—11%
- 25 livers—8%
- 18 kidneys—6%
- 7 pancreases—43%

There were no deaths or complications in the children receiving nonoperative treatment.

AXIOM If a child requires no more than half the calculated blood volume as transfusions, one can continue with nonoperative management of spleen or liver injuries.

In hemodynamically stable adults with injuries involving the spleen, liver, or kidney, there is an increasing tendency toward nonoperative treatment but with careful observation for several days.

AXIOM If an adult requires more than two units of blood to maintain stable vital signs or if there is clinical evidence of peritonitis, an exploratory celiotomy is indicated.

Surgical Management

Indications for Laparotomy

Significant intraabdominal bleeding or hollow viscus injury are the main indications for laparotomy following trauma. Intraabdominal bleeding should be strongly suspected if the patient comes to the hospital in severe shock or if mild to moderate shock is persistent or recurs despite aggressive fluid resuscitation.

Pelvic Fractures

If the patient has an unstable pelvic fracture and is hemodynamically unstable despite aggressive fluid and blood resuscitation, an immediate celiotomy should be performed. If the major intraabdominal bleeding can be controlled but the patient remains hypotensive, the pelvis should be packed and the abdomen should be closed. An external fixator should then be applied. If the bleeding continues despite pelvic fixation, the patient should be taken to the arteriogram suite immediately for embolization of the arterial bleeders.

If the patient has an open pelvic fracture and is exsanguinating, the perineal wound should be packed and a pneumatic antishock garment can be applied. With large perineal wounds associated with a pelvic fracture, a diverting sigmoid colostomy should be performed after the major bleeding is controlled.

Urethral or Bladder Tears

If the patient has an emergency urethrogram or cystogram, and it reveals a tear in the urethra or bladder, no further diagnostic studies are indicated because suprapubic drainage of the bladder should be carried out in the operating room, and a thorough exploration of the abdomen can be carried out at the same time.

Perforations or Peritonitis

If there is any clinical or radiologic evidence of bowel perforation or peritonitis, the abdomen should be explored promptly. If a duodenal perforation is missed for more than 24 to 48 hours, the mortality rate may exceed 50% (17). Diagnosis of perforations of the stomach or duodenum can be facilitated by the oral contrast on the CT scan. Distal colon injuries may be detected by a contrast CT enema. With the remaining bowel, the first evidence of injury may be an elevated WBC count on DPL.

AXIOM Bowel or mesentery injury should be suspected if the DPL after blunt trauma shows more than 25,000 RBC/mm^3 and there is no solid organ injury apparent on the CT scan.

Preoperative Preparation

Once the decision to perform an exploratory laparotomy for trauma has been made, the surgery should not be delayed. Before surgery, electrolyte or acid-base imbalance or hyperglycemia should be corrected, if possible, but preoperative delays may cause deterioration of the clinical situation and increase the operative risk.

Anesthesia

Most general anesthetics reduce cardiac contractility, cause systemic vasodilation, and increase vascular capacitance, thereby increasing the tendency to hypotension. Consequently, trauma patients must be closely monitored as the general anesthetic is induced. Rapid replacement of blood and other fluids may be required before, during, and after induction of the anesthetic to reduce the chances of severe hypotension.

Body Preparation and Placement

Before exploring the abdomen for trauma, especially gunshot wounds, the skin should be prepped and draped widely from the chin to the knees and laterally as far as possible, so that the surgeon can gain access to any body cavity or the groin expeditiously and can properly place drains and chest tubes as needed.

If it is known before the operation that it is likely that a thoracotomy will also be needed, it is sometimes helpful to elevate the patient's hip and shoulder on the involved side on sand bags. This allows a more lateral extension of an anterior thoracotomy incision if needed.

Incision

Stab wounds in the flanks or lateral abdomen with well-localized signs or symptoms can sometimes be approached satisfactorily through a transverse or oblique incision. In general, however, a midline incision is preferred because it is relatively bloodless, can be performed rapidly, and allows good exposure to virtually all parts of the abdomen.

For gunshot wounds, the midline incision is particularly desirable because the bullet may have ricocheted unpredictably and cause widely separated injuries. Occasionally, the incision may have to be extended into the left or right side of the chest to obtain adequate exposure to structures immediately under the diaphragm or to treat concomitant thoracic injuries. In severe hepatic trauma involving the hepatic veins or retrohepatic vena cava, extension of the midline incision into the chest by splitting the sternum is a quick and effective approach to these structures, especially if an atriocaval shunt is to be inserted.

If the patient has a very distended abdomen and is in profound shock despite rapid infusions of large quantities of fluid and blood, the incision into the abdominal cavity may be followed by torrential bleeding. Consequently, only the top part of the incision is opened initially so that the surgeon can reach in and compress the abdominal aorta at the diaphragm. An aortic compressor can then be positioned and held in place while the rest of the incision is opened and the abdomen is explored. Another alternative is to perform a prelaparotomy thoracotomy and clamp the descending thoracic aorta above the diaphragm.

Prelaparotomy Thoracotomy with Aortic Clamping

A prelaparotomy thoracotomy with thoracic aortic cross-clamping can help to

1. Maintain blood flow to the heart and brain;
2. Reduce the amount of intraabdominal blood loss;
3. Reduce the duration of central hypotension; and
4. Reduce the number of blood transfusions (18).

In patients with high-risk abdominal vascular injuries, (admission systolic BP less than 70 mm Hg and four or more associated injuries) if the shock duration was kept to less than 30 minutes and the number of blood transfusions was kept to less than 10 units, the mortality rate was zero (0 of 12 patients); however, if one of these conditions was present, the mortality rate was 92% (24 of 26 patients) (18).

AXIOM For patients arriving at the operating room with massive intraabdominal bleeding and a systolic BP less than 70 mm Hg, a prelaparotomy cross-clamping of the thoracic aorta should be considered.

If, following thoracic aortic cross-clamping and aggressive fluid resuscitation, the systolic BP does not increase to at least 90 mm Hg within 5 minutes, the patient has terminal cardiovascular failure and will almost certainly die in the operating room (18). Prolonged surgical efforts for many hours using multiple units of blood in such patients have been uniformly futile. If the systolic BP proximal to the clamp is allowed to exceed 160 to 180 mm Hg, the resultant left ventricular dilation can cause acute cardiac failure to develop within a few minutes.

Following laparotomy, the thoracic aortic clamp should be moved to the abdominal aorta as soon as possible.

Initial Control of Bleeding

When a major intraabdominal injury is expected because of continued severe hypotension, the abdominal incision should be extended from the xiphoid to below the umbilicus to gain adequate exposure. Free blood and clot are removed rapidly, and the small bowel is eviscerated as needed so that each quadrant of the abdomen can be inspected rapidly for bleeding. Packs can be placed temporarily to absorb excess free blood and apply pressure to any suspected bleeding areas.

If the patient becomes severely hypotensive, the aorta should be compressed at the diaphragm and packs should be used to help control the bleeding until the anesthesiologist can resuscitate the patient adequately.

AXIOM Once the major bleeding has been controlled, further abdominal surgery should be delayed until the systolic BP increases to 100 mm Hg or more, the urine output is at least 0.5 mL/kg/h, and the core (esophageal) temperature is at least 34°C to 35°C.

Operative Techniques

Abdominal Exploration

When all significant bleeding has been controlled and the patient has been adequately resuscitated, an orderly exploration of the abdomen should be performed. As intestinal injuries are encountered, they can be controlled temporarily with Babcock clamps or rapid-running absorbable sutures.

AXIOM The number one priority during a celiotomy for trauma is to control bleeding. A second consideration is keeping intestinal contamination to a minimum.

If one has a fairly good idea of the main source of the patient's blood loss and it is controlled by packs, the other areas of the abdomen can be explored first. If the packs are not controlling the bleeding, the suspected source should be explored first. If the site of the major blood loss is not known, one can start in the left upper quadrant. The retractors are placed to provide optimal exposure and the packs are removed one by one, looking carefully for bleeding sites, especially the spleen.

Spleen. If the spleen is bleeding, a decision must be made immediately as to whether to remove the spleen promptly or control the bleeding temporarily with local pressure. If this appears to be the major site of bleeding, one can mobilize the spleen carefully while controlling the bleeding to determine whether repair or partial splenectomy is possible. If there are other causes of major blood loss in the abdomen, the spleen should be removed promptly.

Liver. If there is obvious injury to the liver with gross hemorrhage, proper application of packs can often control the bleeding. If this does not stop the hemorrhage, compression of the liver between two hands often suffices. If this is also unsuccessful, a Pringle maneuver (clamping of the hepatoduodenal ligament, which encloses the hepatic artery and portal vein at the foramen of Winslow) may help. If there is still continued bleeding from the depths of a liver laceration, one should suspect a major injury to a hepatic vein.

If the bleeding appears to be coming from the back of the liver, injury to the retrohepatic inferior vena cava or attached hepatic veins should be strongly suspected. This area should be compressed manually or repacked while consideration is given to possible use of an atriocaval shunt, a venous bypass of the inferior cava, packing as definitive treatment, or clamping the infradiaphragmatic aorta, portal triad, and suprahepatic and intrahepatic inferior vena cava to gain control of the bleeding.

Intestine

AXIOM After the major hemorrhage has been controlled and obvious intestinal leaks contained, a thorough exploration of the abdomen cavity should be performed.

A Kocher maneuver is done to facilitate exploration of hematomas or bile staining of the upper central retroperitoneum. A perirenal hematoma resulting from blunt trauma is usually not explored unless it is expanding or radiologic studies have identified a problem that needs to be addressed. Pelvic hematomas should not be explored if they are due to blunt trauma.

Access to central retroperitoneal hematomas above the pelvic brim is best achieved by taking down the attachments of the right colon (as part of an extended Kocher maneuver to examine the duodenum and head of the pancreas) or left colon with mobilization of the corresponding viscera to the midline (to examine the aorta and the origins of its major branches).

The bowel must be inspected systematically and meticulously. If a penetrating injury is present, one should demonstrate an even number of holes or attempt to prove that the injury to the small intestine was tangential.

⊘ PITFALL

If an odd number of holes in the intestine is attributed to a tangential injury, small wounds on the mesenteric aspect can easily be overlooked.

When an intestinal injury is recognized, it should be closed temporarily by a nontraumatic clamp, rapid suturing, or staples until the initial inspection of the abdomen is completed. Allowing continuing escape of intestinal contents into the peritoneal cavity can result in later severe peritonitis or abscess formation.

If there is any suspicion of injury in the lesser sac, the gastrocolic omentum should be opened. The transverse colon, posterior wall of the stomach, and pancreatic region can then be thoroughly inspected.

Blood Vessels. Single holes in blood vessels should always be viewed with skepticism. If a second hole is missed, subsequent hemorrhage, a false aneurysm, or an arteriovenous fistula may develop. A search should also be made to ensure that the missile has not migrated down an injured vessel.

AXIOM At the conclusion of the operation, it is advisable to reexplore the abdomen carefully, to ensure that no area of injury has been overlooked (19).

Peritoneal Irrigation

Once the bleeding and all intestinal leaks have been controlled, one should lavage the peritoneal cavity carefully with saline to reduce the bacterial load from any contamination and to remove any residual free blood or blood clots. Excessive irrigation, however, may adversely affect resident macrophages, and all residual fluid should be removed from the peritoneal cavity.

Addition of antibiotics to the last liter of irrigant is recommended by some surgeons, but its usefulness remains to be proven. Furthermore, if neomycin or another aminoglycoside is added to the irrigating solutions, prolonged postoperative respiratory depression may result.

Drains

The indications, numbers, and types of drains used for any particular intraabdominal injury vary greatly from surgeon to surgeon. Drains can be extremely beneficial by removing any bile or pancreatic secretions that may continue to leak from an injured liver, biliary tract, or pancreas; however, they can also cause problems by (1) serving as a conduit for bacteria to enter the peritoneal cavity or (2) eroding into adjacent vessels or organs.

Drains should be of the closed type (i.e., not directly open to the air) whenever possible. They should be soft, accurately placed, and brought out through stab wounds of adequate size in the abdominal wall away from the surgical incision. They should also be carefully dressed and adjusted intermittently.

AXIOM Drains generally should not be left in situ after they cease functioning; however, with pancreatic or liver injuries, the drains should not be removed until it is clear that there is no drainage and the patient is tolerating an oral diet.

Planned Reoperations

Planned reoperations are being used increasingly in the management of critically injured patients. At the first "damage control" operation, measures are taken to rapidly stop all bleeding and prevent further spillage of intestinal contents or urine (20). The patient is then warmed and resuscitated in the intensive care unit. The patient is usually returned to the operating room within 24 to 48 hours, when the patient appears to be sufficiently stable to tolerate definitive repair of all injuries.

Occasionally, more bleeding is encountered at the second operation, requiring repeat packing and another reoperation.

An increasing tendency to do staged surgery for severe abdominal injuries seems to stem from the growing realization that the mortality rate increases abruptly in patients who are allowed to maintain the "terrible triad" of hypothermia, acidosis, and coagulopathy for prolonged periods in the operating room.

Closure of Abdominal Incisions

In patients who have had extensive trauma and in whom peritonitis, severe ileus, or respiratory failure is likely to develop, large full-thickness retention sutures tied over dental rolls or rubber tubing may add considerable strength to an otherwise tenuous abdominal wall closure. If the abdomen cannot be closed except under some tension, but it is important to make the closure watertight, the skin can be closed and the fascia left open temporarily. If the skin also cannot be closed, one can suture in plastic material (as from sterile 3-L plastic bags) to skin or fascia to produce a watertight closure.

Measuring Intraabdominal Pressure

If the abdomen is closed and there is concern about continued intraabdominal bleeding, edema, or bowel dilatation, the IAP should be monitored closely. This is usually done via a Foley catheter in the bladder. To measure the IAP, the drainage portion of the Foley catheter is clamped a few inches downstream and a central venous pressure (CVP) manometer is hooked up to the proximal portion of the Foley catheter via a needle in its side. After instilling 25 to 50 mL of sterile saline into the bladder, the pressure inside the bladder, which reflects IAP, can then be measured with a CVP manometer with the zero point at the level of the midaxillary line. If the IAP exceeds 20 to 30 mm Hg (26 to 39 cm H_2O) and there is severe oliguria despite more than adequate BP and cardiac output, then development of an abdominal compartment syndrome should be suspected and the abdomen should be opened promptly. Ideally, any coagulopathy that was present should have been corrected by that time by warming the patient and infusing platelets and fresh frozen plasma (FFP) or cryoprecipitate, as needed. For severe coagulopathies, more than 8 to 12 units of FFP may have to be infused fairly rapidly.

Leaving the Abdomen Open

In patients with severe abdominal trauma, infusions of large quantities of intravenous fluid may result in excessive swelling of bowel, the mesentery, and the retroperitoneal tissues. In addition, increased edema can make the abdominal wall less compliant. Under such circumstances, closing the abdominal fascia may result in increased intraperitoneal pressure with a resultant decrease in hepatic, renal, and intestinal mucosal blood flow. Use of a plastic intravenous bag to provide a temporary abdominal wall silo closure has also been reported (21).

Leaving the Skin and Subcutaneous Tissue Open

If there has been gross contamination of the peritoneal cavity and subcutaneous tissue, as with massive colonic wounds, the fascia can be closed, but the skin and subcutaneous tissue should be left open for at least several days.

AXIOM One of the best ways to prevent wound infections after abdominal trauma with severe contamination is to leave the skin and subcutaneous tissue open.

⊘ FREQUENT ERRORS

1. ***Failure to recognize the need for emergency abdominal surgery at an early stage.***

2. ***Failure to repeatedly reexamine the patient with possible intraabdominal injuries.***
3. ***Concentrating on an abdominal injury to the extent that serious extraabdominal injuries are overlooked.***
4. ***Insistence on "routine" preoperative radiologic studies in hemodynamically unstable patients.***
5. ***Failure to insert a gastric decompression tube in patients who have an injury that may cause vomiting or a severe ileus.***
6. ***Failure to resuscitate the patient's blood volume and core temperature adequately once the major bleeding has been controlled.***
7. ***Unsystematic examination of the abdomen during laparotomy, thereby increasing the likelihood of missing lesions.***
8. ***Insistence on performing a one-stage operation, including skin closure, when a staged procedure (i.e., a damage control initial procedure) might be much safer.***
9. ***Failure to repeat needed antibiotic therapy after massive bleeding has been controlled.***
10. ***Removal of "nonfunctioning" drains from around hepatic or pancreatic injuries before the patient is eating.***

SUMMARY POINTS

1. One should never assume that bullets travel in a straight line. The bullet or secondary missiles can often injure structures far outside the presumed trajectory.

2. Because of the unpredictable path and possible blast effect of bullets, all abdominal gunshot wounds (except those proven to only be tangential and only involve abdominal wall) require surgical exploration.

3. The initial resuscitation of patients with severe trauma should rapidly ensure an adequate airway and the maintenance of a minute ventilation that is at least 1.5 to 2.0 times normal.

4. Patients who are bleeding rapidly should have their hemorrhage controlled promptly before being aggressively resuscitated with fluids.

5. The failure of 2,000 to 3,000 mL of Ringer's lactate given over 10 to 15 minutes to restore adequate blood pressure and tissue perfusion strongly suggests that the patient is bleeding rapidly and requires urgent surgical exploration to control the sites of hemorrhage.

6. One should avoid nasal tubes in patients who may have fractures of the midface.

7. Before inserting a Foley catheter in patients with severe blunt trauma, one should examine the penis and perineum for bleeding or hematomas and do a rectal exam to check the position of the prostate, look for any rectal blood, and check sphincter tone.

8. Intravenous prophylactic antibiotics that cover enteric gram-negative aerobes and anaerobes should be given as soon as possible if intraabdominal contamination is suspected.

9. Careful repeated examination of the patient are important in the early diagnosis of hollow viscus injuries.

10. Narcotics generally should not be given to patients who are hypovolemic or who are being observed for possible central nervous system or abdominal injuries; multiple, small intravenous doses, however, may relieve severe pain and make the patient more cooperative without altering physical signs.

11. If a trauma patient has signs of peritonitis, a prompt celiotomy is generally indicated.

12. If there is doubt regarding whether abdominal rigidity or tenderness is due to intraabdominal trauma or to an injury to the abdominal wall, one should assume that an intraabdominal injury is present.

13. If a child requires more than half the calculated blood volume as transfusions, then nonoperative management of spleen or liver injuries should be discontinued.

14. If an adult requires more than 2 units of blood to maintain stable vital signs or if there is clinical evidence of peritonitis, an exploratory celiotomy is indicated.
15. The presence of bowel sounds is a reassuring indicator of peristalsis, but it is not reliable for ruling out visceral injuries.
16. A hemoglobin level less than 10.0 g/dL may not provide adequate oxygen transport during anesthesia if the patient has cardiac or pulmonary dysfunction.
17. Many false-positive and false-negative results occur when using serum amylase levels to diagnosis pancreatic injury.
18. The delay and extra movement caused by an insistence on "routine" radiologic examinations can be extremely dangerous in patients with severe abdominal trauma.
19. Free air is most reliably seen if a patient remains upright or on his or her side for at least 10 minutes before the radiologic examination.
20. Up to 25% of patients with renal injuries requiring a nephrectomy have no hematuria because the renal pedicle or ureter is completely torn.
21. The safest policy with stab wounds is to explore the abdomen if there is any question of whether a visceral injury exists.
22. The accuracy of abdominal ultrasonography and CT scans is largely determined by the expertise of the individuals performing and interpreting the studies.
23. The clearest indication for DPL is continued hemodynamic instability in a patient with multiple injuries, especially if physical examination of the abdomen cannot be performed reliably.
24. Of the patients with intraabdominal trauma who reach a hospital alive, 20% to 30% of those who die do so because of delayed, inadequate, or inappropriate treatment.
25. Massive bleeding from an unstable pelvic fracture should necessitate prompt external fixation or therapeutic angiography.
26. One should suspect bowel or mesentery injury if the DPL after blunt trauma shows more than 25,000 RBC/mm^3 (or there is significant peritoneal fluid on US or CT) and there is no solid organ injury on the CT scan.
27. General anesthesia can cause a severe decrease in BP and cardiac output if the patient is hypovolemic.
28. Patients with massive hemoperitoneum and continued severe hypotension (systolic BP less than 70 mm Hg) often benefit from a prelaparotomy thoracotomy and aortic cross-clamping.
29. If the aorta is cross-clamped, the proximal aortic pressure in previously normal individuals should not be allowed to exceed 160 to 180 mm Hg.
30. When major bleeding is controlled, further abdominal surgery should be delayed until aggressive resuscitation increases the systolic BP to 100 mm Hg or more, the urine output to at least 0.5 mL/kg/h, and the core (esophageal) temperature to at least 34°C to 35°C.
31. If an odd number of holes in the intestine is attributed to a tangential injury, small wounds on the mesenteric aspect may be easily overlooked.
32. At the conclusion of the operation, it is advisable to explore the abdomen again carefully, to ensure that no area of injury has been overlooked.
33. One of the best ways to prevent wound infections after abdominal trauma causing severe contamination is to leave the skin and subcutaneous tissue open.

REFERENCES

1. Wilson RF, Walt AJ. General considerations in abdominal trauma. In: *Management of trauma: pitfalls and practice,* 2nd ed. Philadelphia: Williams & Wilkins, 1996:411.
2. Livingston DH, Lavery RF, Passannante MR, et al. Admission or observation is not necessary after a negative abdominal computed tomographic scan in patients with suspected blunt abdominal trauma: Results of a prospective, multi-institutional trial. *J Trauma* 1998;44:273.
3. Dowe MF, Shanmuganathan K, Mirvis SE. CT findings of mesenteric injury after blunt trauma: implications for surgical interventions. *AJR Am J Roentgenol* 1997;168:425.

4. Brasel KJ, Olson CJ, Stafford RE, et al. Incidence and significance of free fluid on abdominal computed tomographic scan in blunt trauma. *J Trauma* 1998;44:889.
5. Cunningham, MA, Tyroch AH, Kaups KL, et al. Does free fluid on abdominal computed tomographic scan after blunt trauma require laparotomy? *J Trauma* 1998;44:599.
6. Kinnunen J, Kivioja A, Poussa K, Laasonen EM. Emergency CT in blunt abdominal trauma of multiple injury patients. *Acta Radiol* 1994;35:319.
7. Trunkey DD, Federle MP. Computed tomography in perspective. [Editorial]. *J Trauma* 1986;26:660.
8. Rozycki GS, Ochsner MG, Frankel HL, et al. A prospective study of surgeon-performed ultrasound as the initial diagnostic modality for injured patient assessment [Abstract]. *J Trauma* 1994;37:160.
9. Petersen FR, Sheldon GF. Morbidity of a negative finding at laparotomy in abdominal trauma. *Surg Gynecol Obstet* 1979;148:23.
10. Moore JB, Moore EE, Markovchick VJ, et al. Diagnostic peritoneal lavage for trauma: superiority of the open technique at the infraumbilical ring. *J Trauma* 1981;21:570.
11. Ivatury RR, Simon RJ, Stahl WM. A critical evaluation of laparoscopy in penetrating abdominal trauma. *J Trauma* 1993;34:822.
12. Diebel LN, Saxe JM, Dulchavsky SA, et al. Hepatic perfusion responses to increased intra-abdominal pressure. *J Trauma* 1991;31:1714.
13. Josephs LG, Este-McDonald JR, Birkett DH, Hirsh EF. Diagnostic laparoscopy increases intracranial pressure. *J Trauma* 1994;36:815.
14. Koehler RH, Smith RS. Thoracoscopic repair of missed diaphragmatic injury in penetrating trauma: case report. *J Trauma* 1994;36:424.
15. Morrison JE, Wisner DH, Bodai BI. Complications after negative laparotomy for trauma: long-term follow-up in a health maintenance organization. *J Trauma* 1996;41:509.
16. Haller JA Jr, Papa P, Drugas G, Colombani P. Nonoperative management of solid organ injuries in children. Is it safe? *Ann Surg* 1994;219:615.
17. Lucas CE. Diagnosis and treatment of pancreatic and duodenal injury. *Surg Clin North Am* 1977;57:49.
18. Wilson RF, Wiencek RG Jr, Balog M. Factors affecting mortality rate with iliac vein injuries. *J Trauma* 1990;30:320.
19. Sung CK, Kim KH. Missed injuries in abdominal trauma. *J Trauma* 1996;41:276.
20. Hirshberg A, Wall MJ, Mattox KL. Planned reoperation for trauma: a two year experience with 124 consecutive patients. *J Trauma* 1994;37:365.
21. Fernandez L, Norwood S, Roettger R, et al. Temporary intravenous bag silo closure in severe abdominal trauma. *J Trauma* 1996;40:258.

21. DIAPHRAGMATIC INJURIES[1]

Diaphragmatic injuries can be extremely important. They are often associated with severe abdominal or thoracic injuries, and the mortality rates with this injury may be as high as 40% with blunt trauma and 15% for penetrating trauma (2,3). In addition, if the injury is not recognized and bowel herniates into the chest and later strangulates, the resultant sepsis is frequently fatal.

INCIDENCE

AXIOM Diaphragmatic injuries should be suspected with all penetrating wounds of the lower chest and with severe blunt abdominal trauma.

The diaphragm is lacerated in at least 10% to 15% of penetrating wounds to the chest in most series. If the chest wound is anterior and below the nipple line, the diaphragm is injured up to 50% of the time (4). Between 1980 and 1992, the incidence of diaphragmatic injuries at Detroit Receiving Hospital was 20% (273 of 1,358) with gunshot wounds of the abdomen and 15% (119 of 810) with stab wounds.

It is estimated that 2% to 3% of all patients with blunt chest trauma have a diaphragmatic injury (4). In those hospitalized for multiple injuries following motor vehicle accidents, the incidence doubles to about 4% to 8%. Over the 12-year period of 1980 to 1992, 420 patients were admitted to Detroit Receiving Hospital with diaphragmatic injuries, and only 28 (6.7%) of the injuries were due to blunt trauma. Of 573 patients with blunt trauma to intraabdominal organs, only 4.9% involved the diaphragm.

ANATOMY

The word *diaphragm* comes from the Greek and means a partition or wall. The thoracoabdominal diaphragm is a large fan or dome-shaped sheet of skeletal muscle and fascia separating the chest and abdominal cavities. It is attached anteriorly to the xiphoid cartilage and to the inner surface of the cartilages and bony portions of the six lowest ribs where it interdigitates with the transversalis muscle. Posteriorly it is attached to two aponeurotic arches (the internal and external arcuate ligaments) and to the lumbar vertebrae.

Two crura, or pillars, lie on the bodies of the lumbar vertebrae on either side of the aorta. The right crus is larger and longer than the left and arises from the anterior surface of the upper three or four lumbar vertebrae. The left crus arises from the first two lumbar vertebrae. The tendinous portions of the crura converge slightly to the left of the midline to form an arch, beneath which pass the aorta, azygous vein, and thoracic duct.

There are three large and several smaller openings in the diaphragm. The aortic opening, at the level of the eleventh thoracic vertebra, is the lowest and most posterior of the three large openings. The aortic opening also contains the azygous vein and thoracic duct. The esophageal opening at the level of the tenth thoracic vertebra contains the esophagus, vagus nerves, and some small esophageal arteries. The opening for the inferior vena cava is at a level between the eighth and ninth thoracic vertebra at the junction of the right and middle leaflets of the central tendon.

The left and right halves of the diaphragm are innervated primarily by the ipsilateral phrenic nerves. The phrenic nerves arise from the third, fourth, and fifth anterior cervical nerve roots and course along the mediastinum on the pericardial surface. Each phrenic nerve inserts into the diaphragm at the junction of the

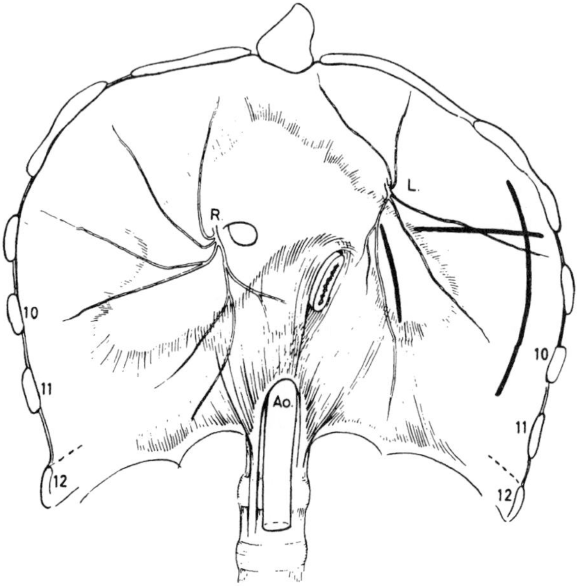

FIG. 21-1. Inferior aspect of the diaphragm, showing its origins, the course of the phrenic nerves, and the relation of three common incisions to the phrenic nerve branches (From Gibbon JH, ed. *Surgery of the chest.* Philadelphia: WB Saunders, 1962:526.)

pericardium and central tendon, at which point a crow's foot configuration of four to five branches splays laterally (Fig. 21-1).

PHYSIOLOGY

During quiet inspiration, the diaphragm provides 75% of the tidal volume. When larger intrathoracic volumes are needed, the accessory muscles of inspiration (the scalenes, sternocleidomastoid, and external oblique muscles) provide progressively more help. During passive exhalation, the right leaflet rises anteriorly to the fourth intercostal space and the left leaflet rises anteriorly to the fifth intercostal space. With forced inspiration and expiration, the total excursion of the top of the diaphragm may exceed 10 cm.

ETIOLOGY OF DIAPHRAGMATIC INJURIES

Penetrating Injuries

Because the diaphragm normally rises to the level of the fourth and fifth ribs, it is frequently perforated by stab wounds to the anterior chest below the nipple line. Gunshot wounds can traverse the diaphragm in virtually any direction from almost any entrance site in the chest or abdomen. Wounds from knives and bullets usually produce small (1 to 2 cm) holes in the diaphragm.

Because of the pressure gradient between the negative pressure in the thorax and positive pressure in the abdomen, many holes in the diaphragm will not heal spontaneously, and abdominal viscera can gradually herniate into the chest. Marchand (5) has pointed out that the pressure gradient between the pleural and peritoneal cavities varies between 7 and 20 cm H_2O normally, and with maximal inspiration, it may exceed 100 cm H_2O.

Blunt Trauma

During blunt abdominal trauma, intraperitoneal pressure may increase from a normal of 2 to 10 cm H_2O to more than 1,000 cm H_2O (6). The fusion lines of the individual leaflets during the development of the diaphragm running posterolaterally out from the central tendon seem most predisposed to rupture. When a tear occurs as a result of blunt trauma, it is usually at least 5 cm long, and one or more intraabdominal organs usually herniate through the defect into the chest. With blunt trauma, the rupture is in the left diaphragm in 65% to 85% of injuries, in the right diaphragm in 15% to 35%, and bilateral in 1% of the injuries (7).

The left diaphragm is more often torn because the liver protects the right side. Kearney et al. (8) have noted that diaphragmatic injuries caused by motor vehicle accidents seem to result more from lateral impact than from frontal collisions and that right lateral impact accounts for the majority of right-sided diaphragmatic injuries.

In most series, only one organ is herniated into the chest, and the stomach is involved more than half the time. The other organs that tend to herniate into the left chest are, in decreasing order of frequency, the colon, omentum, spleen, and small bowel.

AXIOM Blunt disruptions of the diaphragm are usually associated with herniation of all or part of the liver into the right chest and stomach into the left chest.

PATHOPHYSIOLOGY

Hemodynamic Changes

The hemodynamic instability so often seen with blunt diaphragmatic injury is usually a result of associated injuries; however, the herniated viscera can cause a reduction in venous return. At the Montreal General Hospital, roughly one-third of the patients with diaphragmatic injury were hypotensive while in the emergency department (9). In addition, in the rare instances in which the diaphragmatic pericardium is torn, displacement of visceral organs into the pericardial cavity can interfere with ventricular filling and produce hypotension by a mechanism similar to pericardial tamponade (6,10).

AXIOM A clinical picture of pericardial tamponade and bowel obstruction after blunt abdominal trauma should suggest the presence of an intrapericardial rupture of the diaphragm.

Pulmonary Changes

As an increasing volume of abdominal viscera enters the chest, vital capacity progressively decreases and the injured diaphragm may not work as efficiently. Indeed, in the Angood and Mulder series (9), all of the hypotensive patients were hypoxic to varying degrees, and almost one-third required emergency department endotracheal intubation and ventilatory support as part of their initial management.

AXIOM In older individuals with a delayed diaphragmatic hernia, symptoms of dyspnea, chest pain, and fatigue may be presumed erroneously to be myocardial in origin.

Bowel Obstruction or Strangulation

Hollow viscera in the chest eventually become incarcerated and obstructed. The diaphragmatic opening often acts as a one-way valve, causing the bowel to distend progressively in the chest, until it ruptures. Leaking gastric contents can cause a severe chemical pleuritis, which usually becomes infected within 12 to 24 hours.

Spillage of colon contents into the chest almost invariably causes a rapidly progressive sepsis.

ASSOCIATED INJURIES

In the 1980–1992 Detroit Receiving Hospital series of diaphragmatic injuries, the incidence of associated liver injuries was 48% (57 of 119) with stab wounds and 69% (128 of 273) with gunshot wounds. The next most common associated injuries with penetrating diaphragmatic trauma were the stomach (30%, 116 of 392) and spleen (26%, 102 of 392). The pulmonary injuries associated with penetrating wounds of the diaphragm are often located peripherally and usually require no treatment except placement of a chest tube. However, in Wiencek's series, 18% required a thoracotomy for repair of a lung injury (2).

In one series, more than 50% of the patients with blunt diaphragmatic trauma also had a pelvic fracture (11). Most of the associated injuries were orthopedic, and Wiencek's series noted an average of 3.2 associated injuries per patient (2).

DIAGNOSIS

In 1951, Carter et al. (12) divided the initial presentation of traumatic diaphragmatic hernias into three phases: acute, interval or latent, and obstructive.

It has been estimated that a correct diagnosis of *acute* diaphragmatic injury is made in only 40% to 60% of patients with blunt trauma within 24 to 48 hours of injury (3,12). If the injury is not diagnosed during the acute phase, the latent phase begins. The patient may either be completely asymptomatic during this phase or have only vague, nonspecific complaints, which are often attributed to problems with other organ systems (e.g., biliary or coronary artery disease).

The obstructive phase may occur weeks to years after the original injury and starts when an abdominal organ becomes incarcerated in the diaphragmatic defect.

History and Physical Examination

Any stab or gunshot wound of the chest below the nipple, especially anterior, should be suspected of injuring the diaphragm. Even "trivial" knife wounds can result eventually in strangulation of herniated bowel. With blunt trauma, any history of sudden severe deceleration or crushing should make one suspect a diaphragmatic injury.

The symptoms in a patient with an acute diaphragmatic tear are usually nonspecific (shortness of breath or vague abdominal or chest pain) (13) or are related to obvious associated injuries. Occasionally, a patient has top-of-shoulder pain (Kehr's sign) with an injury to the diaphragm.

There are no external signs that are pathognomonic for diaphragmatic injury; however, if there are decreased breath sounds in the left chest, if the abdomen is scaphoid, and if bowel sounds are heard high in the chest, a diaphragmatic injury should be suspected. Patients with a large diaphragmatic injury who require urgent surgery are usually tachycardic, hypotensive, and dyspneic to a greater degree than the magnitude of the apparent injuries would suggest.

If sudden severe respiratory distress develops when the abdominal portion of a pneumatic antishock garment is inflated, the abdominal portion should be deflated immediately and the possibility of a diaphragmatic injury investigated.

Radiologic Studies

Chest Film

AXIOM The single most useful noninvasive technique for diagnosing diaphragmatic injury is an upright chest radiograph.

In Wiencek's series, 56% of the patients with penetrating diaphragmatic injuries had a hemothorax or pneumothorax (2). In patients with entrance wounds in the chest, this is a nonspecific finding; however, in the 65 patients in Wiencek's series with abdominal entrance wounds, x-ray evidence of a hemopneumothorax in 22 (34%) was considered diagnostic.

Although the chest radiograph is almost always abnormal with blunt diaphragmatic injury, the radiologic findings are diagnostic in only about 16% to 30% of the cases. Radiographic findings strongly suggestive of a diaphragmatic injury include a very high diaphragmatic shadow (Fig. 21-2), the presence of herniated bowel in the chest, or the nasogastric tube passing from the abdomen high up into the left hemithorax.

AXIOM Any abnormal shadows in the left lower lung fields after trauma should make one suspect a diaphragmatic injury.

With opacification of the lower hemithorax and slight shifting of the mediastinal structures to the opposite side, it is easy to assume that a hemothorax is present. Caution, however, must be taken when inserting a chest tube until diaphragmatic rupture has been ruled out. This can be done by obtaining lateral decubitus films or overpenetrated radiographs, which may reveal a typical bowel gas pattern in the chest.

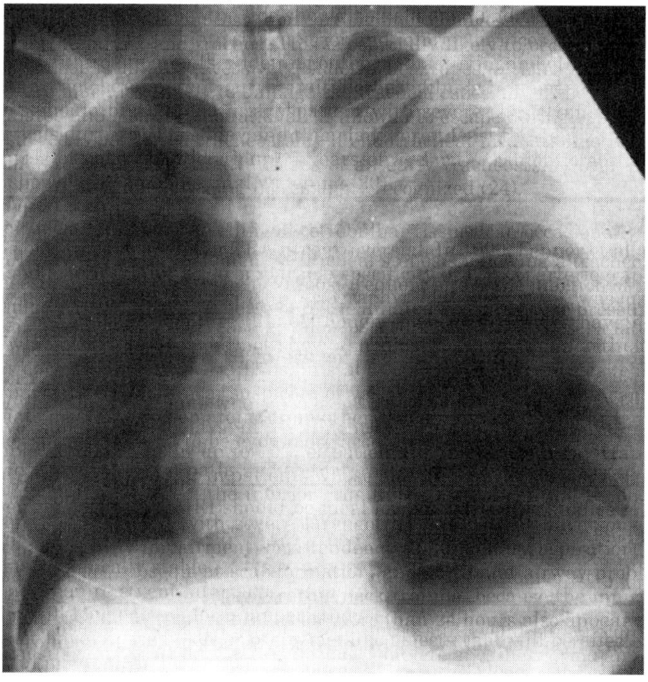

FIG. 21-2. Traumatic rupture of the diaphragm. Plain chest radiograph showing displacement of air-filled viscera, especially the stomach, into the left lower chest (From Orringer MB, Kirsh MM. Traumatic rupture of the diaphragm. In: Kirsh MM, Sloan H, eds. *Blunt chest trauma—general principles of management.* Boston: Little, Brown and Company, 1977;6:134.

With an injured diaphragm on the right, all that is usually seen on chest radiograph is an apparently elevated diaphragm because of the herniated dome of the liver; however, separate inspiratory and expiratory chest radiographs may demonstrate a stationary lateral diaphragmatic leaflet with movement of the herniated liver.

If positive-pressure ventilation is provided soon after admission, it may prevent herniation of abdominal viscera into the chest through a diaphragmatic defect. The injury may become apparent only when the patient begins to breathe spontaneously and the intrathoracic pressure decreases below that of the abdominal cavity.

If a diaphragmatic injury is suspected, a nasogastric tube should be carefully inserted and connected to low continuous suction. If the nasogastric tube enters the abdomen normally and then curls up into the left chest above the diaphragm, this is virtually diagnostic of a ruptured diaphragm.

Contrast Studies

AXIOM A contrast study of the upper gastrointestinal tract is the most accurate radiologic test for diaphragmatic ruptures on the left.

The stomach, small bowel, spleen, liver, and colon are the organs most likely to herniate into the chest. Contrast material delivered through an indwelling nasogastric tube can usually clearly demonstrate displacement of the stomach into the chest. Follow-through films may also show small bowel that has herniated through the diaphragm. A barium enema may be helpful if colon has herniated into the chest.

Computed Tomography Scans

The integrity of the diaphragm on computed tomography (CT) scan is largely inferred by examining the relationship of the organs above and below it. Thus, a diaphragmatic hernia is usually diagnosed positively with CT only if there is protrusion of abdominal viscera above the remaining visualized portions of the diaphragm.

Magnetic Resonance Imaging

The unique ability of magnetic resonance imaging (MRI) to visualize the body in all planes allows easier coronal and sagittal depiction of the diaphragm. The drawback to using MRI is that patients must be remarkably stable to have an MRI, and this is difficult to ensure immediately after severe trauma.

Ultrasound

A properly performed ultrasound study can detect organs herniated above diaphragmatic injuries and may be helpful in patients whose condition is too poor to permit safe transportation to the radiology department. Echocardiography may also detect an intrapericardial diaphragmatic hernia (14).

Thoracoscopy and Laparoscopy

Ochsner et al. (15) described the use of thoracoscopy to rule out diaphragmatic injury in 14 patients with penetrating injuries of the lower chest. The diaphragmatic injuries found in nine of the patients were repaired at laparotomy, but there were two major complications including a subphrenic abscess and empyema in one patient and bleeding from a laceration of the lung in another.

Ivatury and colleagues (16) reported on diagnostic laparoscopy performed in 23 patients with a total of 17 stab wounds and six gunshot wounds of the lower chest or upper abdomen. Unsuspected diaphragmatic injury was found in five of these eight patients.

Using diagnostic laparoscopy, Salvino et al. (17) found that 3 of 15 patients with stab wounds had injuries to the diaphragm. All three had less than 10,000 red blood cells (RBC)/mm^3 on diagnostic peritoneal lavage (DPL), but the injury was easily seen on diagnostic laparoscopy.

Diagnostic Peritoneal Lavage

AXIOM A negative DPL does not rule out diaphragmatic injury. False-negative DPLs have been noted in up to 36% of blunt diaphragmatic disruptions and in up to 40% of penetrating diaphragmatic injuries (18).

The number of red cells that constitutes a positive DPL for a penetrating diaphragmatic injury varies considerably from author to author. Even with greatly reduced RBC criteria of 5,000 to 20,000/mm^3, diaphragmatic perforations can still be missed by DPL.

Other evidence suggesting a diaphragm injury during DPL is increasing dyspnea, reduced return of the lavage fluid, or DPL fluid coming out a previously placed chest tube.

Diagnosis at Surgery

AXIOM Most penetrating injuries of the diaphragm are discovered incidentally during exploratory surgery (3).

To reduce the incidence of missed diaphragmatic injury, Madden et al. (19) reported on 95 patients who had a laparotomy for penetrating injury to the lower chest or upper abdomen. Eighteen (19%) had diaphragmatic injury, but only one had any evidence of herniation on preoperative x-ray examination. On the basis of their findings, the authors proposed that stab wounds of the epigastrium or of the left chest in the "D-zone" (below the fourth intercostal space anteriorly, the sixth intercostal space laterally, and the eighth interspace posteriorly) require celiotomy until a reliable nonoperative method is described.

Patients have had diaphragmatic injuries missed at laparotomy. Proper inspection involves pulling the spleen and the fundus of the stomach down on the left and the liver down on the right. Blind palpation of the diaphragm is not adequate.

TREATMENT OF ACUTE INJURIES

Patients with diaphragmatic injuries frequently have associated intraabdominal or thoracic injuries. The associated abdominal injuries may result in significant blood loss and the associated thoracic injuries may add to the cardiorespiratory dysfunction. Bagging with a mask can increase the amount of bowel distension and herniation into the chest.

⊘ PITFALL

Nitrous oxide should be avoided in patients with a possible diaphragmatic hernia, because it can greatly increase the volume of gas within entrapped viscera.

Virtually all acute diaphragmatic injuries can be repaired from within the abdomen through a midline vertical incision. This approach also affords exposure for the repair of the associated intraabdominal injuries, which are frequently present. If a thoracotomy incision is used, a double-lumen endotracheal tube and one-lung anesthesia can assist in providing optimal conditions for exposing the diaphragmatic injury.

Simple lacerations of the diaphragm with wounds less than 2.0 cm in length can be securely repaired by 0 or 2-0 slowly absorbable or nonabsorbable interrupted horizontal mattress sutures. Because the sutures at the medial end of the tear can inadvertently include branches of the phrenic nerve, they should be placed very carefully.

With defects larger than 2 cm, a two-layer closure should be considered because diaphragm muscle can tear easily. An initial layer of horizontal mattress sutures can be used to evert the torn edges of the diaphragm toward the abdomen, and this can be reinforced with a running suture.

Chest Tubes

Even if a hemopneumothorax is not already present, exposure and repair of a tear in the diaphragm almost always allow entry of significant amounts of air into the chest. The resultant pneumothorax should be evacuated following the repair. This can be accomplished sometimes by placing a tube through the tear and then removing it after the repair is completed; however, we prefer to leave a chest tube in place for at least 24 to 48 hours in case there is any unrecognized injury causing continued bleeding or an air leak. The chest tube also evacuates any residual air or blood more completely.

Postoperative Morbidity and Mortality

Postoperative complications are frequent with diaphragmatic injury and most commonly include atelectasis and pneumonia. These patients may require prolonged postoperative ventilator support because of the diaphragmatic injury as well as the high incidence of associated injuries to the lung and chest wall.

The mortality rate for blunt diaphragmatic rupture ranges from 16% to 41% (2,3,18). In the 12-year Detroit Receiving Hospital series, it was 25% (7 of 28) for blunt trauma, 8% for stab wounds, 21% for gunshot wounds, and 42% for shotgun wounds.

DELAYED RECOGNITION OF DIAPHRAGMATIC INJURY

Incidence

The frequency of missed diaphragmatic injuries and subsequent late presentation is difficult to estimate, but de la Rocha et al. (20) have estimated that about 30% of diaphragmatic injuries are diagnosed late. If strangulation of herniated bowel develops, it occurs within 3 years of the initial injury in about 85% of cases.

AXIOM Absence of a history of trauma does not rule out a delayed traumatic diaphragmatic hernia.

Diagnosis

Stab wounds are the most common cause of delayed traumatic diaphragmatic hernias, and the risk of strangulation is high because the defects are generally small. In more than 85% of patients with a delayed diagnosis of a diaphragmatic hernia, symptoms of intestinal obstruction develop as a result of incarceration of bowel in the hernia. Without prompt therapy, this can rapidly progress to strangulation and necrosis.

Signs and Symptoms

AXIOM Signs and symptoms of a bowel obstruction after previous trauma are usually due to adhesions, but one should also look for hernias, especially in the diaphragm.

As abdominal viscera increasingly herniate into the chest, vague symptoms of abdominal cramping and nausea may develop, suggesting the presence of an incomplete bowel obstruction. In some instances, chest pain or shortness of breath may develop, suggesting pulmonary or cardiac disease.

Occasionally, massive dilatation of the stomach or intestine in the chest can produce severe dyspnea with what we have referred to as a “tension enterothorax.” Perforation of bowel can produce a similar picture with pneumothorax and a large pleural effusion. Rarely, abdominal contents herniate into the pericardial cavity and cause a clinical picture of acute pericardial tamponade (10).

Radiologic Studies

The chest radiograph usually remains normal in the presence of old penetrating injuries of the diaphragm until significant abdominal contents have herniated into the chest. Once bowel has herniated into the chest, upper or lower intestinal contrast studies can be very sensitive (21). Right-sided diaphragmatic injuries can be particularly difficult to visualize, even on CT scan, because the torn portion of the diaphragm blends into the liver contour.

AXIOM Once a delayed presentation of a traumatic diaphragmatic hernia is suspected, barium studies of the gastrointestinal tract are the most reliable means of confirming the diagnosis (21).

It can be extremely difficult at times to differentiate a traumatic diaphragmatic hernia from an eventration of the diaphragm. A pneumoperitoneum may be helpful in making this differentiation; however, this test may be negative if adhesions have sealed the hole in the diaphragm (21).

Treatment

If bowel obstruction is not present, patients undergoing surgery after the acute phase of injury should undergo a full cathartic and antibiotic bowel preparation. This can help reduce the incidence and severity of sepsis if an enterotomy is inadvertently performed during the release of bowel that has become adhered to the lung and other structures.

AXIOM Surgery for a diaphragmatic hernia caused by remote trauma is usually best done through a posterolateral thoracotomy incision.

Diaphragmatic injuries away from the pericardium that are repaired more than 1 week following trauma are often approached best through a thoracotomy incision, particularly if there is a significant amount of herniated bowel in the chest. Herniated bowel quickly adheres to the lung because there is no peritoneal hernia sac, and release of these adhesions through a laparotomy incision can be extremely difficult.

Caution must also be taken when manipulating herniated abdominal organs back into the peritoneal cavity. Unrecognized injury to the herniated organs can lead to severe complications. In some instances, a separate abdominal incision may be required to facilitate return of the organs to the abdomen. In some cases the herniated organs are damaged so badly that they have to be resected. After the bowel and any other herniated abdominal viscera are returned to the peritoneal cavity, a standard two-layer diaphragm closure is performed.

Occasionally, long-standing large diaphragmatic hernias require closure of the defect with prosthetic material, such as Marlex, Dacron, or Prolene mesh. This is most common following chronic rents in which large portions of the liver or bowel have herniated into the chest for several months, leaving a defect that may exceed 10 to 15 cm in diameter. Experience with latissimus dorsi or external oblique muscle flaps and omentum for reconstruction has also been good.

Outcome

Correction of a chronic diaphragmatic hernia in the absence of strangulation or a bowel leak is usually tolerated well. However, the mortality rate may be as high as 20% for late incarceration and ranges from 25% to 66% if the bowel becomes strangulated (13,18). Indeed, Hegarty et al. (22) noted mortality rates as high as 80% when bowel strangulation progressed to gangrene.

⊘ FREQUENT ERRORS

1. ***Failure to suspect a diaphragmatic injury with penetrating trauma to the lower chest or upper abdomen or with severe blunt thoracoabdominal trauma.***
2. ***Failure to suspect a diaphragmatic injury if a chest radiograph shows abnormal shadows in the lower lung fields or does not show the diaphragms well.***
3. ***Failure to rule out herniated viscera in patients who appear to have a loculated lower pneumothorax after thoracoabdominal trauma.***
4. ***Ruling out a diaphragmatic injury because a diagnostic peritoneal lavage is negative.***
5. ***Use of nitrous oxide for anesthesia in patients with a traumatic diaphragmatic hernia.***
6. ***Failure to be aware of the possibility of catching phrenic nerve branches with the sutures used to repair the medial portion of a large diaphragmatic tear.***

SUMMARY POINTS

1. One should suspect diaphragmatic injuries with all penetrating wounds of the lower chest and with severe blunt abdominal trauma.

2. No injury to the diaphragm is so small that it can be considered safe from later herniation.

3. Blunt disruptions of the diaphragm are usually associated with herniation of all or part of the liver into the right chest and stomach into the left chest.

4. The phrenic nerve is more likely to be injured during the repair of a diaphragmatic tear than by the original trauma.

5. If it is necessary to widen a diaphragmatic defect to facilitate reduction of herniated organs into the abdomen, the incision in the diaphragm should be extended laterally away from the phrenic nerve branches.

6. A clinical picture of pericardial tamponade and bowel obstruction after blunt abdominal trauma should suggest the presence of an intrapericardial rupture of the diaphragm.

7. In older individuals with a delayed diaphragmatic hernia, symptoms of dyspnea, chest pain, and fatigue may be erroneously presumed to be myocardial in origin.

8. The single most frequently abnormal noninvasive method for diagnosing diaphragmatic injury is an upright chest radiograph.

9. Any abnormal shadows in the left lower lung field after trauma on chest x-ray study should make one suspect a diaphragmatic injury.

10. A contrast study of the upper gastrointestinal tract is the most accurate radiologic test for diaphragmatic rupture on the left.

11. A negative DPL does not rule out diaphragmatic injury.

12. Most penetrating injuries of the diaphragm are discovered incidentally during exploratory surgery.

13. The most common reason for missing diaphragmatic tears during laparotomy is failure to inspect the leaflets thoroughly, especially posteriorly.

14. Nitrous oxide should be avoided in patients with a possible diaphragmatic hernia because it can greatly increase the volume of gas within entrapped viscera.

15. Signs and symptoms of a bowel obstruction after prior trauma are usually due to adhesions, but one should also look for hernias, especially in the diaphragm.

16. Rapid dilatation of bowel herniated into the chest can cause severe shortness of breath, and the radiographic appearance occasionally resembles a pneumothorax.

17. If a diaphragmatic hernia is not diagnosed until herniated bowel becomes strangulated and perforated, the mortality rate is very high.

18. Surgery for a diaphragmatic hernia resulting from old trauma is usually best done through a posterolateral thoracotomy incision.

REFERENCES

1. Wilson RF, Bender J. Diaphragmatic injuries. In: Wilson RF, Walt AJ, eds. *Management of trauma,* 2nd ed. Philadelphia: Williams & Wilkins 1996:432.
2. Wiencek RG, Wilson, RF, Steiger Z. Acute injuries of the diaphragm. An analysis of 165 cases. *J Thorac Cardiovasc Surg* 1986;92:989.
3. Symbas PN, Vlasis SE, Hatcher CR Jr. Blunt and penetrating diaphragmatic injuries with or without herniation of organs into the chest. *Ann Thorac Surg* 1986;42:158.
4. Beeson A, Popovici Z. Diaphragmatic injuries. Invited Comment in Thoracic Surgery: Surgical Management of Chest Injuries. In: Webb WR, Beeson A, eds. St. Louis: Mosby–Year Book, 1991:317–322.
5. Marchand P. A study of the forces productive of gastro-oesophageal regurgitation and herniation through the diaphragmatic hiatus. *Thorax* 1957;12:189.
6. Van Loenhout RM, Schiphurst TJ, Wittens CH, et al. Traumatic intrapericardial diaphragmatic hernia. *J Trauma* 1986;26:271.
7. Humphreys TR, Abbuhl S. Massive bilateral diaphragmatic rupture after an apparently minor automobile accident. *Am J Emerg Med* 1991;9:246–249.
8. Kearney PA, Rouhana SW, Burney RE. Blunt rupture of the diaphragm mechanism; diagnosis and treatment. *Ann Emerg Med* 1990;18:105.
9. Angood PB, Mulder DS. Rupture of the diaphragm. In: Cameron JL, ed. *Current surgical therapy.* Philadelphia: BC Decker, 1989:657–661.
10. Nelson RM, Wilson RF, Huang CL, et al. Cardiac tamponade due to an iatrogenic pericardial-diaphragmatic hernia. *Crit Care Med* 1985;13:607.
11. Rodriquez-Morales G, Rodriquez A, Shatney CH. Acute rupture of the diaphragm in blunt trauma. *J Trauma* 1986;26:438.
12. Carter BM, Giuseffi J, Felson F. Traumatic diaphragmatic hernia. *AJR Am J Roentgenol* 1951;65:56.
13. Saber WL, Moore EE, Hopeman AR, et al. Delayed presentation of traumatic diaphragmatic hernia. *J Emerg Med* 1986;4:1.
14. Colliver C, Oller DW, Rose G, et al. Traumatic intra-pericardial diaphragmatic hernia diagnosed by echocardiography. *J Trauma* 1997;42:115.
15. Ochsner MG, Rozycki GS, Lucente F, et al. Prospective evaluation of thoracoscopy for diagnosing diaphragmatic injury in thoracoabdominal trauma: a preliminary report. *J Trauma* 1993;34:704.
16. Ivatury RR, Simon RJ, Weksler B, et al. Laparoscopy in the evaluation of the intrathoracic abdomen after penetrating injury. *J Trauma* 1992;33:101.
17. Salvino CK, Esposito TJ, Marshall WJ, et al. The role of diagnostic laparoscopy in the management of trauma patients: a preliminary assessment. *J Trauma* 1993; 34:507.
18. Root HD. Injury to the diaphragm. In: Moore EE, Mattox KL, Feliciano DV, eds. *Trauma,* 2nd ed. Norwalk, CT: Appleton & Lange, 1991;427–439.
19. Madden M, Paull D, Shires GT, et al. Occult diaphragmatic injury from stab wounds to the lower chest and abdomen. *J Trauma* 1989;29:292.
20. de la Rocha AG, Creel RJ, Mulligan GW, et al. Diaphragmatic rupture due to blunt abdominal trauma. *Surg Gynecol Obstet* 1982;154:175.
21. McHugh K, Ogilvie BC, Brunton FJ. Delayed presentation of traumatic diaphragmatic hernia. *Clin Radiol* 1991;43:246.
22. Hegarty MM, Bryer JV, Angorn IB, et al. Delayed presentation of traumatic diaphragmatic hernia. *Ann Surg* 1978;188:229–233.

22. INJURIES TO THE LIVER AND BILIARY TRACT[1]

ANATOMY

The liver, with its name derived from the old English "life," is indeed vital to human existence, and survival without it is impossible for more than a few hours except under very unusual circumstances. Its average weight is about 1,400 to 1,700 g in men and 1,200 to 1,500 g in women. Its average largest dimensions are 22 cm transversely, 17 cm vertically, and 12 cm in the anteroposterior dimension.

Anatomic studies of the hepatic vessels and bile ducts have demonstrated that the right and left lobes of the liver are separated by a plane (Cantlie's line) running from the gallbladder fossa to the inferior vena cava. This cleavage plane is devoid of major branches of the portal vein, hepatic artery, and bile ducts, but it frequently contains a portion of the middle hepatic vein. The lobes in turn can be divided into a total of eight segments (Fig. 22-1).

Virtually all of the blood perfusing the gastrointestinal tract in the abdomen drains into the liver via the portal vein. The hepatic artery supplies about 25% of the liver blood flow and almost 50% of its oxygen, with the portal vein providing the remainder. Hepatic artery anomalies are frequent and occur in about 10% to 28% of patients. These include an anomalous origin of the common or right hepatic artery from the superior mesenteric artery in about 8% to 18% of patients and an anomalous origin or accessory left hepatic artery off the left gastric artery in about 4% to 8% of cases.

The three main hepatic veins are primarily intraparenchymal structures, and their extrahepatic length before entering the cava is only about 1 to 2 cm. The right and

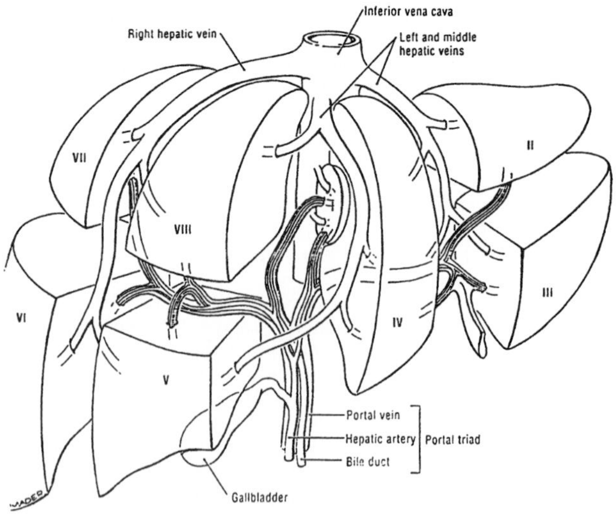

FIG. 22-1. Segmental and vascular anatomy of the liver: Each segment of the liver is supplied by a branch of the hepatic artery, bile duct, and portal vein. The hepatic veins do not follow the structures of the portal triad and are considered intersegmental in that they drain portions of adjacent segments (From Agur AMR, Lee MJ, eds. *Grant's atlas of anatomy,* 9th ed. Baltimore: Williams & Wilkins, 1991:115.)

left hepatic veins enter the cava directly, but 84% of the time the middle hepatic vein drains into the left hepatic vein near its junction with the inferior vena cava (2). There are also about 10 to 20 small hepatic veins draining directly from the caudate lobe into the retrohepatic inferior vena cava. The short extrahepatic length of the major hepatic veins and the relatively inaccessible retrohepatic cava can make exposure and control of these vessels, when they are injured, extremely difficult.

ETIOLOGY OF LIVER INJURIES

Penetrating Trauma

Of 2,168 patients with penetrating abdominal trauma admitted to Detroit Receiving Hospital (1980–1992), 750 (35%) involved the liver. Of those that involved the liver, 475 (63%) were caused by gunshot wounds (GSWs), 251 (34%) by stab wounds, and 24 (3%) by shotgun wounds (SGWs). The only abdominal organ injured more frequently by penetrating trauma was the small bowel (jejunum and ileum), which was injured in 1,001 cases (46%).

For the 750 patients with penetrating liver trauma, the most frequent associated abdominal injuries were of the diaphragm (32%), abdominal vessels (24%), stomach (23%), colon (19%), and jejunum and ileum (15%). Only 162 (18%) of the patients had isolated penetrating liver injuries.

Blunt Trauma

Of 573 patients having laparotomies at Detroit Receiving Hospital from 1980 to 1992 for blunt abdominal injuries, 160 (28%) had liver trauma, making liver injury second only to spleen injury (30%). Typically, more than 90% of blunt hepatic injuries are accompanied by damage to other intraabdominal organs, especially the spleen, kidney, and intestine. For the 160 patients with blunt liver trauma seen at Detroit Receiving Hospital from 1980 to 1992, the most frequent associated abdominal injuries were the spleen (24%), abdominal vessels (14%), and kidney (13%).

DIAGNOSIS OF LIVER INJURIES

Patients with GSWs to the abdomen undergo exploration routinely and do not generally present any diagnostic problem. Blunt abdominal trauma, however, may be a diagnostic challenge even for the most experienced clinicians, particularly when patients are inebriated or have concomitant head or high spinal cord injury.

Clinical Examination

Any recent history of trauma to the right upper quadrant of the abdomen or right lower chest should signal the presence of a possible hepatic injury. Pain referred to the right shoulder may also be caused by a liver injury.

Any patient with a stab wound to the abdomen and hypotension, abdominal distension, or tenderness requires immediate operative intervention without any diagnostic tests.

Diagnostic Peritoneal Lavage

Diagnostic peritoneal lavage (DPL) can be helpful for evaluating patients with suspected intraabdominal injuries when (1) suspicion is high and clinical signs are lacking or (2) patients have an altered sensorium as a result of drugs, alcohol, or head trauma. If a tractotomy reveals the abdominal fascia has been penetrated by a stab wound, DPL can be performed with an accuracy rate of 90% to 95%; however, a hemodynamically stable patient with a positive DPL resulting from increased red cells from what is probably just an isolated solid organ injury often can undergo nonoperative treatment.

Computed Tomography Scans

If an isolated liver injury is strongly suspected in a hemodynamically stable patient, computed tomography (CT) scanning is often the only diagnostic test required. The CT scan can also be used to classify the severity of the liver injury (Table 22-1).

TABLE 22–1. *Liver Injury Scale*

	Grade[a]	Injury Description[b]	AIS[c] 90
I.	Hematoma	Subcapcular, nonexpanding, <10% surface area	1
	Laceration	Capsular tear, nonbleeding, <1 cm parenchymal depth	
II.	Hematoma	Subcapsular, nonexpanding, 10%–50% surface area	2
		Intraparenchymal, nonexpanding, <2 cm in diameter	
	Laceration	Capsular tear, active bleeding, 1–3 cm parenchymal depth, <10 cm	
III.	Hematoma	Subcapsular, >50% surface area or expanding	3
		Ruptured subcapsular hematoma with active bleeding	
		Intraparenchymal hematoma >2 cm or expanding	
	Laceration	>3 cm parenchymal depth	3
IV.	Hematoma	Ruptured intraparenchymal hematoma with active bleeding	4
	Laceration	Parenchymal disruption involving 25%–50% of hepatic lobe	4
V.	Laceration	Parenchymal disruption involving >58% of hepatic lobe	5
	Vascular	Juxtahepatic venous injuries; i.e., retrohepatic vena cava/major hepatic veins	5
VI.	Vascular	Hepatic avulsion	6

[a]Advance one grade for multiple injuries to the same organ.
[b]Based on most accurate assessment at autopsy, laparotomy, or radiologic study.
From Moore EE, Shackford SR, Pachter HL, et al. Organ injury scaling: spleen, liver, kidney. *J Trauma* 1989;29:1664.
[c]AIS—abbreviated injury score.

CT scans are accurate for determining the presence and severity of liver injuries; however, they are *not* very accurate for excluding injuries to the small bowel, especially past the proximal jejunum. In addition, some diaphragmatic and pancreatic injuries can be missed. Consequently, if a liver injury is diagnosed on the CT scan but there is an equivocal abdominal examination or inability to closely monitor the patient, such as during prolonged nonabdominal operations, a DPL should be performed.

AXIOM DPL and abdominal CT scanning should be considered complementary (not competing) diagnostic tests in patients with abdominal trauma.

TREATMENT

Nonoperative Management of Blunt Hepatic Injuries

In patients with blunt abdominal trauma who have evidence of liver injury by CT scan but who do not demonstrate clinical evidence of significant continuing hemorrhage or peritoneal irritation, nonoperative management with close observation has been shown to be safe, particularly in children.

Transfusion Requirements

AXIOM Need for more than 2 units of blood in adults or replacement of more than half of the estimated blood volume in children to maintain stable vital signs is generally an indication for surgery in patients with isolated splenic or hepatic injuries.

If there is a progressive decrease in the hemoglobin levels in a hemodynamically stable patient, arteriography often reveals bleeding from one or more small hepatic artery branches. These can usually be controlled angiographically.

Success of Nonoperative Treatment

In one report, 30 (50%) of 60 patients with blunt hepatic injury were designated for nonoperative therapy (4). The grades of liver injury in the nonoperative group were I-3, II-7, III-14, IV-6, and V-0. There were no deaths, delayed laparotomies, or missed intraabdominal injuries in the nonoperative group; however, one patient required angiographic embolization of her hepatic injury 8 hours after admission because of continued bleeding. The time for resolution of the liver injuries as evidenced by CT scanning ranged from 18 to 88 days with a mean of 57 days.

In a multiinstitutional study (5) from 15 level I trauma centers, 40% of the adults with blunt liver injuries were managed nonoperatively. Of the patients initially selected for nonoperative therapy, only six required surgery (three for bleeding, two for missed enteric injuries, and one for persistent sepsis) and only two (0.4%) deaths could be attributed to the liver injuries.

Biliary Complications

AXIOM Even if the bleeding stops, some deeper liver injuries treated nonoperatively may require drainage of bile collections.

Of 106 patients with blunt liver trauma reported by Sugimoto et al. (6), 64 (60%) underwent nonoperative treatment. Of these 64 patients, a biloma requiring drainage developed in five. Consequently, patients with severe liver injuries treated nonoperatively should be considered for endoscopic retrograde cholangiography if there is any clinical or laboratory evidence of a bile duct injury.

In-Hospital Observation

When a nonoperative approach to blunt liver trauma is pursued, close in-hospital observation of the patient for at least several days is recommended. If serial hematocrit determinations (after fluid resuscitation) show no evidence of continued bleeding, the patient can be discharged on limited activity. Physical activity is slowly increased over the next 6 to 8 weeks. The patient should not participate in contact sports until a CT scan shows healing of the liver wounds.

Operative Management of Liver Injuries

The overwhelming majority of hepatic injuries are minor (grades I and II) and require no therapy or only simple sutures, electrocautery, or topical hemostatic agents. Complex hepatic injuries, on the other hand, often are still bleeding at the time of laparotomy and can be a challenge to the trauma surgeon.

AXIOM Once the major bleeding has been controlled, the patient should be fully resuscitated and warmed to at least 34°C to 35°C before the definitive surgery is performed.

Mobilization of the Liver

When bleeding hepatic wounds cannot be seen clearly, proper mobilization of the liver is extremely important. Such mobilization is usually begun by division of the round ligament anteriorly and then the falciform ligament over the anterior and superior aspect of the liver. Further mobilization of the individual hepatic lobes is achieved by division of the right or left triangular ligaments, leading to exposure of the anterior and superior surfaces of the respective lobes.

The left triangular ligament can usually be divided under direct vision. The right triangular ligament may have to be divided blindly, and, at times, ongoing hemorrhage may obscure the area. Care must be taken to palpate the tips of the scissors with the opposite and retracting hand to protect the inferior vena cava and right hepatic vein from injury during the posterior portion of the dissection. One must also be careful to avoid injury to the inferior phrenic vessels coursing along the underside of the diaphragm.

Controlling Bleeding from the Liver

Pringle Maneuver

The Pringle maneuver should be considered when bleeding from the injured liver continues despite the use of packs or if it resumes when the packs are removed later. The Pringle maneuver refers to occlusion of the portal triad at the foramen of Winslow, usually by application of a "soft" vascular clamp to the margin of the hepatoduodenal ligament. Failure of such inflow occlusion to adequately control hemorrhage suggests either an anomalous blood supply to the liver or the possibility of retrohepatic caval or juxtahepatic venous injury.

Traditionally, the clamp on the portal triad is released every 15 to 20 minutes for at least 5 minutes to allow intermittent hepatic perfusion. More recently, periods of complete inflow occlusion have been extended to more than an hour without evidence of ischemic damage to the liver.

The upper limit of normothermic occlusion of the liver in humans is presently unknown. Reports from France (7) have documented occlusion times up to 1 hour during elective hepatic cancer surgery without untoward effects. Indeed, a study by Delva et al. (8) reported normothermic liver ischemia times up to 90 minutes without subsequent complications.

Protecting the Ischemic Liver

Hypothermia. Experimental work by Bernhard et al. (9) demonstrated that dogs subjected to normothermic portal triad occlusion for greater than 40 minutes always died. When the dogs were made hypothermic (28°C–32°C), portal triad occlusion for up to 1 hour was tolerated by all the dogs. Thus, if the portal triad is anticipated to be clamped for more than 20 to 30 minutes, it may be wise to attempt topical hypothermia, preferably before portal triad occlusion, by applying cold saline "slush" directly onto the liver surface. Ideally, an intrahepatic temperative probe should be used to ensure that the liver is cooled to 27°C to 32°C. If central liver temperature readings exceed 32°C, additional "slush" should be applied around the liver to lower the temperature to the desired range (2).

Steroids. The rationale for using large doses of corticosteroids to prolong the safe hepatic ischemia time is based on the reports of Figueroa and Delpin (10). By pretreating experimental animals with methylprednisolone sodium succinate (Solu-Medrol), they were able to decrease the mortality rate from 100% to 10% when the portal triad was occluded for 30 minutes and to only a 50% mortality rate if the portal triad was occluded for 60 minutes.

Steroids Plus Hypothermia. Pachter et al. (11) reported on 44 patients with complex hepatic injuries in whom a combination of topical hypothermia and intravenous corticosteroids was used to prevent hepatic ischemic damage when the portal triad was occluded. Seventy percent of these patients had their portal triad cross-clamped for more than 20 minutes, 40% for longer than 30 minutes, and 7% for more than 1 hour. Serial measurements of liver function tests revealed an increase in hepatic enzymes corresponding to the length of ischemia time; however, all of the laboratory values returned to virtually normal levels before hospital discharge, and no patient experienced clinical hepatic dysfunction.

AXIOM If it appears that the portal triad may have to be occluded for more than 20 to 30 minutes, one should consider the use of topical hypothermia and possibly also massive intravenous corticosteroids.

Liver Suturing

Hepatic suturing is the most frequently used technique for achieving hemostasis from severe liver wounds. The careful placement of sutures, usually 2-0 or 1-0 chromic or Vicryl, on a long blunt-tipped liver needle in a mattress fashion, preferably with pledgets, across the site of injury frequently provides hemostasis. Care must be taken to avoid undue tension when tying the sutures because they can easily tear through the enclosed hepatic tissue or cause it to necrose.

Cogbill et al. (12) have also noted that liver sutures can control hemorrhage, but they can also cause liver necrosis and increase the risk of subsequent hepatic abscess formation. Deep liver sutures were used in 25% of the grade III injuries in their multicenter study. Of the 23 patients who had this type of treatment, a 30% morbidity rate followed. Abscesses developed in two patients, one patient hemorrhaged, and bile leaks developed in four patients.

Finger-Fracture Hepatorrhaphy

AXIOM Persistent bleeding from deep hepatic wounds is usually best managed with hepatorrhaphy so that the bleeding vessels can be controlled under direct vision. If this is not practical or successful, packing the wound with viable omentum should be considered.

When the depth of the liver wound precludes safe use of direct vessel ligation or simple hepatic sutures, the wound should be opened further to permit direct ligation of the injured vessels and biliary radicles. With portal triad occlusion achieved by an atraumatic vascular clamp, the injuries can be approached by incising Glisson's capsule with electrocautery and then finger-fracturing the hepatic parenchyma in the direction of the injury. The blood vessels and bile ducts encountered are ligated or clipped under direct vision. When using the finger-fracture technique, the position of the main right and left hepatic ducts should be kept in mind, so that they are not injured inadvertently (2).

After hemostasis has been achieved, the vascular clamp occluding the portal triad is slowly released. Any additional points of hemorrhage are then ligated or clipped. Once adequate hemostasis is obtained, the margins of the wound may then be reapproximated with liver sutures. The liver closure should begin at the bottom of the wound so that no dead space is left. If the hepatic wound cannot be closed without leaving dead space, the wound should be packed with omentum.

Viable Omental Pack

When using an omental pack, it is important that the omentum be freed up enough and the opening to the liver be made large enough for the omentum to be pushed well down into the bottom of the liver wound. Some of the advantages of using a viable omental pedicle to fill hepatic dead space include

1. The ability of the omentum to tamponade bleeding (13);
2. The decreased chance of abscess development; and
3. The rich supply of macrophages to reduce the incidence of infection.

Selective Hepatic Artery Ligation

AXIOM Hepatic artery ligation should only be considered if arterial bleeding from a deep hepatic wound cannot be controlled by any other means.

Hepatic artery ligation should be reserved for those instances in which intrahepatic arterial bleeding can be controlled only by clamping a right or left hepatic artery. If necessary, the proper hepatic artery may be ligated, but this entails a risk of hepatic necrosis, particularly if used in combination with placement of perihepatic packs.

Following hepatic artery ligation, subsequent hyperbilirubinemia and enzymatic derangements are generally only moderate and seldom persist for more than 1 week (14); however, strenuous efforts must be made to maintain a normal or increased blood pressure, cardiac output, and oxygen delivery.

Hepatic Resection

Only rarely does bleeding from a hepatic injury require a major liver resection. Except for the left lateral segment, a formal hepatic lobar or segmental resection in the presence of continuing hemorrhage or hypotension can be extremely difficult, and it is usually much safer to continue to attempt control with perihepatic or intrahepatic packing and other maneuvers (15).

AXIOM Hepatic resections should be reserved for situations in which the trauma has almost completed the dissection or there is no other reasonable way to control the bleeding.

Pelton et al. (16) have noted that patients undergoing hepatic resections show a characteristic laboratory value profile postoperatively. With lobectomies, the prothrombin time (PT) increased within 48 hours to a mean high of 16.0 seconds, then returned to normal by postoperative day (POD) 4. Partial thromboplastin time levels remained normal. Total bilirubin increased to a mean high of 2.6 mg/100 ml, then returned to normal by POD 14. Aspartate transaminase and lactate dehydrogenase levels increased abruptly to very high levels, then returned rapidly to normal by POD 5. Total protein and albumin both decreased to approximately 50% of normal, gradually increasing to normal by POD 14. Alkaline phosphatase remained normal initially, then showed a progressive elevation to a high of 288 mg/100 ml on POD 14. Although patients undergoing lesser (wedge) resections did not show the same increase in total serum bilirubin, there were similar smaller trends in all of the other tests.

Liver Transplantation

AXIOM If bilateral severe liver trauma is the only significant injury and there is continued massive bleeding that cannot be controlled in any other way, total hepatic resection with liver transplantation may be considered (17).

Ginzburg et al. (18) have reviewed the role of liver transplantation following severe liver trauma in the United States. Only one liver transplant operation had been performed previously for trauma at the University of Pittsburgh. Reasons to account for this lack of use of liver transplantation for acute severe liver trauma include the lack of predictable donor availability, intolerance of anhepatic periods, and the demand for donor livers by patients in metabolic end-stage liver failure. Candidates need to be free from sepsis and have no other major organ injuries.

Adjunctive Hemostatic Agents

Topical hemostatic agents are useful adjuncts for achieving complete hemostasis once the major hemorrhage has been controlled. These agents are manually compressed against the bleeding surface with lap pads for a period of 10 to 15 minutes. After the compression is released, the area is inspected for further bleeding. Any continuing spots of bleeding can then usually be controlled with additional applications of a hemostatic agent, sutures, or cautery.

AXIOM If a topical hemostatic agent controls hemorrhage from a large area of denuded liver, the portion of hemostatic agent attached to the liver wound can be left in place, especially if bleeding tends to recur after its removal.

Localized surface bleeding that persists despite surgical efforts and other topical agents frequently can be controlled by applying fibrin gel, which works best when applied to a surface that is at least temporarily dry.

Fibrin gel can be formed by using 2 to 4 units of cryoprecipitate in one syringe and 5 to 10 mL of concentrated thrombin solution plus 2 to 4 mL of calcium chloride in another syringe and applying them as a mixture to the bleeding surface. The bleeding should be controlled by local pressure or some other technique to keep the surface dry until the fibrin gel "sets." This can often be accomplished by applying pressure to the bleeding area over a topical hemostatic agent containing the fibrin gel.

Perihepatic Mesh

Absorbable mesh wrapped around severely injured, bleeding livers has been reported in several clinical cases. In a report by Brunet et al. (19), 35 liver injuries (grade II–V) were wrapped with a polyglactin mesh. There were only two (6%) deaths (one from hepatic coma and one from an inferior vena cava avulsion). No hemobilia and no liver abscesses developed. The authors also noted that early use of the mesh resulted in saving large amounts of blood.

Balloon Tamponade

If a patient has a deep penetrating wound to the liver and it is causing severe, continuing bleeding despite all other attempts to control it, one can insert a Foley catheter with a 30-cc balloon into the depths of the wound (20). The balloon is inflated just enough to control the hemorrhage. Hemostatic agents, such as fibrin gel, can also be injected into the depths of the wound through the lumen of the Foley catheter.

Perihepatic Packing

If other techniques have failed to achieve adequate hemostasis from liver wounds, the surgeon should consider placing perihepatic packs and then closing the abdomen to prevent death from exsanguination. Primary indications for perihepatic packing include

1. Transfusion-induced coagulopathy;
2. Presence of extensive bilobar injuries in which bleeding cannot be controlled surgically;
3. Large expanding or ruptured subcapsular hematomas; and
4. Profound hypothermia and hemodynamic instability.

Perihepatic packing can be accomplished in a variety of ways. A relatively effective technique of perihepatic packing has been described by Pachter et al. (2). A Steri-Drape, with the adhesive bands removed, is folded upon itself and placed directly on the surface of the involved portion of liver. Lap pads are then applied until there is no space under the ipsilateral hemidiaphragm. The interposition of the plastic drape between the injured liver and the lap pads helps to keep the packs relatively dry to maintain their effectiveness.

AXIOM Perihepatic packs can cause severe ischemia to portions of the liver that have lost their arterial supply.

The patient may be returned to the operating room for pack removal after 24 to 48 hours, but all hemodynamic, acid-base, core temperature, and coagulation-abnormalities should be corrected first. At the time the packs are removed, one should also

1. Debride any nonviable hepatic tissue;
2. Control any active bleeding points or lacerated bile ducts;
3. Irrigate the abdomen of any clots or bile; and
4. Establish new perihepatic drainage.

A recent review of 145 patients with complex hepatic injuries treated with perihepatic packing from seven different centers revealed that 105 patients (72.4%) survived (2). Because this maneuver was generally used only in the most desperate circumstances, the salvage rate of 72% suggests that perihepatic packing should be considered more than just a "last ditch effort" to control bleeding.

Debridement

AXIOM After hemostasis is obtained, nonviable liver tissue should be debrided to reduce the incidence of later septic complications.

Debridement should be limited to obviously nonviable tissue and should not stir up bleeding. This can usually be accomplished with electrocautery or blunt finger-fracture techniques. Precise anatomic resection is seldom indicated except in unusual instances in which hepatic artery ligation or the injury leads to obvious severe lobar or segmental necrosis.

Drains

AXIOM Even a relatively small collection of bile in contact with a hematoma increases the risk of later sepsis.

Perihepatic drainage of a liver with a grade I or II injury is unnecessary if the patient is hemodynamically stable, hemostasis has been adequate, and no apparent bile leaks exist. Major complex hepatic injuries, on the other hand, should be drained to prevent the accumulations of bile or blood that would otherwise develop. There has been an increasing tendency to use closed (Jackson-Pratt) drainage systems rather than open (Penrose) drainage systems for perihepatic damage. Bender et al. (21) showed that patients with grade I, II, or III hepatic injuries who had open (Penrose) drainage had a 10% incidence of intraabdominal abscesses whereas patients with similar injuries but either no drainage or closed drainage had no postoperative abscesses.

AXIOM Drains are left in place after severe liver trauma until the output is negligible, there is no gross evidence of bile in the drainage fluid, and the patient is taking an enteral diet.

Biliary Tract Drainage

AXIOM Drainage of the common bile duct does not reduce the incidence of hepatic bile leaks or postoperative infections after liver trauma.

In a prospective randomized study of 189 patients with moderate to severe hepatic trauma and no extrahepatic biliary tract injury, Lucas and Walt (22) demonstrated that the presence of a T tube in the common bile duct was associated with a significant increase in morbidity. In many of these patients, the common bile duct was small and insertion of a T tube was often difficult and hazardous. Furthermore, it did not appear to reduce the tendency for injured intrahepatic ducts to leak.

OUTCOME

Death

The overall mortality rate from hepatic trauma continues to be approximately 10% to 15% (3); however, in the Detroit Receiving Hospital series, it was 20% (182 of 910); 144 (78%) of the deaths occurred within 48 hours of admission, and about two-thirds of those early deaths were primarily due to bleeding from associated injuries. Of 162 patients with isolated hepatic injuries, only six (4%) died. In contrast, of 358 patients with three or more associated injuries, 113 (32%) died. The mortality rates for stab wounds, GSWs, and blunt trauma were 8%, 22%, and 35%, respectively.

Complications

Most patients with severe liver trauma have complications, especially if operative therapy is required. Knudson et al. (23) noted complications in 52% of their patients with Grade IV–V liver injuries resulting from penetrating trauma.

Bleeding

Continued postoperative bleeding from severe liver injuries is not uncommon; however, the incidence of significant postoperative hemorrhage should not exceed 3% of all hepatic injuries. For the most severe liver injuries, the postoperative hemorrhage rate may exceed 7% (12).

Even if a coagulopathy cannot be excluded, recurrent bleeding in the early postoperative period is usually due to inadequate surgical hemostasis. If the patient's condition is reasonably stable, reoperation and definitive control of specific bleeding sites is the procedure of choice, preferably after first correcting any hypothermia or coagulopathy that may be present. Recently, De Toma et al. (24) have emphasized the value of selective or superselective angiographic hepatic artery embolization for control of continued bleeding after surgery for liver trauma.

Fever

AXIOM Fever or jaundice soon after major liver trauma is probably related to localized hematomas or hepatic necrosis; fever after 7 days is usually the result of an infection.

The mechanism of fever after major liver trauma is often unclear, but it is probably related to resorption of nonviable hepatic tissue and usually resolves within 3 to 5 days. Fevers that persist beyond 6 to 7 days usually reflect the presence of an infection (12). If pneumonitis can be excluded, intraabdominal sepsis should be strongly considered and a CT scan of the abdomen and pelvis should be performed; however, up to 5% to 10% of fairly large pus collections may be missed on CT scans.

The need to move patients to the operating room and perform a major operation to drain an established abdominal abscess has been reduced by the increasing expertise of interventional radiologists (2). Success rates with CT or ultrasound-guided percutaneous drainage of perihepatic abscesses have approached 95%; however, if the patient's sepsis does not respond promptly to percutaneous drainage, surgical exploration should be considered.

If surgery is necessary to drain a subphrenic abscess, an extraperitoneal approach is generally preferred (2). If the abscess is anterior, a new subcostal incision is generally best.

Biliary Fistulas

Biliary fistulas can be defined as the persistence of more than 50 mL of biliary drainage daily for at least 2 weeks (2). The reported incidence of biliary fistulas following liver trauma varies but should generally not exceed 10%. The patients most susceptible to development of this complication are those with major parenchymal destruction.

AXIOM If adequate drainage of the hepatic injury is accomplished at the initial surgery and the flow of bile into the duodenum is unimpeded, virtually all adequately drained biliary fistulas close spontaneously.

Persistent drainage of more than 300 mL of bile per day for more than 4 to 5 days should lead to the performance of a fistulogram to determine its anatomy. If it is found that a major intrahepatic duct has been completely lacerated, spontaneous closure is unlikely. Occasionally, one can provide internal drainage via endoscopic retrograde cholangiopancreatography (ERCP) and this may obviate the need for urgent surgery. Such drainage can, at times, be therapeutic, and it can serve as an invaluable "road map" in case a Roux-en-Y hepaticojejunostomy is later required.

Liver Failure

Enough hepatic regeneration to maintain normal liver function is possible if at least 20% of the normal liver tissue remains following elective resection. In liver trauma, with its associated shock, multiple transfusions, or gross bacterial contamination, the results of large liver resections are far less satisfactory. Efforts to prevent failure of a severely damaged liver include maintenance of optimal hepatic perfusion, adequate perihepatic drainage, prompt control of sepsis, and provision of intestinal rest and adequate oxygen and glucose. If the liver failure cannot be reversed, liver transplantation may be the only solution.

Hemobilia

Hemobilia, sometimes referred to as hematobilia, is the result of a fistula between a biliary duct and a branch of a hepatic artery. It is uncommon and was seen in only 0.3% of patients with liver trauma at Detroit Receiving Hospital.

AXIOM Gastrointestinal bleeding after liver trauma in a patient with a normal esophagogastroduodenoscopy (EGD) and colonoscopy is due to hemobilia until proven otherwise.

Up to one-third of the patients with hemobilia have the classic triad of hemorrhage, colicky right upper quadrant pain, and jaundice (25). Bleeding may occur as early as the fourth day after injury or it may occur more than 1 month later. In most patients, hemobilia presents as gastrointestinal bleeding without an apparent source. Endoscopy and upper gastrointestinal contrast studies are usually negative. The diagnosis is generally confirmed by angiography.

The efficacy of angiographic embolization to treat hemobilia has clearly been established (25). Surgical intervention is seldom necessary, except in the rare instances when hemobilia is associated with a large intrahepatic cavity.

INJURY TO THE RETROHEPATIC VENA CAVA OR HEPATIC VEINS

AXIOM Injury to a hepatic vein or the retrohepatic vena cava is often lethal. Frequently, the bleeding is only moderate initially, but it may become exsanguinating as the liver is mobilized to provide better exposure of the injury.

When the Pringle maneuver fails to arrest major hemorrhage from behind the liver, a juxtahepatic venous injury should be suspected (2). Major venous injury is also suggested by retrohepatic bleeding after the liver is compressed manually or with packs. Indeed, the usual practice of placing packs on the diaphragmatic surface of the liver to achieve compression may occasionally exacerbate such bleeding.

Treatment

Attempts to expose the source of bleeding behind an injured liver may result in massive exsanguinating hemorrhage. Under such circumstances, extension of the abdominal incision into the chest to provide better exposure while the area is compressed may be necessary. Extension of the incision as a median sternotomy is the preferred approach if one plans to insert an atriocaval shunt.

Extension into a Right Thoracotomy

One approach to retrohepatic injuries involves extension of the midline abdominal incision obliquely across costal cartilages into the right thorax via the seventh or eighth intercostal space. This thoracoabdominal approach with division of the right hemidiaphragm can provide excellent access to the posterior aspect of the right lobe of the liver and juxtahepatic veins, but it is more painful postoperatively than a median sternotomy, and it has a higher incidence of pulmonary complications. It also does not provide optimal exposure of the heart if an atriocaval shunt becomes necessary.

Atriocaval Shunts

The optimal method of managing juxtahepatic venous injuries remains controversial. Although a number of surgeons have had experience with atriocaval shunts, mortality rates reported with their use may exceed 70% to 80% (26).

Atriocaval shunts can be inserted via the right atrium or via the inferior vena cava above the renal veins. Typically, a 28- to 32-French chest tube is inserted via the R. atrial appendage where it is secured with a pursestring suture. The chest tube is passed down through the inferior vena cava until its tip lies below the renal veins. The inferior vena cava is cinched tightly around the chest tube just proximal to its distal holes. The inferior vena cava is also cinched just below the right atrium. Blood then flows through the chest tube from below the lower cinch and out a hole that has been made in the chest tube just inside the R. atrium.

If an endotracheal tube is inserted via the R. atrium, the blown up distal balloon (rather than the caval cinch) can provide the distal occlusion.

AXIOM For atriocaval shunts to be successful, they must be inserted early, before prolonged hypotension, hypothermia, acidosis, and coagulopathy develop.

Saphenofemoral Shunts

Pilcher et al. (27) have reported achieving vascular isolation with balloon-tipped shunts inserted through the saphenofemoral junction up into the retrohepatic inferior vena cava. The appealing aspect of these shunts is that neither a thoracotomy nor sternotomy with cannulation of the right atrial appendage is necessary; however, the number of patients in whom balloon shunts have been inserted through the groin is relatively small. Nevertheless, Cogbill et al. (12) were not able to discern any difference in survival rate between a group of 21 patients receiving an atriocaval shunt and a comparable group of 17 patients receiving the Moore-Pilcher shunt inserted through the groin.

Vascular Isolation of the Liver

One can also attempt to control bleeding from the retrohepatic vena cava by vascular isolation of the liver. This involves sequential vascular clamping of the upper abdominal aorta (above the celiac artery), the porta hepatis, the suprarenal inferior vena cava, and the suprahepatic inferior vena cava. This should eliminate most bleeding from liver and retrohepatic vascular injuries to allow precise repairs or ligations as needed. In many respects, this may be the most expeditious method for controlling retrohepatic bleeding. Grazi et al. (28) have also noted the value of total vascular exclusion of the liver during hepatic surgery in patients with lesions closely adherent to or infiltrating the retrohepatic vena cava or large hepatic veins.

Transhepatic Exposure of Retrohepatic Vessels

Survival of patients with juxtahepatic venous injuries treated without a shunt has been reported in children by Coln et al. (29). Such excellent results may, in part, be due to the fact that the hepatic veins and the retrohepatic cava in children are substantially more extrahepatic than in adults. Nevertheless, based on these results, Pachter et al. (2) managed five consecutive adult patients with portal triad occlusion (mean occlusion time 46 minutes) and finger-fracture of normal hepatic parenchyma down to the site of the vascular injury for primary repair or ligation.

INJURY TO THE PORTA HEPATIS

Injuries to the porta hepatis are best treated by direct repair of the involved structures. This may be facilitated by a Pringle maneuver during the initial dissection. In patients with severe hypotension and a technically difficult repair of a very small hepatic artery, it may be preferable to ligate the artery if the portal blood flow is intact and liver viability is not otherwise compromised from prolonged hypotension or cirrhosis. The patient, however, may not tolerate ligation of the proper hepatic artery distal to the gastroduodenal and right gastric artery branches.

Injury to the portal vein can cause massive hemorrhage and is often fatal. Lateral repair or reconstruction with a patch or panel vein graft should be attempted whenever possible. Simple ligation of the injured portal vein may be associated with a high mortality rate and is generally used only as a final attempt at treatment; however, early ligation with continuing aggressive fluid resuscitation to make up for fluid accumulating in the intestine is occasionally successful.

EXTRAHEPATIC BILIARY TRACT INJURIES

Injuries to the extrahepatic biliary tract may be present in up to 10% to 15% of patients with liver trauma. Most such injuries are penetrating, with the gallbladder being the structure involved most often. In the Detroit Receiving Hospital series, the extrahepatic biliary tract was injured in only 3 of 573 blunt abdominal trauma patients having surgery.

The common bile duct is more susceptible to blunt injury than hepatic ducts and is most likely to be injured at its junction with the pancreas. This is typically caused by a sudden, severe deceleration or compression of the right upper quadrant of the abdomen, causing the liver to move upward and the pancreas and duodenum to move downward, stretching and tearing the bile duct (30).

Mild gallbladder contusions usually resolve spontaneously, but severe contusions may cause necrosis of the wall or fill the lumen with blood. Blood in the gallbladder can cause hematobilia or block the cystic duct. The resulting stasis with secondary bacterial proliferation can result in acute cholecystitis.

Diagnosis

Diagnosis of an extrahepatic bile tract injury is seldom made preoperatively. Peritoneal lavage is often falsely negative for bile, and even if bile is found in the lavage fluid, it can also come from the injuries to the liver or small bowel.

AXIOM Free bile anywhere in the abdomen suggests injury to the liver, extrahepatic bile ducts, or duodenum and necessitates a thorough exploration of these structures.

If there is bile staining of tissues in the right upper quadrant of the abdomen without an obvious source after thorough exploration, one should consider performing an intraoperative cholangiogram and EGD.

Treatment

Although cholecystectomy is the preferred maneuver for almost all gallbladder injuries, this technique may not be desirable in (1) patients with a coagulopathy or (2) hemodynamically unstable patients with minor damage to the gallbladder. In unstable patients with a mild gallbladder injury, a cholecystostomy may be preferred.

AXIOM The subhepatic space should be drained in most patients with a gallbladder injury.

For a simple laceration involving less than 50% of the common duct circumference, treatment usually consists of primary repair, T-tube placement, and external drainage. If possible, the T tube should be brought out at least 1 to 2 cm from the site of the repair. Although no evidence exists that placement of a T tube is mandatory in bile duct trauma, the tube permits early postoperative decompression of the biliary tree when edema might otherwise restrict drainage into the distal common duct. It also provides a ready access for postoperative cholangiography. When confronted with an extremely small duct, a ureteral catheter brought out through the duodenum, then the omentum, and then the abdominal wall can be used as a substitute for a T tube.

AXIOM Construction of a biliary Roux-en-Y enteric anastomosis and external drainage is the treatment of choice for complex, extrahepatic bile duct injuries.

With damage to the right or left hepatic duct, it may be necessary to use the finger-fracture technique through liver parenchyma to expose and identify the right and left ductal system. The optimal repair is a biliary-enteric (Roux-en-Y) anastomosis performed over a stent (such as a ureteral catheter), which may be left in place for several months. One must be careful to preserve the tenuous blood supply of the bile duct during the dissection and to keep the anastomosis tension-free (31).

Complications

Major late morbidity from bile duct trauma is usually in the form of a biliary stricture, which may not become apparent until months or years later (2). If a stricture develops, reoperation with anastomosis to a Roux-en-Y loop of jejunum is almost always necessary to prevent recurring cholangitis or biliary cirrhosis. Balloon dilatation of traumatic strictures by an interventional radiologist is a technique that has occasionally proved successful, but the follow-up period is short in most reports. Prolonged stenting, usually for at least 3 to 6 months, may improve the long-term patency rate of the bile duct following reoperation.

⊘ FREQUENT ERRORS

1. ***Prolonged occlusion of the portal vein and hepatic artery in a hypotensive patient when the bleeding could be controlled by more localized means.***
2. ***Attempting to control bleeding from deep hepatic wounds with superficial closure of the injury tract.***
3. ***Performing a major hepatic resection for bleeding that might be controlled by simpler techniques.***
4. ***Delaying performance of an atrial-caval shunt until the patient has had prolonged hypotension and is hypothermic.***
5. ***Inadequate debridement after successful control of bleeding in a patient who is hemodynamically stable.***
6. ***Drainage of minor hepatic wounds and open (Penrose) drainage of moderate-severe hepatic wounds.***
7. ***Failure to adequately evaluate a patient for sepsis if jaundice develops more than 6 to 7 days after hepatic trauma.***
8. ***Direct repair of a greater than 50% circumference common bile duct injury in a hemodynamically stable patient.***

SUMMARY POINTS

1. Definitive surgery should not be performed until the major bleeding is controlled, the resuscitation is completed, and the hypothermia is corrected to at least 34°C to 35°C.

2. A hemodynamically stable patient with a positive DPL because of increased red cells from an isolated solid organ injury can generally undergo nonoperative treatment.
3. DPL and abdominal CT scanning should be considered complementary, rather than competing, diagnostic tests in patients with abdominal trauma.
4. The need for more than 2 units of blood in adults or replacement of more than half of the estimated blood volume in children to maintain stable vital signs is generally an indication for surgery in patients with isolated splenic or hepatic injuries.
5. Nonoperative management of liver injuries is not advisable in uncooperative patients.
6. If it appears that the portal triad may have to be occluded for more than 20 to 30 minutes, one should consider the use of topical hypothermia (and possibly massive intravenous corticosteroids).
7. If sutures incorporating a great deal of liver tissue are used to control bleeding, the incidence of later liver necrosis and abscesses is increased.
8. Persistent bleeding from deep hepatic wounds is usually best managed by opening the liver wound so that the bleeding vessels can be controlled under direct vision. If this is not practical or successful, packing the wound with viable omentum should be considered.
9. Hepatic artery ligation should only be considered if arterial bleeding from a deep hepatic wound cannot be controlled by any other means.
10. Hepatic resections should be reserved for situations in which the trauma has almost completed the dissection or there is no other reasonable way to control the bleeding.
11. If a topical hemostatic agent controls hemorrhage from an area of "denuded" liver, the hemostatic agent can be left in place.
12. Localized bleeding from small vessels that persists despite surgical efforts and use of other topical agents can frequently be controlled by applying fibrin gel.
13. Perihepatic packs can cause necrosis of portions of the liver that have had their arterial supply ligated.
14. Compression of the suprahepatic inferior vena cava by perihepatic packs should be avoided in hypovolemic patients because the abrupt decrease in venous return to the heart can cause a cardiac arrest.
15. After hemostasis is obtained, obviously nonviable liver tissue should be debrided to reduce the incidence of later septic complications.
16. Even if a relatively small collection of bile is in contact with a hematoma, there is an increased risk of later sepsis.
17. Minor liver injuries do not require drainage.
18. Closed drainage systems are associated with fewer postoperative abscesses after trauma than open (Penrose) systems.
19. Drains are left in place after severe liver trauma until the output is negligible and the patient is taking an enteral diet.
20. Drainage of the common bile duct with a T tube does not reduce the incidence of hepatic bile leaks or postoperative infections after liver trauma.
21. The most frequent cause of postoperative bleeding is inadequate technical control of bleeding vessels.
22. Fever caused by liver trauma is usually related initially to localized hematomas or hepatic necrosis; fever after 5 to 7 days is usually due to an infection.
23. If adequate drainage of the hepatic injury is accomplished at the initial surgery and the flow of bile into the duodenum is unimpeded, virtually all adequately drained biliary fistulas close spontaneously.
24. Gastrointestinal bleeding after liver trauma in a patient with a normal EGD and colonoscopy is due to hemobilia until proven otherwise.
25. Hemobilia is best diagnosed and treated angiographically.
26. Failure of properly placed perihepatic packs to control bleeding from the posterior liver should strongly suggest injury to retrohepatic veins.
27. Attempts to expose the source of bleeding behind an injured liver may result in massive exsanguinating hemorrhage if a retrohepatic venous injury is present.
28. For atriocaval shunts to be successful, they must be inserted early, before prolonged hypotension, hypothermia, acidosis, and coagulopathy develop.

29. Free bile anywhere in the abdomen suggests an injury to the liver, extrahepatic bile ducts, or duodenum and necessitates a thorough exploration of these structures.
30. Cholecystectomy is the preferred treatment for trauma to the gallbladder or cystic duct.
31. Construction of a biliary Roux-en-Y anastomosis and external drainage is the treatment of choice for an extensive, extrahepatic bile duct injury (3).
32. Ischemia sufficient to cause a later bile duct stricture may occur just from excessive freeing up of the common bile duct from surrounding tissue.

REFERENCES

1. Wilson RF, Walt AJ. Injuries to the Liver and Biliary Tract. In: Wilson RF, Walt AJ, eds. *Management of trauma—pitfalls and practice,* 2nd ed. Philadelphia: Williams & Wilkins, 1996:449.
2. Pachter HL, Liang HG, Hofstetter SR. Liver and biliary tract trauma. In: Moore EE, Mattox KL, Feliciano DV, eds. *Trauma,* 2nd ed. Norwalk, CT: Appleton & Lange, 1991:441–463.
3. Shanmuganthan K, Mirvis SE. CT evaluation of the liver with acute blunt trauma. Crit Rev Diagn Imaging 1995;36:73.
4. Sherman HF, Savage BA, Jones LM, et al. Non-operative management of blunt hepatic injuries: safe at any grade? *J Trauma* 1994;37:616.
5. Pachter HL, Knudson MM, Esrig B, et al. Status of nonoperative management of blunt hepatic injuries in 1995: a multicenter experience with 404 patients. *J Trauma* 1996;40:31.
6. Sugimoto K, Asari Y, Sakaguchi T, et al. Endoscopic retrograde cholangiography in the non-surgical management of blunt liver injury. *J Trauma* 1993;35:192.
7. Huguet C, Nordlinger B, Bloch P. Tolerance of the human liver to prolonged normothermic ischemia. *Arch Surg* 1978;113:1448.
8. Delva E, Camus Y, Nordlinger B, et al. Vascular occlusions for liver resections: operative management of tolerance to hepatic ischemia: 142 cases. *Ann Surg* 1989;209:211.
9. Bernhard WF, McMurrey JD, Curtis GW. Feasibility of partial hepatic resection under hypothermia. *N Engl J Med* 1955;253:159.
10. Figueroa I, Delpin EA. Steroid protection of the liver during experimental ischemia. *Surg Gynecol Obstet* 1975;140:368.
11. Pachter HL, Spencer FC, Hofstetter SR. Experience with the finger-fracture technique to achieve intrahepatic hemostasis in 75 patients with severe injuries to the liver. *Ann Surg* 1983;197:771.
12. Cogbill TH, Moore EE, Jurkovich GJ, et al. Severe hepatic trauma: a multicenter experience with 1,335 liver injuries. *J Trauma* 1988;28:1433.
13. Fabian TC, Stone HH. Arrest of severe liver hemorrhage by an omental pack. *South Med J* 1980;73:1487.
14. Mays ET, Wheeler CS. Hepatic artery ligation. *N Engl J Med* 1974;290:993.
15. Moore FA, Moore EE, Seagraves A. Non-resectional management of hepatic trauma: an evolving concept. *Am J Surg* 1985;50:725.
16. Pelton JJ, Hoffman JP, Eisenberg BL. Comparison of liver function tests after hepatic lobectomy and hepatic wedge resection. *Am Surg* 1998;64:408.
17. Esquivel CO, Bernardos A, Makowka L, et al. Liver replacement after massive hepatic trauma. *J Trauma* 1987;27:800.
18. Ginzburg E, Shatz D,Lynn M, et al. The role of liver transplantation in the subacute trauma patients. *Am Surg* 1998;64:363.
19. Brunet C, Sielezneff I, Thomas P, et al. Treatment of hepatic trauma with perihepatic mesh in 35 cases. *J Trauma* 1994;37:200.
20. Thomas SV, Dulchavsky SA, Diebel LN. Balloon tamponade for liver injuries. *Case Report* 1993;34:448.
21. Bender JS, Geller ER, Wilson RF. Intra-abdominal sepsis following liver trauma. *J Trauma* 1989;29:1140.
22. Lucas CE, Walt AJ. Analysis or randomized biliary drainage for liver trauma in 189 patients. *J Trauma* 1972;12:925.

23. Knudson MM, Lim RC, Olcott EW. Morbidity and mortality following major penetrating liver injuries. *Arch Surg* 1994;129:256.
24. De Toma GD, Mingoli A, Modini G, et al. The value of angiography and selective hepatic artery embolization for continuous bleeding after surgery in liver trauma: case reports. *J Trauma* 1994;37:508.
25. Czerniak A, Thompson JN, Hemingway AP, et al. Hemobilia: a disease in evolution. *Arch Surg* 1988;123:718.
26. Kudsk KA, Sheldon GF, Lim RC Jr. Atrial-caval shunting (ACS) after trauma. *J Trauma* 1982;22:81.
27. Pilcher DB, Harman PK, Moore EE. Retrohepatic vena cava balloon shunt introduced via the sapheno-femoral junction. *J Trauma* 1977;17:837.
28. Grazi GL, Mazziotti A, Jovine E, et al. Total vascular exclusion of the liver during during hepatic surgery. *Arch Surg* 1997;132:1104.
29. Coln D, Crighton J, Schorn L. Successful management of hepatic vein injury from blunt trauma in children. *Am J Surg* 1980;140:858.
30. Thal AP, Wilson RF. A pattern of severe blunt trauma to the pancreas. *Surg Gynecol Obstet* 1964;119:773.
31. Feliciano DV. Biliary injuries as a result of blunt and penetrating trauma. *Surg Clin North Am* 1994;74:897.

23. INJURIES TO THE SPLEEN[1]

IMPORTANCE OF THE SPLEEN

Injury to the spleen is important, not only because it occurs frequently but also because the spleen is vital immunologically. Splenectomy is associated with an increased incidence of postoperative abdominal abscesses and later with rapidly fatal overwhelming postsplenectomy infection (OPSI). The risk is greatest in children younger than 2 years of age, especially those who have their spleens removed for nontraumatic reasons (2,3), but adults who have had a splenectomy for trauma are also vulnerable.

In 1952, King and Shumacker (2) reported a syndrome of OPSI in five infants who had splenectomies for congenital hemolytic anemia. This was followed in 1973 by a review of 2,795 patients from the literature by Singer (3) who noted an overall incidence of sepsis was 1.6%, with a mortality rate of 65% in those who become septic. Subsequent reports estimated the risk of OPSI in adults to be about 1% to 2% (4). As a consequence, increasing efforts have been made to save the injured spleen, even to the point of avoiding surgical exploration for isolated splenic injuries when possible.

ANATOMY

The normal spleen in an adult is about 10 to 14 cm long, 6 to 10 cm wide, 3 to 4 cm thick, and weighs 80 to 300 g. Accessory spleens have been reported in 14% to 35% of patients and are much more common in patients undergoing surgery for hematologic disorders.

The arterial blood supply of the spleen, which is about 5% of the cardiac output, is provided by the splenic artery and the short gastric vessels. Gupta et al. (5) demonstrated that 84% of adult human spleens have two major lobes (superior and inferior), whereas the remainder have three (superior, intermediate, and inferior). Each of these is divided into two segments with essentially no vascular communication between these segments.

The arterial pedicle at the splenic hilum has a "Y" shape in 70% to 80% of patients with the splenic artery dividing into two or three major vessels 2 to 5 cm away from the hilum; these two branches divide into smaller segmental branches at the edge of the spleen itself.

The spleen's internal architecture or stroma is a rich vascular network consisting of white pulp (which contains lymphocytes and macrophages), red pulp (which is a storage area for red blood cells [RBCs], granulocytes, and platelets), marginal zones (containing additional macrophages and plasma cells where cellular interactions take place), and ellipsoids (which contain dense periarteriolar concentrations of phagocytes).

PHYSIOLOGY

Normal Circumstances

The total circulation of the spleen is estimated at about 250 mL per minute. Blood passes first through the central arteries of the germinal centers, bringing particulate matter into contact with the lymphocytes there for antigen processing. More than 90% of the blood is then forced through the cords of Billroth. During this process, the fixed macrophages actively phagocytose aged blood cells and any bacteria that may be present.

If the spleen is absent, the spleen's filtration function must be performed largely by the reticuloendothelial system in the liver. As a general rule, encapsulated organisms require much greater opsonization to be removed by hepatic macrophages. As a consequence, patients with liver disease are more susceptible to development of postsplenectomy infections.

AXIOM Although it is often more difficult to repair the injured spleen or save part of it in patients with cirrhosis, it is particularly important in those patients.

The other major role of the spleen is immunologic. It is a major producer of immunoglobulins (especially IgM), and it may produce all of the tuftsin and most of the properdin (6). As the first antibody formed in response to an antigen, the primary role of IgM is initiation of other immune mechanisms.

Complement activation in the spleen, largely via properdin, is also vital to host defense. It increases vascular permeability and promotes chemotaxis, phagocytosis, and intracellular killing. Tuftsin is a substance made predominantly by the spleen (7). This tetrapeptide binds to leukokinin, which coats circulating neutrophils, inducing a nonspecific enhancement of phagocytosis.

Asplenic Physiology

AXIOM Asplenic patients have low levels of IgM, properdin, and tuftsin; these deficiencies contribute to an increased susceptibility to OPSI.

The spleen contains 25% of the total lymphoid mass of the body, and it is important for maintaining T and B lymphocyte numbers and function (8). As a consequence, the asplenic state is characterized by (4,6):

1. Impaired capacity for clearance of bloodborne particles;
2. Decreased phagocytic activity directed against encapsulated bacteria;
3. Decreased antibody response to specific antigens;
4. Decreased opsonization of bacteria;
5. Absence of circulating tuftsin;
6. Decreased antibody responses; and
7. Decreased properdin.

AXIOM Asplenic patients with lower respiratory infections caused by encapsulated organisms are particularly susceptible to development of OPSI.

The microorganisms most often found in OPSI are typically encapsulated and include *Streptococcus pneumoniae* (also referred to as pneumococcus) (50%), meningococcus (12%); *Escherichia coli* (11%), *Haemophilus influenzae* (8%); staphylococci (8%), and other streptococci (7%) (4,6). The remarkable virulence of the pneumococcus is related to its rapid multiplication and its capsule, which resists opsonization and phagocytosis. The incidence of OPSI in asplenic patients is estimated to be 50 to 200 times more than in the normal population and mortality rates vary from 40% to 70% (18). Early recognition and aggressive treatment with antibiotics are necessary. Although 50% of OPSIs occurs within 2 years of splenectomy, the syndrome has been reported to occur as late as 37 years after splenectomy.

Healthy individuals splenectomized for trauma appear to be at slightly lower risk than those who are splenectomized for hematologic disease, and young children, especially those younger than 2 years of age, seem to fare worse than older children and adults (9). In addition to an increased tendency to overwhelming bacterial sepsis, asplenic patients also seem to have an increased susceptibility to viral infections.

SPLEEN TRAUMA

Etiology

Blunt Trauma

In a 12-year period at Detroit Receiving Hospital (1980–1992), the spleen was injured in 345 patients. Of 573 patients admitted with blunt abdominal injuries, the spleen was injured in 172 (30%), usually in motor vehicle accidents, making it the abdominal organ most commonly injured by blunt trauma. Enlarged spleens (e.g., as a result of infectious mononucleosis, hemolytic anemia, leukemia, agnogenic myeloid metaplasia) are thought to be more susceptible to injury.

Because of the increasing efforts to treat splenic injuries nonoperatively, the incidence and types of associated injuries are extremely important. In adults, Fisher et al. (10) found a 27% incidence of gastrointestinal disruption (versus 7% in children). Buckman et al. (11), however, found that of 142 patients with blunt splenic injuries, only 16 (11.2%) had associated injuries that would require laparotomy. This included 12 (8.4%) diaphragmatic ruptures, four (2.8%) bowel perforations, and one (0.7%) bowel ischemia.

Of 172 adults with blunt splenic injury seen at Detroit Receiving Hospital during a 12-year period, 13 (7.6%) also had a major vascular injury, 12 (6.9%) had a diaphragmatic injury, and 12 (6.9%) had a gastrointestinal injury. Thus, it is important in adults to look carefully for other organ injuries, using computed tomography (CT) scans, diagnostic peritoneal lavage (DPL), or ultrasound (US) techniques.

Penetrating Trauma

The incidence of splenic injury in patients having a celiotomy for penetrating abdominal trauma is generally less than 10%. In the 1980 to 1992 Detroit Receiving Hospital series, it was almost 5% for stab wounds and 10% for gunshot wounds. Mortality rates with penetrating splenic trauma vary with the mechanism of injury and have ranged from 0% to 1% with stab wounds to 4% to 10% with gunshot wounds (6,12). Most patients with penetrating splenic trauma have associated injuries that require surgical correction, thereby justifying the universal consensus that penetrating splenic trauma demands operative intervention.

AXIOM Delayed rupture of the spleen, which is usually only a result of a delayed diagnosis of a significant splenic injury, is one of the most common causes of preventable death following blunt trauma.

An increasingly aggressive diagnostic approach to abdominal injuries may explain the marked reduction in the incidence of "delayed rupture" of the spleen, previously reported to occur in up to 40% of splenic injuries, to less than 2% in more recent series (13). The possibility of a delayed rupture of the spleen should always be explained to patients with unoperated splenic trauma and their families before they are discharged from the hospital.

Diagnosis

Symptoms and Signs

Abdominal pain is common following splenic injury. Pain localized to the left upper quadrant is reported in about 30% of patients. The reported incidence of pain over the top of the left shoulder when the patient lies down (Kehr's sign) varies from 15% to 75%, but averages about 20% and can be enhanced by placing the patient in the Trendelenburg position.

Fractures of the ninth, tenth, or eleventh rib are frequent in adults with splenic trauma. Up to 25% of adults with fractures of these three ribs from blunt trauma have a splenic injury. In children, because of the flexibility of their rib cage, the chest wall injury may be minimal.

AXIOM Children, in contrast to adults, may have a severe splenic injury with little or no evidence of chest or abdominal wall trauma.

On occasion, a large perisplenic hematoma may cause a positive Ballance's sign, which is an area of "fixed" dullness to percussion over the left lower posterolateral ribs when the patient is put in one and then the other lateral decubitus positions.

Laboratory Evaluation

With an appropriate history of trauma, a declining hematocrit, and an increasing white blood cell (WBC) and platelet count, one should suspect an injury to the spleen. The WBC count usually increases rapidly after severe splenic injury, and a leukocytosis of 12,000 to 30,000/mm^3 may be present within 12 to 72 hours; however, the hemoglobin level may not decrease significantly for 6 to 12 hours, even with fairly substantial blood loss, unless large quantities of intravenous fluids are given.

AXIOM Splenic injury should be suspected in patients with abdominal or left lower chest trauma if the patient has a declining hematocrit plus an increasing WBC or platelet count.

Diagnostic Peritoneal Lavage

AXIOM An RBC count greater than 100,000/mm^3 in the DPL aspirate is positive for intraabdominal bleeding, but it does not necessarily mean that a laparotomy is required, especially in children.

One of the major limitations of DPL in the assessment of splenic trauma has been its lack of specificity as to exactly what organ might be injured and whether there is continued bleeding. With stable patients, many physicians rely primarily on CT scans of the abdomen to diagnose intraabdominal injuries.

Radiologic Evaluation

AXIOM DPL and CT scans should be viewed as complementary and not competing examinations in patients with suspected intraabdominal injuries.

Plain chest radiographs may be abnormal in up to half the patients with splenic injury, but none of the changes are specific. Up to 40% of patients with blunt trauma to the spleen have fractures of the ninth, tenth, or eleventh ribs on the left. A left pleural effusion, elevated left hemidiaphragm, and left lower lobe pulmonary contusion are additional evidence of significant left upper abdominal trauma.

Seven radiographic signs considered to be relatively characteristic of a ruptured spleen on plain radiographs of the abdomen are

1. Increased density or a mass in the left upper quadrant of the abdomen;
2. Displacement of the gastric bubble to the right;
3. Distortion of the left side of the gastric bubble;
4. Increased space between the top of the gastric bubble and the diaphragm;
5. Elevated left diaphragm with a pleural effusion;
6. Loss of definition of the normal outline of the left kidney; and
7. Indentation of the splenic flexure of the colon.

One or more of these signs are present in about 50% of patients with splenic trauma (14). Fractures of the left transverse processes of the upper lumbar vertebrae should also suggest possible splenic injury.

Computed Tomography

AXIOM A properly performed CT scan with intravenous and upper gastrointestinal contrast often can provide a good anatomic description of the splenic injury.

Computed tomography is usually accurate enough to grade most splenic injuries (Table 23-1).

TABLE 23–1. ***Splenic Injury Scale***

	Grade	Injury Description	AIS 90
I.	Hematoma	Subcapsular, nonexpanding <10% surface area	1
	Laceration	Capsular tear, nonbleeding, <1 cm parenchymal depth	—
II.	Hematoma	Subcapsular, nonexpanding, 10%–50% surface area	2
		Intraparenchymal, nonexpanding, <2 cm in diameter	—
	Laceration	Capsular tear, active bleeding; 1–3 cm parenchymal depth, which does not involve a trabecular vessel	2
III.	Hematoma	Subcapsular, >50% surface area or expanding; ruptured subcapsular hematoma >2 cm or expanding; intraparenchymal hematoma >2 cm or expanding	3
	Laceration	>3 cm parenchymal depth or involving trabecular vessels	3
IV.	Hematoma	Ruptured intraparenchymal hematoma with active bleeding	4
	Laceration	Laceration involving segmental or hilar vessels producing major devascularization (>25% of spleen)	4
V.	Laceration	Completely shattered spleen	5
	Vascular	Hilar vascular injury, which devascularizes spleen hematoma >2 cm expanding	5

From Moore EE, Shackford SR, Pachter HL, et al. Organ injury scaling: spleen, liver, kidney. *J Trauma* 1989;29:1664.

Recently, Schurr et al. (15) have reported on the value of a "CT vascular blush," which represents a false aneurysm that apparently keeps enlarging and ruptures. Of 17 patients (8.0%) who had this CT sign, none were successfully treated nonoperatively. Subcapsular hematomas are often seen as low-density perisplenic masses, and intraparenchymal injuries are frequently seen as intrasplenic accumulations of contrast. Free intraperitoneal blood may also be identified.

Arteriography

AXIOM Trauma patients having an arteriogram for possible injuries in the thoracic aorta, pelvis, or extremities should also have a splenic arteriogram if there is any chance that the spleen has been injured.

Ultrasound

US is popular because it can be performed rapidly at the patient's bedside in the emergency department (ED). Free intraperitoneal blood can often be identified, but in one controlled study comparing US to CT for abdominal trauma in children, US had a false-negative rate of 50% (16).

Laparoscopy

Diagnostic laparoscopy is increasingly used to evaluate patients with possible abdominal injuries. Townsend et al. (17) reported on the use of diagnostic laparoscopy in 15 hemodynamically stable patients with nine spleen injuries and eight liver injuries on CT scan. The diagnostic laparoscopy revealed ongoing hemorrhage in four patients and poor visualization in another patient. These problems prompted laparotomy, which resulted in four splenorrhaphies and one hepatorrhaphy. Conservative management was used in the remaining eight patients, all of whom had adequate hemostasis.

Treatment

Emergent celiotomy is clearly appropriate for acutely injured patients who are hemodynamically unstable despite resuscitative efforts. In patients with blunt trauma who have potential sites of bleeding outside the abdomen, DPL may be extremely helpful for confirming a clinical suspicion of intraabdominal bleeding.

Individual management of hemodynamically stable patients is based largely on the injury mechanism and its site. Gunshot wounds to the anterior abdomen are explored routinely, whereas stab wounds can be managed selectively by local wound exploration and DPL or laparoscopy. Penetrating injuries of the lower chest, with the possible exception of minor stab wounds, should probably also undergo DPL or laparoscopy.

Nonoperative Treatment

In hemodynamically stable patients sustaining major blunt trauma, if a CT scan shows that only the liver or spleen is injured, nonoperative treatment may be attempted, especially in young children. Increasingly, pediatric surgeons do not perform a laparotomy for splenic injury unless the blood transfusions to maintain stable vital signs exceed 40 mL/kg. In addition, anything that precludes a reliable abdominal examination, such as an altered level of consciousness, is an indication for prompt laparotomy.

An increasing number of surgeons have been accumulating favorable data on adults receiving nonoperative treatment for isolated splenic or liver injuries (13). Brasel et al. (18) recently reported on 164 patients with blunt splenic injuries treated from July 1, 1991, to June 30, 1996. Overall, successful nonoperative management occurred in 84% of patients (73 of 87) and was successful in five of seven patients older than 55 years of age and in 14 of 15 patients with Glasgow Coma Scale scores less than 13.

AXIOM If more than 2 units of blood are needed to maintain hemodynamic stability in an adult, operative or angiographic management of splenic or liver injuries is indicated.

Operative Treatment

Cathey et al. (19) recently found that clinical variables suggestive of the need for urgent surgical intervention for splenic trauma include hypotension (systolic blood pressure less than 90 mm Hg) in the prehospital setting or ED; tachycardia (heart rate greater than 100 beats/min) in the ED; hematocrit less than 30% or a prothrombin time greater than 14 seconds in the ED; multiple injuries; or blood transfusion in the ED. Abdominal symptoms or signs did not identify patients requiring urgent operative management.

Celiotomies for acute severe trauma are usually performed via an upper midline incision. In patients appearing late after injury with what is almost certainly an isolated splenic injury, a left subcostal incision may be preferred.

With acute trauma, the abdomen is explored rapidly, and bleeding sites are compressed or packed while the anesthesia team resuscitates the patient. More definitive control of bleeding sites and bowel injuries can be provided after the patient is fully resuscitated and warmed to at least 34°C to 35°C.

Following careful manual extraction of blood and clots from the left upper quadrant, one should assess the spleen and the extent of any ongoing hemorrhage. The finding of either a totally shattered spleen or one avulsed from the splenic pedicle leaves the surgeon no alternative but to gain immediate control of the bleeding by manual compression of the splenic pedicle and perform splenectomy.

Splenic Mobilization

AXIOM If the spleen is not bleeding significantly, care must be taken to avoid making any existing injury worse during the mobilization.

Except for extremely simple tears or avulsions of the anterior capsule of the spleen, effective splenic repair demands a complete mobilization to thoroughly assess the extent and severity of the injury. The phrenicolienal and lienorenal ligaments are generally avascular, but the lienocolic ligament may contain sizable blood vessels, and the gastrolienal ligament contains the short gastric vessels (Fig. 23-1).

When possible, the lienocolic ligament is visualized and divided first after displacing the splenic flexure of the colon downward to visualize this area more clearly. Following division of the lienorenal and phrenicolienal ligaments, a plane can generally be developed posterior to the pancreas with its attached splenic artery and vein by blunt finger dissection.

The superior pole of the spleen sometimes cannot be mobilized adequately without transection and ligation of the upper short gastric vessels. The spleen should then be rotated medially up into the incision. If there is resistance to this maneuver, the stomach may have to be mobilized more.

When the spleen is adequately mobilized, it is helpful to place several large packs in the splenic bed to help support the elevated spleen. These packs may also help to tamponade any oozing from small posterior vessels that were injured while the spleen was being mobilized.

Splenorrhaphy

There is little disagreement that, if operative intervention is indicated for splenic trauma, then splenorrhaphy, rather than splenectomy, is preferred; however, this

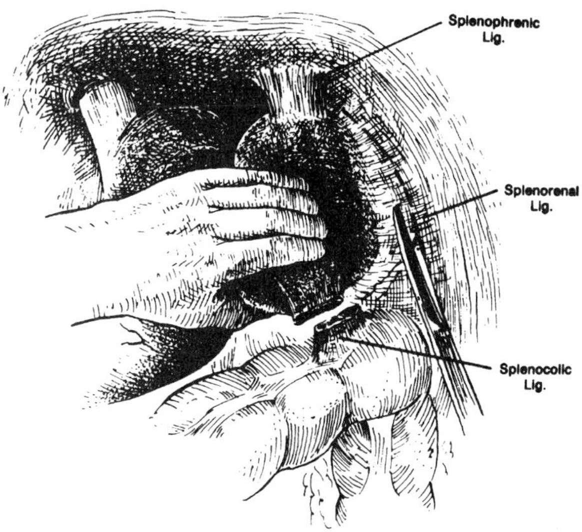

FIG. 23-1. Techniques for transecting the ligamentous attachments of the spleen. (From Schwartz SI. Spleen. In: Schwartz SI, Ellis H, eds. *Maingot's abdominal operations.* 9th ed, vol II. East Norwalk, CT: Appleton & Lange 1990;81:1692)

should only be done if the patient is hemodynamically stable, does not have other life-threatening injuries, and the splenic injury is not too severe to repair.

Most superficial injuries stop bleeding with one or two applications of microcrystalline collagen (Avitene), Surgicel, Gelfoam, topical thrombin, or fibrin gel. Electrocautery can sometimes be effective on tiny areas of bleeding, but one must be careful because it is easy to penetrate the splenic parenchyma with the cautery tip. Moore et al. (6) and others have found the Argon Beam Coagulator (Bard Electro Medical Systems, Englewood, CO) can be effective for controlling bleeding from superficial lesions of the spleen, liver, and other organs. Others have advocated ultrasonic scalpels. Currently, we have been applying fibrin gel (made by combining cryoprecipitate, thrombin, and calcium) to the bleeding sites while the splenic vessels are manually compressed.

Actively bleeding vessels in a parenchymal laceration are ligated or controlled with mattress sutures. Loose or devitalized tissue should be gently debrided, but this must be done with great care so as not to cause more bleeding. In children, the relatively thick capsule permits more direct suturing, In the adult, pledgets are recommended to reduce the tendency for the horizontal mattress sutures to pull through the splenic tissue. Recently, a technique for using mattress sutures to hold omentum over the cut surface has been described (20).

Temporary control of the splenic artery is advisable for complex injuries with active bleeding. Permanent splenic artery ligation may be associated with a significant loss of immunologic function and should be avoided if possible (21). If the splenic artery cannot be found or dissected out readily, one may have to use a wide vascular clamp on the splenic hilum itself until the bleeding sites are controlled.

One should not hesitate to abandon repair if, in the surgeon's judgment, adequate splenic hemostasis cannot be obtained.

Partial Splenectomy

AXIOM In the absence of other life-threatening problems, an injured spleen that cannot be repaired should be considered for partial splenectomy.

To perform an anatomic partial resection of the spleen, the segmental arteries to the devascularized segments of the spleen are identified and ligated. This should help demarcate the location of the avascular intersegmental plane in the parenchyma (6). The ischemic portion of the spleen can then be removed. We have seldom been successful with this technique unless the trauma has almost completed the dissection.

If one does attempt a partial resection, it is generally thought that at least half of the splenic mass along with its usual blood supply should be salvaged; however, Resende and Petroianu (22) have reported six cases of severe trauma of the spleen and its pedicle treated by subtotal splenectomy, preserving only the upper pole, which is supplied by splenogastric vessels. Postoperative scintigraphy confirmed the preservation of the splenic filtering function as reflected by macrophage capture of sulfur colloid labeled with ^{99m}Tc.

Splenic Artery Ligation

Splenic artery ligation, either alone or in combination with topical hemostatic agents or suture techniques, has been proposed for injuries causing continued bleeding despite attempts at hemostasis and when the only other alternative would be a splenectomy; however, without adequate pulsatile flow, the spleen is probably of relatively little immunologic value.

Splenic Wrapping

Moore et al. (6) have successfully managed a number of patients with major splenic injuries by application of topical microfibrillar collagen and splenic wrapping. Self-made buttressing Vicryl ladders have also been described for holding the injured spleen together and compressing the bleeding areas (6). More recently, Lange et al. (23) have used commercial woven polyglycolic acid (Dexon) mesh like a hair net to hold the pulverized pieces of spleen together.

Splenic Artery Embolization

Recently Firstenberg et al. (24) described successful treatment of delayed splenic rupture with splenic artery embolization. Several reports have also described splenic artery embolization as an adjunct to the nonoperative management of selected blunt splenic injuries (25,26).

Splenectomy

Total splenectomy should be performed promptly if

1. The spleen is pulverized;
2. The patient has other life-threatening injuries; and
3. Hemostasis cannot be secured after splenorrhaphy or partial splenectomy (6).

Before clamping the splenic artery and vein, one should clearly identify the tail of the pancreas and its relationship to the splenic hilum. In 90% of cases, it lies adjacent to the caudal part of the spleen and, therefore, is easily injured during splenectomy (6).

Splenic Autotransplantation

If a splenectomy is required, it is advisable to take time to autotransplant some thin slices of the spleen into the omentum (6). Experimental studies have confirmed the viability of autotransplanted splenic tissue and its capability of phagocytosing pneumococcal organisms and contributing to a higher level of antibody formation following pneumococcal vaccination (27). It is doubtful, however, whether such implants significantly reduce the incidence or later OPSI (6).

Drainage of the Splenic Bed

If there is any concern about possible injury to the adjacent pancreas, Pachter et al. (28) have demonstrated that there are no apparent increased complications in patients in whom closed drain systems (Jackson-Pratt or Hemovac) are used. They also noted that stiff drains left in place for excessively long periods probably accounted for the high complication rates associated with drains in earlier studies.

Postoperative Care

Some surgeons maintain nasogastric tube decompression of the stomach for a minimum of 4 to 5 days after splenic injury to avoid distension of the stomach; however, most surgeons see little need for prolonged gastric decompression unless there are associated pancreatic or gastrointestinal injuries or a fairly severe ileus.

The practice of routinely checking platelet counts at specific intervals following a splenectomy to recognize significant thrombocytosis as a guide for institution of prophylactic anticoagulation has also fallen into disrepute. Nevertheless, if the platelet count exceeds 1 million/mm^3, we give the patient a baby aspirin (75 to 85 mg) per day by mouth or by rectum.

Prophylaxis against OPSI

Pneumovax

AXIOM All patients having a splenectomy for trauma should be given Pneumovax before they leave the hospital.

Asplenic patients have an increased lifetime likelihood of development of overwhelming infections, particularly in the lungs and particularly with encapsulated organisms. *S. pneumoniae* (the pneumococcus) is cultured in more than half of the serious infections that develop in asplenic individuals. The currently available vaccines (Pneumovax 23 from Merck and Pnu-Immune 23 from Lederle) contain 23 serotypes of pneumococci, which account for 90% of the pneumococcal infections (29). The antibody response to vaccination of an otherwise normal asplenic patient is nearly equal to that of controls, but the duration of elevated titers is unknown (30). Shatz et al. (31) have found that postvaccination immunoglobulin G serum antibody concentrations were not significantly different from normal control subjects regardless of the time of vaccination relative to splenectomy (1, 7, or 14 days). However, although serum concentrations approached normal, functional antibody activity was significantly lower in splenectomized patients. Better functional antibody responses against the serogroup and serotypes studied seemed to occur with delayed (14-day) vaccination.

The question of the timing of the administration of the vaccination is controversial. Our tendency is to give the Pneumovax on the day of discharge from the hospital and warn the patients that they will probably have some fever over the next 5 to 10 days.

Other Vaccines

H. influenzae type 2b conjugate and meningococcal polysaccharide vaccines are available, and although the risk of these bacteria causing overwhelming postsplenectomy sepsis is relatively low, increasing numbers of clinicians are giving these vaccines to splenectomized patients, particularly children.

Penicillin Prophylaxis

AXIOM All postsplenectomy children younger than 2 years of age should receive long-term penicillin prophylaxis, and older children and adults should receive such prophylaxis before any invasive procedure and with almost any upper respiratory infection.

Because pneumococcal sepsis can occur despite vaccination, long-term oral penicillin prophylaxis has been recommended, especially in splenectomized children younger than 2 years of age; however, the documented compliance rate with penicillin prophylaxis programs is probably less than 50%. Antibiotics should also be given at the first signs of any respiratory infection that causes fever, sore throat, or a cough.

Postoperative Complications

Infections

Patients who have had splenic repairs or resections have an increased risk of development of intraabdominal infections in the area of the spleen. This is particularly true if there has been enteric contamination and use of foreign material for bolsters, pledgets, or wrapping.

Broad-spectrum antibiotics are usually given for at least 5 days after a splenic injury requiring repair or resection. Any evidence of sepsis that is not clearly due to some other cause should make one suspect an infection in or near the splenic bed. CT scans can be helpful for diagnosis and for percutaneous draining of such collections.

Bleeding

AXIOM Early postsplenorrhaphy bleeding is usually due to technical problems (32).

Recurrent intraperitoneal bleeding following splenic surgery is usually a result of failure to adequately secure short gastric or splenic hilar vessels. Any evidence of active bleeding is an indication for a prompt exploration. Any coagulation abnormality should be corrected simultaneously with platelets or fresh frozen plasma as needed; however, a mild to moderate progressive drop in hemoglobin levels is not unusual in patients who have had multiple blood transfusions and are not bleeding.

Pancreatitis

Pancreatitis following splenic surgery may occur either from operative trauma or from the initial injury. Intraoperative pancreatic trauma can be minimized by ligating the hilar vessels near the splenic capsule and by avoiding any blind clamping or suturing near the pancreas.

Splenosis

Splenosis occasionally results from the implantation and subsequent growth of fragments of disrupted splenic tissue upon various peritoneal surfaces and organs. Although splenosis is usually harmless, intestinal obstruction may occur if the implants on adjacent loops of bowel become adherent (14).

Posttraumatic Cysts

Pachter et al. (33) reviewed the literature on posttraumatic cysts (pseudocysts) of the spleen in 1993 and concluded that small, asymptomatic cysts (<4 cm) are likely to resolve, whereas larger cysts (>5 cm) have a risk of rupture of at least 25%.

OUTCOME OF SPLENIC INJURY

Mortality Rate

The overall mortality rate for splenic injury at Detroit Receiving Hospital in a 12-year period (1980–1992) was 18% (61 of 345). The mortality rate in patients having nonoperative therapy (5%; 2 of 43) or splenorrhaphy (8%; 12 of 151) was much lower than for the patients requiring a splenectomy (31%; 47 of 151). The mortality rate also increased with the grade of splenic injury from 10% (23 of 227) for grade 1-2 injuries, to 26% (21 of 82) for grade 3 injuries, to 47% (17 of 36) for grade 4-5 injuries.

The mortality rate was influenced greatly by the number and type of associated injuries. The mortality rate with up to none, one, or two associated injuries was 6% (12 of 185), but for three or more associated injuries, the mortality rate was 31% (49 of 160). The more lethal associated injuries and their mortality rates were

- Major vessels 56% (31 of 55)
- Small bowel 43% (12 of 28)
- Liver 34% (34 of 101)
- Pancreas 33% (26 of 80)
- Pelvic fractures 33% (8 of 24)

Follow-Up Studies

Patients who have undergone nonoperative management should have a repeat CT scan 3 to 4 weeks after injury, particularly if there is any risk of recurrent injury. If the CT scan shows a normal spleen with no disruptions, the patient may resume normal activity. If the scan shows a persistent defect, rescanning should be done at 6 to 8 weeks and then monthly as needed. Patients should probably not return to full physical activity until complete healing of the spleen is confirmed.

⊘ FREQUENT ERRORS

1. ***Inadequate search for associated injuries in a patient who has splenic trauma and is hemodynamically stable.***
2. ***Assuming that a CT scan can reliably rule out associated injuries to the pancreas or small bowel.***
3. ***Transfusing more than 2 units of bank blood in an effort to continue nonoperative management of a splenic injury.***
4. ***Failing to gently mobilize the spleen when attempting to examine it.***
5. ***Prolonged efforts to save a mild to moderately injured spleen in an adult with other life-threatening injuries.***

6. ***Allowing an unreliable patient to leave the hospital after a splenectomy without first receiving Pneumovax.***
7. ***Inadequate attention to "minor" respiratory infections in patients who have had splenectomy.***
8. ***Failure to "cover" splenectomized patients with antibiotics during invasive procedures.***

SUMMARY POINTS

1. The spleen is an important immunologic organ, especially in children younger than 2 years of age.

2. Although the risk of OPSI is only about 1% to 2%, it is 50 to 200 times higher than in nonsplenectomized individuals, and the risk of death from OPSI is about 30% to 70%.

3. Asplenic patients have low levels of IgM, properdin, and tuftsin, and these deficiencies contribute to an increased susceptibility to OPSI.

4. Asplenic patients in whom lower respiratory infections caused by encapsulated organisms develop are particularly susceptible to OPSI.

5. An enlarged, abnormal spleen is much more susceptible to accidental trauma than a normal spleen.

6. If there is evidence of a splenic injury, one must look carefully for associated intraabdominal injuries, especially in adults, before considering nonoperative treatment in hemodynamically stable adults.

7. Virtually all patients with acute penetrating splenic trauma should have a surgical exploration because of the high incidence of associated injury requiring treatment.

8. Delayed rupture of the spleen, which is usually only a delayed diagnosis of a significant splenic injury, is one of the most common causes of preventable death following blunt trauma.

9. Children, in contrast to adults, may have a severe splenic injury with little or no evidence of chest or abdominal wall trauma.

10. Splenic injury should be suspected in patients with abdominal or left lower chest trauma if the patient has a declining hematocrit and an increasing WBC or platelet count.

11. An RBC count greater than 100,000/mm^3 in the DPL fluid is positive for intraabdominal bleeding, but it does not necessarily mean that a laparotomy is required, especially in children.

12. A properly performed CT scan with intravenous and upper gastrointestinal contrast often can usually provide a good anatomic description of injuries to the spleen and most other intraabdominal organs, except the pancreas and distal small bowel.

13. Trauma patients having an arteriogram for possible injuries in the thoracic aorta, pelvis, or extremities should also have a splenic arteriogram if there is any chance that the spleen has been injured.

14. Criteria for nonoperative management of splenic injuries documented by imaging techniques include (1) hemodynamic stability and (2) absence of serious associated intraabdominal injury.

15. If more than 2 units of blood are needed to maintain hemodynamic stability in an adult, operative or angiographic management of splenic or liver injuries is indicated.

16. Gentle, adequate mobilization and exposure are the keys to safe and successful surgery on the spleen.

17. When possible, repair rather than splenectomy should be the goal of surgery to control bleeding from the spleen.

18. If bleeding is persistent, one should abandon prolonged efforts to repair or save a substantial part of an injured spleen, especially in older patients.

19. A spleen without a patent splenic artery or intact short gastric vessels is probably of relatively little immunologic use to the patient.
20. One should avoid damage to the tail of the pancreas while ligating the splenic vessels in the hilum of the spleen.
21. Although splenic implants may be viable and may grow, it is not completely clear that they are of much immunologic benefit to the patient.
22. Unless there is damage to the adjacent pancreas, splenic injuries should not be drained.
23. Postsplenectomy thrombocytosis probably does not require any treatment unless the platelet count exceeds 1 million/mm^3. Then, 75 to 85 mg of aspirin daily is probably adequate prophylaxis.
24. All patients having a splenectomy for trauma should be given Pneumovax and vaccines for the meningococcus and *H. influenzae* before they leave the hospital.
25. All postsplenectomy children younger than 2 years of age should receive long-term penicillin prophylaxis, and older children and adults should receive antibiotic prophylaxis before any invasive procedure and as early treatment for almost any upper respiratory infection.
26. Patients who have had a splenectomy should be watched carefully for development of delayed infections in the left subphrenic space.
27. Early postsplenorrhaphy bleeding is usually due to technical problems.

REFERENCES

1. Wilson RF, Steffes CP, Tyburski J. Injury to the spleen. In: Wilson RF, Walt AJ, eds. *Management of trauma—pitfalls and practice.* 2nd ed. Philadelphia: Williams & Wilkins 1996:473.
2. King H, Shumacker HB Jr. Splenic studies: I. Susceptibility to infection after splenectomy performed in infancy. *Ann Surg* 1952;136:239.
3. Singer DB. Postsplenectomy sepsis. In: Rosenberg HS, Bolande RP, eds. *Perspectives in pediatric pathology.* Chicago: Year Book, 1973;285.
4. Green JB, Shackford SR, Sise MJ, et al. A prospective analysis of late septic complications in adult patients following splenectomy for trauma. *J Trauma* 1986;26: 999.
5. Gupta CD, Gupta SC, Arora AK, Jeya SP. Vascular segments in the human spleen. *J Anat* 1976;12:613.
6. Moore FA, Moore EE, Abernathy CM. Injury to the spleen. In: Moore EE, Mattox KL, Feliciano DV, eds. *Trauma.* 2nd ed. East Norwalk, CT: Appleton & Lange, 1991;30:465–483.
7. Likhite VV. Opsonin and leukophilic gamma-globulin in chronically splenectomized rats with and without heterotopic autotransplanted splenic tissue. *Nature* 1975;253:742.
8. Amsbaugh DF, Prescott B, Baker PJ. Effect of splenectomy on the expression of regulatory T cell activity. *J Immunol* 1978;121:1483.
9. Holschneider AM, Kreiz-klimeck H, Strasser B, et al. Complications of splenectomy in childhood. *Z Kinerchir* 1982;35:130.
10. Fisher RP, Miller-Crotchett P, Reed RL. Gastrointestinal disruption: the hazard of nonoperative management with blunt abdominal injury. *J Trauma* 1988;28: 1445.
11. Buckman RF Jr, Piano G, Dunham CM, et al. Major bowel and diaphragmatic injuries associated with blunt spleen or liver rupture. *J Trauma* 1988;28:1317.
12. Feliciano DV, Bitondo CG, Mattox KL, et al. A four year experience with splenectomy versus splenorrhaphy. *Ann Surg* 1985;201:568.
13. Mucha P, Daly RC, Farnel MB. Selective management of blunt splenic trauma. *J Trauma* 1986;26:970.
14. Walt AJ, Wilson RF. Specific abdominal injuries. In: Walt AJ, Wilson RF, eds. *Management of trauma: pitfalls and practice.* Philadelphia: Lea & Febiger, 1975;23:348–374.
15. Schurr MJ, Fabian TC, Woodman G, et al. Management of blunt splenic trauma: CT vascular blush predicts failure of nonoperative management. *J Trauma* 1994; 37:164.

16. Kaufman RA, Towbin R, Babcock DS, et al. Upper abdominal trauma in children: imaging evaluated. *AJR Am J Roentgenol* 1984;142:449.
17. Townsend MC, Flancbaum L, Choban PS, et al. Diagnostic laparoscopy as an adjunct to selective conservative management of solid organ injuries after blunt abdominal trauma. *J Trauma* 1993;35:647.
18. Brasel KJ, DeLisle CM, Olson CJ, et al. Splenic injury: trends in evaluation and management. *J Trauma* 1998;44:283.
19. Cathey KL, Brady WJ, Butler K, Blow O, et al. Blunt splenic trauma: characteristics of patients requiring urgent laparotomy. *Am Surg* 1998;64:450.
20. Sarmiento JM, Yugueros P. An atraumatic technique to fix the omentum after partial splenectomy. *J Trauma* 1996;41:140.
21. Horton J, Ogden ME, Williams S, et al. The importance of splenic blood flow in clearing pneumococcal organisms. *Ann Surg* 1982;195:172.
22. Resende V, Petroianu A. Subtotal splenectomy for treatment of severe splenic injuries. *J Trauma* 1998;44:933.
23. Lange D, Zaert PH, Merlotti GJ, et al. The use of absorbable mesh in splenic trauma. *J Trauma* 1988;28:269.
24. Firstenberg MS, Plaisier B, Newman JS, et al. Successful treatment of delayed splenic rupture with splenic artery embolization. *Surgery* 1998;123:584.
25. Sclafani SJA, Shaftan GW, Scalea TM, et al. Nonoperative salvage of computed tomography-diagnosed splenic injuries: utilization of angiography for triage and embolization for hemostasis. *J Trauma* 1995;39:818.
26. Hagiwara A, Ukioka T, Ohta S, et al. Nonsurgical management of patients with blunt splenic injury: efficacy of transcatheter arterial embolization. *AJR Am J Roentgenol* 1996;167:159.
27. Steely WM, Satava RM, Brigham RA, et al. Splenic autotransplantation: determination of the optimal amount required for maximal survival. *J Surg Res* 1988; 45:327.
28. Pachter HL, Hofstetter SR, Spencer FC. Evolving concepts in splenic surgery: splenorrhaphy versus splenectomy and postsplenectomy drainage; experience in 105 patients. *Ann Surg* 1981;194:262.
29. *The Medical Letter on Drugs and Therapeutics.* New Rochelle, NY, November 1985;27:97.
30. Giebink GS, Foker JE, Kim Y, et al. Serum antibody and opsonic response to vaccination with pneumococcal capsular polysaccharide in normal and splenectomized children. *J Infect Dis* 1980;141:404.
31. Shatz DV, Schinsky MF, Pais LB, et al. Immune responses of splenectomized trauma patients to the 23-valent pneumococcal polysaccharide vaccine at 1 versus 7 versus 14 days after splenectomy. *J Trauma* 1998;44:760.
32. Moore FA, Moore EE, Moore GE, et al. Risk of splenic salvage following trauma: analysis of 200 adults. *Am J Surg* 1984;148:800.
33. Pachter HL, Hofstetter SR, Elkowitz A, et al. Traumatic cysts of the spleen: The role of cystectomy and splenic preservation. Experience with seven consecutive patients. *J Trauma* 1993;35:430.

24. INJURIES TO THE STOMACH AND SMALL BOWEL[1]

INCIDENCE

In the literature, the incidence of gastric injury from blunt trauma is low, averaging between 0.9% and 1.8%. The incidence of small bowel injury resulting from blunt trauma ranges from 5% to 15% (2,3). In a 12-year period (1980–1992) at Detroit Receiving Hospital, 573 patients were admitted with blunt intraabdominal injuries. This included injury to the stomach in only six (1.0%) and jejunum or ileum in 58 (10.1%).

Reports from other centers indicate that the incidence of gastrointestinal injury secondary to gunshot wounds may exceed 80% and the incidence of hollow viscus injury secondary to stab wounds that penetrate the peritoneum is about 30% (4). Over the 12-year period (1980–1992) at Detroit Receiving Hospital, 2,168 patients had abdominal organs injured by penetrating trauma. The small bowel was injured in 701 (32%) of these cases, and the stomach was injured in 334 (15%). The small bowel was also the organ most frequently injured by gunshot wounds.

DIAGNOSIS

Diagnosis of stomach or small bowel injury is no problem with gunshot wounds that clearly enter the abdomen because exploration is mandatory. With stab wounds and no signs of significant blood loss or peritoneal irritation, one may elect to explore the wound to see if the tract penetrates the anterior abdominal fascia. If it does but the patient is essentially asymptomatic, one may elect to do a diagnostic peritoneal lavage (DPL) and explore the abdomen if results are positive. Diagnosis is even more difficult with blunt trauma and often requires some combination of findings on physical examination, DPL, computed tomography (CT) scan, ultrasound, or laparoscopy.

Physical Examination

Physical examination can be extremely helpful for diagnosing intraabdominal injuries in patients who are awake and alert. The early signs of intestinal perforation are often variable and nonspecific, and waiting for signs of peritonitis or sepsis tends to increase morbidity and mortality rates; however, in children undergoing nonoperative treatment for blunt spleen or liver trauma, the 5% who have coincident small bowel injury and require later surgery do not appear to suffer from the delay. In adults, the incidence of hollow viscus injury with liver or spleen trauma is at least two to three times greater.

Patients with marks made by a seat belt on the abdomen are much more likely to have small bowel or mesenteric injuries, especially if there is a "Chance" (transverse) fracture of a lumbar vertebra.

AXIOM One should be suspicious of a characteristic tetrad of injuries caused by seat belts in motor vehicle accidents. These include abdominal wall contusions, small bowel ruptures, mesenteric tears, and lumbar spine fractures.

Laboratory Evaluation

A progressive elevation in serum amylase levels and the white blood cell (WBC) count, especially with a shift to the left, should alert the surgeon to the possibility of an intraabdominal injury to the pancreas or gastrointestinal tract.

Radiography

Plain Films

In general, plain radiographs of the abdomen are not helpful for diagnosing gastric or small bowel injuries but, occasionally, intraperitoneal air allows visualization of both sides of the bowel wall clearly. An erect chest radiograph or left lateral decubitus film is more likely to reveal free intraperitoneal air, especially if the patient is kept in that position for 15 to 30 minutes before the radiographs are obtained.

AXIOM Intestinal injuries do not commonly cause free air to be visible on plain radiographs of the abdomen.

Contrast Studies

Gastrografin studies of the stomach and proximal small bowel usually show a leak if one is present, but false-negative studies do occur. Occasionally, a contrast study shows occlusion of the small bowel lumen (especially the duodenum) caused by a hematoma or late ischemic stenosis. Injuries to the distal small bowel generally require a barium follow-through study to demonstrate a leak or obstruction.

AXIOM A falsely negative Gastrografin study is possible if a hole in the bowel has become sealed by clot or omentum.

Computed Tomography

CT scanning of the abdomen with gastric and intravenous contrast demonstrates most gastric, duodenal, and proximal jejunal perforations (4). Dowe et al. (5) have also noted that the CT finding of mesenteric bleeding or bowel wall thickening associated with mesenteric hematomas or infiltration in blunt trauma patients indicates a high likelihood of a mesenteric or bowel injury requiring surgery. The finding of focal mesenteric hematomas or infiltration without adjacent bowel wall thickening is nonspecific and can occur both in mesenteric or bowel lesions that require surgery and those that do not.

AXIOM One cannot rely on abdominal CT scans to detect injuries to the small intestine distal to the ligament of Treitz.

Diagnostic Peritoneal Lavage

Using standard DPL criteria, Harrison and Whelan (6) did not miss a case of perforation or other serious injury to the stomach or small bowel in 77 patients. The DPL in such cases is generally positive because of an increased red blood cell or WBC count. Bile and food fibers are seldom found; however, if the DPL is performed less than 3 hours after the injury, there may not be enough of an inflammatory response to increase the WBC in the DPL aspirate to above $500/mm^3$.

AXIOM If one suspects a bowel injury and the initial DPL results are equivocal, the catheter can be left in place for a repeat DPL 3 to 6 hours later.

Some authors have reported using alkaline phosphatase levels in the lavage effluent as a means of diagnosing small bowel injuries (7); however, its value is controversial.

Laparoscopy

Laparoscopy is being used increasingly to diagnose and treat a wide variety of traumatic and nontraumatic problems in the abdomen. Frantzides et al. (8) recently described their use of laparoscopy to diagnose and treat two stab wounds of the anterior wall of the stomach. In a similar manner, Brams et al. (9) used a new gasless laparoscopic technique to evaluate and repair a traumatic gastric perforation with success.

TREATMENT

Nonoperative Treatment

In certain very high risk patients with a gastric perforation, nonoperative management may be considered if the stomach is decompressed well with a nasogastric tube and signs and symptoms of peritonitis are minimal and not getting worse (10).

Initial Operative Management

AXIOM The traditional techniques-ƒprompt exploration, debridement, and repair of bowel, followed by irrigation and removal of any contamination-ƒremain the cornerstones of the treatment of bowel injuries.

After the patient is given a dose of prophylactic antibiotics directed at enteric pathogens, including gram-negative aerobes (such as *Escherichia coli*) and anaerobes (such as *Bacteroides fragilis*), the operative approach is through a generous midline incision. The abdomen is opened expeditiously and, if multiple injuries are present, they are usually managed in the following order:

1. Control of hemorrhage;
2. Control of contamination;
3. Complete resuscitation; and
4. Thorough exploration and definitive control of all injuries.

Examination of the Stomach

During the examination of the stomach, one should pay particular attention to the lesser curvature, the esophagogastric-gastric junction, the lower third of the esophagus, and the top of the fundus. All injuries should be controlled as they are encountered to prevent continued contamination of the peritoneal cavity. The posterior wall of the stomach is inspected by division of the gastrocolic omentum along the greater curvature of the stomach up to the short gastric vessels. Care must be taken not to injure the middle colic artery, which can pass very close to the stomach about midway along the greater curvature.

If only one hole is found, the anesthesiologist can be asked to insufflate air into the stomach via the nasogastric tube. If a second hole still cannot be found, one should consider performing a gastrotomy to inspect the entire stomach thoroughly. One needs to look with particular care along the lesser curvature and the "bare area" high on the posterior wall of the stomach.

AXIOM If two holes in bowel are close to each other, one should join the holes to ensure that there is no mucosal bleeding between the holes.

Examination of the Jejunum and Ileum

The small bowel is eviscerated and inspected carefully throughout its entire length. Small nonexpanding hematomas of the mesentery are carefully inspected at intervals throughout the operative procedure to ensure their stability. If seromuscular rupture of intestine is found in young children, one should suspect child abuse.

Injuries to the base of the mesentery associated with large hematomas should make one suspect a superior mesenteric artery (SMA) or vein (SMV) injury. Complete occlusion of the SMA distal to the middle colic artery can cause severe ischemia to the bowel, and such ischemia may extend from the ligament of Treitz down to the mid-transverse colon. If the superior mesenteric vessels are injured, they should be repaired. In some instances, an interposition graft or patch graft may be necessary.

Access to the proximal portions of the SMA and SMV can be difficult and is best gained by mobilizing the entire left colon and left-sided viscera to the midline so that the aorta and the origin of its major visceral branches can be visualized clearly. The involved vessels should then be dissected and repaired.

Avulsed areas of mesentery can cause later bowel necrosis resulting in a leak or stenosis. Bowel associated with large mesenteric tears should be resected and the remaining bowel joined by a primary anastomosis. Some authors believe that only 50 cm of distal small bowel needs to be left to maintain near normal small bowel absorptive function, but this appears to be highly variable from patient to patient, and it is probably much safer to leave at least 100 cm of distal small bowel.

AXIOM Hematomas that are large, are expanding, or are at the base of the mesentery should be explored.

Repair of the Stomach

If properly mobilized, the stomach is easily repaired. Its walls are generally thick, well vascularized, able to hold sutures well, and redundant in most areas, so that large defects usually can be closed without tension. This contributes to quick healing and minimizes the chance of breakdown.

Gastric injuries should be debrided if needed and then closed with absorbable, inverting sutures for an inner layer and nonabsorbable sutures for the seromuscular second layer. All particulate matter and gastric juice that entered the peritoneal cavity should be removed and the surrounding area should be irrigated thoroughly. Particular attention should be given to cleaning and irrigating the subhepatic and subphrenic spaces, the pelvis, and the lesser sac.

Repair of Small Bowel Injuries

Small perforations of the bowel wall are debrided as needed and closed primarily by lateral sutures. Adjacent through-and-through holes are joined to be sure the intervening bowel is not bleeding or ischemic (Fig. 24-1). Areas of necrosis are removed or,

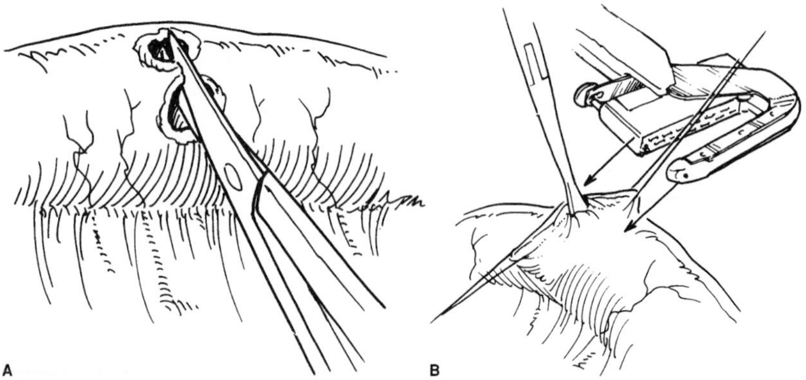

A B

FIG. 24-1. Intestinal perforations in close proximity should be joined, thereby producing a single larger perforation. The enterotomy exposes any bleeding or ischemic bowel that may lie between two wounds. In certain instances, if the defect in the intestinal wall does not exceed one-third of the circumference, a stapled closure can be effected rapidly. (From Maull KI. Stomach, small bowel and mesentery injury. In: *Rob & Smith's Operative Surgery; Trauma Surgery.* 4th ed. London: Butterworth, 1989:406.)

if small, they can be invaginated. The use of either a single-layer or double-layer suturing technique is not crucial and is left to the discretion of the operating surgeon (3). Recently, Fansler et al. (11) reported on the use of biofragmentable anastomotic rings to establish continuity between injured loops of bowel in 18 patients. Using a one-way analysis of variance, the authors found no difference in a comparison with 63 historical controls who had sutured or stapled anastomoses.

AXIOM Several small bowel holes in close proximity are best treated by a segmental resection and primary anastomosis.

The limits of resection of badly injured bowel are determined primarily by the gross appearance of the bowel and its vascular supply. Short segments of bowel of questionable viability should be resected; however, if most of the small bowel is of marginal viability, its color and peristalsis should be evaluated repeatedly. Intravenous fluorescein and examination under a Wood's light have been used to clarify the condition of questionable areas (12). If any doubt still exists at the end of the operation, a "second-look" operation should be performed within 24 hours.

AXIOM The surgeon should make every attempt to leave at least 150 cm of proximal small bowel or 100 cm of distal small bowel to prevent short bowel syndrome.

Abdominal Irrigation

After the bowel repairs are completed, the abdomen should be irrigated copiously with warm saline solution to remove any remaining clots, foreign debris, and intestinal contents (3). The use of antibiotics in the last liter of irrigant is controversial, but we believe that it may be beneficial.

Feeding Jejunostomy

AXIOM Before closure, all patients with severe abdominal injuries should be considered for operative placement of an enteral feeding device.

Schwab et al. (3) perform a needle catheter jejunostomy in virtually all patients with major abdominal injuries before closure, except in those who will be returning for relaparotomy within 24 to 48 hours. We agree with this approach but generally use a larger (peritoneal dialysis) Tenckhoff catheter. Ideally, these conduits are placed approximately 40 cm distal to the ligament of Treitz. The jejunum at the site of the jejunostomy is sutured securely and widely (6 to 8 cm) to the anterior abdominal wall to prevent twisting at that site. Accurate placement of the jejunal catheter can be confirmed postoperatively by aspirating intestinal contents or obtaining an abdominal radiograph after injection of 20 to 30 mL of Gastrografin through the J tube.

Abdominal Closure

Closure of the abdomen can be difficult if the bowel becomes very dilated or edematous. The bowel wall is particularly likely to swell after a major vascular injury because of reperfusion edema. Because most of the edema fluid is intramural or interstitial, an enterotomy to remove the fluid is seldom useful, and any enterotomy is another area that might leak postoperatively. Large intraluminal fluid or gas accumulations can be removed by either retrograde milking of the fluid back into the stomach, where it may be aspirated via the nasogastric tube, or by passing a long intestinal tube.

Despite the use of these techniques, primary closure of the abdominal fascia may still not be possible. In such circumstances, one can sometimes close the skin and subcutaneous tissue and then repair the ventral hernia at a later date. Very large fascial defects may sometimes be bridged with prosthetic mesh. If there has been much contamination, it is best to pack the abdominal opening with moist dressings after covering the anterior bowel surfaces with silk or rayon cloth. An adhesive steridrape covered with an abdominal binder may then be placed across the opening to hold the dressings in the abdomen.

AXIOM Closing the abdominal wall under tension increases the risk of abdominal wall and intestinal complications.

If intraabdominal pressure increases above 30 mm Hg, the resulting abdominal compartment syndrome can cause severe oliguria plus ischemia to the liver and bowel mucosa.

"Second-Look" Operative Management

When the viability of large areas of bowel is in question because of a major vascular injury, it may become necessary to close the abdomen without 100% assurance that all the remaining bowel is viable. In such circumstances, the surgeon makes a commitment to perform a second-look operation 24 to 48 hours later. If a relaparotomy is to be performed, ancillary procedures, such as a gastrostomy or a feeding jejunostomy, should usually be delayed until the time of the relaparotomy.

Postoperative Care

Gastric Decompression

AXIOM With gastric or intestinal injuries, gastric decompression should be continued until bowel activity has returned and the bowel is no longer distended.

Gastric decompression is generally continued until good bowel sounds are heard, the abdomen is not tender except at the incision, there is little or no distension, and the patient is passing flatus or has had a bowel movement.

Enteral Nutrition

Jejunal feedings distal to any upper gastrointestinal injuries can often be begun as soon as tube placement has been confirmed by aspiration of bile-stained intestinal contents or by radiologic contrast studies. Liberal and early use of the feeding jejunostomy has greatly reduced the use of parenteral hyperalimentation (13). With distal small bowel injuries, it is probably wise to wait at least 4 to 5 days before beginning jejunostomy feedings.

Isotonic jejunal feedings at about 10 mL/h are generally tolerated well. The isotonic tube feedings can then be increased about 10 mL/h every 12 hours as long as there is no bloating or cramping. Incremental advances are made until the patient's nutritional goal of at least 25 to 35 nonprotein calories/kg/day are achieved.

Antibiotics

AXIOM Prophylactic antibiotics are usually needed for only one or two doses after most gastric or small intestinal injuries.

Prophylactic preoperative antibiotics are continued for at least 24 to 48 hours if bowel perforation has occurred. Wounds with low infectious potential (i.e., uncomplicated stomach or proximal small bowel perforations) may require only one or two doses of antibiotics. In patients who are at high risk for infection because of severe peritoneal contamination, multiple injuries, prolonged hypotension, or multiple blood transfusions, therapeutic antibiotics for at least 4 to 5 days may be warranted.

Although this is controversial, intraperitoneal antibiotic irrigation may also be of some benefit in cases with severe peritoneal contamination (14).

COMPLICATIONS

Hemorrhage

Postoperative bleeding is particularly likely to occur following a gastric repair if excess or prolonged traction was applied to the stomach to enhance exposure. Probably the single most common site of postoperative intraabdominal bleeding after gastric surgery is an injury to the spleen. Bleeding into the gastric lumen can occur at suture lines or areas of bowel wall contusion.

AXIOM In critically ill or injured patients, the gastric pH should be monitored and kept above 4.5 to 5.0 until the patient is eating properly.

Bleeding from the stomach after 2 to 3 days may be due to stress gastritis. Postoperative bleeding from injured small bowel is unusual.

Bowel Obstruction

Small bowel obstruction is not unusual following intestinal injuries. Although the obstruction is usually caused by adhesions, it can also be a result of edema at an anastomosis or an intussusception. Early postoperative small bowel obstruction can be difficult to differentiate from the usual postoperative ileus, and often it is not diagnosed until there is clinical evidence of strangulated or leaking bowel.

AXIOM Early postoperative bowel obstructions tend to have a high mortality rate because they often are not diagnosed until strangulation or peritonitis occurs.

Suture Line Disruption

Suture line disruption is much more likely to occur in the small bowel than in the stomach; however, regardless of its source, it can be a catastrophic event. Any gastric anastomosis that leaks should be excised and reclosed. With small bowel leaks, the involved bowel should be resected and clean, uninvolved bowel can be reanastomosed. If the distal ileum is the site of the leak and severe peritonitis is present, the proximal end of the involved bowel should be brought out as an ileostomy. The distal end can also be brought out, or simply stapled off and left in situ.

In polytraumatized patients, a leak at a suture line may be difficult to diagnose without reoperation. In some instances, the only way to make the diagnosis is prompt exploration of patients who have increasing signs of sepsis or are not improving as they should. If the intraabdominal infection is severe enough to warrant temporary diversion with an end-jejunostomy or ileostomy, total parenteral nutrition for metabolic support and meticulous stomal care are essential.

Occasionally, a suture line disruption is not recognized until there is an enterocutaneous fistula. If the patient is not septic, a small-volume enterocutaneous fistula without distal obstruction usually heals spontaneously after 2 to 3 weeks of parenteral hyperalimentation and bowel rest (3). If an enterocutaneous fistula is associated with a distal obstruction, operative relief of the distal obstruction is essential as soon as the patient's condition allows. Such obstructions may be caused by intestinal adhesions or interloop abscesses.

Metabolic Complications of Small Bowel Resection

Resection of large amounts of small bowel may lead to a malabsorption or short bowel syndrome caused by a loss of absorptive segments or alterations in bacterial flora. Generally, at least half of the small bowel can be removed without serious disability (3). Length for length, removal of the distal ileum leads to far more serious complications than removal of equal portions of the jejunum.

AXIOM If large amounts of small bowel must be removed, special efforts should be made to preserve the distal ileum.

In patients with short bowel syndromes, the absorption of fat is usually a much greater problem than carbohydrate uptake. Despite massive resections of small bowel, ingested disaccharides can induce changes in enzyme secretion in the remaining ileum or jejunum, so that after a relatively short time, intestinal adaptation occurs, and carbohydrate absorption may approach normal. Fluid and most electrolyte losses can be compensated to some degree by the kidneys, but large losses of calcium, magnesium, and zinc may be much more difficult to manage.

Removal of jejunum may be associated with lactose intolerance, which is often self-limited. Removal of the distal ileum often causes vitamin B_{12} and bile salt deficiencies, fat malabsorption, and bacterial overgrowth that compounds the other metabolic deficiencies. Interference with the absorptive capacity for fat leads to bile salt deficiencies, which can cause further reductions in the bowel absorption of vitamins A, D, K, and E. Vitamin B_{12} deficiencies also tend to occur if the distal ileum is diseased or resected.

An unusual syndrome, usually seen only with short bowel syndromes, is D-lactic acidosis, which can cause patients to exhibit bizarre behavior and various neurologic findings, including ataxia and confusion (3). This problem is caused by an overgrowth of colonic bacteria that produce the D-isomer of lactic acid, which cannot be metabolized by the patient. The diagnosis of D-lactic acidosis should be suspected if the patient has an increased anion gap metabolic acidosis in the absence of usual causes such as uremia, ketoacidosis, or tissue ischemia. Treatment is directed at suppression of colonic bacterial overgrowth with appropriate enteral antibiotics (15).

⊘ FREQUENT ERRORS

1. ***Inadequate exploration of the abdomen because of an assumption that a particular organ could not possibly have been injured by a bullet apparently passing through another area of the abdomen.***
2. ***Inadequate search for another hole if one can find only an odd number of openings in the bowel after a gunshot or stab wound.***
3. ***Assuming that an abdominal injury has not occurred because a CT scan and an early DPL are negative.***
4. ***Failure to explore a hematoma at the base of the small bowel mesentery adequately.***
5. ***Failure to perform a second-look procedure in 24 to 48 hours if the bowel is marginally ischemic.***
6. ***Failure to consider placement of an enteral feeding tube in a patient who has severe injuries and is not apt to be eating by mouth within 4 to 5 days.***
7. ***Closure of the abdomen under tension when it is not really necessary, particularly if there is a risk of the abdominal compartment syndrome.***
8. ***Delay in reoperating for a possible small bowel suture leak.***

SUMMARY POINTS

1. Taken together, the stomach and small bowel are the most frequently injured organs in penetrating abdominal trauma.

2. One should be suspicious of a characteristic tetrad of injuries caused by seat belts, which includes abdominal wall contusion, small bowel rupture, mesenteric tears, and lumbar spine fractures.

3. Signs of peritonitis after blunt intestinal trauma to small bowel may be delayed for hours or days.
4. Intestinal injuries do not commonly cause free air to be visible on plain radiographs of the abdomen.
5. One cannot rely on abdominal CT scans to detect injuries to the small intestine distal to the ligament of Treitz.
6. DPL is the most reliable method for diagnosing injury to intraperitoneal hollow viscera; however, if done within 2 hours of injury, there may not have been enough time for an adequate WBC response.
7. If one suspects a bowel injury or the initial lavage results are equivocal, the catheter can be left in place for a repeat DPL 3 to 6 hours later.
8. If two holes in bowel are close to each other, one should join the holes to ensure that there is no mucosal bleeding between the holes.
9. In suspicious cases, celiotomy is the safest course to follow, even in the face of little or no confirming data of an intraabdominal injury.
10. The traditional techniques of prompt exploration, debridement, and repair of the bowel followed by irrigation and removal of any contamination are the cornerstones of the treatment of bowel injuries.
11. Access to the proximal SMA is best done from a lateral retroperitoneal approach after mobilizing the left-sided abdominal viscera to the right.
12. Hematomas that are large or expanding at the base of the mesentery should be explored.
13. Several small bowel holes in close proximity are best treated by a segmental resection and primary anastomosis.
14. Bowel of questionable viability should be left in situ only if the patient's survival may be threatened by "short-gut syndrome."
15. Any deterioration in a patient with mesenteric trauma should be considered to be due to intestinal ischemia or perforation until proven otherwise.
16. Before closure, all patients with severe abdominal injuries should be considered for operative placement of an enteral feeding device.
17. Closing the abdominal wall under tension increases the risk of abdominal wall and intestinal complications.
18. With gastric or intestinal injuries, gastric decompression should be continued until bowel activity has returned and the bowel is no longer distended.
19. Prophylactic antibiotics are usually needed for only one or two doses after most gastric or small intestinal injuries.
20. In critically ill or injured patients, the gastric pH should be monitored and kept above 4.5 to 5.0 until the patient is eating properly.
21. Early postoperative bowel obstructions tend to have a high mortality rate because they often are not diagnosed until strangulation or peritonitis occurs.
22. If large amounts of small bowel must be removed, special efforts should be made to preserve the distal ileum.

REFERENCES

1. Wilson RF, Walt AJ. Injury to the stomach and small bowel. In: Wilson RF, Walt AJ, eds. *Management of trauma—pitfalls and practices.* 2nd ed. Philadelphia: Williams & Wilkins, 1996:497.
2. Fabian TC, Patterson CR. Injuries of the stomach, duodenum, pancreas, and small intestine. In: Kreis DJ, Gomez GA, eds. *Trauma management.* Boston: Little, Brown and Company, 1989:229–230.
3. Schwab CW, Shaikhra, Talucci RC. Injury to the stomach and small bowel. In: Moore EE, Mattox KL, Feliciano DV, eds. *Trauma.* 2nd ed. Norwalk, CT: Appleton & Lange, 1991;31:485–497.
4. Roberts JL. CT of abdominal and pelvic trauma. Semin Ultrasound CT MR 1996; 17:142.
5. Dowe MF, Shanmuganathan K, Mirvis SE, et al. CT findings of mesenteric injury

after blunt trauma: implications for surgical intervention. *AJR Am J Roentgenol* 1997;168:425.
6. Harrison AW, Whelan P. Bowel injury from blunt abdominal trauma. In: McMurtry RY, McLellan BA, eds. *Management of blunt trauma.* Baltimore: Williams & Wilkins, 1990;265–271.
7. Bosworth BM. Perforation of the small intestine from nonpenetrating abdominal trauma. *Am J Surg* 1948;76:472.
8. Frantzides CT, Ludwig KA, Aprahamian C, Salaymeh B. Laparoscopic closure of gastric stab wounds. A case report. *Surg Laparosc Endosc* 1993;3:63.
9. Brams DM, Cardoza M, Smith RS. Laparoscopic repair of traumatic gastric perforation using a gasless technique. *J Laparoendosc Surg* 1993;3:587.
10. Low LL, Ripple GR, Bruderer BP, et al. Non-operative management of gastric perforation secondary to cardiopulmonary resuscitation. *Intensive Care Med* 1995;20:442.
11. Fansler RF, Mero K, Steinberg SM, et al. Utility of the biofragmentable anastomotic ring in traumatic small bowel injury. *Am Surg* 1994;60:379.
12. Bulkley GB, Perler BA, Zuidema GD. Mesenteric vascular disease. In Cameron JL, ed. *Current surgical therapy.* 5th ed. St Louis: Mosby, 1995:126.
13. Moore EE, Jones TN. Benefits of immediate jejunostomy feeding after major abdominal trauma. *J Trauma* 1986;26:874.
14. Ablan CJ, Olen RN, Dobrin, et al. Efficacy of intraperitoneal antibiotics in the treatment of severe fecal peritonitis. *Am J Surg* 1991;1562:453.
15. Cerise EJ, Schully JH. Blunt trauma to the small intestine. *J Trauma* 1970;10: 46.

25. INJURIES TO THE PANCREAS AND DUODENUM(1)

ANATOMY

The pancreas and the duodenum, except for the first part of the duodenum, are retroperitoneal structures and are protected by the thick paraspinal muscles posteriorly. Consequently these organs are usually injured only with deeply penetrating wounds or forceful blunt trauma (2,3).

AXIOM Associated injuries are the major cause of the high mortality rates seen with pancreatic and duodenal trauma.

Because the duodenum lacks a complete serosal covering for most of its length, repairs to it have an increased tendency to leak. In addition, normal pancreas has limited tensile strength, so that sutures tend to cut through it easily. It is also difficult to penetrate the pancreas deeply at any point with sutures without passing through some ductal structures.

The head of the pancreas is nestled into the curve of the duodenum and shares its blood supply. In addition, both of the pancreatic ducts (the main duct of Wirsurg and accessory duct of Santorini) penetrate the wall of the duodenum to allow pancreatic juices to enter the intestinal lumen. The tail of the pancreas nestles against the hilum of the spleen, and the spleen shares its blood supply with the body and tail of the pancreas.

PHYSIOLOGY

Duodenal Contents

Because there is little absorption in the stomach, the duodenum receives virtually all of the ingested food as well as 500 to 1,000 mL of salivary secretions, 500 to 1,500 mL gastric secretions, 600 to 1,000 mL of bile, 800 to 1,500 mL of pancreatic juice, and some duodenal secretions.

AXIOM The total volume of fluid passing through the duodenum may exceed 3 to 6 L per day, and a fistula in this area can cause serious fluid and electrolyte problems.

Stimuli to Secretion

Secretin, which is secreted by duodenal mucosa primarily as a response to acid contents, stimulates secretion of pancreatic juice that is high in volume and bicarbonate and low in enzyme content. Cholecystokinin, which is secreted in response to the presence of breakdown products of food in the duodenum, stimulates contraction of the gallbladder and passage of bile into the duodenum. It also stimulates the exocrine pancreas to secrete a relatively low volume of pancreatic juice that has a high concentration of enzymes that usually become activated after they enter the duodenum.

AXIOM Dehiscence of a duodenal suture line can be especially dangerous because of the large amounts of activated enzymes that may be rapidly liberated into the abdomen.

MECHANISMS OF INJURY

In a 12-year period at Detroit Receiving Hospital (DRH) ending in June 1992, 2,741 patients were admitted with abdominal injuries. The incidence of pancreatic injuries with blunt trauma was 6%, and that of gunshot wounds, 10%, and stabs, 5%. Of 177 penetrating pancreatic injuries seen at DRH, 128 (72%) were caused by pistols or rifles, 12 (7%) were caused by shotguns, and 37 (21%) were caused by knives.

Associated Injuries

With Pancreatic Trauma

Blunt Trauma

Although the pancreas may be ruptured over the spine at the neck of the pancreas by blunt trauma, and there may be lacerations of the head of the pancreas, most of the deaths are caused by the frequent associated injuries. In the DRH series, the most frequent associated injuries with blunt pancreatic trauma were

- Liver, 36%
- Spleen, 30%
- Kidney, 18%
- Colon, 18%
- Major vessels, 9%

Jordan (2) also noted that injuries to large arteries and veins, which are the major cause of death in patients with pancreatic trauma, occur in about 9% of these patients.

Penetrating Trauma

Jordan (2) noted that up to 45% of patients with penetrating pancreatic trauma had associated injuries of major arteries or veins. In the DRH series, the most frequent associated injuries with penetrating pancreatic trauma were

- Stomach, 54%
- Liver, 49%
- Kidneys, 44%

In the DRH series, the mortality rate with penetrating pancreatic injuries was 25% (45 of 177). Mortality rates were largely related to the number of associated injuries, and the patients with none or only one associated injury had a mortality rate of only 4%.

With Duodenal Injuries

Blunt Trauma

Duodenal injury in motor vehicle accidents is usually ascribed to crushing the duodenum against the vertebral column or causing blow-out of the duodenal loop because it is partially closed at the pylorus and at the ligament of Treitz.

Although blunt duodenal injuries are most common in the second part of duodenum, about 25% are found in the fourth part, close to the ligament of Treitz (4). Consequently this latter area must be carefully inspected by incising the peritoneum and dissecting gently under the lower border of the pancreas.

In the DRH series, the mortality rate from blunt duodenal trauma was 30%. All of the patients in the DRH series who died with blunt duodenal trauma had four or more associated injuries. About 40% to 50% of the patients with duodenal injuries have associated pancreatic damage (5). Associated pancreatic injuries increase the mortality rate of duodenal injuries from about 5% to 10% to almost 40% (6).

Penetrating Trauma

Of the 167 patients with duodenal injuries diagnosed at laparotomy at DRH in the 12-year period, 157 (94%) were caused by penetrating trauma. With penetrating trauma, the most frequent associated injuries were

- Liver, 54%
- Major blood vessels, 52%
- Small bowel, 50%
- Colon, 49%

DIAGNOSIS

Signs and Symptoms

AXIOM The clinical changes in isolated pancreatic or duodenal injury may be extremely subtle until severe, life-threatening peritonitis develops.

Although isolated retroperitoneal injuries occasionally can produce signs of frank peritonitis, the vast majority initially produce only a mild tenderness. By the time that there are clear signs of a problem, severe peritonitis is usually present.

Laboratory Evaluation

Serum Amylase

AXIOM A consistently increased or increasing serum or urinary amylase should make one suspect a pancreatic injury.

Jordan (2) noted that serum amylase concentrations are increased in only about 25% of patients sustaining penetrating injury to the pancreas; however, they may be increased in up to 80% of patients with pancreatic injuries due to blunt trauma. It should be remembered that perforation of the duodenum or any portion of the upper gastrointestinal tract also may lead to increased serum amylase levels as a result of spillage of intraluminal amylase into the peritoneal cavity.

Radiologic Studies

Plain Films

Plain films of the abdomen with the patient in the recumbent and upright positions may be helpful in patients suspected of having an intraabdominal injury. Lucas (5) described scoliosis or obliteration of the right psoas shadow in 18 (90%) of 20 patients with duodenal rupture. In 50% of the patients, retroperitoneal air bubbles could be seen along the right psoas muscle or around the right kidney. The presence of retroperitoneal air is sufficient evidence to compel exploration, but an upper gastrointestinal (GI) series with water-soluble contrast is recommended in patients with scoliosis or blurring of the psoas margin.

Contrast Swallow

An upper GI series using water-soluble contrast material can provide positive results in 50% of patients with duodenal perforations (6). If a duodenal injury is suspected, the meglumine (Gastrografin) swallow should be done with the patient in the right lateral position. Some surgeons believe that barium is more accurate and can provide more positive results, but barium also tends to cause more peritoneal and retroperitoneal inflammation if a leak is present. Upper GI studies with contrast also are indicated in patients with a suspected hematoma of the duodenum, because these may demonstrate the classic "coiled-spring" appearance of complete obstruction by the nematoma (2).

Computed Tomography

Computed tomography (CT) scans may demonstrate a high percentage of duodenal injuries. Kunin et al. (7) reported that, in seven patients with blunt trauma, resulting in a duodenal hematoma in four and perforation in three, all seven were diagnosed correctly by the CT scan. Extraluminal gas or extravasated contrast was seen in the right anterior prerenal space in all three perforations. In another study of 10 patients with pancreatic injury proven by surgery or autopsy after blunt abdominal trauma, the CT scans of all 10 patients showed abnormalities suggesting pancreatic injury (8); nevertheless, it is generally believed that many pancreatic injuries are missed on CT scans.

AXIOM All techniques used to diagnose injuries of the pancreas or duodenum may be characterized as reliable only when they identify an injury; a "normal" study has relatively little negative predictive value.

Although ultrasonography in the hands of an experienced examiner may demonstrate some pancreatic injuries, because of overlying bowel gas that is often present, a CT scan is generally the more useful modality.

Diagnostic Peritoneal Lavage

Although virtually all patients with blunt duodenal injury will eventually have increased white blood cells and amylase levels in diagnostic peritoneal lavage (DPL) fluid, DPL has a low sensitivity for duodenal perforations.

Endoscopic Retrograde Cholangiopancreatography

Endoscopic retrograde cholangiopancreatography (ERCP) can demonstrate injury to the main pancreatic ducts. It also can provide a helpful road map for the operative surgeon if the normal anatomy is obscured by hematoma or inflammation; however, this technique has been used in relatively few cases, with the largest series containing only nine patients (2).

Gholson et al. (9) suggested that ERCP may be particularly helpful in evaluating patients with chronic abdominal pain after blunt trauma to the abdomen. The authors described three patients with chronic distal pancreatitis who had severe abdominal pain after an asymptomatic latent period of 3 months to 1 year after their blunt trauma. The ERCP showed ductal stenosis or obstruction in the midbody of the pancreas in all three patients, and in all three, distal pancreatectomy was curative.

Intraoperative Evaluation

All patients with trauma to the upper abdomen having a celiotomy should have a careful exploration of the pancreas and duodenum, particularly if there is a hematoma overlying any portion of these structures.

AXIOM Upper midline retroperitoneal hematomas should be explored to rule out underlying duodenal, pancreatic, or vascular injuries.

A wide Kocher maneuver (opening the right lateral peritoneal reflection of the duodenum) generally will allow investigation of the first, second, and third portions of the duodenum and the posterior portion of the head of the pancreas over to the abdominal aorta. If the Kocher maneuver does not provide adequate exposure of the first three portions of the duodenum and head of the pancreas, one can add the Cattell maneuver. This involves reflecting the right colon medially to the origin of its mesenteric vessels. This technique also allows full exposure of the duodenum except in its most distal portions.

The cause of even minimal bile staining of paraduodenal tissues must be sought carefully. Some surgeons have suggested performing a needle cholecystocholangiogram if no duodenal or biliary tract injury is found on exploration.

An overlying hematoma is the most common intraoperative indication of pancreatic or duodenal injury. All upper central retroperitoneal hematomas should be explored, and if the hematoma is large, a major vascular injury should be suspected. The body and tail of the pancreas can generally be well visualized by opening the lesser sac and then reflecting the stomach superiorly and the traverse colon inferiorly. The plane posterior to the superior margins of the pancreas can be entered bluntly along its entire length, thus allowing bimanual palpation of the entire organ. If indicated, the peritoneum along the entire inferior border of the pancreas also may be incised to allow elevation of the inferior margin of the body and tail of the pancreas to inspect the posterior surface.

AXIOM Severe edema, crepitance, or bile staining of periduodenal tissues implies a duodenal injury until proven otherwise.

After inspection of the entire duodenum, the common bile duct can be exposed by incision of the peritoneum and areolar tissue on the inferolateral border of the hepatoduodenal ligament.

If the exploration seems to be negative, but one is still suspicious of a duodenal injury, Brotman et al. (10) recommended instillation of methylene blue through the nasogastric tube. Rapid staining of periduodenal tissues with this blue–green dye is irrefutable evidence of an intestinal rupture in this area, and the lack of staining, in their hands, has proven reliable in ruling out full-thickness duodenal injury.

Determining the integrity of the main ducts is very important in patients with a suspected pancreatic injury. Some surgeons believe that, if this cannot be accomplished by direct visualization, intraoperative pancreatography should be attempted by intubating the ampulla of Vater through a duodenotomy.

Some surgeons have used secretin to stimulate the pancreas intraoperatively with the hopes of finding leakage of pancreatic secretions from an otherwise undetected ductal injury; however, Jordan (2) would consider doing this only in rare patients.

TREATMENT OF PANCREATIC INJURIES

Grading Pancreatic Injuries

The organ injury scaling (OIS) Committee of the American Association for the Surgery of Trauma (AAST) graded pancreatic injuries from I to V (11).

Grade I Simple contusion of the pancreas
Grade II Major contusion or laceration without tissue loss or involvement of the main pancreatic duct
Grade III Complete transection of the pancreas or a parenchymal injury with involvement of the major duct to the left of the SMV
Grade IV Ductal transection or a major parenchymal injury to the right of the SMV
Grade V Massive disruption of the head of the pancreas

Specific Injuries of the Pancreas

Pancreatic Duct

Wounds that do not involve the main pancreatic duct are generally successfully managed by external drainage alone. Some authors advocated the use of capsular sutures in addition to sump drainage. Such sutures also may aid in hemostasis.

The most serious pancreatic wounds are those that transect a major pancreatic duct so that there is continued uncontrolled leakage of pancreatic exocrine secretions into the peritoneal cavity and retroperitoneum. Wounds involving the main duct in the distal body and tail of the pancreas can be treated with resection of the distal pancreas. Occasionally efforts are made to leave the splenic artery and vein intact to preserve the spleen; however, this can be very time consuming and difficult.

After a distal pancreatectomy is completed, the distal end of the proximal pancreas can be stapled or a series of interlocking U-sutures of polypropylene can placed at close intervals (3). An apron or tongue of viable omentum is then secured over the resected end of the pancreas. A closed suction drain is placed near, but not on, the resected edge of the pancreas. If, for some reason, one is anxious to preserve the body and tail of the pancreas, the injured end can be anastomosed to a Roux-en-Y loop of jejunum (3).

AXIOM Because 80% to 90% of the normal pancreas can generally be resected without significant endocrine or exocrine deficiency, complex preservation procedures are rarely indicated.

Kopelman et al. (12) recently reported a case of late diagnosis of blunt pancreatic head injury with ductal transection. Treatment of this problem included intraoperative ERCP with internal transpancreatic stent drainage of the distal duct.

Head of the Pancreas

Wounds to the head of the pancreas are usually the result of penetrating trauma, and these are often associated with major vascular injuries, which can be rapidly fatal. Once the bleeding is controlled, one should try to determine whether there is damage to the major pancreatic duct (2). If it can be ascertained that the duct is not injured, the treatment of wounds of the head of the pancreas is no different from that of wounds of the body and tail. If the main duct is injured, one must make a major decision.

Fabian and Patterson (3) managed major ductal injuries in the head of the pancreas by drainage. If a pancreatic fistula developed, it was managed as a chronic fistula. Many surgeons believe that one should place an onlay Roux-en-Y loop of jejunum over the injured area. This may be done with or without some type of pyloric exclusion to direct gastric secretions away from the duodenum for at least 3 weeks.

AXIOM Severe injuries to the duodenum or head of the pancreas are usually managed best by some type of duodenal diverticulization or pyloric exclusion procedure (Figs. 25-1 and 25-2).

Pancreaticoduodenectomy (Whipple procedure) is thought by some surgeons to be the treatment of choice for injury to the main duct in the head of the pancreas, especially if the duodenum or common bile duct or both also are severely injured. In some instances, this may have to be done in two steps with the resection performed in the first stage, and the anastomoses performed 24 to 48 hours later.

Enteral Feeding

AXIOM A jejunostomy catheter should be inserted about 60 cm beyond the ligament of Treitz at the time of definitive pancreatic or duodenal surgery to allow early enteral feeding.

Complications of Pancreatic Injuries

Fistula

A fistula is the most common complication of pancreatic injury (2); it develops in nearly one third of patients with pancreatic wounds. Most surgeons expect some drainage from a pancreatic wound and do not consider it a complication unless the drainage is of large volume or persists for more than several days or both. When such a definition is used, the incidence of pancreatic fistula is quite small.

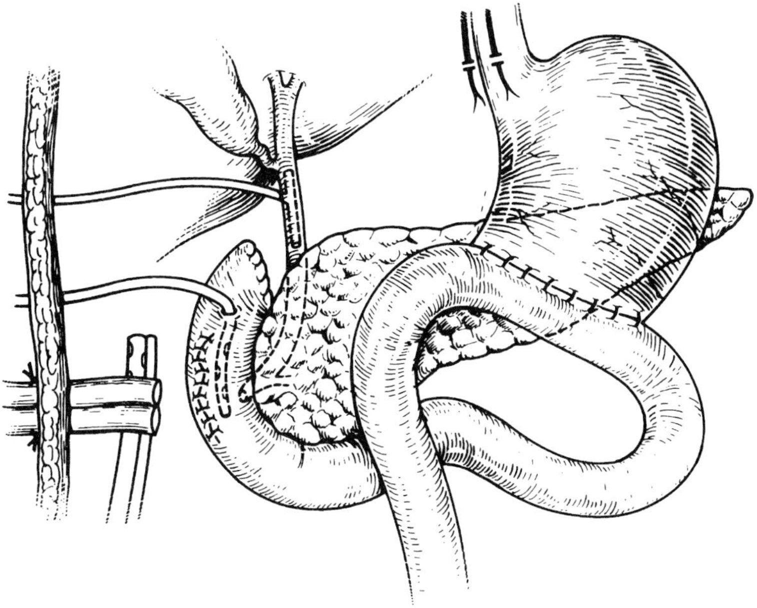

FIG. 25-1. Duodenal diverticulization. For extensive injury of the duodenum and pancreas or severe injury of the duodenum alone, Berne et al. (13) described a duodenal diverticulation procedure that included **(A)** suture repair of the primary injury, **(B)** antrectomy, **(C)** tube duodenostomy, and **(D)** generous drainable of the area. Truncal vagotomy and biliary decompression may also be advisable. From ref. 15, with permission.

Major fistulas are more likely to occur after wounds of the head of the pancreas than after wounds of the body and tail (2). When the major pancreatic duct is injured, a fistula can be anticipated unless the ductal wound is repaired.

Pure pancreatic juice usually has an amylase concentration of approximately 50,000 U/mL, but the amylase concentration in some fistulas exceeds 1,000,000 U/mL. With lesser values in the range of 5,000 to 10,000 U/mL, the amount of pancreatic juice draining may be quite small, and such fistulas usually close relatively quickly (2).

Initial Treatment

AXIOM The initial treatment of pancreatic fistulas should be conservative because most fistulas heal spontaneously within 2 to 4 weeks.

The treatment of posttraumatic pancreatic fistulas includes

- Adequate drainage
- Prevention of infection
- Protection of the skin

The enzymes are usually not activated and consequently produce little problem with skin excoriation (3).

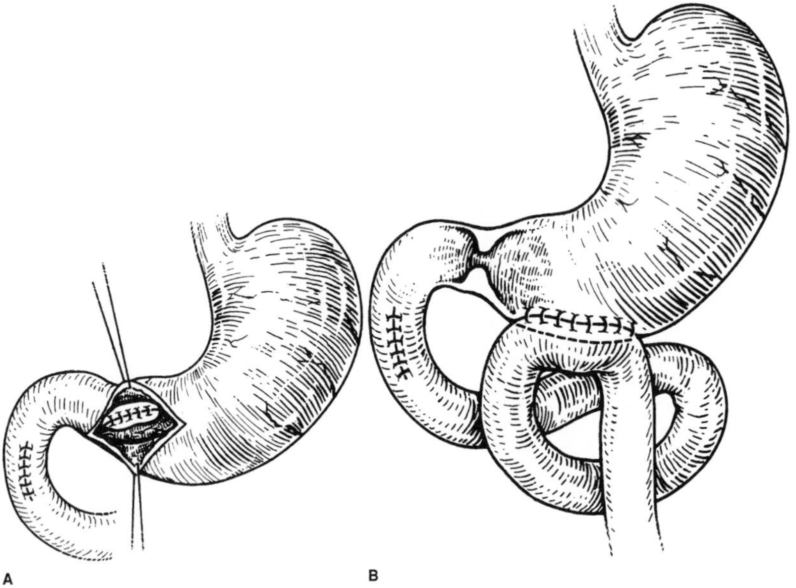

FIG. 25-2. Pyloric exclusion. With severe duodenal or duodenal and pancreatic injuries, an alternative method of management is to obstruct the pylorus temporarily and perform a gastrojejunostomy without antrectomy. The duodenal wound is repaired primarily, followed by a gastrotomy on the greater curvature of the antrum at a site selected for gastrojejunostomy. Truncal vagotomy is not routinely performed, although a small incidence of marginal ulcers has been reported. From ref. 15, with permission.

AXIOM Drains should be left in place after pancreatic trauma until the patient is eating a full diet and there is little or no drainage, or until the drainage tract is well established.

Frequently there is little or no pancreatic drainage until the patient resumes eating by mouth. If the drains have already been removed, a major pancreatic leak can accumulate in the abdomen and can cause severe complications.

Once a chronic tract has developed, the drains should be withdrawn 1 to 2 inches. Drains left too close to the pancreas may impede healing of the fistula. A sinogram can also be obtained to determine the size and course of the fistula.

Fluid, electrolyte, and nutritional balance should be maintained throughout the treatment of large pancreatic fistulas. In the early period, this is accomplished by intravenous fluids and intravenous hyperalimentation. Jejunal tube feedings should be started as soon as small bowel activity has resumed.

AXIOM Somatostatin and its analogs significantly decrease the volume of pancreatic secretions in some patients, and they may help provide a more rapid closure of some fistulas.

The surgical treatment of choice for a persistent large pancreatic fistula is anastomosis of the fistula tract at the surface of the pancreas to a Roux-en-Y loop of jejunum (2). Once a fistula has been present for more than 6 weeks, there is usually enough fibrosis of the surrounding tissue so that it can be sutured to bowel safely.

Pancreatic Abscesses

Intraabdominal abscesses develop in approximately 5% of patients with pancreatic injuries, but in most patients, they are caused primarily by associated injuries of the liver, colon, or small bowel. Hematomas or devitalized tissue or both contaminated by gastrointestinal contents are particularly prone to infection (3). Aerobic gram-negative rods and gram-positive cocci are the usual infecting organisms, and antibiotics covering these should be started as soon as possible after the trauma. A true pancreatic abscess is usually the result of inadequate debridement of necrotic pancreas at the time of surgery.

AXIOM Pancreatic necrosis or an abscess should be suspected in anyone who becomes toxic or develops multiple organ failure after a major pancreatic injury.

With the use of CT scans, the presence of pancreatic or peripancreatic abscesses or fluid collections can usually be confirmed quite accurately. If percutaneous drainage does not improve the patient's condition rapidly, a laparotomy should be performed to provide adequate drainage.

Posttraumatic Pancreatitis

Many patients with pancreatic trauma develop abdominal or back pain with increased serum or urine amylase levels or both (2). If the patient is doing well clinically, he or she can be treated conservatively; however, a patient occasionally can develop severe posttraumatic pancreatitis with a persistent increase in serum amylase levels and increasing deep abdominal or midback pain.

Traumatic pancreatitis will usually resolve within 1 or 2 weeks with symptomatic therapy (3). Occasionally the serum amylase and lipase levels remain moderately increased even though the symptoms have completely resolved. If pain develops or if the amylase or lipase levels increase markedly with feeding, bowel rest can be reinstituted. If a jejunostomy tube is in place, feedings through it will not usually disturb the pancreas. If the patient is not eating adequately within 5 days, one should consider starting total parenteral nutrition (TPN).

Pseudocysts

Pseudocyst formation (fluid collection with a fibrous capsule) is uncommon after pancreatic trauma unless there has been a major ductal injury without proper drainage. Although some series reported an incidence of pseudocysts as high as 20%, for most series in which the initial pancreatic operation was undertaken promptly, the incidence is in the range of 1.5% to 5% (2).

AXIOM Development of a pancreatic pseudocyst should be suspected in anyone with an upper abdominal mass or persistent increase of serum amylase levels after pancreatic trauma (1).

Traumatic pancreatic pseudocysts that occur after peripheral duct injury may resolve spontaneously, and those associated with distal main duct injuries can be treated by percutaneous aspiration or catheter drainage. Proximal duct injuries generally require surgical intervention, usually with internal drainage.

AXIOM ERCP should be performed before the treatment of traumatic pancreatic pseudocysts to aid in the selection of the most appropriate procedure (3).

Delayed Postoperative Hemorrhage

Pancreatic wounds seldom bleed massively after the initial 24 to 48 hours after surgery; however, if a fistula or an abscess develops, erosion into a large adjacent vessel can cause delayed massive hemorrhage (2). In such instances, angiographic localization and occlusion of the bleeding site is generally preferable to surgery.

Malabsorption

Most patients sustaining pancreatic injury have a normal pancreas at the time of the traumatic episode, and exocrine insufficiency is unlikely to develop unless 80% to 90% or more of the pancreas is removed. Alcoholic patients or patients with prior recurrent pancreatitis who have pancreatic trauma may, however, require administration of pancreatic enzymes with their food, especially if a pancreatic resection is performed.

TREATMENT OF DUODENAL INJURIES

Grading Duodenal Injuries

The OIS Committee of the AAST developed a system classifying duodenal injuries (11):

Type I Include serosal tears or hematomas involving a single portion of the duodenum

Type II Include hematomas involving more than one portion of the duodenum or a laceration involving less than 50% of the circumference

Type III Include lacerations involving 50% to 75% of the circumference of the second part of the duodenum or a 50% to 100% disruption of any other part of the duodenum

Type IV Include disruptions involving more than 75% of the second part of the duodenum or lacerations involving the ampulla of Vater or the distal common bile duct

Type V Include massive disruptions of both the duodenum and pancreas or pancreatic damage combined with devascularization of the duodenum

Specific Duodenal Injuries

Duodenal Hematomas

An uncommon but special type of duodenal injury after blunt trauma is an intramural hematoma, usually in the second or third portion, that results in partial or complete obstruction of the lumen. In many patients, this is the only injury, and the symptoms of abdominal pain and bilious vomiting may not be impressive soon after injury. The diagnosis may be suspected on the basis of a CT scan, but it is usually confirmed by an upper GI study with barium showing a characteristic "stack of coins" or coiled spring with partial or complete obstruction of the duodenum.

Treatment of duodenal hematomas with nasogastric suction and hyperalimentation usually allows resolution of the hematoma within 1 to 3 weeks. If the duodenal occlusion is complete, one can generally anticipate a prolonged period of intravenous hyperalimentation, and early surgical drainage may be preferable (2).

Duodenal Lacerations

Wounds to portions of the duodenum that have a serosal surface can usually be managed successfully by simple primary closure; however, the retroperitoneal duodenum has no serosal covering and is, therefore, at greater risk of leak from a primary repair (3).

If a penetrating injury on the anterior surface of the duodenum is encountered, it is critical that the posterior and medial (pancreatic) surfaces also be examined very carefully (2). These wounds can usually be repaired by simple suture after adequate debridement. Debridement is usually not necessary for simple knife wounds, but with high-velocity missiles, some debridement is usually appropriate. Covering the completed repair with omentum or an onlay patch of jejunum should reduce the leak rate somewhat.

AXIOM Gunshot wounds or blunt trauma to the duodenum should be repaired carefully after debridement as needed. The repaired area also should be buttressed with well-vascularized uninjured tissues, such as omentum.

Duodenal Decompression

If primary repair of the duodenum is possible but there is significant concern about the wound closure, several special techniques have been advocated (2). The simplest of these is the placement of a duodenal drainage catheter, to keep the duodenum decompressed so that the suture line is less likely to be placed under tension. For the most severe injuries, pyloric exclusion or duodenal diverticulization is preferred.

Duodenal Wall Loss

If there loss is of duodenal tissue, but it is only on the lateral wall, a transverse primary repair should be attempted, even though some narrowing of the duodenal lumen may occur. In some instances, primary repair is impossible without creating too much tension on the suture line (2). Under such circumstances, a duodenojejunostomy can be performed.

Patients with extensive damage to the third and fourth portions of the duodenum also can be managed by distal duodenectomy and an end-to-end duodeno-Roux-en-Y-jejunostomy (3).

One can also repair the defect by suturing intact proximal jejunum as a patch over the defect (2,3).

Duodenal Transections

When the duodenum is totally transected, the preferred treatment is usually a primary anastomosis of the two ends after appropriate debridement; however, if a large amount of tissue is lost, approximation of the duodenum may not be possible without producing undue tension on the suture line (2). When such injuries occur distal to the ampulla of Vater, they should be repaired by resection or closure of the distal duodenum and an anastomosis of the proximal duodenum to a loop of jejunum.

If a total transection occurs in the first portion of the duodenum, an antrectomy should be performed with closure of the duodenal stump, completing the procedure as a Billroth II gastrojejunostomy (2). With complicated injuries involving the ampulla of Vater, an occasional successful primary repair of the ampulla has been accomplished; however, more complicated procedures, including pancreatoduodenectomy, may be required (1).

Duodenal Diverticulization or Pyloric Exclusion

In patients with severe duodenal injuries, many surgeons use some modification of the diverticulization procedure described by Berne et al. in 1974 (13). This technique, as originally described, includes a distal gastrectomy, closure of the duodenal stump, closure of the duodenal wound, a gastrojejunostomy, and placement of a decompressive catheter into the duodenum. A vagotomy is generally not performed at the time of the duodenal diverticulization (2).

Jordan's (2) modification of the diverticulization technique consists of closure of the pylorus and creation of a gastrojejunostomy to divert the flow of GI contents away from the injured duodenum. The closure of the pylorus originally was performed with a running suture of catgut through the opening in the stomach created for the gastrojejunostomy. Currently, Prolene suture is used more commonly, and closure of the pylorus also has been performed with a stapler.

As originally designed by Jordan, it was anticipated that in a few weeks, the catgut would dissolve, and the pylorus would reopen with reinstitution of the flow of gastric contents into the duodenum (2). In fact, it was found that it is very difficult to occlude the pylorus permanently by any technique.

Drainage of Duodenal Injuries
Although pancreatic injuries should be drained, placing external drains close to an isolated duodenal repair is not encouraged.

Duodenal Fistulas
Fistula formation is the worst complication of duodenal wounds (2). In a collected series of 1,563 patients with duodenal injuries, fistulas developed in 3% to 12% (14). Without diverticulization or pyloric exclusion, these are all "side fistulas," which usually have a much greater fluid loss and are generally much more difficult to treat than "end fistulas."

If a duodenal fistula develops, and drains have been properly placed, the leaking duodenal contents will exit along the drain tract to the skin, and severe peritonitis will be usually avoided. Keeping the patient on a regimen of nothing by mouth (NPO), removing all gastric secretions with a nasogastric tube, and use of TPN and somatostatin also may help the management of duodenal fistulas.

Once a duodenal fistula has become well established, a sinogram should be performed to determine the location of the opening into the duodenum and to determine whether the GI tract is patent distal to the fistula (2). After the drainage tract has developed a strong fibrous wall (usually within 3 to 4 weeks), spontaneous closure usually occurs.

⊘ FREQUENT ERRORS

1. ***Reliance on isolated serum amylase determinations to diagnose or rule out pancreatic injuries.***
2. ***Failure to examine plain radiograph films of the abdomen closely for retroperitoneal air in patients with severe blunt trauma.***
3. ***Assuming that a normal DPL and abdominal CT can completely rule out pancreatic and duodenal injuries.***
4. ***Failure to open upper central retroperitoneal hematomas over the pancreas and duodenum.***
5. ***Failure to adequately expose the pancreas if there is any suspicion that it may be injured.***
6. ***Failure to adequately search for the cause of any bile staining near the duodenum or head of the pancreas.***
7. ***Attempting complex reconstruction of a transected pancreas in patients with other high-risk injuries.***

SUMMARY POINTS

1. Associated injuries are the major cause of the high mortality rates seen with pancreatic and duodenal trauma.

2. Pancreatic parenchymal injuries are difficult to repair and generally leak for at least several days after injury.

3. Severe injuries to the duodenum or head of the pancreas are usually managed best by some type of duodenal diverticulization or pyloric exclusion procedure.

4. The total volume of fluid passing through the duodenum normally exceeds 5 to 6 L per day, and a side fistula as opposed to an end fistula in this area can cause serious fluid and electrolyte problems.

5. Dehiscence of a duodenal suture line can be especially dangerous because of the large amounts of activated enzymes that may be rapidly liberated into the abdomen.

6. One should look very closely for an associated pancreatic injury whenever the duodenum is damaged.
7. A consistently increased or increasing serum or urinary amylase level should make one suspect a pancreatic injury.
8. All techniques used to diagnose injuries of the pancreas or duodenum are reliable only when they identify an injury; a "normal" study has relatively little negative predictive value.
9. A DPL may be completely negative with severe injuries of retroperitoneal organs, such as the pancreas and duodenum.
10. In a patient with a suspected pancreatic ductal injury, an ERCP can help to determine the need for surgery and to determine the exact site of a major ductal injury.
11. Upper midline retroperitoneal hematomas should be explored to rule out underlying duodenal, pancreatic, or vascular injuries.
12. The presence of any bile staining or crepitation in the periduodenal area after trauma mandates a very careful search for injuries of the bile ducts and duodenum.
13. Splenic salvage should be attempted for traumatic rupture of the pancreas requiring distal pancreatectomy if the patient is young and hemodynamically stable and there are no other life-threatening injuries.
14. Because 80% to 90% of the normal pancreas can generally be resected without significant endocrine or exocrine deficiency, complex procedures to preserve pancreas are rarely indicated.
15. All pancreatic injuries should be drained because there will be some leakage of pancreatic enzymes in almost all cases.
16. The initial treatment of pancreatic fistulas should be conservative because most of them heal spontaneously within 2 to 4 weeks.
17. Peripancreatic drains should be left in place until the patient is eating a full diet and there is little or no drainage.
18. Fluid, electrolyte, and protein losses from large pancreatic fistulas can be especially dangerous in malnourished patients.
19. Somatostatin and its analogues can significantly decrease the volume of pancreatic secretions, and they may help provide a more rapid closure of some fistulas.
20. Pancreatic necrosis or an abscess should be suspected in anyone who becomes toxic or develops multiple organ failure after a major pancreatic injury.
21. Persistent posttraumatic pancreatitis is frequently the harbinger of complications such as a pseudocyst or pancreatic abscess.
22. Development of a pancreatic pseudocyst should be suspected in anyone with an upper abdominal mass or a persistent increase of serum amylase levels after pancreatic trauma.
23. Endoscopic retrograde pancreatography should be performed before the treatment of traumatic pancreatic pseudocysts to aid in the selection of the most appropriate procedure.
24. Delayed bleeding from pseudocysts or injured pancreas is generally best treated angiographically.
25. Diabetes mellitus is uncommon after pancreatic trauma unless 80% or more of the pancreas is resected.
26. Most deaths within the initial 48 hours in patients with pancreatic injuries are the result of associated vascular injuries, and the later deaths are usually caused by sepsis.
27. Duodenal obstruction due to an intramural hematoma can usually be treated nonoperatively.
28. Lacerations of the duodenum should be carefully repaired, and the repaired area should be buttressed with well-vascularized tissues, such as omentum or jejunum.
29. A simple duodenostomy drainage tube may be the most effective method for reducing the tendency to leak from the repair of a badly torn duodenum.
30. Severe duodenal or head of the pancreas injuries should have duodenal diverticulization.
31. A gastrojejunostomy to divert gastric juice from an injured duodenum does not necessitate a vagotomy because a marginal ulcer develops only rarely in these circumstances.

32. Placing a drain near an intestinal suture line increases the likelihood that it will leak.
33. If duodenal obstruction appears to be present after a repair, an initial period of nonsurgical treatment is appropriate and often successful.

REFERENCES

1. Wilson RF. Injury to the pancreas and duodenum. In: Wilson RF, Walt AJ, eds. *Management of trauma: pitfalls and practice.* 2nd ed. Philadelphia: Williams & Wilkins, 1996:510.
2. Jordan GJ Jr. Injury to the pancreas and duodenum. In: Moore EE, Mattox KL, Feliciano DV, eds. *Trauma.* 2nd ed. Norwalk, CT: Appleton & Lange, 1991: 498–510.
3. Fabian TC, Patterson CR. Injuries of the stomach, duodenum, pancreas, and small intestine. In: Kreis DJ, Gomez GA, eds. *Trauma management.* Boston: Little, Brown, 1989:215–229.
4. Lucas CE, Ledgerwood AM. Factors influencing outcome after blunt duodenal injuries. *J Trauma* 1975;5:839.
5. Lucas CE. Diagnosis and treatment of pancreatic and duodenal injury. *Surg Clin North Am* 1977;57:49.
6. Adkins RB, Keyser JE. Recent experiences with duodenal trauma. *Am Surg* 1985;51:121.
7. Kunin JR, Korobkin M, Ellis JH, et al. Duodenal injuries caused by blunt abdominal trauma: value of CT in differentiating perforation from hematoma. *Am J Roentgenol* 1993;160:1221.
8. Lane MJ, Mindelzun RE, Sandhu JS, et al. CT diagnosis of blunt pancreatic trauma: importance of detecting fluid between the pancreas and the splenic vein. *Am J Roentgenol* 1994;163:833.
9. Gholson CF, Sittig K, Favrot D, et al. Chronic abdominal pain as the initial manifestation of pancreatic injury due to remote blunt trauma of the abdomen. *South Med J* 1994;87:902.
10. Brotman S, Cisternino S, Myers RA, Crowley RA. A test to help diagnosis of rupture in the injured duodenum. *Injury* 1981;12:464.
11. Moore EE, Cogbill TH, Malangoni MA, et al. Organ scaling II: pancreas, duodenum, small bowel, colon, and rectum. *J Trauma* 1990;30:1427.
12. Kopelman D, Suissa A, Klein Y, et al. Pancreatic duct injury: intraoperative endoscopic transpancreatic drainage of parapancreatic abscess. *J Trauma* 1998;44: 555.
13. Berne CJ, Donoval AJ, White EJ, et al. Duodenal "diverticulation" for duodenal and pancreatic injuries. *Am J Surg* 1974;127:503.
14. Martin TD, Feliciano DV, Mattox, et al. Severe duodenal injuries. *Arch Surg* 1983; 118:631.
15. Thal ER. Duodenal injuries. In: Champion HR, Robbs JV, Trunkey DD, eds. *Rob and Smith's operative surgery.* London: Butterworth, 1989:934.

26. INJURIES TO THE COLON AND RECTUM[1]

COLON INJURIES

Types of Trauma

Penetrating Trauma

The presence of colon in all quadrants of the abdomen places it at risk with almost all penetrating abdominal wounds, and the high concentrations (10^9 to 10^{12} per mL) of bacteria in the colon make sepsis a threat whenever it is injured.

In the 12-year period from 1980 to 1992, 2,168 patients with gunshot, shotgun, or stab wounds of abdominal organs were admitted to Detroit Receiving Hospital (DRH). Of these, 620 (28.6%) involved the colon, and 75 (3.5%) involved the rectum.

With any gunshot wound, efforts should be made to assure the viability of adjacent tissues before performing a primary repair, and debridement of the colon for 1 or 2 cm beyond the immediate area of injury may be necessary. Close-range shotgun injuries may destroy and contaminate large amounts of colon and adjacent tissues, greatly increasing the likelihood of sepsis.

With endoscopic perforations, early repair is essential if one is to minimize the morbidity associated with such accidents. Because the bowel has usually been cleansed before study, if repair is accomplished within 6 hours, virtually no complications should occur; however, if surgery is delayed for more than 24 hours, high morbidity and mortality rates may result.

Blunt Trauma

Blunt trauma to the colon and rectum is unusual. Of 736 colon and rectal injuries seen from 1980 to 1992, only 51 (6.9%) were caused by blunt trauma, and 34 (67%) of the blunt injuries were a result of automobile accidents. Because the blunt force required to produce a colonic injury is great, associated organ injury was noted in more than 90% of these patients.

Blunt colonic injuries most frequently involve the transverse colon, followed by the right and left colon, respectively. Transverse colonic injuries are most commonly serosal or intramural hematomas; right and left colonic injuries are frequently full thickness. Bursting injuries of the colon usually involve the cecum.

AXIOM Because contused and devitalized colon may extend beyond the area of obvious injury, primary repair of blunt colon injuries can be risky (2).

Insufflation Injuries

Insufflation injuries are often the result of a prank when an air-pressure hose is pushed between the buttocks of the victim. Even though the end of the pressure hose may be several inches from the anus, severe lacerations of the intraabdominal colon may result. It has been estimated that a pressure exceeding 4 lb/in^2 is needed to rupture bowel, and compressed air jets may generate up to 125 lb/in^2 (2). The laceration of the bowel usually occurs in the rectosigmoid area and may extend for 10 cm or more.

Diagnosis

Most colon injuries are diagnosed at laparotomy (3). One of the biggest pitfalls in the present trend to treat hemodynamically stable adults with blunt trauma to the liver or spleen nonoperatively is the risk of missing an unsuspected bowel injury.

Physical Examination

Skin abrasions or tears of the rectus abdominis muscle, which may be caused by a seat belt, should be noted, especially because the underlying bowel lesions may have a prolonged and deceptive clinical course. Bowel sounds often disappear after a few hours if bowel perforation has occurred. Nance (4) found that loss of bowel sounds is an ominous finding, and that it is frequently associated with bowel perforation or other serious abdominal injuries.

With penetrating wounds near the pelvis, the anal and gluteal regions should always be carefully inspected because small wounds may be hidden. Even apparently minor penetrating wounds in this area may be associated with critical internal injuries.

A rectal and pelvic examination should accompany the physical examination of all patients with blunt or lower abdominal penetrating injury. Gross blood found on the digital rectal examination strongly suggests a rectal or colonic injury, and an endoscopic evaluation should be performed preoperatively if the patient's clinical condition permits taking the time. Evaluation of sphincter tone also should be noted during the rectal examination.

Radiologic Examinations

Plain Films

Plain radiographs of the abdomen, with the entrance and exit wounds covered with opaque markers, may be helpful in demonstrating the tract of a missile. Associated fractures also may provide some clues as to the severity of the trauma.

⊘ PITFALL

One should never assume that the path of a bullet is a straight line from its entrance to its exit wound or to its current position in the body.

Loss of psoas shadows may suggest retroperitoneal injury, but this is not a reliable finding. Air collections, either under the diaphragm (on an erect film) or in the flanks (on decubitus films), are usually a reliable sign of a perforated viscus, but they are seldom present with colon or rectal injuries. Because air is used to distend the colon lumen during colonoscopy, free intraperitoneal air is frequently present after endoscopic perforation of the colon.

Contrast Studies

Cautious contrast roentgenographic studies via the rectum can be helpful in the evaluation of patients with a potential colonic injury, particularly if there is no other reason to explore the abdomen. Water-soluble contrast material should be used in most cases because free barium in tissues or the peritoneal cavity increase the tendency to severe infections and later fibrosis with scar contracture.

Computed Tomography

The diagnostic sensitivity of the computed tomography (CT) scan for hollow viscus injuries is relatively poor, with a false-negative rate of up to 13% (4,5). Triple-contrast CT examinations, which include intravenous, gastric, and rectal (enema) instillation of water-soluble contrast, greatly increase the likelihood of diagnosing a colonic injury.

Diagnostic Peritoneal Lavage

Bacterial or fecal material found on diagnostic peritoneal lavage (DPL) allows the diagnosis of an intestinal injury to be made readily; however, the white blood cell count in DPL fluid may not become increased until 4 to 6 hours after injury.

Consequently, in suggestive cases, if a negative DPL is obtained soon after injury, one may wish to leave the catheter in place and repeat the lavage 3 to 6 hours later.

AXIOM A negative DPL does not reliably rule out gastrointestinal injuries, especially if the DPL was performed soon after the trauma or if the injury is retroperitoneal.

Endoscopy

In preparation for endoscopy for suspected rectal or colon injury, many surgeons are reluctant to use enemas to clean out the feces because of the potential risk of increasing contamination of damaged pericolonic or perirectal tissues; however, a careful Fleet's enema is not likely to cause much contamination and may greatly improve visibility.

Laparoscopy

Laparoscopy is being used increasingly in trauma patients because it may allow early, organ-specific diagnosis after penetrating or blunt abdominal trauma. Furthermore, more advanced laparoscopic techniques may permit the repair of simple gastrointestinal and colonic injuries without laparotomy. Exquisite judgment must be exercised in these patients because complete laparoscopic visualization of the colon, especially its retroperitoneal portions, is not possible. Any suspicion of an injury in these areas mandates laparotomy.

Laparotomy

The diagnosis of colonic injury, especially after blunt trauma, is often made during a laparotomy for associated organ injuries that have caused peritoneal signs or hypotension. In patients with blunt colon injury seen at DRH, concomitant injuries occurred in almost 90%. The associated injuries included

- Spleen, 26%
- Liver, 23%
- Jejunum, 17%
- Ileum, 14%
- Blood vessels, 11%
- Kidney, 9%
- Pancreas, 9%

Treatment

Nonsurgical Management

Partial-thickness colon injuries produced by endoscopy, enema tips, or thermometers can be cautiously observed. In an extensive review of iatrogenic injuries of prepared bowel, Thomson et al. (6) noted that these patients generally do well by simply being kept without food by mouth (NPO), given antibiotics, and carefully observed; however, some of these patients may not show any signs or symptoms for 2 to 3 days and then progress from minimal signs or symptoms to severe sepsis in another 12 to 24 hours.

Surgical Management

Indications for Operation

With a stab to the abdomen, any hemodynamic instability or signs of peritoneal irritation indicate a need for an emergency laparotomy.

AXIOM Stab wounds of the flank have a 15% to 25% chance of causing an intraabdominal organ injury, whereas wounds in the back have a 5% to 10% chance of damaging these organs (3,4).

Penetrating wounds to the flank or back may have to penetrate 6 to 8 cm or more to cause significant damage to the retroperitoneal right or left colon. During exploration for wounds of the back and flank, the retroperitoneal colon must be fully mobilized to exclude any posterior or intramesenteric injuries.

Patients with stable vital signs and abdominal stab wounds proven to penetrate into the peritoneal cavity can have either an immediate laparotomy, a DPL, or careful observation for 24 to 48 hours. If the DPL is positive because of the red blood cell count, one can still elect to observe the patient. If the DPL is positive for other criteria, the patient should be explored. With gunshot wounds of the abdomen, a laparotomy should be performed unless it is clear that the GSW was only tangential.

Preoperative Management

Patients with suspected colon or rectal injuries should receive preoperative parenteral antibiotics to cover gram-negative aerobes (such as *Escherichia coli*) and anaerobes (such as *Bacteroides fragilis*), so that adequate blood levels can be achieved by the time the laparotomy incision is made. Addition of ampicillin to cover for possible enterococcus involvement is generally unnecessary.

Many surgeons administer antibiotics in the emergency room during the initial resuscitation of patients with penetrating abdominal injuries. If there is much blood loss during the operation, the antibiotics should be administered again after the bleeding is controlled. If no hollow viscus injury is identified at operation, the antibiotics can be discontinued. If stomach or proximal small bowel is injured, one or two additional doses of the antibiotics can be given. If a colon perforation is identified, antibiotics may be continued for 2 to 5 days according to the extent of the injury, the patient's host defenses, and the personal preferences of the surgeon.

Initial Dissection

After bleeding has been controlled and hemodynamic stability established, a rapid examination of the bowel should be performed, looking for obvious intestinal perforations. Such injuries should be identified and controlled promptly with noncrushing clamps or running sutures to prevent further contamination. If an injury requiring resection is found, proximal and distal occlusive clamping of the bowel with Kelly or Kocher clamps will help prevent further fecal contamination.

When all bleeding sites and bowel leaks have been controlled, all peritoneal contamination should be removed by irrigation and suction. If there is any suggestion of a retroperitoneal colon injury, it is mandatory that that portion of the colon be completely exposed by division of its lateral peritoneal attachments. Any hematoma, staining, or air in the retroperitoneum is an indication of a possible colonic injury.

AXIOM Retroperitoneal injuries of the large bowel are easily missed unless the colon is fully mobilized.

Care must be taken when evaluating the splenic flexure to avoid iatrogenic injury to the spleen by gently cutting the splenocolic ligament before performing the dissection. The lesser sac should be entered, and the entire length of the transverse colon should be examined carefully from all sides.

The examination of the colon should extend distally down to the peritoneal reflection in the pelvis; however, dissecting farther into the pelvis to search for a rectal injury is generally not recommended.

In desperately ill patients with exsanguinating hemorrhage, coagulopathy, acidosis, and hypothermia, the colon can be stapled just proximal and distal to the injured areas. The colon can then be dropped back into the peritoneal cavity. The abdominal cavity is packed as needed for hemostatic control, and then the incision is closed rapidly.

Options in Colon Repair

In general, the four options available for management of colon injuries are

1. Primary repair or resection of the right colon without a proximal colostomy or ileostomy;
2. Primary repair with a proximal colostomy;
3. Definitive colostomy at the area of injury; and
4. Exteriorization of the repaired colon.

The specific therapy chosen depends largely on the amount of damage to the colon, the patient's other injuries, and the hemodynamic stability of the patient. Factors that may influence the success or failure of primary colon repairs include (7)

- Presence of shock
- Age of the patient
- Extent of the colon injury
- Number and types of associated injuries
- Time from injury to surgery
- Degree of fecal contamination

The anatomic, physiologic, and bacteriologic differences between the right and left colon have probably been overemphasized.

AXIOM If a colon resection is performed, a colo–colonic anastomosis, except in prepared bowel, is generally not recommended; small bowel–colonic anastomoses generally heal much better.

Primary Repair. The ideal indications for a primary repair of a colon injury include

1. A hemodynamically stable patient;
2. A wound involving less than one third of the circumference of the bowel;
3. Little or no involvement of the mesentery of the bowel;
4. A good blood supply;
5. An injury less than 6 to 8 hours old; and
6. Little or no contamination.

In addition, the primary repair should not prolong the intraoperative management of patients with severe or multiple associated injuries.

AXIOM All things considered, older patients tend to do better with a single operation than with two or three separate procedures of similar cumulative duration.

Fecal contamination. Patients with much fecal spillage, especially when cleansing of the peritoneal cavity is delayed beyond 6 to 8 hours, are certainly at an increased risk for developing septic complications. Nance (4) emphasized, however, that there are no objective data to indict primary closure as producing greater morbidity than a colostomy with civilian injuries. Indeed, there is some question whether a colostomy is really necessary for any penetrating colon injuries (4,8).

AXIOM Although the great majority of colon injuries can be safely treated with a primary anastomosis, in the presence of severe contamination or overt peritonitis, a colostomy is probably the safest choice.

Left colon versus right colon. Although the concept that the left colon heals less readily than the right colon is now seriously questioned by many, caution still prevails. Between 1980 and 1988 at DRH, surgeons performed primary repair on 43 (59%) of 73 lesions of the right colon and only 23 (26%) of 88 lesions of the left colon (3). Even the trauma centers with the largest experience remain slightly hesitant to perform primary left colo–colonic anastomoses. Although Burch et al. (9) had only 13 fecal fistulas in 592 primary repairs, the incidence of fistulas with colocolostomy [three (21.4%) of 14] was 12 times higher than that in the other 578 primary repairs.

Techniques of primary repair. Clean stab wounds and low-velocity gunshots generally need little or no debridement. The anastomosis or repair should be tension free. An inner row of interrupted 3-0 or 4-0 slowly absorbable sutures incorporating all layers of the bowel and providing hemostasis and an outer layer of inverting (Lembert) 4-0 interrupted silk sutures is used by most surgeons. A transverse orientation for the closure should be attempted whenever possible to reduce the tendency for the repair to narrow the lumen. In recent years, stapling devices have been used increasingly for expeditious closure of colonic injuries.

Right colon resections. Resection of injured colon and primary anastomosis is used most frequently to manage extensive wounds of the right colon. A right colectomy with ileocolostomy can usually be performed rapidly with a very low leak rate in the majority of patients; however, if there has been massive contamination or there is already established sepsis, a proximal ileostomy and end-colonic fistula is safer.

Colostomy. Colostomy is generally indicated for colon injuries when

1. A resection of the left colon is needed for an extensive injury;
2. Uncertainty exists about the quality of the colonic repair;
3. An exteriorized repair breaks down or cannot be returned to the abdomen; or
4. There is established peritonitis.

If, after resection of a left colon injury, the conditions for a primary repair do not seem optimal, it is considered much safer to exteriorize the proximal bowel as an end colostomy. The distal bowel can then be brought out as a mucous fistula, or it can be closed and returned to the abdominal cavity as a Hartmann's pouch.

AXIOM Performing a colostomy is not always the safest way to manage a colon injury.

The use of colostomy for treating colon injuries has a number of drawbacks. Among the obvious disadvantages are its esthetic unpleasantness, the difficulty that many patients have in caring for it, associated complications, prolonged hospitalization, the need for readmission and another anesthetic for colostomy closure, the morbidity associated with both the establishment of the colostomy and the subsequent closure, the economic loss to the patient for time away from work, the prolonged convalescence, the cost to society of the hospitalizations, and the loss of productivity.

AXIOM It is increasingly recognized that patients who have colostomies have appreciably higher intraperitoneal and abdominal wound-infection rates than do patients who have primary closure.

A loop colostomy, while popular, has the disadvantage of being relatively bulky and more difficult for the patient to manage postoperatively. Its advantage relates to the fact that when the colostomy is closed, the repaired loop can be gently replaced in the peritoneal cavity, usually without extensive dissection. Dissecting out a previous Hartmann's pouch can be extremely difficult at times.

Exteriorized Primary Repair. An alternative to protecting a primary repair of injured colon with a proximal colostomy is a primary repair with exteriorization of the sutured segment of colon over a tongue of fascia (10). The exteriorized colon is kept moist and should be examined daily. If a leak occurs, the loop is converted to a colostomy with little risk of peritonitis. Otherwise, after 7 to 10 days, the repaired segment is surgically returned to the abdomen.

AXIOM Because primary repair of colon injuries is feasible and they heal well in the majority of patients, there seems to be little place for exteriorized primary anastomosis today.

Adjuvant Measures

Drains. Drains are now seldom used in the management of intraperitoneal colonic wounds. Drains placed close to colonic suture lines are thought to lead to an increased number of anastomotic leaks.

Intraperitoneal Antibiotics. Intraperitoneal antibiotic irrigation was pioneered by Isidore Cohn Jr., and was shown by Noon et al. (11) in a prospective randomized study to be effective in reducing the incidence of intraperitoneal infections after trauma. Many surgeons, however, believe that the efficacy of the antibiotic irrigant is doubtful when compared with the protective effect of adequate blood levels of appropriate antibiotics. For many years, Nance and others used a 1% kanamycin solution or a solution of 80 mg of tobramycin in 100 mL of saline to irrigate the peritoneal cavity after completion of a copious saline lavage (4). Most of the antibiotic irrigant was then aspirated. About 50 mL of the antibiotic solution was saved for lavage of the fascia and subcutaneous tissue just before closure.

RECTAL INJURIES

Introduction

Because of its extraperitoneal location, injuries of the rectum are generally considered to be serious injuries. In addition, because the rectum is surrounded by poorly vascularized fatty tissue without fixed anatomic boundaries, a perirectal infection can spread rapidly throughout the pelvis.

Serious associated injuries can greatly increase the morbidity and mortality of rectal injuries. The four most frequent associated injuries and their incidence in 92 patients with rectal injuries at DRH were

- Small bowel, 27%
- Colon, 24%
- Bladder, 21%
- Abdominal vessels, 13%

There were no deaths in the 80 patients who did not have associated vascular injuries.

Diagnosis

Rectal injuries must be sought diligently in all patients with penetrating injuries of the pelvis or lower abdomen. Blunt rectal trauma also should be suspected in anyone with severe pelvic fractures or perineal injuries. A meticulous examination of the anus, rectum, and vagina is essential in such patients. Any trauma patient with blood in the rectum should be assumed to have a rectal injury.

Sigmoidoscopy may be helpful when the rectum is clear of feces, but the examination is frequently hampered by an inability to adequately prepare the bowel.

AXIOM Rectal injuries can easily be missed at laparotomy and should be diagnosed preoperatively whenever possible.

Because the rectum is extraperitoneal, routine exploration at laparotomy may fail to demonstrate some injuries. Consequently, stable patients with penetrating wounds of the perineum, buttocks, or lower abdomen should have a careful preoperative examination of the retrosigmoid area, including proctosigmoidoscopy. Endoscopy also can be performed in the operating room with the abdomen open, if needed.

Treatment

Repair of the Rectum

Repair of the rectal injury itself should be done only if it can be visualized and performed easily, either transanally or at laparotomy, without extensive dissection. Indeed, easily visualized, partial-thickness injuries of the rectum can be repaired without proximal diversion (12). Usually the extent of the damage is virtually impossible to assess adequately at the initial operation, and in many cases, the situation is further complicated by associated genitourinary or sacral injuries.

Sigmoid Colostomy

AXIOM The treatment of most rectal injuries includes a diverting sigmoid colostomy and presacral drainage.

A sigmoid-loop colostomy is the preferred method of fecal diversion for rectal injuries for most surgeons. An end-sigmoid colostomy with a Hartmann's pouch is preferred by some surgeons to ensure complete diversion of fecal material away from the injured rectum. Reestablishment of bowel continuity later, however, is much more difficult than with a loop colostomy.

Saline Irrigation of the Rectum

Saline irrigation of the defunctionalized rectum to wash out the feces is not absolutely necessary, but in theory, it should reduce the amount of continuing contamination of perirectal tissues. This maneuver may be particularly important if the rectal vault is full of stool. Dilatation of the anus to three or four fingers also may be a useful adjunct at the conclusion of the case to allow any fluid in the rectum to come out through the anus rather than escape into perirectal tissues.

AXIOM If much fecal matter is present in an injured rectum, it should be removed as carefully as possible to avoid increasing the contamination of the perirectal tissues.

Presacral Drainage

Adequate drainage of the presacral space posterior to the rectum can be extremely important. Many surgeons prefer a sump or closed suction catheter placed in the retrorectal space and brought out just anterior to the coccyx (Fig. 26-1).

If no significant leak is apparent at the end of 5 days, the presacral drain can usually be removed. If a leak becomes apparent, closure of the fistula usually occurs spontaneously if fecal diversion was properly performed.

Other Types of Rectal Injury

Rectal Foreign Bodies

Retained rectal foreign bodies are only rarely the result of violence; however, patients usually seek medical attention late, after making multiple attempts of their own to remove the object. The majority of these objects will be lodged in the sacral hollow, and they can usually be removed transanally once the anal sphincter has been relaxed.

Before removal of the foreign body, appropriate antibiotics and antitetanus prophylaxis should be administered. In some patients, the foreign body can be removed in the emergency room under sedation and local anesthesia. If this is unsuccessful, removal in the operating room under general anesthesia will be required. A careful proctosigmoidoscopy should be performed after removal of the foreign body to rule out a perforation.

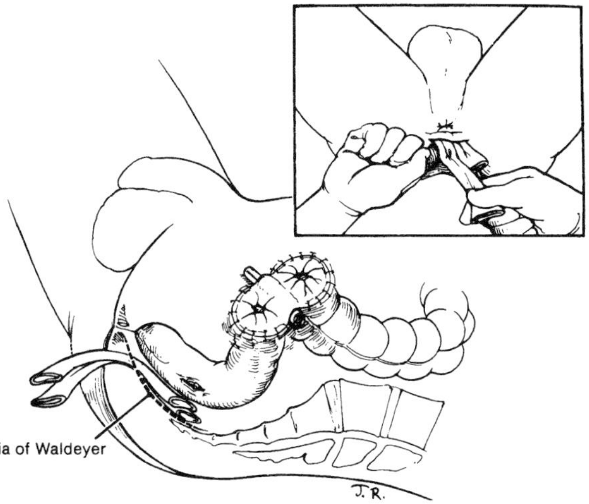

FIG. 26-1. To obtain presacral drainage, the perineum is incised about halfway between the anal verge and tip of the coccyx. The presacral space is then bluntly dissected until one is certain that the space is opened up to the level of the rectal injury. From ref. 18, with permission.

Impalement Injuries

True impalement wounds are the result of violent insertion of a foreign body into the rectum. Because of the anatomic relation of the rectum and bladder, the impaling device also can penetrate the anterior rectal wall and enter the urinary bladder. Consequently, associated injury to the urinary bladder should be searched for in these patients (13).

Patients with an impalement injury of the rectum require a laparotomy to look for associated injuries. If a full-thickness rectal injury is present, it should be treated with a diverting colostomy, and the distal sigmoid colon and rectum should be irrigated clean. If the tear is in the intraperitoneal colon, is small, and is without gross fecal spillage, a primary repair can be attempted.

Small perianal and anal disruptions may be primarily repaired without fecal diversion. If the anal and perianal injury is large or is seen after infection has developed, the wounds should be left open and protected from further soiling with a proximal colostomy.

Colostomy Closure

Standard Techniques

AXIOM The closure of a posttraumatic colostomy can be extremely difficult and may be associated with a number of serious complications.

A colostomy for trauma can be closed as soon as the colon or rectal injuries and all incisions and drainage sites have healed and the patient has achieved a positive nitrogen balance. This usually takes at least 4 to 8 weeks, but many surgeons prefer to wait at least 3 months. Most surgeons examine the colon with a barium enema (BE) or endoscopy before scheduling closure of a colostomy performed for trauma. Atweh et al. (14) suggested that this is particularly important for rectal injuries not visualized at the first operation. Conversely, Sola et al. (15) believe that BE before colostomy closure for colonic injuries provides little useful information.

Once it has been decided that a colostomy can be closed safely, the colon and rectum must be completely cleaned preoperatively. Appropriate prophylactic parenteral antibiotics should be given about 30 minutes before the incision.

Divided stoma colostomies and colostomies with a distal Hartmann's pouch require a formal laparotomy. The small bowel and colon to be used for the anastomosis often have extensive adhesions, which must be taken down very carefully. After an adequate length of proximal bowel and distal colon are freed, they should be trimmed back to normal tissue and anastomosed in a standard fashion. Postoperatively these patients must be watched very carefully because it is not unusual to have leaks occur after colostomy closures. Daily dilating rectal exams may be helpful.

In a study by Sola et al. (16), 86 trauma patients underwent colostomy closure. There were no deaths after colostomy closure, but there was a total morbidity of 24%. There were 11 anastomotic complications (two of which required repeated laparotomy) and nine wound infections. Interestingly, the morbidities were most likely to occur in patients who had complications during their initial hospitalization. This was especially true if these patients underwent closure earlier than 3 months after injury.

AXIOM Fever, leukocytosis, or abdominal pain within 2 weeks of a colostomy closure should be considered to be caused by a leaking anastomosis until proven otherwise.

If a colon leak occurs, and the patient has any evidence of infection or intraperitoneal contamination, the anastomosis should be exteriorized as a colostomy; however, if the leak is small and relatively well contained, a proximal colostomy may suffice. The leaking anastomosis has an increased chance of developing a stricture later. If a small colocutaneous fistula develops, and there is no evidence of a distal obstruction or infection, the fistula will usually heal spontaneously without a proximal colostomy.

Same-Admission Colostomy Closures

In a report by Renz et al. (17), 30 consecutive patients with rectal wounds (RWs; 90% of which were caused by gunshot wounds) were entered into a prospective study to determine whether same-admission colostomy closure (SACC) could be performed safely if the rectal wound was healed on contrast enema (CE). The first CE was performed 5 to 10 days after injury in 29 patients. At 7 and 10 days after injury, 55% and 75% of the RWs were healed radiologically. Sixteen patients with rectal healing underwent SACC 9 to 19 days after injury (mean, 12.4 days). There were two (29%) fecal fistulas after simple suture closure of seven of the colostomies, but there were no complications after resection of the stoma with end-to-end anastomosis in nine patients. Thus SACC was performed without complications in 88% of the patients with radiologically healed rectal wounds.

OUTCOMES OF COLON AND RECTAL INJURIES

Patients with colon injuries die primarily because of hemorrhage from associated severe injuries. Even patients dying of sepsis usually have other injuries. The patients dying of colon or rectal injuries at DRH had an average of two associated visceral injuries per patient, and those who died in the operating room received an average of 13 units of blood before death. During the past 12 years at DRH, the mortality rate was 6% in patients with stab wounds, 14% in patients with gunshot wounds, and 16% in those with shotgun injuries of the colon. Of the patients with no or only one associated injury, only 15 (5%) of 318 died. Of those with two or more associated injuries, 68 (20%) of 345 died ($p < 0.0001$). If the patients with associated abdominal vessel injuries (who had a mortality rate of 40%) are excluded, the mortality rate was only 4% (22 of 509).

Wound infections after rectal injuries have a frequency of about 5% to 15% but can be avoided most of the time by leaving the skin and subcutaneous tissue open (4).

⊘ FREQUENT ERRORS

1. ***Failure to adequately examine the perineum and gluteal creases in patients with penetrating wounds of the lower abdomen, lower back, or pelvis.***
2. ***Failure to completely examine all portions of the colon (including the lesser sac and retroperitoneum) after gunshot wounds of the abdomen because the trajectory suggests that a colon injury would be extremely unlikely.***
3. ***Failure to perform an early exploratory laparotomy if one suspects a colon injury.***
4. ***Complete reliance on a negative DPL to rule out a bowel injury.***
5. ***Failing to perform a colostomy or ileostomy on patients who have colon injuries due to high-velocity missiles or close-range shotgun blasts.***
6. ***Closing the skin and subcutaneous tissue of the incision if there has been recognizable contamination from a colon injury.***
7. ***Extensive dissection in the pelvis in an attempt to identify a suspected low rectal injury.***
8. ***Failure to perform a diverting colostomy for a severe perianal or suspected rectal injury.***
9. ***Delay in exploring a patient who is not doing well after a colostomy closure.***

SUMMARY POINTS

1. Because contused and devitalized colon may extend beyond the area of obvious injury, primary repair of blunt colon injuries is somewhat risky.

2. Insufflation injuries of the colon can occur even without direct contact of the patient with the air hose.

3. Loss of bowel sounds may be the earliest evidence of bowel injury after blunt trauma to the abdomen.

4. Whenever possible, a proctosigmoidoscopic examination should be performed preoperatively in any patient suspected of having a rectal or colonic injury.

5. A negative DPL does not rule out gastrointestinal injuries reliably, especially if the DPL was done soon after the trauma or if the injury is retroperitoneal.

6. Stab wounds in the flank have a 15% to 25% incidence of causing an intraabdominal organ injury, whereas wounds in the back have a 5% to 10% chance of damaging these organs.

7. Retroperitoneal injuries of the large bowel are easily missed unless the colon is fully mobilized.

8. Dissecting deep into the pelvis to look for possible rectal injuries may cause much more harm than good.

9. If a colon resection is performed, a colo–colonic anastomosis, except in prepared bowel, is generally not recommended; small bowel–colonic anastomoses generally heal much better.

10. Transient hypotension is not a contraindication to primary repair of colon injuries.

11. Performing a colostomy is not always the safest way to manage a colon injury.

12. Patients who have colostomies generally have appreciably higher infection rates than do patients who have primary closures.

13. Closure of a loop colostomy is often much safer and easier than closure of a colostomy with a Hartmann's pouch, especially if there has been any intraperitoneal infection.

14. Because primary repair of colon injuries is feasible and will heal well in the majority of patients, there seems to be little place for exteriorized primary anastomoses today.
15. Intraperitoneal drains are seldom indicated in patients with colonic injuries.
16. After irrigation of the peritoneal cavity, the fluid should be removed as completely as possible.
17. Rectal injuries can easily be missed at laparotomy and should be diagnosed preoperatively whenever possible.
18. The treatment of most rectal injuries includes a diverting sigmoid colostomy and presacral drainage.
19. If there is much feces in an injured rectum, the rectum should be cleaned out as carefully as possible to reduce continuing contamination of perirectal tissues.
20. After a foreign body is removed from the rectum, endoscopy should be performed to rule out a perforation.
21. A careful search for a bladder perforation should be made in patients with an impalement injury of the rectum.
22. Patients with colonic injuries and any visible fecal spill should generally not have the skin and subcutaneous tissues of their incisions closed at the time of surgery.
23. Intraperitoneal closure of a posttraumatic colostomy can be difficult because of the adhesions that may be present, and the procedure may be associated with a number of complications.
24. Fever, leukocytosis, or abdominal pain within 2 weeks of a colostomy closure should be considered to be caused by a leaking anastomosis until proven otherwise.

REFERENCES

1. Wilson RF, Walt AJ, Dulchavsky SA. Injuries to the colon and rectum. In: Wilson RF, Walt AJ, eds. *Management of trauma: pitfalls and practice.* 2nd ed. Philadelphia: Williams & Wilkins, 1996:534.
2. Walt AJ, Wilson RF. Specific abdominal injuries: colon, rectum, and anus. In: Walt AJ, Wilson RF, eds. *Management of trauma: pitfalls and practice*. Philadelphia: Lea & Febiger, 1975:365.
3. Levison MA, Walt AJ. Colonic trauma in current therapy. In: Faxio V, ed. *Therapy in colon and rectal surgery.* Philadelphia: BC Decker, 1989:329–333.
4. Nance FC. Injuries to the colon and rectum. In: Moore EE, Mattox KL, Feliciano DV, eds. *Trauma*. 2nd ed. Norwalk, CT: Appleton & Lange, 1991:521–532.
5. Walt AJ. Injuries and iatrogenic disorders of the colon and rectum. In: Berk JE, ed. *Bockus gastroenterology*. 4th ed. Philadelphia: WB Saunders, 1985: 2575–2582.
6. Thomson SR, Fraser M, Stupp C, et al. Iatrogenic and accidental colon injuries; what to do? *Dis Colon Rectum* 1994;37:496.
7. Stone HH, Fabian TC. Management of perforating colon trauma. *Ann Surg* 1979;190:430.
8. Gonzalez RP, Merlotti GJ, Holevar MR. Colostomy in penetrating colon injury: is it necessary? *J Trauma* 1996;41:271.
9. Burch JM, Martin RR, Richardson RJ, et al. Evolution of the management of the injured colon in the '80s. *Arch Surg* 1991;126:979–984.
10. Kirkpatrick JR. The exteriorized anastomosis: its role in surgery of the colon. *Surgery* 1977;82:362–365.
11. Noon GP, Beall AC, Jordon GL, et al. Clinical evaluation of peritoneal irrigation with antibiotic solution. *Surgery* 1967;62:73.
12. Vitale GC, Richardson JD, Flint LM. Successful management of injuries to the extraperitoneal rectum. *Am J Surg* 1983;49:159.
13. Franko ER, Ivatury RR, Schwalb DM. Combined penetrating rectal and genitourinary injuries: a challenge in management. *J Trauma* 1993;34:347.
14. Atweh NA, Vieux EE, Ivatury R, et al. Indications for barium enema preceding colostomy closure in trauma patients. *J Trauma* 1989;29:641–642.
15. Sola JE, Buchman TG, Bender JS. Limited role of barium enema examination preceding colostomy closure in trauma patients. *J Trauma* 1994;36:245.

16. Sola JE, Bender JS, Buchman TG. Morbidity and timing of colostomy in trauma patients. *Injury* 1993;24:438.
17. Renz BM, Feliciano DV, Sherman R. Same admission colostomy closure (SACC): a new approach to rectal wounds: a prospective study. *Ann Surg* 1993;218:279.
18. Burch JM, Feliciano DV, Mattox KL. Colostomy and drainage of civilian rectal injuries: is that all? *Ann Surg* 1989;209:600.

27. ABDOMINAL VASCULAR TRAUMA[1]

INCIDENCE

It is estimated that patients with penetrating stab wounds to the abdomen will sustain a major abdominal vascular injury about 10% of the time (2), and patients with gunshot wounds to the abdomen will have injury to a major vessel about 25% of the time (3). In the Detroit Receiving Hospital (DRH) series, the incidence of abdominal vessel injury was 6.5% in 810 patients examined for abdominal stab wounds and 18.9% in 1,358 patients who had surgery for abdominal gunshot wounds.

The incidence of injury to major abdominal vessels in patients sustaining blunt abdominal trauma is much lower, estimated at about 5% to 10% (2). In the DRH series, it was 4.0% (23 of 573). Although significant vascular injury occurs less frequently in blunt abdominal trauma, these injuries are frequently more complex and more likely to be fatal. In the DRH series, the mortality rates with abdominal vascular injuries due to blunt trauma were 70%; gunshot wounds, 53%; and stab wounds, 32%.

PATHOPHYSIOLOGY

Knife wounds typically cause clean transections or lacerations that are readily amenable to arteriorrhaphy or venorrhaphy. Injuries created by gunshot wounds depend on the trajectory and energy transferred to the vessel. Because the energy transmitted to tissues is proportional to the square of the velocity of the missile, high-velocity missiles (greater than 2,000 ft/s) can cause 16 times more destruction than a similar bullet traveling at only 500 ft/s. With high-velocity missiles, the vessel can be badly damaged for several centimeters beyond the bullet tract, even if the tissues appear to be grossly normal.

AXIOM Tissues damaged by high-velocity missiles may require extensive debridement to ensure that the remaining tissue is normal and will heal properly.

Blunt injuries damage blood vessels primarily by deceleration, producing shear injuries, or by crushing. Deceleration-type traumas such as those sustained in motor vehicle accidents can cause avulsion of branches off major vessels or intimal tears or flaps with secondary thrombosis of vessels. Burst injuries also may occur if intravascular pressure increases high enough.

A frequent mechanism of blunt abdominal aortic injury is compression against the lumbar spine by the steering wheel in a road traffic accident (4). The infrarenal segment is most commonly involved (92% of reported cases), with the most common injury being intimal disruption with ensuing aortic thrombosis.

AXIOM Blunt abdominal aortic contusion may not cause signs and symptoms for days or weeks until the aorta becomes thrombosed.

DIAGNOSIS

Signs and Symptoms

Increasing abdominal pain and tenderness associated with hypotension after abdominal trauma should raise suspicion of bleeding or bowel injury within the abdomen. Shoulder pain or pain with breathing may be referred pain from blood or intestinal fluid irritating the diaphragm.

AXIOM Severe hypotension with a poor response to aggressive fluid resuscitation is usually the result of continued bleeding, which should be controlled rapidly in the operating room (OR).

Loss of pulses to the legs may be seen with aortic injuries, whereas loss of the femoral pulses in only one leg occurs with an injury to the ipsilateral common or external iliac artery. A mass palpable within the abdomen, especially if it is pulsating and enlarging, may be seen with an enlarging hematoma from a major arterial injury.

Acute arteriovenous fistulas may be difficult to detect preoperatively because the prominent bruit or thrill that is often present after several weeks or months may not be present initially.

The symptoms and signs of blunt infrarenal aortic injury may include peripheral neuropathy or anterior spinal artery syndrome. Other suggestive findings include abdominal or bilateral femoral bruits, diminished or absent femoral pulses, and coldness, cyanosis, or weakness of the lower extremities.

Radiologic Evaluation

AXIOM After trauma, nonvisualization of one kidney on computed tomography (CT) in a stable patient is usually an indication for renal arteriography or surgery.

Absence of excretion of intravenous contrast in the presence of a cortical-rim sign on CT scan is virtually diagnostic of blunt thrombosis of the renal artery, and arteriography is generally not necessary before corrective surgery if this radiologic sign is present (5).

A CT scan also may identify abnormal mass effects, which may represent hematomas. Large amounts of peritoneal fluid in a patient who was hypotensive most likely represent blood. The intravenous contrast also may demonstrate local collections of opacified blood, clots in vessels, or lack of opacification of some vessels.

Preoperative abdominal aortography is seldom used to diagnose intraabdominal vascular injuries after penetrating trauma. In patients with blunt trauma, aortography can be used to diagnose deep pelvic arterial bleeders associated with fractures or to diagnose unusual injuries such as intimal tears with thrombosis in the infrarenal aorta, iliac artery, or renal artery.

Occasionally, isolated bleeding vessels, especially in solid organs or in the internal iliac system, can be occluded during the angiography.

Diagnostic Peritoneal Lavage

A diagnostic peritoneal lavage (DPL) will reveal gross blood in the majority of patients with significant abdominal vascular injury; however, retroperitoneal bleeding will occasionally be missed.

Surgical Evaluation

AXIOM The diagnosis of major abdominal vascular injury is most frequently made during a laparotomy for severe hemorrhagic shock.

During a laparotomy performed for trauma, control of active bleeding is obtained initially with pressure applied digitally or with packs; later dissection can allow definitive treatment. Frequently, major retroperitoneal vascular injuries are well contained by surrounding structures and will not be bleeding actively at the time of exploration.

⊘ PITFALLS

Assuming that only a mild intraabdominal injury is present if the patient's initial hypotension is reversed by modest amounts of intravenous fluids.

TREATMENT

Resuscitation

Fluid Therapy

The majority of patients with significant intraabdominal vascular injuries will be hypotensive on arrival to the emergency department (ED). After two large peripheral i.v. lines are inserted, these patients should be brought to the OR as expeditiously as possible.

AXIOM Lower extremity intravenous access should be avoided whenever possible in patients with suspected major abdominal vascular injuries.

Resuscitative ED Thoracotomy

An ED resuscitative thoracotomy for a prehospital cardiac arrest caused by intraabdominal bleeding is rarely successful (6); however, if cardiac arrest occurs in the ED, an ED thoracotomy with cross-clamping of the descending thoracic aorta can be used to maintain cerebral and coronary flow until a celiotomy can be performed to obtain vascular control. This may provide the patient's only chance for survival.

Prelaparotomy Thoracotomy

Although the results of an ED thoracotomy for cardiac arrest from intraabdominal bleeding are poor (6), there is a definite role for prelaparotomy thoracotomy, preferably in the OR, for proximal aortic control in patients with massive hemoperitoneum and continued severe hypotension [systolic blood pressure (BP) less than 70 mm Hg; 7]. Patients with significant intraabdominal bleeding from an abdominal vascular injury appear to have a tamponade effect produced by the intact abdominal wall. Release of the tamponade by the laparotomy incision may cause a hypovolemic cardiac arrest before the bleeding sites can be controlled.

In one study, prelaparotomy thoracotomy with thoracic aortic cross-clamping helped to keep shock duration to less than 30 minutes and the number of blood transfusions to less than 10 units (7). In patients at high risk for dying (admission systolic BP less than 70 mm Hg plus four or more associated injuries), if shock was kept to less than 30 minutes and blood transfusions to less than 10 units, the mortality rate was reduced from 92% (24 of 26) to 0 (0 of 12).

Care must be taken not to let the systolic BP in the proximal aorta exceed 160 to 180 mm Hg. If proximal hypertension develops, left ventricular dilation can cause acute cardiac failure to develop rapidly. After the bleeding is controlled and hypovolemia corrected, the cross-clamp can usually be gradually removed.

Abdominal Exploration

The abdominal exploration is performed through a long midline incision. The incision should not violate the peritoneum until the fascia is divided over the entire length of the incision. The peritoneum is then rapidly opened, and the supraceliac aorta is compressed if the patient is hypotensive or develops hypotension on opening the abdominal cavity.

As soon as the abdomen is opened, easily removed blood and clots are rapidly evacuated, and lap pads are aggressively packed into the areas of suspected injury to tamponade the bleeding sites. Continued bleeding despite packing usually indicates a major vascular injury requiring definitive control, often with proximal clamping of the aorta in the chest or the supraceliac area.

Operative Exposure of Blood Vessels

Several authors, including Fry et al. (8), found it helpful to divide the abdomen into four anatomic vascular zones.

Zone 1 Includes the suprarenal aorta, the celiac axis, the superior mesenteric artery (SMA), and the left renal artery. Surgical exposure of these vessels can be achieved by dividing the peritoneal reflection of the descending colon, the splenic flexure, and the peritoneum that attaches the spleen to the diaphragm and then moving all these viscera to the right side of the abdomen.

Zone 2 Includes the entire infrahepatic inferior vena cava (IVC), right renal artery, the right side of the suprarenal aorta, the proximal right side of the SMA, and the common hepatic artery. Exposure of these vessels involves incision of the peritoneal reflections of the right colon, hepatic flexure, and the second and third parts of the duodenum, with displacement of these structures to the left.

Zone 3 Includes the infrarenal aorta and proximal common iliac arteries. The small bowel is rotated to the right upper quadrant to provide exposure in the midabdomen. The peritoneal reflection over the inferior aspect of the third and fourth portions of the duodenum is then incised, and the duodenum and pancreas are mobilized cephalad. The incision into the retroperitoneum is made directly over the infrarenal aorta.

Zone 4 Includes the common, external, and internal iliac arteries and veins. To expose the right iliac system, the cecum is mobilized cephalad. The bifurcation of the left common iliac artery is best exposed by reflecting the distal descending and sigmoid colon medially to the right.

Specific Injuries

Retroperitoneal Hematomas

Retroperitoneal hematomas are found in about 44% of patients who have a laparotomy for blunt abdominal trauma. Because a significant vascular injury may be hidden in a retroperitoneal hematoma, no effort to open this should be made until the patient is adequately resuscitated, and proximal and distal control of the potentially involved vessels is obtained.

AXIOM If a retroperitoneal hematoma is not expanding or actively bleeding, other intraabdominal injuries take precedence.

Midline retroperitoneal hematomas above the pelvis are routinely explored; however, lateral nonexpanding perirenal hematomas after blunt trauma are simply observed unless the patient has been in shock or that kidney had not been visualized on intravenous pyelogram (IVP). Perirenal hematomas after penetrating traumas are routinely explored by some surgeons; however, routine exploration of these hematomas may lead to an increased nephrectomy rate; if one can rule out an injury to major renal vessels or the renal pelvis, renal exploration is unnecessary.

AXIOM Pelvic hematomas after blunt trauma are usually the result of bleeding from pelvic fracture sites and should not be opened.

If a pelvic retroperitoneal hematoma is expanding rapidly during exploratory laparotomy, the pelvis should be packed and the patient transported rapidly to the arteriography suite for embolization. Ligation of internal iliac arteries seldom, if ever, helps to control bleeding deep in the pelvis.

Supraceliac Aortic Injuries

Penetrating injuries to the aorta as it enters the abdominal cavity carry a mortality rate exceeding 60% because of the difficulties in exposing and controlling the injury (9). Injuries to this vessel should be suspected in patients with midline upper abdominal penetration and massive bleeding on exploration. A large midline, supramesocolic hematoma also suggests proximal aortic injury.

Surgical exposure of the suprarenal aorta, the celiac axis, and the origins of the SMA and left renal artery is best achieved by dividing the left lateral peritoneal reflections and mobilizing of the spleen, stomach, and left colon to the midline. The left kidney also can be mobilized, but generally, it is left within Gerota's fascia (Fig. 27-1).

To provide control of the thoracic aorta at a higher level, the midline laparotomy incision can be extended into the left chest along the seventh or eighth interspace. If the diaphragm is incised about 2 cm from its attachments to the ribs in a circumferential manner, the diaphragmatic blood supply and its innervation are preserved.

If a proximal aortic clamp has been in place for more than 30 minutes, the anesthesiologist should be warned at least 5 to 10 minutes before removing the clamp, so

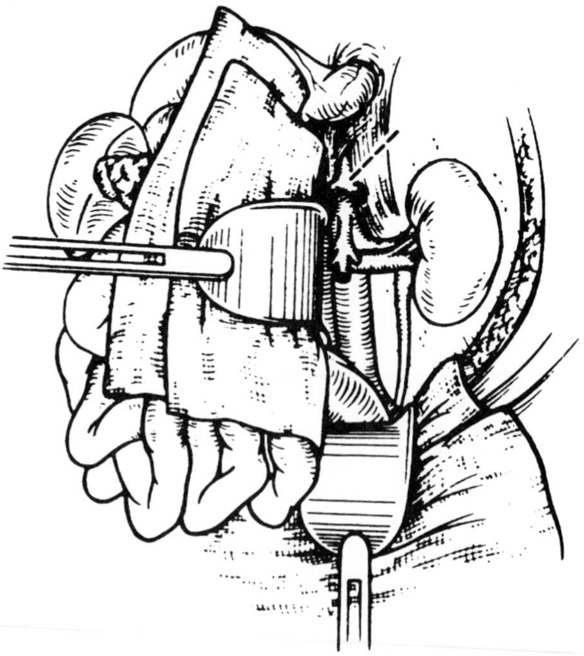

FIG. 27-1. Exposure of zone 1 abdominal arteries, including the suprarenal and supraceliac aorta, the celiac axis, the superior mesenteric artery, and the left renal artery. To expose this zone adequately, the left colon, small bowel, and retroperitoneal gastric fundus are mobilized to the right. If the left kidney is mobilized to the right, the posterolateral surface of the aorta also can be visualized. From ref. 8, with permission.

that additional fluid and blood can be given. The declamping should then be done slowly to prevent central hypotension. Prophylactic administration of intravenous bicarbonate may be helpful to reverse the "washout acidosis" from the relatively ischemic lower limbs after the aorta is unclamped.

Celiac Axis Injuries

AXIOM The celiac artery can be ligated and divided at its origin to provide improved exposure of aortic injuries in that area.

Injuries to the celiac axis and the proximal portions of its branches are difficult to repair because of the dense neural and lymphatic tissue in this area. Because of the technical difficulties of dissecting in this area and the excellent collateral blood supply of the branches of the celiac axis, the injured vessels can be ligated rather than making prolonged efforts to repair isolated injuries. Injuries to the hepatic artery proximal to the gastroduodenal artery generally also can be ligated without incident.

Superior Mesenteric Artery Injuries

Injuries to the superior mesenteric artery (SMA) near its origin may be approached by rotation of the left-sided abdominal viscera to the right to facilitate exposure of the aorta and the origin of the SMA and its proximal 2 to 3 cm. With injuries to the SMA beneath the pancreas, transection of the neck of the pancreas may be required to gain vascular control.

If a saphenous vein interposition or prosthetic graft is required to repair an injury to the proximal SMA, it is safest to run the graft from the infrarenal aorta to the underside of the proximal SMA to avoid exposing the vascular anastomosis to secretions from a possibly injured adjacent pancreas.

Injuries of the SMA between the pancreaticoduodenal artery and the middle colic artery are difficult to repair because of the proximity of the pancreas and the usual large coexistent mesocolic hematoma. With severe injuries to the SMA in this area, the SMA may be ligated; however, postoperatively, the patient should be given enough fluid to ensure an adequate collateral blood flow to the intestines (10).

Injuries to the distal SMA beyond the middle colic branch and at the level of the enteric branches require repair because the injury is distal to the collateral blood supply. If the arterial injury cannot be repaired, a bowel resection may be required. If bowel of questionable viability is not resected, a "second look" within 24 to 48 hours is important.

Renal Artery Injuries (see Chapter 29)

Infrarenal Aorta Injuries

Access to the infrarenal aorta, the inferior mesenteric artery (IMA), and the proximal common iliac arteries can be gained by rotating the small bowel to the right upper quadrant. The midline retroperitoneum is opened directly over the aorta from the aortic bifurcation up to the left renal vein. The peritoneal reflection at the inferior aspect of the duodenum is then divided close to the duodenum, where a relatively avascular plane exists. This is carried cephalad along the fourth portion of the duodenum with division of the ligament of Treitz. The duodenum and pancreas can then be mobilized cephalad above the left renal vein (Fig. 27-2).

The left renal vein can be divided at its origin from the IVC, if necessary, to gain more proximal exposure of the aorta. If the left renal vein is divided, it should be done as close to the vena cava as possible to avoid interrupting the collateral venous drainage of the left kidney.

The most common blunt abdominal aortic lesion is an intimal disruption. The intimal flap is then dissected downward by the blood flow. Thrombosis can then occur, causing acute arterial insufficiency. If all layers of the aorta are ruptured, this will lead to false aneurysm formation or frank rupture. If the intimal dissection is not extensive, thromboendarterectomy with intimal flap suture can be performed, but if

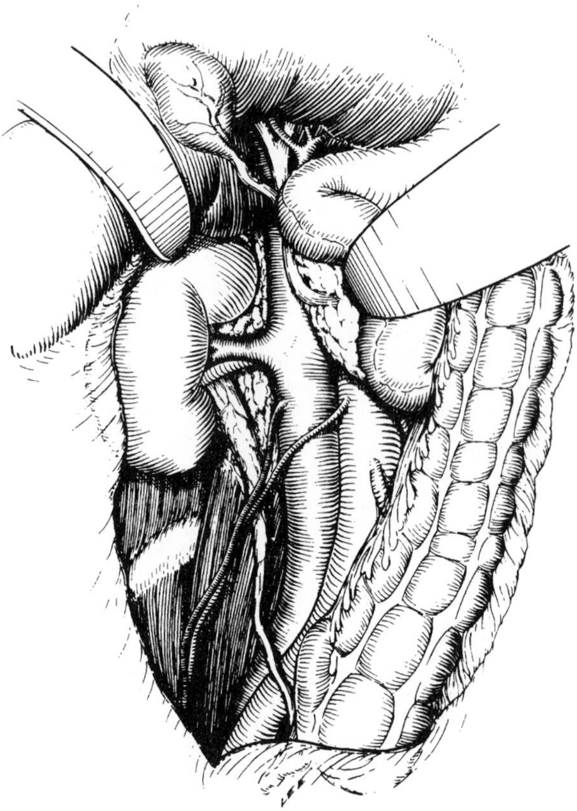

FIG. 27-2. Exposure of zone 2 arteries, including the infrarenal aorta, inferior mesenteric artery, and proximal iliac arteries, can be accomplished by mobilizing the right colon and hepatic flexure. A full Kocher maneuver is then performed to mobilize the duodenum and head of the pancreas medially to expose the origins of the right renal artery and vein. This exposure also provides access to the inferior vena cava below the liver. From ref. 10, with permission.

extensive injury has occurred, a prosthetic graft should generally be inserted (11). All vascular repairs and prosthetic grafts should be covered by omentum or mesentery whenever possible.

Inferior Mesenteric Artery Injuries

Injuries to the IMA are suspected in patients with midline hematomas in an infrarenal location without aortic injury. An injured IMA should generally be ligated as close to the aorta as possible.

Iliac Artery Injuries

With blunt trauma, great efforts are made to not disturb the pelvic hematoma unless absolutely necessary to revascularize the lower extremities. If the patient has intact femoral pulses but is bleeding excessively into the pelvis, and it is not controlled with external stabilization of unstable pelvic fractures, arteriography is indicated. The bleeding arteries are usually branches of the internal iliac artery, and they generally can be embolized radiographically.

Care must be exercised when looping the proximal common iliac artery to avoid iliac vein injury, especially in older individuals in whom vascular reaction to atherosclerosis may cause the common iliac artery and vein to be tightly adherent. Distal control is then attempted in the abdomen where the external iliac artery exits the abdomen. In distal external iliac artery injuries, distal control may have to be obtained on the common femoral artery or through an inguinal incision.

Injuries to the common or external iliac artery should be repaired, preferably with a primary anastomosis. Ligation of either of these two vessels after trauma can result in 40% to 50% amputations. If there is extensive pelvic contamination from associated bowel injuries, the artery should be ligated and divided, and the suture lines in the ends of the divided vessels placed retroperitoneally. A femoral graft may then be placed if the extremity appears to be in jeopardy at the completion of the procedure. In patients with prolonged lower extremity ischemia, the development of compartment syndrome should always be suspected.

Hepatic Artery Injuries (see Chapter 22)

Inferior Vena Cava Injuries

From 1980 to 1992 at DRH, 124 patients had IVC injuries with a 55% mortality rate. The mortality rates for each portion of the IVC were

- Infrarenal, 28 (48%) of 58
- Pararenal, six (60%) of 10
- Infrahepatic, 19 (48%) of 40
- Retrohepatic, 18 (90%) of 20

These results are worse than those reported by Ombrellaro et al. (12).

Hemorrhage from the IVC can usually be controlled fairly easily by packing of the area or by manual pressure. As better exposure is obtained, more precise control can be provided by localized pressure with fingertips or with sponge sticks.

Retrohepatic Inferior Vena Cava and Hepatic Vein Injuries (see Chapter 22)

Suprarenal Inferior Vena Cava Injuries

The IVC inferior to the liver and more than 1 to 2 cm superior to the renal veins is called either the suprarenal or infrahepatic IVC. Small injuries to the anterior surface of the IVC below the liver are usually easy to expose, control, and suture. Care must be exercised to avoid occluding the IVC while controlling the bleeding because, even with hepatic venous flow continuing, complete occlusion of the infrahepatic IVC can cause hypovolemic patients to have a cardiac arrest.

Posterior wounds in the suprarenal IVC can be very difficult to expose and repair. If the posterior wound is not bleeding, occasionally it may be prudent to leave it undisturbed to heal spontaneously. Posterior wounds that are actively bleeding may be controlled by anterior pressure above and below the lesion while the anterior caval wound is enlarged enough to expose the posterior wound from inside. The repair can then be accomplished transcavally. Alternatively, the IVC can be freed from surrounding tissue. Vascular clamps can then be placed in an anteroposterior plane and the IVC gently rotated until the posterior surface of the midsuprarenal cava is exposed. In some cases, the right kidney has to be mobilized anteriorly out of its bed to be able to rotate the IVC adequately. Ligation and cutting of a few lumbar veins is often necessary to provide enough mobility to expose and repair a posterior injury.

AXIOM Ligation of the suprarenal IVC should not be done unless there is no other alternative to control bleeding.

If ligation of the suprarenal cava is contemplated because of an injury that cannot be repaired, the portion to be ligated should be occluded temporarily with a vascular clamp to evaluate the degree of venous hypertension that will develop and the amount of renal function that will remain (13). If urine output continues to be good (greater than 0.5 mL/kg/h) and the distal IVC pressure remains less than 30 cm H_2O, the IVC can be ligated relatively safely. Otherwise, ligation is contraindicated.

An alternative to suprarenal IVC ligation is a substitute vascular conduit. Another technique involves a reversed IVC interposition. If an autogenous or prosthetic graft does not seem appropriate, the injury can be managed by a splenorenal or portocaval anastomosis.

Pararenal Inferior Vena Cava Injuries

The portion of the IVC between the renal veins and 1 to 2 cm proximal and distal is sometimes referred to as the renal portion of the IVC. Injuries in this area are handled as are those in the suprarenal IVC, but control of the renal veins must usually also be obtained, and the right kidney often must be mobilized from its bed to expose and repair posterior injuries. The left renal vein can generally be ligated and cut at its junction with the IVC because it has extensive collaterals.

AXIOM Care must be taken to ligate, and not avulse, the first lumbar vein on the right, because in many cases, it enters the junction of the right renal vein and IVC.

Infrarenal Vena Cava Injuries

Optimal exposure of the infrarenal IVC is obtained by mobilizing the right colon, hepatic flexure, and duodenum toward the midline. This permits wide exposure of the IVC from the liver down to the iliac veins.

AXIOM Injuries to the IVC can often be controlled better and more safely with digital pressure or with sponge sticks than with vascular clamps.

Anterior wounds to the IVC can usually be repaired with a running suture of 5-0 or 6-0 polypropylene, preferably everting the edges. Everting the edges of veins when they are repaired ensures intima-to-intima approximation and lessens the tendency to thrombosis at the suture line.

AXIOM Excessive efforts to mobilize the IVC to repair a small posterior wound may cause significantly more bleeding and more damage than the original injury.

Ligation of the infrarenal IVC is usually tolerated well hemodynamically, unless the patient is hypovolemic, and may be safer than repair in patients with complex injuries.

AXIOM Long-term venous sequelae after infrarenal ligation of the IVC can usually be minimized by careful prevention of lower extremity edema and appropriate follow-up care.

Iliac Vein Injuries

Injured common or external iliac veins are exposed by using techniques similar to those described for injuries to the iliac arteries. It is not usually necessary to pass umbilical tapes around these vessels because they are readily compressible digitally or with sponge sticks. Even if there is extensive bilateral injury, the internal iliac veins do not have to be repaired.

Injuries to the common or external iliac veins are best treated with either lateral or end-to-end repair by using 5-0 or 6-0 everting polypropylene suture. In young patients, ligation of the common or external iliac veins is relatively well tolerated if precautions are taken to prevent leg edema.

AXIOM If bleeding sites in the pelvis cannot be controlled during one or two inspections, and the patient becomes hypotensive during these inspections, one should pack the pelvis and close the abdomen.

The mortality rate of patients with injuries to the iliac veins is variable, but it was 25% in 141 patients compiled by Feliciano (2) from three large series. If patients with other vascular injuries, especially to the iliac arteries, were excluded, the survival rate in 56 patients was 95%.

The mortality rates for iliac vein injuries reported by Wilson et al. (14) were much higher and included

- Common iliac veins, 40% (6 of 15)
- Internal iliac veins, 65% (9 of 14)
- External iliac veins, 29% (4 of 14)
- Two or more iliac veins, 100% (6 of 6)

Several of these deaths might have been prevented by earlier control of bleeding and a more rapid resuscitation, including restoration of core temperature to above 35°C. In several patients, early packing of the pelvis and closing of the abdomen, rather than persistent efforts to achieve definitive control of specific bleeding vessels, would probably have been better tolerated.

Renal Vein Injuries (see Chapter 29)

Superior Mesenteric Vein Injuries

The proximal superior mesenteric vein (SMV) lies just to the right of the SMA, and injuries to this structure should be suspected when there is major bleeding at the base of the mesocolon. Treatment of proximal SMV injuries is complicated by the overlying pancreas, the proximity of the SMA, and its junction with the splenic vein. With some proximal SMV injuries, the pancreas may have to be transected to achieve adequate exposure.

Injuries to the more distal SMV can usually be sutured while the vein is compressed proximally and distally by the surgeon's fingers or noncrushing clamps. If multiple abdominal injuries are present, or the injury is impossible to repair, ligation may be the safest procedure. Severe splanchnic congestion may develop, and the patient's blood-volume status must be watched carefully for at least 3 days (15). In three recent series, ligation of the SMV was performed in 27 patients, and 22 (82%) survived (2).

Portal Vein Injuries (see Chapter 22)

Hypothermia

Patients requiring massive fluid resuscitation and blood transfusions will almost routinely have a core body temperature of less than 35°C. Hypothermia, particularly with core temperatures less than 32°C, is frequently associated with poor cardiac performance and myocardial irritability. Furthermore, hypothermia greatly contributes to the development of coagulopathies.

Maneuvers to help prevent and correct hypothermia in the OR include

1. Covering the patient's head with transparent plastic;
2. Placing the patient on a heating blanket;
3. Covering the lower extremities with plastic bags or a "space" blanket;
4. Use of a heating cascade on the anesthesia machine;
5. Irrigation of the nasogastric tube with warm (42°C) saline;
6. Irrigation of thoracostomy tubes with warm saline; and
7. Irrigation of open body cavities with warm saline.

Coagulopathies

The majority of patients who arrive in the OR with active hemorrhage from a major abdominal vascular injury will require massive transfusions. If more than 10 units of blood is required, the patient will frequently develop a transfusion-induced coagulopathy (17). Clinical coagulopathies often do not correlate well with laboratory clotting studies or platelet counts, and patients with excessive microvascular bleeding should be given platelet transfusions and fresh frozen plasma (FFP) without waiting for the results of coagulation tests. The use of "prophylactic" FFP or platelet transfusions (just because a certain number of blood transfusions have been given), however, should be discouraged.

Hemostatic Adjuvants

Biologically based hemostatic agents can enhance native coagulatory mechanisms and improve local hemostasis. Fibrin-based compounds have the added advantage of independence from the usual requirements for platelets or coagulation factors for hemostasis, and they can be effective during heparinization, thrombocytopenia, and various other coagulopathies.

AXIOM Localized bleeding in spite of surgical efforts frequently can be controlled by applying fibrin glue.

Fibrin glue mimics the last step in the natural coagulation cascade. Factor XIII and fibrinogen are activated by thrombin in the presence of calcium ion, converting fibrinogen to fibrin. Activated factor XIII then polymerizes fibrin to form a stable clot. Although anaphylaxis to the bovine protein is a theoretic possibility, it is rarely of clinical importance, especially if care is taken to avoid intravascular application.

We prepare fibrin gel from cryoprecipitate, which is mixed with thrombin and calcium as it is being injected over the injured surface and the bleeding is being controlled with pressure. This material has been remarkably effective and seems to resist infection.

Planned Reoperation

Planned reoperations after an initial "damage control" operation are increasingly used in the management of critically injured patients (16). The initial damage-control operation includes measures to

1. Control bleeding;
2. Prevent continued spillage of intestinal contents and urine; and
3. Close the abdomen or chest.

The patient is then warmed and resuscitated in the intensive care unit until he or she is physiologically stable enough for a planned reoperation with definitive repair of the injuries. Coagulopathies also should be corrected before reoperation.

Complications

Vascular Occlusion or Ischemia

The complications of vascular repairs in the abdomen include vessel thrombosis, ischemia to abdominal organs, dehiscence of suture lines, and infection. Vessel occlusion is not uncommon in the trauma situation when vasoconstricted vessels undergo lateral arteriorrhaphy or reanastomosis.

AXIOM If there is any question about the adequacy of a vascular repair, a completion arteriogram should be performed. If there is any question about intestinal viability, a second-look operation should be performed within 12 to 24 hours.

Postoperatively, the diagnosis of ischemic bowel should be suspected if there is excessive abdominal pain or tenderness, increased arterial lactate, or excessive uptake of intravenous fluids.

Infections

The high incidence of infection after intraabdominal vascular injury is probably related to the frequent occurrence of three main factors:

1. Prolonged shock;
2. Massive transfusions; and
3. Associated bowel injuries, especially colon, requiring a colostomy.

In a recent series of 210 patients with abdominal vascular injuries, the incidence of serious infection in those who survived 48 or more hours was 37% (41 of 111) (7). Of the 41 patients with infections, 23 (50%) had intraabdominal infections, and the mortality rate in these patients was 35% (eight of 23).

⊘ FREQUENT ERRORS

1. ***Delaying surgery that is needed to control intraabdominal bleeding in an attempt to improve blood pressure preoperatively or perform urologic studies for hematuria.***
2. ***Reliance on only one intravenous line or on lower-extremity veins for intravenous access when an abdominal injury with hypotension is present.***
3. ***Opening a pelvic retroperitoneal hematoma due to blunt trauma if the femoral pulses are satisfactory.***
4. ***Failure to take active early steps to prevent or rapidly to correct hypothermia, especially after the major bleeding sites have been controlled.***
5. ***Allowing proximal aortic pressure to increase above 160 to 180 mm Hg after the thoracic or abdominal aorta is cross-clamped.***
6. ***Taking time to repair nonvital injuries when bleeding or other major trauma is present.***
7. ***Inadequate debridement after a high-velocity missile injury.***
8. ***Failure to interpose adequate tissue between vascular and intestinal repairs.***
9. ***Exploring a perirenal hematoma before obtaining adequate control of the renal vessels.***
10. ***Failure to look for increased lower-extremity compartment pressures after aortic or iliac artery occlusion.***
11. ***Compressing or clamping the retrohepatic IVC in a hypovolemic patient without first clamping the abdominal or lower thoracic aorta.***

SUMMARY POINTS

1. Tissues damaged by high-velocity missiles may require extensive debridement to ensure that the remaining tissue is normal and will heal properly.

2. Blunt aortic contusion may not cause signs or symptoms for days or weeks until the aorta becomes thrombosed.

3. Severe hypotension with a poor response to aggressive fluid resuscitation is usually the result of continued bleeding, which should be controlled rapidly in the OR.

4. Lower-extremity intravenous access should be avoided whenever possible in patients with suspected major abdominal vascular injuries.

5. Hypothermia is a major cause of morbidity and mortality in patients with abdominal vascular injury and should be prevented or rapidly corrected.

6. An inflated pneumatic antishock garment (PASG) can reduce bleeding from fractures in the lower extremities or pelvis, but may increase bleeding in areas not compressed by the PASG.

7. Patients with massive hemoperitoneum and continued severe hypotension should have a prelaparotomy thoracotomy with thoracic aortic cross-clamping.

8. If the aorta is cross-clamped, the proximal aortic pressure should not be allowed to exceed 160 to 180 mm Hg.

9. Contained retroperitoneal hematomas should not be opened until actively bleeding intraperitoneal vessels and gastrointestinal leaks are controlled and the patient is adequately resuscitated.

10. Pelvic hematomas after blunt trauma are usually due to bleeding from the pelvic fracture sites and should not be opened.
11. Reflection of the left colon and abdominal viscera to the right is generally the best way to rapidly expose the superceliac abdominal aorta.
12. The celiac artery should be ligated, rather than repaired, if it is injured, and it can be ligated and divided at its origin to provide improved exposure of aortic injuries in that area.
13. Efforts should be made to limit aortic clamping to less than 30 minutes whenever possible.
14. Contained hematomas of the pelvis due to blunt trauma should not be disturbed unless the blood supply to the lower extremities is compromised.
15. Isolation of a proximal common iliac artery can easily cause injury to an adherent iliac vein in older individuals.
16. Compartment syndrome should be suspected in any patient who has had prolonged lower-extremity ischemia.
17. Ligation of the suprarenal IVC should not be done unless there is no other alternative to control bleeding.
18. Care must be taken to ligate, and not avulse, the first lumbar vein on the right if posterior exposure is needed in that area, because it often enters the junction of the right renal vein and IVC.
19. Injuries to the IVC can often be controlled better and more safely with digital pressure or with sponge sticks than with vascular clamps.
20. Excessive efforts to mobilize the IVC to repair a small posterior nonbleeding wound may cause significantly more bleeding and damage than the original injury.
21. Long-term venous sequelae after infrarenal ligation of the IVC can usually be minimized by careful long-term prevention of lower-extremity edema.
22. If bleeding sites in the pelvis cannot be controlled during one or two inspections, and the patient becomes hypotensive during each inspection, one should simply pack the pelvis and close the abdomen.
23. In patients with extensive injuries, ligation of an injured SMV may be much safer than a repair, but may take up large amounts of fluid.
24. Localized bleeding in spite of surgical efforts can frequently be controlled by applying fibrin glue or fibrin gel.
25. If there is any question about a vascular repair, a completion arteriogram should be performed; if there is any question about intestinal viability, a second-look operation should be performed within 12 to 24 hours.
26. The combination of massive transfusions, prolonged shock, and intestinal spill will result in serious postoperative infections in at least a third of the patients who survive more than 48 hours.
27. Patients with prolonged shock tend to be anergic. Consequently, they are more apt to become infected and may not show any evidence of infection until multiple organ failure develops.

REFERENCES

1. Wilson RF, Dulchavsky SA. Abdominal vascular trauma. In: Wilson RF, Walt AJ, eds. *Management of trauma: pitfalls and practice.* 2nd ed. Philadelphia: Williams & Wilkins, 1996:554.
2. Feliciano DV, Burch JM, Graham JM. Abdominal vascular injury. In: Moore EE, Mattox RL, Feliciano DV, eds. *Trauma.* 2nd ed. East Norwalk, CT: Appleton & Lange, 1991:533–552.
3. Feliciano DV, Burch JM, Spjut-Patrinely V, et al. Abdominal gunshot wounds: an urban trauma center's experience with 300 consecutive patients. *Ann Surg* 1988; 208:362.
4. Lassonde J, Laurendeau F. Blunt injury of abdominal aorta. *Ann Surg* 1981;194: 745.
5. Sclafani SJA. The diagnosis of bilateral renal artery injury by computed tomography. *J Trauma* 1986;26:295.
6. Washington BC, Wilson RF, Steiger Z. Emergency thoracotomy for penetrating trauma. *J Trauma* 1983;23:672.

7. Wiencek RG, Wilson RF. Injuries to the abdominal vascular system: how much does aggressive resuscitation and prelaparotomy thoracotomy really help? *Surgery* 1987;102:731.
8. Fry WR, Fry RE, Fry WL. Operative exposure of the abdominal arteries for trauma. *Arch Surg* 1991;126:289.
9. Accola KD, Feliciano DV, Mattox KL, et al. Management of injuries to the suprarenal aorta. *Am J Surg* 1987;154:613.
10. Smith GJ, Holcroft JW. Mesenteric vascular trauma. In: Champion HR, Robbs JV, Trunkey DV, eds. *Rob and Smith's operative surgery: trauma surgery*. 4th ed. London: Butterworth, 1989:539.
11. Reisman JD, Morgan AS. Analysis of 46 intra-abdominal aortic injuries from blunt trauma: case reports and literature review. *J Trauma* 1990;30:1294.
12. Ombrellaro MP, Freeman MB, Stevens SL, et al. Predictors of survival after inferior vena cava injuries. *Am Surg* 1997;63:178.
13. Starzl TE, Groth CG, Brettschneider L, et al. Extended survival in three cases of orthotopic homotransplantation of the human liver. *Surgery* 1968;63:549.
14. Wilson RF, Wiencik RG Jr, Balog M. Factors affecting mortality rate with iliac vein injuries. *J Trauma* 1990;30:320.
15. Stone HH, Fabian TC, Turkleson ML. Wounds of the portal venous system. *World J Surg* 1982;6:335.
16. Hirshberg A, Wall MJ, Mattox K. Planned reoperation for trauma: a two year experience with 124 consecutive patients. *J Trauma* 1994;37:365.
17. Wilson RF, Dulchavsky SA, Soullier G, Beckman B. Problems with 20 or more transfusions in 24 hours. *Am Surg* 1987;53:410.

28. PELVIC FRACTURES(1)

INCIDENCE

AXIOM Second to fractures of the skull, pelvic fractures are the commonest skeletal injury associated with death in patients with multiple injuries.

The overall incidence of pelvic fractures in the United States is 37 per 100,000 person-years, with a gradual increase with age to a maximal incidence of 446 per 100,000 person-years in women aged 85 years or older (2). These elderly women often have pelvic fractures with minimal falls because of an underlying severe osteoporosis. Most of the mortality and disabling morbidity with pelvic fractures is due to major blood loss or injury to adjacent nerves and the genitourinary and distal gastrointestinal organs. Late mortality from pelvic fractures is usually caused by sepsis and multiorgan failure from retroperitoneal hematomas or associated intestinal, genitourinary, or soft tissue injuries or a combination of these.

MECHANISMS OF INJURY

Bone and Joint Injuries

The most severe pelvic fractures result from forces that disrupt the pelvic ring by three different mechanisms or forces:

1. Opening the ring at the symphysis pubis;
2. Crushing the pelvis in anteroposterior or lateral directions; and
3. Disrupting the sacroiliac joints with forces applied from the perineum upward.

AXIOM The posterior ligaments are by far the strongest and most important structures for maintaining pelvic stability.

Direct anterior-impact injuries tend to cause fractures of the pubic symphysis and dislocations of the sacroiliac joints. This can result in a classic "open book" diastasis at the pubic symphysis plus a high rate of bladder or male urethral injuries or both. Straddle injuries, which can cause bilateral superior and inferior pubic rami fractures, also have a high incidence of associated lower urinary tract injuries.

AXIOM Forceful crushing, axial compression, or vertical shear injuries have a high incidence of associated injuries to adjacent structures.

Trauma striking the pelvis at an angle tends to cause vertical shearing forces, which can produce unilateral disruptions of the pelvic ring known as Malgaigne fractures. Posterior injuries can cause sacroiliac joint dislocation and disruption of posterior nerves and blood vessels (3).

Acetabular fractures with femoral head dislocations tend to occur when force is applied to the hip from the front or the rear, such as when an unrestrained motorist hits the dashboard with the knees in a deceleration injury. Central acetabular fracture and dislocation can occur when the hip is hit from a lateral direction.

Soft-Tissue Injuries

When the rectum tears, it is most commonly just inside the anus where the rectum is fixed and less distensible. The rectum and vagina also may be injured by forceful compression against the sacral promontory or by perforation from bony spicules.

AXIOM A full bladder is much more susceptible to injury than one that is empty.

A full bladder may shear off the urethra at the pubis because of severe deceleration, or it may burst because of excessive compression. Management of bladder ruptures is determined to some extent by whether they occur intraperitoneally or extraperitoneally.

AXIOM Open pelvic fractures with extensive perineal, rectal, or vaginal involvement can have a 40% to 50% mortality rate if not treated properly (3).

INITIAL EMERGENCY MANAGEMENT

Hemodynamic Status

Pelvic fractures are usually associated with damage to multiple small vessels; only 6% to 18% of pelvic hemorrhage is primarily from the arterial system (3). In addition, the retroperitoneal space can accommodate up to several liters of blood before any appreciable tamponade of bleeding sites occurs. Grimm et al. (4) noted that in cadaveric specimens with a normal pelvis, pressures rapidly increased to an average of 30 mm Hg after infusion of 5 L of fluid into the retroperitoneal pelvic soft tissues. After fracture of the pelvis, up to 20 L of fluid could be infused at pressures not exceeding 35 mm Hg. External fixation increased pressures approximately 3 mm Hg at low fluid volumes, and approximately 11 mm Hg at the highest fluid volumes. Thus low-pressure venous hemorrhage may be tamponaded by an external fixator. However, external fixation may not be adequate to stop arterial bleeding.

AXIOM Unstable pelvic fractures greatly increase the amount of bleeding that can occur in the pelvis.

Mucha (6) noted that the mortality rate for pelvic fractures in patients who were hypotensive on admission was 42%, but in patients who were hemodynamically stable, the morbidity rate was only 3%. Although 10% to 15% of patients with pelvic fractures are hemodynamically unstable initially, in almost two thirds of these, spontaneous tamponade of the pelvic fracture hemorrhage occurs, and the patient becomes hemodynamically stable with the usual resuscitation (7).

Approximately 75% to 85% of pelvic-fracture victims are hemodynamically stable and have a relatively uncomplicated course. Another 15% to 25% are an intermediate hemodynamic group, usually with varying degrees of hypotension (3,7). These patients usually respond to aggressive infusions of crystalloid initially, but subsequently they may require relatively large amounts of blood and other fluid to maintain a normal blood pressure and urine output.

Very severe bleeding occurs in about 0.5% to 1.0% of patients with pelvic fractures (3,7). These patients have severe hypotension and respond poorly to aggressive intravenous fluids. One must determine rapidly if there is blood loss from associated abdominal injuries that requires immediate surgical control. If the bleeding sites are all in the pelvis, the vessels causing the bleeding must be compressed or embolized rapidly.

Fluid Administration

As a general rule, lower-extremity routes for fluid administration should be avoided in patients with suspected pelvic fractures because of the possibility of associated iliac or femoral vein injury. If fluids are administered rapidly (2 to 3 L in 10 to 15 minutes) and there is little or no hemodynamic improvement or it is only transient, one should consider a prompt diagnostic peritoneal lavage (DPL), application of external fixators, angiography with embolization of bleeding pelvic arteries, or a combination of these. One may also consider application of a pneumatic antishock garment (PASG).

AXIOM Chest radiograph, DPL, and physical examination will rule out most extrapelvic sources of blood loss in patients with pelvic fractures.

Emergency Laparotomy

If the DPL is positive, the patient should be brought to the operating room (OR) promptly. The patient should be placed in the lithotomy position, as for an abdominoperineal resection. This will allow the perineum and abdomen to be explored simultaneously by two teams if needed. In females, the vagina also should be cleansed for careful examination.

If no intraperitoneal bleeding sources are found, but there is a rapidly expanding or ruptured pelvic hematoma, it should be packed and arrangements made for immediate bony pelvic fixation or angiographic embolization of the bleeding vessels or both.

External Fixation of the Pelvis

External fixation of pelvic fractures limits pelvic hemorrhage by reducing the volume of the pelvic retroperitoneal space. Because the bleeding in the majority of patients is mainly from small vessels on the edges of the fractured bones, external fixators that approximate and occlude exposed bleeding bone can be extremely helpful.

AXIOM The major disadvantages of external fixators are that they do not stabilize posterior pelvic fractures adequately, and they introduce the possibility for pin-tract infections.

Interventional Angiography

Percutaneous angiographic localization of pelvic fracture hemorrhage followed by therapeutic embolization is successful in more than 80% of patients (7). If the patient has had an exploratory laparotomy, and massive pelvic bleeding is found, this is an indication for angiographic embolization. A transfusion requirement greater than 4 to 6 units within the first 12 to 24 hours, according to many authors, is also an indication for angiography and embolization of bleeding vessels (7).

Pneumatic Antishock Garments

If there is evidence of continued blood loss in the emergency department, and external pelvic fixation or interventional angiography is not readily available, apposition of the disrupted pelvic fracture fragments by the application of a PASG can help reduce external and internal bleeding (7,8). Even in hemodynamically stable patients, low-pressure inflation of the PASG can provide some splinting of the pelvis and lower-extremity fractures while the patient's evaluation is continuing.

AXIOM If application of a PASG causes severe respiratory distress, one should look carefully for a diaphragmatic injury.

DIAGNOSIS

Physical Examination

Pelvic fractures with massive bleeding can cause ecchymosis in the external genitalia, medial thigh, and flanks. Ecchymosis about the pubis, perineum, or scrotum or the presence of blood in the urethral meatus also is highly suggestive of lower genitourinary trauma.

Part of the examination of an injured pelvis is determination of its stability. Bilateral pressure on the anterior iliac spines or iliac crest, looking and feeling for opening and closing of the pelvis, can usually detect any instability present. Pushing and pulling gently on a leg may reveal vertical instability.

AXIOM Once it is determined that the patient has an unstable pelvic fracture, checking for instability should not be repeated because it can greatly increase pelvic bleeding.

Another extremely important part of the physical examination of an injured pelvis is a check for hematuria or blood in the vagina or rectum.

AXIOM Lacerations of the perineum, groin, or buttock after blunt trauma indicate an open pelvic fracture until proven otherwise.

Even when urethral laceration in men is treated optimally, urethral stricture, incontinence, and impotence are frequent complications. A careful search for signs of urethral injury should be made during the initial examination, before a urethral catheter is inserted. These signs include

1. Blood at the urethral meatus;
2. Perineal hematoma; and
3. Displaced or "floating" prostate found on rectal examination.

In the female patient, the pelvic examination should also include palpation of the posterior pubis and lateral pelvic walls. The presence of rectal blood is usually due to a rectal injury. A lax anal sphincter and lack of a response to perianal pain or to a request to tighten the anal sphincter often indicates a major neurologic injury.

Radiologic Evaluation

Plain Films and Computed Tomography Scans

A minimal radiographic examination of the pelvis is the anteroposterior view, which is a standard study taken in all patients with severe blunt trauma. More precise evaluation of the pelvis requires additional views or a computed tomography (CT) scan of the pelvis or both. Routine CT scanning is not needed for every pelvic fracture, but it does provide invaluable information for assessment of the sacroiliac joints and fractures of the acetabulum.

AXIOM The possibility of early pregnancy should be considered in women of childbearing age with pelvic trauma; however, radiographs needed for management should not be delayed because of pregnancy.

Genitourinary Tract Evaluation

Retrograde contrast urethrography is performed if there is any clinical evidence of urethral injury.

With a large pelvic hematoma, cystography frequently discloses a characteristic "teardrop" deformity of the urinary bladder as a result of compression and elevation by the surrounding blood. Empty ("washout" or "post-evac") views are important and sometimes provide the only clear evidence of a bladder injury.

Angiography

Angiography may be extremely helpful in determining the site of continuing blood loss in the pelvis. Posterior branches of the internal iliac artery are a common location for persistent bleeding in these patients, and these can usually be embolized radiologically.

Diagnostic Peritoneal Lavage

If there is concern about intraperitoneal bleeding or intestinal injury in a patient with a fractured pelvic bone, a DPL may be performed. In the presence of a pelvic fracture, the DPL should be performed as an open procedure above the umbilicus.

AXIOM In a patient with a pelvic fracture, a negative DPL is generally a highly accurate indicator that significant intraperitoneal injury is not present; however, the DPL is often false positive if a large pelvic hematoma is present.

The main difficulty with DPL in pelvic fractures is the increased false-positive rate, which may be as high as 40%. Further complicating the problem is the increased mortality rate (up to 30%) for patients undergoing an unnecessary laparotomy in the presence of a pelvic fracture (3). Some surgeons say that the number of red blood cells for a positive DPL in patient with pelvic fractures should be increased to 200,000/mm^3. Others believe that severe bleeding from an intraperitoneal source is probably not present unless 20 mL or more of gross blood is aspirated.

TREATMENT

Techniques of Fracture Management

Open reduction and internal fixation of pelvis fractures are increasing in popularity. Typical indications for internal fixation are widely displaced anterior lesions, unstable posterior lesions, and acetabular fractures.

Skeletal traction is frequently used as a provisional modality in patients with unstable pelvic or acetabular fractures. It is usually applied through a femoral pin and is discontinued when the definitive treatment is performed.

Management of Associated Injuries

AXIOM Almost 90% of patients with major pelvic fractures have significant associated injuries to other body regions (3).

Associated injuries to the lower extremities have been reported in more than 60% of patients with major pelvic fractures (3), and these can seriously complicate orthopedic management of the pelvis.

Bladder Injuries

More than 75% of bladder ruptures seen with pelvic fractures are extraperitoneal, and most of these can be managed with just good bladder drainage via a Foley catheter in female patients and a suprapubic catheter in male patients. Intraperitoneal bladder tears usually produce signs of peritonitis and are generally managed at laparotomy. The bladder repair is performed in two to three layers by using absorbable sutures. Continuous drainage of the bladder is then provided with a Foley or suprapubic catheter.

Urethral injuries are extremely rare in female patients, and in male patients are usually treated initially with suprapubic drainage.

Vagina, Uterus, Adnexa Injuries
Injuries to the vagina, uterus, and adnexa are treated with debridement, repair, and drainage as needed.

Liver, Spleen, Intestine, or Kidney Injuries
Injuries to the liver, spleen, mesentery, intestine, or kidneys are present in at least 5% to 10% of patients with severe pelvic fractures. In hemodynamically stable patients with pelvic fractures, many centers now use contrast-enhanced CT scans for assessment of both the pelvic and intraabdominal contents. If one relies on CT, however, injuries to the intestine are easily missed; except for surgery, the most objective means of excluding intestinal injuries is DPL.

Rectal Injuries
Patients with a pelvic fracture plus a rectal injury or severe perineal lacerations should be given a sigmoid colostomy. It is also worthwhile digitally to extract and irrigate out any feces present in the defunctionalized rectum because it might act as an ongoing source of contamination. Irrigation of the rectum with broad-spectrum antibiotic solutions [neomycin, 0.5%, or povidone–iodine (Betadine), 5%] also has been recommended (6).

Neurologic Injuries
Associated neurologic injuries, particularly to the lumbosacral plexus, may have very important long-term consequences (9). Neuropathies resulting from hematoma compression, unrelated to pelvic fractures, may be alleviated by early operative decompression. With persistent neurologic deficits, electromyography (EMG) is recommended 3 to 4 weeks after injury to serve as a baseline for determining eventual prognosis.

AXIOM Even in the absence of clinically apparent neurologic signs, injury to the lumbosacral plexus is demonstrated by EMG abnormalities in up to 64% of patients with sacral fractures and sacroiliac separation (10).

An aggressive rehabilitation program with early attention to passive range of motion and maintenance of motor tone offers the patient the best chance for a functional return to society.

MANAGEMENT OF COMPLICATIONS
Complications of particular concern with pelvic fractures include pelvic sepsis, posttraumatic pulmonary insufficiency, deep venous thrombosis, impotence, hyperbilirubinemia, and physical disabilities.

Pelvic Sepsis

AXIOM The most common cause of death more than 48 hours after a pelvic fracture is sepsis (3).

Appropriate debridement and irrigation of all open wounds and diversion of the fecal stream, when indicated, are extremely important in patients with pelvic fractures. The antibiotics used should be effective against gram-negative enteric bacilli (such as *Escherichia coli*) and anaerobes (such as *Bacteroides fragilis*). Although it is not clear how long such antibiotics should be given, unless there is continued contamination, 4 to 6 days should be more than adequate.

Posttraumatic Pulmonary Insufficiency (see Chapter 40)
Pulmonary insufficiency in patients with pelvic fractures may be caused by associated chest or diaphragm injuries, aspiration of oral or gastric contents, fat emboli,

acute respiratory distress syndrome (ARDS), or later pulmonary emboli. Aggressive pulmonary toilet, careful pain control, rapid mobilization out of bed, and early deep venous thrombosis (DVT) preventive measures are important; however, if arterial blood gases or ventilatory mechanics are borderline, early ventilatory assistance should be strongly considered.

Deep Vein Thrombosis

Because of the venostasis and the associated soft-tissue injuries, the incidence of DVT after severe pelvic fractures is at least 15% to 20% (11).

AXIOM Because of the high incidence of DVT, weekly duplex ultrasonography of the lower extremities should be considered in patients with pelvic fracture who are not ambulatory.

Prophylaxis for DVT in patients with pelvic fractures can be extremely difficult. Early ambulation is not possible in many of these patients because of their multiple injuries. Subcutaneous heparin also can increase the risk for bleeding. Sequential compression stockings have been liberally used by the authors in this setting. Treatment for DVT in patients with pelvic fractures is anticoagulation if possible; however, many times it is not, and early placement of a vena caval filter is appropriate (12).

AXIOM If anticoagulation is not possible in a patient who is immobilized with a severe pelvic fracture, a prophylactic vena cava filter should be considered.

Impotence

Impotence, as a result of damage to portions of the parasympathetic nervous system, is a well-established complication of membranous urethral injury, which commonly occurs in association with anterior pelvic disruptions (3). Impotence also has been described in association with pelvic hemorrhage treated by angiographic embolization (13); however, in such cases, associated injuries to the lumbosacral nervous plexus are more likely to have caused the impotence. Retrograde ejaculation, a result of damage to portions of the sympathetic nervous system, is also frequent with severe anterior pelvic fractures, especially if the urethra is injured.

AXIOM Evidence of impotence should be sought in all sexually active males with pelvic fractures so that the psychosocial aspects of this problem can be dealt with as early as possible.

OUTCOMES OF PELVIC FRACTURES

Patients with severe pelvic fractures often have severe disabilities and require extensive physical therapy and rehabilitation. Even with rather simple avulsion fractures, physical disability persists for an average of 19 weeks (3). Major disabilities usually last for more than 6 to 9 months, and many are permanent.

Late complications of pelvic fractures include chronic pain from malunion or nonunion, posttraumatic sacroiliac arthritis, and permanent nerve root injuries. Accurate early reduction of posterior vertical shear injuries and sacroiliac joint disruptions appears to decrease the incidence of late chronic pain. Early decompression of sacral fractures that may be compressing nerve roots also should be considered (14).

⊘ FREQUENT ERRORS

1. ***Failure to look carefully for associated injuries in patients with pelvic fractures.***
2. ***Failure to be aggressive in determining and controlling the cause of continuing large fluid and blood requirements.***
3. ***Reliance on plain radiographs to rule out pelvic fractures in patients with suggestive symptoms or signs.***
4. ***Failure to appreciate the high mortality and morbidity of pelvic fractures that have associated perineal lacerations.***
5. ***Opening a pelvic hematoma due to blunt trauma.***
6. ***Failure to perform a diverting sigmoid colostomy in a patient with a pelvic fracture and a laceration in or very near the rectum.***
7. ***Failure to thoroughly evaluate the lower genitourinary tract in patients with severe anterior pelvic fractures.***

SUMMARY POINTS

1. Second to fractures of the skull, pelvic fractures are the most common skeletal injury associated with death in patients with multiple injuries.

2. The main cause of early deaths in patients with pelvic fractures is uncontrolled bleeding.

3. The posterior ligaments are by far the strongest and most important structures for maintaining pelvic stability.

4. Open pelvic fractures with extensive perineal, rectal, or vaginal involvement can have a 40% to 50% mortality rate if not treated properly.

5. Once it is determined that the patient has an unstable pelvic fracture, checking for instability should not be repeated because it can greatly increase pelvic bleeding.

6. Suprapubic pain, low back pain, or lower-extremity weakness or diminished sensation after trauma should suggest the presence of a pelvic fracture.

7. Neurologic injuries to the cauda equina or the sciatic or femoral nerves are easily missed in patients with severe trauma.

8. Angiography of the abdominal aorta and iliac arteries can be used to diagnose and treat continued intraabdominal or pelvic bleeding.

9. In a patient with a pelvic fracture, a negative DPL is generally a highly accurate indicator that significant intraperitoneal injury is not present; however, the DPL is often falsely positive if there is a large pelvic hematoma.

10. The possibility of early pregnancy should be considered in women of childbearing age with pelvic trauma; however, radiographs needed for management should not be delayed because of pregnancy.

11. One should always anticipate significant blood loss with unstable pelvic fractures, especially if the patient is hypotensive on admission.

12. Chest radiograph, DPL, and physical examination will rule out most extrapelvic sources of blood loss in patients with pelvic fractures.

13. If a rapidly expanding or ruptured pelvic hematoma is found at laparotomy, it should be packed, and arrangements made for prompt external pelvic fixation or angiographic embolization of the bleeding vessels or both.

14. If pelvic packing is successful, a second-look operation 24 to 48 hours later is recommended if the patient's core temperature and coagulation and bleeding studies can be returned to normal.

15. Hemipelvectomy for otherwise uncontrollable pelvic bleeding should be performed only if most of the dissection has already been accomplished by the trauma.

16. The most important disadvantages of external fixators are that they do not stabilize posterior pelvic fractures adequately.

17. More than 80% of pelvic arterial injuries can be controlled by appropriate arterial embolization.
18. Because of the high incidence of DVT, weekly duplex ultrasonography of the lower extremities should be considered in patients with pelvic fractures who are not ambulatory.
19. Severe bladder injuries should be ruled out by retrograde cystography if there is hematuria or a severe anterior pelvic fracture.
20. If the patient with a pelvic fracture has rectal, vaginal, or extensive perineal wounds, the fecal stream should be diverted with a sigmoid colostomy.
21. Even in the absence of clinically apparent neurologic signs, injury to the lumbosacral plexus is demonstrated by EMG abnormalities in up to 64% of patients with sacral fractures or sacroiliac joint separation or both.
22. If anticoagulation or sequential-compression devices for the legs are not possible in a patient who is immobilized with a severe pelvic fracture, a vena cava filter should be inserted.
23. Evidence of impotence or retrograde ejaculation should be sought in all sexually active male patients with pelvic fractures so that the psychosocial aspects of this problem can be dealt with as early as possible.

REFERENCES

1. Wilson RF, Tyburski JG, Georgiadis GM. Pelvic fractures. In: Wilson RF, Walt AJ, eds. *Management of trauma: pitfalls and practice.* 2nd ed. Philadelphia: Williams & Wilkins, 1996:578.
2. Melton LJ III, Sampson JM, Morrey BF, et al. Epidemiologic features of pelvic fractures. *Clin Orthop* 1981;155:43.
3. Mucha P. Pelvic fractures. In: Moore EE, Mattox KL, Feliciano DV, eds. *Trauma.* 2nd ed. Norwalk, CT: Appleton & Lange, 1991:553.
4. Grimm MR, Vrahas MS, Thomas KA. Pressure-volume characteristics of the intact and disrupted pelvic retroperitoneum. *J Trauma* 1998;44:454.
5. Richardson JD, Harty J, Amin M, Flint LM. Open pelvic fractures. *J Trauma* 1982;22:533.
6. Mucha P Jr. Pelvic fractures. In: McIlrath DC, Farnell MB, eds. *Problems in general surgery.* Philadelphia: JB Lippincott, 1984:154.
7. Mucha P Jr, Farnell MB. Analysis of pelvic fracture management. *J Trauma* 1984;24:379.
8. Mucha P Jr, Welch TJ. Hemorrhage in major pelvic fractures. *Surg Clin North Am* 1988;68:757.
9. Conway RR, Hubbell SL. Electromyographic abnormalities in neurologic injury associated with pelvic fracture: case reports and literature review. *Arch Phys Med Rehabil* 1988;69:539.
10. Weis EB Jr. Subtle neurological injuries in pelvic fractures. *J Trauma* 1984;24:983.
11. Consensus Development Conference, National Institutes of Health. Prevention of venous thrombosis and pulmonary embolism. *JAMA* 1986;256:744.
12. Webb LX, Rush PT, Fuller SB, Meredith JW. Greenfield filter prophylaxis of pulmonary embolism in patients undergoing surgery for acetabular fracture. *J Orthop Trauma* 1992;6:139.
13. Ellison M, Timberlake GA, Kerstein MD. Impotence following pelvic fracture. *J Trauma* 1988;28:695.
14. Denis F, Davis S, Comfort T. Sacral fractures: an important problem. *Clin Orthop* 1988;227:67.

29. TRAUMA TO THE URINARY TRACT[1]

Urologic injuries occur in approximately 3% to 4% of patients admitted to a hospital with trauma (2,3). The kidney is injured 80% to 90% of the time, and the bladder and urethra are injured about 5% to 10% of the time.

RENAL INJURIES

Although the kidneys are well protected by the ribs, vertebrae, back muscles, and abdominal viscera, they are among the most commonly injured abdominal organs in blunt trauma. In addition, up to 83% of patients with blunt renal trauma have associated injuries (2,3).

AXIOM Abnormal kidneys, such as those with congenital anomalies, tumors, or hydronephrosis, are much more susceptible to injury than are normal kidneys.

Five grades of renal injury are generally recognized (Table 29-1).

Table 29-1. ***Renal Injury Scale***[a]

Grade[b]		Injury description[c]	AIS 90[d]
I	Contusion	Microscopic or gross hematuria; urologic studies normal	2
	Hematoma	Subcapsular, nonexpanding without parenchymal laceration	2
II	Hematoma	Nonexpanding perirenal hematoma confined to renal retroperitoneum	2
	Laceration	<1.0 cm parenchymal depth of renal cortex without urinary extravasation	2
III	Laceration	>1.0 cm parenchymal depth of renal cortex with collecting system rupture or urinary extravasation	3
IV	Laceration	Parenchymal laceration extending through the renal cortex medulla, and collecting system	4
	Vascular	Main renal artery or vein with contained hemorrhage	4
V	Laceration	Completely shattered kidney	5
	Vascular	Avulsion of renal hilum, which devascularizes kidney	5

[a]This classification scheme for acute renal injury has been devised by the Organ Injury Scaling Committee of the American Association for the Surgery of Trauma.
[b]Advance one grade for multiple injuries to the same organ.
[c]Based on most accurate assessment at autopsy, laparotomy, or radiologic study.
[d]AIS 90, 1990 version of the Abbreviated Injury Score.

Diagnosis

AXIOM The keystone to the diagnosis of renal injuries is a high index of suspicion based on the type of trauma and its location.

Signs and Symptoms

With blunt abdominal, pelvic, or lower thoracic trauma, the presence of flank or abdominal pain should make the physician suspicious of a genitourinary (GU) tract injury. The pain of serious renal injury is often described as a "dull ache." The associated retroperitoneal bleeding may also cause nausea, vomiting, and paralytic ileus.

Physical Examination

Flank or upper abdominal tenderness is a frequent finding after renal injury, and in some patients, a flank mass may be palpable. An expanding mass indicates that the injury is severe enough to cause continuing extravasation of blood or urine or both into perirenal tissues.

Occasionally, a bruit heard in the posterior midline near the first or second lumbar vertebrae may be the only indication of damage to renal vessels (2). With penetrating injuries in the flank, a bruit suggests the presence of a renal arterial injury.

Laboratory Evaluation

Urinalysis

Because the insertion of a urethral catheter can cause hematuria, the urine to be examined should, whenever possible, be a midstream specimen collected without catheterization; however, seriously injured patients often cannot urinate within the first 15 to 30 minutes. Consequently, a Foley catheter should be promptly inserted in patients with severe blood loss so that the urine output can be monitored properly. In menstruating women, a catheterized specimen is generally much more accurate than a spontaneously voided specimen.

AXIOM Although hematuria (more than 50 red blood cells/high-power field) suggests the presence of a urologic injury, the absence of hematuria is of little diagnostic value.

Hematuria is present in 90% of renal injuries; however, up to 30% of major renal injuries may have a normal urinalysis (3), and up to one third have only microscopic hematuria. Conversely, Krieger et al. (4) found that 40% of patients with gross hematuria had only contusions or simple lacerations of the kidney.

AXIOM With renal dysfunction, creatinine clearance (Cl_{Cr}) tends to decrease long before there is any increase in the blood urea nitrogen (BUN) or serum creatinine.

An increasing BUN or serum creatinine generally indicates impaired renal function after trauma; however, these changes are not often apparent for at least 24 to 48 hours. Furthermore, the BUN may increase without renal disease or damage. Blood in the intestinal tract, for example, may increase the BUN up to 50 mg/dL, even with normal renal function. The serum creatinine varies far less, but normal values can vary widely depending on age, muscle mass, and activity.

AXIOM In elderly individuals with minimal muscle mass and activity, a serum creatinine exceeding 0.6 to 0.8 mg/dL often indicates significant renal impairment.

Radiologic Evaluation

AXIOM The patients who are usually in most need of complete radiologic evaluation of the GU tract are often those who can least tolerate it because of multiple other injuries.

So-called kidney–ureter–bladder (KUB) plain films may provide important information concerning the retroperitoneum and associated skeletal structures. The films should be examined for fractures of the lower ribs, lumbar spine (especially L1–3 transverse processes) and pelvis, which may suggest possible adjacent urinary tract injury.

A soft-tissue mass, loss of the psoas shadow (especially upper third), and scoliosis suggest the presence of blood, urine, or pus in the retroperitoneum (5). Displacement or abnormal size of the kidneys may indicate trauma or a preexisting abnormality or disease process. Hessel and Smith (5) found that only 30% of patients with renal injuries had plain film findings that correlated well with the type and extent of renal damage present.

With penetrating wounds, particularly those caused by bullets, radiopaque markers should be placed over the entrance and exit wounds; however, one should not assume that the path of the bullet will be in a straight line between the entrance and exit wounds.

Intravenous Urography

Patients with severe GU injuries are often hemodynamically unstable and in need of immediate resuscitation or operation or both. In such cases, there may be no time for a detailed radiologic GU evaluation. Nevertheless, it is important to assess the integrity of the urinary tract before major renal surgical intervention. Although not optimal, a "one-shot intravenous pyelogram (IVP)" can be performed in the resuscitation suite or on the operating table to evaluate the presence and function of the contralateral kidney before removal of a severely damaged kidney.

The accuracy of an IVP is highly dependent on the use of sufficiently high doses of contrast and optimal technique. The recommended technique for the so-called one-shot IVP calls for bolus administration of 60% urographic contrast in a dose of 1 mL/lb (up to 150 mL), and a single abdominal film taken 3 to 5 minutes after injection. If at all possible, a flat plate of the abdomen should be obtained before the IVP. Thus any changes in the radiograph after the intravenous contrast is given can be assumed to be the result of excreted contrast material. An extra 50 mL of 60% contrast should be given to get better renal visualization if

1. A great deal of intravenous fluid has been given,
2. Renal function is probably good, and the
3. Urine output is more than 1.0 mL/kg/h.

In an evaluation of 239 one-shot IVPs done because evaluation in the radiology suite was thought to be unsafe, it was found that 8% of the patients with a normal one-shot IVP had renal injuries (i.e., were falsely negative), and 26% with an abnormal one-shot IVP had no intraoperative evidence of renal injury (i.e., were falsely positive) (6).

AXIOM Delaying definitive therapy to obtain a preoperative one-shot IVP in an unstable patient is generally not warranted.

In "allergic-type" patients (asthma, food allergies, etc.) who have no known iodine sensitivity, a low-osmolality, nonionic agent (e.g., iohexol) is recommended. If there is history of a previous allergic reaction (urticaria, edema, etc.) to iodinated contrast or iodine-containing foods (e.g., shellfish), noncontrast computed tomography (CT), ultrasound (US), or radionuclide imaging may be reasonable substitutes. If nothing but iodinated contrast will do, steroid pretreatment should be instituted.

AXIOM If an IVP or CT scan indicates that an injury to a ureter or the collecting system may be present, cystoscopy with insertion of catheters into the ureters and retrograde urography should be considered.

Computed Tomography

It is now widely accepted that CT provides significantly more detailed and reliable information about renal injuries and with less variability in technique and quality than does IVP; however, it may not be possible to obtain a CT scan because the patient is hemodynamically unstable.

If an IVP has been performed, a CT scan of the abdomen should not be performed for at least 3 to 4 hours (7). If a CT scan must be performed before the IVP contrast has cleared, it is done after only a 50-mL intravenous contrast bolus. Whereas more information will be gained with the post-IVP CT than with the IVP, a CT will yield significantly more information if it is done as the primary examination.

AXIOM Injured kidneys tend to retain contrast longer than noninjured kidneys, and contrast may still be visible in some injured kidneys up to 24 hours later.

Renal Arteriography

If no renal function is apparent on urography or CT, arteriography may be indicated. In patients who have sustained other injuries, it may also be possible to embolize bleeding vessels during the angiography, thereby obviating the need for an operation (8). Findings strongly suggesting major vascular injury on CT usually warrant immediate surgical intervention rather than delaying surgery to get an arteriogram.

⊘ PITFALL

The 4 to 6 hours of warm ischemia that a kidney can tolerate can be lost while obtaining various studies, including an arteriogram.

Ultrasound

Acute parenchymal, perinephric, or pelvic hematomas and urinomas may be seen as anechoic collections on US; however, injured parenchyma and hematoma may be isoechoic, making it very difficult to distinguish them from normal parenchyma and perinephric fat (9). Sonography also may identify renal fragments or clots or both in the collecting system or bladder. The presence of the two kidneys and their sizes also may be assessed.

Treatment

Nonsurgical Management

AXIOM Most renal injuries heal well without surgical intervention.

Contusions and mild to moderate lacerations, which make up the majority of renal injuries, usually heal very well without surgical intervention. Goff and Collin (10) recently reemphasized that the nephrectomy rate among patients who undergo laparotomy as part of their initial management of renal injuries was 20% (vs. 3% for those patients initially managed nonoperatively).

AXIOM If the collecting system and renal pedicle are intact and there is no ongoing bleeding, kidneys with penetrating injuries do not require exploration.

Surgical Management

Even if early operative intervention is unnecessary, later renal surgery may be necessary if

1. Uncontrollable sepsis develops;
2. The involved kidney stops functioning; or
3. The patient develops severe hypertension.

If the patient has only one kidney, treatment should be even more conservative, and every effort should be made to salvage the solitary kidney, even if it is severely damaged or bleeding.

Although multiple severe renal lacerations often require nephrectomy, sometimes a severely injured kidney may be treated with a partial nephrectomy. However, this may add 1 to 2 hours to the surgery, and a partial nephrectomy should not be attempted in a critically injured patient with an intact contralateral kidney.

AXIOM If a devascularized kidney is to be saved, its blood supply should be restored within 4 to 6 hours of the injury, and the amount of functional recovery is usually inversely proportional to the duration of normothermic ischemia (11).

The decision as to whether a devascularized kidney can be salvaged depends largely on the appearance of the kidney at the time of exploration and how easily the bleeding is controlled. If the kidney is very dark, it is probably infarcted, and nephrectomy is usually necessary.

Failure to recognize a rupture of the renal pelvis or ureter generally leads to development of a urinoma. This pseudoencapsulated enlarging sac of urine usually develops inferior and medial to the kidney and tends to push the kidney superiorly and laterally. Urinomas are sometimes not identified for several days or weeks after the injury and can become quite large.

If a retrograde pyelogram indicates a leak from the renal pelvis but the ureteropelvic junction (UPJ) is intact, simple drainage of the perirenal space with a Jackson–Pratt or similar catheter is generally the easiest and most effective method of management in acute situations when a laparotomy is required for other injuries. If a laparotomy is not indicated for other injuries or if the diagnosis is made later, cystoscopy with insertion of a ureteral stent should be attempted. Alternatively, percutaneous, image-guided drainage, rather than an operative approach, may be used.

Surgical Exploration of the Kidneys

AXIOM The function of a kidney cannot be evaluated by its size, gross appearance, or by the way it feels on palpation.

Techniques. Exploration of the abdomen for trauma generally should be carried out through a midline abdominal incision. This provides the best exposure to most intraabdominal injuries. If there is little or no bleeding, a Kocher maneuver followed by dissection and retraction of the ascending and right transverse colon to the left can expose the right renal artery between the vena cava and the aorta; however, one must be careful not to disturb the perirenal hematoma until the renal vessels have been controlled.

⊘ PITFALL

Failure to control the renal vessels before opening a perirenal hematoma can result in severe bleeding and an unnecessary nephrectomy.

If there is ongoing bleeding from the kidney, it is usually safer to get control of the renal arteries by incising the peritoneum over the aorta at the base of the transverse mesocolon and then dissecting upward along the aorta until the renal arteries are found (12). The right renal artery usually can be found going posterior to the inferior vena cava. The inferior vena cava above and below the renal veins can usually be controlled with local pressure until the renal veins are found.

The left renal artery can usually be found by entering the lesser sac and incising the posterior peritoneum over the aorta. If the bleeding is too great to be controlled by any of these techniques, occlusion of the aorta at the diaphragm should be considered. If this still does not adequately control the bleeding, a left thoracotomy and clamping of the descending thoracic aorta just above the diaphragm should be considered.

After the renal vessels are controlled, the hematoma can be opened and evacuated and the kidney carefully inspected. If the kidney appears to be salvageable, one can repair the renal vein(s) and then the artery. Renal artery injuries, however, can be very difficult to manage. They are often deeply embedded in the retroperitoneum and are closely surrounded by dense lymphatics, neural fibers, and connective tissue. Nevertheless, repairs of the main renal artery can usually be accomplished by lateral arteriorrhaphy or mobilization of the kidney with primary anastomosis.

AXIOM Complex renal artery injuries requiring more than 30 minutes of vascular clamping require protection of the kidney from warm ischemia.

Protection from warm ischemia may include packing in saline slush with or without perfusion or the renal vessels with ice-cold irrigant. Kidney excision with benchtop repair and then transposition to a pelvic location has also been used to reduce the ischemic damage. Nevertheless, nephrectomy may be required for severe renal arterial injuries, especially in patients with multiple injuries and severe continuing blood loss.

After all dead or macerated tissue has been debrided, injuries in the collecting system are repaired with continuous slowly absorbable sutures. The remaining portions of the kidney are then carefully closed to control hemorrhage and decrease the risk of leakage of urine. Horizontal mattress sutures tied over Teflon pledgets reduce the chance of sutures tearing the capsule and can be very useful for this purpose. Perirenal fat or omentum also can be used for pledgets.

Delayed Recognition of Renal Artery Occlusion

Controversy exists regarding the role of renal revascularization after delayed recognition of thrombosis of the renal artery from contusion or intimal flap disruption (11). The interval from occlusion to repair appears to be a critical factor. In one review of the problem, there was an 80% chance of restoring some renal function if the kidney was revascularized before 12 hours. This decreased to 57% if the kidney was not revascularized before 18 hours. The low salvage rate and the 37% chance of delayed nephrectomy for postrevascularization complications, such as hypertension, have caused many surgeons to try to save the kidney surgically only if less than 12 hours have elapsed since injury (13); however, Chambers et al. (3) noted that even a delay of only 3 hours in revascularization is often associated with severe tubular necrosis.

AXIOM An ischemic kidney should be revascularized within 3 to 6 hours if at all possible.

There are now five separate case reports in the literature that document spontaneous revascularization or recovery of one or both kidneys after presumed blunt thrombotic occlusion of the renal artery (14). These authors suggested that attempts at late revascularization may occasionally be rewarding, and they advised that early nephrectomy is unnecessary because of the low incidence of chronic hypertension.

AXIOM If renal artery occlusion cannot be relieved within 6 to 12 hours, an immediate nephrectomy is not necessary because occasional spontaneous revascularization can occur.

Postoperative Management

After any surgery on the kidney for trauma, the perirenal space should be drained adequately, preferably with closed (Jackson–Pratt) drains brought out through a stab wound in the flank. These drains should be left in place for at least 5 to 7 days. If urine leakage persists beyond 5 to 7 days, an IVP or CT should be obtained to rule out obstruction of the collecting system or ureter.

When the gross hematuria has resolved, the patient can get out of bed (7). Hourly urine output and daily serum creatinine levels should be monitored until the viability of the injured kidney is assured.

Postoperative Complications

Some of the complications that may develop in the first few days after renal injury include recurrent hemorrhage, urinary fistulas or urinomas, infection, and nonfunction. Some of the delayed problems occurring weeks, months, or even years later include hydronephrosis, renal calculi, and renovascular hypertension.

Follow-up

Follow-up examinations after serious renal injuries should include BUN, serum creatinine, urinalysis, and blood pressure. For severely damaged kidneys, an imaging procedure every 3 to 6 months for at least 2 years may be helpful (5). Although late postoperative hypertension due to renal artery stenosis or partial renal infarction occurs in fewer than 5% of patients with renal injuries, it can have important consequences (3).

AXIOM Hypertension due to an injured kidney may not develop until 1 to 2 years after the initial trauma.

URETER INJURIES

Ureteral injuries due to accidental trauma are usually the result of gunshots or stabs (3). Blunt abdominal trauma rarely involves the ureter and, when it does, there is usually disruption at the ureteropelvic junction.

Gunshot wounds can cause contusions of a ureter, and the blast effect can severely damage the intima of small blood vessels in the ureteral wall. Blunt injuries of the ureter usually take the form of rupture or avulsion of the UPJ or of a tear of the renal pelvis. They are most likely to be caused by hyperextension injuries.

AXIOM Injuries of the UPJ are the most frequent ureteral injuries found in children.

Diagnosis

Signs and Symptoms

The first evidence of a urinary tract injury is often leakage of urine from the incision. Postoperatively, an IVP may show that extravasation from a torn ureter, and cystoscopy with retrograde pyelography can identify the site of leakage more clearly.

A ureter lacerated or severed by external trauma may produce a mass, abdominal distention, vomiting, paralytic ileus, and cellulitis (3). In contrast, a contusion often will show no immediate signs except some hematuria. Microscopic hematuria is present in 90% of patients with ureteric trauma. If the ureter is completely severed and the blood and urine are draining into the retroperitoneum, hematuria is usually absent (15).

⊘ PITFALL

Failure to adequately explore the ureters if they are not seen clearly on IVP or CT scan when there is a penetrating wound near them.

Treatment

Surgical Management

Techniques

When dissecting out a ureter, one should disturb its blood supply as little as possible. The ureter obtains its blood supply from the renal artery and from segmental vessels from the aorta, common iliac, and hypogastric vessels. The segmental vessels can be sacrificed as long as the longitudinal vessels running in and along the adventitia coming from either the lower or upper ureter are intact. If more than 1 to 2 cm of the adventitia is disturbed during the dissection or trauma, a segment of the ureter may necrose and form a ureteral fistula.

With injuries involving the upper two thirds of the injured ureter, the ends of the ureter should be debrided as needed, spatulated for about 1 cm, and then sutured end-to-end. The ureteral repair is usually performed with two running 5-0 absorbable sutures. It is important to try to obtain a watertight anastomosis. It is particularly important that no tension be allowed on the suture line because this almost invariably leads to a breakdown of the anastomosis (15; Fig. 29-1).

Repairs can be difficult when the ureter is injured in its lower third. If the ureter is damaged just above or near the bladder, it usually best to reimplant it in the anterolateral bladder, preferably by using a submucosal antireflux type of insertion. If the ureter is injured somewhat higher, near the pelvic rim, it may be necessary to use a pedicled flap of bladder known as a Boari or Ockerblad flap; however, it may be possible to obviate the need for a bladder flap by mobilizing the bladder and fixing it to the psoas muscles and the pelvic rim (3). The ureter can then be reimplanted into the mobilized bladder. This operation is known as a psoas-hitch type of ureteral reimplantation.

Autotransplantation of the kidney to the iliac fossa (3) or a transureteroureterostomy (suturing the lacerated end of the proximal ureter into the side of the uninjured ureter) also may be considered in selected instances when the lower ureter is severely injured and no other treatment seems adequate. Cutaneous ureterostomy may be used as a last resort if it is impossible to provide ureterobladder continuity, and especially if the functional status of the other kidney is in question. If it is certain that the contralateral kidney and urinary tract are normal, removal of the kidney and the injured ureter is generally preferred to a cutaneous ureterostomy.

Whenever possible, a ureteral stent should be used with all ureteral injuries (15). The stent should be small enough so that it will not cause pressure on the ureter walls, and it should extend from the renal pelvis down into the bladder, where it can later be retrieved by cystoscopy.

AXIOM With all ureteral injuries, a drain should be left in the periureteral area and brought out through a stab wound in the flank to remove any urine or blood that may leak into that area (15).

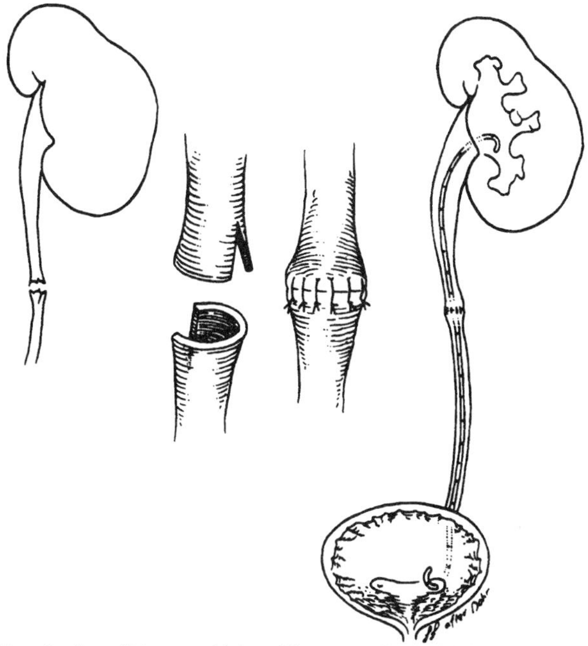

FIG. 29-1. Repair of a mild ureteral injury. The upper and middle thirds of the ureter are best repaired with a primary ureteroureterostomy. The injured ends of the ureter should be adequately debrided and should be dissected proximally and distally to make the anastomosis tension free. The ends of the ureter are spatulated to prevent stenosis at the site of the repair, which is performed with fine interrupted absorbable sutures. A silicone stent of the double-J type can be passed via a guidewire from the site of the repair proximal to the renal pelvis and distal to the bladder. From ref. 25, with permission.

Delayed Recognition of Ureteral Injuries

Most ureteral injuries that are missed initially are picked up on a later IVP or CT scan with intravenous contrast. Ureterectasis, pyelectasis, a dense nephrogram, or delayed or absent opacification of the collecting system usually indicates obstruction, whereas a mass effect suggests leakage.

Although CT scanning is probably unnecessary in most cases, it can often precisely locate a urine collection and suggest its cause. Retrograde pyelography will usually reveal the exact site of injury. If a complete obstruction or a complete tear of the ureter is found, a percutaneous nephrostomy tube can be inserted to drain the kidney while a definitive treatment approach is being selected.

BLADDER INJURIES

Bladder injuries are often associated with fractures of the pelvis. Predisposing factors include bladder distention, fixation by tumor or scar, and obstruction.

Bladder injuries can be classified as ruptures or contusions (3). About 50% to 80% of bladder ruptures are extraperitoneal, and approximately 10% of patients with bladder ruptures have both types. Intraperitoneal ruptures usually occur on the posterior superior wall as a result of blunt trauma to a full bladder. Extraperitoneal ruptures are usually on the anterior or anterolateral bladder wall near the bladder neck and are almost always associated with pelvic fractures. It has been estimated that about 5% of patients with pelvic fractures have an extraperitoneal rupture of the bladder. Intraperitoneal rupture of the bladder leads to peritonitis, which is worse if the urine is infected (7). Extraperitoneal extravasation of infected urine can lead to spreading pelvic cellulitis and sepsis.

The adult bladder is a pelvic organ (16), whereas in the infant and young child, the bladder is primarily intraabdominal. Consequently, children are more susceptible to blunt bladder injury than are adults.

Diagnosis

Signs and Symptoms

AXIOM The classic triad of bladder injury includes lower abdominal pain, gross hematuria, and inability to void. If the bladder rupture is intraperitoneal, the patient also may have signs and symptoms of peritonitis.

Bladder injuries should be suspected with any trauma to the lower abdomen or pelvis, especially if there is a fracture of the pubic rami or separation of the pubic symphysis. If a bladder injury is suspected, careful rectal and vaginal examination should be done in search of an enlarging pelvic mass or an injury extending into the vagina or rectum.

Diagnostic Tests

Cystogram

Retrograde cystograms are obtained by emptying the bladder with a catheter and then filling it by gravity with at least 300 to 400 mL of a standard cystographic contrast medium. Full bladder distention with contrast is imperative to avoid false-negative studies (7). Filling should be performed under fluoroscopic control to avoid filling the entire peritoneal cavity with contrast through a tear.

The cystogram should include films taken in the anteroposterior, lateral, and both posterior oblique projections, before and after contrast enters the bladder. This is followed by postdrainage films of the pelvis, occasionally after the bladder is "rinsed" with saline (7).

AXIOM The "post-evac" film may be the only film to demonstrate a small amount of extravasation, particularly posteriorly, and should not be omitted.

Intraperitoneal rupture is characterized radiologically by failure of the bladder to fill on cystography and the appearance of contrast material between loops of intestine above the bladder. The typical cystography findings in extraperitoneal rupture are a flame-like extravasation of contrast outside the bladder and a teardrop appearance of the bladder because of compression by hematoma.

AXIOM In about one third of the patients with a bladder injury, there is no extravasation on the cystogram because the hole is tamponaded by blood clot; even tears 2 to 4 cm long may be sealed by hematoma.

Patients with pelvic fractures should be watched carefully for delayed extravasation from a missed bladder injury after the Foley catheter has been removed.

Surgical Exploration

If there is a high index of suspicion of bladder injury and the patient is unable to void, suprapubic catheterization should be done. A simultaneous cystogram and direct examination can be performed, but extraperitoneal injuries may be impossible to see without opening the bladder.

Treatment

Surgical Management

Techniques

Foley catheter drainage may be the treatment of choice for an intraperitoneal bladder injury if there is minimal extravasation, no infection or disruption of visceral structures, and no other abdominal injury (16); however, most patients with intraperitoneal injuries to the bladder should undergo exploration. After the entire bladder is inspected, the mucosa and muscle in the laceration are closed. This is done with a running 4-0 or 5-0 absorbable suture, followed by a second or even a third layer closing the muscle and serosa. Postoperatively, the bladder and the perivesical space are drained until it has been shown that the bladder has healed.

AXIOM Most extraperitoneal bladder injuries can be treated with simple catheter drainage of the bladder.

About 80% of extraperitoneal bladder injuries seal quite readily with only Foley or suprapubic catheter drainage (16). Extraperitoneal injuries that are extremely large or associated with bony fragments will generally not seal without surgical closure.

If surgery is performed, these injuries are best repaired from within the bladder. The bladder is entered anteriorly through a midline incision, and the area of rupture located. The muscularis is closed with either an interrupted or a running 4-0 absorbable suture. The mucosa is then closed with a running 5-0 absorbable suture. The midline surgical incision in the bladder is then closed in three layers.

If a penetrating wound of the urinary bladder is near a ureteral orifice, cystoscopy and a retrograde urethrogram can be performed on the table. If a ureterogram is not possible at that time, passage of a ureteral stent through the area of ureter in question may facilitate healing (16).

AXIOM Adequate drainage of a mildly-to-moderately injured bladder is best done with a urethral Foley catheter; however, with severe trauma in a male patient, prolonged bladder drainage should be done with a suprapubic cystostomy tube.

Postoperative Management

Once it is clear, postoperatively, that the cystostomy tube drains the bladder adequately, the Foley catheter can be removed. The cystostomy tube should be left in place for at least 8 to 10 days and then clamped if there is no evidence of a urine leak. If there are no complications after it has been clamped for 24 hours and the patient can empty his bladder well, the cystostomy tube can be removed. If there is any question about bladder integrity, a cystogram should be performed before removal of the cystostomy tube.

URETHRAL INJURIES

Types of Injuries

The male urethra is divided anatomically by the urogenital diaphragm into three parts (Fig. 29-2).

1. Prostatic urethra between the bladder and the superior leaf of the urogenital diaphragm;
2. Membranous urethra, which traverses the urogenital diaphragm; and
3. Anterior urethra distal to the inferior leaf of the urogenital diaphragm.

The anterior urethra may be further subdivided into the bulbous (perineal) urethra (extending to the penoscrotal junction) and the distal penile (pendulous) urethra.

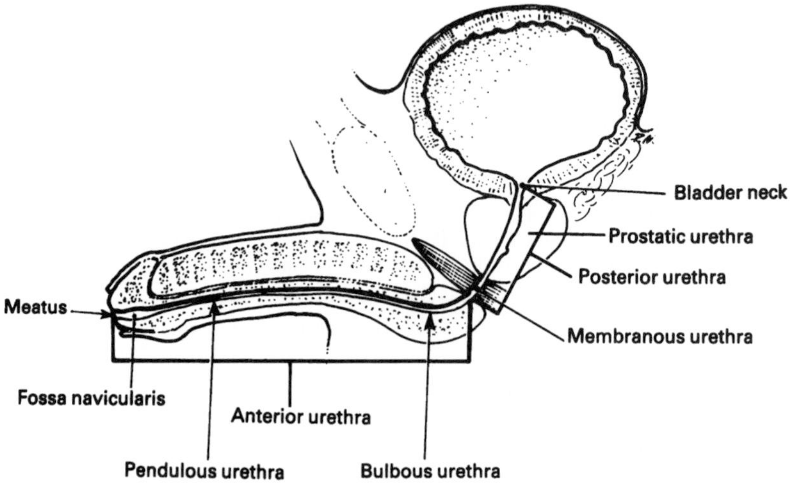

FIG. 29-2. Urethral anatomy. The urethra can be divided into the anterior and posterior urethra. The anterior urethra extends from the inferior edge of the urogenital diaphragm to the external urethral meatus. The posterior portion of the urethra extends from the bladder neck to the inferior edge of the urogenital diaphragm. From ref. 21, with permission.

Urethral injuries are extremely rare in female subjects. Serious urethral injuries in the male patient from blunt trauma are most often associated with pelvic fractures, especially anterior pubic arch fractures with displacement. The incidence of urethral and bladder injury accompanying pelvic fractures ranges from 0.7% to 25% (7,17). In approximately half of these lower urinary tract injuries, only the urethra is injured. In female patients, pelvic fractures are seldom associated with urethral injuries unless vaginal lacerations also are present.

Injuries of the male urethra affect the membranous (posterior) portion three times as often as the bulbous and penile (anterior) portion (18). Severe blunt trauma to the lower abdomen and pelvis, causing fractures of the pubic rami, characteristically tears the prostatic urethra just above the superior leaf of the urogenital diaphragm. Rarely, the tears extend into the membranous urethra.

With tears of the prostatic urethra, blood or urine extravasates into the periprostatic and perivesical spaces and, if the urogenital diaphragm is badly damaged, also into the perineum. Continued extravasation of urine can lead to cellulitis and sepsis, and urethral stricture is a common long-term problem. Urinary incontinence also may occur if the sphincter is injured. Approximately one third of the patients will also have impotence (16).

AXIOM With straddle injuries, the bulbous urethra, just below the urogenital diaphragm, is crushed against the ischial rami and may rupture.

Diagnosis

AXIOM If there is a suspicion of a urethral injury, a urethral catheter should not be passed until a retrograde urethrogram has excluded a tear.

Signs and Symptoms

The symptoms of urethral injury are pain in the perineum and lower abdomen and inability to void. Attempts to micturate are painful and can cause increased perineal or penile swelling.

Frequent signs include urethral bleeding and gross hematuria (7). A tender suprapubic mass may represent a distended bladder or extravasated blood and urine. If Buck's fascia around the corpora of the penis remains intact, only discoloration and edema of the penis will be seen. If Buck's fascia is disrupted, the extravasation of urine and blood can be extensive and is contained only by Colles' fascia, which extends posteriorly around the anterior half of the anus and a short distance laterally to the fascia lata of the thighs. Anteriorly, the blood can spread up over the entire abdomen and chest.

On rectal examination of the patient who has had a separation of the prostatic urethra from the membranous urethra, the prostate may be felt to be riding higher than usual or one may feel only a large boggy mass of extravasated fluid.

AXIOM A periprostatic and perivesical hematoma may make the prostate feel as though it is higher than normal even when no separation is actually present.

Diagnostic Tests

If there has been a partial urethral laceration with an incomplete separation and a Foley catheter is passed into the bladder, the injury may be completely missed, with the catheter being removed before urethral healing is adequate. The catheter also may enter the tear and be advanced submucosally, turning a small, unobstructing tear into a large, obstructing injury.

AXIOM If a Foley catheter is inserted into a patient with severe pelvic or perineal trauma before a urethrogram is performed, it is wise to obtain a urethrogram alongside the Foley catheter before it is removed.

A retrograde urethrogram is obtained by gentle injection of 10 to 25 mL of sterile 30% iodinated contrast material into the urethra with a bulb syringe or soft catheter. If a Foley catheter is already in place, it should not be removed because it may be difficult or impossible to reinsert. A small catheter can be placed alongside it, at the urethral meatus, to obtain the urethrogram. The patient should be placed in a posterior oblique position and gentle traction applied to the penis. The contrast instillation and filming is performed under direct fluoroscopic guidance. If an injury is found, special efforts should be made to determine whether the extravasation is below or above the urogenital diaphragm.

Treatment

Nonsurgical Management

In most patients with multiple trauma and a complete urethral rupture, other injuries take precedence, and the urologist's efforts may be confined to inserting a suprapubic cystostomy tube. Treatment of the urethral injury may have to be delayed until the orthopedic surgeons have reduced the pelvic fractures, which may bring the severed ends of the urethra closer together.

Opinion is divided on whether urethral continuity should then be restored by open end-to-end anastomosis or use of interlocking sounds or catheters passed through the urethra and the bladder neck simultaneously or whether suprapubic drainage with later urethroplasty is optimal (16). Delayed urethroplasty has become more appealing with the demonstration that urethral continuity can often be reestablished by a combination of transurethral and endoscopic means without open operation.

Partial ruptures of the posterior urethra are managed by a combination of suprapubic cystostomy and perivesical drainage or by urethral catheter drainage (5). Only an experienced urologist should attempt to pass a urethral catheter in these patients, as there is considerable risk of converting a partial rupture into a complete one.

AXIOM If a transection of the urethra is incomplete, it is important not to increase the extent of the injury by attempting to pass a Foley catheter.

If a rupture of the anterior urethra is incomplete, and if it is confined by the fascial covering of the corpus spongiosum so that there is no extravasation of blood and urine into the perineum, treatment may involve only splinting of the urethra with a urethral catheter for 5 to 7 days. If a urethral catheter cannot be passed, a suprapubic cystostomy with a 30F Pezzar catheter should be performed.

If a Foley catheter is left in place, its management is extremely important. The catheter should be taped onto the anterior abdominal wall or medial thigh and cleansed frequently at the point where it enters the urethra. This cleansing is extremely important because one of the complications of urethral catheter drainage is purulent urethritis, which can cause urethral stricture. Mechanical cleansing of the catheter with soap and water or povidone–iodine (Betadine) solution 5 or 6 times per day is very effective. The bladder-drainage system should be kept completely closed to reduce the chance of contamination.

Surgical Management

Complete ruptures of the anterior urethra are repaired by end-to-end anastomosis with evacuation of the hematoma, suprapubic cystostomy drainage, and adequate antibiotic coverage. If there is evidence of extravasation into the perineum or anterior abdominal wall or both, it also may be necessary to open and drain the involved areas for at least 5 to 7 days.

If the urethral injury is extensive and more than 2 cm of urethra has been destroyed, the distal and proximal ends as well as other areas involved are sutured to the penile skin with 4/0 polyglycolic acid sutures (19).

Strictures

For most types of urethral injury, the resulting strictures can often be corrected by cold-knife urethrotomy. If the stricture is less than 2 cm long, this technique is successful in more than 90% of patients, obviating the need for repeated urethral dilatations.

PENIS INJURIES

Blunt injuries to the penis are usually caused by direct trauma and are generally diagnosed quite readily. Some injuries occur because excessive stress has been placed on the penis while it is in the erect state (20). The patient will often report a loud cracking sound and immediate pain and detumescence.

Associated Injuries

Urethral injury is present in approximately 20% of penile injuries and is usually evidenced by a small amount of bloody urethral discharge (21). Urethrography is indicated with all major penile injuries, and operative repair should be undertaken. The most common severe injury is penile fracture (rupture of the corpora cavernosa), frequently with an associated rupture of the suspensory ligaments.

Treatment

Immediate surgical evacuation of the hematoma and primary repair of the torn structures appears to produce better long-term results than conservative management. Penetrating penile injuries from gunshots or stab wounds require urethrography and operative exploration.

Cline et al. (22) found that 38% of tested individuals with penetrating trauma to the male external genitalia were positive for hepatitis B, C, or both; although the high prevalence of hepatitis B and C in this group emphasizes the importance of universal precautions in these patients. Debridement should be minimal because of the excellent blood supply of the penile tissues. Injuries to the glans penis are carefully reconstructed, and bullet openings are simply managed by approximation of the wound edges.

Traumatic amputation of the penis is best treated by reattachment if the distal segment is in good condition, if the ischemia time is less than 12 to 18 hours, and if expertise in microvascular repair is available (3,7); however, the results with replantation are usually less than optimal. As a result, some urologists favor repairing the remaining tissues and suturing the urethral mucosa to the skin to form a neourethrostomy.

TESTES INJURIES

Testicular rupture usually results from severe blunt scrotal trauma. The actual mechanism is usually a direct blow with impingement of the testis against the symphysis pubis. Patients with testicular injuries usually have a large scrotal hematoma on the injured side and severe pain as a result of the swelling and intracapsular testicular edema. The surrounding hematoma often prevents palpation of the testicle, but real-time ultrasonography can be extremely reliable in detecting testicular rupture (23); however, if there is a large scrotal hematoma, significant testicular ruptures can be missed by US, CT, and physical examination.

AXIOM All large traumatic scrotal hematomas should be explored.

Treatment

If the tunica albuginea of the testis is not ruptured, the initial treatment should include bed rest, scrotal support, analgesics, and cold applications for 24 to 48 hours. If the tunica vaginalis sac is filled with blood (hematocele) resulting in a large, swollen, tender, blue scrotal mass, the testicle should be explored, the hematoma evacuated, the area debrided, and the tunica albuginea reapproximated with sutures (7).

Postoperatively, if the testicle maintains its normal size, it has probably maintained its viability (24). Hormonal and spermatogenic function is difficult to assess if the contralateral testicle is normal. Orchidectomy is seldom necessary if diagnosis and reconstruction are prompt.

SCROTAL AVULSION

If at all possible after scrotal avulsion, the remaining scrotal skin should be reconstructed around the testes, even if the closure is under considerable tension (7). The scrotal skin can grow rapidly, and the scrotum usually regenerates to nearly its normal size within a few months. If scrotal reconstruction is impossible, the testicles should be placed in thigh pockets superficial to the subcutaneous fat, where the temperature is similar to that inside the scrotum.

⊘ FREQUENT ERRORS

1. ***Neglect of the patient's general condition and other injuries while investigating the urinary tract.***
2. ***Failure to give a hemodynamically stable patient an opportunity to void spontaneously before a Foley catheter is inserted.***
3. ***Failure to obtain an early IVP or CT scan in patients who might have renal injury. (If the patient is hemodynamically stable, a CT scan is preferred).***
4. ***Failure to obtain a CT scan or an arteriogram promptly if a kidney is not visualized on IVP.***
5. ***Assuming that the uninjured kidney is normal because it looks and feels normal.***
6. ***Failure to obtain control of the renal vessels before opening a perirenal hematoma.***

7. ***Excessive mobilization of the ureter while examining or repairing it.***
8. ***Vigorous attempts to pass a Foley catheter in a patient who may have a urethral or bladder injury.***

SUMMARY POINTS

1. Abnormal kidneys, such as those with congenital anomalies, tumors, or hydronephrosis are much more susceptible to injury than are normal kidneys.
2. Although hematuria (more than 50 RBC/HPF) suggests the presence of a urologic injury, the absence of hematuria is of much less diagnostic value.
3. With renal dysfunction, urine creatinine and creatinine clearance (Cl_{Cr}) tend to decrease before there is any increase in the BUN or serum creatinine.
4. In elderly individuals with minimal muscle mass and activity, a serum creatinine exceeding 0.6 to 0.8 mg/dL often indicates significant renal impairment.
5. The patients who are usually most in need of complete radiologic evaluation of the GU tract are often those who can least tolerate it because of multiple other injuries.
6. Excretory urography is seldom needed in blunt trauma victims if they have no associated major intraabdominal injuries, no microscopic hematuria, and no hypotension.
7. Delaying definitive therapy to obtain a preoperative one-shot IVP in an unstable patient is probably not warranted.
8. If an IVP or CT scan indicates that an injury to a ureter or the collecting system may be present, cystoscopy with insertion of catheters into the ureters and retrograde urography should be considered.
9. An abdominal CT scan with intravenous contrast is the most accurate technique for visualizing a kidney that may be injured.
10. Injured kidneys tend to retain contrast longer than the noninjured kidneys, and contrast may still be visible in some injured kidneys up to 24 hours later.
11. Most renal injuries heal well without surgical intervention.
12. If the collecting system and renal pedicle are intact and there is no ongoing bleeding, kidneys with penetrating injuries do not need to be explored.
13. If a devascularized kidney is to be saved, its blood supply should be restored within 3 to 6 hours of the injury, and the amount of functional recovery is usually inversely proportional to the duration of normothermic ischemia.
14. The function of a kidney cannot be evaluated by its size or appearance or by the way it feels on palpation.
15. Complex renal artery injuries requiring more than 30 minutes of vascular clamping require protection of the kidney from warm ischemia.
16. Before a nephrectomy is performed, it is important to know that there is a functioning contralateral kidney. Evidence that the contralateral kidney is functional includes visualization on IVP or CT or continued good urine output after the pedicle of the injured kidney is occluded.
17. If the patient has a contralateral functioning kidney, a partial nephrectomy should be considered only if the patient is hemodynamically stable and will not be jeopardized by 1 to 2 hours of additional surgery.
18. If renal artery occlusion cannot be relieved within 6 to 12 hours, an immediate nephrectomy is not necessary because occasional spontaneous revascularization can occur.
19. Hypertension due to an injured kidney may not develop until 1 to 2 years after the initial trauma.
20. Injuries of the ureteropelvic junction are the most frequent type of ureteral injury in children.
21. Ureteral stents greatly improve the chances for a ureteral repair to heal without complications.

22. With all ureteral injuries, a drain should be left in the periureteral area and brought out through a stab wound in the flank to remove any urine or blood that may leak into that area.
23. The bladder is much more easily ruptured when it is full.
24. The classic triad of bladder injury includes lower abdominal pain, gross hematuria, and inability to void. If the bladder rupture is intraperitoneal, the patient also may have signs and symptoms of peritonitis.
25. The "post-evac" cystogram film is the view most likely to show bladder injuries.
26. In about one third of the patients with a mild to moderate bladder injury, there is no extravasation on the cystogram because the hole is tamponaded by blood clot; even tears that are 2 to 4 cm long may be sealed by hematoma.
27. Most extraperitoneal bladder injuries can be treated by simple catheter drainage of the bladder.
28. Adequate drainage of a mildly-to-moderately injured bladder is best done with a urethral Foley catheter; however, with severe bladder trauma in a male patient, one should drain the bladder with a suprapubic cystostomy.
29. If there is a suspicion of a urethral injury, a urethral catheter should not be passed until a retrograde urethrogram has excluded a tear.
30. A periprostatic and perivesical hematoma may make the prostate feel as though it is higher than normal even when no separation is actually present.
31. If a Foley catheter is inserted into a patient with severe pelvic or perineal trauma before a urethrogram is performed, it is wise to obtain a urethrogram alongside the Foley catheter before it is removed.
32. If a transection of the urethra is incomplete, it is important not to increase the extent of the injury by attempting to pass a Foley catheter.
33. All large trauma scrotal hematomas should be explored.

REFERENCES

1. Wilson RF, Smith JB, McCarroll KA. Trauma to the urinary tract. In: Wilson RF, Walt AJ, eds. *Management of trauma: pitfalls and practice.* 2nd ed. Philadelphia: Williams & Wilkins, 1996:600.
2. Peterson NE. Genitourinary trauma. In: Feliciano DV, Moore EE, Mattox KL, eds. *Trauma.* 3rd ed. Stamford, CT: Appleton & Lange, 1996:661–664.
3. Chambers RJ Jr, Champion HR, Edson M. Ureteric and renal trauma. In: Champion HR, Robbs JV, Trunkey DV, eds. *Rob and Smith's operative surgery: trauma surgery.* 4th ed. Boston: Butterworth, 1989:466–475.
4. Kreiger JN, Algood CB, Mason JT, et al. Urological trauma in the Pacific Northwest: etiology, distribution, management and outcome. *J Urol* 1984;132:70.
5. Hessel SJ, Smith EH. Renal trauma: a comprehensive review and radiologic assessment. *CRC Crit Rev Clin Radiol Nucl Med* 1974;5:251.
6. Stevenson J, Battistella FD. The one-shot intravenous pyelogram: is it indicated in unstable trauma patients before celiotomy? *J Trauma* 1994;36:828.
7. Cass AS. Genitourinary trauma. In: Kreis DJ, Gomez GA, eds. *Trauma management.* Boston: Little, Brown, 1989:265–280.
8. Reilly KJ, Shapiro MB, Haskal ZJ. Angiographic embolization of a penetrating traumatic renal arteriovenous fistula. *J Trauma* 1996;41:763.
9. Furtschegger A, Egender G, Jaske G. The value of sonography in the diagnosis and follow-up of patients with blunt renal trauma. *Br J Urol* 1988;62:110.
10. Goff CD, Collin GR. Management of renal trauma at a rural, level I trauma center. *Am Surg* 1998;64:226.
11. Dean RH. Management of renal artery trauma. *J Vasc Surg* 1988;8:89.
12. McAninch JW, Carroll PR, Armenakas NA, et al. Renal gunshot wounds: methods of salvage and reconstruction. *J Trauma* 1993;35:279.
13. Spirnak JP, Resnick MI. Revascularization of traumatic thrombosis of renal artery. *Surg Gynecol Obstet* 1987;164:22.
14. Greenholz SK, Moore EE, Paterson NE, et al. Traumatic bilateral renal artery occlusion: successful outcome without surgical intervention. *J Trauma* 1980;26: 941.

15. Brandes SB, Chelsky MJ, Buckman RF, et al. Ureteral injuries from penetrating trauma. *J Trauma* 1994;36:766.
16. Edson M. Injury to the bladder. In: Champion HR, Robbs JV, Trunkey DV, eds. *Rob and Smith's operative surgery: trauma surgery*. 4th ed. London: Butterworth, 1989:481–484.
17. Palmer JK, Benson GS, Corriere JN Jr. Diagnosis and initial management of urological injuries associated with 200 consecutive pelvic fractures. *J Urol* 1983; 130:712.
18. MacMahon R, Hosking D, Ramsey EW. Management of blunt injury to the lower urinary tract. *Can J Surg* 1983;26:415.
19. Corriere JN Jr, Rudy DC, Benson GS. Voiding and erectile function after delayed one-stage repair of posterior urethral disruptions in 50 men with a fractured pelvis [Abstract]. *J Trauma* 1993;35:160.
20. Mansi MK, Emran M, El-Mahrouky A, et al. Experience with acute penile fractures in Egypt: long-term results of immediate surgical repair. *J Trauma* 1993; 35:67.
21. Edson M. Injuries to the urethra. In: Champion HR, Robbs JV, Trunkey DV, eds. *Rob and Smith's operative surgery: trauma surgery*. 4th ed. London: Butterworth, 1989:476–480.
22. Cline KJ, Mata JA, Venable DD, et al. Penetrating trauma to the male external genitalia. *J Trauma* 1998;44:492.
23. Anderson KA, McAninch JW, Jeffrey RB, et al. Ultrasonography for the diagnosis and staging of blunt scrotal trauma. *J Urol* 1983;130:933.
24. McAninch JW. Genital injury. In: Champion HR, Robbs JV, Trunkey DV, eds. *Rob and Smith's operative surgery: trauma surgery*. 4th ed. London: Butterworth, 1989:486–491.
25. McAninch JW. Injuries to the urinary system. In: Blaisdell WF, Trunkey DD, eds. *Trauma management: abdominal trauma*. New York: Thieme-Stratton, 1982:216.

30. GYNECOLOGIC AND OBSTETRICAL TRAUMA[1]

GYNECOLOGIC INJURIES IN NONPREGNANT WOMEN

With the exception of sexual assault and domestic violence, injuries to female reproductive organs in the nonpregnant state are uncommon unless the organs are enlarged or diseased.

Vulvovaginal Injuries

AXIOM Vulvovaginal injuries are easily missed in trauma patients because of the patient's modesty or the doctor's reluctance to examine the perineum (unless there is severe pain, bleeding, or an obvious wound; 2).

Because the patient history can be inaccurate or frankly deceptive, accurate diagnosis of vulvovaginal injuries depends primarily on careful complete examination. Severe injuries of the perineum, vagina, urethra, bladder, and rectum can be easily overlooked during the initial examination of a struggling, anxious patient.

⊘ PITFALL

An adequate examination may not be possible in some uncooperative patients with suspected gynecologic injuries without general anesthesia.

The vulva and vagina are considered contaminated areas and should be carefully cleaned before any examination. The bladder should be emptied with a sterile catheter before the examination, and the urine submitted for urinalysis. In the adult, digital and speculum examination is mandatory, especially if the vagina may be injured. If there is a possibility of rectal damage, proctosigmoidoscopy also is indicated. In the child, a rectal examination plus vaginal endoscopy will usually suffice.

Vulvar Hematomas

Most vulvar hematomas are less than 5 cm in diameter and resolve spontaneously without surgical intervention. Hematomas that are progressively enlarging or are more than 5 cm in diameter require evacuation of the clots (3). If bleeding continues despite application of local pressure, the hematoma is opened, and bleeding sites are controlled directly with figure-of-eight sutures around the periphery of the hematoma as needed, followed by tight packing of the hematoma cavity. Concomitant packing of the vagina may facilitate hemostasis.

Vaginal Fistulas

If less than 12 hours old, traumatic rectovaginal and vesicovaginal fistulas can usually be closed, and injuries to the anal sphincter can be carefully repaired. If a large perineal or rectal laceration or a rectovaginal fistula is present, a proximal colostomy is recommended (2).

Rape

⊘ PITFALL

Failure to perform a complete initial examination on an alleged rape victim increases not only the risk of complications but also the possibility of gross injustice.

Rape is not always easily confirmed. The examining physician can describe specific areas of obvious trauma. Material from the vagina obtained during the speculum examination should be studied microscopically as a wet-mount and analyzed for acid phosphatase. If the vagina appears to be empty, it can be irrigated with saline, which can then be removed and examined microscopically.

If the victim is a virgin, rape may cause multiple hymenal and vaginal lacerations with severe bleeding, which occasionally requires ligation of bleeding vessels. All alleged rape victims should also be examined for extrapelvic injuries. The level of consciousness and sobriety should be noted, and a blood alcohol level and drug screen also should be determined.

All suspected or proven victims of rape should be protected from pregnancy by the oral administration of some form of estrogen. Estrogen/progestin (Ovral) is effective and has a low incidence of side effects when taken in the usual dose of 2 tablets within 72 hours (preferably 12 to 24 hours) of coitus and 2 tablets again 12 hours later (4).

Vaginal Foreign Bodies

AXIOM Vaginal drainage in a child should be considered the result of a foreign body and possible sexual abuse until proven otherwise (5).

Trauma to the vulva or vagina from foreign bodies is most common in young children. If hemorrhage does not occur immediately after insertion of the foreign body, there is often a delay of days or weeks before the child is brought to the physician because of a purulent vaginal discharge. Rectal examination with simultaneous insertion of a uterine sound into the vagina may detect a metallic foreign body. Because of the associated pain, general anesthesia is often necessary to perform an adequate examination and to remove the foreign body.

Open Pelvic Fractures

AXIOM Blood coming from the vagina after blunt trauma should serve as a warning of a possible open pelvic fracture into the genital tract.

Pelvic fractures are often associated with severe blunt injuries to the external genitalia, and these fractures commonly involve the perineum, vagina, bladder, or a combination of these (6).

AXIOM If the pelvic examination in a patient with a pelvic fracture is not performed very gently, a closed pelvic fracture can easily be converted into an open one.

The risk of pelvic abscesses in patients with pelvic fractures increases if a vaginal laceration is not recognized promptly. Vaginal lacerations should be closed transvaginally with slowly absorbable suture after the vagina is gently but thoroughly cleansed with an antiseptic solution. Deep perineal tears, with or without rectal injury, usually require a proximal diverting colostomy plus irrigation of the distal defunctionalized segment of bowel (7). Preoperative and perioperative antibiotics also are indicated.

Internal Gynecologic Injuries

Internal gynecologic injuries with blunt trauma are extremely rare if the patient is not pregnant and is otherwise normal. If an exploratory laparotomy is performed on a female patient with pelvic fractures, the gynecologic structures should be evaluated carefully, but caution should be taken not to release an associated retroperitoneal hematoma.

Treatment of penetrating uterine injuries in young women depends on whether or not the uterus can be reconstructed well enough to make a future pregnancy reasonably safe. If this cannot be accomplished, or if the patient is beyond childbearing years, hysterectomy is the treatment of choice.

Penetrating injuries to uterine adnexa may occasionally cause extensive hemorrhage from disruption of the ovarian or uterine arteries.

TRAUMA TO PREGNANT WOMEN

Incidence and Consequences

Trauma is the leading cause of death in pregnant women and accounts for more than twice as many deaths in women as do all other causes of maternal mortality combined (7). It is estimated that about 6% to 7% of the 8,000,000 pregnancies occurring in the United States annually are complicated by trauma. In one study, approximately 64% of the pregnant trauma patients were injured in motor vehicle accidents, 16% were burn victims, 8% were assaulted, 8% were victims of penetrating injuries, and 4% were injured in falls (8).

In a review of 103 cases of blunt maternal trauma, eight of 10 women first seen in shock had an unsuccessful pregnancy outcome (9). Other factors contributing to fetal loss included prematurity, specific pelvic visceral injuries, and direct fetal injury. Among mothers who survive their injuries, placental abruption is the most common cause of fetal loss.

AXIOM Maternal death is the most frequent cause of fetal death after trauma.

Among pregnant women who die as a result of trauma, head injury and hemorrhagic shock account for most deaths (9). Increased risks of splenic rupture and retroperitoneal hemorrhage due to blunt abdominal trauma during pregnancy also have been reported.

AXIOM For all injured pregnant women, the possibility of chemical dependency must be considered in the initial assessment.

In 80% of the serious female trauma victims seen at Detroit Receiving Hospital (DRH), alcohol or an illicit drug has been present in the blood or urine or both at the time of admission.

Physiologic Changes in Pregnancy

Blood Volume

Blood volume increases steadily during pregnancy from 20% to 25% above normal at the end of the first trimester to 30% to 50% above normal near term (10). There is a greater increase in plasma volume than red cells, and this results in a slight-to-moderate decrease in hematocrit from a normal mean of 40% to an average of about 32% to 34% by week 32 or 34. Some hyponatremia also may be present.

Cardiac output increases by 30% to 40% from a normal average of 4.5 L/min to 6 to 7 L/min from week 10 until the end of the pregnancy. This occurs despite a decrease in the average central venous pressure from 9 mm Hg in nonpregnant women to about 4 mm Hg in the third trimester. This is accompanied by a 10 to 15 beat/min increase in the heart rate throughout pregnancy (Table 30-1).

During pregnancy there is a modest decrease in systolic and diastolic blood pressure (8 to 15 mm Hg) from an average normal of 110/70 mm Hg to about 102/55 mm Hg at the end of the second trimester. At term, the blood pressure often returns to normal.

AXIOM After trauma, as much as 30% of the maternal blood volume may be lost with little change in maternal vital signs; however, there may be a severe reduction in placental blood flow, causing fetal distress or death.

The placenta is extremely reactive to hypovolemia or sympathetic stimulation. Even relatively mild decreases in maternal blood flow can cause severe decreases in placental perfusion.

During pregnancy, a relative leukocytosis occurs, increasing the white blood cell (WBC) count from a previous mean of 7,200/mm^3 to about 9,800/mm^3 in the third trimester. Indeed, a WBC up to 12,000 to 15,000/mm^3 may be "normal" in some pregnant women. The differential count is usually unaffected.

Blood also becomes "hypercoagulable" with increases in factors VII, VIII, IX, X, and XII. Plasma fibrinogen levels may almost double, and the plasma levels of plasminogen activator tend to decrease (11).

AXIOM Normal concentrations of coagulation factors in a critically ill pregnant woman should make one suspicious of the presence of disseminated intravascular coagulation (DIC).

Table 30-1. *Physiologic and Anatomic Changes of Pregnancy*

Cardiovascular	Plasma volume increases by 40% to 50%
	Hct decreases from a mean of 40% to 32%
	Cardiac output increases by 30% to 40%
	Heart rate increases by 10 to 15 beats/min
	Sys blood pressure decreases slightly (10 to 15 mm Hg)
	Peripheral vascular resistance decreases
	CVP falls from a mean of 9 to 4 mm Hg
	ECG shows L. axis deviation (10% to 15%)
Respiratory	Minute ventilation increases by 40% to 50%
	Tidal volume increases by 40% to 50%
	Respiratory rate is unchanged
	P_aCO_2 decreases to 30 to 32 mm Hg
	Functional residual capacity decreases 20%
	Oxygen reserve decreases
Hematologic	Hematocrit decreases to about 32%
	A white blood cell count of 12,000 per mm^3 may be normal
	Fibrinogen increases to 400 mg/dL
	Coagulation factors VII, VIII, IX, X, and XII all increase
	Coagulation times decrease
Anatomic	Pituitary gland doubles in size
	Heart is pushed upward and rotates
	Diaphragm elevates 4 cm
	Uterus becomes the largest intraabdominal organ
	Bladder is displaced into the abdominal cavity
	Pelvic joints loosen

From ref. 25, with permission.

Lungs

As the uterus enlarges and encroaches on the upper abdomen, the diaphragms rise about 4 cm, and the functional residual capacity of the lungs is reduced about 20%. Tidal volume and minute ventilation increase approximately 50%, causing a chronic state of compensated respiratory alkalosis.

Intestines

AXIOM Although all trauma patients are at increased risk for vomiting and aspiration of gastric contents, pregnant women are especially susceptible because of the decreased gastrointestinal motility that accompanies pregnancy.

Compression by the gravid uterus and an overall reduction in smooth-muscle tone cause delays in gastric emptying and prolonged intestinal transit times.

AXIOM Because the peritoneum has a decreased sensitivity during pregnancy, there is less pain and tenderness, and it can be much more difficult to diagnose intraabdominal injury or disease (12).

Ureter

Increased progesterone during pregnancy tends to cause ureteral dilation, which can be increased by compression by ovarian vessels and the uterus. There is also delayed urinary bladder emptying that can lead to bacteremia and pyelonephritis.

Pituitary Gland

The pituitary gland gets 30% to 100% heavier during pregnancy. As a consequence, shock may cause necrosis of the anterior pituitary, resulting in postpartum pituitary insufficiency (Sheehan's syndrome).

Uterus and Placenta

The uterus grows from a 7-cm long, 70-g organ in the adult nonpregnant state to a 36-cm long, 1,000-g organ at term, and the combined weight of the uterus, fetus, placenta, and amniotic fluid at term is about 4,500 g (13). Blood flow to the uterus increases from 60 mL/min to 600 mL/min at term. This predisposes pregnant women to massive blood loss if the uterine vasculature is disrupted.

AXIOM At about 26 weeks, when the delivery of a viable fetus is possible, the top of the uterus is about halfway from the umbilicus to the xiphoid process.

During the first trimester, the uterus is a thick-walled structure confined within the safety of the bony pelvis. During the second trimester, the uterus leaves its protected intrapelvic location, but the small fetus is still relatively well protected because it is cushioned by a relatively large amount of amniotic fluid. By the third trimester, the uterus is large and thin walled, and during the last 4 weeks of gestation, the fetus slowly descends as the fetal head engages in the pelvis.

The placental vasculature exists in a state of maximal vasodilatation throughout gestation, but it is exquisitely sensitive to catecholamine stimulation so that mild to moderate maternal hypovolemia can cause severe placental vasoconstriction and hypoperfusion.

Direct trauma to the placenta or uterus can release high concentrations of placental thromboplastin (a plasminogen activator) from the myometrium into the circulation and can cause DIC (6).

Supine Hypotension

AXIOM At least 10% of women in late pregnancy will develop hypotension if placed in the supine position.

Hypotension from compression of the inferior vena cava by the gravid uterus in the third trimester can be corrected rapidly by turning the patient about 10 to 15 degrees to the left. If the patient has had blunt trauma and there is any concern about the spine, the patient's backboard can be turned or one can displace and try to hold the uterus manually to the left. Vena caval compression by the uterus also can increase venous pressure in the lower part of the body and increase bleeding from injuries to the pelvis and lower extremities.

Types of Injuries

Pelvic Fracture

Pelvic fracture in the mother after severe blunt trauma may cause intrauterine death by three mechanisms:

1. Maternal shock;
2. Placental separation; or
3. Direct fetal injury.

Of the direct fetal injuries, skull fracture with intracranial bleeding is the leading cause of death.

Placental Separation

AXIOM Placental separation (abruptio placentae) is the leading cause of fetal death when the mother survives major trauma.

Abruptio placentae from direct trauma is caused by maldistribution of shearing forces between the elastic and flexible uterine wall and the inelastic placenta. Disruption of 25% or less of the placenta from the uterus is compatible with fetal survival but often causes intrauterine bleeding and premature labor. Disruption of 50% or more of the placenta is almost always fatal to the fetus (6).

Uterine Rupture

Uterine rupture after blunt trauma most often occurs at the site of a previous cesarean section (14). Without prior operation, the most likely site of rupture is the posterior uterine wall. The urinalysis frequently shows hematuria because of concomitant bladder injury.

Penetrating Wounds of the Uterus

Penetrating wounds to the midabdomen during the late second and all of the third trimester are very likely to involve the uterus and its contents. Gunshot wounds to the gravid uterus involve the fetus 60% of the time and have a fetal mortality approaching 80% if wounding is sustained preterm versus 40% if the fetus is near term (15). If the fetus is less than 26 weeks' gestation or is dead, and the uterine injury is small, the uterus can be sutured and the mother left to deliver the fetus vaginally. Although fetal mortality is high with low-velocity gunshot wounds of the uterus, maternal mortality from such trauma is uncommon. This is related to the high density of the uterine contents and the rapid dissipation of kinetic energy by the muscular uterine wall, the fetus, and the amniotic fluid.

Management of lower midline abdominal stab wounds is controversial. Careful local wound exploration may identify superficial injuries, and peritoneal lavage is helpful in ruling out significant intraperitoneal bleeding or bowel injury. Retrograde cystography can generally rule out a bladder injury, and external fetal monitoring will determine how the fetus is doing.

Burns

Burns exceeding one third of the total body-surface area usually result in termination of the pregnancy within 1 week (12). Even if the fetus survives the first week of such a burn, eventual fetal loss from sepsis can be expected. During the third trimester with such injuries, an occasional fetus is saved by delivery or cesarean section within the first 5 days.

Noncatastrophic Maternal Trauma

The high pressures that can be generated during deceleration injuries may cause relatively little extrauterine damage, but may create marked uterine distortion and a shearing effect on the placental insertion site. Consequently, abruption and fetal injury can occur with little or no external sign of trauma to the abdominal wall. Vaginal bleeding is likewise often absent, and fetal distress is frequently the initial sign (16).

Initial Emergency Management

AXIOM The initial approach to severely injured pregnant women should probably be more aggressive than that for nonpregnant women.

Even if the initial vital signs are normal, the physician should remain concerned about significant maternal visceral or fetal injury. The mother's prenatal history also is important, and the trauma physician should be particularly concerned about the presence of diabetes mellitus, preeclampsia, or vaginal spotting before the accident.

AXIOM Resuscitation of the mother takes precedence over that of the fetus.

Oxygen

Fetal blood functions on a different oxygen–hemoglobin dissociation curve, and a higher than normal maternal Po_2 may be required to provide an adequate fetal hemoglobin saturation (17). The more oxygen reserve a distressed fetus has, the better the fetal outcome is likely to be.

AXIOM Injured pregnant women with a marginal airway or ventilation must be rapidly intubated, ventilated, and oxygenated.

Fluid Resuscitation

Fluid resuscitation should be very aggressive in third-trimester patients with even minimal evidence of hypovolemia. Even with mild to moderate maternal hypovolemia, uterine blood flow to the fetus can be severely compromised by the placental vasoconstriction (18). In like manner, vasopressors are to be avoided because they further decrease placental blood flow.

AXIOM Inflation of the abdominal portion of the pneumatic antishock garment (PASG) is usually contraindicated in the pregnant patient after the first trimester because it might damage the fetus and compromise maternal venous return.

Gastric and Bladder Decompression

A nasogastric tube (or an orogastric tube if major facial trauma is present) is passed to empty the stomach and reduce the chances of aspiration of gastric contents. A urinary catheter should be passed to record urinary output as an additional guide to the adequacy of tissue perfusion. It also may help to assess the possibility of urinary tract trauma.

Fetal Monitoring

AXIOM Fetal monitoring is essential during the evaluation of all pregnant women with trauma.

Evaluation of the fetus and uterus includes checking fetal heart rate, fetal movement, uterine size and irritability, and observing the vagina for amniotic fluid or blood. Early signs of fetal distress include decreased variability of heart rate, bradycardia of 110 beats/min or less (18), and late fetal deceleration.

Determining fetal age and maturity is critical to deciding whether and when to deliver the fetus of a woman who is apt to remain hypotensive or die. However, such determinations can be very difficult. Measuring fundal height by palpation of the abdomen is probably the quickest way to estimate fetal age. If the top of the uterus is more than halfway from the umbilicus to the xiphoid process, the fetus may be viable.

Diagnosis of Injuries in Pregnant Women

History and Physical Examination

While instituting immediate life-saving resuscitation procedures and monitoring maternal vital signs and fetal heart tones, a history concerning the pregnancy also should be elicited, if possible. The date of the last menstrual period, the expected date of confinement, the first perception of fetal movement, the most recent maternal perception of fetal movement, and the status of previous pregnancies all are important.

AXIOM Nagele's rule calculates the predicted day of labor by subtracting 3 months from the first day of the last menstrual period and adding seven days.

As part of the complete physical examination, there should be a vaginal speculum examination to detect any dilatation of the cervix or bleeding from the cervical os.

AXIOM Vaginal bleeding is absent in 20% of patients with abruptio placentae, and the uterus may fill with as much as 2,000 mL of blood with little external evidence of bleeding.

Laboratory Evaluations

The initial laboratory studies in severely injured pregnant women should include

1. Complete blood count with a differential;
2. Type and cross-match;
3. Arterial blood gases;
4. Serum electrolytes;
5. Serum amylase;
6. Blood alcohol and toxicology studies;
7. Urinalysis; and
8. Indirect Coombs' test.

Nitrazine paper pH analysis of any vaginal discharge also is done. Amniotic fluid has a pH of about 7, whereas normal vaginal fluid has a pH of about 5 (6). Bleeding from the fetus into the maternal circulation is identified by using the Kleihauer–Betke stain (19). If this test is strongly positive and the fetus is alive and of appropriate gestational age, immediate cesarean section may be indicated. With severe trauma, serial coagulation studies also should be performed.

AXIOM Decreasing fibrinogen levels are the most sensitive indicator of DIC in the pregnant woman with a placental injury and are an indication for prompt induction of labor.

If delivery does not follow within 6 to 8 hours of diagnosis of a suspected DIC or if the maternal condition worsens, evacuation of the uterine contents is required and should be performed promptly.

If the patient is not obviously pregnant (i.e., does not have a uterus greater than 16 to 20 weeks in size), a qualitative (rapid) pregnancy test should be performed immediately, and serial levels determined.

AXIOM If a quantitative β-human chorionic gonadotropin (βhCG) is not as high as expected from the historic duration of the pregnancy or size of the uterus or if it does not at least double every 2 days, the viability of an existing pregnancy is in question.

Kleihauer–Betke Test

The incidence of fetal hemorrhage into the maternal circulation after trauma is about 26% compared with 6% for controls (20) and is more common if the placenta has an anterior location or if there is uterine tenderness after the trauma (18). The Kleihauer–Betke acid elution assay to detect fetomaternal hemorrhage in cases of maternal trauma is used to determine the need for Rh immunoglobulin in Rh-negative mothers and to help identify abruptial bleeding that could lead to fetal distress. Goodwin and Breen (21) pointed out that the amount of fetomaternal hemorrhage needed to sensitize some Rh-negative mothers is far below the sensitivity of the Kleihauer–Betke test. Consequently, they recommend routine treatment of all Rh-negative mothers with abdominal trauma. Nevertheless, the Kleihauer–Betke test may indicate who requires increased doses of Rho (D) immune globulin.

The ultrasound can be very beneficial at determining the presence of a pregnancy, fetal viability, placental position, and the presence of a moderate or large abruption or other obstetric problems (8). With proper use and experience, pregnancy as early as 5 weeks can be documented. However, ultrasound may miss a small abruption, and it gives only limited information regarding maternal trauma, except for fluid in the cul de sac of Douglas.

Ultrasound

AXIOM Ultrasound of the abdomen, uterus, and fetus should be performed on all gravid patients with moderate-to-severe abdominal trauma.

Radiologic Evaluations

AXIOM A diagnostic modality considered necessary for proper evaluation of an injured gravid woman should not be withheld for fear of potential hazard to the fetus.

The risk of congenital defects below a 10-rad exposure to the fetus at any stage of pregnancy is similar to the 4% to 6% incidence of congenital defects seen with no history of irradiation (20). When medically appropriate, consideration should be given to minimizing fetal irradiation by limiting the scope of the examination plus appropriate shielding and collimation.

The presence of bloody urine mandates cystography as well as evaluation of the upper urinary tracts, preferably through contrast-enhanced computed tomography (CT). Computed tomography of the abdomen may obviate multiple studies, such as intravenous pyelography (IVP), and consultation with the radiologist can help minimize the number of radiation exposures.

Diagnostic Peritoneal Lavage

Because of the relative insensitivity of abdominal examination in pregnant trauma victims, early consideration should be given to performing a diagnostic peritoneal lavage (DPL). Some believe that a DPL is contraindicated in pregnancy; however, a DPL can be done with reasonable safety if it is performed in a supraumbilical location superior to the enlarged uterus with inspection of the peritoneum and opening of the peritoneum under direct vision.

Fetal/Placental Monitoring

Pregnant women with major injuries and a viable fetus should be monitored closely for at least 48 hours. If the fetus is doing well after 48 hours, it is unlikely that a significant placental separation is present.

Fetal compromise is generally manifested by fetal bradycardia or tachycardia, loss of accelerations, and prolonged or late decelerations (18). Fetal monitoring also is of benefit to the mother because the fetal heart rate is a much more sensitive indicator of decreases in maternal blood flow and oxygenation than maternal hemodynamic and blood gas changes.

AXIOM Cardiotocographic monitoring after the week 20 of pregnancy is very sensitive at predicting adverse outcome and can predict abruptio placentae at an early stage, allowing timely diagnosis and intervention (18).

The second most common cause of fetal death from trauma (after maternal death) is placental abruption, which complicates about 1% to 5% of minor blunt abdominal trauma. In "severe" trauma, the incidence of abruption is between 7% and 66%, and fetal mortality from abruption ranges from 30% to 68% (13,18). If more than half of the placental surface separates from the uterus, the fetal mortality rate approaches 100%. Factors that increase the risk of traumatic abruption include hypertension, cocaine, preeclampsia/eclampsia, smoking, diabetes mellitus, advanced maternal age, and multiparity.

Clinical findings of abruption can include vaginal bleeding, uterine tenderness, abdominal pain, amniotic fluid leakage, maternal signs of hypovolemia out of proportion to visible bleeding, a uterus larger than expected for the gestational age, increasing uterine size, or a change in the fetal heart rate (9).

AXIOM If no fetal heart sounds or activity are identified after trauma, fetal nonviability should be confirmed by real-time and B-mode ultrasonography.

Treatment

Uterine Trauma

The risk of uterine injury in the face of a pelvic fracture increases with the length of gestation (2,6). Stable pelvic fractures usually do not interfere with vaginal delivery. Unstable fractures may predispose the patient to bony displacement and urinary tract injuries if vaginal delivery is attempted.

The indications for laparotomy for trauma in pregnancy include evidence of significant intraabdominal bleeding or injury to a hollow viscus. If the uterus is involved, selective observation can be advocated if

1. The entry wound is below the fundus of the uterus;
2. The mother is hemodynamically stable with a fetus that is either dead or without injury or compromise; and
3. There is no evidence of injury to the genitourinary or gastrointestinal tracts.

The presence of a gravid uterus should not be a deterrent to needed operative intervention, and the surgery itself is unlikely to lead to premature labor unless there is extensive manipulation of the uterus.

AXIOM General anesthesia is preferred for all pregnant patients with multisystem injuries requiring operative management.

The risk of spontaneous abortion after trauma or surgery is greatest during the first trimester and is least toward the end of the second trimester.

Dead Fetus

If the fetus is doing well and there is no bleeding, the patient can be watched. If the fetus is dead, spontaneous evacuation of the uterus can be anticipated within 1 week. If DIC or sepsis seems to be developing, the uterus should be evacuated promptly.

Tocolysis

AXIOM If there is evidence of uterine contractions and progression of cervical dilatation in an injured mother who is not at term, tocolysis should generally be used to allow time for full fetal evaluation.

Some contraindications to tocolysis include

1. Active vaginal bleeding;
2. Suspected placental abruption (because blood will further accumulate inside a relaxed uterus);
3. Preeclampsia or eclampsia;
4. Uncontrolled diabetes mellitus;
5. Serious cardiac disease; and
6. Maternal hyperthyroidism.

Cesarean Section

AXIOM If the fetus is viable, but in distress despite resuscitative measures, or if the mother is not considered to be salvageable, urgent cesarean section is recommended.

Cesarean section usually prolongs a laparotomy done for other injuries by about 1 hour and increases blood loss by at least 1,000 mL (22). In general, the critically injured mother who has her injuries treated and then delivers vaginally within 24 hours will generally tolerate the stress of vaginal delivery better than emergency prolonged surgery right after admission; however, if the fetus continues to be distressed and it is thought that the mother can withstand the extra operating time at the initial operation, a cesarean section should be performed. Other reasons for cesarean section include uterine rupture and situations in which the uterus mechanically limits repair of maternal injuries.

If a decision is made to pronounce the mother dead, salvage of the fetus must be considered. The likelihood of fetal survival with postmortem cesarean delivery depends on fetal maturity and the time since the mother's death. Ritter's review of 250 years of literature documented 120 successful postmortem cesarean sections (23). Of all the children who survived postmortem cesarean section from 1900 to 1985, 70% were delivered within 5 minutes of the mother's death, and all of these infants were neurologically normal; after 15 minutes, the survival rate was only 2% to 3%, and 67% to 100% of the survivors had severe neurologic sequelae.

AXIOM Inadequate placental circulation to the placenta, because of severe shock or death, for more than 5 to 10 minutes, makes it unlikely that the fetus delivered by cesarean section will live and have normal neurologic function.

If it is decided that a cesarean section is appropriate, it should be done while cardiopulmonary resuscitation (CPR) or open heart massage (without aortic cross-clamping) is continued on the mother. A classic midline vertical incision is made from the epigastrium to the symphysis pubis and rapidly carried down through all layers of the abdomen to the peritoneal cavity. A vertical incision is then made in the anterior uterus from the fundus to the upper bladder reflection. If an anterior placenta is encountered as the uterus is entered, it should be incised to reach the fetus promptly. The umbilical cord should be promptly clamped and cut after delivery of the child.

Complications of Pregnancy

Eclampsia

AXIOM Any traumatized pregnant patient with seizures or coma may have a trauma-induced intracerebral bleed, but such central nervous system (CNS) changes also may be due to preeclampsia or eclampsia.

Eclampsia in pregnancy has a predilection for the young primigravida, the older multigravida, diabetics, and women with chronic hypertension (20). Hypertension, edema, proteinuria, and hyperactive reflexes are usually present. Postpartum eclamptic seizures usually occur within the first 48 hours after delivery.

In any suspected eclamptic with significant trauma, intravenous magnesium sulfate ($MgSO_4$) should be started promptly, and an immediate cesarean section considered. A loading dose of 4 g of $MgSO_4$ solution is given intravenously, followed by either 2 to 3 g intravenously per hour or 5 g intramuscularly in each buttock immediately after the loading dose, and then every 4 hours as long as the deep tendon reflexes are still present. Because administration of $MgSO_4$ can cause vasodilation and hypotension, careful monitoring is essential. The $MgSO_4$ treatment should continue for at least 24 hours postpartum or 24 hours after the last seizure.

Thrombophlebitis

Overall, pregnancy is associated with a 5.5-fold increase in the risk of thromboembolism, especially in the postpartum period (24). Increasing age and parity also are important risk factors associated with an increased risk of fatal pulmonary embolism during or after pregnancy.

⊘ FREQUENT ERRORS

1. ***Reluctance to thoroughly examine the perineum of a girl or woman with possible pelvic trauma.***
2. ***Failure to use general anesthesia to examine a girl's or woman's vagina or perineum if that is the only way a proper examination can be performed.***

3. ***Failure to perform a complete physical examination and obtain all proper specimens in an alleged rape victim.***
4. ***Failure to look carefully for a foreign body and sexual abuse in a young girl with a vaginal discharge.***
5. ***Failure to correct hypovolemia adequately and promptly in traumatized pregnant women, even if they are not hypotensive.***
6. ***Failure to promptly push the uterus off the inferior vena cava in a hypotensive traumatized pregnant woman.***
7. ***Failure to monitor the fetus closely in a pregnant traumatized woman.***
8. ***Failure to provide prompt ventilatory assistance to pregnant women with marginal ventilation or blood gases.***
9. ***Failure to obtain a needed radiologic test because of its possible effect on the fetus.***
10. ***Failure to perform, or delay in performing, needed surgery in a pregnant woman because of the possibility of causing an abortion or premature delivery.***

SUMMARY POINTS

1. Vulvovaginal injuries are easily missed in trauma patients because of the patient's modesty or the doctor's reluctance to examine the perineum.

2. Ecchymoses about the perineum may be the only evidence of severe hemorrhage into the ischiorectal fossa.

3. Vaginal drainage in a child is due to a foreign body and possible sexual abuse until proven otherwise.

4. Patients with vaginal tears associated with pelvic fractures have open fractures and an increased incidence of septic complications.

5. If the pelvic examination in a patient with a pelvic fracture is not performed very gently, a closed pelvic fracture can easily be converted into one that is open.

6. Maternal death is the most frequent cause of fetal death after trauma.

7. After trauma, as much as 30% of the maternal blood volume may be lost with little change in maternal vital signs. However, there may be a severe reduction in placental blood flow, causing fetal distress or death.

8. Normal concentrations of coagulation factors in a critically ill pregnant woman should make one suspicious of the presence of DIC.

9. Traumatized pregnant women are especially susceptible to vomiting and aspiration because of their decreased gastrointestinal motility.

10. Because the peritoneum has a decreased sensitivity during pregnancy, there is less pain and tenderness, and it can be much more difficult to diagnose intraabdominal injury.

11. At about 26 weeks, when the delivery of a viable fetus is possible, the top of the uterus is about halfway from the umbilicus to the xiphoid process.

12. At least 10% of women in late pregnancy will develop hypotension if placed in the supine position.

13. Placental separation is the leading cause of fetal death when the mother survives major trauma.

14. If a full evaluation rules out life-threatening injuries to both the mother and the fetus, pregnant women with lower abdominal stab wounds can be managed with careful observation.

15. Cardiotocographic monitoring after week 20 of pregnancy is very sensitive at predicting adverse outcomes and can predict abruptio placentae at any early stage.

16. Resuscitation of the mother takes precedence over that of the fetus.

17. Oxygen may be of benefit in all injured patients, but especially for the fetus in pregnant women.

18. Injured pregnant women with a marginal airway or ventilation should be rapidly intubated, ventilated, and oxygenated.

19. Hypovolemia must be rapidly corrected, and vasopressors should be avoided in pregnant women.
20. Fetal monitoring is essential in all pregnant women with trauma.
21. Nagele's rule calculates the predicted day of labor by subtracting 3 months from the first day of the last menstrual period and adding 7 days.
22. Vaginal bleeding is absent in 20% of patients with abruptio placentae, and the uterus may fill with as much as 1,000 to 2,000 mL of blood with little external evidence of exsanguination.
23. Decreasing fibrinogen levels are the most sensitive indicator of DIC in the pregnant woman with a placental injury, and DIC is an indication for prompt induction of labor.
24. If a quantitative βhCG is not as high as expected from the historic duration of the pregnancy or size of the uterus or if it does not at least double every 2 days, the viability of an existing pregnancy is in question.
25. The fetus is most vulnerable to developing deformities if more than 10 to 15 rads of irradiation are given during the period from day 10 through week 10 after conception.
26. Ultrasound of the abdomen, uterus, and fetus should probably be performed on all gravid patients with abdominal trauma.
27. If a DPL is indicated in an injured pregnant woman after week 12, it should be done as an open technique above the umbilicus and uterus.
28. One should look for placental injury in all traumatized pregnant women, especially if there is any fetal distress.
29. Disruption of 25% or less of the placental–uterine surface is compatible with fetal survival, but separations greater than 50% generally result in fetal death.
30. If no fetal heart sounds are identified after trauma, fetal nonviability should be confirmed by real-time and B-mode ultrasonography.
31. If there is evidence of uterine contractions and progression of cervical dilatation in an injured mother who is not at term, tocolysis should generally be used.
32. General anesthesia is preferred for all pregnant patients with multisystem injuries requiring operative management.
33. If the fetus is viable but in distress despite resuscitative measures, and the mother is not considered to be salvageable, urgent cesarean section is recommended.
34. The best protection for the fetus after trauma is an early and aggressive restoration of normal maternal oxygenation and perfusion.
35. Inadequate placental circulation to the placenta, because of severe shock or death, for more than 5 to 10 minutes makes it unlikely that the fetus delivered by cesarean section will live and have normal neurologic function.
36. Fetal death is not an indication for cesarean section.
37. If fetal delivery is accomplished within 5 minutes of cardiac arrest or the onset of severe shock, there is about a two thirds chance of survival of a mature fetus without neurologic sequelae.
38. Any traumatized pregnant patient with seizures or coma may have a trauma-induced intracerebral bleed, but these CNS changes may also be due to preeclampsia or eclampsia.

REFERENCES

1. Wilson RF, Vincent C. Gynecologic and obstetrical trauma. In: Wilson RF, Walt AJ, eds. *Management of trauma: pitfalls and practice.* Philadelphia: Williams & Wilkins, 1996:621–642.
2. Evans TN, Teshima J. Gynecologic and obstetric trauma. In: Walt AJ, Wilson RF, eds. *Management of trauma: pitfalls and practice*. Philadelphia: Lea & Febiger, 1975:393–402.
3. Stone NN, Ances IG, Brotman S. Gynecologic injury in the nongravid female during blunt abdominal trauma. *J Trauma* 1984;24:626.
4. Yuzpe A, Smith R, Rademaker A. A multicenter clinical investigation employing ethinyl estradiol combined with dl-norgestrel as a postcoital contraceptive agent. *Fertil Steril* 1982;37:508.

5. Herman-Giddens ME. Vaginal foreign bodies and child sexual abuse. *Arch Pediatr Adolesc Med* 1994;148:195.
6. Maull KI, Pedigo RI. Injury to the female reproductive system. In: Moore EE, Mattox KL, Feliciano DV, eds. *Trauma*. 2nd ed. Norwalk, CT: Appleton & Lange, 1991:587–595.
7. Fildes J, Reed L, Jones N, et al. Trauma: the leading cause of maternal death. *J Trauma* 1992;32:643.
8. Drost TF, Rosemurgy AS, Sherman HF, et al. Major trauma in pregnant women: maternal/fetal outcome. *J Trauma* 1990;30:574.
9. Rothenberger D, Quattlebaum FW, Perry JF, et al. Blunt maternal trauma: a review of 103 cases. *J Trauma* 1978;18:173.
10. Hytten FE, Leitch I. *The physiology of human pregnancy*. 2nd ed. Oxford, England: Blackwell Scientific Publications, 1971:18.
11. Biland L, Duckert F. Coagulation factors of the newborn and his mother. *Thromb Diath Haemorrh* 1973;29:644.
12. Lavin JP, Polsky SS. Abdominal trauma during pregnancy. *Clin Perinatol* 1983; 10:423.
13. Pearlman MD, Tintinalli JE, Lorenz RP. Blunt trauma during pregnancy. *N Engl J Med* 1990;373:1609.
14. Schrinsky DC, Benson RC. Rupture of the pregnant uterus: a review. *Obstet Gynecol Surv* 1978;33:217.
15. Iliya FA, Hajj SN, Buchsbaum HJ. Gunshot wounds of the pregnant uterus: report of two cases. *J Trauma* 1980;290:90.
16. Kettel LM, Branch DW, Scott JR. Occult placental abruption after maternal trauma. *Obstet Gynecol* 1988;71:449.
17. Shaw DB, Wheeler AS. Anesthesia for obstetric emergencies. *Clin Obstet Gynecol* 1984;27:112.
18. Pearlman MD, Tintinalli JE, Lorenz RP. A prospective controlled study of outcome after trauma during pregnancy. *Am J Obstet Gynecol* 1990;162:1502.
19. O'Brien JA, Coustan DR, Singer DB, et al. Prepartum diagnosis of traumatic fetal-maternal hemorrhage. *Am J Perinatol* 1985;2:214.
20. Neufeld JDG, Moore EE, Marx JA, et al. Trauma in pregnancy. *Emerg Med Clin North Am* 1987;5:623.
21. Goodwin TM, Breen MT. Pregnancy outcome and fetomaternal hemorrhage after noncatastrophic trauma. *Am J Obstet Gynecol* 1990;116:665.
22. Strong TH, Lowe RA. Perimortem caesarean section. *Am J Emerg Med* 1989; 7:489.
23. Ritter JW. Postmortem caesarean section. *JAMA* 1961;175:715.
24. Bolan JC. Thromboembolic complications of pregnancy. *Clin Obstet Gynecol* 1983; 26:913.
25. Pimentel L. Mother and child: trauma in pregnancy. *Emerg Med Clin North Am* 1991;9:549.

31. MUSCULOSKELETAL TRAUMA (1)

INITIAL MANAGEMENT

Fracture healing is unique because it results in the reconstitution of normal tissue (i.e., bone) as opposed to scar tissue. The most important prerequisites for healing are close proximity of the fracture fragments with adequate stability and maintenance of good blood supply.

Diagnosis

AXIOM The most obvious injuries are often not the most important.

In patients with multiple injuries, severe deformities of the extremities are often so striking that they tend to receive much of the initial attention, with possible neglect of other, more serious injuries. Maintenance of an adequate airway and ventilation, control of hemorrhage, and correction of hypovolemia take priority over injured bones. Nevertheless, open fractures are surgical emergencies and, after proper resuscitation, should receive operative intervention within 6 hours of injury to have the best chance for a favorable outcome (2). Fractures and dislocations, when associated with neurovascular compromise, also are surgical emergencies requiring prompt attention.

History

The history from patients with musculoskeletal injuries should include

1. Mechanism of injury;
2. Location of pain;
3. Limitation of motion; and
4. Neurovascular function.

It is important to remember that pain from fractures is occasionally referred to more distal portions of the extremity; hip fractures, for example, commonly cause pain in the thigh or knee.

AXIOM If a major fracture occurs as a result of a minor injury, the presence of a pathologic fracture should be suspected.

Physical Examination

All obvious deformities of the extremities should be recorded, as should the location and size of any contusions, abrasions, swellings, or lacerations. All extremities should be gently palpated, noting the location and severity of any tenderness. In comatose patients, areas of deformity or crepitation may be the only objective evidence of a fracture. Joints also should be evaluated for range of motion, tenderness, or effusion.

AXIOM Child abuse should be suspected whenever the history is inconsistent with the physical examination or radiographs, or when there are multiple fractures at different stages of healing.

Radiographs

The radiograph request should contain as much pertinent information about the injury as possible, and should list all areas that might require radiographs. The physician that examined the patient should carefully review the radiographs when they become available and correlate them with the physical findings.

AXIOM In patients who are otherwise stable, poor-quality radiographs should not be accepted, and radiographs should be repeated until satisfactory.

Despite a conscientious initial evaluation, it is inevitable that some injuries will be missed in some patients with multiple injuries. In a recent study from a busy Level I trauma center, as many as one in five patients with severe multiple trauma had at least one orthopaedic injury that was not initially appreciated (3). Only repeated, comprehensive physical examinations after admission with appropriate radiographs will detect these missed injuries in a reasonable period.

Descriptions of fractures should include

1. Location within the bone: epiphyseal, metaphyseal, diaphyseal;
2. Description of any articular involvement;
3. Fracture pattern: transverse, oblique, segmental, comminuted;
4. Any bone loss if present; and
5. Whether the fracture is open (any loss of skin integrity near the fracture) or closed.

Splinting

Any splints that were applied before the patient reached the hospital must be inspected carefully to be sure that they are adequate, are not causing excessive pressure, and are not hiding any neurovascular problems or open fractures.

AXIOM Fractures that have not been immobilized by the time the patient reaches the hospital should be splinted as soon as possible after arrival at the hospital.

With shoulder and most arm injuries, the extremity is placed in a sling, with the elbow usually at a right angle, and is bound to the chest with a bandage. Padded commercial metal splints or inflatable air splints may be used for forearm and wrist injuries. The addition of a sling with the elbow at a right angle often adds to the patient's comfort.

If an injured elbow is in extension, no attempt should be made to flex it to a right angle. A posterior splint or an inflatable air splint may be used.

Fixed traction splinting in a hinged half-ring splint or Hare splint, by using a hitch about the foot and ankle, is effective for hip, thigh, and knee injuries. The hitch may be applied over a shoe if it is not easily removed.

An alternative to fixed traction is the use of padded board splints along the medial and lateral sides of the lower extremity. For injuries at the knee, a long inflated air splint may be used.

An inflated air splint can provide excellent emergency splinting of lower leg and foot injuries. For fractures at the ankle, a pillow wrapped securely with tape around the lower leg, ankle, and foot can be effective. The foot should be included in the splint to prevent rotation during transport.

AXIOM A bone fragment protruding through an open wound should be covered with a sterile dressing and left undisturbed until definitive care is provided.

If there is neurovascular impairment, deformities should be corrected by traction, even if a protruding fragment is pulled back into the wound.

For neck injuries, the patient should be supine on a firm surface such as a long spine board, and a rigid collar is applied with the head and neck in the neutral midline position.

For thoracic and lumbar spine injuries, the patient should be kept supine on a firm surface, such as a long spine board, but with a small roll under the lumbar spine. If turning is necessary, the patient is rolled "like a log" by two or three individuals.

Treatment of Open Fractures

Classification

In the Gustilo classification system (4), grade I open fractures are those with a wound less than 1 cm long and without any significant soft-tissue damage. Grade II fractures have larger wounds with some underlying tissue damage. Grade IIIA fractures have extensive lacerations or soft-tissue flaps, but delayed primary closure is feasible. Grade IIIB fractures have major wounds that require local or free microvascular tissue transfers for closure. Grade IIIC open fractures have an associated arterial injury that requires repair. Reported infection rates of open fractures range from 0% to 9% for grade I, 1% to 12% for grade II, and 9% to 55% for grade III (4).

Limited Manipulation

Manipulation of open fracture wounds should be limited to whatever is necessary to control major hemorrhage or to relieve neurovascular impairment until definitive treatment can be carried out in the operating room. Tscherne et al. (5) showed that the infection rate after open fractures was 4 times lower in patients who had a sterile dressing in place from the scene of the accident to the operating room, compared with those who did not.

Antibiotics

With open fractures, parenteral antibiotics should be started as soon as possible in the emergency room. The antibiotic of choice is a cephalosporin, typically 1 or 2 g of cefazolin every 6 to 8 hours. For grade III injuries, an aminoglycoside is added. For *Clostridia*-prone wounds (e.g., farm injuries), 2 to 4 million units of penicillin every 2 to 4 hours should be added. The duration of antibiotic therapy remains controversial, but most orthopedic surgeons treat for at least 3 days. Antibiotics also should be given during any subsequent operative procedures.

In severe open fractures, antibiotics also can be delivered locally in polymethylmethacrylate (PMMA) beads impregnated with gentamicin or tobramycin (6).

With tetanus-prone injuries, human tetanus immune globulin and antibiotics should be given in addition to a tetanus toxoid booster.

Debridement

A thorough surgical debridement of all crushed or devitalized skin and soft tissue is essential in the treatment of open fractures. Muscle that does not bleed when cut or does not twitch when pinched is dead and should also be removed. All foreign bodies, with the exception of inaccessible missile fragments, should be removed.

Dirty or contaminated essential structures (such as nerves, tendons, large blood vessels, and ligaments) that cannot be adequately debrided should be cleansed mechanically with voluminous irrigation under pressure. Use of antiseptic solutions, such as povidone–iodine (Betadine), in open wounds can eradicate microorganisms, but it also damages local natural host-defense mechanisms (7). In most cases, irrigation with sterile saline is adequate.

AXIOM Bone fragments completely free of any soft-tissue attachment generally should be removed.

Fracture Stabilization

After debridement and wound cleansing, the fracture should be stabilized. External fixation is often a good option, as it can stabilize the fracture without adding more foreign material to the wound. Internal fixation may be preferred for certain articular injuries, but it tends to be associated with increased infection rates.

Wound Management

After thorough debridement of the wound and stabilization of the fractures, grade I wounds can be closed, but grade II or III wounds are usually left open initially.

Patients with grade II or III open fractures are returned to the operating room within 24 to 72 hours for further debridement or closure. Delayed primary closure should be performed, when possible, within 3 to 5 days by using skin grafting, local muscle flaps, or free tissue transfers, as needed (8).

Associated Nerve Injuries

AXIOM The neurovascular status of an injured extremity should be evaluated both before and after any manipulation.

The most common mechanism of peripheral nerve injury with fractures is neuropraxia, in which the axon and nerve sheath remain intact, but there is functional impairment due to stretching or compression by fractures and hematomas. Peripheral nerves also can have ischemic damage due to compartment syndromes.

AXIOM Closed fractures and dislocations seldom disrupt nerves completely, and contusion or stretching is the usual cause of neurologic deficits.

Trauma to peripheral nerves is relatively common with certain extremity fractures. Up to 12% of humeral shaft fractures are accompanied by paralysis of the radial nerve (9). Other neurologic lesions frequently seen with musculoskeletal injuries in the upper extremities include

1. Axillary nerve or brachial plexus in dislocations of the shoulder;
2. Median or ulnar nerve in supracondylar fractures or posterior dislocations of the elbow; and
3. Median nerve in fractures about the wrist.

In the lower extremity, injury to the sciatic nerve, especially its peroneal portion, can be seen in up to 13% of posterior dislocations of the hip, and nerve injuries are reported in 18% of knee dislocations (10). The peroneal nerve is especially likely to be involved with tears of the lateral collateral ligament or fractures of the proximal fibula.

If a well-localized nerve disruption is found at the time of the initial wound exploration, it can often be repaired. If there is much contamination or if the extent of the nerve damage is not clear, nerve repair should be delayed until the wound has healed.

About 3 to 4 weeks after the fracture has been treated, nerve function can be evaluated both clinically and by electromyographic (EMG) and conduction studies. If there is no evidence of reinnervation after 6 to 8 weeks, the nerve should be explored.

Associated Vascular Injuries

The blunt upper-extremity injuries most likely to damage major vessels include dislocations of the shoulder, compressing or contusing the axillary artery; midshaft humeral fractures, bruising or tearing the brachial artery; and dislocations of the elbow or supracondylar fractures of the humerus, compressing the brachial artery, particularly if the elbow is flexed.

Blunt lower-extremity injuries particularly likely to involve major vessels include fractures of the middistal femoral shaft (tearing or contusing the superficial femoral artery) and dislocations of the knee (causing intimal flaps in the popliteal artery). Fractures of the tibia and fibula can produce compartment syndromes compressing the tibial or peroneal arteries.

In many instances, reduction of a dislocation relieves neurovascular compression in an extremity, but an arteriogram should still be performed. Otherwise, a large intimal flap, which may cause later occlusion, may be missed.

In patients with a fracture of the shaft of the femur associated with a lacerated superficial femoral artery, reperfusion of the distal limb can usually be accomplished fairly quickly with an intravascular shunt. After fixation of the femur, the shunt can be removed, and the artery can be definitively repaired out to its proper length.

Early Postreduction Care

The first 24 to 72 hours after fracture reduction is a period of increasing swelling and danger of soft-tissue complications. The integrity of the circulation and peripheral nerve function should be checked immediately postoperatively and intermittently for the next 24 to 72 hours. Radiographs confirming the reduction also should be taken.

If a circular cast is used for immobilization, it should be bivalved or removed if the patient complains of increasing pain or if there is any question of vascular impairment.

No patient should be allowed to leave the hospital without receiving specific instructions to return immediately if (a) the fingers or toes distal to a cast or splint become white, blue, cold, or insensitive; or (b) if there is increased pain. Patients who complain of increasing pain should not be given more analgesics, as this may prevent the early diagnosis of serious complications.

AXIOM A well-reduced and immobilized fracture should not cause severe pain; increasing or excessive pain often indicates tissue pressure or ischemia that requires urgent correction.

The patient with a cast also should be given advice concerning elevation of the injured part and detailed instructions in finger or toe exercises to be carried out at frequent intervals.

FRACTURES AND DISLOCATIONS OF THE UPPER EXTREMITIES

Scapula

⊘ PITFALL

Failure to look carefully for intrathoracic injuries in patients with a fractured scapula can lead to delayed diagnosis of important injuries.

Fractures of the scapula usually require great force and can be associated with severe damage to underlying ribs and thoracic viscera. The fractures themselves usually can be treated symptomatically with a "sling-and-swathe" for a few days, followed by early motion of the arm in a sling, so that a frozen shoulder does not result.

Clavicle

Sling application is suggested for all age groups until the full range of motion at the shoulder is painless. A figure-of-eight dressing is popular for use in children; however, these bandages seldom reduce the overriding fragments. In bedridden patients, a rolled towel placed vertically between the shoulders may help relieve some of the discomfort from these injuries.

Acromioclavicular Separations

The initial treatment of acromioclavicular separations is immobilization in a sling, until the patient is asymptomatic (usually 1 or 2 weeks). Surgical repair of the ligaments is occasionally performed for grade III injuries.

Dislocations of the Shoulder

Dislocation of the glenohumeral joint is the most common dislocation of a major joint. Up to 98% of all traumatic shoulder dislocations are anterior. The elbow cannot be made to touch the side of the chest and the hand cannot be placed on the opposite shoulder unless there is an associated fracture of the humerus.

Transient damage to the axillary nerve by the humeral head as it leaves the shoulder joint occurs in up to 15% of dislocations. The nerve injury can cause anesthesia over the outer shoulder and paralysis of the deltoid muscle. Occasionally, signs of trauma to the axillary vessels and large nerves of the brachial plexus also are present.

Reduction of the dislocation usually can be accomplished by using only intravenous analgesia, but general anesthesia makes the reduction easier and minimizes the risk of producing a fracture of the surgical neck of the humerus.

Techniques for shoulder reduction typically involve either traction or leverage. Leverage or manipulative techniques are associated with an increased incidence of complications, especially neurovascular injury and fracture.

Once the shoulder dislocation has been reduced, it is typically immobilized in a sling for at least 3 to 4 weeks. Pendulum exercises can be started when the patient is comfortable, but external rotation should be avoided, as it can lead to redislocation. Recurrent shoulder dislocations may require operative repair.

Fractures of the Proximal Humerus

Fractures of the proximal humerus involving the anatomic or surgical neck usually result from a fall on the outstretched hand or elbow in elderly individuals. The majority of these fractures are impacted, and the best functional results are usually obtained by accepting the position of impaction and beginning early motion.

Pain can often be alleviated by supporting the extremity in a sling, with or without a swathe, for a few days. Relaxed circumduction or pendulum exercises in and out of the sling should be initiated within 1 week of the injury.

Fractures of the Greater Tuberosity

Isolated fractures of the greater tuberosity of the humerus may occur after a fall on the point of the shoulder or after forcible abduction. Undisplaced or minimally displaced fractures require only a sling for comfort and early active exercises.

Fractures of the Shaft of the Humerus

The radial nerve in the spiral groove of the humerus is particularly susceptible to injury by fractures of the shaft. If the nerve palsy was there before any manipulations, it usually recovers spontaneously over the course of 2 to 3 months. If recovery is not seen at that point, EMG studies should be performed.

The majority of humeral shaft fractures respond well to a sling or hanging arm cast. Early use of functional bracing allows movement of adjacent joints and has a high success rate.

Supracondylar Fractures

Supracondylar fractures of the humerus occur most often in children and usually result from a fall on an extended, outstretched arm. Because there are occasional injuries to the median, radial, or ulnar nerves or brachial artery with these fractures, it is important to carefully assess the neurovascular status of the arm before any manipulation. An absent pulse can often be restored by extending the arm at the elbow, but if this fails, arteriography should be considered. If arteriography cannot be obtained in a timely fashion, and the extremity is ischemic, prompt closed or open reduction of the fracture with internal fixation plus surgical exploration of the brachial artery is appropriate.

AXIOM Elbow flexion to reduce supracondylar fractures of the humerus can occlude the brachial artery, and if not promptly corrected, this can cause Volkmann's ischemic contracture.

Comminuted Fractures of the Lower Humerus

Adults with these fractures have a painful, swollen elbow and varying degrees of comminution in the distal humerus. Undisplaced condyle fractures in children require only a plaster cast or posterior splint for a few weeks; however, careful follow-up is important because late displacement can occur. With fractures of the medial epicondyle in adults, the best treatment is support of the extremity in a sling for 7 to 10 days. If the fragment is widely displaced, operative fixation is performed. In young or middle-aged patients with displaced fragments, open reduction and internal fixation is recommended. If the patient is elderly or the fracture is severely comminuted, continuous traction by using a Kirschner wire through the olecranon with the arm elevated anteriorly may be preferable.

Fractures of the Olecranon

The best treatment of an undisplaced fracture of the olecranon is immobilization of the elbow in moderate extension with a posterior molded splint for 7 to 14 days. Thereafter, a sling may be substituted and removed for frequent active exercises.

Displaced olecranon fractures are reduced anatomically and fixed internally. If the fragment is comminuted or cannot be reduced, it is excised, and the triceps mechanism is reattached more distally on the ulna.

Dislocations of the Elbow

AXIOM Anterior dislocations of the elbow do not occur without an accompanying fracture of the olecranon.

Circulation and nerve function should be checked and recorded before reduction is attempted. If the patient is neurovascularly intact, radiographs, including oblique views, should be taken (before the attempted reduction) to rule out associated fractures, particularly of the radial head.

Reduction can usually be accomplished by application of longitudinal traction under regional or general anesthesia. If the reduction is not complete, it is impossible to flex the elbow freely. After reduction, the elbow is immobilized for about 7 to 10 days at an angle of about 90 degrees in a posterior molded splint and sling. Thereafter, only a sling is required.

Dislocation of the ulna with an associated fracture or dislocation of the head of the radius can severely compromise function of the elbow. The fracture of the head of the radius may be treated in a wide variety of ways, but loss of motion relative to the radial head is frequent.

Fractures of the Head of the Radius

A fracture of the radial head should be suspected if there is localized tenderness and restricted supination. If there is an undisplaced fracture, oblique, anteroposterior, and lateral views may be needed to see the fracture line. A posterior fat-pad sign indicates intraarticular swelling and can be present when there are nondisplaced fractures about the elbow.

If a fracture is not seen, treatment may include aspiration of the elbow joint and rest in a sling for about 48 hours, followed by gradually increasing active exercises. Radiographs made 2 to 3 weeks later may then demonstrate a fracture line.

With minimal displacement of the fracture fragments or with a fragment of less than one third of the articular surface of the proximal radius, a brief period of immobilization in a sling or posterior splint is usually all that is indicated.

If the fracture of the radial head involves more than one third of the articular surface, if there is significant comminution, or if a block to pronation and supination is present, then excision in an adult may be indicated. If the fractured radial head is excised, insertion of a polymeric silicone (Silastic) radial head spacer may prevent late proximal translation of the radius.

Fractures of the Shaft of the Ulna

A Monteggia fracture is a fracture of the shaft of the ulna plus a dislocation of the head of the radius. In children, these are best treated by closed reduction of the ulna. The radial-head dislocation will usually reduce spontaneously at the same time. The arm is then casted or splinted in this position.

In adults, the preferable treatment is open reduction of the ulnar fracture followed by plating to provide rigid fixation.

Isolated fractures of the shaft of the ulna are usually the result of a direct blow to the forearm and are sometimes referred to as "nightstick" fractures. They are usually minimally displaced and are now being treated with brief periods of short-arm splinting or functional bracing (11).

Fracture of the Shaft of the Radius

Galeazzi's fracture is the eponym used for a radial shaft fracture combined with a dorsal or volar dislocation of the distal ulna. Open reduction and internal fixation of the radius is almost always required. The distal radioulnar joint disruption can be treated with closed reduction and casting or pinning.

Combined Fractures of the Shafts of the Radius and Ulna

In children, one or both of the fractures may be incomplete (greenstick), and completion of the fracture(s) is often required to prevent recurrent angular deformity after closed reduction and casting, with careful early follow-up.

In adults, the treatment of displaced radius and ulna fractures is internal or plate fixation of both bones.

AXIOM Anatomic reduction and fixation of both bone fractures of the forearm is needed to maintain the interosseus space to allow normal pronation and supination.

Fractures of the Distal Radius

Fractures of the distal radius are the most frequent fractures of the upper extremity. Eponyms such as Colles' (dorsal angulation of the distal fragment), and Smith's (volar angulation of the distal fragment) fracture continue to be used to denote specific fracture patterns.

Treatment is closed reduction by manipulation with immobilization in a cast for 5 to 6 weeks. For fractures at risk for loss of fixation in a cast, percutaneous fixation of the distal fragment is an option. In young, active patients, open reduction may be required to provide precise reduction of intraarticular fragments.

AXIOM With all wrist fractures, exercise of the fingers to maintain their range of motion throughout the period of immobilization is extremely important.

Fractures of the Carpus

The most frequent fracture of the wrist is that of the carpal navicular (scaphoid), especially in young adult men. The scaphoid usually has a precarious blood supply, which enters the bone distally. If a displaced fracture is sustained across the waist of the scaphoid, the proximal fragment loses most of its blood supply and may develop avascular necrosis.

The diagnosis of a scaphoid fracture can be very difficult. Clinically, there is pain and swelling in the wrist with moderate-to-severe tenderness in the anatomic snuff box. Oblique, ulnar deviation, anteroposterior, and lateral views may be required to see the fracture. Some fractures will not be visible on any of the initial radiographs.

AXIOM A "wrist sprain" that does not resolve quickly may represent a scaphoid fracture.

If there is localized tenderness in the anatomic snuff box, but all of the radiographs are negative, good practice calls for plaster immobilization in a thumb spica cast for 10 to 14 days and then repeated roentgenograms (without the cast; 12). If the fragments are displaced, surgical intervention is generally required.

The majority of nondisplaced scaphoid fractures will unite if the fragments are properly immobilized early and for a long enough period. Some orthopedic surgeons believe that if progress toward healing is not evident by 6 to 10 weeks, open reduction and bone grafting may significantly speed union. If avascular necrosis of the proximal fragment occurs, nonunion is common, and posttraumatic arthritis of the wrist joint is the result.

Dislocation of the Lunate

When the lunate dislocates, it is generally extruded anteriorly, where it can interfere with median nerve function. Closed reduction should be attempted as soon as possible. If efforts at closed reduction are not successful, open reduction is indicated. A high incidence of avascular necrosis is associated with this injury.

In perilunate dislocations, the lunate retains its normal relation with the radius, but the remaining carpal bones are displaced. This is treated in the same manner as lunate dislocations. There is a high association with scaphoid fracture, in which case, the injury is termed a "transscaphoid, perilunate, fracture dislocation."

FRACTURES AND DISLOCATIONS OF THE LOWER EXTREMITIES

Hip Fractures

Fractures of the hip are the most frequent serious fractures in elderly patients. They usually occur after a fall, which is often provoked by one of the patient's medical problems. The injured lower extremity typically appears shortened and falls into external rotation.

These patients frequently develop complications, including progression of cardiovascular and renal disease, pneumonia, and pulmonary embolism. Mortality in trochanteric fractures is higher than with intracapsular fractures (30% vs. 15%), even though fractures of the trochanteric region almost always unite, whereas fractures of the femoral neck often result in nonunion and avascular necrosis.

Fractures of the Neck of the Femur

The blood supply to the femoral head comes primarily from small vessels running along the femoral neck, and it is easily disrupted when a displaced fracture occurs, especially if the deplaced femoral head is not promptly reduced. Internal fixation with multiple pins or screws is recommended for nondisplaced, minimally displaced, or impacted femoral neck fractures, and the prognosis for these fractures is generally good.

Displaced femoral neck fractures are typically treated operatively unless the patient is nonambulatory. In younger patients, early anatomic reduction, followed by multiple pin or screw fixation, is mandatory, but the complication rates of nonunion and avascular necrosis are high. In older patients, excision of the femoral head and prosthetic hemiarthroplasty replacement is a frequent treatment option.

AXIOM As a general rule, the earlier a fractured hip is reduced and fixated, the less likely the patient is to develop cardiopulmonary complications.

Intertrochanteric Fractures of the Femur

The fragments in intertrochanteric (IT) fractures have an excellent blood supply and almost always unite after internal fixation. The high mortality rate with these fractures is due to the advanced age (70 to 85 years) of these patients and preexisting cardiopulmonary problems. In addition, more blood is lost with this fracture and during operative fixation than with other hip fractures.

Dislocations of the Hip

In about 90% of hip dislocations, the head of the femur comes to rest posterior to the acetabulum. This injury is usually sustained while the thigh is flexed and adducted, as in an automobile collision when the knee strikes the dashboard. The posteriorly dislocated hip remains flexed, adducted, and internally rotated, and the extremity appears shortened. The peroneal portion of the sciatic nerve may be injured, resulting in inability to dorsiflex the foot.

AXIOM Hip dislocations are orthopaedic emergencies and should be reduced as soon as possible to reduce the incidence of aseptic necrosis of the femoral head.

After reduction, radiographs should confirm a concentric reduction of the hip joint. A nonconcentric reduction may be due to fracture debris trapped inside the hip joint, and this is an indication for open reduction.

If there is a big fracture defect in the posterior acetabular wall, the hip will tend to dislocate or subluxate repeatedly. Consequently, large fragments should be reduced and fixed.

Anterior dislocation of the hip may be distinguished clinically from a fracture of the hip because of the increased rather than decreased length and the mild flexion. Obliteration of the femoral pulse may accompany this injury, and prompt reduction is imperative under such circumstances.

Reduction of anterior dislocation of the hip can usually be achieved rather easily, often without anesthesia, by traction in the axis of the thigh, followed by internal rotation and adduction. Only a few days of bed rest (with avoidance of abduction, external rotation, and hyperextension), followed by about 4 weeks on crutches is needed.

Fractures of the Shaft of the Femur

Considerable force is required to break the femoral shaft, and there is often local blood loss exceeding 1.0 to 1.5 L. In addition, the bone fragments can injure large adjacent blood vessels.

AXIOM If the knee and hip are not evaluated carefully in patients with femoral shaft fractures, serious proximal or distal joint problems may not be appreciated until they are very difficult to treat.

Femur fractures in children are most often treated closed with hip spica casting. They also can be treated with skin or skeletal traction. Older children or adolescents can be treated with conventional reamed nailing or flexible nails (13). Adults are usually treated with closed, reamed intramedullary nailing to allow early mobilization and better fracture alignment.

Fractures of the Distal End of the Femur

Displaced supracondylar fractures of the femur are best treated with open reduction and internal fixation. The joint surface must be anatomically reduced. Postoperative management includes early passive and active motion and delayed weight leaning until bony healing is present.

Patellar Dislocations

Patellofemoral (patellar) dislocations are relatively common and may occur as a result of a congenital deformity, usually in adolescent girls, or as a result of relatively mild trauma to the knee from the side (14).

Reduction is accomplished by direct pressure over the deformity with the knee passively extended, followed by 4 to 6 weeks of immobilization. Spontaneous reduction before being seen by a physician is not uncommon, but postreduction radiographs should be carefully examined for the presence of osteochondral fractures.

Knee Dislocations

AXIOM Knee dislocations are orthopaedic emergencies. They require immediate reduction and assessment of the vascular status of the extremity.

Tibiofemoral (knee) dislocations are associated with extensive ligamentous disruption and an increased incidence of severe neurologic and vascular injuries. For the knee to dislocate, the collateral and cruciate ligaments are often torn. Dislocations of the knee may occasionally reduce spontaneously. In such instances, the only clues to the true nature of the injury may be the history, a gross instability of the knee, a hemarthrosis, a neurovascular injury, or a combination of these.

Complications of complete dislocation of the knee include damage to the popliteal artery and to the peroneal or posterior tibial nerves (14). If a major neurologic defect with no evidence of recovery persists for more than 6 to 12 weeks, surgery may be considered after appropriate EMG studies. The prognosis for recovery is poor, and bracing or tendon transfers are usually necessary.

The incidence of popliteal artery injury is quite high (25% to 30%) with knee dislocations and may include contusions, tears, or intimal flaps, with or without thrombosis (14). Even if normal pedal pulses return after reduction, early arteriography is indicated to rule out a large intimal flap or other lesions that are likely to result in thrombosis. If anything worse than a small intimal tear is found, the vascular injury should generally be repaired.

AXIOM An arteriogram of the knee should be considered in all patients with a knee dislocation.

Meniscal Injuries

The medial and lateral menisci of the knee are relatively avascular structures that have an essential role in stress distribution across the knee joint; however, they can be torn with forceful twisting motions. In the majority of instances, the diagnosis of a torn meniscus is made on the history of a twisting injury to the knee, and subsequent repeated episodes of painful slipping, catching, or near-locking sensations or both on the inner side of the knee. Physical examination is not completely reliable, and confirmatory tests such as magnetic resonance imaging (MRI) or diagnostic arthroscopy are often needed.

The main indications for surgery are repeated locking or chronic pain and effusion. An arthroscopic partial meniscectomy, leaving a smooth and stable rim of cartilage, is generally performed. Occasionally, one can successfully repair tears near the meniscal rim, where there is some blood supply (15).

AXIOM The meniscus cartilages of the knee have a poor blood supply, and tears frequently do not heal.

Torn Collateral Ligaments

Tears of the collateral ligaments result from varus (pushing the knees apart) or valgus (pushing the knees together) forces on the extended knee. The patient is unable to tolerate weight-bearing. Pain and tenderness are localized over the torn collateral ligament, and a hemarthrosis can develop rapidly. Within 12 to 24 hours, the skin overlying the torn ligament often becomes discolored from underlying hemorrhage.

The diagnosis is confirmed by stressing the injured knee in a varus and valgus direction in both the fully extended and a 30-degree flexed position. Lack of a firm end point often indicates complete ligament tears.

Medial collateral ligament injuries, which are more common, can be treated nonoperatively with a hinged knee brace that provides medial and lateral support but allows flexion and extension at the knee. Operative treatment may be considered for complete tears of the lateral ligament complex or for multiple ligamentous injuries.

Torn Cruciate Ligaments

The anterior cruciate ligament runs from the posterior portion of the lateral femoral condyle to the anterior aspect of the tibial spines and prevents anterior displacement of the tibia on the femur. Conversely, the posterior cruciate ligament runs from the anterior aspect of medial femoral condyle to the posterior tibial spine and prevents posterior displacement of the tibia on the femur.

The cruciate ligaments are stretched or torn in injuries that cause excessive movement of the tibia on the femur in an anteroposterior direction. The anterior cruciate ligament tends to be torn with twisting hyperextension injuries. The posterior cruciate ligament is torn when the upper portion of the flexed tibia is driven backward on the femur. With anterior cruciate injuries, which are more common, the patient experiences a sense of the knee giving way with attempts to plant the extremity and pivot.

On physical examination, there is excessive movement of the tibia on the femur. For anterior cruciate tears, the most reliable test is the Lachman maneuver, which is performed with the knee flexed about 20 degrees and the tibia directed straight ahead. The femur is held steady with one hand, while the other attempts to bring the tibia forward. The so-called anterior drawer sign, in which the knee is flexed to 90 degrees, and anterior translation of the tibia on the femur is tested, is considered a less reliable test for anterior cruciate insufficiency. The posterior drawer sign can be used to detect posterior cruciate ligament tears. This is performed with the knee flexed to 90 degrees, to see if the tibia can be pushed posteriorly on the femur.

If swelling and pain make a good clinical evaluation impossible, an examination under anesthesia or an arthroscopic examination of the knee can be considered. MRI also is used increasingly for diagnosing ligamentous injuries about the knee.

Older, sedentary patients may be treated without surgery in many cases, whereas younger patients often have surgical reconstruction. Isolated posterior cruciate ligament tears are more likely to be treated nonoperatively.

AXIOM Anterior cruciate tears often occur with other knee injuries, especially medial meniscal and medial collateral ligament tears, producing the "terrible triad."

Osteochondral Fractures

Osteochondral fractures of the femoral condyles or patella cause pieces of articular cartilage with accompanying subchondral bone to be broken off inside the knee joint. These fractures should be suspected in any patient with a traumatic knee hemarthrosis and can result in severe posttraumatic arthritis. If loose bodies are suspected in the knee joint, arthroscopy is indicated.

Fractures of the Patella

Fractures of the patella can occur indirectly from severe contracture of the quadriceps mechanism or from a direct blow to the flexed knee. They are characterized clinically by a hemarthrosis, and when they are displaced, there is a palpable defect and an inability to extend the knee actively.

If the patellar fragments are not separated, aspiration of the hemarthrosis, a compression dressing, splinting, and use of crutches for several weeks is often all that is needed.

Fractures with separation require accurate open reduction and fixation, often with a tension band–wiring technique and repair of the defects of the quadriceps expansion on both sides of the patella. If the fracture is extensively comminuted, a partial or complete patellectomy may be required (16).

Fractures of the Proximal End of the Tibia

AXIOM Fractures of the proximal tibia usually cause massive hemarthrosis and deformity.

Fractures of the Lateral Tibial Plateau

Large displaced fractures of the lateral tibial plateau require open reduction and internal fixation. For depressed fractures, elevation of the tibial plateau and autologous bone grafting also may be required. Immediate continuous passive motion and early active exercises are important to maintain the range of motion of the knee. Non–weight bearing, progressing slowly to protected weight bearing, is required for 2 to 3 months.

Fractures of the Medial Tibial Plateau

Treatment of medial tibial plateau fractures is analogous to those of the lateral plateau, but they often have a worse prognosis, especially if associated with a "fracture–dislocation" of the knee.

Tibial Shaft Fractures

Closed Fractures

Diagnosis of fractures of the tibia or fibula or both is usually established easily by the clinical symptoms and signs, but it is important that the entire shafts of both the tibia and fibula be well visualized on the radiographs.

When a stable reduction of a closed tibial shaft fracture can be achieved, long-leg casting followed by early conversion to a short-leg walking cast or a weight-bearing functional brace can produce excellent results.

Indications for internal fixation include fractures with significant shortening or malalignment or an associated compartment syndrome. Intramedullary nailing, if technically possible, is generally preferred. Interlocking nails have increased the spectrum of fractures that can be stabilized with intramedullary techniques and decrease the need for postoperative immobilization.

Open Tibial Fractures

Open tibial fractures are the most common open fractures in the lower extremity. The most important factor in achieving successful healing is prompt surgical debridement of all necrotic or devitalized tissue. Once bony stability has been achieved, early soft-tissue coverage is essential to decrease the rates of infection and complications. With very severe soft-tissue damage, some open tibial fractures might be better treated with a primary amputation, especially if protective nerve function is lost (17).

Primary external fixation of the fracture is often necessary to protect otherwise precarious wound edges and to facilitate mobilization of the patient. Less severe open fractures can be stabilized with intramedullary nails.

If open reduction appears preferable but is contraindicated because of the injured skin, the poor general condition of the patient, or inadequate equipment, one can use continuous traction via a pin or Kirschner wire through the os calcis or lower tibia until the conditions for surgery are favorable.

Bony union after open tibial fractures may be delayed or may not occur at all because of the severe injury. In some situations, prophylactic autogenous cancellous bone grafting, usually at 6 weeks or once the soft tissues have healed, has resulted in high union rates for open tibial fractures (18). Recently, bone transport involving corticotomy and traction osteogenesis also has been popularized as a method to treat tibial bone loss (19).

AXIOM With severe tibial shaft fractures, one should look for a compartment syndrome, even if the fracture is "open."

Fractures and Dislocations about the Ankle

Uncomplicated Injuries

A clear history of the mechanism of injury helps distinguish direct from indirect fractures and gives the physician an idea of the magnitude of the force involved. When a displaced ankle fracture is first examined, any subluxation or dislocation should be promptly reduced and splinted. Once this has been performed, three radiographic projections (anteroposterior, lateral, and mortise views) are obtained.

Best results after displaced ankle fractures have been produced by accurate open reduction of the medial and lateral malleoli. Displaced posterior malleolar fragments also are being reduced and fixed.

Special Ankle Problems

Tibial "pilon" or "plafond" fractures involve the weight-bearing articular surface of the distal tibia. These fractures can involve all three malleoli and can produce considerable comminution of the joint surface. Optimal care generally involves surgical reconstruction of the articular surface of the distal tibia and early motion.

Open ankle fractures should be treated with debridement plus an immediate open reduction and internal fixation. Higher complication rates can be expected, but the alternatives are poor.

Ankle "sprains" usually involve the lateral collateral ligament complex, especially the anterior talofibular ligament. Most of these injuries are treated nonoperatively; however, chronic posttraumatic instability often requires operative reconstruction.

Fractures of the Bones of the Foot

AXIOM A swollen foot after trauma should be assumed to be fractured until proven otherwise.

Foot injuries are often unrecognized or underestimated in multiply injured patients. As a consequence, definitive therapy is often delayed, resulting in increased disability.

Open fractures of the foot are treated with debridement, repair of critical structures, and fixation of fractures as necessary to prevent further loss of skin. Loss of dorsal or plantar skin is a serious complication. The dorsal skin contains virtually all of the venous drainage of the foot, and the weight-bearing plantar skin is unlike any other skin in the body and cannot be fully replaced.

Fractures of the Calcaneus

AXIOM Fractures of the heel due to a fall from a height are often associated with compression fractures of the lumbar spine at T-12 to L-1.

Fractures of the calcaneus often result in marked swelling and discoloration as a result of hemorrhage, which may be severe enough to cause massive bleb formation and even spotty necrosis of the skin on the sides of the heel.

Computerized tomography is increasingly used to identify the three-dimensional nature of these fractures and has caused increasing interest in surgical treatment aimed at restoring the subtalar joints (20).

Patients are treated typically with bed rest and elevation until the swelling resolves and wrinkles return to the skin (wrinkle test). This often takes 7 to 14 days. In some severely comminuted fractures, in which surgical intervention is not thought to be technically possible or prudent, satisfactory results may be obtained by omitting immobilization altogether and starting non–weight-bearing and active exercises immediately.

Fractures of the Talus

AXIOM Fracture–dislocations of the talus often result in aseptic necrosis.

Fractures of the talus usually result from trauma that produces excessive dorsiflexion of the foot. Because the major nutrient arteries for the talus enter through the distal portion of the bone, a fracture through the neck of the talus destroys the major blood supply to the proximal bone and is very likely to cause avascular necrosis, especially if there is any delay in reduction. If aseptic necrosis of the talus develops, disabling traumatic arthritis of the ankle is very common.

Fractures of the Midtarsal Bones

Midtarsal fractures involving the navicular, cuboid, or cuneiforms, or a combination of these, result from side-to-side crushes or from a heavy weight falling on the foot. After these fractures have healed, there is often considerable disability from loss of motion in the midtarsal joints. The fragments can usually be reduced by manual manipulation, but open reduction and internal fixation often produces better results.

Tarsometatarsal (Lisfranc) Fracture–Dislocations

Fracture–dislocations of the tarsometatarsal joints (Lisfranc's) either are a result of a dorsiflexion stress to the foot or are associated with a high-energy trauma and other foot injuries. Open reduction and internal fixation is usually required for best results.

Fractures of the Metatarsals

Fractures of the metatarsals may be grouped into (a) fractures of the shafts or necks of the metatarsals, (b) fractures of the base of the fifth metatarsal, and (c) stress fractures. Undisplaced fractures of the shafts or necks of the metatarsals require only a compression dressing and crutches for 4 to 6 weeks. A walking boot cast with a long plantar slab to protect the toes may be preferable because it makes the patient ambulatory without crutches. Displaced fractures of the first and fifth metatarsals require accurate reduction so that the weight-bearing heads of these bones are in their normal position.

Proximal diaphyseal fractures of the fifth metatarsal ("Jones fracture") typically occur in young male athletes and have a higher propensity for nonunion. Treatment is generally a non–weight-bearing cast for 6 to 8 weeks.

Stress (fatigue or "march") fractures of the shafts of the second, third, or fourth metatarsals result from prolonged strain. In many instances, they can be managed with only a metatarsal pad in the shoe combined with restricted activity. If pain or disability is excessive, a walking cast for several weeks may be required.

Fractures of the Toes

The only treatment necessary for undisplaced fractures of the toes, including the great toe, is protection from additional injury. Strapping of the injured toe to the adjacent toe or toes with small strips of adhesive tape affords some protection and tends to minimize discomfort. Crutches may be needed for comfort during the first 7 to 10 days. A metatarsal bar applied to the shoe may permit patients to resume activity more quickly. In displaced fractures of the great toe, particularly in the proximal phalanx, closed reduction and pinning may be necessary.

FRACTURES IN CHILDREN

Fractures in children (21) are unique in many ways:

1. Incomplete or greenstick fractures are much more common;
2. The periosteum is much thicker, making initial displacement less, and allowing easier closed reductions;
3. The blood supply from the thick periosteum makes nonunions uncommon;
4. Fractures involving growth plates can cause abnormal growth, limb-length inequality, or angular deformities;
5. Because the bones in the joints may not be completely ossified, comparison films with the contralateral extremity are often needed; and
6. Physical therapy is seldom needed.

Remodeling and Growth

AXIOM In children, angulation and overriding of fracture fragments will often be corrected by growth, but rotation will not.

The younger the child and the closer the fracture to the growth center of the bone, the greater the degree of remodeling that will take place with healing, and the greater the degree of deformity and angulation that can be accepted. This is especially true if the fracture angulation is in the plane of motion of that joint. Overriding with bayonet apposition also is acceptable in a child. The shortening that occurs will usually correct itself because of overgrowth of the involved extremity.

Epiphyseal Injuries

General Considerations

Epiphyseal plate injuries are most common during periods of rapid skeletal growth, especially during the prepubertal growth spurt (9 to 12 years for girls and 12 to 14 for boys). When an epiphysis is separated from the rest of the bone by injury, it tends to occur through the weakest area of the epiphyseal plate, which is the zone of calcifying cartilage. In long-bone epiphyses, the blood vessels penetrate the side of the epiphysis at a point remote from the epiphyseal plate so that they usually are not injured by epiphyseal separation. A notable exception is the proximal femoral epiphysis, where the blood vessels enter the epiphysis by traversing the rim of the plate.

The distal radial epiphyseal plate is by far the most frequently separated. Other frequent sites of epiphyseal injuries are the distal humerus (including the epicondyles), proximal radius, distal femur, and distal tibia. An epiphyseal injury should be suspected clinically in any child who shows evidence of pain, swelling, tenderness, and spasm at a joint.

Accurate interpretation of radiographs for epiphyseal injuries requires a knowledge of their normal appearance at various ages. Two views at right angles to each other are essential, and comparable views of the opposite uninjured extremity can be invaluable.

AXIOM A positive radiograph confirms the diagnosis, but a negative radiograph does not exclude epiphyseal injury in a child.

Epiphyseal plate injuries are not usually associated with disturbance of growth unless there is severe crushing or separation. If the entire epiphyseal plate ceases to grow, the result is progressive shortening, usually without angulation. If the involved bone is one of a parallel pair (such as tibia and fibula or radius and ulna), progressive shortening of one bone can produce a severe angular deformity. A similar problem can occur if growth ceases in one part of the epiphyseal plate but continues in the rest of the plate.

Classification of Epiphyseal Plate Injuries

The Salter–Harris classification of epiphyseal plate injuries is based on the relation of the fracture line to the growing cells of the epiphyseal plate (21; Fig. 31-1).

With a type I injury, the epiphysis is transiently separated from the metaphysis without a bone fragment, and the growing cells remain with the epiphysis. This type is more common in early childhood when the epiphyseal plate is relatively thick. The prognosis for future growth is usually excellent.

With type II injuries, the epiphysis is separated along the epiphyseal plate and out through the metaphysis, leaving a characteristic triangular fragment attached to the epiphysis. This is the most common type of epiphyseal injury. The growing cartilage cells remain with the epiphysis, the circulation remains intact, and the prognosis is usually good.

With type III injuries, there is an intraarticular fracture through the epiphysis, extending from the articular surface to the epiphyseal plate and then along the plate to its periphery. This usually occurs at the upper or lower tibial epiphysis. Accurate reduction is essential, and open reduction may be necessary.

With type IV fractures, an intraarticular fracture extends from the joint surface across the full thickness of the epiphyseal plate and through a portion of the metaphysis to produce a complete split. It most commonly occurs at the lateral condyle of the humerus. Perfect reduction is essential to prevent growth disturbances and to provide a smooth joint surface.

With type V injuries, a severe force crushes the epiphysis and may result in severe growth retardation. Treatment consists of splinting and no weight-bearing for 3 weeks or until the epiphyseal tenderness disappears.

Special Pediatric Fractures

Most children's fractures can be treated with closed reduction and a plaster cast with excellent results, but some require special management.

Greenstick Fractures

With greenstick fractures, one cortex remains unbroken but there is often some angulation. This type of fracture is seen most frequently in the forearm bones of older children. The fracture must often be completed to allow accurate reduction.

Torus Fractures

A torus fracture (usually in or near the distal third of the radius) is a form of greenstick fracture in which neither cortex appears broken on radiograph examination; the bone is merely bent slightly from an impacting force. No attempt at reduction should be made. Only 2 to 3 weeks of protection by a splint or plaster cast is required.

Supracondylar Fractures of the Humerus

Supracondylar fracture of the humerus is the most frequent elbow fracture in children. Proper reduction of the distal fragment often requires flexion to 90 degrees at the elbow; however, there is often much swelling at the elbow, and flexion to 90 degrees may cause compression of the brachial artery and can be a serious threat to the circulation of the forearm and hand. If improperly treated, this can lead to Volkmann's ischemic contracture of the flexor muscles of the forearm.

Fracture of the Distal Humeral Condyles

Fractures of the medial or lateral condyles in children are epiphyseal injuries, which carry late complications of malunion, nonunion, arrest of normal growth, and late

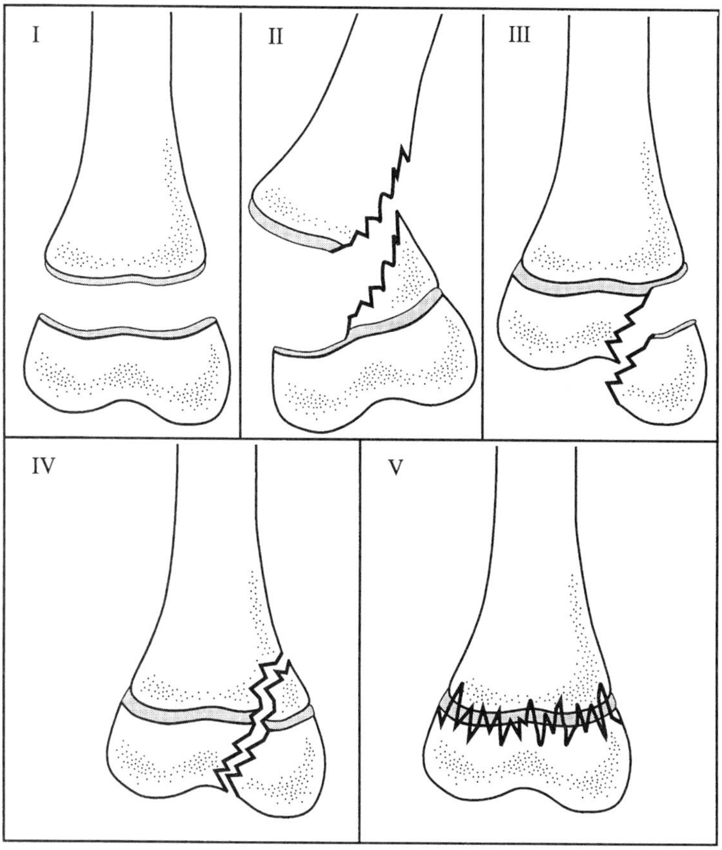

FIG. 31-1. Salter–Harris classification of fractures through the growth plate.

ulnar nerve palsy (22). Closed reduction of displaced fractures is extremely difficult, and anatomic open reduction by direct visualization with smooth pins placed across the epiphysis is often required. Pin removal at 3 to 4 weeks, followed by early motion, is suggested if radiographs show healing.

Subluxation of the Radial Head ("Pulled Elbow")

Dislocation of the head of the radius, often called pulled elbow or "nursemaid's elbow," is a common injury in children between the ages of 2 and 6 years. The mechanism of the injury is a sudden pull, jerk, or lift on the child's wrist or hand. This results in the radial head being pulled distally and jammed into the annular ligament, which grips it tightly, or catching of a portion of the annular ligament between the radial head and capitellum.

The main symptoms are pain and refusal to use the elbow and arm. Flexion and extension at the elbow are usually not limited but are painful. Supination is definitely limited. The child holds the arm extended, but little swelling or deformity is seen or felt. Radiographic examination is of no value except to rule out other bony injury.

Reduction is accomplished with the patient's elbow flexed and with the examiner's thumb placed over the radial head. The forearm is slowly supinated and thumb pressure applied to the radial head. A snap or click is usually heard. The forearm is again tested to make certain that full supination has been regained. The elbow should then be moderately flexed and rested in a sling. The child usually begins to use the arm spontaneously within a few hours. The prognosis is excellent; however, this injury may be recurrent up to the age of 4 to 5 years.

Slipped Capital Femoral Epiphysis

An acute slipped capital femoral epiphysis represents a displaced Salter I fracture of the growth plate of the proximal femur. Occasionally, the child complains primarily of knee pain, and with negative knee radiographs, the diagnosis can be greatly delayed. This injury requires prompt accurate reduction followed by internal fixation. The rate of avascular necrosis after such an injury, no matter how well it is treated, is extremely high.

A chronic slipped capital femoral epiphysis results in an abnormal tilting of the proximal femur that is typically seen in overweight boys who are age 10 to 12 years. It is usually differentiated from an acute slip in that symptoms have been present for at least 3 weeks. This is frequently treated with pinning of the hip with a single cannulated pin under image intensification.

⊘ FREQUENT ERRORS

1. ***Concentration on the most obvious injuries first in patients with multiple trauma.***
2. ***Failure to provide proper early immobilization of extremities with possible fractures.***
3. ***Failure to accurately document a careful and complete neurovascular examination on all possibly injured extremities.***
4. ***Failure to check carefully for frequent associated injuries, such as the lumbar spine with calcaneus fractures or the pelvis with severe lower-extremity fractures.***
5. ***Accepting radiographs that are of poor quality or that do not completely show both ends of a possibly fractured bone.***
6. ***Failure to perform a complete orthopedic reexamination within 24 to 48 hours of admission.***
7. ***Failure to properly protect open fracture wounds before adequate cleaning and debridement.***
8. ***Not promptly seeking the cause of increased pain after splinting or casting an extremity.***
9. ***Failure to obtain accurate reduction of fractures involving joint surfaces, especially in the legs.***
10. ***Prolonged immobilization of joints, especially in the upper extremities, particularly in elderly patients.***
11. ***Failure to ensure adequate motion of fingers or toes when the limb is casted.***
12. ***Failure to watch for development of compartment syndromes with elbow and tibial fractures, especially if there has been any ischemia to the limb.***

SUMMARY POINTS

1. The most obvious injuries are often not the most important.

2. If the trauma causing a fracture is very mild, a pathologic fracture should be suspected.

3. Child abuse should be suspected whenever the history is inconsistent with the physical examination or radiographs, or when there are multiple fractures at different stages of healing.

4. Repeated orthopaedic examinations are mandatory in the early hospital course of all trauma patients to detect injuries that may be missed during the initial examinations.

5. Fractures that have not already been immobilized should be splinted as soon as possible after arrival at the hospital.
6. A bone fragment protruding through an open wound should be covered with a sterile dressing and left undisturbed until definitive care is provided.
7. Grade IIIC open fractures (with associated vascular injuries requiring repair) have an infection rate 3 times higher than those without an ischemic component.
8. Although early fixation of fractures of the lower extremity permits earlier mobilization and results in fewer pulmonary complications, if infection develops at the fracture site, the result can be disastrous.
9. Delayed wound closure is safer than primary closure in grossly contaminated open fractures.
10. The neurovascular status of injured extremities should be evaluated before and after any manipulation.
11. Closed fractures and dislocations seldom disrupt nerves completely, and contusion or stretching of the nerve (i.e., neuropraxia) is the usual cause of neurologic deficits.
12. Increasing or excessive pain at the site of a well-reduced and immobilized fracture often indicates tissue pressure or ischemia that requires urgent correction.
13. Elbow flexion to reduce supracondylar fractures of the humerus can occlude the brachial artery, and if not promptly corrected, this can cause Volkmann's ischemic contracture.
14. Anatomic reduction of both bone fractures of the forearm is needed to maintain the interosseous space to allow normal pronation and supination.
15. With all wrist fractures, exercise of the fingers to maintain their range of motion throughout the period of immobilization is extremely important.
16. A wrist sprain that does not resolve quickly may represent a scaphoid fracture.
17. The majority of nondisplaced scaphoid fractures will unite if the fragments are properly immobilized for a long enough period.
18. Hip dislocations are orthopaedic emergencies and should be reduced as soon as possible, to reduce the incidence of aseptic necrosis of the femoral head.
19. If the knee and hip are not evaluated carefully in patients with femoral shaft fractures, serious problems may not be appreciated until they are very difficult to treat.
20. Knee dislocations are orthopaedic emergencies. They require immediate reduction plus clinical and radiologic assessment of the vascular status of the extremity.
21. The meniscus cartilages of the knee have a poor blood supply, and tears frequently do not heal.
22. Anterior cruciate tears often occur with other knee injuries, especially medial meniscal and medial collateral ligament tears, producing the "terrible triad."
23. A swollen foot after trauma should be assumed to be fractured until proven otherwise.
24. Fractures of the heel are often associated with compression fractures of the thoracolumbar spine.
25. In children, angulation and overriding of fracture fragments will often be corrected by growth, but rotation will not.
26. Any injury near a joint in a child should be assumed to involve the epiphysis until proven otherwise.
27. Passive joint motion or manipulation should be avoided in children; it usually does more harm than good.
28. Open reduction and internal fixation (ORIF) is rarely indicated in long-bone fractures in children.
29. With severe tibial shaft fractures, one should look for a compartment syndrome, even if the fracture is "open."
30. Fracture–dislocations of the talus often result in aseptic necrosis.

REFERENCES

1. Georgiadis GM, Wilson RF. Musculoskeletal trauma. In: Wilson RF, Walt AJ, eds. *Management of trauma: pitfalls and practice.* 2nd ed. Philadelphia: Williams & Wilkins, 1996:643.

2. Dellinger EP. Prevention and management of infection. In: Moore EE, Mattox KL, Feliciano DV, eds. *Trauma*. 2nd ed. East Norwalk, CT: Appleton & Lange, 1989:236.
3. Ward WG, Nunley JA. Occult orthopaedic trauma in the multiply injured patient. *J Orthop Trauma* 1991;5:308.
4. Gustilo RB, Mendoza RM, Williams DN. Problems in the management of type III (severe) open fracture: a new classification system of type III open fractures. *J Trauma* 1984;24:742.
5. Tscherne H, Oestern HJ, Sturm J. Osteosynthesis of major fractures in polytrauma. *World J Surg* 1983;7:80.
6. Henry SL, Ostermann PAW, Seligson D. The antibiotic bead pouch technique: the management of severe compound fractures. *Clin Orthop* 1993;295:54.
7. Rodeheaver G, Bellamy W, Kody M, et al. Bactericidal activity and toxicity of iodine-containing solutions in wounds. *Arch Surg* 1982;117:181.
8. Byrd HS, Spicer TE, Cierny G. Management of open tibial fractures. *Plast Reconstr Surg* 1985;76:719.
9. Pitts LH, Rosegay H. Peripheral nerve injury. In: Moore EE, Mattox KL, Feliciano DV, eds. *Trauma*. 2nd ed. East Norwalk, CT: Appleton & Lange, 1989:663–673.
10. Gurdjian ES, Smathers HM. Peripheral nerve injury in fractures and dislocations of long bones. *J Neurosurg* 1945;2:202.
11. Rockwood CA, Thomas SC, Matsen FA. Subluxations and dislocations about the glenohumeral joint. In: Rockwood CA, Green DP, Bucholz RW, eds. *Fractures in adults*. 3rd ed. Philadelphia: JB Lippincott, 1991:1021.
12. Gellman H, Caputo RJ, Carter V, Aboulafia A, McKay M. Comparison of short and long thumb spica casts for non-displaced fractures of the carpal scaphoid. *J Bone Joint Surg Am* 1989;71:354.
13. Bucholz RW, Jones A. Current concepts review: fractures of the shaft of the femur. *J Bone Joint Surg Am* 1991;73:1561.
14. Rosenthal RE. Lower extremity fractures and dislocations. In: Moore EE, Mattox KL, Feliciano DV, eds. *Trauma*. 2nd ed. East Norwalk, CT: Appleton & Lange, 1989:623–638.
15. DeHaven KE, Black KP, Griffiths HT. Open meniscus repair technique and two to nine year results. *Am J Sports Med* 1989;17:788.
16. Saltzman CL, Goulet JA, McClellan RT, Schneider LA, Matthews LS. Results of treatment of displaced patellar fractures by partial patellectomy. *J Bone Joint Surg Am* 1990;72:1279.
17. Georgiadis GM, Behrens FF, Joyce MJ, et al. Open tibial fractures with severe soft tissue loss: limb salvage versus below knee amputation. *J Bone Joint Surg Am* 1993;75:1431.
18. Blick SS, Brumback RJ, Lakatos R, et al. Early prophylactic bone grafting of high energy tibial fractures. *Clin Orthop* 1989;240:21.
19. Paley D, Catagni MA, Argnani F, et al. Ilizarov treatment of tibial nonunion with bone loss. *Clin Orthop* 1989;241:146.
20. Sanders R. Intra-articular fractures of the calcaneus: present state of the art. *J Orthop Trauma* 1992;6:252.
21. Bright RW. Physeal injuries. In: Rockwood CA Jr, Wilkins KE, eds. *Fractures in children.* Philadelphia: JB Lippincott, 1991:87–186.
22. McCoy RL, Dec KL, McKeag DB, Honing EW. Common injuries in the child or adolescent athlete. *Primary Care* 1995;22:117.

32. AMPUTATIONS AFTER TRAUMA[1]

GENERAL CONSIDERATIONS IN THE MANAGEMENT OF MANGLED EXTREMITIES

It can be extremely difficult at times to determine which severely injured extremities to amputate primarily, and which to attempt to save. Nevertheless, in cases of irreparable major peripheral neurologic injury, or severe crush injuries in combination with prolonged ischemia or life-threatening injuries, or both, primary amputation is indicated.

AXIOM One should not attempt to save a marginal limb if it will be of little use to the patient and salvage is achieved only at great cost.

All too often, physicians have considered an amputation a last resort and an acknowledgment of failure; however, in some instances, early amputation is preferred because it can greatly speed up the rehabilitation of severely injured patients. In addition, outcome studies have shown that the quality of life of traumatic below-knee amputees is better than that of many patients with salvaged, but abnormal, limbs (2).

AXIOM Although no prosthesis can ever function as well as a normal extremity, most prostheses function better than painful, insensate limbs.

Before the surgeon embarks on a prolonged series of complicated operations to save a severely injured limb, it should be understood that long hospitalizations and numerous surgeries can have negative medical, economic, social, and psychological effects and can cause a patient to become a disabled, nonproductive citizen. The amount of time lost from work, number of procedures, pain and inconvenience, and final functional outcome of the salvaged limb all should be considered. Independent reviews by other orthopaedic, plastic, and general surgeons, with the aim of establishing a prognosis for successful salvage, may be very useful (3). Ideally, the patient should make the final decision, but this will not always be possible in life-threatening or multiple-trauma situations.

EARLY INDICATIONS FOR AMPUTATION

Management of Completed Amputation

With completed traumatic amputations in older adults, bleeding is controlled, and wound toilet is performed with the aim of producing a useful viable stump; however, in children, a relatively clean, noncrushing accidental amputation, especially of the upper extremity, can often be replanted successfully. Nevertheless, a combination of multiple fractures, nerve disruption, warm ischemia time greater than 6 hours, extensive crush injury involving muscle and skin, or a combination of these is not compatible with restoration of useful function.

Severe IIIC Open Fractures

Quirke et al. (3) found that with type IIIC open extremity fractures (with vascular injuries requiring repair), early revascularization was successful in 13 (93%) of 14; however, contraindications to aggressive attempts at revascularization include

1. Poor patient health before injury;
2. Completely severed limb;
3. Segmental tibial loss greater than 8 cm;
4. Ischemia time greater than 6 hours; and
5. Severance of the posterior tibial nerve.

With severe crush injuries of limbs, hyperbaric oxygen can improve transcutaneous Po_2, and resulted in complete healing in 17 of 18 patients in whom it was used (vs. 10 of 18 when it was not used; $p < 0.01$) (4).

Scoring Systems

General Considerations

A number of scoring systems have been developed in an effort to help predict the need or lack of need for amputation of a severely injured limb (5,6). Each of these scoring systems has its shortcomings. For example, some of them combined mangled upper and lower extremities, even though the salvage implications for these are significantly different. Indeed, preservation of protective sensation, anatomic continuity of major nerves, and avoidance of limb-length discrepancy are of less importance in upper extremities. Furthermore, prosthetic limbs [especially for below-knee amputations (BKAs)] are much more advanced for lower extremities than for upper extremities.

Some studies have used "functional" limb salvage as the end point. Patient motivation, delayed appearance of chronic causalgia or dystrophy, and development of overwhelming infections complicate such attempts at functional assessment, and none of these factors is predictable at the time of the initial evaluation.

The MESS System

The MESS (mangled extremity severity scoring) system developed by Johansen et al. (5) has four components, each with a higher score for less-favorable circumstances (Table 32-1):

1. Skeletal/soft tissue injury with 1 to 4 points;
2. Limb ischemia with 1 to 6 points;

Table 32-1. ***MESS (Mangled Extremity Severity Score) Variables***

A. Skeletal/soft-tissue injury	
Low energy (stab, simple fracture, "civilian" GSW)	1
Medium energy (open or multiple Fxs, dislocation)	2
High energy (close-range shotgun or "military" GSW, crush injury)	3
Very high energy (above + gross contamination, soft-tissue avulsion	4
B. Limb ischemia	
Pulse reduced or absent but perfusion normal	1*
Pulseless, paresthesias, diminished capillary refill	2*
Cool, paralyzed, insensate, numb	3*
C. Shock	
Systolic BP always >90 mm Hg	0
Hypotensive transiently	1
Persistent hypotension	2
D. Age (y)	
<30	0
30–50	1
>50	2

*Score doubled for ischemia >6 h

3. Shock with 0 to 2 points; and
4. Age with 0 to 2 points.

Johansen et al. (5) found in both retrospective and prospective studies that all limbs with a MESS of 6 or less were salvaged, whereas all limbs with a MESS of 7 or higher were amputated.

Protective Neurologic Function

As a general rule, when four of the five main components or structures of a limb—skin, bone, muscles, vessels, nerves—are injured, but there is little or no nerve injury, efforts to reconstruct and salvage the extremity can be considered; however, if is unlikely that the extremity will have any protective sensation, the most prudent course to follow is immediate amputation and early fitting with a prosthesis.

AXIOM If protective nerve function to an extremity is lost, that limb is essentially useless.

A detailed neurologic assessment (e.g., sciatic or brachial plexus) at the time of acute injury may be difficult, especially in patients with impaired levels of consciousness or severe pain and anxiety. It also can be difficult to identify nerve integrity clearly at operation in the presence of severe associated soft-tissue trauma. Under such circumstances, it is advisable to treat the vascular and soft-tissue injuries and defer final assessment of the extent of the nerve injury and the possible reconstruction and recovery of the limb.

Crush Syndrome

In some patients, early amputation may be indicated for a severe life-threatening crush syndrome, which refers to the systemic signs and symptoms resulting from the products of severely damaged tissue entering the circulation. These problems can include sudden severe hyperkalemia with possible arrhythmias and acute oliguric renal failure resulting from myoglobinuria, with or without hemoglobinuria.

Maintenance of a high urine output, at least 100 and preferably 200 mL/h, will help prevent renal failure. Maintaining an alkaline urine by infusing sodium bicarbonate intravenously (1 to 2 mEq/kg/h until the urine pH is 6.5 or higher) increases the urine solubility of myoglobin and hemoglobin and thereby reduces the likelihood of these pigments occluding renal tubules. Alkalemic urine also reduces the formation of ferrihemate, which is toxic to tubule cells.

Later Indications for Amputation

AXIOM Late indications for amputation of a mangled extremity include severe infection, persistent severe causalgia, and severe deformities, resulting in limb dysfunction or repeated skin breakdown.

GENERAL PRINCIPLES

Once a decision to amputate has been made, several principles can help the rehabilitation and return of the patient to an active and productive life (6).

1. The first amputation does need not be definitive, especially if infection is present.
2. One should consider the patient's potential ability to use a prosthesis.
3. One should know the level of residual limb that will allow optimal prosthetic use.
4. Rehabilitation, both mental and physical, begins at the time of amputation.
5. One should not close the amputation wound if infection is present or likely to occur.

AXIOM For best results, an amputation should be considered part of a total rehabilitation program.

Open (Guillotine) Amputations

AXIOM It is generally ill advised to attempt a primary definitive amputation on a severely injured or infected extremity.

If an amputation is an interim life-saving procedure, it is often unwise to approximate the remaining tissues. In particular, one should not close an amputation site if nonviable or contaminated tissue is present.

A guillotine amputation should provide maximal open drainage of the tissues while preserving as much length as possible. The wound should be covered with a sterile dressing. The amputation site is reassessed and debrided as needed at 24- to 48-hour intervals until the wound is clean and stable. At that time, a definitive, closed amputation can be performed.

Closed (Flap) Amputations

In the absence of infection and nonviable tissue, primary closure of the amputation may be performed. The incisions are made to produce two flaps of skin, attempting, except perhaps with above-knee amputations (AKAs), to keep the scar from the end or weight-bearing portion of the stump. The flap with the tougher skin and better blood supply is fashioned longer. Ideally, large arteries and veins should be ligated separately to prevent arteriovenous (A-V) fistula formation. Hemostasis is achieved with fine ligatures. Cautery is avoided as much as possible. The nerves are divided under traction so they will not adhere to the scar and produce stump pain. The deep fascia is sutured to allow proper muscle attachment to the bone and to prevent muscle ends from adhering to the skin.

Ideal Amputation Stumps

Requirements for the ideal amputation stump include

1. The stump must be durable, adequately perfused, and capable of wear over pressure areas.
2. There should be neither neuromas nor increased tenderness at pressure areas.
3. Bone should be covered with muscle or fascia without residual prominent spicules or protuberances.
4. Proximal joints should retain full mobility with strong balanced muscle action.
5. The length and shape of the stump should allow placement into a prosthetic socket and application of sufficient leverage to produce motion without the stump disengaging or "popping out."

AXIOM Exercise to strengthen and prevent contracture of the muscles of the extremity at the amputation site should be begun early, even before the extremity has healed completely.

SPECIFIC AMPUTATIONS

Lower-Extremity Amputations

The main goals in rehabilitation of the patient with a lower-extremity amputation include

1. Preservation of the knee, whenever possible;
2. Salvage of an end-weight-bearing stump; and
3. Reliance, if possible, on full-thickness covering of the stump.

The energy cost of walking for lower-extremity amputees is many times greater with AKAs than with BKAs.

AXIOM With amputations, every effort should be made to salvage a functional knee or elbow.

Digital (Toe) Amputations

Toe amputation is indicated when gangrene, infection, or unreconstructable trauma is limited to a digit distal to the metatarsophalangeal joint. In patients with proximal vascular disease or trauma, distal perfusion pressures should be determined (7). An ankle–brachial systolic blood pressure (BP) index (ABI) below 0.45 (0.55 to 0.60 in a diabetic) generally indicates that perfusion will not be adequate to heal an open wound.

Amputations of the four lesser toes generally cause little disturbance of gait. Amputation of the great toe produces loss of push-off strength and causes instability of the medial longitudinal arch of the foot, but routine gait is fairly normal (8).

Transmetatarsal (Forefoot) Amputations

With transmetatarsal amputations, some spring and resilience of the foot is lost, but there is little disability in routine gait, and a good plantar flap is necessary. It is the highest level of amputation at which no special prosthesis is required.

Midfoot Amputations (Lisfranc's, Chopart's, Boyd's, Pirogoff's)

Midfoot amputations have the advantage of preserving length and a weight-bearing stump. They are used infrequently in trauma settings because of other damage in the injured foot and the problem of equinus deformity (9). Lisfranc's amputation is performed at the tarsometatarsal level, and Chopart's amputation is performed at the midtarsal joint. Boyd's amputation involves talectomy and calcaneotibial fusion. Pirogoff's amputation involves calcaneotibial fusion after rotation and vertical sectioning of the calcaneus (Fig. 32-1).

Syme's Amputation (Ankle Disarticulation)

AXIOM Syme's amputation is considered a reasonable alternative to BKA if there is a good heel pad to use as a base.

Syme's amputation involves disarticulation of the ankle with preservation of the heel pad. Unlike a classic BKA, it offers an end-bearing stump. It may be attempted whenever the talus and calcaneus and the overlying soft tissue are normal. The major advantage is that short distances (such as to the bathroom at night) can be covered without the necessity of a prosthesis. It can also provide a better cosmetic result in female patients than a BKA.

One of the biggest problems with Syme's amputation is excessive mobility of the heel pad; however, immediate application of a short-leg cast after surgery can decrease the incidence and severity of this problem.

Below-Knee Amputations

When an amputation must be performed above the ankle, the site should generally provide a stump that extends 5 to 7 inches below the knee joint. Longer stumps are more difficult to fit to a prosthesis. With this amputation, it is possible for many rehabilitated persons to achieve an active lifestyle (2). In doubtful cases, the "gamble" to preserve a below-knee stump is usually worthwhile; however, one should, if possible, avoid wounds or skin grafts lying on the anterior border of the tibia.

In the absence of significant contamination or a marginal stump in patients who are candidates for a prosthesis, some surgeons prefer immediate casting and appli-

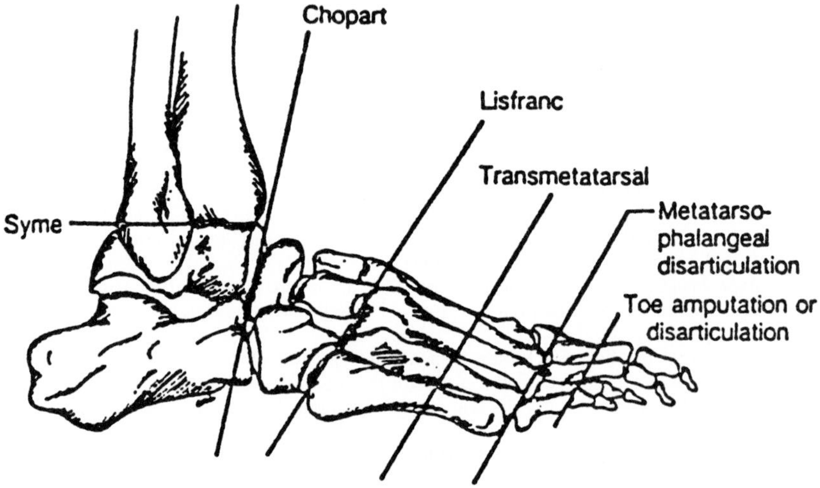

FIG. 32-1. Midfoot amputation sites. With amputation through the metatarsal-tarsal joint, one should try to preserve the insertion of the tibialis anterior on the medial cuneiform and distal first metatarsal to allow dorsiflexion at the ankle. Chopart's amputation at the junction of the tarsal bones and the talus and calcaneus is rarely used now. From ref. 10, with permission.

cation of a prosthesis with early ambulation. This can greatly speed the patient's mental, psychological, and physical rehabilitation.

Through-Knee Amputations

Amputations through the knee joint are unpopular with many prosthetists because the added length of femur hinders construction of a cosmetically pleasing functional knee prosthesis. Many prosthetists prefer an above-knee stump that provides adequate space for the knee-joint mechanism and thus provides a better cosmetic and functional result; however, amputation through the knee provides a weight-bearing stump that is functionally superior to an AKA.

Above-Knee Amputations

Above-knee amputation should be reserved for patients who have one or more of the following:

1. Traumatic amputations above the level of the knee;
2. Frank gangrene extending above the knee; or
3. Documented lack of ambulation before the injury.

The optimal length is approximately two thirds the length of the femoral shaft, as measured from the greater trochanter. This is approximately 35 to 40 cm in the average individual. If circumstances dictate a more proximal amputation, a femur length of 10 to 12 cm from the greater trochanter is the shortest that allows use of a conventional prosthesis. Shorter stumps require the use of the cumbersome "tilting table" prosthesis. If ambulation is not thought likely, midfemur amputation provides better healing than more distal sites.

Hip Disarticulation

True hip disarticulation is rarely required in the trauma patient except with severe avulsions in pedestrian accidents or when a patient develops a severe necrotizing infection. Even when disarticulation of the hip seems necessary, one should still try to make do with a high AKA. The femoral head and proximal femur also should be retained whenever possible because they help preserve buttock contour and provide for better sitting balance and comfort.

Upper-Limb Amputations

General Principles

Weight bearing is not an issue in upper-extremity amputation stumps, and one can use residual unconventionally based flaps to obtain soft-tissue cover of bone ends. It is, however, important to have protective sensation. Partial-thickness skin grafts should be avoided whenever possible because of their friability.

Wrist Disarticulation

If the hand is unreconstructable, preservation of any part of the wrist confers no advantage because the added length makes prosthetic fitting difficult.

Forearm Amputations

Amputations through the forearm are performed with the extremity in supination. The optimal length is at the junction of the middle and distal thirds of the forearm. This allows adequate leverage and space to accommodate the usual prosthesis. In addition, there is sufficient muscle at this level to provide good soft-tissue coverage of the bone ends.

Above-Elbow Amputations

AXIOM The primary concerns with above-elbow amputations are obtaining healing and preserving shoulder function.

The optimal length of humerus to accommodate a prosthetic elbow is provided by an amputation site about 9 cm above the medial and lateral humeral epicondyles. The shortest stump that will allow some useful function with a prosthesis is 6 cm below the anterior axillary fold.

On occasion, it may prove necessary to amputate proximal to the ideal prosthesis level. Under these circumstances, it is important not to disarticulate the humerus, but to divide the bone through its neck. This preserves the shoulder contour and enables the patient to wear a cosmetic prosthesis with some comfort.

IMMEDIATE POSTSURGICAL PROSTHESIS

The term "immediate postsurgical prosthesis fitting" is usually synonymous with BKAs because (a) BKAs are the most common type of amputations in which this technique is used, (b) the rigid dressing is easiest to apply at this level, and (c) early ambulation is best achieved in the below-knee amputee. After the amputation is completed, a rigid dressing is applied to the stump, and then a walking pylon is added to the dressing in the operating room.

Many highly motivated patients can begin crutch walking the night of surgery. By the first or second postoperative day, all patients are encouraged to begin crutch walking, applying up to 25 pounds of weight bearing on the amputated side. By the fifth day, they are walking between parallel bars and progressively increasing the amount of weight bearing.

COMPLICATIONS OF AMPUTATIONS

Infected amputation sites with gross pus should be opened as soon as possible for incision, drainage, and debridement as needed. Other local complications after amputation include wound hematomas and skin necrosis, which may require reoperation. Later stump problems may include neuromas, phantom pain, chronic sores or stump pain, and problems with prosthetic fit, which may require formal late stump revision.

With any late amputation on a nonfunctional extremity, especially the leg, deep venous thrombosis (DVT) is often present. If DVT is present, some anticoagulation or an inferior vena cava filter or both should be considered before surgery.

⊘ FREQUENT ERRORS

1. ***Making exceptional efforts to salvage a marginal, nonfunctional extremity, particularly in an elderly individual.***
2. ***Performing a definitive amputation (i.e., closing the skin) on a badly mangled or infected extremity.***
3. ***Delaying physical therapy and rehabilitation of a patient with an amputation.***

SUMMARY POINTS

1. One should not attempt to salvage a severely injured limb if it will be of little use to the patient and if salvage is achieved only at great cost.
2. Although no prosthesis can ever function as well as a normal extremity, most prostheses function better than painful or insensate limbs.
3. Scoring systems for determining need for primary amputation of mangled extremities provide only guidelines, not mandates.
4. A badly injured lower extremity with division of the sciatic or posterior tibial nerve in adults should have immediate amputation.
5. Severe tissue damage with a warm ischemia time exceeding 6 hours as a result of vascular injury is generally an indication for a primary amputation.
6. Late indications for amputation of a mangled extremity include severe infection, persistent severe causalgia, and severe deformities resulting in limb dysfunction or repeated skin breakdown.
7. For best results, an amputation should be considered as part of a total rehabilitation program.
8. During the initial surgery, a guillotine or open amputation should generally be performed at the most distal level at which tissues are assessed to be viable, but not where a definitive (closed) amputation would be made.
9. Exercises to strengthen and prevent contracture of the muscles of the extremity at the amputation site should be begun early, even before the extremity has healed completely.
10. With amputations, every effort should be made to salvage a functional knee or elbow.
11. A good plantar flap is necessary for a useful transmetatarsal amputation.
12. Rehabilitation with a below-knee prosthesis is much better than with an above-knee prosthesis, which requires much more energy to operate.
13. One should make a great effort to keep below-knee amputation incisions away from pressure and weight-bearing areas.
14. It is worthwhile to attempt to preserve the knee in "doubtful" cases in young trauma victims.
15. The primary concerns with above-elbow amputations are obtaining healing and preserving shoulder function.

REFERENCES

1. Wilson RF, Georgiadis GM. Amputation after trauma. In: Wilson RF, Walt AJ, eds. *Management of trauma: pitfalls and practice.* 2nd ed. Philadelphia: Williams & Wilkins, 1996:672.
2. Georgiadis GM, Behrens FF, Joyce MJ, et al. Open tibial fractures with severe soft-tissue loss: limb salvage compared with below-the-knee amputation. *J Bone Joint Surg Am* 1993;75:1431.

3. Quirke TE, Sharma PK, Boss WK, et al. Are type IIIC lower extremity injuries an indication for primary amputation? *J Trauma* 1996;40:992.
4. Bouachour G, Cronier P, Gouello JP, et al. Hyperbaric oxygen therapy in the management of crush injuries: a randomized double-blind placebo-controlled clinical trial. *J Trauma* 1996;41:333.
5. Johansen K, Daines M, Howey T, et al. Objective criteria accurately predict amputation following lower extremity trauma. *J Trauma* 1990;30:568.
6. Kirkpatrick JR, Wilson RF. Amputations following trauma. In: Walt AJ, Wilson RF, eds. *Management of trauma: pitfalls and practice*. Philadelphia: Lea & Febiger, 1975:270–284.
7. Schwartz JA, Schuler JJ, O'Connor RJA, et al. Predictive value of distal perfusion pressure in healing of the digits and the forefoot. *Surg Gynecol Obstet* 1982;154: 865.
8. Mann RA, Poppen NK, O'Konski M. Amputation of the great toe: a clinical and biomechanical study. *Clin Orthop* 1988;226:192.
9. Lieberman JF, Jacobs RL, Goldstock L. Chopart amputation with percutaneous heel cord lengthening. *Clin Orthop* 1993;296:86.
10. Robbs JV. Amputation for trauma. In: Champion HR, Robbs JV, Trunkey DD, eds. *Rob and Smith's operative surgery: trauma surgery, part 2*. London: Butterworth, 1989:599.

33. COMPARTMENT SYNDROME[1]

INTRODUCTION

Definition

Compartment syndrome was defined by Matsen as "a condition in which increased pressure within a limited space compromises the circulation and function of the tissues within that space" (2). Although compartment syndrome may occur anywhere that muscles are enclosed by fascia, it is most common in the lower leg. The forearm is the next most common site, and the thigh is a distant third (3). There has also been increasing awareness of abdominal compartment syndrome (4).

Etiology

Most compartment syndromes are associated with fractures and related bleeding or muscle damage. Compartment syndromes also can be seen with any condition that interferes with blood flow to muscle enclosed within a fascial space (5).

Lower Extremity

Compartment syndrome of the lower leg is most frequent and most severe in the anterior compartment. It is particularly likely to occur after fractures of the tibia, combined arterial and venous injuries at the knee, prolonged compression, or severe muscle contusions.

Patman et al. (6) reported a compartment syndrome incidence of 32% with arterial injuries and 14% with venous injuries. In our own experience, at least 50% of combined popliteal artery and vein injuries have required a fasciotomy (2). Abouezzi et al. (8), in a recent reappraisal of the indications for fasciotomy after extremity vascular trauma, found that fasciotomy was performed for 30% of their isolated arterial injuries, 15% of their isolated venous injuries, and 32% of combined arterial and venous injuries. The incidence of compartment syndrome was not related to venous repair or ligation; however, the highest incidence of fasciotomy was for combined popliteal artery and vein injuries (61%).

AXIOM The incidence of compartment syndrome is often higher with open tibial fractures than with closed fractures.

The incidence of compartment syndrome with open tibial fractures has been reported to be between 6% and 9% (7), whereas the incidence in closed fractures has been reported to be about 1%. The true incidence may be much higher, especially because some of the late sequelae of compartment syndrome in the leg can be quite subtle and may include varying degrees of joint stiffness, claw toes, and cavus or equinus deformities.

Other problems that can cause compartment syndrome include infection, inadvertent intraarterial injection of drugs, and localized pressure by casts, circular dressings, burn eschar, or pneumatic antishock garments (PASGs). A report of 27 cases of compartment syndrome after application of a PASG suggests that systemic hypotension and increased external pressure may be important factors in etiology (9).

Watson and Kelikian (10) noted that although the ankle-traction Thomas splint can effectively control femur fractures for patient transport, vigilant monitoring of the neurovascular status of the leg and periodic relief of the cuff are essential. The cuff of an ankle-traction Thomas splint can further compromise arterial inflow to the foot, resulting in ischemia or compartment syndrome or both.

Upper Extremity

Development of compartment syndrome in the upper extremities, especially the forearm, has been attributed to a multitude of causes including supracondylar fractures, fractures of the forearm, brachial artery puncture for arterial blood gases or for arteriography, subfascial intravenous infiltrations, hemophilia, crush injuries, drug overdose, replantations, and gunshot wounds (3). The deep volar compartment of the forearm is particularly vulnerable because it is nourished by the anterior interosseous artery, which has no significant collateral flow.

Abdominal Compartment Syndrome

An abdominal compartment syndrome (ACS) exists when there is abdominal organ dysfunction because of increased intraabdominal pressure. The most frequent causes of increased intraabdominal pressure are ruptured aortic aneurysms and intraabdominal bleeding. Diebel et al. (11) showed that intraabdominal pressures more than 20 to 30 mm Hg can drastically reduce renal, hepatic, and intestinal mucosal blood flow. Of 2,500 intensive care unit (ICU) admissions during a 6-year period, Widergren and Battistella (12) reported on 46 patients with abdominal compartment syndrome. The overall mortality was 41%. The most important physiologic changes occurring after relieving the intraabdominal pressure were a decline in peak inspiratory pressure from 52 ± 12 to 44 ± 11 cm H_2O and an increase in the P_aO_2/FIO_2 ratio from 159 ± 105 to 215 ± 119 mm Hg.

PATHOPHYSIOLOGY

Ischemia and Reperfusion

Ischemic or damaged muscle and other tissues tend to swell. If the muscle or tissue is confined to a tight fascial space, the resultant increased intracompartmental pressure can retard venous return and capillary blood flow, causing even more ischemia.

Ames et al. (13) described the "no-reflow phenomenon" occurring after a period of severe ischemia. Although there is a transient period of increased perfusion to most tissues, over the next 30 to 60 minutes after the circulation is restored, subsequent blood flow to the ischemic tissues may decrease almost to zero. They ascribed the delayed but progressively worse hypoperfusion to narrowing of the lumens of arterioles and capillaries by various factors including swollen endothelial cells. This group also demonstrated a secondary type of capillary narrowing associated with formation of intravascular blebs on the capillary endothelium. More recent studies showed that clumps of leukocytes also can plug capillaries after prolonged hemorrhagic shock (14).

AXIOM Cessation of capillary blood flow can occur at tissue pressures of 20 to 30 mm Hg, which is much less than normal arterial pressure.

Reperfusion injury plays a major role in many cases of compartment syndrome, and compartment pressure often begins to increase precipitately only after the blood supply has been reestablished in ischemic muscles.

Some of the accelerated tissue changes with reperfusion may result from the formation of increased quantities of free radicals. These free radicals can cause lipid peroxidation of cell membranes and other intracellular and extracellular structures.

AXIOM Partial ischemia (with blood flows less than 30% of normal) is capable of causing more cell damage than that caused by complete ischemia (15). Partial ischemia prevents adequate adenosine triphosphate (ATP) production for normal cell function, but it provides enough oxygen to allow the formation of free radicals.

Compartmental Perfusion Pressure

Heppenstall et al. (16) emphasized the importance of the compartmental perfusion pressure (CPP), which is the mean arterial blood pressure (mBP) minus the compartment pressures (CP). An increasing CP and decreasing systemic pressure can quickly reduce the CPP to ischemic levels. Perfusion pressures to muscles that might be developing compartment syndrome should be kept above 70 to 80 mm Hg, if possible, without causing fluid overload.

The Vicious Cycle

Holden (17) suggested that the "vicious cycle" of compartment syndromes begins with vascular damage or tissue hemorrhage. Vascular damage causes ischemia and increased intracellular and interstitial edema, and this plus any tissue hemorrhage increases local pressure and reduces capillary blood flow. The enclosed muscle becomes ischemic and swells even more, further reducing compartment blood flow. As the vicious cycle continues, intracompartment pressures become higher and higher, and tissue ischemia gets worse and worse.

⊘ PITFALL

Failure to consider the possible need for a fasciotomy on an extremity that has had severe blunt trauma, prolonged ischemia, or compression can lead to delayed diagnosis of compartment syndrome.

DIAGNOSIS

Clinical Examination

History

A history of severe trauma to the lower leg, thigh, or forearm should raise suspicion of a compartment syndrome, particularly if fractures were present and if blood flow to the muscles in those areas was reduced for prolonged periods by hypovolemia, proximal vessel injury, or external pressure.

The earliest symptoms and signs of compartment syndrome in the extremities are increasing pain and paresthesias. The pain from an early compartment syndrome is often more severe than one would expect from the injury, and it continues to get worse despite increased narcotic use and splinting. Paresthesias are subtle but important early symptoms, because the sensory nerves in a compartment are especially sensitive to ischemia. A proximal nerve injury or an unconscious patient may mask both these symptoms. Distinguishing ischemic pain from the pain of muscle injury, fracture, or contusion, however, can be extremely difficult at times.

AXIOM The most characteristic symptom of developing compartment syndrome is deep, throbbing, unrelenting pain that is usually much greater than expected from the physical signs (2).

Physical Examination

Increased tenseness and swelling of the muscles in question can be helpful signs. However, these are subjective and may be relatively late signs in the leg because they primarily assess the superficial posterior compartment, and this is the least likely compartment to be involved.

AXIOM Palpable distal pulses do not rule out the presence of compartment syndrome.

A crushed, swollen, painful hand held in an intrinsic minus position (metacarpophalangeal joints in extension and interphalangeal joints in flexion) plus pain on passive abduction and adduction of the fingers suggest the presence of interosseous compartment syndrome in the hand (18).

Serial Examinations Versus Prophylactic Fasciotomy

In patients requiring major vascular surgery, the prolonged anesthesia can make physical examination unreliable for several hours after surgery. After recovery from anesthesia, the clinical findings may be obvious, requiring a second anesthetic for fasciotomy.

Feliciano et al. (19) emphasized this fact and pointed out that 19% of the fasciotomies performed at Houston's Ben Taub Hospital were done at reoperation. In certain patients who are at continued risk for 24 to 48 hours after surgery, careful and continuous monitoring may be impractical or impossible, and prophylactic fasciotomies may be indicated. Prophylactic fasciotomies are recommended if

1. Arterial supply to a limb is interrupted for more than 4 to 6 hours;
2. Patient is unconscious or has peripheral nerve injuries; or
3. Open fracture reduction is being carried out near a compartment at risk.

Signs of Ischemia

⊘ PITFALL

Not diagnosing compartment syndromes until the "seven Ps" of ischemia are present causes unnecessary time lost until treatment is begun.

The findings associated with compartment syndromes or ischemia have been described as the seven Ps. These include

1. Increased compartment pressure;
2. Pulselessness, usually a very late sign of compartment syndrome;
3. Paresis or paralysis;
4. Paresthesias or anesthesia;
5. Loss of a normal pink color;
6. Pain, especially with stretch; and
7. Poikilothermia (coolness).

It can be difficult at times to distinguish between compartment syndrome, arterial injury, and nerve injury. These conditions frequently coexist, and all three problems may have associated motor or sensory deficits and pain. Arterial injury is usually associated with absent pulses, whereas patients with compartment syndrome usually have intact peripheral pulses, at least initially. Nerve injuries often cause relatively little pain. Nevertheless, Doppler flow determinations or arteriography and compartment-pressure measurements may be required to differentiate between these three conditions.

Neuromuscular Function

In the leg, the deep peroneal (anterior tibial) nerve runs the length of the anterior compartment. It innervates the muscles of that compartment and supplies sensation to the dorsal web space between the first and second toes. When checking for extension of the toes, active effort at extension must be confirmed by feeling the tightened tendons of the extensor hallucis longus and extensor digitorum longus muscles.

The superficial peroneal (musculocutaneous) nerve traverses the lateral compartment and innervates the peroneus longus and brevis muscles, which pronates (abducts and everts) and plantar flexes the foot. It also supplies sensation to the dorsum of the foot, except for the first web space.

The tibial nerve lies within the deep posterior compartment of the calf and supplies motor branches to the posterior muscles of the lower leg and sensation to the plantar surface of the foot. Because the deep posterior compartment is smaller and less accessible, its involvement can be missed very easily.

The superficial posterior compartment is the largest compartment of the lower leg, and it is the least likely to be involved in a compartment syndrome. The sural nerve traverses the proximal portion of this compartment and perforates the fascia to supply sensation to the lateral border of the foot. It has no muscular branches.

Laboratory Evaluation

Severely increased levels of creatine phosphokinase (CPK) often reflect severe muscle trauma or ischemia. High levels that continue to increase suggest increasing muscle ischemia, as in compartment syndromes; however, CPK levels may decline after there is complete loss of circulation to an involved compartment.

Compartment Pressures

AXIOM Measurement of compartment pressure is the most accurate technique for diagnosing compartment syndrome, especially in the early phases when a fasciotomy produces the best results.

In the Extremities

Patman described the use of a central venous pressure manometer, which is filled with sterile saline and attached to an extension tube and a regular 18-gauge needle that is inserted directly into the compartment in question, with the extremity positioned level with the heart (20). The manometer is positioned so that initially the top of its fluid level is slightly below the compartment being tested. The stopcock is then opened and the manometer gradually raised until the meniscus falls. Matsen proposed using a small-needle catheter with a continuous slow infusion for long-term surveillance (2).

Development of a solid-state transducer small enough to fit in a catheter tip has simplified measurements of compartment pressures. This hand-held, inexpensive solid-state transducer allows rapid, repeatable, or continuous pressure monitoring (2).

Measuring Intraabdominal Pressure

To measure intraabdominal pressure, one can use a nasogastric tube, but a Foley catheter in the urinary bladder is usually preferred. The usual technique, first described by Kron et al. (21) in 1984, involves clamping the Foley catheter just distal to the aspiration port. A variable amount of sterile saline (30 to 90 mL) is then instilled into the urinary bladder via a needle in the catheter proximal to the clamp on the collection tubing. The needle is then connected to an electric transducer or a filled water manometer with the midaxillary line of the patient or the pubic tubercle as the zero point. The water level in the manometer falls until the pressure in the bladder (which is essentially the same as the intraabdominal pressure) equals the pressure reflected by the water level in the manometer.

INITIAL MANAGEMENT TO PREVENT COMPARTMENT SYNDROME

Any vascular problem causing distal ischemia must be corrected promptly. Warm ischemia time must be kept to a minimum, preferably less than 3 to 4 hours. Cardiac output and BP should be kept at the upper limits of normal or slightly higher to maintain the best possible collateral circulation.

AXIOM If any evidence of ischemia persists distal to a fracture after attempts at traction or closed reduction, immediate arteriography or surgical exploration is indicated.

AXIOM One should look for compartment syndrome in any patient who has had external compression or a PASG inflated for more than 30 minutes.

Although BP and cardiac output should be kept at levels slightly to moderately above normal to maintain optimal perfusion to injured or ischemic tissues, one should not overhydrate the patient. In patients treated with diuretics, compartment pressures have fallen about 25% over 24 hours, with a 40% decrease by the third day (24).

TREATMENT OF COMPARTMENT SYNDROMES

If compartment syndrome is suspected, one should remove any potential constricting circumferential dressing (i.e., release or bivalve circular bandages or casts).

AXIOM If compartment pressures are marginally increased, hypotension can cause severe ischemic damage to the intracompartmental muscles.

Fasciotomy

Indications for Fasciotomy

Prophylactic Fasciotomy

Many surgeons believe that a prophylactic fasciotomy should be carried out, even if the patient can be monitored closely, when

1. There has been a significant delay between the onset of ischemia or injury and reperfusion;
2. There has been prolonged hypotension;
3. Massive tissue swelling occurs before or during the operative procedure;
4. There is combined proximal arterial and venous injury;
5. The major veins in the popliteal area or distal thigh are ligated; or
6. There is a severe crush injury.

AXIOM In patients with a warm ischemia time of more than 4 to 6 hours distal to a vascular injury, a fasciotomy should be performed before the vascular repair.

Using Compartment Pressures

Muscle compartment pressures in the leg are normally about 5 to 10 mm Hg. With absent or equivocal clinical signs, Patman and others (20) suggested that fasciotomy be performed if the pressure exceeds 40 mm Hg. There is no consensus regarding these measurements, and Matsen et al. (2) described patients in whom compartment pressure exceeded 40 mm Hg, yet no untoward effects resulted from continued observation. We agree with Perry et al. (22) that compartment pressures greater than 30 mm Hg, when associated with appropriate clinical findings, are a firm indication for fasciotomy, yet totally asymptomatic, alert, and cooperative patients with compartment pressures of 30 to 40 mm Hg can probably continue to be observed without fasciotomy (3). Based on animal studies, Heckman et al. (23) suggested that fasciotomies be performed if compartment pressures increase to a level that is within 10 to 20 mm Hg of the diastolic BP.

AXIOM If unequivocal signs of compartment syndrome are present, one should proceed with fasciotomy without waiting for measurements of compartment pressures.

Abdomen

AXIOM A decline in urine output in spite of normal or higher cardiac output and BP after abdominal trauma or a laparotomy or both should make one suspect an abdominal compartment syndrome.

If measured intraabdominal pressures are 20 mm Hg or higher and there is oliguria in spite of a good BP and cardiac output, the abdomen should be opened. If intraabdominal pressure is greater than 30 mm Hg, one should probably open the abdomen even if the urine output has been relatively well maintained.

Techniques of Fasciotomy

Lower Leg

Most authorities suggest that a four-compartment fasciotomy should be performed in the calf in almost all patients with suspected compartment syndrome, even though the symptoms, signs, or increased pressures may be confined to the anterior compartment (Fig. 33-1).

Fibulectomy Fasciotomy. Some surgeons favor doing a four-compartment fasciotomy in the lower leg through a single incision anterolaterally with excision of the mid and upper shaft of the fibula (25). Removing most of the shaft of the upper fibula plus its periosteum and fascial connections provides relatively good decompression of all four compartments.

Single-Incision Fasciotomy Without Fibulectomy. Rollins et al. (26) described a single incision four-compartment fasciotomy without fibulectomy. This involves a long lateral skin incision made directly over the fibula, extending from just below the neck of the fibula to a point 3 to 4 cm above the lateral malleolus. The dissection then continues in back of the fibula into all four fascial compartments.

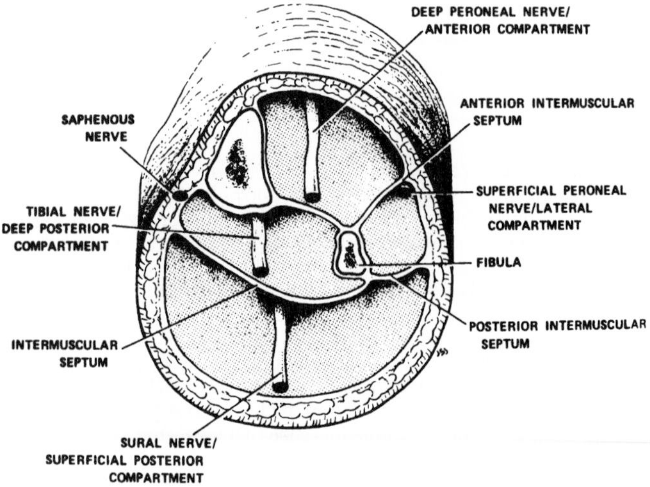

FIG. 33-1. Cross section at junction of middle and distal thirds of the leg, illustrating the four fascial compartments and their respective nerves. From ref. 27, with permission.

Two-Incision Fasciotomy. Most trauma surgeons use the two-incision, four-compartment fasciotomy popularized by Mubarak and Owen (27) because it can be performed quickly and safely. Although it is often possible to decompress all four compartments fairly well through limited skin incisions, the skin itself can sometimes cause significant constriction, and a small incision does not allow one adequately to evaluate the entire muscle mass within those compartments.

AXIOM The skin incisions for decompressive fasciotomies should be long enough to ensure that none of the underlying muscle is still compressed.

The anterior and lateral compartments are exposed by an anterolateral incision that begins between the fibular shaft and the crest of the tibia at midleg level. The intermuscular septum is identified by making a transverse incision through the fascia. The compartments are then released by longitudinal incisions with scissors.

AXIOM During anterior and lateral compartment fasciotomies, the superficial peroneal nerve should be visualized to avoid injuring it.

The superficial and deep posterior compartment can be decompressed through a posteromedial incision approximately 2 to 3 cm posterior to the posterior margin of the tibia. The greater saphenous vein and nerve can usually be protected by keeping them with the tissues anterior to the incision.

The superficial posterior compartment is decompressed first. The posterior fasciotomy should extend the entire length of the compartment proximally and distally to a point near the medial malleolus.

The deep posterior compartment is released distally and then proximally under the soleus. If the soleus muscle is attached to the tibia, this attachment has to be released to enter the deep posterior compartment. Occasionally the soleus muscle extends almost to the ankle, completely covering the fascia of the deep posterior compartment. In such cases, the deep posterior compartment will not be decompressed until the soleus is freed from the back of the tibia.

Response to Decompression. After decompression of a compartment, it is useful to quantify and document the changes in compartment pressures, thereby verifying adequate decompression.

Thigh

Compartment syndromes in the thigh are unusual except with severe crushing injuries. A fracture of the femur is often present, and this can cause loss of more than 1 to 2 L of blood into the deep tissues.

In most instances, only the quadriceps compartment must be decompressed in the thigh, but the adductor and flexor compartment pressures also should be checked and monitored.

Foot

Patients with calcaneus fractures or other severe foot trauma can develop foot compartment syndromes. Surgical techniques for decompression typically involve dorsal or medial incisions or both (28).

Forearm

In the forearm, the volar and dorsal compartments are the major confined areas. The compartment containing the mobile wad, which includes the brachioradialis and extensor carpi radialis longus and brevis muscles, can usually be approached through the volar incision (Fig. 33-2).

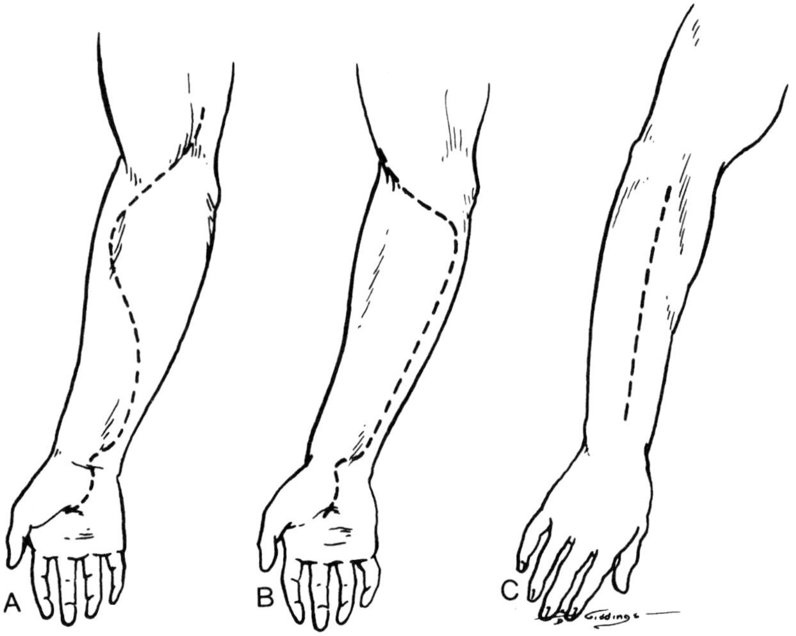

FIG. 33-2. Fasciotomy incisions in the forearm. **A:** Volar fasciotomy incision. **B:** Volar–ulnar fasciotomy incision. **C:** Dorsal fasciotomy incision. From ref. 31, with permission.

Volar Incision. The volar incision for decompressing the muscle compartments of the forearm begins proximal to the antecubital fossa and extends to the midpalm. The incision allows division of the volar and brachial fascia and the transverse carpal ligament, as well as exposure of the arteries and nerves of the forearm and the mobile wad (29). The incision is generally in the form of a "lazy" double S. It should start near the medial epicondyle at the elbow and then course distally and obliquely toward the pronator teres insertion at the radial margin of the forearm at the junction of the middle and proximal thirds. The incision should then gently curve back toward the ulnar border of the forearm at the junction of the distal and middle thirds of the forearm. Then it gently curves in a radial direction again to the midportion of the wrist flexion crease and into the palm.

Skin flaps are then raised, and a complete fasciotomy of all compartments is performed from elbow to wrist. The superficial flexors are decompressed, and then the space between the flexor carpi ulnaris and the flexor digitorum sublimis is opened to expose the deep flexor compartment muscles. Some believe that the individual muscles within each compartment also should be decompressed.

Some surgeons believe that the median and ulnar nerves should also be carefully explored and freed from any constrictions when performing a fasciotomy.

Dorsal Incision. If it is necessary to open the dorsal compartment, this is usually done through a separate longitudinal incision directly over the extensor muscles. The dorsal skin incision begins 2 cm lateral and 2 cm distal to the lateral epicondyle, and extends approximately 10 cm distally toward the wrist. The skin edges are undermined and the dorsal fascia incised throughout the length of the forearm. Individual muscles are freed as needed.

Hand

There is some controversy over the need for decompressing the hand if there is forearm compartment syndrome; however, if there is any question about the status of the hand, the volar incision in the forearm should be extended into the palm, and the carpal tunnel should be released. In addition, the four interosseous muscle compartments should be opened via incisions on the dorsum of the hand over the second and fourth metacarpals (18).

Abdomen

When the abdomen has been closed tightly to control a coagulopathy, the patient should be rapidly warmed to a core temperature of 35°C or higher. The platelet count, plasma thromboplastin (PT), and partial thromboplastin times (PTT) also should be corrected with infusions of platelet concentrates or fresh frozen plasma or both as needed before reopening the abdomen.

Ideally, the abdomen should be opened in the operating room (OR) so that any residual bleeding sites can be controlled with cautery or ligatures. The bowel is then protected with moist rayon or nylon, and moist dressings are applied and held in place with retention sutures or with an abdominal binder over the dressings.

Debridement of Nonviable Tissue

All obviously necrotic or nonviable tissue should be removed at the time of fasciotomy. Tissue that looks relatively healthy and bleeds when cut but does not contract when stimulated can probably be left behind, but it must be examined carefully, preferably in the OR, at least every 24 to 48 hours.

AXIOM If the patient is becoming septic, any marginally ischemic tissue should be removed.

Postfasciotomy Care

Fasciotomy incisions are packed open with saline-soaked dressings and covered with a dry, bulky bandage. The limb is kept elevated. If there is any question about muscle viability, the wound is examined carefully in the OR every 24 to 48 hours.

Patients requiring a fasciotomy should be given broad-spectrum antibiotics at the time of the procedure, and for at least 24 to 48 hours after surgery, especially if any marginally viable tissue is present. Although some believe that the incidence of infection may be reduced if the fasciotomy incisions are closed early, early closure may cause death of additional tissue if the closure is tight and there is any residual marginally ischemic muscle.

Once the edema resolves, which usually takes at least 5 to 10 days, a delayed primary closure can be accomplished in most patients. If the skin edges have been widely separated, the large central portion of the fasciotomy wound may require a split-thickness skin graft.

AXIOM Early physical therapy is essential to prevent contractures after a fasciotomy.

After fasciotomy, passive and active exercises with the leg or arm elevated are maintained throughout convalescence to ensure joint mobility and to improve venous and lymphatic drainage. If a split-thickness skin graft is applied, the exercises are discontinued for 5 to 7 days and then reinstituted.

Complications of Fasciotomy

Proponents of fasciotomy for the treatment of compartment syndromes stress the importance of providing decompression before tissue death occurs. If muscle dies because of a delay in treatment and then is exposed by a fasciotomy, infection is almost certain to develop unless adequate debridement is obtained.

Accidental injury to nerves is always a risk when performing fasciotomies. On occasion, causalgia follows compartment syndrome, but this is usually a result of the initial trauma or ischemic nerve damage rather than operative injury during the fasciotomy.

Some patients have viable muscle but become disabled because of neuropraxia from the initial injury, the compartment syndrome, or fasciotomy. This usually resolves over 2 to 3 months; in the meantime, these patients need optimal physical therapy to prevent muscle atrophy and contracture.

Adjunctive Therapy

The major, immediate complications of compartment syndrome result from the presence of devitalized muscle and include hyperkalemia and renal failure (secondary to myoglobinuria). In patients with hyperkalemia or myoglobinuria or both, restoration of normal or increased blood volume and administration of mannitol to enhance urine flow to at least 100 to 200 mL/h are important to improve renal blood flow and urine output and thereby increase potassium excretion and prevent acute renal failure. Alkalinization of the urine to a pH of at least 6.5 with intravenous sodium bicarbonate (0.5 to 2.0 mEq/min) may help prevent the precipitation of myoglobin within the renal tubules. Alkalinization can also help to reduce serum potassium levels if arrhythmias develop because of hyperkalemia; one also can administer calcium gluconate and glucose and insulin.

Buchbinder et al. (30) demonstrated that the reperfusion syndrome can be prevented in some patients by the administration of mannitol. The salutary effects of mannitol were initially thought to be a result of osmotic activity, but it is now clear that mannitol also is a potent scavenger of toxic hydroxyl ions. Other scavengers of free radicals (superoxide dismutase, catalase, and dimethyl sulfoxide) may also be of some benefit in the treatment of compartment syndromes.

Problems with Inadequate or Delayed Treatment

The final clinical state of the untreated limb with compartment syndrome is a replacement of the involved muscle with scar tissue. In the forearm, this can produce a severe flexion contracture of the wrist and fingers (Volkmann's contracture). A "strangulation neuropathy" of the median and ulnar nerve can also occur where the nerves pass through the fibrous tissue, resulting in a hand that has no intrinsic muscle function and is completely numb over the median and ulnar nerve distributions.

Reconstructive surgery after scarring or loss of muscle tissue usually includes excision of all fibrotic muscle, multiple tendon transfers, and neurolysis and epineurolysis of the entrapped nerves. When wide debridement of muscle is required, some disability is inevitable; however, physical therapy and proper splinting and bracing can help preserve function of the limb.

⊘ FREQUENT ERRORS

1. ***Failure to recognize that compartment syndrome can occur with any type of compression of an extremity, even with a PASG.***
2. ***Failure to anticipate the development of compartment syndrome in a limb that has been ischemic, especially after reestablishment of perfusion.***
3. ***Allowing a patient with possible compartment syndrome to become even marginally hypotensive.***
4. ***Assuming compartment syndrome cannot be present in the lower leg if the calf feels soft or if a distal pulse or open fracture is present.***
5. ***Failure repeatedly to check deep peroneal nerve function (sensation in the first dorsal web space and extension of the big toe) in a patient at risk for developing compartment syndrome in the lower leg.***
6. ***Failure to promptly and adequately assess the reason for excessive or increasing lower leg pain after trauma or ischemia.***

7. ***Failure to adequately incise skin and fascia to relieve the pressures in all possible compartments completely in a patient with either diagnostic clinical findings or increased compartment pressures.***
8. ***Failure to check for and treat myoglobinuria in a patient with suspected or proven compartment syndrome.***
9. ***Failure to promptly and adequately debride nonviable tissue resulting from compartment syndrome.***

SUMMARY POINTS

1. Any prolonged compression of an extremity can cause compartment syndrome.
2. Hand injuries, especially metacarpal fractures, occasionally cause compartment syndrome localized to the hand.
3. Delayed repair of combined injuries to the popliteal or lower femoral artery and veins is likely to cause compartment syndrome, especially if the vein is ligated.
4. Cessation of capillary blood flow to muscle in extremities or bowel mucosa in the abdomen can occur at tissue pressures exceeding 20 to 30 mm Hg, which is much less than normal arterial pressures.
5. Compartment pressures are likely to increase precipitately shortly after reestablishing blood flow to ischemic tissues.
6. Partial ischemia (especially less than 30% of normal; because it allows production of free radicals but not ATP) tends to cause more cell damage than is caused by complete ischemia.
7. Palpable distal pulses do not rule out the presence of compartment syndrome.
8. Excessive pain in an injured or previously ischemic extremity is often the first indication of compartment syndrome.
9. Frequent and thorough sensory and motor examinations are required on any extremity that may develop compartment syndrome.
10. High or increasing CPK levels may reflect extensive muscle damage and may indicate the presence of an otherwise unsuspected compartment syndrome.
11. Measurement of compartment pressure is the most accurate technique for diagnosing compartment syndrome, especially in the early phases when fasciotomy produces the best results.
12. If unequivocal symptoms or signs of compartment syndrome are present, one should perform a fasciotomy without waiting for measurements of compartment pressures.
13. If any evidence of ischemia persists distal to a fracture after attempts at traction or closed reduction, immediate arteriography or surgical exploration or both is indicated.
14. If compartment pressures are marginally increased, hypotension can cause severe ischemic damage to intracompartment muscles.
15. In patients with a warm ischemia time of more than 4 to 6 hours distal to a vascular injury, fasciotomies should be performed before the vascular repair.
16. A decline in urine output in spite of normal or higher cardiac output and BP after abdominal trauma or a laparotomy should make one suspect an abdominal compartment syndrome.
17. The skin incisions for decompressive fasciotomies should be long enough to ensure that none of the underlying muscle is still compressed by skin or fascia.
18. A complete forearm fasciotomy may require decompression of each nerve and muscle.
19. If the patient is becoming septic, any marginally ischemic tissue should be excised.
20. Early physical therapy is essential to prevent contractures after a fasciotomy.
21. The severe contractures that can result from compartment syndrome can be prevented only by early, continued, vigorous physical therapy.

REFERENCES

1. Wilson RF, Georgiadis GM. Compartment syndrome. In: Wilson RF, Walt AJ, eds. *Management of trauma: pitfalls and practice.* 2nd ed. Philadelphia: Williams & Wilkins, 1996:687.
2. Matsen FA, Winquist RA, Krugmire RB. Diagnosis and management of compartmental syndromes. *J Bone Joint Surg Am* 1980;62:286.
3. Perry MO. Compartment syndromes and reperfusion injury. *Surg Clin North Am* 1988;68:853.
4. Eddy VA, Key SP, Morris JA. Abdominal compartment syndrome: etiology, detection, and management. *J Tenn Med Assoc* 1994;87:55.
5. Mubarak SJ, Hargens AR. Acute compartment syndromes. *Surg Clin North Am* 1983;63:539.
6. Patman RD. Compartmental syndromes in peripheral vascular surgery. *Clin Orthop* 1975;113:103.
7. Blick SS, Brumback, Poka A, Burgess AR, Ebraheim NA. Compartment syndrome in open tibial fractures. *J Bone Joint Surg Am* 1986;68:1348.
8. Abouezzi Z, Nassoura Z, Ivatury RR, et al. A critical reappraisal of indications for fasciotomy after extremity vascular trauma. *Arch Surg* 1998;133:547.
9. Aprahamian C, Gessert G, Banoyk DF, et al. MAST-associated compartment syndrome (MACS): a review. *J Trauma* 1989;29:549.
10. Watson AD, Kelikian AS. Thomas splint, calcaneus fracture, and compartment syndrome of the foot: a case report. *J Trauma* 1998;44:205.
11. Diebel LN, Wilson RF, Dulchavsky SA. Effect of increased intra-abdominal pressure on hepatic arterial, portal venous and hepatic microcirculatory blood flow. *J Trauma* 1992;33:279.
12. Widergren JT, Battistella FD. The open abdomen: treatment for intra-abdominal compartment syndrome. *J Trauma* 1994;37:158.
13. Ames A III, Wright RL, Kowada M, et al. Cerebral ischemia: the no-reflow phenomenon. *Am J Pathol* 1968;52:437.
14. Ernst E, Hammerschmidt DE, Bagge U, et al. Leukocytes and the risk of ischemic diseases. *JAMA* 1987;257:2318.
15. Roberts JP, Perry MO, Hariri RJ, et al. Incomplete recovery of muscle cell function following partial but not complete ischemia. *Circ Shock* 1985;17:253.
16. Heppenstall RB, Sapega AA, Scott R, et al. The compartment syndrome: an experimental and clinical study of muscular energy metabolism using phosphorous nuclear magnetic resonance spectroscopy. *Clin Orthop* 1988;226:138.
17. Holden CE. Compartment syndromes following trauma. *Clin Orthop* 1975;113:95.
18. Wolfort FG, Cochran TC, Filtzer H. Immediate interossei decompression following crush injury of the hand. *Arch Surg* 1973;106:826.
19. Feliciano DV, Cruse PA, Spjut-Patrinely V, et al. Fasciotomy after trauma to the extremities. *Am J Surg* 1988;156:533.
20. Patman RD. Fasciotomy: indications and technique. In: Rutherford RR, ed. *Vascular surgery.* Philadelphia: WB Saunders, 1984:513.
21. Kron IL, Harman PK, Nolan SP. The measurement of intra-abdominal pressure as a criterion for abdominal re-exploration. *Ann Surg* 1984;199:28.
22. Perry MO, Shires GT III, Albert SA. Cellular changes with graded limb ischemia in reperfusion. *J Vasc Surg* 1984;1:536.
23. Heckman MM, Whitesides TE Jr, Grewe SR, et al. Histologic determination of the ischemic threshold of muscle in the canine compartment syndrome model. *J Orthop Trauma* 1993;7:199.
24. Christenson JT, Wulff K. Compartment pressure following leg injury: the effect of diuretic treatment. *Injury* 1985;16:591.
25. Ernst CB, Kaufer H. Fibulectomy fasciotomy: an important adjunct in the management of low extremity arterial trauma. *J Trauma* 1971;11:365.
26. Rollins DL, Bernhard VM, Towne JB. Fasciotomy: an appraisal of controversial issues. *Arch Surg* 1981;116:1474.
27. Mubarak SJ, Owen CA. Double-incision fasciotomy of the leg for decompression in compartment syndromes. *J Bone Joint Surg Am* 1977;59:184.

28. Manoli A II, Weber TG. Fasciotomy of the foot: an anatomical study with special reference to release of the calcaneal compartment. *Foot Ankle* 1990;10:267.
29. Gelberman RH, Zakaib GS, Mubarak SJ, et al. Decompression of forearm compartment syndromes. *Clin Orthop* 1978;134:225.
30. Buchbinder D, Karmody AM, Leather RP, et al. Hypertonic mannitol: its use in the prevention of revascularization syndrome after acute arterial ischemia. *Arch Surg* 1981;116:414.
31. Moore EE, Eisman B, Van Way CW. *Critical decisions in trauma.* St. Louis: CV Mosby, 1984.

34. FAT EMBOLISM SYNDROME[1]

INTRODUCTION

Definition

Posttraumatic fat embolism syndrome (FES) is a clinical condition characterized by pulmonary or central nervous system dysfunction or both resulting from fat microemboli to the lungs, brain, skin, and other tissues, usually after fractures of long bones or the pelvis or both. The symptoms may develop rapidly but classically begin 12 to 48 hours after injury in about 2% to 4% of patients with long-bone fractures (2).

AXIOM A subclinical form of fat embolism with a reduced platelet count and increased $P_{(A\text{-}a)}O_2$ occurs after almost all fractures.

Source of Fat Emboli

The mechanical theory on the source of fat emboli in the FES has been proposed since the time of Zenker and von Bergmann, when it was assumed that the marrow of fractured long bones produced the fat emboli which then embolized to the lung.

The alternative (chemical) theory is that fat emboli are mobilized from fat stores because of the lipolytic effects of stress hormone. Indeed, catecholamine-induced mobilization of lipids greatly increases free fatty acid (FFA) levels in the blood after trauma. Although the small amount of free fat found in the marrow of large long bones favored a chemical source for fat emboli, Peltier (3) was able to show, on the basis of extraction of fat from entire human tibias and femurs, that a large amount of fat was contained within the metaphyseal sponge of these bones, rather than in the marrow, and this could enter the blood after fractures.

AXIOM Both mechanical and biochemical mechanisms are probably involved in the development of most cases of FES.

When lipase acts on a neutral fat, the fat is broken down into glycerol, which is an innocuous water-soluble substance, and fatty acids, which can rapidly cause severe pulmonary changes. Peltier's classic studies showed that intravenous injection of neutral fat did not cause pulmonary changes for at least 24 to 48 hours. Intravenous injection of fatty acids, however, produced immediate effects on the lung, closely resembling those of clinical fat emboli (4). Thus the lag period to development of clinical signs and symptoms is probably a result of the time it takes pulmonary lipase to break down the neutral fat emboli into fatty acids.

PATHOPHYSIOLOGY

Phases of Fat Embolism

FES can be divided into two phases:

1. Initial phase in which the mechanical obstruction of capillaries and other small vessels by neutral fat emboli is most important; and
2. Later chemical phase, as fatty acids are formed from neutral fat (5).

Platelet Changes

Severe trauma causes a massive release of tissue thromboplastin and other platelet activators, which results in platelet adhesion to any abnormal surface, including fat droplets in the blood. The activated platelets attached to fat emboli in the lung release vasoactive amines (which can cause pulmonary vascular dysfunction) and cause the formation of thrombin (which can result in intravascular coagulation), all of which can cause hypoxemia.

Coagulation Changes

Within minutes of experimental fractures, there is an abrupt decline in the plasma concentrations of fibrinogen and factors V and VIII (6), reflecting an increase in intravascular clotting. Some of the clotting obviously occurs at the site of the fracture where multiple vessels are torn; however, this is not adequate to explain the tremendous consumption of these factors.

Increasingly, it appears that the platelet activation caused by tissue thromboplastin and the subsequent platelet aggregation occurring at multiple sites in the body, particularly in the pulmonary capillaries, may stimulate the intrinsic clotting pathway.

AXIOM Disseminated intravascular coagulation (DIC) is a component of the FES, and there appears to be a correlation between the severity of the intravascular coagulation and the blood gas changes.

Pulmonary Changes

The vast majority of the fat emboli released from fractured bone lodge in the lung. Initially, the pulmonary microemboli mechanically block small pulmonary vessels. The lung responds to the presence of neutral fat particles by secreting lipase, which hydrolyzes the neutral fat into FFAs and glycerol. The FFAs damage the local capillaries and alveoli and inactivate surfactant (4). Both the mechanical and chemical effects of the fat emboli on the lung can seriously impair the ability of the lung to oxygenate blood.

Cerebral Changes

Hypoxemia resulting from lung injury can explain the brain dysfunction of FES in some cases, but not all (7). In some fatal cases, cerebral symptoms occur early and seem to reflect direct brain injury. Histologic examination of the brain in these cases reveals many fat emboli and associated hemorrhage and necrosis.

Petechiae

The reason for the transient petechiae occurring around the second to fifth day in FES is not known. Damage to the skin capillaries by fatty acids may be an important contributing factor. In some patients, the thrombocytopenia may be quite severe and appears to be associated with other laboratory evidence of DIC (5); however, there is no explanation for the striking localization of the petechiae to the pectoral regions, axillae, and conjunctivae.

DIAGNOSIS

AXIOM Some degree of FES should be expected in all patients with major fractures, and these changes can contribute significantly to the pulmonary and central nervous system (CNS) dysfunction that may develop 12 to 48 hours after major trauma.

FES is most likely to occur in patients with multiple severe long-bone fractures plus hypovolemic shock or any other process causing increased catecholamine release (5). Damage to a fatty liver also can be a source of fat emboli. Indeed, it is not unusual to find emboli of bone marrow or liver in the lungs at autopsy in patients who have died of severe blunt trauma.

Gurd's Criteria

Gurd's criteria, which may be used to diagnose FES, are divided into major and minor criteria (8):

Major criteria include

- Axillary or subconjunctival petechiae
- Hypoxemia
- CNS depression (disproportionate to the hypoxemia or head injury)
- Pulmonary dysfunction

Minor criteria include

- Tachycardia (more than 110 beats/min)
- Pyrexia (temperature more than 38.5°C)
- Retinal changes on fundoscopic exam (fat or petechiae)
- Urinary changes (fat globules with or without oliguria)
- Sudden decreases in hemoglobin or platelet levels
- High erythrocyte sedimentation rate
- Fat globules in the sputum

At least one of the major criteria and at least four of the minor criteria are used by Gurd to make the diagnosis of FES.

Clinical Findings

Pulmonary Changes

The characteristic clinical pulmonary changes with FES include an initial tachypnea and increased minute ventilation plus hypoxemia. Radiographic changes usually appear after 24 to 48 hours and are typically a diffuse microatelectasis and congestion (2,9). Despite the hyperventilation and low arterial P_{CO_2}, which is usually present in FES, the arterial P_{O_2} in young adults with fat emboli tends to be 70 mm Hg or less, so that the $P_{(A\text{-}a)}O_2$ on room air is usually at least 45 to 55 mm Hg.

Neurologic Changes

Neurologic manifestations are common in FES, and may occur in up to 84% of patients (10). Indeed, many of the patients with encephalopathy develop their CNS changes before there is any clinical evidence of pulmonary failure.

One third of patients with CNS changes have focal neurologic abnormalities that tend to occur at the same time as the most severe impairment of the level of consciousness (10). Some of the more common focal features include apraxia, hemiplegia, scotomata, anisocoria, and conjugate eye deviation. Occasionally, fat emboli can be seen on fundoscopic examination.

Petechial

A transient petechial rash may develop in 50% to 60% of patients with FES on the skin of the chest, axilla, and neck, and on the conjunctivae. The petechiae can easily be missed because they may be present for less than 4 to 6 hours.

Laboratory Evaluation

AXIOM There are no specific laboratory tests for FES; however, a combination of thrombocytopenia and low P_aO_2 (or high $P_{[A-a]}O_2$) occurring within 24 to 48 hours of major fractures is almost diagnostic of FES.

Hypoxemia

It has been suggested by Moed et al. (11) that pulse oximetry is an effective technique to screen for FES in patients with fractures of long bones or the pelvis or both. Of 43 fracture patients screened with this technique, 15 (35%) had a pulse oximetry saturation of less than 94%. These patients were managed with an intensive pulmonary-care regimen, and the hypoxemia resolved in all patients within 48 hours of their initial therapy.

Thrombocytopenia

AXIOM A normal platelet count after long-bone fractures generally rules out the presence of FES.

An early thrombocytopenia less than 100,000/mm^3 is almost diagnostic of FES if the patient has not had massive transfusions, severe prolonged shock, or another cause of platelet consumption. The decrease in the platelet counts usually correlates fairly well with the increases in $P_{(A-a)}O_2$ on room air (2,9).

Fat in the Urine

Other tests that might be helpful in diagnosing FES include examinations of urine, sputum, cerebrospinal fluid (CSF), and blood for fat. Lipuria occurs in about half of all patients with significant bony injury, most of whom have no other findings suggestive of FES. Examination of frozen peripheral blood via a cryostat test for fat droplets also may be too sensitive to be of clinical value.

Hemoglobin Decrease

Hemoglobin levels may decline by as much as 3 to 5 g/dL with FES; however, one should look carefully for other injuries before attributing this change to FES alone.

Consumptive Coagulopathy

Complete coagulation studies in full-blown cases of FES may reveal varying degrees of a consumptive coagulopathy with decreased levels of platelets, fibrinogen, prothrombin, factor V, and factor VIII.

AXIOM Almost all of the laboratory tests for FES are too sensitive and nonspecific to be of great diagnostic value; however, if multiple tests are positive in the appropriate clinical setting, the diagnosis is likely.

Radiologic Examinations

Chest Radiographs

AXIOM The chest radiograph findings of FES tend to lag at least 12 to 24 hours behind the clinical, blood gas, and platelet changes.

The clinical and arterial blood gas (ABG) changes usually become clinically obvious at least 12 to 24 hours before any radiologic abnormalities appear. When radiographic changes become apparent, they resemble those of other types of acute respiratory distress syndrome (ARDS) and include early congestion and diffuse infiltrates. If the radiologic changes occur before clinical respiratory changes, one should suspect pulmonary contusion.

Computed Tomography Scan and Magnetic Resonance Imaging of the Head

AXIOM Before it is assumed that the neurologic changes occurring after major trauma are a result of FES, a computed tomography (CT) scan of the head is needed to rule out space-occupying lesions.

In studying a patient with cerebral fat embolism, Erdem et al. (12) found that the brain CT showed no abnormality. Differentiating the changes of FES from diffuse axonal injury may be very difficult. A magnetic resonance imaging (MRI) scan performed after recovery from the trauma may demonstrate multiple abnormalities in the white matter.

INITIAL MANAGEMENT TO PREVENT FAT EMBOLISM SYNDROME

Early Aggressive Correction of Hypovolemia and Hypotension

The incidence of FES increases in patients with hypovolemic shock (5). Nevertheless, one should be careful not to overload the circulation and cause cardiogenic pulmonary edema, especially if there has been coincident chest trauma.

Early Fixation of Fractures

AXIOM Although transesophageal echocardiography has detected fat emboli entering the heart in approximately 40% of patients undergoing major orthopaedic procedures (13), early fixation of long-bone fractures is thought to be one of the best ways to prevent or treat FES.

Early operation on fractures and decompressing and evacuating the associated hematoma should reduce the amount of fat entering the circulation.

Avoiding Heparin?

Heparin, in the past, was recommended for its lipolytic and anticoagulant properties; however, heparin actually increases the formation of FFAs and may make the FES worse. Heparin antibodies occasionally also can cause significant platelet aggregation.

Reduction of Platelet Aggregation with Corticosteroids, Aspirin, or Both

The use of corticosteroids has been extremely controversial since they were first reported to be beneficial in the treatment of FES by Ashbaugh and Petty in 1966 (14).

Shier et al. (2) found that aspirin (300 mg every 6 hours during the first 24 to 48 hours by mouth or by rectum) also caused less platelet aggregation and maintained a significantly higher platelet count and lower $P_{(A\text{-}a)}O_2$ on room air than did controls (2).

Administration of Albumin

The amount of lung damage in FES appears to be related primarily to the levels of FFAs. Fatty acids are bound primarily by albumin, and low levels of plasma albumin increase the concentration of FFAs (4). Although very low albumin levels are often associated with a poor prognosis in many types of trauma, excessive administration of albumin can increase the tendency to heart failure and ARDS.

Early Glucose Administration

Inadequate caloric intake increases the mobilization of fat from tissue stores, and hypertonic glucose has been thought to reduce the incidence and severity of FES. In a prospective randomized study, early aggressive administration of glucose did not alter the platelet count or ABG changes from those in control patients (4).

TREATMENT OF FAT EMBOLISM SYNDROME

Oxygen or Ventilatory Assistance or Both

AXIOM Because most of the symptoms of FES appear to be associated with hypoxemia, pulse oximetry and ventilator assistance should be instituted early.

It has become increasingly evident that fat embolism is largely a pulmonary problem and that oxygen or ventilatory support or both should be begun early to maintain the PO_2 at about 80 to 90 mm Hg.

Positive end-expiratory pressure (PEEP) may reduce the need for high concentrations of inspired oxygen and should be considered if an FIO_2 greater than 0.4 or 0.6 is needed. Increased PEEP may increase the intracranial pressure (ICP) in patients with CNS changes.

Neurologic Dysfunction

The initial approach to patients with posttraumatic neurologic dysfunction should be to exclude intracranial hemorrhage that might require a craniotomy (10). If this and other primary CNS problems can be ruled out, the CNS changes should be considered a result of FES until proven otherwise. In such patients, early aggressive ventilation and maintenance of normal or increased cerebral perfusion with well-oxygenated blood should provide the best overall results.

OUTCOME

Reported mortality rates for FES have been as high as 29%, but these data are difficult to interpret because many of the patients had associated injuries to the head, chest, and abdomen. More recent studies have tried to exclude patients with associated injuries, and under such circumstances, the mortality rate from FES itself tends to be less than 10%.

⊘ FREQUENT ERRORS

1. ***Failure to consider the possible presence of fat emboli in a patient with major fractures, especially if there are pulmonary or neurologic changes that are not clearly due to direct trauma.***
2. ***Failure to promptly and adequately resuscitate patients with major fractures.***
3. ***Failure to check the platelet count in patients with hypoxemia after major fractures.***
4. ***Delay in checking for hypoxemia with blood gases or pulse oximetry or both after major fractures.***
5. ***Delaying rigid fixation of major fractures in trauma patients, especially if there is any evidence of pulmonary dysfunction.***
6. ***Failure to obtain CT scans of the head in trauma victims with impaired CNS function that appears to be due to fat embolism.***

SUMMARY POINTS

1. A subclinical form of fat embolism with a reduced platelet count and increased $P_{(A-a)}O_2$ occurs after almost all fractures.

2. Both mechanical and biochemical mechanisms are probably involved in the development of most cases of FES.

3. DIC is a component of the FES, and there appears to be a correlation between the severity of the intravascular coagulation and the blood-gas changes.
4. FES can be divided into an initial phase in which the mechanical obstruction of capillaries and other small vessels by neutral fat emboli is most important, and a later chemical phase, when FFAs are formed from the neutral fat.
5. Despite the hyperventilation and low arterial P_{CO_2} usually present in FES, the arterial P_{O_2} in young adults with fat emboli tends to be 70 mm Hg or less.
6. A transient petechial rash develops in up to 50% to 60% of patients with FES.
7. There are no specific laboratory tests; however, a combination of thrombocytopenia and low P_aO_2 (or high $P_{(A-a)}O_2$) occurring within 24 to 48 hours of major fractures is almost diagnostic of FES.
8. A normal platelet count after long-bone fractures generally rules out the presence of FES.
9. Increased fat in blood, sputum, and urine is a relatively nonspecific finding after major trauma.
10. Almost all of the laboratory tests for FES are too sensitive and nonspecific to be of great diagnostic value; however, if multiple tests are positive in the appropriate clinical setting, the diagnosis is very likely.
11. The chest radiograph findings of FES tend to lag at least 12 to 24 hours behind the clinical, blood-gas, and platelet changes.
12. Before it is assumed that the neurologic changes occurring after major trauma are a result of FES, a CT scan of the head is needed to rule out space-occupying lesions.
13. Rapid correction of hypotension and hypovolemia in patients with long-bone fractures may reduce the incidence and severity of FES.
14. Because most of the symptoms of FES appear to be associated with hypoxemia, pulse oximetry and ventilator assistance should be instituted early.

REFERENCES

1. Wilson RF, Georgiadis GM. Fat embolism syndrome. In: Wilson RF, Walt AJ, eds. *Management of trauma: pitfalls and practice.* 2nd ed. Philadelphia: Williams & Wilkins, 1996:703.
2. Shier MR, Wilson RF. Fat embolism syndromes: traumatic coagulopathy with respiratory distress. *Surg Ann* 1980;12:139.
3. Peltier LF. Fat embolism I: the amount of fat in human long bones. *Surgery* 1956; 40:657.
4. Peltier LF. Fat embolism III: the toxic properties of neutral fats and fatty acids. *Surgery* 1956;40:665.
5. Peltier LF. Fat embolism: a perspective. *Clin Orthop* 1988;232:263.
6. Bergentz SE, Nilsson IM. Effect of trauma on coagulation and fibrinolysis in dogs. *Acta Chir Scand* 1961;122:21.
7. Scopa M, Magatti M, Rossitto P. Neurologic symptoms in fat embolism syndrome: case report. *J Trauma* 1994;36:906.
8. Gurd AR. Fat embolism: an aid to diagnosis. *J Bone Joint Surg Br* 1970;52:732.
9. Wilson RF, McCarthy B, LeBlanc LP, et al. Respiratory and coagulation changes after uncomplicated fractures. *Arch Surg* 1973;106:395.
10. Jacobson DM, Terrence CF, Reinmuth OM. The neurologic manifestations of fat embolism. *Neurology* 1986;36:847.
11. Moed BR, Boyd DW, Andring RE. Clinically inapparent hypoxemia after skeletal injury: the use of the pulse oximeter as a screening method. *Clin Orthop* 1993; 293:269.
12. Erdem E, Namer IJ, Saribas O, et al. Cerebral fat embolism studied with MRI and SPECT. *Neuroradiology* 1993;35:199.
13. Pell ACH, Keating JF, Christie J, et al. Use of transesophageal echocardiography to predict patients at risk of the fat embolism syndrome following traumatic injuries. *J Am Coll Cardiol* 1993;21(suppl):264A.
14. Ashbaugh DG, Petty TL. The use of corticosteroids in the treatment of respiratory failure associated with massive fat embolism. *Surg Gynecol Obstet* 1966;123: 493.

35. VASCULAR INJURIES[1]

INTRODUCTION

Many isolated vascular injuries, particularly in the extremities, can be easily managed; however, correct diagnosis and treatment of vessel damage when it is associated with multiple other injuries can be extremely challenging.

⊘ PITFALL

Delay in definitive repair of an arterial injury beyond 4 to 6 hours increases the incidence of severe complications.

ETIOLOGY

Penetrating Wounds

Stabs of vessels are usually cleanly incised, and a primary repair is almost always possible. High-velocity bullets, however, can create special problems. With a muzzle velocity of 3,000 feet/s, the bullet creates a cavitational effect on impact that can cause massive destruction of soft tissues for several centimeters around the missile tract. In contrast, low-velocity hand-gun missiles (500 to 1,000 feet/s) cause much less soft-tissue injury, and no debridement of injured vessels is usually needed.

Close-range shotgun blasts also can cause extensive soft-tissue damage. Furthermore, the wad and plastic caps used to separate the powder charge from the shot also may penetrate the wound. If the wad is not recovered during the initial debridement, severe infection is likely to develop.

Blunt Trauma

Blunt arterial injury is usually the result of automobile accidents. Such injuries are associated frequently with fractures or dislocations of major bones or joints.

The more common sites of combined vascular and orthopaedic trauma include

1. Fractured femoral shaft and superficial femoral artery;
2. Knee dislocation and popliteal artery;
3. Fractured clavicle and subclavian artery;
4. Dislocated shoulder and axillary artery; and
5. Supracondylar fracture of the humerus and brachial artery (5).

PATHOPHYSIOLOGY

Ischemic Changes

Acute cessation of arterial flow can produce regional ischemia to the organs or limb perfused by the artery. The vulnerability of tissue to ischemic insult depends on its basal energy requirements and substrate stores. Skeletal muscle is much more tolerant of ischemia than are peripheral nerves. Extremity tissues can often survive without nutrient blood flow up to 4 hours without developing any permanent changes due to ischemia.

AXIOM A limb that has been ischemic for 6 hours or longer is at risk for sustaining tissue changes that may not be reversible with reperfusion (7).

Bleeding

After complete transection, severed arterial ends retract, and thrombosis usually occurs before there is extensive blood loss. Exsanguination is more likely with partial transections, which prevent vessel retraction. Blood loss also may be reduced if the bleeding is contained within the perivascular tissues. Such blood may clot and lead to a pulsatile hematoma, often called a false aneurysm. If there are contiguous wounds to both an artery and an adjacent vein, an arteriovenous fistula may develop.

Arteriovenous Fistulas

Arteriovenous (AV) fistulas tend to enlarge with time and can eventually produce a significant increase in pulse rate, pulse pressure, and cardiac output. If the fistula becomes large enough, high-output cardiac failure may result. This may be associated with an increased incidence of bacterial endocarditis. Compression of a large fistula often causes a characteristic decrease in pulse rate (Nicoladoni/Branham sign).

Contusions

Contusion of a vessel may be caused by direct trauma, which produces hemorrhage or edema in the wall of the vessel and "spasm." Subsequent fibrosis also can cause narrowing or partial occlusion of the lumen weeks or months later.

Vessel Spasm

AXIOM Narrowing of the arterial lumen at an injury site is seldom caused by spasm; in most instances, an area of persistent narrowing on arteriogram is actually an area of significant vascular injury.

INITIAL EMERGENCY MANAGEMENT

Control of Bleeding

Active external bleeding should be controlled as completely and rapidly as possible, preferably by digital pressure or a compression dressing directly over the bleeding site.

AXIOM Blind placement of clamps in the depths of an actively bleeding wound should never be done, especially in patients with dislocations or fracture–dislocations and absent distal pulses.

Reduction of Dislocations

Dislocations or fractures causing neurovascular problems should be reduced immediately. Traction on the injured limb also may help to relieve arterial kinking, compression, or entrapment.

AXIOM Failure to reduce a dislocation promptly to restore the circulation to an extremity may result in extensive tissue necrosis and need for a later amputation.

The most frequent dislocations causing loss of arterial circulation include anterior dislocations of the shoulder and posterior dislocations of the knee. Early reduction of these dislocations often leads to rapid restoration of perfusion to the distal extremity. If possible, an immediate radiograph of the involved joint should be done to identify any associated fractures before attempting to reduce the joint.

DIAGNOSIS

The workup for a possible major vascular injury should be expeditious with the goal to reestablish perfusion of the ischemic limb in less than 3 to 4 hours.

Clinical Examination

A history of pulsatile, bright red blood spurting from a wound strongly suggests a major arterial injury, whereas the history of a steady flow of dark blood from the wound often indicates a venous injury (2). A history of extensive blood loss at the scene, hypotension, or syncope also can be helpful.

The Six "Ps"

Six Ps that may suggest a vascular injury include

1. Pulselessness;
2. Pain;
3. Pallor;
4. Poikilothermia;
5. Paresthesias; and
6. Paralysis or paresis.

All of these signs may be helpful, but they are not foolproof. For example, peripheral pulses may be seen in up to 25% of the patients with extremity arterial injuries (3). The neurologic signs of paresthesias and paralysis are particularly important because peripheral nerves can be relatively tolerant of ischemia for up to 6 hours. There is relatively little risk of gangrene if neurologic function is intact.

In hypotensive patients, it may not be possible to determine whether or not an arterial or venous injury is present until shock has been corrected by infusion of fluids and the peripheral pulses in the uninjured limbs have returned.

"Hard" Signs of Vascular Injury

Signs directly indicative of ischemia or severe bleeding are commonly referred to as hard signs of vascular injury (2). These include

1. Pulsatile bleeding;
2. Expanding hematoma;
3. Palpable thrill;
4. Audible bruit;
5. Severe rest pain;
6. Pallor;
7. Paralysis;
8. Paresthesia;
9. Poikilothermia; and
10. Pulselessness.

AXIOM Careful auscultation over the area of trauma is an important part of the physical examination.

"Soft" Signs of Vascular Injury

Signs suggestive of vascular injury, but without definite evidence of ischemia or hemorrhage, are called soft signs. These include

1. History of moderate hemorrhage;
2. Injury (fractures or penetrating wounds) in proximity to major vessels;
3. Diminished but palpable pulses;
4. Peripheral nerve deficits; and
5. Knee dislocation.

These soft signs indicate a need for diagnostic imaging or noninvasive studies of flow and pressure or both.

Diagnostic Studies

Noninvasive Studies

Doppler techniques for the determination of segmental blood pressures and for arterial waveform analysis have been used increasingly to diagnose peripheral vascular trauma. Shah et al. (3) considered any decrease in ankle pressure greater than 20 torr (compared with the uninjured limb) or an abnormal waveform to be indicative of arterial injury. It also was suggested that an ABI less than 0.9 should arouse suspicion of an arterial injury.

The combination of ultrasound imaging with spectral analysis (duplex scanning) may be useful in the diagnosis of traumatic arterial or venous thrombosis, arterial pseudoaneurysm, and AV fistulas (2). The image resolution is usually not sufficient to display intimal injury unless the disruption is severe enough to produce a major disturbance in flow.

Arteriography

Single-Stick Arteriography

If a patient with an extremity wound is hemodynamically unstable or has a threatened distal extremity, immediate transportation to the operating room (OR) for exploration of the involved vessel is appropriate. If threatened ischemia from inadequate circulation is reversed in the OR, intraoperative angiography can be used as needed, especially if there are multiple possible sites of vascular injury. Another alternative in marginally perfused limbs is "single-stick" arteriography in the resuscitation area.

Formal Angiography

Patients with clinical signs and symptoms of an arterial injury without threatened ischemia are candidates for studies in the angiography suite to identify the site of the injury and to provide a road map for the surgeon. Another indication of arteriography is altered or absent distal pulses associated with long-bone fractures or fracture–dislocations, even if the pulses return to normal with reduction and splinting.

AXIOM The significance of abnormal findings on arteriography is determined by the surgeon who coordinates the clinical and roentgenographic findings.

The incidence of arterial injury in patients in whom proximity of either a fracture or a penetrating wound to a major artery was the sole indication for arteriography have ranged from 0% to 6.7%. Frykberg et al. (4) found only 16 (10.5%) arteriographic abnormalities in major arteries in 152 proximity wounds. They concluded that arteriography was not cost effective in evaluating patients who had penetrating proximity wounds but no other evidence of arterial injury.

Although major arterial injuries are rarely missed, clinically occult, nonocclusive "minimal" injuries such as focal narrowing, intimal flaps, small pseudoaneurysms, or arteriovenous fistulas may be present. Dennis et al. (5), however, showed that nonoperative management of these clinically occult arterial injuries is safe and effective.

AXIOM Angiography is not without risks; complications occur in at least 2% to 4% of patients (6).

Intraarterial Digital Subtraction Arteriography. Intraarterial digital subtraction arteriography (IADSA) has a sensitivity and specificity similar to those of arteriography and has several advantages, including a shorter time to complete the examination, less exposure to radiation, reduced cost, reduced dye load, and less discomfort (7). Because a smaller catheter is used, IADSA may lessen the chances of an iatrogenic injury. Its usefulness is limited in shotgun injuries, in which metallic fragments may distort the images.

Venography. Venography may be useful in certain circumstances for identifying reparable venous injuries. Probably the main indication for preoperative venography after trauma is signs and symptoms of arterial injury in a nonthreatened distal limb with a normal arteriogram.

TREATMENT

Nonoperative Treatment

The treatment of some angiographic defects, such as intimal irregularity, focal narrowing, and small pseudoaneurysms, is controversial (4). Recent experience suggests that these injuries have a benign course and can be safely observed. Frykberg et al. (4) followed up 20 such injuries documented arteriographically and found that 53% resolved, 16% improved, and 26% remained unchanged. One patient required operation for enlargement of a brachial artery pseudoaneurysm.

Follow-up of any vascular injury should include physical examinations and objective assessment of both the anatomy and the flow characteristics of the injured artery and the distal arterial bed with duplex imaging. Similarly, observation can be advocated in asymptomatic injuries of arterial segments that are difficult to expose or control, such as high lesions in the carotid or vertebral arteries (8).

Operative Treatment

General Principles

Control of Bleeding

External bleeding should be controlled with digital pressure or compressive bandages until the involved vessels can be controlled proximally and distally. Occasionally, one can expose the involved area and directly control the bleeding site with a single curved vascular clamp, but such efforts should generally be done in the OR.

Temporary Shunts

Rapid restoration of perfusion is the goal of treatment of injuries to major peripheral arteries. In some instances, a temporary shunt can be used while other procedures, such as reduction and fixation of fractures, are performed.

Antibiotic and Tetanus Prophylaxis

Broad-spectrum antibiotics should be started as soon as possible after injury and continued through the first postinjury day. Extensive soft-tissue injury or contamination that requires repeated aggressive debridement and irrigation may necessitate longer antibiotic therapy. Tetanus prophylaxis should also be provided.

Positioning and Draping

AXIOM The position and draping for emergency vascular surgery should allow rapid securing of proximal and distal control of the injured vessels and an autologous vein graft if needed.

AXIOM Whenever a vascular patch or graft is needed, the injured patient's own veins generally provide the most suitable material.

Intraoperative Techniques

Incisions and Vascular Control

The incision in most patients with extremity wounds should follow the course of the neurovascular bundle and remain between natural anatomic planes to reduce the chance of causing inadvertent injury to adjacent structures. When the injury is at the junction of anatomic compartments, the incision may have to be carried into the more proximal compartment to achieve proper exposure and control of the vessels.

⊘ PITFALL

Failure to obtain proximal and distal control before exposing the site of injury of a large vessel may convert a careful anatomic dissection into a frantic attempt to stop massive hemorrhage.

After obtaining proximal and distal vascular control, one can gradually dissect along the vessel toward the site of injury and at the same time replace the vascular tapes closer to the injury until the distance between the proximal and distal tapes is reduced to the area of injury plus 1 or 2 cm at each end.

Combined Major Vascular and Orthopaedic Injuries

If the definitive vascular repair is to be delayed for more than 30 minutes to fixate an associated fracture, temporary restoration of blood flow can be achieved with a Javid or similar shunt placed in the proximal and distal ends of the injured vessel and secured with shunt clamps or umbilical tapes (9). While the Javid shunt is in place, a surgeon should remain on the scene to check the circulation and prevent inadvertent kinking or compression of the shunt during the orthopaedic procedure. Johansen et al. (9) documented shunt "dwell" times for these temporary intraluminal shunts of up to 6 hours, with an average of 3.7 hours without morbidity.

Occasionally the soft-tissue injury around the associated fracture is too extensive for definitive internal fixation and stabilization. In such circumstances, the vascular repair is protected best by the use of external skeletal fixators that will keep the bone fragments from inadvertently disrupting the vascular repair.

Distal Thrombectomy

Before definitive arterial repair, one must be assured that any clots that may have formed proximally or distally have been removed. Proximal extraction of a clot can often be achieved by just releasing the proximal vascular clamp and allowing fresh blood to flow through the vascular wound.

AXIOM Good back-bleeding from the distal artery does not ensure the absence of intravascular thrombus beyond the first patent collateral vessel.

The distal extraction of clots is best achieved with Fogarty balloon catheters passed distally until resistance is met. As the catheter is being slowly extracted, the balloon is inflated just enough to cause a slight resistance to its withdrawal. Overinflation must be avoided because it can produce intimal injury. The Fogarty balloon catheter is passed as many times as necessary to ensure that the last passage produces no clot.

Heparinization

After clot extraction, local heparinization can be obtained with a heparin solution containing 100 U/mL. Local heparinization is much safer if the patient has other injuries that can bleed during this systemic heparinization. A Fogarty irrigating catheter is used to instill at least 10 to 20 mL of the "local heparin solution" distally and 3 to 5 mL proximally.

If systemic heparinization seems preferable and is safe, it can be obtained with 50 to 100 units heparin/kg body weight. This has the advantage of producing a more complete and effective anticoagulation; however, if there is little or no distal blood flow, additional heparin will have to be injected into the injured vessel to prevent distal thrombosis.

After the vascular anastomosis has been completed, the heparin is allowed to metabolize. Giving protamine to counteract the remaining heparin is generally unnecessary and probably unwise because it may cause a rebound hypercoagulability.

Debridement

Damaged tissue should be thoroughly debrided to avoid incorporating it into the suture line. Debridement, however, should generally not extend beyond the point of gross injury.

Arterial Repair

If an arterial repair is performed, atraumatic vascular clamps and fine synthetic monofilament sutures on small atraumatic needles should be used. This includes 5-0 polypropylene sutures for the femoral, axillary, popliteal, and brachial arteries.

Performing the Anastomosis. To help achieve the desired length of proximal and distal vessel, major collaterals can be dissected free of surrounding tissue, but they should not be interrupted just to achieve sufficient length for a primary anastomosis. If flexion of the joint is used during exposure of the vascular injury, the extremity should be returned to a straight position before repair to ensure adequate proximal and distal length to perform an end-to-end anastomosis without undue tension. During the actual repair, the extremity can be flexed to suture the ends of the vessel more easily.

With smaller vessels, especially those less than 5 mm in diameter, some surgeons prefer to use the spatulated technique in which the artery on each end is cut in an elongated "spatulated" manner with the length of the spatulated extension approximately equal to the diameter of the distal vessel.

The most critical technical aid in performing the anastomosis is keeping the two ends of the artery approximated without tension. Consequently, the second assistant must hold the two vascular clamps to approximate the ends of the vessel perfectly while the first assistant provides the correct position to expose the artery properly.

Vascular Grafts. Close-range shotgun blasts, rifle wounds, some blunt injuries, and deep avulsion injuries often cause extensive arterial disruption, thereby precluding end-to-end anastomosis after appropriate debridement of the damaged vessel. Consequently, the vascular reconstruction requires interposition grafting. The saphenous vein, taken from an uninjured lower extremity, usually provides the most readily available and safest graft for arterial interposition (10).

If autologous vein is not available or is of inadequate luminal size or quality, both dacron and polytetrafluoroethylene (PTFE) have been used successfully as synthetic vascular conduits. Whereas the long-term patency rate is less than with autologous vein, particularly distal to the knees or elbows, previous concerns about the potential for infection with prosthetic grafts were probably exaggerated (11).

"Venting" the Anastomosis. Most surgeons vent the artery of air or clots or both before the last one or two sutures are tied. The distal clamp is released first and then the vessel is occluded just distal to the suture line to allow proximal air or clots or both to be vented. After this has been accomplished, the suture is tied.

Controlling Postrepair Bleeding. A nonbleeding anastomosis requires no additional sutures. Oozing through needle holes or between sutures can usually be controlled by gentle digital pressure and a topical thrombotic agent placed directly over the site of oozing for 5 to 10 minutes.

AXIOM Properly placed digital pressure on small bleeding points at a completed vascular anastomosis, with a little patience, will usually obviate the need for repair sutures.

Covering Exposed Vessels or Grafts. When arterial injury is associated with massive soft-tissue loss, the muscle and subcutaneous tissue normally overlying the neurovascular bundle may be gone. If a vein graft is exposed or covered only by ischemic or contaminated muscle, it will necrose and rupture (12). If a prosthetic graft becomes infected, a false aneurysm can develop at the site of repair or sometimes in the artery just proximal or distal to the anastomosis where clamps had been applied (11).

One technique that may be used to preclude the need for primary amputation in such patients is rerouting the vascular bypass graft through an extraanatomic plane. If a safe extraanatomic bypass is precluded because the injury involves all the muscle compartments of the involved limb, the graft must be covered by a biologic dressing.

Oxygenation of vein grafts is provided not from the red cells that flow through the lumen, but from oxygen dissolved in the interstitial fluid bathing the outside of the vein. Consequently, some technique must be used to permit oxygen-containing fluid to bathe all portions of the walls of the vein (13). This can be achieved by the placement of biologic dressings, such as split-thickness porcine skin grafts, over the exposed arterial or vein graft wall (14). This is likely to succeed as long as one wall of the vein is lying on healthy muscle with oxygenated interstitial fluid that flows by capillary action between the exposed vein wall and the covering split-thickness porcine graft. The porcine graft can be changed every 48 hours at the bedside if the patient has no associated long-bone fractures and does not require general anesthesia to facilitate the dressing change.

Over a period of 4 to 6 weeks, the "exposed" vein graft will gradually become covered with pink granulation tissue, after which the vein wall can no longer be seen. At this time, the vein graft and the covering granulation tissue will accept an autologous split-thickness skin graft.

Completion Arteriography

After proper and timely vascular reconstruction, excellent distal flow should be apparent by the restoration of normal peripheral pulses. If there is any question about the successful restoration of flow, as may occur in patients with peripheral vasoconstriction from prolonged ischemia, intraoperative "completion arteriography" is needed. If an anatomic problem is noted at the site of injury, the anastomosis should be redone or bypassed as needed. Occasionally, distal pulses are absent immediately after proximal arterial repairs as a result of hypothermia and vasoconstriction. Once the extremities are warmed, distal pulses should be present. If pulses are absent, arteriography should be obtained, and any abnormalities corrected.

Distal Arterial Spasm. For a short time after an injured artery has been repaired, some degree of spasm may persist, not only at the site of the injury, but also in the distal vessels, particularly if there has been a prolonged period of ischemia. Under these circumstances, local stripping of the adventitia 1 to 2 cm above and below the repair or local application of papaverine or lidocaine (Xylocaine) or both may improve flow. Increasing the patient's blood pressure and cardiac output to levels greater than normal also may be helpful. Injection of dilute papaverine or lidocaine plus some heparin into the vessel lumen with temporary inflow occlusion also may improve distal blood flow.

Multiple Distal Thrombi. If there is clinical or radiologic evidence of multiple distal thrombi, infusions of urokinase may be helpful (15). If the patient has no other injuries that might bleed, one can infuse 250,000 units of urokinase plus 1,000 plus units of heparin in 250 mL of saline intraarterially distal to an occluding clamp over a period of 30 minutes. If one drains the venous effluent, one can give up to 1,000,000 units of urokinase in 45 to 60 minutes.

Closure of Incisions

After successful vascular repair, one should ascertain that all devitalized tissue and foreign material have been removed to reduce the risk of postoperative infection. The soft tissue over the vascular repairs can then be approximated with interrupted absorbable sutures to allow egress of blood and fluid from associated soft-tissue injury and hematoma. With severe soft-tissue injury, temporary drainage with a sump catheter for 12 to 36 hours may be helpful.

Postoperative Management

Prompt replacement of all blood and fluid losses will help maintain flow through the vascular repair and ensure adequate perfusion of the injured extremity. Hypothermia, which frequently accompanies prolonged operative procedures, also can cause peripheral vasoconstriction, making it more difficult to assess the distal pulses. In such instances, the distal circulation can be evaluated by examining the Doppler signal and comparing segmental Doppler pressures in the injured and uninjured limbs.

If there is an abrupt decrease in distal blood flow at any time postoperatively, reoperation may be required, even if the anastomosis is patent on arteriography. If the skin temperature is only slightly reduced and motor and nerve function are adequate, the limb may be carefully observed while attempting to improve blood flow by infusing additional fluids, blood, or low-molecular-weight dextran.

If there is any suspicion of a compartment syndrome, a fasciotomy should be performed. If all of these efforts fail to provide adequate distal blood flow, a repeated arteriogram should be performed. If a surgically correctible obstruction or narrowing is noted, reoperation is indicated. If small distall thrombi are present and they cannot be removed with a Fogarty catheter, intraarterial urokinase may be helpful (15).

Complications

Infection

Infection at the site of vascular repair is a dreaded complication that may require complete excision of the infected graft plus ligation of the involved vessels and an extraanatomic bypass to maintain the viability of the distal tissues.

When performing an extraanatomic bypass, it is essential that the proximal and distal artery be dissected well away from the site of infection, which should be draped out of the surgical field. The graft, preferably autologous vein, can be placed subcutaneously or brought through a viable muscular tunnel.

Delayed Complications

Delayed complications of repaired vascular injuries include stenosis, late thrombosis, and infections. Delayed problems with vein grafts include aneurysmal changes and intimal hyperplasia.

AXIOM The potential for late complications and symptomatic missed injuries emphasizes the need for prolonged follow-up of patients with vascular injuries.

The use of noninvasive tests, such as duplex scanning, has lessened patient discomfort and allows rapid and objective assessment of the structure and dynamics of flow at the area of injury (2).

VENOUS INJURIES

Primary Venous Repair

Venous injury is usually diagnosed during surgical exploration for a known arterial injury or by venography obtained in patients with signs and symptoms of a vascular injury but a normal arteriogram. With moderately severe venous injuries, a primary repair should be attempted if the patient is stable, the overall operative time is relatively short, and the venous repair can be accomplished with reasonable likelihood for long-term patency.

The type of venous repair used varies with the extent of the injury. Most stab wounds of veins need only a simple primary closure. Patients with small-caliber through-and-through gunshot wounds often can be treated by combining the entrance and exit sites into one larger opening, which is then repaired by simple venorrhaphy by using a running everting suture of 5-0 polyethylene suture.

Venous Ligation

When patients with moderate or severe venous injuries do not meet the criteria for a repair, primary venous ligation is recommended. With extensive injury to a major systemic vein, venous ligation also may be preferred because of the likelihood that a long suture line will thrombose and occlude or be a source of pulmonary emboli.

Postoperative Management

When a major vein is ligated in patients with a concurrent arterial injury, compartment syndrome may develop, and compartment pressures should be monitored closely or a prophylactic fasciotomy should be performed. Continuous postoperative elevation of the involved limb may circumvent the need for fasciotomy in up to 80% of patients with venous ligation.

Whether or not fasciotomy is needed, the limb in which the major venous return has been ligated should be elevated until the postoperative edema has resolved completely (16). Once this has been achieved, the patient may be started on trials of ambulation to see if the edema returns. Recurrent edema with ambulation necessitates rest and elevation of the leg for another 3 days before another trial at ambulation. Once the patient can ambulate without edema, discharge is planned. If the patient has refractory edema in spite of elevation, support hose designed to maintain the tissue pressure at 25 to 35 mm Hg is applied before discharge.

A compulsive approach to preventing peripheral edema after venous ligation minimizes long-term problems with venous insufficiency and prevents postphlebitic limb syndrome. If this program is carefully followed, fewer than 10% of the patients develop edema after venous ligation, and only 2% develop severe edema (16).

Goff et al. (17) also noted that long-term follow-up of patients with deep venous injuries is necessary to avoid complications from chronic venous insufficiency. They also reported a case of recurrent ulceration from chronic venous insufficiency that was treated successfully with an axillary vein–valve transfer.

PEDIATRIC VASCULAR INJURIES

The incidence of pediatric vascular trauma is increasing as a result of more invasive diagnostic and therapeutic procedures and because children are more frequently the victims of domestic violence (18). Attempts at diagnosis should initially be made noninvasively because arteriography has a high potential for causing further injury, especially if the vessels are small. Even if the extremity is viable, injured major arteries should be repaired.

INTRAARTERIAL INJECTION INJURIES

Drug addicts occasionally will inadvertently inject narcotics or amphetamines intraarterially, causing a severe necrotizing angiitis (19). The classic clinical syndrome of an intraarterial injection at the wrist includes sudden, constant, burning pain in the hand, particularly in the thumb, index finger, and long finger. Blanching of the involved fingers also is often seen. This appears to be due to a combination of arterial spasm and small-vessel occlusion by injected particulate matter. The result often is ischemic dry gangrene of the thumb and one or more adjacent fingers.

Treatment with intraarterial injection of vasodilators, sympathetic blocking agents, or anticoagulants or a combination of these has not been helpful in palliating this syndrome; however, in patients with marginally viable hand and severe constant pain, a stellate ganglion block or a dorsal sympathectomy will usually relieve some of the ischemia. This approach, however, seldom completely alleviates the pain that usually persists for many weeks. Occasionally, late amputation of a viable distal phalanx is the only way to control refractory pain so that patient can be restored to normal function (19).

OUTCOME OF VASCULAR INJURIES

The mortality rate after isolated peripheral vascular trauma is low, and some series reported no mortalities. Feliciano et al. (10) reported a mortality rate of 2.7% in a series of 220 patients with vascular injuries of the lower extremities. Four of the six deaths occurred within 72 hours and were attributed to complications of hemorrhagic shock. Of the two late deaths, one was a result of sepsis, and the other, a pulmonary embolus.

AXIOM Poor outcome after peripheral vascular injury is usually a result of prolonged ischemia, shock, or severe damage to other structures.

Early postoperative amputation is usually performed for tissue necrosis due to prolonged ischemia. Late amputation is done primarily for severe disability and pain or continued infection (10). Although most reported series have low early rates of amputation, there are few data on return of function, late amputations, or long-term complications.

AXIOM Nerve blocks to correct spasm after trauma to a vessel generally should be condemned because the time lost with such procedures may allow tissue changes caused by ischemia to become irreversible.

If blood flow distal to the repair still seems inadequate, an arteriogram should be performed in the OR. Any evidence of partial or complete blockage at the site of injury mandates correction, even if a new end-to-end anastomosis must be done or an autologous vein graft inserted.

⊘ FREQUENT ERRORS

1. ***Failure to look closely for vascular injuries in patients with fractures and dislocations.***
2. ***Assuming that inadequate circulation after trauma or vascular catheterization is a result of spasm rather than mechanical occlusion of the vessel.***
3. ***Delay of definitive repair to obtain arteriography when the need for vascular exploration is obvious.***
4. ***Failure to prepare and drape the entire involved extremity and to make provisions for obtaining an autologous vein for grafting from an uninvolved leg if needed.***
5. ***Failure to obtain adequate proximal and distal control before exposing the site of a major vascular injury.***
6. ***Failure to perform an adequate thrombectomy after vascular repair because there is "good back-bleeding."***
7. ***Failure to heparinize the proximal and distal portions of an injured vessel adequately while it is occluded during vascular repair.***
8. ***Delay in performing an adequate fasciotomy in patients with compartment syndrome.***

SUMMARY POINTS

1. A high-velocity missile can severely damage tissues up to several centimeters beyond the apparent missile tract.

2. A limb that has been ischemic for 4 to 6 hours or longer is at risk for sustaining tissue changes that may not be reversible with reperfusion.

3. Narrowing of the arterial lumen after trauma is seldom caused by "spasm"; in most instances, an area of persistent narrowing on arteriogram is actually an area of vascular injury.
4. Failure to promptly reduce a dislocation to restore the circulation to an extremity may result in extensive tissue necrosis and need for a later amputation.
5. Because peripheral pulses may be present in up to 25% of the patients with extremity arterial injuries, a history suggesting vascular injury may be the most important part of the initial evaluation.
6. Careful auscultation over the area of trauma is an important part of the physical examination.
7. Patients with unstable vital signs plus suspected vascular injury or threatened limbs should be taken directly to the OR.
8. The significance of abnormal findings on arteriography should be determined by the surgeon.
9. Proximity as a sole indication for angiography has an extremely low yield for revealing an injury that requires prompt surgical correction.
10. Angiography is not without risks; complications occur in at least 2% to 4% of patients.
11. Venography is seldom helpful and may be hazardous if it delays treatment of more severe injuries.
12. The position and draping for emergency vascular surgery should allow rapid securing of proximal and distal control of the injured vessels and for obtaining an autologous vein graft if needed.
13. Whenever a vascular patch or graft is needed, the injured patient's own veins generally provide the most suitable material.
14. Refractory external bleeding from leg or forearm injuries can often be controlled (before surgical control) by a sphygmomanometer inflated well above systolic pressure on the proximal thigh or arm.
15. Good back-bleeding from the distal artery does not ensure the absence of intravascular thrombus beyond the first patent collateral vessel.
16. Properly placed digital pressure on small bleeding points at a completed vascular anastomosis, with a little patience, will usually obviate the need for repair sutures.
17. The immediate aims of postoperative management after repair of a vascular injury are to maintain a normal or increased intravascular volume and cardiac output and to rewarm the patient.
18. If the survival of a limb begins to appear doubtful any time after a vascular repair, immediate arteriography or reoperation or both should be performed with correction of any anastomotic problem and distal thrombectomy with Fogarty catheters.
19. Poor outcome after a peripheral vascular injury is usually a result of prolonged ischemia or underlying vascular disease.
20. Whenever venous ligation is deemed necessary, care must be taken to prevent postoperative edema, which may go on to the development of the postphlebitic limb syndrome.

REFERENCES

1. Ledgerwood AM, Lucas CE. Vascular injuries. In: Wilson RF, Walt AJ, eds. *Management of trauma: pitfalls and practice.* 2nd ed. Philadelphia: Williams & Wilkins, 1996:711.
2. Shackford SR, Rich NH. Peripheral vascular injury. In: Moore EE, Mattox KE, Feliciano DV, eds. *Trauma.* 2nd ed. Norwalk, CT: Appleton & Lange, 1991:639.
3. Shah DM, Naraynsingh V, Leather RP, et al. Advances in the management of acute popliteal vascular blunt injuries. *J Trauma* 1985;25:793.
4. Frykberg ER, Vines FS, Alexander RH. The natural history of clinically occult arterial injuries: a prospective evaluation. *J Trauma* 1989;29:577.
5. Dennis JW, Frykberg ER, Veldenz HC, et al. Validation of nonoperative management of occult vascular injuries and accuracy of physical examination alone in penetrating extremity trauma: 5- to 10-year follow-up. *J Trauma* 1998;44:243.

6. Reid JD, Weigelt JA, Thal ER, et al. Assessment of proximity of a wound to major vascular structures as an indication for arteriography. *Arch Surg* 1988;123:942.
7. Howard CA, Thal ER, Redman HC, et al. Intra-arterial digital subtraction angiography in the evaluation of peripheral vascular trauma. *Ann Surg* 1989; 210:108.
8. Hiatt JR, Martin NA, Machleder HI. The natural history of a traumatic vertebral artery aneurysm: case report. *J Trauma* 1989;29:1592.
9. Johansen K, Bradyk D, Thiele B, et al. Temporary intraluminal shunts: resolution of a management dilemma in complex vascular injuries. *J Trauma* 1982;22: 395.
10. Feliciano DV, Herskowitz K, O'Horman RB, et al. Management of vascular injuries in the lower extremities. *J Trauma* 1988;28:319.
11. Feliciano DV, Mattox KL, Graham JM, et al. Five-year experience with PTFE grafts in vascular wounds. *J Trauma* 1985;25:75.
12. Rich NM, Baugh JH, Hughes CE. Acute arterial injuries in Vietnam: 1,000 cases. *J Trauma* 1970;10:359.
13. Artz CP, Rittenbury MS, Yarbrough DR III. An appraisal of allografts and xenografts as biological dressings for wounds and burns. *Ann Surg* 1972;175:934.
14. Ledgerwood AM, Lucas CE. Biological dressings for exposed vascular grafts: a reasonable alternative. *J Trauma* 1975;15:567.
15. Comerota AS, White JV. Intraoperative, intra-arterial thrombolytic therapy as an adjunct to revascularization in patients with residual distal arterial thrombi. *Semin Vasc Surg* 1992;5:110.
16. Mullins RJ, Lucas CE, Ledgerwood AM. The natural history following venous ligation for civilian injury. *J Trauma* 1980;20:737.
17. Goff JM, Gillespie DL, Rich NM. Long-term follow-up of a superficial femoral vein injury: a case report from the Vietnam Vascular Registry. *J Trauma* 1998;44: 209.
18. Shaker IJ, White JJ, Singer RD, et al. Special problems of vascular injuries in children. *J Trauma* 1976;16:863.
19. Johnson JE, Lucas CE, Ledgerwood AM. Infected venous pseudoaneurysm: a complication of drug addiction. *Arch Surg* 1984;119:1097.

36. INJURIES TO THE HAND[1]

The hand is a uniquely specialized organ. It contains what may be the largest number and variety of integrated structures found in the body (2). It is capable of perception and a wide variety of movements with strength and precision. Injuries to the hand and upper extremity account for almost one third of all trauma emergency room visits in many hospitals, making them among the most common injuries seen by physicians (2,3).

FUNCTIONAL ANATOMY AND BIOMECHANICS

Rather than numbering the fingers, the digits should be referred to by their common names: thumb, index, middle, ring, and small or little fingers. The sides of a digit should be described as "radial" or "ulnar" rather than "medial" and "lateral" to reduce confusion further. "Flexion" and "extension" of the thumb refer to motion occurring at the metacarpophalangeal (MP) or interphalangeal (IP) joints. "Adduction" of the thumb occurs when the extended thumb moves toward the palm, and with "abduction" the extended thumb moves away from the hand. "Opposition" is the rotational motion of the extended thumb toward the tips of the other fingers to form an "O."

Extrinsic Muscles

Flexors

The extrinsic flexor muscles lie on the volar side of the forearm and are arranged in three layers. The most superficial group includes the pronator teres, flexor carpi radialis (FCR) and ulnaris (FCU), and the palmaris longus (PL). The intermediate layer includes the flexor digitorum superficialis (FDS), the four tendons of which move independently to flex the proximal interphalangeal (PIP) joints.

The deep flexors include two muscles. The flexor pollicus longus (FPL) lies on the radius and flexes the interphalangeal (IP) joint of the thumb. The flexor digitorum profundus (FDP) lies on the ulna, and it has a common muscle belly to the middle, ring, and little fingers in the forearm; the index finger flexor is usually independent. These deep (profundus) muscles produce flexion of the distal interphalangeal (DIP) joints.

The tendons of the hand on the flexor or volar surface at the wrist are classically arranged in three layers as they enter the carpal canal (Fig. 36-1). Starting on the radial side and moving to the ulnar side, the most superficial layer includes the FCR, PL, and FCU. The middle layer includes the tendons of the FDS with the middle and ring-finger tendons lying superficial to those of the tendons to the index and small fingers. The deepest layer includes the tendons of the four FDP muscles and the FPL on the radial side (see Fig. 36-1).

Extensors

The extrinsic extensor muscles are located dorsally in the forearm and may be divided into three subgroups. The most radial (lateral) subgroup of extensors (often termed the "mobile wad") include the brachioradialis, extensor carpi radialis longus, and extensor carpi radialis brevis. The second subgroup of extensors include the extensor carpi ulnaris, the extensor digitorum communis, and the extensor digiti quinti minimi. The deep subgroup of extensors consists of five muscles, all of which act on the thumb and index finger and include the abductor pollicus longus, extensor

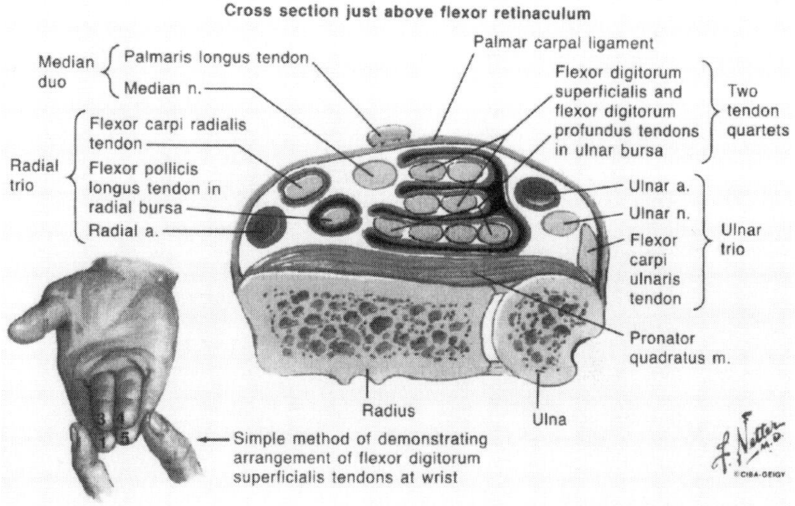

FIG. 36-1. The flexor tendons at the wrist. The tendons of the flexor pollicis longus, flexor digitorum superficialis, and flexor digitorum profundis muscles pass through the carpal tunnel. The tendons of the flexor digitorum superficialis muscle destined for the ring and middle fingers lie superficial to the tendons for the index and little fingers. Still deeper in the compartment are the four tendons of the flexor digitorum profundus muscle, lined up side by side. The tendon of the flexor pollicis longus muscle passes through the carpal tunnel deeply on the radial side. The median nerve passes into the hand through the carpal tunnel radial to the superficial row of flexor tendons. From ref. 8, with permission.

pollicus brevis, extensor pollicus longus, the extensor indicis proprius, and the supinator.

On the dorsal aspect of the wrist are six extensor compartments (Fig. 36-2).

Intrinsic Muscles

Lumbricals

The lumbricals originate from the FDP tendons and insert on the radial side of the extensor mechanism on the dorsum of the fingers, providing flexion at the MP joint and extension at the PIP and DIP joints. The first and second lumbricals (on the radial side of the hand) are innervated by the median nerve. The third and fourth lumbricals (on the ulnar side of the hand) are innervated by the ulnar nerve.

Interosseous Muscles

Four dorsal interosseous muscles originate from the sides of the metacarpal bones and insert on the sides of the extensor mechanisms. These act to abduct the other fingers away from the middle finger. The three volar interosseous muscles insert on the other sides of the extensor mechanism so that they can “adduct” the fingers toward the middle finger. All of the interosseous muscles are innervated by the ulnar nerve. They assist the lumbricals in flexing the digits at the MP joints and extending at the PIP and DIP joints.

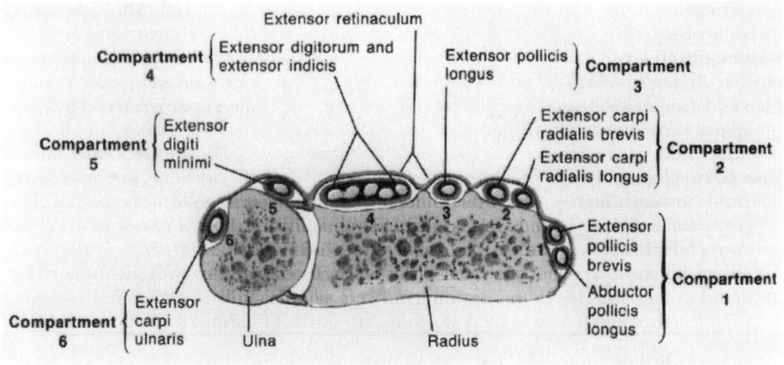

FIG. 36-2. The extensor tendons at the wrist. The extensor tendons at the wrist are arranged in six separate compartments. The tendons of the abductor pollicis longus and extensor pollicis brevis muscles occupy the first (radialmost) compartment, which is located at the styloid process of the radius. The second compartment, which lies over the rather smooth area of the radius, radial to its dorsal tubercle, contains the tendons of the extensor carpi radialis longus and extensor carpi radialis brevis. The third compartment is occupied by the tendon of the extensor pollicis longus. This tendon, passing obliquely to its insertion in the distal phalanx of the thumb, forms the prominent dorsal border for the anatomic snuff-box. The fourth compartment, over the smooth ulnar third of the dorsum of the radius, contains the four tendons of the extensor digitorum muscle and the tendon of the extensor indices. The small fifth compartment is located directly over the distal radioulnar point and transmits the tendon of the extensor digiti minimi muscle. The sixth compartment, which overlies the head of the ulna, contains the tendon of the extensor carpi ulnaris. From ref. 8, with permission.

Nerves

Radial Nerve

As the radial nerve travels between the brachioradialis and the extensor carpi radialis longus and brevis muscles, it supplies innervation to the supinator muscle and then divides into the posterior interosseous and the superficial radial nerves. The posterior interosseous nerve is motor to the long extensors of the hand and sensory to the wrist joint. The superficial radial nerve provides sensation to the dorsal skin of the thumb, the proximal and middle phalanges of the next radial 2½ digits, and the associated portion of the dorsum of the hand.

Ulnar Nerve

The ulnar nerve enters the forearm through the cubital tunnel at the elbow. In the forearm, it provides motor innervation to the FCU and the two ulnar FDP muscles. Proximal to the wrist crease, it gives off a dorsal sensory branch that innervates the ulnar side of the dorsum of the hand and 1½ fingers.

In the hand, the deep motor branch of the ulnar nerve innervates the two ulnar lumbricals, the three volar interossei (which adduct the fingers), and the four dorsal interossei (which abduct the fingers). It also innervates the adductor pollicus brevis and the deep head of the flexor pollicis brevis of the thumb, as well as the three hypothenar muscles (abductor, opponens, and flexor brevis digiti minimi).

Median Nerve

The anterior interosseous nerve is a branch of the median nerve in the forearm, and it is motor to the FPL, pronator quadratus, and the radial half of the FDP. One of the signs of damage to this nerve is the inability to "oppose" to (make an "O") with the tips of the thumb and index finger.

The median nerve in the palm divides into a motor branch to the thenar muscles and into common (sensory) digital nerves. The motor branch supplies the abductor pollicus brevis, opponens pollicus, and superficial head of the FPB. Other branches innervate the two radial lumbricals.

Arteries

The two main vessels to the hand are the radial artery (which forms the superficial palmar arch) and the ulnar artery (which forms the deep palmar arch). In most instances, the branches of these vessels communicate so well with each other that excellent hand perfusion is maintained even if one of the two vessels is completely occluded.

Branches from the common digital arteries give off branches into mesenteries called "vincula," which supply the flexor tendons. There are two vincula (longus and brevis) to each flexor profundus tendon and two vincula (longus and brevis) to each flexor superficialis tendon.

DIAGNOSIS OF HAND INJURIES

⊘ PITFALL

Failure to perform a careful systematic examination of the hand, even with apparently minor injuries, can lead to major errors in diagnosis and treatment.

A detailed history of the mechanism of the trauma coupled with a thorough examination of the hand will generally lead to a fairly accurate diagnosis.

Patient History

The pertinent medical history also includes previous surgery on the extremity, cigarette use, medical disorders, and medications.

Physical Examination

AXIOM With hand injuries, one should perform as complete a functional assessment as possible before taking off the bandage or manipulating the wound. The function of the hand is as informative as the wound itself.

As a general rule, the obviously injured areas should be examined last. This helps one to perform a more complete and systematic examination.

AXIOM When there is a finger laceration, tenderness over a flexor tendon sheath may indicate a partial tendon tear, even if the finger can move properly.

Evaluating Tendons

Each tendon should be evaluated separately. The superficialis flexor tendons are evaluated by blocking (holding) three of the four fingers with their DIP joints extended. This will allow flexion only at the PIP joint of the unheld finger by the superficialis.

The FDP is tested by blocking the other fingers in extension at the PIP joint and asking the patient to flex the DIP joint of the finger in question. The FPL is tested by blocking the MP joint in extension and asking the patient to flex the IP joint of the thumb.

Evaluating the long extensors can be accomplished by testing each compartment. For dual extensors (i.e., the indicis proprius and digiti minimi), the patient makes a fist while one looks for greater extension of the index and small fingers (to zero degrees), compared with the middle and ring fingers.

AXIOM Painful extension against resistance may be the only clinical evidence of partial extensor tendon lacerations.

Evaluating Nerve Function

Sensation

The sensory component of the radial nerve can be evaluated in the relatively autonomous area it innervates in the first dorsal web space between the thumb and index finger. Sensory function of the median nerve is best tested over the distal pulp of the index finger. For the ulnar nerve, the best area to test sensation is over the distal pulp of the small finger. Differentiating between "sharp" and "dull" is frequently used to determine if sensation is intact (Fig. 36-3).

In children, sensory nerve damage may be reflected by a loss of sweating of the skin in the distribution of the nerve. If neural function to an area of skin is intact, beads of sweat can be seen readily through an ophthalmoscope. With the wrinkle

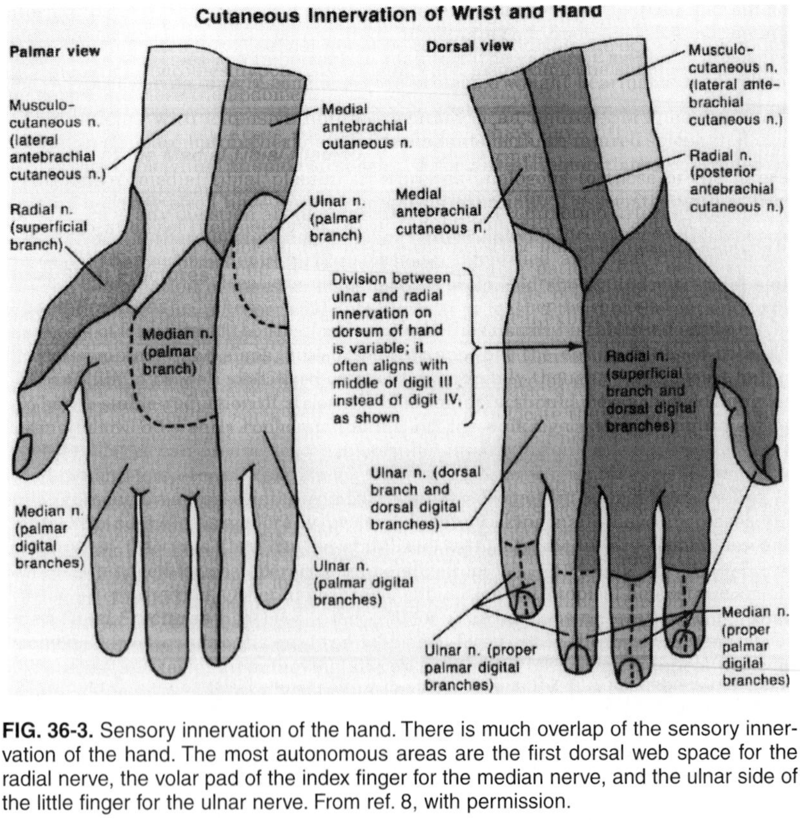

FIG. 36-3. Sensory innervation of the hand. There is much overlap of the sensory innervation of the hand. The most autonomous areas are the first dorsal web space for the radial nerve, the volar pad of the index finger for the median nerve, and the ulnar side of the little finger for the ulnar nerve. From ref. 8, with permission.

test, the area in question is immersed under water for 10 to 20 minutes; normal skin tends to wrinkle, whereas denervated skin will not.

Motor Function

For evaluation of motor function of the thumb, abduction by the abductor pollicis brevis so that the thumb is at right angles to the palm is an action unique to the median nerve. The ability to spread the fingers apart while they are extended at the IP and MP joints uses the dorsal interosseus muscles innervated solely by the ulnar nerve. Simultaneous extension at the wrist and MP joints is an action specific to the radial nerve. In a similar manner, the ability to cross the fingers requires ulnar nerve function, and snapping of the fingers requires median nerve function.

Blood Vessels

The patency of the radial and ulnar arteries at the wrist can be determined by Allen's test, which involves the patient raising the hand high above the head. The fist is clenched several times, and then clenched again firmly while the examiner occludes the ulnar and radial arteries. The patient's hand is then lowered and the fist opened. The hand should look quite pale. The pressure on the ulnar artery is then released. If the hand does not "pink up" within 3 seconds, Allen's test is considered positive, and there is some concern about the adequacy of ulnar artery blood flow to the hand. The hand can then be raised and the test repeated for the patency of the radial artery.

Radiologic Evaluation

Radiographic examinations are part of the wound assessment in any case in which there may be fractures or retained foreign bodies. Stone, tooth, metal, and many forms of glass are radiopaque. Most wood and some types of glass are radiolucent.

Whenever possible, radiographs should be taken before making any attempts at reduction of dislocations to determine the presence of associated fractures. Postreduction radiographs also are necessary to determine the adequacy of reduction.

AXIOM Dislocations associated with distal ischemia should be reduced immediately without waiting for radiographs.

Three views of any hand or wrist bone thought to be fractured are mandatory. If there is an amputated part, it also should be radiographed. Arteriography may be useful in patients with previous severe hand injuries, prior shunts for dialysis, or congenital deformities. Doppler ultrasound can be used to assess arterial patency and the competency of the collateral circulation.

TREATMENT

Routine initial management of open hand wounds includes appropriate prophylaxis against bacterial infections (usually at least one dose of a first-generation cephalosporin) and tetanus.

AXIOM Ideally, hand injuries should be repaired in an OR, where the wounds can be examined completely and the environment is sterile.

Priorities

In general, the priorities in surgical care of hand injuries are

1. Provision of an adequate blood supply;
2. Establishment of a clean wound;
3. Skin coverage, especially over bones, joints, and tendons;
4. Bone alignment and stability;

5. Tendon repairs; and
6. Nerve repairs.

Anesthesia

In children and uncooperative patients, general anesthesia is preferred. In cooperative individuals, one can use a regional or local anesthetic. Many procedures on the digits can be performed under local anesthesia. The most commonly used form of local anesthesia is the digital block. Marcaine (bupivacaine hydrochloride, 0.25% to 0.50%) or 1% to 2% lidocaine, without epinephrine, is injected through a 25-, 27-, or 30-gauge needle. The needle is introduced into the dorsal aspect of the hand approximately 1 to 2 cm proximal to the web. A small wheal of lidocaine may be introduced at the site of the skin penetration, but this is not essential. The tip of the needle is advanced proximally and volarly just dorsal to the palmar fascia on either side of the metacarpal bone of that finger. The syringe is aspirated to avoid an intravascular injection. Approximately 2.0 mL of lidocaine or bupivacaine, without adrenaline, is then injected slowly. The adjacent web space is infiltrated in a similar manner, and if surgery is required on the dorsum of the finger, a small amount of anesthetic can be injected over the extensor tendon to block the terminal branches of the nerves.

AXIOM An excessive volume of local anesthetic in a finger can cause venous congestion and vascular compromise.

Exploration

Use of a Proximal Tourniquet

Proper inspection of a hand wound requires a bloodless field, which can usually be provided only with a proximal tourniquet. To apply a tourniquet properly on the upper arm, padding is placed under a wide blood-pressure cuff, the arm is elevated, blood is squeezed out of the arm with an elastic bandage, unless infection or tumor is suspected, and the cuff pressure is then increased to 100 mm Hg above the systolic pressure, usually to at least 250 to 280 mm Hg. The cuff should be deflated for 15 to 20 minutes every 1.5 to 2.0 hours and the process repeated as needed. Thorough hemostasis must be accomplished after the cuff pressure is released.

Incisions

Adequate surgical exposure frequently requires proximal and distal extension of the wound and may also require a proximal counterincision for tendon retrieval. Basic principles of extending incisions include

1. Preservation of local circulation;
2. Extension along nonpinch surfaces whenever possible; and
3. Crossing flexion creases at angles less than 90 degrees to avoid scar-related flexion contractures.

Debridement

All devitalized and severely contaminated tissues should be removed from open wounds, and a thorough irrigation of exposed structures must be performed. Controlled pulsating lavage can be quite effective for removing surface contamination.

Fasciotomies

Fasciotomies in the forearm and hand are often indicated after severe roller injuries, crush injuries, high-pressure injection injuries, and prolonged ischemia.

AXIOM If there is any question about the need for a fasciotomy, either it should be done or compartment pressures should be measured serially. Open fractures can still have compartment syndrome.

TREATMENT OF COMMON INJURIES

Contaminated Wounds

AXIOM Hand wounds caused by contact with another individual's teeth have a high risk of severe infection, and they should be explored in the OR but should not be closed.

Although most hand wounds can be closed primarily, if there is contamination from human or animal bites, or from soil or grease, it is best to leave the wound open after thorough debridement.

Fractures and Dislocations

General Principles

Closed Fractures

Nondisplaced fractures are often stable, but they should be carefully evaluated for subtle rotational deformities. This can be done by passive motion of the wrist and fingers, thereby allowing the tenodesis effect to show malrotation. The digits are then accurately splinted or casted to prevent any movement of the fragments. Follow-up physical examination and timely radiographs are essential.

Displaced fractures should be treated closed whenever possible. Accurate reduction is essential for intraarticular fractures if good joint motion is to be preserved. One also should attempt to correct any angulation or malrotation.

Fixation of fractures is indicated if a satisfactory and stable reduction cannot be maintained with a cast or splint. Spiral, oblique, or displaced fractures are often quite unstable unless they have rigid fixation by small pins.

AXIOM Unstable hand and wrist fractures need fixation, not an aluminum splint.

Open Fractures

Open fractures generally require antibiotics and surgical exploration as soon as possible. Extensive cleansing, irrigation, and meticulous debridement are mandatory. A combination of penicillin plus an antistaphylococcal antibiotic is adequate for most hand wounds; however, one should not hesitate to use a combination of high doses of penicillin with an aminoglycoside and clindamycin in severely contaminated wounds.

Dislocations of Digits

Most dislocations of digits, when seen within 12 hours of injury, can be reduced under local anesthesia.

Dorsal dislocation of the PIP joint of a finger is the most common dislocation in the hand. With complete dislocation, the volar plate is torn, and the collateral ligament mechanism is torn to some degree. Manipulative reduction is accomplished by longitudinal traction on the finger and digital pressure distally against the dislocated joint surface. A proper digital anesthetic block usually renders this procedure painless and allows unimpeded testing of stability in anteroposterior and lateral planes after reduction. Because the volar plate is ruptured, there is almost always some hyperextension instability.

After reduction, the stability of the collateral ligaments and the palmar plate should be assessed by applying lateral and medial tension against the joints. If the ligaments are unstable, they should be repaired; this is especially important for an unstable thumb, but it is not as necessary for unstable PIP collateral ligaments. Unstable carpal–metacarpal joint dislocations require percutaneous Kirschner wire fixation.

Once the joint is reduced and if the collateral ligaments are stable, the digit can be moved immediately, but it should be protected with buddy-taping in 30 degrees of flexion for approximately 2 weeks, after which a guided-motion therapy program can be instituted.

Immobilization of the Hand

Whenever the hand will be immobilized for more than a few days, it should be placed in the "safe position," also called the "intrinsic plus" position. In this position, the wrist is neutral or slightly extended, and there is 90° MP joint flexion and 165° IP joint extension.

AXIOM A stiff hand in the intrinsic plus position is easier to mobilize than a stiff hand in a claw or intrinsic minus position.

Immobilization for fractures should include one joint above and one joint below the fracture. Three weeks of immobilization usually allows adequate healing of most phalangeal and metacarpal fractures. Rigid internal fixation with plates and screws will allow mobilization within the first few days postoperatively.

The entire injured extremity should be elevated to reduce edema. If the patient is hospitalized, the extremity can be secured to an intravenous pole or a Carter foam pillow. At home, the extremity can be elevated above the heart by using pillows at night and a sling during the day.

Tendon Injuries

General Principles

Whenever primary healing of skin lacerations can be expected, one should strive for primary tendon repairs. If large soft-tissue defects are present, the use of free or local flaps for coverage also may allow primary tendon repair. If this is not possible, delayed tendon repair, up to 4 weeks later, can provide satisfactory results (2,3).

Extensor Tendons

Although circulation to the extensor tendons is usually good, factors conspiring against a good outcome are

1. The flat, thin tendon distal to the MCP joint is easily frayed with improper handling;
2. The repaired tendon is easily ruptured by the much stronger flexors; and
3. The structure of the extensor system is quite complex, particularly at the level of the PIP joints.

Extensor tendons should be repaired in the OR with proper anesthesia and vascular control with a tourniquet. The wound is extended sufficiently to expose the ends of the tendon and accomplish repair. For lacerations involving the extensor mechanism on the fingers, additional exposure can be obtained with angled longitudinal incisions on the dorsum of the finger.

The tendons are repaired with 4-0 nonabsorbable suture by using a modified Kirchmayr (Kessler), figure-of-eight, or other techniques (4). The area of repair can be tidied up with interrupted or continuous finer sutures in the epitenon.

Postoperative care includes immobilization in a position that minimizes tension on the repair (i.e., immobilization with the wrist in extension, MP joints in slight flexion, and IP joints in full extension) for approximately 3 weeks, followed by 2 to 3 weeks of dynamic splinting and protected digital motion.

Boutonniere Deformity

Disruption of the central portion of the extensor mechanism over a proximal phalanx without proper repair can result in a boutonniere deformity. This deformity occurs if the lateral bands of the extensor mechanism are allowed to become volar to the PIP joint. This causes flexion at the PIP joint and a compensatory hyperextension at the DIP joint.

An early boutonniere deformity resulting from a closed injury may be corrected by dynamic splinting of the PIP joint in extension, allowing the DIP joint to flex. This is followed by intermittent removal of the splint and active and passive exercises for an additional 3 weeks.

Mallet Finger

A mallet finger is an acute interruption of the extensor tendon at its insertion into the distal phalanx, resulting in an inability to extend the DIP joint. Treatment requires sutures of the tendon plus immobilization with the DIP joint in slight hyperextension for 6 to 8 weeks. If an associated avulsion fracture involves more than 33% of the joint surface, open reduction is required.

Flexor Tendons

General Principles

If the condition of the wound allows, it is preferable to perform a primary repair of the flexor tendons, followed by immediate controlled mobilization. Otherwise, a delayed repair can be performed 3 to 10 days later when wound inflammation has subsided and there is no risk of infection.

Flexor tendons are repaired in the operating room (OR) under adequate extremity anesthesia, by using magnification as needed, and vascular control with a proximal tourniquet. Flexor tendons are usually repaired with nonabsorbable 3-0 or 4-0 material, by using a modified Kirchmayr (Kessler) suture (Fig. 36-4).

No Man's Land

AXIOM Combined profundis and superficial flexor tendon lacerations in "no-man's land" can be repaired early, but the procedure must be done extremely carefully (Fig. 36-5).

No-Man's Land refers to the area of the hand where the superficial and deep flexor tendons are in a common tendon sheath, between the distal palmar crease and the

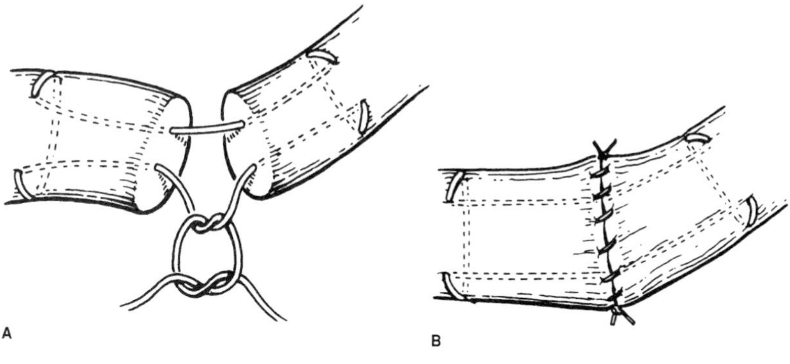

FIG. 36-4. Flexor tendon repairs. Flexor tendon repairs are accomplished with intratendinous placement of a core 4-0 nylon modified Kessler suture when there is adequate length of the distal stump. A running, shallow epitendinous suture of 6-0 nylon is added to smooth the surface of the repair so that the tenorrhaphy site can glide freely within the tendon sheath system. From ref. 9, with permission.

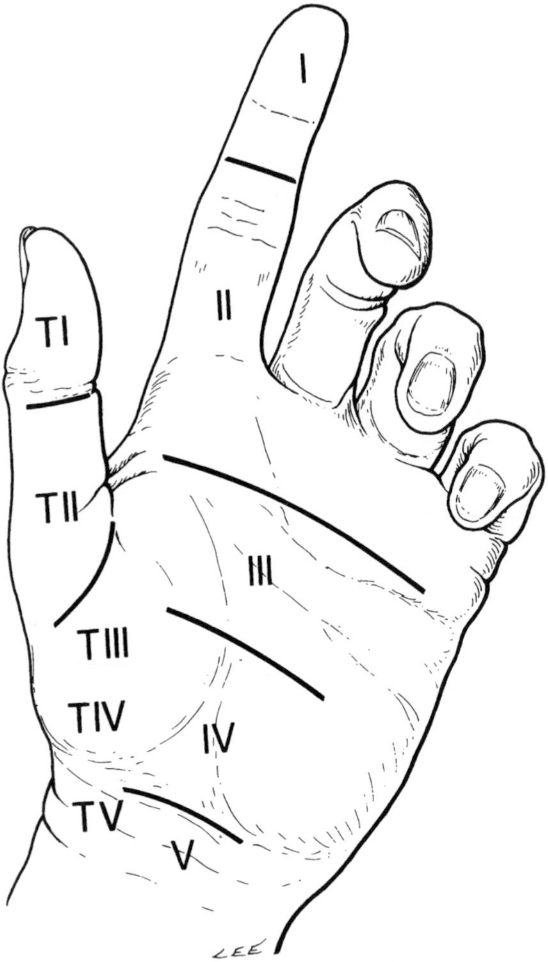

FIG. 36-5. Zones of flexor tendon injuries. International agreement among hand surgeons has resulted in a standard nomenclature to describe the zones of flexor tendon injury. The region of the fibroosseous sheath through which both the deep and superficial flexor travel to the finger was previously called no-man's land and is now referred to as zone II. From ref. 9, with permission.

proximal end of the middle phalanx. With tendon injuries in this area, the tendon sheath is opened between the annular pulleys as needed to effect the repair. Both the profundus and superficialis tendons are repaired with an intratendinous suture without exposed knots. The pulley systems are preserved as much as possible, and early controlled passive mobilization is begun (5).

AXIOM Proper tendon repairs include careful reconstruction of the tendon sheath pulleys.

With early controlled passive mobilization, two rubber bands are sewn to the fingernail or to a hook glued on the tip of the involved digit(s) at the end of the operation. A circumferential short-arm plaster dressing is then applied past the PIP joints, keeping the wrist in 30 degrees of flexion and the MCP joints in 45 degrees of flexion to allow relaxation of the repaired tendons (5). A safety pin is fixed in position to a cast or splint at the level of the scaphoid.

Two to three days after surgery, the rubber bands are attached to the safety pin. This draws the finger(s) into flexion and allows motion of the tendon juncture(s) within the sheath(s). The patient is instructed to extend the finger actively to the limits of the extensor splint and then allow the rubber band to bring the finger back into flexion. The exercise is repeated 50 times, 3 to 4 times a day. No active flexion is permitted for 3 to 4 weeks.

After 3 to 4 weeks, the dressing is removed, and the patient is encouraged to squeeze an ordinary sponge gently in warm water for 5 to 10 minutes, 3 to 4 times per day. No power gripping is permitted for an additional 2 to 3 weeks. Between exercises, a splint holding the wrist and hand in a position of function is applied for an additional week or 2. The pull-through buttons and tie-over sutures are removed at 6 weeks.

Vascular Injuries

AXIOM Even if the hand is obviously viable, major arteries in the hand or wrist should be repaired whenever possible to maintain optimal blood flow.

Nerve Injuries

Acute nerve injuries resulting from blunt trauma can be divided into neuropraxia (in which there is functional impairment but no anatomic disruption of the nerve), axontmesis (in which the axons, but not the nerve sheaths, are torn), and neurontmesis (in which both the axons and nerve sheaths are torn). Electrodiagnostic studies are usually postponed for 3 weeks after the initial trauma to be more accurate. They are then repeated at 3 months as indicated.

AXIOM If there is a reasonable likelihood that injury to a nerve is only functional (neuropraxia), early exploration is not required; however, careful follow-up examinations are extremely important.

Penetrating injuries with nerve dysfunction require examination of all possibly involved nerves at the time of surgery. It is important to reestablish nerve integrity by repair or grafting during the first 2 weeks whenever possible because the hand cannot function optimally without sensation. Lacerated nerves to the hand should have a grouped fascicular repair performed under an operating microscope whenever possible.

Nail Injuries

Injury to the germinal or sterile matrix or both is virtually assured if there is a subungual hematoma associated with a distal tuft fracture from a crush injury. It is essential with these injuries to remove the nail plate and to repair the nail bed accurately. The nail plate can then be replaced to protect the nail bed.

If the eponychium and nail bed are both cut, they should be sutured separately. A small wick of paraffin mesh or vaseline gauze should then be inserted under the eponychium to ensure that adhesions do not develop between it and the nail bed. The paraffin mesh or vaseline gauze wick is extruded from under the eponychium as the fresh nail advances.

Fingertip Injuries

If the loss of skin is less than 1 cm^2 with a fingertip injury, the pulp can be allowed to granulate and heal by secondary intention. Larger defects without exposed bone can be covered with full-thickness skin grafts.

Whenever possible, one should try to maintain finger length after amputations. Excising bone to close the soft tissue at the tip is often easier, but generally it is not optimal therapy. If bony length is desirable for function, especially when the DIP joint or fingernail can be preserved, flap reconstruction is indicated.

With proximal digital amputations, the tendon ends should not be secured over the end of the bone.

Injuries from Pressure Injections

Pressure-injection injuries can be very deceptive, and the entrance may be difficult to find. Nevertheless, they can cause severe tissue loss, dysfunction, and deformities and must be treated as an emergency. Immediate exploration and meticulous debridement are required (6).

Loss of Skin

Small skin defects on the dorsum of the hand or fingers can often be closed primarily after mobilization of the skin. If a large defect is present but the tendon sheaths are still present, a split-thickness skin graft can often be used successfully. If bare tendon is exposed, rotational or transposition flaps are indicated. Occasionally, a reverse cross-finger flap can be used.

Skin grafts on the volar surface of the fingers or palm should be of similar color and texture, especially for patients with darker pigmented skin. Potential donor sources are the hypothenar eminence and dorsum or sides of the foot.

Avulsed skin flaps that have been defatted may be used as full-thickness skin grafts as long as only minimal crush occurred during the injury.

Large defects with exposed tendon, bone, joint, and blood vessels require flap coverage. Local pedicle flaps may be sufficient if the size and the location of the wounds permit; however, a microvascular free-flap transfer may be preferred.

Specific Techniques

Fasciotomies

Crush injuries should be treated with early fasciotomy unless hand function and compartment pressures are normal and can be measured frequently. The first symptom of compartment syndrome is often a subjective decrease in sensation or pain with passive stretch.

Replantations

Indications

Replantation is the restoration of viability to a totally amputated part of the body (7). Replantation should be attempted only if experienced surgeons are available, if the wound ends are optimal, and microsurgical technique and careful follow-up care can be provided.

Some of the more common indications for replantation include multiple amputations of digits and amputation of the thumb, especially in children; however, some patients are better served in terms of function with a primary amputation than with multiple subsequent operations, decreased sensation, and pain and cold intolerance. In order of importance, the priorities for replantation of amputated digits are the thumb, middle, ring, small, and index finger.

Technical Considerations

Cooling of the amputated part before replantation is accomplished by completely covering it with a sterile sponge that has been lightly moistened with lactated Ringer's solution. It is then placed in a sealed, plastic, watertight envelope in a large container of regular ice. Dry ice should not be used.

During replantation, all nerves, arteries, and veins are labeled with sutures. Bony fixation is then accomplished, often with about 5 mm of shortening, and the flexor tendons are usually repaired first. The hand is then turned over, and the extensor tendons are repaired. Last, the veins, arteries, nerves, and skin are repaired in that order. The replanted parts are then covered with a dressing and noncompressive protective casting or splinting.

Postoperative Care

The replanted part must be constantly watched for several days for the adequacy of perfusion. The surgeon(s) undertaking replantation must be prepared to reexplore the hand if vascular compromise becomes evident. Some anticoagulation, preferably with aspirin or dextran or both, may be indicated if the amputation was produced by means other than a clean cut.

POSTTRAUMATIC INFECTIONS

Volar infections in the hand can often cause significant dorsal swelling, and one may be fooled into thinking that the process is actually dorsal rather than volar in origin.

Kanavel described four classic signs of tenosynovitis in the fingers: flexed position, fusiform swelling, tenderness along the flexor tendon sheath, and pain on passive extension. These infections usually require surgical drainage of the tendon sheath plus intravenous antibiotics.

Any laceration over a knuckle should be considered a human bite injury until proven otherwise. If it is a suspected human bite, antibiotics should be started promptly and the depths of the laceration explored and thoroughly debrided in the OR. The wound is left open.

⊘ FREQUENT ERRORS

1. ***Assuming a tendon is not injured because the finger moves properly.***
2. ***Repair of tendon or deep soft-tissue injuries of the hand outside the OR.***
3. ***Exploration of hand injuries without a proximal tourniquet or adequate anesthesia.***
4. ***Failure to check sensation before giving an anesthetic block.***
5. ***Attempts to fixate unstable finger fractures with splints.***
6. ***Immobilization of joints for a prolonged period after tendon repairs, fractures, or dislocations in elderly patients.***
7. ***Failure to accurately repair nail-bed lacerations.***
8. ***Failure to suspect human bite wounds with lacerations over knuckles.***

SUMMARY POINTS

1. With hand injuries, one should perform a complete functional assessment before taking off the bandage or manipulating the wound.

2. The function of each tendon should be evaluated separately, but it must be remembered that a partially lacerated tendon that needs repair may seem to function relatively well.

3. When there is a finger laceration, tenderness over a flexor tendon sheath or painful extension against resistance may indicate a partial tendon tear, even if the finger can move properly.

4. Ideally, hand injuries should be repaired in an OR with proximal tourniquet applied to provide maximal visibility of all structures that might have been injured.

5. There is no substitute for thorough surgical debridement and lavage for preventing wound infections after trauma.

6. If there is any question about the need for a fasciotomy, either it should be done or compartment pressures should be measured serially.
7. Hand wounds caused by contact with another individual's teeth have a high risk of severe infection, and they should be explored in the OR but should not be closed.
8. Unstable hand and wrist fractures need fixation, not an aluminum splint.
9. Patients with open fractures in the hand should receive antibiotics against gram-positive cocci (such as streptococci, *Staphylococcus aureus*), aerobic gram-negative bacilli (such as *Escherichia coli*), and mouth anaerobes.
10. A stiff hand in the intrinsic plus position is easier to mobilize than a stiff hand in a claw or intrinsic minus position.
11. Combined profundus and superficial flexor tendon lacerations in no-man's land can be repaired early, but the procedure must be done extremely carefully with reconstruction of the tendon sheath pulleys plus early passive motion.
12. Even if the hand is obviously viable, major arteries in the hand or wrist should be repaired whenever possible to maintain optimal blood flow to the hand.
13. The first symptom of compartment syndrome is often a subjective decrease in sensation or pain with passive stretch.
14. If there is a reasonable likelihood that injury to a nerve is only functional (neuropraxia), early exploration is not required; however, careful follow-up examinations are extremely important.
15. Aggressive, precise, early repair of an injured nail bed is the key to optimal healing.
16. Whenever possible, one should try to maintain finger length after amputations.
17. Replantation should be attempted only if experienced surgeons are available, if the wound ends are optimal, and microsurgical technique and careful follow-up care can be provided.
18. Preservation of life should not be jeopardized to try to save a limb.
19. Because ischemic tissue easily develops frostbite, amputated parts to be replanted should not come directly into contact with ice.
20. One should assume that all injection injuries are severe and require prompt extensive debridement and exploration in the OR.

REFERENCES

1. Zidel P, Wilson RF. Injuries to the hand. In: Wilson RW, Walt AJ, eds. *Management of trauma: pitfalls and practice.* 2nd ed. Philadelphia: Williams & Wilkins, 1996:736.
2. Kleinert HE, Freund RK. Hand injury. In: Moore EE, Mattox KL, Feliciano DV, eds. *Trauma.* 2nd ed. Norwalk, CT: Appleton & Lange, 1991:607–621.
3. Angermann P, Lohmann M. Injuries to the hand and wrist: a study of 50,272 injuries. *J Hand Surg [Br]* 1993;18:642.
4. Greenwald DP, Hong HZ, May JW. Mechanical analysis of tendon suture techniques. *J Hand Surg [Am]* 1994;19:641.
5. Karlander LE, Berggren M, Larsson M, et al. Improved results in zone 2 flexor tendon injuries with a modified technique of immediate controlled mobilization. *J Hand Surg [Br]* 1993;18:26.
6. Pinto MR, Turkula-Pinto LD, Cooney WP, et al. High-pressure injection injuries of the hand: review of 25 patients managed by open wound technique. *J Hand Surg [Am]* 1993;18:125.
7. Kleinert HE, Jablon M, Tsai TM. An overview of replantation and results of 347 replants in 245 patients. *J Trauma* 1980;20:390.
8. Netter FH. *The CIBA collection of medical illustrations. Vol. 8: musculoskeletal system. Part I: anatomy, physiology, and metabolic disorders.* Summit, New Jersey: Ciba-Geigy Corp., 1987:61.
9. Markinson RE. Tendon injuries in the hand. In: Champion HR, Robbs JV, Trunkey DD, eds. *Rob and Smith's operative surgery: trauma surgery, part 2.* 4th ed. Boston: Butterworth, 1989:734.

37A. THERMAL INJURIES[1]

INDICATIONS FOR BURN CENTER CARE

Of the 2 million people burned each year in the United States, approximately 70,000 require hospital treatment. Of these, 80% can be managed in a general hospital setting; however, burn center care may be of benefit for the remaining 20% who have

1. More than 10% total body surface area (TBSA) burns and are younger than 10 years or older than 50 years;
2. More than 20% TBSA burns and are age 10 to 50 years;
3. Significant burns of the face, hands, feet, genitalia, perineum, or over major joints;
4. Full-thickness burns more than 5% TBSA;
5. Significant electric injury, lightning injury, or chemical burns;
6. An inhalation injury;
7. Burns associated with significant preexisting illness;
8. Burns associated with a need for special social or emotional support or rehabilitation; or
9. Burns due to possible child abuse or neglect (2).

PREHOSPITAL EMERGENCY MANAGEMENT

Burn Wounds

Burn wounds (other than those caused by chemicals) require minimal early care. The patient should be moved immediately from the source of heat. Clothing should be removed promptly from the involved areas because garments may continue to smolder or retain sufficient heat to extend the area and depth of the wound. Prompt application of cold water or towels to small burns affords some relief of pain and may lessen the degree of injury. Covering the patient with a clean dry sheet will decrease pain from air contact. More elaborate dressings or topical agents will interfere with assessment of the wound at the burn center.

⊘ PITFALL

Wet dressings and cold compresses applied to large burn wounds for prolonged periods may cause hypothermia.

Chemical Burns

Chemical burns represent a special situation in which prompt action is essential to prevent additional tissue injury and systemic toxicity from continued absorption of the chemical (3). The victim's clothing should be removed immediately, but care should be taken not to spread the chemical on bystanders. Identification of the offending agent is important to determine proper decontamination procedures.

AXIOM One should not irrigate chemical burns with neutralizing acid or alkali solutions because the heat of reaction that can occur may cause further tissue damage.

Hydrofluoric acid is unique in that therapy consists of immediate decontamination by water lavage or a quaternary ammonia solution followed by specific treatment.

Topical application of 2.5% calcium gluconate gel forms an insoluble calcium salt with the fluoride ion. Alternatively, a 5% solution of calcium gluconate may be injected into the involved area in a dose not to exceed 0.05 mL/cm^2. Recurrence of pain is an indication that additional injections may be necessary. Intraarterial calcium gluconate also has been used in the treatment of hydrofluoric acid burns of an extremity.

INITIAL HOSPITAL MANAGEMENT

Endotracheal Intubation

Patients who have major burns involving the head and neck and require large volumes of fluid for resuscitation and patients with oropharyngeal burns should be promptly intubated, preferably via the nasotracheal route, before significant edema develops. Extubation can be performed safely when the edema of the head and neck has receded, usually 3 or 4 days later.

Initial Cleansing and Debridement

All involved areas should be cleansed gently with a mild detergent. The wounds also should be debrided to remove loose, nonviable epidermis and bullae more than 2 cm in diameter. Hair should be clipped from the wound and from a generous margin of adjacent unburned skin.

Proper tetanus immunization should be provided to all burn patients.

Estimating the Depth of the Burns

AXIOM Mortality from burn wounds is determined primarily by the extent of burn and the age of the patient.

First-degree injury, such as a sunburn, consists of epidermal damage alone.

Second-degree burns involve the entire epidermal layer and part of the underlying dermis. Superficial partial-thickness injuries are usually quite painful and have an erythematous appearance with blebs and bullae. In deep partial-thickness burns, sensation is impaired to a variable degree.

A third-degree (full-thickness) burn implies destruction of all epidermal and dermal elements. The skin is often charred or leathery and has a pearly white sheen. Typically it is anesthetic, but there may be intermixed areas of partial-thickness injury.

Severe scald injuries may initially appear bright red and may be classified as superficial partial-thickness burns even though the damage is full thickness. Failure to blanch with pressure helps to differentiate them from partial-thickness injuries (4).

Estimating the Body Surface Area (BSA) Involved

The patient should be weighed, and the percentage of BSA involved should be determined. Initially, in the adult, the size of the burn wound can be estimated by using the "rule of nines," which approximates the BSA as follows:

Head and neck, 9%
Chest plus abdomen, 36%
Each arm, 9%
Each leg, 18%
Genitalia, 1%.

A more exact determination also can be made by using a surface-area diagram, such as the Lund–Browder chart adjusted for age. For example, in a 1-year-old infant, the head and neck is 17% to 19% of the total BSA, and each lower extremity is 12% to 14%.

One side of the patient's hand is approximately 1% of the BSA. When calculating the extent of a burn for fluid therapy, only second- and third-degree injuries are included.

Pain Management

During the initial period of resuscitation, general anesthesia should be avoided if possible. Procedures such as wound debridement and escharotomy can generally be performed safely in the intensive care unit by using small doses of intravenous narcotics, preferably morphine, titrated to the patient's needs.

If a patient with a significant burn (i.e., more than 30% TBSA) requires general anesthesia because of concomitant mechanical trauma, a Swan–Ganz catheter should be placed, and invasive cardiac monitoring used to guide fluid therapy and other hemodynamic support measures. Succinylcholine should be avoided in patients with extensive burns, especially after the first 24 to 48 hours, because it may precipitate a severe hyperkalemia.

Fluid Resuscitation

Burn injury more than 20% BSA results in an obligatory loss of substantial amounts of fluid into the burn wound and a resultant decrease in vital organ perfusion (5). This "burn shock," if left untreated, can rapidly result in acute tubular necrosis and other organ failure.

Fluid resuscitation should begin as early as possible by using a large-bore peripheral intravenous line, preferably placed in an area of unburned skin. Lactated Ringer's solution is the fluid of choice for burn resuscitation in the first 24 hours.

Estimating Fluid Needs

The fluid needs for adults can be calculated as 2 to 4 mL/kg body weight/% BSA burned (2 to 4 mL/kg/%). In children weighing less than 30 kg, the usual fluid needs are 3 mL/kg body weight/% BSA burned (3 mL/kg/%) plus maintenance fluids (D5 ½ NS at a rate of 1,500 mL/m^2/day). Half of the burn resuscitation fluids are usually administered within the first 8 hours after injury, and the remainder, over the subsequent 16 hours.

Thus an 80-kg adult with a 50% second- and third-degree burn would theoretically require 8,000 to 16,000 mL of isotonic crystalloid in the first 24 hours. About 4,000 to 8,000 mL should be given in the first 8 postburn hours at a rate of about 500 to 1,000 mL/h. The adequacy of resuscitation is then determined by the urine output and frequent examination of the patient (Table 37A-1).

Table 37A-1. ***USAISR Formula for Estimation of Fluid Resuscitation Needs in Burn Patients***

- First 24 h after burn
  - Adults and children ≥30 kg
    - Lactated Ringer's solution, 2-4 mL/kg/% burn
      - Half given in first 8 h
      - Half given in remaining 16 h
  - Children <30 kg
    - Lactated Ringer's solution, 3 mL/kg/% burn + maintenance fluids*
- Second 24 h after burn
  - 5% albumin in lactated Ringer's solution
    - 30%–50% burn, 0.3 mL/kg/% burn
    - 50%–70% burn, 0.4 mL/kg/% burn
    - >70% burn, 0.5 mL/kg/% burn
  - 5% dextrose in water to maintain urine output at 30 to 50 mL/h‡

*Frequent adjustments to maintain a urine output of 0.5–1.5 mL/kg/h are necessary in children. Increasing the rates calculated above will be necessary in about 50% of patients (13).

‡D5 0.3-0.5 NS is substituted for 5% dextrose in water for maintenance fluids in children <30 kg.

In adult patients, the usual goal is to infuse fluid at a rate that will result in a urine output of 30 to 50 mL/h. If urine output is not adequate, the volume of infusion should be incrementally increased until the desired urine output is achieved. In children weighing less than 30 kg, the desired urine output is 1 mL/kg/h.

Causes of Increased Fluid Needs

Conditions that may result in fluid requirements above those initially calculated include

1. Delay in resuscitation;
2. Drug or alcohol intoxication;
3. Inhalation injury;
4. Electric injuries (because the extent of damage is difficult to assess); and
5. Associated injuries.

AXIOM Occult hemorrhage from associated mechanical trauma should be suspected when fluid requirements that are much greater than those calculated from the apparent extent of the burn.

If no additional injuries can be found to explain fluid needs that are much greater than expected, invasive monitoring and measurements of cardiac output and pulmonary artery wedge pressure (PAWP) should be performed.

Fluid Needs During the Second 24 Hours

Approximately 24 hours after injury, part of the resuscitation fluid, especially in small children, can be changed from Ringer's lactate to a colloid-containing solution. This can be given as 5% albumin in a balanced salt solution in an amount equivalent to 0.3 to 0.5 mL/kg body weight/% BSA burn. Thus a 20-kg child with a 50% burn might be given 600 to 1,000 mL of 5% albumin as part of the second 24-h fluid intake. In addition, electrolyte-free fluid also should be infused as "maintenance fluid" fast enough to maintain a urine output of 30 to 50 mL/h. In children weighing less than 30 kg, 5% dextrose in one half normal saline is administered to maintain a urine output of 1 mL/kg/h.

AXIOM Modest hyponatremia is expected after resuscitation with lactated Ringer's solution because the total body water is generally greatly increased. Consequently, fluid restriction, not sodium administration, is the eventual best method for increasing serum sodium levels back to normal.

Estimating Insensible Water Loss

Patients with increased insensible water loss from burns may need additional intravenous (i.v.) fluids. The formula for estimating insensible water loss (in mL/h) from burns is

$$\text{Insensible } H_2O \text{ loss} = (25 + \%\text{ burn})(\text{m}^2)\text{mL/h} \tag{1}$$

Thus a 50% burn in a patient with a TBSA of 2.0 m^2 would have an insensible water loss of about (25 + 50) (2) or 150 mL/h.

Fluid Needs After 48 Hours

After 48 hours, fluid administration can usually be reduced because edema resorption will occur and the resorbed edema fluid will enter the circulation. A daily loss of 10% to 12% of the weight gained during resuscitation should be permitted until the patient returns to his or her preburn weight by postburn day 7 to 10. The best way to monitor fluid balance in this period is to maintain an accurate log of the patient's intake and output and get daily weights and serum sodium concentrations.

Glucose and Sodium Needs in Infants and Young Children

AXIOM Adult burn patients do not generally require glucose infusions during the first 24 hours after injury. Children, because of their limited glycogen stores, are prone to develop hypoglycemia if dextrose-free i.v. fluids are infused for prolonged periods.

Children also are far more susceptible than adults to cerebral edema as a result of overhydration. Consequently, the serum sodium should be monitored frequently, and rapid shifts in serum sodium should be prevented by avoiding salt-free solutions.

⊘ PITFALL

Adult resuscitation formulas do not take into account the infant's need for glucose, higher maintenance fluid needs, and increased sensitivity to hyponatremia.

Escharotomies

In Extremities

As resuscitation proceeds, vascular compromise may occur in extremities with circumferential full-thickness thermal injury due to tissue swelling inside an unyielding eschar. The Doppler ultrasonic flow probe is useful in assessing the vascular status of burned limbs. As the resuscitation progresses and there is increasing tissue edema, peripheral neurologic changes or diminution of the Doppler signal indicates impaired tissue perfusion and the potential need for an escharotomy.

AXIOM Because the loss of a Doppler signal also can be caused by hypovolemia, the adequacy of resuscitation should always be assessed before performing escharotomies.

Escharotomy should be performed in the midmedial or midlateral lines of the involved limb or both with the patient in the anatomic position (Fig. 37A-1). Escharotomy can be performed at the bedside by using electrocautery and does not usually require anesthesia because the incision is generally made through insensate full-thickness burn injury.

The burn eschar should be incised only down to the unburned superficial subcutaneous fat to allow the edges of the eschar to spread as much as needed to restore adequate perfusion. The escharotomy incisions should be carried across the entire length of the full-thickness injury and extended across involved joints. Pulses and neurologic function should be rechecked after the escharotomy to ensure that blood flow has been restored.

Chest Wall

Chest-wall escharotomies may be required if circumferential deep thermal injury of the chest impairs chest-wall excursion to the point that blood gases are deteriorating or peak airway pressures on a ventilator are increasing (or both) to levels at which barotrauma may occur.

The eschar is incised in the anterior axillary lines. If the eschar continues onto the abdomen, the lateral chest incisions should be connected by another escharotomy at the level of the costal margins to free the anterior chest wall plate.

Fasciotomies

In patients with high-voltage electric injuries, those with associated soft-tissue mechanical trauma, and those with deep thermal injury in whom escharotomy fails

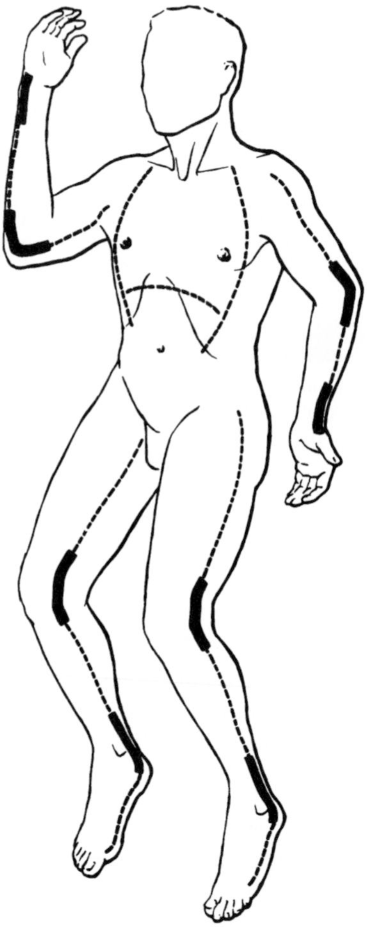

FIG. 37A-1. Preferred sites for escharotomy are the medial and lateral aspects of the extremities.

to restore tissue blood flow, fasciotomy of the involved compartments should be performed. With electrical injuries, the fasciotomies may have to include individual muscles down to the bone.

Initial Management of Carbon Monoxide Poisoning and Inhalation Injury

Carbon Monoxide Poisoning

Carbon monoxide is the leading agent of death by poisoning in the United States. Among survivors, serious complications include both immediate and delayed neurologic syndromes. A history of smoke exposure in an enclosed space plus obtundation should alert one to the possibility of carbon monoxide intoxication. Conventional measurement of arterial blood gases does not exclude carbon monoxide poisoning. Direct measurement of the level of carboxyhemoglobin is the only reliable way to detect carbon monoxide poisoning.

Carbon monoxide levels may normally be up to 10% in smokers, and levels of 10% to 20% may cause no symptoms. Levels of 20% to 40% tend to cause increasing headache and nausea, and levels of 40% to 60% tend to cause increasing neurologic problems. Levels greater than 60% are usually fatal.

The treatment for patients suspected of carbon monoxide poisoning is administration of 100% oxygen via a tight-fitting nonrebreathing face mask or an endotracheal tube. This reduces the half-life of carboxyhemoglobin from 4 to 5 hours on room air to approximately 40 minutes. Treatment should be continued until the carboxyhemoglobin level is less than 10%.

Hyperbaric oxygen (HBO), if available, can reduce the neurologic changes seen with carbon monoxide poisoning, but unless there is a special set-up, HBO therapy entails a period of at least 90 minutes during which the ability to monitor the patient's resuscitation and general condition may be limited. Use of HBO is important, however, if significant neurologic changes persist or develop in a delayed fashion.

Meert et al. (6) treated 106 children who had carbon monoxide poisoning with normobaric oxygen. Fifteen patients died, and seven survivors did not recover their premorbid neurologic state. Although the authors thought that the persistent sequelae were primarily related to asphyxia, the neurologic outcomes might have been improved with hyperbaric oxygen.

Inhalation Injury

Inhalation injury is a chemical tracheobronchitis or pneumonitis or both caused by entry of products of incomplete combustion into the lungs. Except for inhalation of steam under high pressure, there is no direct thermal injury to the lungs. A history of being burned in an enclosed space, the presence of facial burns, or an extensive flame burn should raise the suspicion of inhalation injury. The presence of soot in the nares and mouth, inflamed oropharyngeal mucosa, and carbonaceous sputum are consistent with but not diagnostic of inhalation injury. Patients in whom there is any suspicion of inhalation injury should be treated with 100% oxygen at the scene because of the potential for concomitant carbon monoxide poisoning.

When the patient arrives at the hospital, arterial blood gases and carboxyhemoglobin levels should be promptly obtained. If they are abnormal or there is other evidence of respiratory distress, the patient should be intubated, preferably by the nasotracheal route. Positive findings on bronchoscopy include carbonaceous material below the true vocal cords. Concomitant erythema or ulceration or both in the tracheobronchial mucosa indicate moderate to severe injury.

AXIOM The presence of an inhalation injury increases the mortality rates associated with burns by as much as 20% (7) and may double the initial i.v. fluid needs.

Patients suspected of having inhalation injury who have a negative bronchoscopic examination should have xenon-133 ventilation/perfusion lung scanning (8).

AXIOM Prophylactic antibiotics do not prevent pneumonia and are contraindicated until or unless bacterial pneumonitis is present.

Patients with inhalation injury should undergo daily or every-other-day microscopic examination and surveillance cultures of tracheobronchial secretions to identify the predominant organisms. If the tracheobronchial aspirate reveals more than 20 to 25 polymorphonuclear leukocytes (PMNs) and fewer than 10 squamous cells per high-power field, a diagnosis of tracheobronchitis is made, and antibiotic therapy based on previously obtained surveillance cultures and sensitivity results is begun. Antibiotics also should be started if pneumonia develops, as diagnosed by a new or increasing pulmonary infiltrate on chest roentgenogram in association with fever and tracheobronchial leukorrhea.

AXIOM Corticosteroid use is absolutely contraindicated in inhalation injuries.

TREATMENT OF THE BURN WOUND

Topical Antimicrobial Agents

AXIOM Prophylactic i.v. antibiotics are not given for burn wounds, but bacterial proliferation in the eschar should be suppressed by topical antibiotics until excision and grafting can be performed.

Dries et al. in 1994 (9) showed that INF-γ can reduce infection-related deaths in patients with severe injuries; Wasserman et al. (10) in 1998, however, in a double-blind placebo-controlled study, found that IFN-γ did not protect burn patients from infections or decrease the mortality rate from infection.

Mafenide acetate (Sulfamylon) penetrates eschar well. It is effective against gram-negative organisms, including *Pseudomonas aeruginosa*. The main problems with its use are its inhibition of carbonic anhydrase, which causes an increased loss of bicarbonate in the urine with a resulting metabolic acidosis, and the severe pain that it can cause when applied to wounds with intact sensation.

Silver sulfadiazine (1%) is effective against most gram-negative bacilli, but resistance can develop rapidly. Furthermore, diffusion of this agent into the eschar is limited. Continued application of silver sulfadiazine may cause leukopenia, and neutrophil counts should be monitored. Alternate application of Sulfamylan (days) and Sulfamylon (nights) on a 12-hour schedule reduces the incidence of side effects and realizes the benefits of both.

Silver nitrate–soaked (0.5%) dressings can be applied to wounds of patients with allergies to sulfa-derived agents; however, silver nitrate can leach sodium and chloride from the wound, and it discolors everything with which it comes in contact. The dressings also must be kept moist.

Early Excision and Grafting

Excision and grafting of deep partial-thickness burns (that would otherwise take longer than 3 weeks to heal) and full-thickness burns is begun as soon as resuscitation is complete and mobilization of "third space" fluid is occurring, as evidenced by decreasing daily weights.

Early excision and grafting tends to decrease hospital stay (especially in patients with small full-thickness burns), decrease infectious complications, and improve cosmetic and functional results. Excision of a burn wound, however, may be associated with massive blood loss ranging from one half to one unit of blood per percentage BSA excised, depending on the anatomic location and the maturity of the wound.

In patients with extensive full-thickness burn wounds, excision to the level of the investing fascia results in less blood loss than tangential excision. For burns on an extremity, the blood loss caused by tangential excision can be reduced by using a tourniquet applied proximal to the operative site.

Burn-wound excisions are staged and limited to 20% of the body surface or that which can be accomplished in 2 hours to avoid massive transfusion and hypothermia.

The excised area can then be autografted with available donor sites by using a 3:1 to 4:1 expanded "mesh" graft. Cutaneous allografts are placed over the meshed autogenous tissue to protect the open interstices.

Management of Burn-Wound Infections

Diagnosis

Invasive burn-wound infection remains a risk until all eschar has been excised and the wounds are healed. The burn wound is examined daily for signs of infection, which include focal dark discoloration of the wound, conversion of a partial-thickness injury to full-thickness injury, green discoloration of subcutaneous tissue, early separation of eschar, and vesicular eruption in healing or recently healed partial-thickness injuries. These changes mandate biopsy of the most suggestive areas of the burn wound along with adjacent deep viable tissue. Part of the specimen is sent for culture, and the rest is processed for examination by the pathologist. Biopsies demonstrating progressive eschar colonization indicate loss of microbial control and mandate change in the wound-care regimen.

AXIOM Histologic examination of a burn-wound biopsy is the mainstay in the diagnosis of invasive burn-wound infection.

Treatment

Invasive burn-wound infection is treated immediately with systemic antibiotics appropriate for the organisms identified. For gram-negative bacterial infection, injection of the subeschar space with a broad-spectrum penicillin is performed 6 to 12 hours before urgent surgical excision of the wound (11). Invasive fungal wound infections are excised immediately, and systemic amphotericin B is administered.

Nutrition

Increased Caloric and Protein Needs

The magnitude of the catabolic response after thermal injury is proportional to the burn size. In patients with burns of 50% or more of the body surface, the metabolic rate is approximately 1.5 to 2.0 times the predicted resting energy expenditure. Catecholamines, glucagon, and cortisol are important mediators of the exaggerated metabolic response.

Insulin levels are initially depressed, but they gradually return to normal as catabolism decreases and anabolism increases. Hyperglycemia results from increased tissue resistance to insulin and increased gluconeogenesis (12). Increased glucose demands are generated by the wound, which uses carbohydrates in an obligatory fashion via anaerobic metabolism.

To prevent the erosion of lean body mass that would otherwise occur in unalimented burn patients, nutritional support should provide adequate protein and calories to match the increased metabolic needs. The bulk of the calorie needs is supplied with glucose; however, the capacity for glucose metabolism is limited to 4 to 5 mg/kg/min in most patients, and at higher infusion rates, hyperglycemia can become a problem. The remaining calorie needs must be met with lipids. Nitrogen requirements can be estimated as 1 gram of nitrogen per 150 kilocalories. Whenever possible, estimates of calorie needs in severely burned patients should be based on indirect calorimetry rather than on derived formulas.

Enteral Feeding

At least some enteral feeding is possible in nearly all burn patients after the first 2 to 3 days. It eliminates the risks of central venous catheters, helps maintain gut mucosal integrity, and ameliorates some of the metabolic consequences of the acute inflammatory and hypermetabolic phase. Eaves-Pyles and Alexander (13) found that gut barrier function is impaired as early as 5 minutes after burn in mice and is maximal by 4 hours. Killing of translocated bacteria also is impaired. Khorram-Sefat et al. (14) found that use of a C1-esterase inhibitor in scald burns in pigs significantly decreased the plasma levels of the complement membrane-attack complex (SC5b-9). It also reduced bacterial translocation and the degree of intestinal ischemia in the postburn period compared with that in untreated animals.

Initially, the enteral feeding is done via a nasogastric tube, so that the gastric residual can be checked before each 1- to 4-hour feeding.

Growth Hormone

The effects of recombinant human growth hormone (rhGH) on the enhancement of wound healing and on the improvement of protein metabolism in patients with large burns have been reported in many articles in recent years (15). In addition to its anabolic effect, GH has been described as a stimulator of host defenses against bacterial infections (16).

ELECTRICAL BURNS

High-voltage injuries may cause only small entrance and exit burns, but they can cause severe underlying tissue damage with occasional loss of extremities, hyperkalemia, myoglobinuric renal failure, and need for extensive fasciotomies.

BURN COMPLICATIONS

Gastrointestinal Problems

In patients with burns of 25% or more of the BSA, ileus is virtually universal, and a nasogastric tube is placed to prevent emesis and aspiration. The nasogastric tube also can be used to monitor intragastric pH. A histamine (H_2) antagonist, such as cimetidine, should be started soon after admission. The drug should be given intravenously at first, but it can be given orally once normal bowel function has been restored. Serious gastrointestinal bleeding from erosive gastritis or duodenal ulcers can generally be prevented by maintaining the gastric pH above 5.

The resumption of oral intake as soon as possible is probably the best prophylaxis against upper gastrointestinal stress ulcers.

Hypothermia

AXIOM Patients with major burns should be kept in a warm environment (at least 84°F) that will maintain a core temperature of 100.0°F to 100.5°F.

Failure to maintain extensively burned patients in a warm environment can lead to hypothermia and can greatly increase the stress placed on homeostatic mechanisms. Patients who are already at the limits of their metabolic reserve cannot adapt to further stress, and circulatory collapse may be precipitated if they attempt to maintain body temperature in a cool environment.

Thromboembolism Prophylaxis

Thromboembolic complications in burn patients have been reported to occur with a frequency of 0.4% to 7%. This low incidence of thromboembolism does not justify the risks of routine low-dose heparin prophylaxis, which is associated with a 0.6% to 5% incidence of complications including bleeding, thrombocytopenia, and arterial thrombosis. The high incidence of pulmonary embolism in morbidly obese burn patients, even in the face of heparin prophylaxis, may justify the use of vena cava filter placement for prophylaxis (17).

⊘ FREQUENT ERRORS

1. ***Failure to promptly remove a patient's garments that may still be hot or contaminated with chemicals.***
2. ***Failure to promptly intubate patients with major burns that also involve the face.***
3. ***Underestimating the extent of underlying tissue damage in electrical burns.***
4. ***Excessive reliance on burn formulas to determine the quantity and speed of fluid resuscitation.***
5. ***Failure to anticipate the presence of an inhalation injury in patients with flame burns in a closed environment.***
6. ***Failure to supply adequate glucose during fluid resuscitation of children with major burns.***
7. ***Failure to adequately and promptly explain excessive fluid requirements in a burn patient.***

8. ***Failure to anticipate the need for escharotomy in patients with deep circumferential burns involving the chest, extremities, or both.***
9. ***Excessive blood loss during burn-wound excisions.***
10. ***Relying on clinical criteria to diagnose and treat invasive burn-wound infection.***
11. ***Maintaining patients with severe burns in an environment with a temperature less than 84°F.***

SUMMARY POINTS

1. Removal of the offending agent by removal of clothing and copious irrigation is the mainstay of the early treatment of chemical burns.

2. One should not irrigate chemical burns with neutralizing acid or alkali solutions because the heat of reaction that can occur may cause further tissue damage.

3. Chemical burns may be complicated by systemic toxicity if the agent is absorbed; a history that identifies the causative agent allows specific treatment of systemic effects.

4. Mortality from burn wounds is primarily determined by the extent of burn and the age of the patient.

5. First-degree injuries do not usually require fluid resuscitation, unless they are extensive.

6. The size of the patient and the extent of the burn injury are the most important determinants of the volume of resuscitation fluid required.

7. If there is a significant inhalation injury, the fluid needs and mortality rates are often increased 50% to 100%.

8. Burn-resuscitation formulas provide an estimation of fluid requirements, and adjustments are made as required by frequent assessment of the clinical response, especially urine output.

9. Occult hemorrhage from associated mechanical trauma should be suspected when fluid requirements are much greater than those calculated from the apparent extent of the burn.

10. Adult burn patients do not generally require glucose infusions during the first 24 hours after injury. Children, however, because of their limited glycogen stores, are prone to develop hypoglycemia if dextrose-free i.v. fluids are infused for prolonged periods.

11. Because the loss of a Doppler signal can also be caused by hypovolemia, the adequacy of resuscitation should always be assessed before using the Doppler signal or other indications for performing escharotomies.

12. Blood gas or ventilatory impairment in patients with circumferential deep chest-wall burns indicates a need for escharotomy.

13. Bronchoscopy plus xenon-133 lung scanning is the most reliable method for establishing the diagnosis of inhalation injury.

14. Treatment of inhalation injury consists of providing adequate humidified oxygen and aggressive pulmonary toilet; prophylactic antibiotics and steroids are contraindicated.

15. Excision and grafting of full-thickness and deep partial-thickness burns that will take longer than 3 weeks to heal is begun as soon as resuscitation is complete and mobilization of "third space" fluid is occurring.

16. Expansion of the autograft to ratios greater than 4:1 is frequently associated with desiccation of the recipient bed and failure to obtain closure with autograft.

17. Histologic examination of a burn-wound biopsy is the mainstay in the diagnosis of invasive burn-wound infection.

18. Serious gastrointestinal bleeding from erosive gastritis or duodenal ulcers can generally be prevented by maintaining the gastric pH above 5.

19. The resumption of oral intake as soon as possible is probably the best prophylaxis against upper gastrointestinal stress ulcers.
20. Patients with major burns should be kept in a warm environment (at least 84°F) that will maintain a core temperature of 100.0 to 100.5°F.

REFERENCES

1. Martin RR, Becker WK, Cioffi WG, et al. Thermal injuries. In: Wilson RF, Walt AJ, eds. *Management of trauma: pitfalls and practices.* 2nd ed. Philadelphia: Williams & Wilkins, 1966:760.
2. Committee on Trauma, American College of Surgeons. *Resources for optimal care of the injured patient.* Committee on trauma, American College of Surgeons, Chicago; 1993:64.
3. Mozingo DW, Smith AA, McManus WF, et al. Chemical burns. *J Trauma* 1988;28:642.
4. Heimbach MD, Engrav L, Grube B, et al. Burn depth: a review. *World J Surg* 1992;16:10.
5. Pruitt BA Jr, Mason AD Jr, Moncrief JA. Hemodynamic changes in the early postburn patient: the influence of fluid administration and of a vasodilator (hydralazine). *J Trauma* 1971;11:36.
6. Meert KL, Heidemann SM, Sarnaik AP. Outcome of children with carbon monoxide poisoning treated with normobaric oxygen. *J Trauma* 1998;44:149.
7. Shirani KZ, Pruitt BA Jr, Mason AD Jr. The influence of inhalation injury and pneumonia on burn mortality. *Ann Surg* 1987;205:82.
8. Moylan JA Jr, Wilmore DW, Mouton DE, et al. Early diagnosis of inhalation injury using xenon-133 lung scan. *Ann Surg* 1972;176:477.
9. Dries DJ, Jurkovich J, Maier RV, et al. Effect of interferon gamma on infection-related death in patients with severe injuries. *Arch Surg* 1994;129:1031–1042.
10. Wasserman D, Ioannovich JD, Hinzmann RD, et al. Interferon-γ in the prevention of severe burn-related infections: a European phase III multicenter trial. *Crit Care Med* 1998;26:434.
11. McManus WF, Goodwin CW, Pruitt BA Jr. Subeschar treatment of burn-wound infection. *Arch Surg* 1983;118:291.
12. Jahoor F, Herndon DN, Wolfe RR. Role of insulin and glucagon in the response of glucose and alanine kinetics in burn-injured patients. *J Clin Invest* 1986;78:807.
13. Eaves-Pyles T, Alexander JW. Rapid and prolonged impairment of gut barrier function after thermal injury in mice. *Shock* 1998;9:95.
14. Khorram-Sefat R, Goldmann C, Radke A, et al. The therapeutic effect of C1-inhibitor on gut-derived bacterial translocation after thermal injury. *Shock* 1998;9:101.
15. Ziegler T. Growth hormone administration during nutritional support: what is to be gained? In: Zaloga G, ed. *New horizons: frontiers in critical care nutrition.* Fullerton, CA: Society of Critical Care Medicine, 1994:244–256.
16. Inoue T, Saito H, Fukushoma R, et al. Growth hormone and insulin-like growth factor 1 enhance host defense in a murine sepsis model. *Arch Surg* 1995; 130:1115.
17. Sheridan RL, Rue LW III, McManus WF, et al. Burns in morbidly obese patients. *J Trauma* 1992;33:818.

37B. TEMPERATURE-RELATED (NONBURN) INJURIES[1]

HOMEOTHERMIC REGULATION

Homeothermic (warm-blooded) animals tend to maintain a relatively constant internal (core) temperature that allows free mobility through hostile ambient temperatures, but the body temperature of poikilothermic (cold-blooded) animals tends to take on that of the environment.

Homeothermic regulation begins with detection of the ambient (external) temperature by peripheral thermal receptors and the core temperature by central receptors especially in the preoptic hypothalamus (2). These thermal receptors track directly to the hypothalamic areas concerned with temperature regulation.

Responses to a Cold Environment

The homeothermic responses to a cold environment include

1. Physical thermogenesis (shivering and increased muscle tone);
2. Metabolic thermogenesis (increased secretion of thyroxine and catecholamines);
3. Vasoconstriction; and
4. Conscious responses, such as increased physical activity.

At basal levels, total heat production generally ranges from 40 to 60 kcal/h, but may increase up to 300, 600, or even 900 kcal/h under situations of severe exertion or shivering (3). At core temperatures below 28°C (83°F), however, the homeothermic responses to cold are virtually nonexistent (2).

Responses to a Hot Environment

Besides a basal heat production of approximately 40 to 60 kcal/h, the body may be exposed to up to 150 kcal/h from irradiation from the sun (4). To this load is added the heat produced by any work being performed.

The body's responses to hyperthermia include

1. Cutaneous vasodilation;
2. Sweating; and
3. Decreased physical activity.

Heat conduction from the core of the body to the skin increases linearly eightfold from its vasoconstricted state at an ambient temperature of 24°C (75°F) to its maximally vasodilated state at 43°C (110°F) (4). Sweating can increase heat loss up to 10 times that of basal heat production. Increased humidity or pooling of sweat or both, however, reduces the efficacy of evaporation as a means of heat loss.

AXIOM Heat-stroke syndrome is more likely to occur if there is increased activity and the person is poorly acclimatized.

The physiologic process whereby an individual adapts to work in a hot environment is often referred to as acclimatization. These changes include decreased sweat production, decreased sodium concentration in sweat, increased aldosterone secretion, and a decreased maximal cardiac output, stroke volume, and heart rate. Additionally, acclimatized subjects drink greater quantities of water spontaneously and have baseline increases in their calculated extracellular fluid volumes. The metabolic efficiency of these individuals also increases, thereby decreasing the net heat production for a given unit of work.

Protective homeothermic mechanisms become increasingly impaired if the core temperature exceeds 41°C (106°F) or decreases below 34°C (94°F).

SPECIFIC COLD-INDUCED INJURIES

Nonfreezing Cold Injury

Nonfreezing cold (NFC) injury is caused by tissue chilling and by reduced perfusion of tissues due to cold-induced vasoconstriction. Factors contributing to NFC injury are

1. Immobility;
2. Impaired circulation;
3. Venous stasis;

4. Debilitation;
5. Constrictive footwear or clothing; and
6. Dehydration.

In very cold and wet conditions, NFC injury can develop in hours, but in less extreme conditions, it may require days of exposure.

AXIOM Cold injury is much more likely to occur in areas of the body that are poorly perfused and are not kept dry.

Chilblain refers to the swelling and reddish or violaceous plaques that develop on fingers, toes, or ears after repeated or chronic exposure to dampness at temperatures just above freezing. Burning, itching, and tingling in the involved part may be quite severe after rewarming. In some instances, vesiculations and ulcerations may develop. Treatment consists of careful rewarming of the involved part and protection from further cold or trauma.

Immersion foot occurs with prolonged exposure to a wet and relatively warm environment. It is characterized by white, wrinkled, painful involvement of the soles of the feet. With more prolonged exposure, the dorsum of the foot also may be involved. Some physicians treat immersion foot by warming the feet in water heated to 100 to 105°F and then carefully drying them (2). Others prefer passive rewarming at room temperature because active local rewarming may increase the edema, reactive hyperemia, and pain. Analgesics are often necessary during the rewarming. Although recovery is complete and without major long-term sequelae in most circumstances, severe complications such as nerve and muscle injury, as well as gangrene, may occasionally be seen.

Frostbite

The term frostbite refers to the damage caused by crystallization of water in the skin or subcutaneous tissue due to exposure to temperatures at or below freezing (6). The majority of soldiers who develop frostbite are exposed to temperatures below –12°C (–10°F) for more than 7 hours. Lack of adequate protection to the face, ears, and extremities is a common etiologic factor. The wind-chill factor also is important, and a 30-mph wind can greatly reduce the effective temperature.

Pathophysiology

The pathophysiologic changes of frostbite usually involve at least two factors:

1. Direct tissue damage caused by the cold; and
2. Tissue injury resulting from vasoconstriction and then later vasodilatation with resultant edema, red-cell sludging, and thrombosis of vessels.

Once extracellular freezing begins, unbound intracellular water shifts to the extracellular spaces in response to the hypertonic osmotic gradient surrounding the ice crystals (2). Cellular damage or death from freezing is a complex process involving damage from ice crystals and osmotic gradients, and alterations in intracellular composition (particularly of enzyme systems).

Diagnosis

Sudden blanching or an unusual whiteness of the skin with a pale, glassy appearance may be the first indication of cold injury (6). There is generally also an uncomfortable sensation of coldness followed by numbness. Initially, the depth of frostbite cannot be determined accurately, as all the frozen areas are cold, cadaveric in appearance, and without sensation (2).

The severity of frostbite may be divided into degrees (6).

First-degree (frost nip): Characterized by hyperemia and edema after thawing
Second-degree: Characterized by hyperemia and blisters
Third-degree: Necrosis of the skin and subcutaneous tissue
Fourth-degree: Necrosis of underlying fascia and muscle

Treatment

Rewarming

When the patient with frostbite is in a protected environment where the involved tissues will not be traumatized or cooled again, the frozen tissues should be rapidly rewarmed. Rapid thawing by submerging the frozen areas in water preheated to 38 to 40°C (100.4 to 104°F) is the method of choice for frostbite. Thawing with heat in excess of 40°C (104°F) can increase the loss of tissue. Rewarming is continued until all of the involved tissues are warm and hyperemic. If, after rewarming, third-degree frostbite tissue remains blanched, the patient may benefit from the use of intravenous heparin (6). Analgesics are often required to help reduce the severe pain that can occur during thawing.

AXIOM If systemic hypothermia below 32°C (90°F) accompanies the frostbite, rapid internal rewarming is the treatment of choice (2).

After Rewarming

AXIOM The depth of tissue necrosis in frostbite is usually much less than expected.

The goals of treatment after rewarming are to avoid infection and to minimize loss of tissue (2). Inexperienced observers often incorrectly assume that the black skin of frostbite when the patient is first seen indicates a full-thickness injury with death of the skin and the underlying deep tissue. This assumption has led to unnecessary and an inappropriately high number of early amputations for frostbite. One should wait at least 2 to 3 months, unless infection supervenes, before performing any debridements or amputations.

Prophylactic antibiotics are not used unless indicated for other injuries. The frostbitten areas are treated in an open fashion on sterile padding and under cradles covered by sterile sheets to avoid secondary injury from pressure. Although some surgeons open bullae and then apply a topical antibiotic, most will allow the vesicles and bullae to resolve spontaneously. Sterile cotton is placed between the digits to prevent maceration.

If the tissue becomes infected, the area should be debrided as needed to control the local infection and to prevent systemic sepsis.

Delayed Sequelae

Over a period of weeks or months, the blebs, edema, hyperemia, anhidrosis, and paresthesias largely disappear. In third- or fourth-degree frostbite, however, the patients often remain incapacitated by limitations of motion, pain on walking, hyperhidrosis, hyperesthesias, cold intolerance, and severe vasospastic attacks to even mild cold. Years after suffering deep frostbite, more than two thirds of the patients still complain of cold feet, hyperhidrosis, pain, and numbness, particularly during winter months.

Total-Body Hypothermia

Etiology

AXIOM Hypothermia can occur at virtually any environmental temperature below 80°F.

Impaired Tissue Perfusion

Hypothermia is generally defined as a body core temperature of less than 35°C (95°F). The frequency of posttraumatic hypothermia is unclear, but patients with a reduced cardiac output, in addition to hypotension, are at great risk for developing hypothermia, especially in the operating room (OR). In a group of critically injured adults with head injuries, 40% were hypothermic during resuscitation (2). The incidence of hypothermia in patients who are in shock and require massive transfusions is even higher.

AXIOM One should monitor core temperatures closely in trauma patients, especially those who are in shock, receive massive transfusions, or have prolonged abdominal surgery.

Cold Intravenous Fluids

Hypothermia that develops in the hospital in injured patients is often also related to the amount of cold fluid and blood administered. In one study, hypothermic patients received an average of 8.7 units of blood versus 3.3 units in patients who did not develop hypothermia ($p < 0.01$) (2).

Mechanisms of Heat Transfer

The mechanisms of heat transfer include radiation, conduction, convection, and evaporation.

Radiation, which is the movement of infrared heat rays from the skin at the speed of light, usually accounts for about 50% to 60% of the body's heat loss in a warm room (7). In a cold environment, the radiant heat loss may be much greater.

At room temperature, heat **conduction** accounts for about 20% of the heat loss (15% to the air and 5% to adjacent objects). In water, heat conduction is 24 times faster than that in air (7). Indeed, hypothermia can develop with just 1 or 2 hours of immersion in water as warm as 16°C (65°F).

Convection occurs as warm air next to the skin is replaced by cool air. If there is no wind, convection carries off only about 25% of lost body heat. If the wind velocity is more than a few miles per hour, the heat loss by convection may exceed the body's heat loss by conduction.

Evaporation from the skin accounts for only about 7% of heat loss at rest, but under certain conditions, it can carry off an amount of heat equivalent to 6 times the body's basal metabolic rate. This heat loss increases with exertion or at higher altitudes, especially in cold, dry air. Thus the total heat loss by evaporation from the skin and airways may account for more than 20% of the body's heat loss.

Stages of Hypothermia

The three stages of hypothermia have been described as

1. Responsive;
2. Slowing; and
3. Poikilothermic.

The **responsive phase** (core temperature, 32°C to 35°C) is characterized by an attempt on the part of the patient to maintain a normal body temperature (2). Blood pressure, heart rate, and respiratory rate are initially increased, but later decline as the hypothermia becomes more severe (7). Muscle tone is increased and is frequently accompanied by active shivering. The level of consciousness also may be depressed and is typically manifest as stupor or confusion. Peripheral vasoconstriction is evidenced by diminished pulses, pallor or acrocyanosis, and coolness of the extremities to touch. The increase in central blood volume induced by peripheral vasoconstriction can produce a diuresis (so-called "cold diuresis") that can cause clinically significant hypovolemia. Cardiac output progressively decreases as the heart cools and myocardial contractility decreases, even if the blood volume is maintained at normal levels.

AXIOM The patient has little or no defense against hypothermia during a general anesthetic or if the core temperature decreases to less than 32°C.

During the **slowing phase** (core temperature 23°C to 32°C), enzyme kinetics slow, and shivering, if present, may be manifest only as a fine tremor. The skin vessels become vasodilated, and heart rate, respiratory rate, and blood pressure progressively decrease.

Below 28°C, the patient is usually comatose, and clinically, a core temperature of less than 28°C is considered severe hypothermia. Patients in the **poikilothermic phase** (core temperature less than 23°C) have no effective way of preventing heat loss (2).

Hypothermia produces a decrease in basal metabolic rate and oxygen consumption (VO_2) of approximately 6% to 7% per degree centigrade, so the metabolic rate is 51% of normal at a core temperature of 28°C (7).

Blood viscosity increases with decreased core temperature as a result of an increase in plasma viscosity and an increasing hematocrit (7). Below 32°C, all vital signs tend to be subnormal. Compensatory mechanisms such as shivering tend to disappear below 28°C, but the muscles tend to be quite rigid because of increased muscle tone.

As the core temperature decreases to 28°C, there is progressive slowing of myocardial depolarization. This causes widening of QRS complexes, prolongation of the PR interval, T-wave inversion, J waves, arrhythmias (especially atrial fibrillation), and progressive bradycardia. Osborne (J) waves are slow positive deflections in the latter part of the QRS complex. This abnormality is seen most prominently in aVL, aVF, and in the left chest leads (7).

AXIOM Hypothermic patients are more likely to develop ventricular fibrillation during insertion of a pulmonary artery (PA) catheter.

Physiologic Changes with Hypothermia

Renal

The cold diuresis seen with hypothermia occurs because peripheral vasoconstriction increases the central blood volume and renal perfusion. In addition, there is decreased reabsorption of water and sodium as a result of depressed tubular oxidative activity (7). Renal tubular glucosuria also may result.

AXIOM The diuresis occurring with hypothermia can cause hypovolemia, and this can cause severe hypotension during rewarming.

Pulmonary

Respiratory rate and minute ventilation may initially increase as the core temperature begins to decrease, but at core temperatures below 32°C, the respiratory rate progressively decreases so that below 28°C, the respiratory rate may be less than four breaths per minute. At such temperatures, there is also often an alveolar pattern on radiograph resembling pulmonary edema.

Pulmonary secretions can be greatly increased during hypothermia, especially during rewarming. Additionally, hypothermia decreases the cough reflex and reduces vital capacity (8). All of these processes predispose the patient to severe atelectasis and posthypothermia pneumonitis.

The oxyhemoglobin dissociation curve shifts to the left as a direct effect of reduced temperatures. The PO_2 and PCO_2 decrease about 4% to 5% for each 1°C decrease in temperature.

Laboratory

Electrolyte changes with hypothermia include progressive hyponatremia and either hyperkalemia or hypokalemia. Platelets and leukocytes may be sequestered in the spleen or liver, resulting in thrombocytopenia and leukopenia.

Hyperglycemia during hypothermia may result from

1. Decreased insulin release from the pancreas;
2. Inhibition of peripheral glucose utilization; or
3. Altered hepatic carbohydrate metabolism.

Coagulation

The function of coagulation factors and platelets becomes progressively impaired as the temperature decreases below 34°C to 35°C. Below 28°C to 32°C, a clinical picture of disseminated intravascular coagulation (DIC) may develop.

AXIOM One of the best ways to prevent coagulopathies in trauma patients is to prevent or correct hypothermia rapidly.

Neuromuscular

At 27°C to 32°C (80°F to 89°F) there is usually confusion and decreased deep tendon reflexes, peripheral nerve conduction, and pain sensitivity. Below 26.7°C (80°F), there is usually coma, the pupils are often fixed, and patients are often areflexic. The electroencephalogram is generally flat when the core temperature is lower than 20°C (9).

An oft-quoted dictum in the treatment of hypothermia is that "hypothermic patients are not dead until they are warm and dead." Indeed, all methods of clinical assessment are inaccurate until the patient is adequately rewarmed to at least 32°C, but preferably to 34°C to 35°C (2,7).

Near-Drowning (Diving Response)

Near-drowning in ice-cold water causes a special type of hypothermia. Although the diving response that is seen in marine mammals occurs in most humans to a small extent, in about 15% of the volunteers tested, a profound diving response was noted. This response, which starts immediately on submersion, prevents aspiration of water, redistributes oxygen stores to the heart and brain, slows cardiac oxygen use, and initiates a hypometabolic state. Thus survival from prolonged near-drowning appears to depend on an interplay between the degree of the diving response, the rapidity of development of hypothermia, and the speed with which protective hypometabolism develops.

Monitoring

AXIOM In general, core temperatures are best monitored with an esophageal probe, particularly in the OR.

AXIOM Uncorrected blood gas values in hypothermic patients may be more meaningful than those that are corrected to the patient's temperature.

Arterial blood gases (ABGs) are determined at 37°C. Correction of the Po_2 to the patient's core temperature is acceptable, but the values are difficult to interpret relative to the decreased metabolism occurring while the patient is hypothermic (9). Pulse oximetry and transcutaneous measurement of Po_2 and Pco_2 in severe hypothermia tend to be inaccurate because of the decreased skin perfusion.

Treatment of Hypothermia

Patients with severe hypothermia can often meet their physiologic needs despite significant hypotension, bradycardia, and hypoventilation. Consequently, overly aggressive treatment of hypothermia may cause more harm than good and may even cause ventricular fibrillation.

An important cause of death after rescue may be related to "rewarming shock" (9). Although the patient may be able to maintain adequate perfusion during hypothermia, the vasodilation that occurs during rewarming may cause severe hypotension, and the additional metabolic burden of rewarming may be too great for the cardiovascular system.

If no breathing is present or the respiratory rate is less than four per minute, the hypothermic patient should have endotracheal intubation. Hyperventilation with precipitate changes in arterial pH should be avoided. If there is any cardiac function in a severely hypothermic patient, external cardiac massage is likely to cause more harm (can precipitate ventricular fibrillation) than good.

The indications for the treatment of metabolic acidosis with sodium bicarbonate during cardiac arrest are controversial. Empiric sodium bicarbonate is not generally recommended during the first 10 minutes of CPR; however, it can be given if ABG analysis reveals a severe metabolic acidosis with a pH less than 7.10 or 7.20.

If treatment appears to be indicated for suspected severe metabolic acidosis, most authorities recommend using an initial bolus of 1 mEq $NaHCO_3$/kg of body weight. Further sodium bicarbonate administration should be guided by measurements of the arterial and venous blood gases. Indeed, giving bicarbonate can cause a "paradoxic" cellular acidosis if the increased CO_2 that is produced is not removed adequately by the lungs. The P_{CO_2} should be less than $(HCO_3)(1.5) + 12$ (i.e., if the HCO_3 is 12 mEq per liter, the P_aCO_2 should be 30 mm Hg or less to give bicarbonate).

External Warming

Passive external rewarming consists of adding an insulating layer to the patient (e.g., a blanket) and allowing the patient's own heat-generating mechanisms to restore body temperature (2,7). This increases core temperature approximately 1°C (1.8°F) per hour. Obviously, this method is adequate only in otherwise normal patients with mild hypothermia (Table 37B-1).

Table 37B-1. ***Treatment Options for Rewarming Patients with Hypothermia***

Degree of Hypothermia	Treatment
Mild: Core temperature of 32°–34.9°C (89.6°–94.9°F)	Passive external rewarming Shelter from the environment Remove wet or cold clothes Apply layers of clothing or blankets Provide warm fluids
Moderate: Core temperature of 28.0°–31.9°C (82.4°–89.4°F)	Active external rewarming of truncal areas with Electric warming blankets Hot-water bottles Heating pads Radiant heat sources Warming beds
Severe: Core temperature <28°C (<82.4°F)	Active core rewarming with Warm humidified oxygen Nasogastric lavage Peritoneal lavage Open thoracotomy with myocardial/mediastinal irrigation Cardiopulmonary bypass

Modified from ref. 17, with permission.

Active external warming uses devices that generate their own heat (i.e., hot-water bottles, submersion in a tank of warm water, or heating blankets; 7). Forced-air systems, with disposable plastic covers and a heat source that directs warm air across the skin, can provide simultaneous convective heat transfer plus protection against radiant heat loss (10). This technique can accelerate the rate of rewarming without apparent complications. Active external warming is suitable for patients in the upper range of moderate hypothermia who are without dysrhythmias or significant electrocardiogram (ECG) changes.

Active external warming has some hazards. Blankets or warmers higher than 45°C can burn the patient's skin. Surface warming also causes cutaneous vasodilation. The resulting shift of blood from the core to peripheral vessels may cause a marginally hypovolemic patient to develop rewarming shock. This problem can be avoided if volume repletion is promptly accomplished and maintained during rewarming.

As a result of external rewarming, the cold blood previously trapped in the peripheral circulation of patients with moderate to severe hypothermia can induce core cooling, or "afterdrop," as it enters the central circulation (7). This afterdrop can cause ventricular fibrillation that is unresponsive to pharmacologic or electrical stimuli. Additionally, as the surface temperature increases above that which stimulates shivering, heat production stops, even though an acceptable core temperature has not yet been achieved (2).

The warming method of choice for patients with moderate to severe hypothermia is **active core warming** (2). With these techniques, the heart and brain are rewarmed first. The central thermal receptors regain their previously cold-inhibited function, and homeothermic reflexes can now assist rewarming.

The most effective, easily managed, and readily available method of active core warming is ventilation with heated gases. Because stimulation of the oropharynx may induce cardiac arrhythmias, intubation of severely hypothermic individuals should be attempted only by the individual with the most expertise in this technique. To prevent thermal injury to the respiratory passages, the maximal inspired temperature of the heated gases should be 43.3°C (110°F). In awake patients, the gas temperature must be reduced to approximately 40°C (104°F). With this technique, patients can be warmed at about 1.2°C to 1.4°C (2.2°F to 2.5°F) per hour.

As soon as the major bleeding has been controlled during emergency surgery, the surgeon should irrigate the body cavity being explored with warmed saline until the core temperature is at least 34°C to 35°C.

Warmed peritoneal dialysis and closed pleural lavage, however, are relatively slow and may require large volumes of warmed fluid. Hemodialysis with a blood warmer is especially useful when overdose of certain drugs (e.g., barbiturates) accompanies hypothermia (9).

Extracorporeal circulation with a heart–lung machine [i.e., cardiopulmonary bypass (CPB)] has been used successfully in a number of patients with extreme hypothermia (9). The advantages include extremely rapid rewarming from the core outward, support of the circulation, provision of volume replacement and oxygenation, reversal of hemoconcentration, and decreased stress to the myocardium (11). Core rewarming also shortens the interval during which cardiopulmonary resuscitation (CPR) is required in patients with cardiopulmonary arrest.

Splittgerber et al. (11) showed that CPB rewarms at 4 times the rate of other types of core rewarming. In collective data from 11 studies using CPB for profound hypothermia with a cardiac arrest between 1967 and 1987, the survival rate was 71% (12).

Volume expansion is an essential component of resuscitation from hypothermia. A minimum of 500 mL of isotonic fluid is usually needed for each 1°C temperature increase to maintain an adequate blood volume; however, because cardiac depression often accompanies hypothermia, the rate of the volume replacement should be guided by the response of the central venous pressure (CVP) and cardiac output. Isotonic crystalloid solutions warmed to approximately 40°C can be infused fairly rapidly in doses of 20 mL/kg as often as needed as long as the CVP does not increase abruptly (9).

AXIOM Some glucose should be present in the fluids used to resuscitate hypothermic patients.

Adrenergic medications, especially dopamine in inotropic dosages, can help support blood pressure during hypothermia. Drugs generally not recommended in hypothermic patients include vasoconstrictors, sodium bicarbonate, insulin, corticosteroids, and ethanol (9).

HEAT-OVERLOAD SYNDROMES

Exposure to hot environments may result in a variety of disorders including heat cramps, heat syncope, heat exhaustion, and heatstroke (2).

Heat Cramps

Heat cramps are the most benign type of heat-overload syndrome (2). Athletes participating in strenuous activities are particularly susceptible to this problem. The cramps seem to result primarily from electrolyte imbalances, especially hyponatremia, and are characterized by painful spasms of the voluntary muscles. Occasionally the cramps in abdominal muscles may mimic an acute abdomen. Ingestion of water without electrolytes intensifies the electrolyte imbalance and can make the symptoms much worse.

Heat cramps are usually best corrected by administration of dilute salt solutions after the patient has been placed in a cool environment. Because sweat has 5.0 or more mEq of potassium per liter, excessive sweating, corrected only with water and NaCl, can eventually cause hypokalemia.

Heat Syncope

The symptoms of heat syncope can range from lightheadedness to actual loss of consciousness. The body temperature may be quite elevated, especially if the episode is induced by exercise. In spite of the hyperthermia, the patient is often pale as a result of hypotension from peripheral venous pooling.

Heat syncope is generally self-limiting and often requires no treatment other than removal of the patient from the main heat source and rest in a recumbent position; however, administration of water and salt will usually speed recovery.

Heat Exhaustion

Heat exhaustion, also called heat prostration, is the most common type of heat-overload syndrome (2). Patients typically are seen with weakness, vertigo, headache, and nausea, which may progress to physical collapse. Although recovery from heat exhaustion is usually spontaneous, intravenous saline can speed the process.

Heatstroke

Heatstroke is a medical emergency, with mortality rates ranging from 10% to 80%. It is characterized by a body temperature equal to or greater than 41.1°C (106°F), or by a body temperature of 40.6°C (105°F) or greater with anhidrosis or an altered mental status or both (7).

Types of Heatstroke

Heatstroke syndrome may be either nonexertional ("classic" heatstroke) or exertional. Exertional heatstroke is typically seen in healthy young adults who overexert themselves in high ambient temperatures and humidity. These patients usually stop sweating before the onset of symptoms, and subsequently they may demonstrate hyperpyrexia (2).

Classic heatstroke is nonexertional and is most common in patients with preexisting diseases, such as scleroderma, atherosclerosis, diabetes mellitus, or alcoholism. Other conditions associated with the development of heatstroke syndrome include congestive heart failure, renal insufficiency, chronic obstructive pulmonary disease, cystic fibrosis, and thyrotoxicosis. Although classic heatstroke is most commonly a disorder of the elderly during environmental heat waves, all ages are at risk. Drugs that may increase the risk of heatstroke include diuretics, phenothiazines, anticholinergics, β-blockers, tricyclic antidepressants, and amphetamines (13).

Pathophysiology

Widespread neuronal damage or death can occur rapidly with heatstroke. Irritability or irrationality or both tend to precede any depression in the level of consciousness, and the majority of patients can quickly become unresponsive to painful stimuli. Seizures and signs of cerebellar dysfunction are not uncommon if the process continues.

The pulse in heatstroke is generally weak and thready, and hypotension is common. Cardiac muscle damage occurs frequently in patients with both exertional and classic heatstroke and may develop more rapidly if there is coronary artery disease or hypovolemia or both.

Rhabdomyolysis is common with exertional heat stroke and may contribute to the development of acute renal failure and hyperkalemia. Severe hypocalcemia also may develop as a result of rhabdomyolysis. Exogenous calcium, however, should not be administered unless the patient develops serious ventricular ectopy as a result of the hyperkalemia.

Acute renal failure develops 5 to 6 times more commonly in patients with exertional heatstroke (30% to 35%) than in those with the nonexertional type and appears to be related to dehydration, renal hypoperfusion, and the myoglobinuria of rhabdomyolysis.

DIC in heatstroke may range from an asymptomatic laboratory finding of hypofibrinogenemia and thrombocytopenia to severe clinical bleeding. Patients may also develop melena, hematemesis, hematochezia, or hemoptysis.

Treatment of Heatstroke

AXIOM Survival from heatstroke depends on promptly recognizing the syndrome and immediately reducing the core body temperature, usually with external cooling techniques (7).

Immersion in an ice-water bath is frequently used, but it is not as effective as wetting the skin with tepid water (to prevent cutaneous vasoconstriction) and using fans to facilitate evaporation of the water. If an immersion-cooling technique is used, vigorous skin massage should be used to prevent dermal stasis of cooled blood. Intravenous chlorpromazine (25 to 50 mg every 6 hours) also can be used to help prevent shivering. When the core temperature approaches 39°C, cooling efforts should be terminated because the body temperature will continue to decrease another 1°C to 2°C.

The need for intravascular fluids must be carefully assessed (7). There may be little or no dehydration in patients with underlying cardiac, renal, or hepatic failure, but severe dehydration is common in otherwise normal patients with exertional heat injury.

Early placement of a pulmonary arterial monitoring catheter is recommended in any circumstance in which there is uncertainty regarding the patient's volume status or myocardial function. Dobutamine may be helpful in patients who have an adequate blood pressure but also have myocardial dysfunction and an inadequate cardiac output.

Seizures are commonly seen with heatstroke and should be treated with intravenous diazepam (7). The role of mannitol or furosemide in the management of cerebral edema is unclear; however, they may be of some benefit in patients who have persistent oliguria in spite of adequate fluid loading and blood pressure.

Continuous infusion of heparin at 500 to 800 units per hour may be of some help in patients who develop laboratory evidence of DIC.

EXCESS THERMOGENESIS SYNDROMES

Malignant hyperthermia (MH) and neuroleptic malignant syndrome (NMS) are disorders of body temperature resulting from excessive endogenous heat production, without the influence of ambient temperature (7). The hypothalamic regulation of temperature and the physiologic mechanisms to dissipate heat may be impaired, particularly in NMS. Profound muscle rigidity is often also present.

Etiology

Agents particularly likely to cause MH in susceptible individuals include halothane and succinylcholine (14). Agents that tend to be associated with NMS include phenothiazines, haloperidol, and dopamine-depleting drugs (15). Sudden withdrawal of dopamine agonists, such as levodopa, also may cause this syndrome in susceptible individuals.

MH is a rare genetic myopathy that is estimated to affect approximately 1 in 15,000 children and 1 in 40,000 middle-aged adults. It is the most common cause of death as a direct result of general anesthesia (16). The severest form is autosomal dominant.

Pathophysiology

After muscle contraction, calcium is removed from the contractile apparatus to allow relaxation of the myocytes. Individuals who develop MH tend to have a genetically inherited predisposition for certain drugs to cause increased release of stored calcium from the sarcoplasmic reticulum into the myoplasm plus decreased removal of the calcium from the contractile apparatus. The resultant continued muscle contracture causes rigidity and greatly increased metabolic activity. The resultant thermogenesis can cause the core body temperature to increase 1°C every 5 minutes.

The metabolic consequences of this syndrome include a combined respiratory and metabolic acidosis, plus increased serum potassium, sodium, and calcium levels. If significant myonecrosis develops, serum potassium levels may rapidly increase to life-threatening levels, and plasma ionized calcium may decrease abruptly as calcium moves into injured muscle.

Rhabdomyolysis and hepatic necrosis may develop very rapidly in MH and NMS. The development of ventricular tachydysrhythmias parallels the degree of hypermetabolism and hyperkalemia, but seizures are uncommon. Nevertheless, patients with NMS have an increased tendency to develop aspiration pneumonia because of dystonia and an impaired ability to handle their secretions.

Diagnosis

The classic diagnostic triad includes skeletal muscle rigidity, metabolic acidosis, and increased body temperature. MH also is characterized by the early development of trismus in 50% of patients. The definitive diagnosis can be made in the laboratory by exposing intact muscle fibers to caffeine and halothane in varying concentrations.

NMS should be suspected in patients who are given a neuroleptic drug and subsequently develop signs of muscular rigidity, dystonia, or unexplained catatonic behavior. Laboratory data are variable; however, serum levels of creatine phosphokinase (CPK) and glutamic-oxaloacetic transaminase (GOT) may increase abruptly in patients who develop rhabdomyolysis.

Treatment

Successful treatment of hyperthermic syndromes depends on early recognition. In MH, early discontinuation of the inciting agent is often adequate therapy. Recovery from NMS also may follow discontinuation of the drug; however, the temperature may not return to baseline for 5 to 7 days.

Dantrolene is the drug of choice in hyperthermic syndromes and should be administered to patients in whom hyperpyrexia continues to develop after removal of the inciting agent(s). The recommended dose is 2 mg/kg intravenously, repeated every 5 minutes, up to a total of 10 mg/kg. Dantrolene acts by inhibiting calcium release from the sarcoplasmic reticulum, thereby decreasing the amount of calcium available for ongoing excessive muscle contraction. The role of dantrolene in NMS is less well defined; however, in several case reports, it was shown to reduce thermogenesis.

A number of other drugs, such as bromocriptine, amantadine, and levodopa/carbidopa, have been used to reduce thermogenesis. All of these drugs increase central neurologic dopaminergic tone, thereby altering both the hypothalamic and peripheral mechanisms that increase core body temperature (7).

⊘ FREQUENT ERRORS

1. ***Causing additional injury to frozen tissue by rubbing it with snow or immersing it in excessively hot water in an effort to warm it rapidly.***
2. ***Failure to adequately protect frozen tissues from cold or physical trauma after rewarming.***
3. ***Inadequate fluid administration during rewarming.***
4. ***Failure to detect and treat underlying trauma or systemic diseases, such as hypothyroidism or vascular insufficiency in patients with hypothermia***
5. ***Failure to provide adequate water, salt, and potassium to individuals with excessive sweating.***
6. ***Failure to anticipate severe electrolyte abnormalities, especially hyperkalemia and hypocalcemia, in patients with heatstroke.***
7. ***Failure to anticipate seizures and multiple organ failure in patients with severe heatstroke.***
8. ***Delayed diagnosis and treatment of malignant hyperthermia or neuroleptic malignant syndrome.***

SUMMARY POINTS

1. Impaired mental or cardiovascular function greatly increases the risk of patients developing accidental heat or cold injury.

2. The homeothermic responses to cold are virtually nonexistent at core temperatures below 28°C (83°F).

3. Nonfreezing cold (NFC) injury is caused primarily by cold-induced vasoconstriction.

4. Cold injury is much more likely to occur in areas of the body that become wet.

5. Immersion foot refers to foot injuries caused by prolonged exposure to wet.

6. Nonfreezing cold injuries to the feet frequently result from improperly fitting footwear.

7. Even with what appears to be severe frostbite, a great deal of spontaneous healing eventually occurs.

8. Cold-injured tissues should never be rubbed, especially with snow or cold water.

9. If systemic hypothermia below 32°C (90°F) accompanies frostbite, rapid internal rewarming is the treatment of choice.

10. Surgical debridement or amputations for frostbite should not be performed until the level of mummification or tissue death is clearly demarcated, and this is usually not made clear for least 2 to 3 months.

11. Hypothermia can occur at virtually any environmental temperature below 80°F.

12. One should monitor core temperatures closely in trauma patients, especially those who are in shock, receive massive transfusions, or have prolonged abdominal surgery.

13. Endogenous warming after hypothermia can put a tremendous metabolic and cardiovascular strain on the patient.

14. The patient has little defense against hypothermia if the core temperature decreases to less than 32°C.

15. So-called Osborne (J) waves on an ECG may be the first clue that hypothermia is present, especially in anesthetized patients.
16. Hypothermia increases the likelihood of a patient developing ventricular fibrillation during insertion of a PA catheter.
17. The diuresis occurring with hypothermia can cause hypovolemia, and this can cause severe hypotension during rewarming.
18. Severely hypothermic patients are particularly likely to develop pneumonia after rewarming.
19. One of the best ways to prevent coagulopathies in trauma patients is to prevent or rapidly correct hypothermia.
20. Hypothermic patients with recent loss of signs of life should not be pronounced dead until or unless there are still no signs of life after the patient has been warmed to at least 32°C or preferably 35°C.
21. As soon as the major bleeding has been controlled during emergency surgery, the surgeon should irrigate the body cavity being explored with warmed saline until the core temperature is at least 34°C to 35°C.
22. As long as the hypothermic patient has a pulse and is breathing, treatment should not be overly aggressive.
23. Blood pressure and cardiac filling pressures must be watched carefully during rewarming when there is a strong tendency to develop hypovolemia and hypotension.
24. In hypothermic patients, some ventilation is infinitely better than no ventilation, but hyperventilation can precipitate severe arrhythmias or cardiac arrest.
25. Attempts to restore a perfusing cardiac rhythm, particularly when ventricular fibrillation is present, are unlikely to succeed until the temperature is increased to 32°C to 34°C or higher.
26. Bicarbonate should not be used to treat severe metabolic acidosis until or unless the ventilation is adequate to remove the increased CO_2 that is formed.
27. "Uncorrected" blood gas values in hypothermic patients may be more meaningful than those that are corrected to the patient's temperature.
28. Slow rewarming of patients with moderate to severe hypothermia is not advisable because it allows additional ischemic damage to occur.
29. The most effective, easily managed, and readily available method of active core warming is inhalation of heated gases.
30. If rapidly available, partial CPB is the most rapid, effective method for correcting severe hypothermia.
31. Some glucose should be present in the fluids used to resuscitate hypothermic patients.
32. Vasoconstrictors should not be used in patients with hypotension resulting from hypothermia.
33. Decreased sweating, especially while working in a hot environment, increases the likelihood of a heat-induced injury.
34. Heat cramps are usually best corrected by administration of dilute salt solutions after the patient has been placed in a cool environment.
35. Because sweat has 5.0 or more mEq of potassium per liter, excessive sweating, corrected only with water and NaCl, can eventually cause hypokalemia.
36. Heat syncope often requires no treatment other than removal of the patient from the main heat source and rest in a recumbent position; however, administration of some water and salt will usually speed recovery.
37. Heatstroke usually occurs because of severe exertion or because of severe underlying diseases affecting cardiovascular function or heat loss.
38. Severe hyperkalemia and hypocalcemia can develop during heatstroke.
39. Cooling of patients with heatstroke is best done by wetting the patient's skin with tepid water and facilitating its rapid evaporation with fans.
40. Core temperature should be watched carefully in all patients with severe trauma, particularly during general anesthesia or if the patient has recently taken neuroleptic drugs or both.
41. The keys to successful treatment of excessive thermogenesis are early diagnosis, discontinuance of the inciting agents, administration of dantrolene, cooling of the patient, and carefully monitored cardiopulmonary and metabolic support.

REFERENCES

1. Wilson RF. Temperature-related (non-burn) injuries. In: Wilson RF, Walt AJ, eds. *Management of trauma: pitfalls and practice*. 2nd ed. Philadelphia: Williams & Wilkins, 1996:772.
2. Fisher RP, Souba WW, Ford EG. Temperature-associated injuries and syndromes. In: Moore EE, Mattox KL, Feliciano DV, eds. *Trauma*. 2nd ed. Norwalk, CT: Appleton & Lange, 1991:765–776.
3. Moss JF. Accidental severe hypothermia. *Surg Gynecol Obstet* 1986;162:501.
4. Knochel JP. Heatstroke and related heat stress disorders. *Dis Month* 1989;35:306.
5. Wrenn K. Immersion foot: a problem of the homeless in the 1990s. *Arch Intern Med* 1991;151:785.
6. Vaughn PB. Local cold injury: menace to military operations. *Milit Med* 1980;145:305.
7. Farmer JC. Temperature-related injuries. In: Civetta JM, Taylor RW, Kirby RR, eds. *Critical care*. Philadelphia: JB Lippincott, 1988:693–700.
8. Fitzgerald FT, Jessop C. Accidental hypothermia: a report of 22 cases and review of the literature. *Adv Intern Med* 1982;27:128.
9. Cornelli HM. Accidental hypothermia. *J Pediatr* 1992;120:671.
10. Steele MT, Nelson MJ, Sessler DI, et al. Forced air speeds rewarming in accidental hypothermia. *Ann Emerg Med* 1996;27:479.
11. Splittgerber FH, Talbert JG, Sweezer WP, Wilson RF. Partial cardiopulmonary bypass for core rewarming in profound accidental hypothermia. *Am Surg* 1986;52:407.
12. DaVee TS, Reinberg EJ. Extreme hypothermia and ventricular fibrillation. *Ann Emerg Med* 1980;9:100.
13. Curley FJ, Irwin RS. Disorders of temperature control: hyperthermia, part I. *J Intens Care Med* 1986;1:5.
14. Gronert GA. Malignant hyperthermia. *Anesthesiology* 1980;53:395.
15. Guze GH, Baxter LR. Neuroleptic malignant syndrome. *N Engl J Med* 1985;313:163.
16. Ball SP, Johnson KJ. The genetics of malignant hyperthermia. *J Med Genet* 1993;30:89.
17. Hector MG. Treatment of accidental hypothermia. *Am Family Physician* 1992;45:785.

37C. BITES AND STINGS[1]

MAMMALIAN BITES

Human Bites

Human saliva contains up to 10^{10} bacteria/mL, and plaque on teeth in persons with poor dental hygiene have even greater numbers of bacteria. Common infecting organisms in human bites include *Streptococcus viridans*, *Staphylococcus* spp., *Eikenella corrodens*, *Bacteroides* spp., and microaerophilic streptococci.

AXIOM Lacerations over the knuckles (possibly from a fight) should be considered human bites until proven otherwise.

Serious wound infections can develop in lacerations due to a clenched fist striking the teeth of another person. These wounds are often benign appearing, and involvement of the metacarpophalangeal (MCP) joint may not be apparent unless the patient is examined with his fist clenched. These injuries are usually best treated with exploration and irrigation in the operating room (OR), intravenous antibiotics, and postoperative elevation of the hand and arm.

AXIOM In general, human bites should not be closed, no matter how innocuous they look.

Human bites can be treated with a second-generation cephalosporin, amoxicillin–clavulanic acid, or a combination of dicloxacillin and ampicillin (2). Patients allergic to penicillin can be given ciprofloxacin or erythromycin. Patients seen more than 24 hours after a bite without any signs of infection usually do not need prophylactic antibiotics.

Hepatitis and human immunodeficiency virus (HIV) infections are transmissible by human bites. Hepatitis B requires a much smaller inoculum of blood or saliva and is a much greater risk than HIV. In suggestive cases, serologic testing should be done for HIV and hepatitis B and C, and treatment with γ-globulin and hepatitis B vaccination should be considered. Tetanus prophylaxis is provided as indicated.

Rabies

Rabies causes a viral encephalitis that is almost always fatal. It is caused by a rhabdovirus found in the saliva of animals, and it is transmitted through bites or scratches. The incubation period in humans usually exceeds 10 days but may be much longer; up to 30% of humans who develop rabies cannot recall having had an animal bite (1).

The three phases of rabies include a prodromal phase, with pain or paresthesias at the bite site; an acute neurologic phase, manifested as dysphagia, hydrophobia, hallucinations, or a combination of these; and a late clinical phase, with dysrhythmias, autonomic nervous system dysfunction, and coma (3).

Prevention is the only reasonable approach. Irrigation and cleaning of the bite with soap or a detergent is protective in up to 90% (4). If the bite was unprovoked or the animal was behaving abnormally before the bite, the chance of rabies inoculation is increased.

AXIOM An animal that bites a human, especially if unprovoked, should be considered rabid unless proven otherwise.

Skunks, raccoons, bats, and other wild carnivores that bite a patient should be considered to be rabid. If the responsible dog or cat is healthy and available, it should be observed for 10 days for symptoms. If no symptoms develop, the animal should be considered nonrabid. If the animal was immunized, it should be considered at very low risk for carrying rabies. Rodents, livestock, and rabbits rarely, if ever, harbor the rabies virus.

Passive rabies immunization is obtained with 20 IU/kg of human rabies immune globulin with 50% of the dose injected into the wound and 50% given intramuscularly (i.m.) (3). Active rabies immunization is provided with human diploid cell rabies vaccine given i.m. on the day of the bite and on days 3, 7, 14, and 28.

Cat Bites

Cat bites tend to cause small punctures that become infected in 15% to 50% of the victims (3). Commonly isolated organisms include *Pasteurella multocida* and *Staphylococcus* spp. Ampicillin plus a β-lactamase inhibitor provides reasonable coverage.

AXIOM All animal bites should be copiously irrigated, and preventive antibiotics are recommended for deeper injuries.

Dog Bites

In the United States, an estimated 1 to 2 million dog bites occur annually, accounting for 1% of emergency department visits (2). Infection occurs in about 5% to 15% of cases and typically involve *P. multocida*, *S. aureus*, *S. viridans*, *Bacteroides* spp., *Fusobacteria*, and *Capnocytophaga* (1).

Facial dog-bite wounds can usually be closed after debridement and irrigation, but other wounds should generally be treated with delayed primary closure or allowed to heal by secondary intention.

Patients with low-risk dog bites do not benefit from prophylactic antibiotics unless the hand is involved. Antibiotics recommended for severe dog bites include dicloxacillin or a first-generation cephalosporin (2). Trimethoprim–sulfamethoxazole is an alternative in patients allergic to penicillin.

SNAKE BITES

Snake bites are most common in the southern and southwestern states, and they are responsible for an average of 12 deaths per year in the United States.

Types of Snakes

Venomous snakes indigenous to the United States include crotalids (rattlesnakes, copperheads, and cottonmouths) and elapids (coral snakes).

Crotalids are characterized by a broad triangular head, relatively thick body, elliptical pupils, facial pits, and a single row of subcaudal plates. All but one species of rattlesnake have rattles, which distinguishes them from copperheads and water moccasins.

Coral snakes are small, have nontriangular heads without facial pits, and are brightly colored, with red, yellow, white, and black rings. Their characteristic red bands adjacent to yellow bands distinguish coral snakes from other snakes that are nonvenomous. "Red on yellow, kill a fellow; red on black, venom lack." Coral snakes do not have large fangs, but when they bite, they tend to chew on the bitten area, and one should assume that envenomation has occurred.

Effects of Envenomation

AXIOM Even with the presence of fang marks after a snake bite, approximately 20% to 25% of patients will not have been envenomated (1).

If there are no fang marks, there has not been envenomation. Of the patients with crotalid snake bites, 50% have only minimal to mild envenomation, which should not be a threat to life or limb. Moccasin and copperhead bites tend to be less severe than rattlesnake bites and usually do not require antivenin therapy.

Snake venoms usually contain many enzymes and peptides (5). Damage to the endothelium by peptides increases vascular permeability, which may lead to edema and hypovolemic shock. Proteases cause tissue necrosis; hyaluronidase facilitates the spread of venom through tissues, and phospholipase A damages many cells, but especially erythrocytes and muscle cells. Thus the multiple enzymes present can have deleterious effects on the cardiovascular, pulmonary, renal, coagulation, and neurologic systems.

Coral snakes produce minimal local injury, but systemic signs may include cranial and other nerve dysfunction, which may progress to respiratory depression and paralysis over several hours (6).

AXIOM Rapid onset of pain, edema, and discoloration or bullae at the bite site strongly suggest that significant envenomation has occurred.

Treatment

Local Therapy

Incision and suction have been shown experimentally to remove subcutaneously injected venom; however, unless this is done expertly and very soon after envenomation, the yield of extracted venom is very low, and the risk of damage by the incision is significant.

A properly applied venous tourniquet may delay the onset of systemic symptoms; however, it does not help the affected extremity, and if it becomes too tight, it can cause great harm; nevertheless, application of a compression bandage and immobilization of the bitten extremity can delay systemic absorption of the venom.

Crotalid venoms have very powerful locally destructive effects; however, most envenomations are only subcutaneous. Local excision of envenomated or dead tissue can be helpful, but fasciotomies are often performed unnecessarily.

Antivenin Therapy

Rattlesnake antivenin therapy can limit the amount of tissue damage and systemic action of injected venom if it is administered within 4 hours of envenomation; however, the horse-derived antivenin can cause anaphylaxis in up to 23% of patients, and another 50% or more develop delayed serum sickness (7).

Another commercially available antivenin for *Micrurus fulvius* (the Eastern and Texas coral snake), has little cross-reactivity with the venom of *Micrurus euryxanthus* (the Sonoran coral snake).

All infusions of antivenin from nonhuman sources are started at a very slow rate and are slowed or stopped if an allergic reaction develops. The antivenin should not be administered in any setting in which anaphylaxis cannot be treated (i.e., in the field). One starts with a minimum of five to 10 vials for severe bites and increases the amount as needed.

AXIOM The dose of antivenin is determined by the estimated amount of venom in the patient, not the size of the patient.

The manufacturer recommends skin testing before infusion of the antivenin. If hypersensitivity is demonstrated or if there is known allergy to horse serum, one can premedicate with diphenhydramine hydrochloride (Benadryl; 25 to 50 mg intravenously), and an epinephrine drip (2 to 20 μg/min) can be given during the antivenin administration.

Supportive Therapy

Supportive care for snake bites includes

1. Fluid resuscitation;
2. Tetanus prophylaxis;
3. Appropriate monitoring;
4. Correction of coagulopathies; and
5. Administration of antibiotics.

Organisms likely to be present include *Pseudomonas* spp., *Enterobacteriaceae*, *Staphylococcus* spp., and clostridia. Ticarcillin with clavulanic acid or similar agents provide reasonable empiric coverage.

Coagulopathies should be corrected with fresh-frozen plasma and cryoprecipitate as needed after the antivenin is given. The patient's prothrombin time, partial thromboplastin time, fibrinogen concentration, and platelet count should be monitored and corrected as needed.

Serum Sickness

A high percentage of patients receiving equine antivenin will develop a delayed serum sickness with a severity that parallels the amount of antivenin given. This may occur at any time up to 3 to 4 weeks later, and severe cases are treated with corticosteroids.

MARINE ANIMAL BITES AND STINGS

Coelenterates

Mild envenomations (typically inflicted by fire coral, hydroids, and anemones) can cause immediate pruritus, paresthesias, and throbbing pain with proximal radiation (8). The involved area can develop erythema and edema followed by blisters, which can become infected and ulcerate. Severe envenomations by anemones, sea nettles, and jellyfish can cause fever, nausea, vomiting, malaise, and dysfunction of multiple organ systems. Anaphylaxis also may occur.

AXIOM Fresh-water applications or vigorous rubbing or both can cause attached nematocysts to discharge increased toxin into the patient.

Dilute (5%) acetic acid (vinegar) can inactivate the toxin and should be applied gently for 30 minutes or until the pain is relieved. After the wound has been irrigated copiously with vinegar, the remaining nematocysts can be removed by applying shaving cream or a flour paste and shaving the area with a razor. The affected area should again be irrigated, dressed, and elevated.

AXIOM Medical care providers should wear gloves for self-protection when treating patients who may have embedded nematocysts.

After the toxin is inactivated, one can use cryotherapy, local anesthetics, antihistamines, steroids, or a combination of these to relieve any residual pain. Prophylactic antibiotics are usually unnecessary. Antivenin is available for severe envenomations by the box jellyfish, sea snake, and stonefish (9).

Echinodermata

Starfish, sea urchins, and sea cucumbers have venoms that can cause local and systemic reactions similar to those from coelenterates (8,9). First-aid consists of soaking and rinsing the wound in hot, but tolerable, water. Residual spines can be located with soft-tissue radiographs or magnetic resonance imaging and should be removed if they are easily accessible or if they are close to joints or critical neurovascular structures. Reactive fusiform finger or toe swelling attributed to spines near the metacarpal or metatarsal bones may be alleviated by high-dose corticosteroids given in an oral 14-day taper.

Sting Ray

Sting rays attack defensively by thrusting spines into tissues. Local damage can be severe, with occasional penetration of body cavities (8). The tissue damage in increased by the vasoconstrictive and myonecrotic properties of the venom. Systemic complaints include weakness, nausea, diarrhea, headache, and muscle cramps. Severe envenomation also can cause cardiac arrhythmias, respiratory arrest, seizures, or a combination of these (9).

The wound should be irrigated and then soaked in nonscalding hot water (up to 45°C) for 1 hour (8). Debridement, exploration, and removal of spines should be done during or after the hot water soaking. Radiographic studies should be obtained to locate remaining spines.

Second-generation cephalosporins can provide adequate coverage for most of the gram-positive and gram-negative microorganisms found in ocean water, including the *Vibrio* species (10). Ciprofloxacin, gentamicin, and trimethoprim–sulfamethoxazole also are acceptable.

Shark Bites

Shark bites should be considered infectious and tetanus prone. The wounds should be debrided and irrigated, and antibiotic and tetanus prophylaxis are recommended.

INSECT BITES

Bee and Wasp Stings

Africanized honey bees tend to be aggressive, and persons stung by them are likely to sustain multiple stings. Bees sting with double-barbed lancets, which tend to anchor the bee to the victim's skin. When the bee dislodges itself, it usually leaves its stinging apparatus and attached viscera behind, thereby killing the bee.

Venom from bees and wasps contain histamine and serotonin, which are responsible for the local reaction and pain. Peptides, such as mellitin and various enzymes, primarily phospholipases and hyaluronidase, have been identified as allergens that can elicit an immunoglobulin E (IgE)-mediated response (11).

AXIOM Anaphylactic reactions from bee stings cause more deaths in the United States than all other venomous bites put together.

The most serious problem with bee and wasp stings is the development of an immediate hypersensitivity reaction. Bee-sting anaphylaxis develops in 0.3% to 3% of the general population, causing approximately 40 reported deaths annually (11). Fatalities usually occur within 1 hour of the sting and are more common in adults. Symptoms occur within minutes, ranging from mild urticaria and angioedema to respiratory arrest caused by airway edema and cardiovascular collapse. Unusual reactions to Hymenoptera venom include late-onset allergic reactions (more than 5 hours after the sting), serum sickness, renal disease, neurologic complaints (such as the Guillain–Barré syndrome), and vasculitis.

The venom sac of the bee should be scraped out with a knife, instead of squeezing the skin. Application of an ice pack to the local area tends to reduce associated pain. Some have advocated the local application of papain after removal of the venom sac.

Mild anaphylaxis can be treated with up to 0.3 mL of 1:1,000 subcutaneous epinephrine (0.01 mL/kg in small children), and an oral or intravenous antihistamine. Severe cases may require intravenous fluids, vasopressors, oxygen, bronchodilators, and endotracheal intubation.

Patients who have had an anaphylactic reaction to bee or wasp stings should wear a medical identification bracelet and should carry an emergency kit for the injection of epinephrine and antihistamines after a bee or wasp sting.

Ant Bites

Solenopsis richteri (the black fire ant) has a limited range along the Mississippi–Alabama border (1). *Solenopsis invecta* (the red fire ant) now has a range extending over most of the southeastern United States. The bites can initially cause a vesicle, which is followed by the development of a sterile pustule. Multiple stings can produce a toxic reaction, including vomiting, diarrhea, generalized edema, cardiovascular collapse, and hemolysis, which can be difficult to distinguish from a systemic allergic reaction.

Local therapy includes removing stingers by gentle scraping. Blisters should be left intact. The bite sites should be cleansed, and ice applied. Topical vinegar and salt can decrease pain from the sting. Antihistamines administered orally or topically can decrease pruritus. Treatment of a large envenomation also includes elevation of the extremity, analgesics, and a 5-day course of prednisone (1 mg/kg/day).

Spider Bites

The brown recluse spider (*Loxosceles reclusa*) has three pairs of eyes and a violin-shaped carapace on its body. Usually, there is minimal pain, itching, and erythema at the bite site; however, with a more severe bite, the center turns purple because of thrombosis of local vessels. Later vasoconstriction can create a pale peripheral border. Over the next few days, one may see widening necrosis, which is replaced by an eschar. The eschar eventually separates, leaving an ulcer that usually heals within 2 months but occasionally requires skin grafting (12). Systemic features in children can include headache, nausea and vomiting, fever, malaise, arthralgia, and maculopapular rash. Adults only rarely develop systemic signs or symptoms.

Treatment is usually supportive, but severe lesions may benefit from dapsone, which inhibits neutrophil function if it is given during the first few days after envenomation (13). The recommended adult dose is 100 mg/day.

Bites by the black widow spider (*Latrodectus mactans*) are characterized by a systemic toxic reaction. The female black widow has a black body with a red hourglass on the underside of her abdomen and is much larger than the male. Symptoms of envenomation usually begin within an hour of the bite and can include local pain, muscle rigidity, altered mental status, and seizures. The death rate from severe bites has been reported to be as high as 5%. Treatment is usually only supportive, but dantrolene, calcium gluconate, methacarbamol, and antivenin should be considered for severe cases.

Scorpions

The genus *Centruroides* is responsible for most of the 7,000 scorpion stings that are reported yearly in the United States, with one third of these occurring in Arizona (14). Reactions from scorpion stings vary from mild, local irritation to death. *Centruroides exilicauda*, the scorpion responsible for the rare deaths occurring in the United States, produces a neurotoxin that can prevent sodium channel closure. When stung, a patient typically experiences local paresthesias and burning. Systemic manifestations include cranial nerve and neuromuscular dysfunction, which may progress to respiratory distress. Patients also may develop signs of adrenergic stimulation, accompanied by nausea and vomiting. Stings by other species of scorpions in the United States usually cause only local pain and swelling.

All patients should receive tetanus prophylaxis, ice-pack therapy to the bite site, and analgesics for pain. Patients with signs of systemic envenomation require supportive care, with close monitoring of cardiovascular and respiratory function in an intensive care setting. Administration of antivenin can reverse cranial nerve and neuromuscular symptoms, but it may also cause anaphylaxis and delayed serum sickness.

AXIOM Scorpion bites causing severe systemic symptoms in children should be considered for antivenin therapy.

Administration of antivenin to children can completely reverse the neurologic and cardiopulmonary complications within hours (15). Anaphylaxis seldom occurs, but a large percentage may develop serum sickness. The initial dose is one vial, which should be preceded by skin testing. Patients with positive skin tests should be pretreated with diphenhydramine.

⊘ FREQUENT ERRORS

1. ***Failure to consider the possibility of a human bite as the cause of lacerations over knuckles.***
2. ***Primary closure of animal bites other than for favorable, carefully debrided wounds on the face.***

3. ***Uninformed use of incision-and-suction procedures and improper use of tourniquets for snake bites.***
4. ***Use of antivenin for snake bites with only mild envenomation.***
5. ***Inadequate preparation for treatment of anaphylaxis due to antivenin use.***
6. ***Fasciotomy in snake bites when a compartment syndrome is not really present.***
7. ***Failure to anticipate anaphylactic reactions in patients with bee, hornet, or wasp stings.***
8. ***Failure to provide anaphylaxis kits to patients who have had anaphylactic reactions to insect bites.***

SUMMARY POINTS

1. Lacerations on the back of a hand, near the knuckles, should be considered human bites of an MCP joint until proven otherwise.
2. In general, human bites should not be closed, no matter how good they look.
3. All bite wounds should be copiously irrigated, and preventive antibiotics are recommended for deeper injuries.
4. Animal bites are usually not closed primarily unless they are on the face and can be debrided and cleansed properly.
5. An animal that bites a human, especially if unprovoked, should be considered rabid until proven otherwise.
6. Even with the presence of fang marks after a snake bite, approximately 20% to 25% of patients will not have been envenomated.
7. Rapid onset of pain, edema, and discoloration or bullae, or continued bleeding at a bite site, or a combination of these, strongly suggest that significant envenomation has occurred and antivenin therapy will be needed.
8. Treatment of snake bites at the scene with incision and suction, tourniquets, or ice immersion are apt to cause more harm than good.
9. Snake antivenin is recommended only for systemic signs and symptoms or severe local signs of envenomation.
10. The dose of antivenin is determined by the estimated amount of venom in the patient, not the size of the patient.
11. Fasciotomy is only rarely needed for snake bites and should be reserved for clear evidence of compartment syndrome.
12. Fresh-water applications or vigorous rubbing of marine animal stings can cause nematocysts to discharge venom into the patient or caregiver.
13. Medical care providers should wear gloves for self-protection when treating patients who may have embedded nematocysts.
14. Anaphylactic reactions from bee stings cause more deaths than all other venomous bites put together.
15. Venom sacs from bee stings should be scraped out, not squeezed.
16. Patients who have had an anaphylactic reaction to bee or wasp stings should wear a medical identification bracelet and should carry an emergency kit for the injection of epinephrine and antihistamines after a bee or wasp sting.
17. Early dapsone therapy may reduce the amount of skin necrosis seen with brown recluse spider bites.
18. Dantrolene, calcium gluconate, methacarbamol, and antivenin should be considered if there are severe systemic symptoms from a black widow spider bite.
19. Scorpion bites causing severe systemic symptoms in children should be considered for antivenin therapy.

REFERENCES

1. Stewart RM, Page CP. Wounds, bites, and stings. In: Feliciano DV, Moore EE, Mattox KL, eds. *Trauma.* 3rd ed., Stamford, CT: Appleton & Lange, 1996:928–936.
2. Callaham M, French SP, Tetlow P, Rees P. Bites and injuries inflicted by mam-

mals. In: Auerbach PS, ed. *Wilderness medicine: management of wilderness and environmental emergencies.* 3rd ed. St. Louis: Mosby-Year Book, 1995:943.
3. Groleau G. Rabies. *Emerg Med Clin North Am* 1992;10:361.
4. Dire DJ. Emergency management of dog and cat bite wounds. *Emerg Med Clin North Am* 1992;10:719.
5. Nelson EE, Auerbach PS. Bites and stings. In: Sabiston DC, ed. *The biological basis of modern surgical practice.* 15th ed. Philadelphia: WB Saunders, 1997: 287–295.
6. Gold BS, Wingert WA. Snake venom poisoning in the United States: a review of therapeutic practice. *South Med J* 1984;87:579.
7. Jurkovich GJ, Luterman A, McCullar K, et al. Complications of Crotalidae antivenin therapy. *J Trauma* 1988;28:1032.
8. Auerbach PS. Marine envenomation. In: Auerbach PS, ed. *Wilderness medicine: management of wilderness and environmental emergencies.* 3rd ed. St. Louis: Mosby-Year Book, 1995:1327.
9. McGoldrick J, Marx JA. Marine envenomations. Part 2: invertebrates. *J Emerg Med* 1992;10:71.
10. Auerbach PS, Halstead BW. Injuries from nonvenomous aquatic animals. In: Auerbach PS, ed. *Wilderness medicine: management of wilderness and environmental emergencies.* 3rd ed. St. Louis: Mosby-Year Book, 1995:1303.
11. Reisman RE. Stinging insect allergy. *Med Clin North Am* 1992;76:883.
12. Boyer-Hassen LV, McNally JT. Spider bites. In: Auerbach PS, ed. *Wilderness medicine: management of wilderness and environmental emergencies.* 3rd ed. St. Louis: Mosby-Year Book, 1995:769.
13. King LE, Rees RS. Dapsone treatment of a brown recluse spider bite. *JAMA* 1983;251:889.
14. Connor DA, Seldon B. Scorpion envenomations. In: Auerbach PS, ed. *Wilderness medicine: management of wilderness and environmental emergencies.* 3rd ed. St. Louis: Mosby-Year Book, 1995:847.
15. Bond GR. Antivenin administration for *Centruroides* scorpion stings: risks and benefits. *Ann Emerg Med* 1992;21:788.

38. METABOLIC AND NUTRITIONAL CONSIDERATIONS IN TRAUMA[1]

METABOLIC RESPONSE TO TRAUMA

AXIOM Severe malnutrition following trauma is associated with greatly increased morbidity and mortality rates, primarily resulting from infections and multiple organ failure.

The hypermetabolism caused by multiple injuries and severe stress or sepsis can rapidly lead to severe wasting of lean body mass and impairment of healing and organ function; consequently, early nutritional support is an important part of the management of patients with severe trauma (Fig. 38-1).

Carbohydrate Metabolism

AXIOM Stress carbohydrate metabolism is characterized by increased efforts by the body to provide glucose to injured and healing tissues, so that glycogenolysis and gluconeogenesis are poorly suppressed by exogenous glucose.

The increased glucose production and hyperglycemia seen with stress seem to be driven largely by an increased glucagon:insulin ratio. Glucose uptake into the cell is also depressed in severely stressed individuals (2). The inefficient use of glucose in trauma is primarily due to a limited capacity of the pyruvate dehydrogenase enzyme complex, which is responsible for the formation of acetyl CoA from pyruvate, and not from a failure of oxidative metabolism. This is reflected in an increase in both lactate and pyruvate. This elevation is in contrast with hypovolemic shock, in which lactate levels increase with relatively little change in pyruvate, producing what Huckabee referred to as "excess lactate."

Hepatic gluconeogenesis normally occurs at a rate of approximately 2.0 to 2.5 mg/kg/min, but during stress it can double. This "new glucose" is important to infected and healing tissues as well as the "obligate" glucose-using tissues, including brain.

Fat Metabolism

Fat metabolism in both starvation and stress is characterized by increased lipolysis, which occurs as fat stores are mobilized for energy. Serum triglyceride levels increase, and increased activity of "hormone-sensitive lipase" induced by beta-adrenergic stimulation causes an accelerated release of free fatty acids from fat stores. Although hepatic production of ketones may be increased in stress, plasma ketone levels are low (3). In contrast, during nonstressed starvation or fasting, plasma ketone levels are elevated.

Protein Metabolism

The nitrogen for the increased urine urea nitrogen (UUN) losses after trauma comes from accelerated total body protein catabolism, particularly from skeletal muscle, but also from connective tissue and unstimulated gut. This can rapidly cause marked depletion of lean body mass.

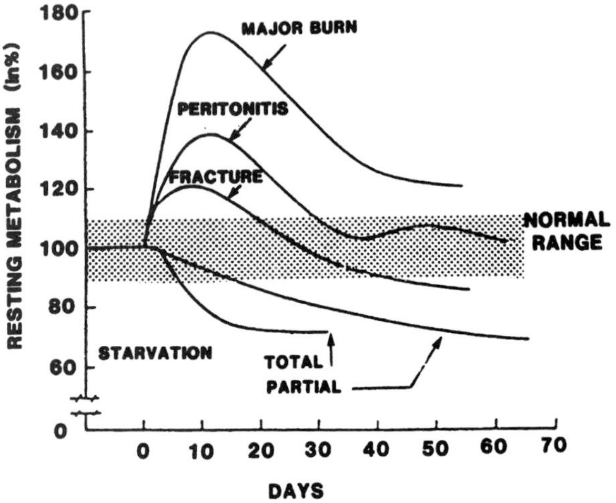

FIG. 38-1. Percent change from normal of resting metabolism as a function of time in patients with major burns, peritonitis, fractures, and total and partial starvation. (From ref. 8, with permission.)

AXIOM UUN losses are usually less than 5 g/day in nonstressed starvation, but in severe stress they often exceed 15 to 30 g/day.

In contradistinction to simple starvation, the excessive protein catabolism seen after injury is not suppressed by exogenous amino acids, fat, or glucose.

One benefit of the increased protein turnover is a greater amino acid availability for hepatic synthesis of acute phase proteins, which are crucial for host survival during severe stress. These liver-derived acute phase proteins include fibrinogen, haptoglobin, ceruloplasmin, C-reactive protein, α-1 acid glycoprotein, and some complement components.

FACTORS AFFECTING METABOLIC CHANGES IN TRAUMA AND SEPSIS

The major identifiable factors that orchestrate the hypercatabolic events following trauma include

1. Metabolic demands of the traumatic wound;
2. Counterregulatory hormones (especially catecholamines, glucagon, and cortisol); and
3. Cytokines.

Metabolic Demands

The metabolic demands of traumatic wounds, especially large burns, can directly increase total body metabolic rate by stimulating regional blood flow and the rate of glucose consumption. Healing tissue has a preference for glycolytic metabolic activity. This can contribute significantly to the total body glucose turnover, especially because glycolysis is a much less efficient energy source than complete glucose oxidation. Additionally, lactate, which is the major end product of glycolytic metabolism, requires disposal, which is done primarily through its reconversion to glucose in the liver. The resulting accelerated lactate recycling also increases energy requirements (4).

Counterregulatory Hormones

Energy availability to the tissues can be viewed in terms of the balance between the effects of insulin, the major storage or anabolic hormone, and the effects of the "counterregulatory hormones"—glucagon, cortisol, and catecholamines. Insulin decreases blood glucose levels primarily by increasing membrane transport and intracellular metabolism of glucose in peripheral tissues, such as skeletal muscle and fat (5). The counterregulatory hormones oppose the effects of insulin (6). They mobilize energy reserves and elevate blood glucose levels, primarily by accelerating body catabolism.

Glucagon is released from the alpha cells of the islets of Langerhans in response to hypoglycemia and beta-adrenergic stimulation. It acts primarily in the liver to promote gluconeogenesis and to enhance hepatic amino acid extraction. Glucagon also acts in concert with cortisol to increase protein catabolism to increase available gluconeogenic substrate.

Cortisol, by promoting hepatic gluconeogenesis, contributes in large part to the hyperglycemia and apparent "insulin resistance" observed in patients with stress (4).

Catecholamines elevate blood glucose levels by stimulating gluconeogenesis and glycogenolysis. Epinephrine, probably through its beta-adrenergic agonist properties, also accounts for some of the reduced peripheral tissue responsiveness to insulin after trauma.

Individually, these hormones—epinephrine, glucagon, and cortisol—induce only mild and short-lived elevations in blood glucose levels and hepatic glucose production; however, the simultaneous infusion of all three causes a sustained synergistic response, which is twofold to fourfold greater than the sum of their individual effects. The concentrations of stress hormones are greatest within 36 hours of injury, and they may be only mildly elevated during the peak period of catabolism, which may occur several days later. Consequently, various cytokines are probably also involved in the hypermetabolic response.

Cytokines

The cytokines are a group of proteins secreted primarily by cells of the immune system (i.e., lymphocytes, macrophages, and reticuloendothelial cells). They are believed to have primarily a local cell-to-cell (paracrine) signaling function within various tissues, but may also exert systemic effects by escaping into the systemic circulation or by altering organ function enough to cause a whole body effect.

Of the numerous cytokines that are produced in increased quantities under stress conditions, interleukin-1 (IL-1), tumor necrosis factor-α (TNFα), and interleukin-6 (IL-6) are considered to be the most important modulators of intermediary metabolism and metabolic rate (6).

Interleukin-1 (IL-1) has a major role in the mobilization of amino acids from skeletal muscle to support increased visceral protein production during stress. IL-1 also appears to elevate plasma glucocorticoids via stimulation of pituitary adrenocorticotropic hormone release, thus creating a hormonal milieu favoring gluconeogenesis.

Tumor necrosis factor (TNF), especially when given with IL-1, can cause the typical endocrine and metabolic responses seen in injury and sepsis. The temporal evolution of the ensuing stress response is identical to that seen with endotoxin, indicating that these cytokines may be primary mediators of the septic/inflammatory response.

Interleukin-6, in conjunction with IL-1 and corticosteroids, has a strong and direct stimulatory effect upon hepatocyte synthesis of acute phase proteins.

GENERAL TREATMENT CONSIDERATIONS

The current basis for the prevention and treatment of multiple organ failure following trauma includes source control (i.e. control of the process, often sepsis, causing the hypermetabolism), plus optimization of oxygen transport and nutritional support.

Source Control

It is increasingly clear that large, open wounds or septic foci may serve as ongoing stimuli of the hypermetabolic response. After major surgery or trauma, some hypermetabolism is a normal, appropriate response pattern and usually is self-limited. Persistence of this response for more than a few days should make one look for a septic focus or any area that needs debridement. Continued hypermetabolism is often a forerunner of increasing organ dysfunction.

Oxygen Transport

Experimental studies have shown that a localized inflammatory focus, which would normally be self-limited, can be converted to a systemic process and organ failure if there is an inadequate systemic oxygen delivery (DO_2) (7). During severe stress, maintaining an "optimal" oxygen delivery often requires maintaining a cardiac output up to 50% greater than normal, a hematocrit of at least 30% to 35%, and an arterial oxygen saturation above 95%.

AXIOM If transport-dependent oxygen consumption or lactic acidosis is seen, it implies that the total body oxygen consumption may be suboptimal and that occult areas of anaerobic tissue metabolism may exist.

When using lactate as a measure of the adequacy of the oxygen delivery, it should be remembered that obesity, sepsis, and hepatic insufficiency can cause elevations of lactate up to 2.0 to 3.0 mmol/L; however, pyruvate also increases to keep a lactate:pyruvate molar ratio of 20:1. If oxygen delivery is inadequate, lactate increases more rapidly than pyruvate, producing increased amounts of "excess lactate."

Calculation of Energy Needs

The need to determine energy requirements is greatest in patients with severe burns, in patients in whom postoperative infections develop, and in patients who are persistently hypermetabolic. All of these patients may require increased caloric and other nutrient support for a prolonged period to avoid excessive loss of body cell mass.

Harris-Benedict Equations

One method for predicting energy needs is the Harris-Benedict equation, which predicts the resting energy expenditure (REE) in kilocalories per day based on height, weight, age, and sex:

$$\text{REE (males)} = 66.47 + 13.75\ (\text{weight}) + 5.0\ (\text{height}) - 6.75\ (\text{age})$$
$$\text{REE (females)} = 655.10 + 9.56\ (\text{weight}) + 1.85\ (\text{height}) - 4.68\ (\text{age})$$

where weight is expressed in kg, height in cm, and age in years. Thus, a 154-lb, 68-inch, 50-year-old man would have the following REE:

$$66.47 + (13.75)(70\ \text{kg}) + 5.0\ (173\ \text{cm}) - (6.75)(50\ \text{yr}) =$$
$$66.47 + 962.5 + 865 - 337.5 = 1{,}556\ \text{kcal/day or about 22 kcal/kg/day.}$$

Likewise, a 132-lb, 64-inch, 50-year-old woman would have the following REE:

$$655.10 + (9.56)(60) + (1.85)(64)(2.54) - (4.68)(50) =$$
$$655.1 + 573.6 + 300.7 - 234 = 1{,}295\ \text{kcal/day or about 22 kcal/kg/day.}$$

To factor in the increases in metabolic rate often associated with trauma, several scaling parameters have been applied to the estimates derived from these equations. For example, to account for the increase in REE resulting from physical activity, the calculated energy expenditure can be multiplied by a factor of 1.1 to 1.2. Additionally, "stress factors" can be used to estimate the increased energy needs with trauma or sepsis. Long et al., using "stress factors" ranging from 1.2 for patients undergoing minor surgery to 2.1 in patients with extensive burns, found that energy expenditure predicted from the Harris-Benedict equations plus these stress factors could estimate energy expenditures within 5% of those measured by indirect calorimetry (8).

Based on population studies, the maintenance caloric requirements in fasting unstressed subjects is about 25 kcal/kg/day. In injured and septic patients, the measured energy expenditure (MEE) tends to be 35 to 50 kcal/kg/day (9). This is similar to estimates derived by multiplying the Harris-Benedict equation by stress factors of 1.2 to 1.6. This wide range leaves considerable room for error, especially in individual patients.

Indirect Calorimetry

AXIOM If indirect calorimetry is not available, it is probably wise to provide about 35 kcal/kg/day to severely hypercatabolic patients because the needs of up to 90% of such patients can be met by this level of caloric support.

Indirect calorimetry involves the measurement of carbon dioxide production and oxygen consumption, which can be converted to energy expenditure. Additionally, the ratio of carbon dioxide produced to oxygen consumed (V_{CO_2}/V_{O_2}), termed the respiratory quotient (RQ), provides an estimate of the relative amounts of glucose and fat that are being oxidized.

Starvation, a state in which fat oxidation is dominant, is characterized by an RQ of 0.7, whereas a glucose-based dietary intake is associated with an RQ of 1.0. RQ values exceeding 1.0 reflect endogenous fat synthesis as a result of excess calories, usually from carbohydrates. Significant hepatic steatosis is likely to develop after 2 to 4 weeks in patients with an RQ persistently exceeding 1.0.

Recently, it was found that, by using indirect calorimetry, the mean MEE averaged 30% higher than the basal energy expenditure calculated from the Harris-Benedict equations, but averaged 11% less than the calculated energy expenditure derived by using an estimated stress factor (10).

AXIOM Current recommendations for caloric support of hypermetabolic injured and septic patients range from 25 to 35 kcal/kg/day.

Despite its apparent advantages, indirect calorimetry is labor intensive and technology intensive, expensive, and not reliably measured in a number of clinical settings, particularly when inspired oxygen concentrations exceed 50% in mechanically ventilated patients and in spontaneously breathing patients on any gas mixture except room air (5). In addition, routine intensive care unit maneuvers (e.g., bronchoscopy, nursing care maneuvers, and respiratory therapy efforts) can increase energy expenditure 20% to 35% above resting levels for up to 1 to 2 hours after completion. In the opposite extreme, patients who have recently been sedated may have significant transient reductions of energy expenditure.

Consequently, repeated or serial determinations of indirect calorimetry are needed to ensure proper caloric needs assessments (11). In addition, the costs associated with the hardware and specialized personnel to perform these tests places some fiscal constraints upon this type of monitoring.

NUTRITIONAL SUPPORT

Timing of Nutritional Support

There are suggestions that early feeding may moderate the metabolic response to injury and improve outcome (12). Mortality rates and the incidence of organ failure in critically ill patients increase substantially when the cumulative negative caloric balance exceeds 10,000 kcal (13), which can develop after only 4 to 5 days in patients receiving only 5% glucose solutions.

Young, previously well-nourished patients who have a simple fracture or a routine, uncomplicated laparotomy and who are expected to eat in 4 to 5 days probably do not benefit from early aggressive nutritional support; however, if the trauma patient was severely malnourished before injury, nutritional therapy should be begun as soon as vital signs are stable.

Standard Nutrients

Glucose

Glucose is generally recommended as the primary energy source for patients receiving intravenous nutritional support. By suppressing hepatic gluconeogenesis, it allows salvage of glucogenic amino acids and suppression of cellular amino acid oxidation; however, the protein catabolism of severe stress is not suppressed by large quantities of glucose. Furthermore, using only glucose to supply the caloric needs of patients can cause a number of complications, including hyperglycemia, hyperosmolar coma, osmotic diuresis, hepatic enzyme elevations, and essential fatty acid deficiency (EFAD) (14).

Current recommendations for the amount of glucose given depend on the level of stress present. Nonprotein caloric intake should range from 25 to 35 kcal/kg/day for most injured patients, and the nutrients to provide this caloric level vary somewhat with the level of stress. In starved, unstressed patients, most of the caloric load can consist of glucose, except for small amounts of fat to prevent EFAD, and relatively small amounts of protein or amino acids. This can be given in a nonprotein calorie:nitrogen ratio of about 150:1. In highly stressed patients, glucose should probably constitute only 60% to 70% of nonprotein calories, with the remainder of the calories supplied as fat. The nonprotein calorie:nitrogen ratio should be about 80–100:1. In highly stressed patients, the initial glucose concentration should probably be 15%.

Fat

Intravenous Fat Emulsions

Use of intravenous (IV) fat emulsions to provide a portion of the nonprotein calories has been fostered by studies indicating that fat clearance and oxidation are relatively normal in most seriously ill, septic patients. Fat has also been shown to have a protein-sparing effect that is equivalent to glucose (15). Indeed, it has been suggested that fat is used in preference to glucose as a metabolic fuel in critically ill, septic patients (16); however, patients with hepatic failure have a decreased capacity to clear lipids from the bloodstream.

AXIOM The daily essential fatty acid requirement is only 1% to 4% of the total caloric need.

Deficiencies of the essential fatty acids (linoleic and linolenic or arachidonic acid) can cause skin scaling, impaired wound healing, increased susceptibility to infection, capillary fragility, thrombocytopenia, fatty infiltration of the liver, and alterations in mental status. The amount of IV fat needed to prevent EFAD is only 500 mL of 10% lipid emulsion once or twice a week.

Although the use of fat calories is increased in postinjury hypermetabolism, excess lipid can also cause complications, particularly when given parenterally. Some of these problems include hypoxemia, neutrophil dysfunction, and decreased phagocytic function of macrophages (17). Additionally, omega-6 fatty acids (the type from plant oils and currently used in IV fat emulsions) are precursors of dienoic prostaglandins and leukotrienes, which may impair host defenses (1). In particular, prostaglandin E_2 suppresses T-cell proliferation, antibody and lymphokine production, and macrophage function. To offset these effects, some authorities have suggested reducing the amount of administered lipid to 5% to 15% of the total nonprotein calories. In addition, if the maximal fat infusion rate exceeds 2.5 g/kg/day, the lipid particles can overload the reticuloendothelial system, causing hepatosplenomegaly, fatty infiltration of the liver, and decreased ability of the reticuloendothelial system to clear bacteria (18). Parenteral omega-6 fatty acids can also increase pulmonary artery pressures and aggravate states of impaired oxygenation in some seriously ill patients (19).

When using intravenous fat preparations, careful attention must be paid to the rate of administration and to monitoring lipid clearance. Lipids are often infused at a rate of 0.5 to 1.0 g/kg/day over 10 to 20 hours, usually beginning after the morning laboratory blood samples are drawn. Serum triglycerides may be monitored two or three times weekly in the early phases of nutritional support, and the lipid infusion rate is decreased if serum triglycerides increase excessively.

AXIOM Triglyceride concentrations exceeding 300 to 350 mg/dL 6 hours after completion of an infusion of 50 g of lipids over a period of 6 to 12 hours suggests that the use of intravenous fat should be limited.

Fish Oils

Experimental studies have shown that marine lipids (fish oils), which contain omega-3 fatty acids, are not immunosuppressive. In a recent report of a multicenter, prospective, randomized clinical trial by Bower et al., which studied the effects of early enteral administration of a formula (IMPACT) composed of arginine, nucleotide, and fish oil, patients who received at least 821 mL/day of the experimental formula had their hospital median length of stay reduced by an average of 8 days (20). In patients stratified as septic, the median length of hospital stay was reduced by 10 days. There was also a major reduction in the frequency of acquired infections. Another recent report demonstrated improved immunologic responses in postoperative patients using an omega-3 fatty acid and arginine supplemented diet (21).

Protein

Standard Amino Acids

Although the accelerated protein catabolism in severe stress is not reduced by exogenously administered calories or amino acids, if enough amino acids are given, the protein synthetic rate can be increased by the exogenously supplied amino acids, and nitrogen balance can be achieved. By achieving nitrogen balance, one can maintain proper immune and reparative function until the source of the neuroendocrine and mediator activation can be eliminated. In low-stress settings, nitrogen balance can be achieved with an amino acid intake as low as 0.5 to 1.0 g/kg/day, as long as the intake of calories is adequate (5). With severe stress, a protein intake of 1.5 to 2.5 g/kg/day (with a nonprotein-calorie:nitrogen ratio of 80–100:1) is needed.

Increased Branched-Chain Amino Acids

Barton and Cerra (5) have favored the use of amino acid preparations enriched in branched-chain amino acids (BCAAs) in settings of high metabolic stress to offset the BCAA deficits that would otherwise occur. Currently available high-BCAA formulations contain 45% to 50% BCAAs, whereas standard amino acid formulations contain only 15% to 33% BCAAs. High-BCAA formulations have been shown to be more efficient than standard formulations at promoting nitrogen retention and supporting hepatic protein synthesis (22). Von Meyenfeldt et al., however, were not able to confirm the reported beneficial effects of BCAA-enriched total parenteral nutrition (TPN) in septic and traumatized patients (23).

Vitamins and Trace Elements

Although the requirements for vitamins and trace elements in hypermetabolic patients are covered by the recommended daily allowance, increased amounts of various vitamins, especially vitamin C, may be of some benefit (5). In oliguric renal failure, the administration of trace elements can usually be decreased to once or twice weekly.

Of the various trace element deficiencies that may occur in patients with severe trauma, those involving zinc, copper, and selenium deserve particular mention. Zinc and copper deficiencies may develop rapidly because of excessive gastrointestinal losses and increased excretion in the urine of hypermetabolic trauma patients. Zinc is particularly important in wound healing, and copper is needed for proper red cell formation. Selenium deficiency, which may cause cardiomyopathy, has also been reported in burn patients. Because selenium and zinc are important in free radical scavenging, anabolism, and immunity, the current recommendations for supplements in severely traumatized patients should probably be increased.

ADMINISTRATION OF NUTRITIONAL SUPPORT

Advantages of Total Parenteral Nutrition versus Total Enteral Nutrition

As a general rule, total enternal nutrition (TEN) is preferable to TPN; however, TPN can be started soon after trauma, its use does not depend on a functional gastrointestinal tract, and it is reliable in the sense that whatever is given will appear in the bloodstream.

TEN requires a functioning small intestine and can be unreliable because the patient may not receive what is ordered or it may not be absorbed. Abdominal distension or excessive diarrhea may also force one to discontinue or alter the enteral nutrition.

Feeding into the stomach increases the risk of aspiration of the enteral feedings into the lungs, particularly if the patient has had a severe head injury and has increased gastroesophageal reflux. Consequently, it is safer to instill the enteral feedings into the proximal jejunum. Placement of a jejunostomy feeding tube at surgery is a reasonable alternative to nasojejunal feeding; however, performing a laparotomy only to insert a jejunostomy tube is not without some risk.

Diarrhea is a problem in at least 20% of enterally fed patients; however, its incidence and severity can be minimized by starting with dilute formulas (usually one-fourth to one-half strength) and increasing concentration and volume slowly. Persistent diarrhea resulting from the enteral formula can usually be controlled by adding dietary fiber or reducing fat content. Before using antidiarrheal agents such as paregoric, diaphenoxylate, or Imodium, one must rule out or treat *Clostridium difficile* enterocolitis, which is more likely to occur with the use of antibiotics. Antidiarrheal agents are contraindicated in *C. difficile* enteritis because reducing bowel motility can increase absorption of the toxin and make the systemic symptoms and bowel damage worse. Empiric administration of 500 mg of metronidazole (Flagyl) every 6 hours into the gastrointestinal tract may control infectious diarrhea while awaiting laboratory studies.

Advantages of Enteral Nutrition over Total Parenteral Nutrition

One of the biggest advantages of enteral nutrition is its ability to stimulate gut mucosal growth. This preserves the gut barrier to translocation of bacteria and bacterial products out of the bowel lumen into the portal vein or bowel lymphatics. The maintenance of small bowel structure and function depends primarily on intraluminal amino acids, particularly glutamine, which is the preferential fuel source.

Enteral nutrition reduces mortality rate (compared to parenteral nutrition) in experimental models of hemorrhagic shock and peritonitis (24) and results in better total lymphocyte counts and significantly fewer major septic complications (4% versus 26%) in trauma patients (25).

Kudsk et al. also noted significantly higher levels of constitutive proteins and lower levels of acute phase proteins in patients randomized to enteral feeding (26). The incidence of septic complications was 15% (5 of 33) with enteral feeding and 41% (14 of 34) with the parenteral route (p=.03).

A metaanalysis combining data from 230 patients from eight prospective, randomized trials showed that significantly fewer TEN patients experienced septic complications (17% versus 44%) (p=.0001) (27).

Additional disadvantages of TPN include

1. It costs much more than enteral feeding.
2. Administration of TPN requires the placement of a central venous catheter.
3. Catheter infections can be a problem.
4. Hyperinsulinemia with TPN tends to reduce mobilization of fat stores for energy.

Providing Enteral Nutrition

Although return of gastric and colonic motility is rather slow after trauma, the small intestine may begin to function adequately for enteral nutrition within 24 to 48 hours of abdominal surgery. Thus, provision of feedings through a jejunostomy or nasojejunal tube permits earlier feedings than would otherwise be tolerated by mouth or through a gastric tube. We usually begin with 10 to 20 mL/h of an isoosmolar solution, which is usually two-thirds IMPACT and one-third Vivonex HN (for increased glutamine). The rate of feeding is increased about 10 mL/h every 12 to 24 hours if abdominal pain, distension, or severe diarrhea does not develop.

Nevertheless, early feeding via a 16- or 18-French nasogastric tube can be effective because gastric residuals can be easily checked, reducing the risk of aspiration of gastric contents. Longer feeding tubes passed into the jejunum are less likely to cause aspiration, but up to 40% to 50% repeatedly retract back into the stomach. A risk of development of sinusitis also exists, especially if the other nostril has a nasotracheal tube. Feedings via a nasogastric tube are begun at 30 to 60 mL every 1 to 2 hours. The nasogastric tube is clamped until 5 to 10 minutes before the next feeding. If the residual volume in the stomach is less than 50 to 100 mL, the feedings can be gradually increased to about 1,800 to 2,400 mL per day.

Percutaneous endoscopic gastrostomy (PEG) catheters avoid nasal and pharyngeal irritation and are less likely to clog than small feeding tubes. PEG is not as accurate for checking gastric residuals; consequently, there is a risk of gastric contents being aspirated. PEG feedings are usually started 24 to 48 hours after insertion as a 50 mL bolus every 4 hours. The amount is increased by 50 to 100 mL for each 4-hourly bolus feeding each day, if there are no excess residuals or other problems, up to a maximum of about 300 mL every 4 hours. Percutaneous endoscopic jejunostomy catheters, in which a catheter inserted through a PEG is advanced into the jejunum, are also available, but many of these catheters keep coming back into the stomach and have to be repositioned frequently.

Providing Total Parenteral Nutrition

After an appropriate central venous line is established and designated for TPN use only, one can start with 15% to 20% glucose mixtures, usually with 4.3% amino acids, at 40 to 80 mL/h. The volume or concentration can be increased as needed and tolerated. Standard additions to each liter of TPN include 50 mEq Na^+, 30 mEq of K^+, 30 to 50 mEq of Cl^-, 4.7 mEq of Ca^{2+}, 4 to 8 mEq of Mg^{2+}, 15 mmol of P, and 60 to 75 mEq of acetate. In addition, standard amounts of trace elements (3.0 mg of Zn, 1.2 mg of Cu, 12 mg of Cr, and 0.3 mg of Mn) and 10 mL of multivitamins are added to the first liter given each day (Table 38-1).

Standard initial TPN monitoring includes monitoring urine every 4 to 6 hours for sugar, acetone, and blood, and daily for electrolytes and glucose. Intravenous lipids may be given as 500 to 1,000 cc of 10% solution daily or only twice weekly depending on clinical needs and triglyceride clearance.

NUTRITIONAL MONITORING

Anthropometric Measurements

Anthropometric measurements, such as midarm circumference and skin fold thickness are measured in only a very few centers, but they can reflect skeletal mass and the amount of fat present; however, because of the increased extracellular water accumulated by critically ill trauma victims patients, a large variance in these anthropometric measurements occurs, making these measurements of little initial use. Weight changes may also be helpful, but these often reflect changes in the extracellular fluid as opposed to true lean body mass.

Table 38-1. *Typical Total Parenteral Nutrition Constituents at Detroit Receiving Hospital for Acute Trauma Patients*

Volume	
2,000–3,000 mL/d	
Nutrients	
Amino acids	4.25%–8.0%
Dextrose	15%–25%
Fat emulsion	500 mL 10%–20% BIW–TIW
MVI	10 mL/d
Electrolytes (per liter)	
Sodium	35 mEq
Potassium	30 mEq
Chloride	35 mEq
Acetate	71 mEq
Phosphate	15 mmol
Calcium	4.7 mEq
Magnesium	5.0 mEq
Trace elements (3 mL)	
Zinc	3 mg
Copper	1.3 mg
Manganese	0.3 mg
Chromium	12 μg

BIW, 2 times a week; TID, 3 times a week

Nitrogen Balance

Twice weekly nitrogen balance determinations are probably the most reliable, readily available, short-term method for ascertaining the adequacy of nutritional support. Nitrogen balance is calculated as nitrogen intake minus nitrogen output from all sources. Nitrogen intake is relatively easy to calculate. Approximately 1 g of nitrogen is provided by every 6.25 g of protein or amino acids given. Nitrogen output includes stool losses (1 to 2 g/day in the absence of gastrointestinal disease), skin losses (0.5 to 1.0 g/day), and urinary losses. Urinary nitrogen has several components, including urea, uric acid, ammonia, amino acids, and creatinine. UUN usually accounts for 80% to 90% of the total urinary nitrogen (TUN), but may account for as little as 65% to 70% in patients with severe stress. In such patients, direct measurements of TUN may provide a much more accurate estimate of urinary nitrogen losses than just adding 3 to 4 g/day to the UUN (28).

Corrections must also be made for increases in the blood urea nitrogen (BUN). A 10 mg/dL increase in the BUN in a 70-kg man is equivalent to a 4,200 mg (4.2 g) loss of N_2 from the lean body mass.

3-Methylhistidine

3-Methylhistidine is an amino acid that comes only from skeletal muscle. It is excreted unchanged in the urine and, therefore, it reflects the rate of muscle proteolysis. Excretion is increased in patients with a larger lean body mass, greater stress, and poorer nutritional intake. Renal failure inhibits the rate of 3-methylhistidine excretion (5).

Evaluating Hepatic Protein Synthesis

Albumin is a plasma protein with a molecular weight of about 65,000 daltons. It is contained in a large body pool (4 to 5 g/kg). In stress, plasma levels may decrease precipitously, but the total body content is often relatively unchanged. Serum albumin levels are also decreased in hepatic failure and burns. Because of its long half-life (20 to 22 days), its plasma levels respond slowly to therapy.

Critically injured patients who are able, by themselves, to maintain hemoglobin levels above 10.0 to 12.0 g/dL and albumin levels above 2.8 g/dL tend to do better than those who require repeated transfusions or have serum albumin levels less than 1.8 g/dL, even with comparable degrees of injury. Girvent et al. (29) found that serum albumin levels less than 35 g/L were virtually always associated with the euthyroid sick syndrome.

Transferrin is present in smaller quantities (220 to 300 mg/dL) than albumin and it has a shorter half-life (8 to 10 days); therefore, it is a more sensitive indicator of the patient's nutritional status. Transferrin, however, is also adversely affected as a nutritional indicator by the same variables as albumin. In addition, iron deficiency can lead to elevations in transferrin levels.

Prealbumin levels are normally 22 ± 7 mg/dL and it has a short half-life (2 days). Therefore, prealbumin can be a sensitive indicator of nutritional status. It is, however, also affected by the state of hydration. In addition, low levels are seen in hyperthyroidism, cystic fibrosis, chronic illness, and acute stress.

Retinol-binding protein is involved in vitamin A transport. It has a very short half-life (12 hours), and it is very sensitive to protein synthesis and utilization changes. Normal serum levels are 5.1 ± 2.5 mg/dL, and these levels increase in patients with renal disease and excess vitamin A administration. Blood levels are reduced in liver disease, cystic fibrosis, hyperthyroidism, and vitamin A deficiency.

Evaluation of Immunocompetence

Delayed Hypersensitivity Skin Testing

At least four antigens should be used simultaneously to perform skin testing for standard recall antigens; a positive test is 5 or more millimeters of induration at 48 to 72 hours. Commonly used skin test antigens are PPD (purified protein derivative, tuberculin), candida, mumps, and trichophyton. Failure to respond positively to any of the four antigens is referred to as "anergy," and response to only one antigen is referred to as "relative anergy." Anergy to recall skin test antigens can be caused by a multitude of factors. It is common for 3 to 4 days after major trauma, but continued anergy usually indicates that the patient is either septic or likely to become septic.

In a report by Meakins et al., more than 50% of anergic surgical patients became septic and a high percentage died (30). The patients with "relative anergy" did almost as badly as those with anergy. A positive response to two or more antigens usually indicates normal immunocompetence, and the patients in this category did very well.

Absolute Lymphocyte Count

The absolute lymphocyte count (ALC) may be helpful in evaluating nutrition and immunocompetence. Normally, the ALC is 2,000 to 2,500/mm^3. An ALC less than 1,500/mm^3 is believed to reflect moderate malnutrition and possible anergy, whereas an ALC less than 800/mm^3 almost always reflects anergy or severe malnutrition. The ALC is also reduced by sepsis, steroids, neoplasia, and transplant immunosuppression.

Ongoing Evaluation of Nutritional Therapy

Standard Laboratory Test

Serum electrolytes are measured daily or every other day for the first week of nutritional support and less often during long-term therapy in stable patients. Magnesium and phosphorus should be checked twice weekly initially and less often during long-term therapy.

Urine glucose is checked every 4 to 6 hours. Blood glucose levels are checked one to two times daily, and then daily after increases or decreases in the rate of TPN or enteral formulas. Patients with poorly controlled diabetes may warrant continued blood glucose levels two to four times daily.

Liver function tests (bilirubin, alkaline phosphatase, AST, and ALT) and serum albumin should be obtained once or twice weekly. During long-term nutritional support, such checks once or twice a month are probably adequate.

In the acute setting, 24-hour urine collections for nitrogen balance should be obtained twice weekly until a persistently positive nitrogen balance is obtained.

Indirect calorimetry should be done at least once or twice weekly until the appropriate nutritional prescription is determined. In hypermetabolic surgical patients, an RQ of 0.80 to 0.85 suggests use of an appropriate mixed fuel source. An RQ of more than 1.0 suggests overfeeding, particularly with carbohydrates.

Prothrombin time should be obtained weekly in the acute setting to monitor the adequacy of vitamin K administration.

Serum triglycerides are checked before and 6 hours after a test dose of triglycerides (usually 500 mL of 10% Intralipid) and then weekly unless increased doses of fat, increased sepsis, or abnormal liver function tests suggests a need for more frequent monitoring.

ORGAN-SPECIFIC NUTRIENT SUPPORT

Pulmonary Failure

Excess calories, particularly excess carbohydrate calories, are associated with an increase in CO_2 production that may be clinically significant in patients with compromised pulmonary function. To minimize CO_2 production, excess carbohydrate calories should be avoided, and up to 50% of the nonprotein calories can be given as fat in hypercarbic patients.

At the opposite extreme, excess intake of fat preparations has been associated with detrimental effects with regard to immune and pulmonary function. Excess serum chylomicrons are believed to be cleared by macrophages, and lipid-laden macrophages appear to have decreased phagocytic function.

Liver Failure

Encephalopathy in cirrhosis may be partially accounted for by accumulation of methionine and aromatic amino acids (tyrosine and phenylalanine) in the plasma and central nervous system (CNS). Because the liver is the major organ system responsible for clearing these amino acids, an increase in their plasma concentration caused by hepatic insufficiency, increased protein intake, or increased gut absorption encourages their transport across the blood-brain barrier. The resultant excess of aromatic amino acids in the CNS may then serve as precursors for the formation of false neurotransmitters, such as octopamine, which can induce encephalopathy (31).

Therapy, in addition to attempts to reduce blood ammonia levels by gut decontamination with lactulose or nonabsorbable antibiotics, includes adequate glucose and amino acids enriched with BCAAs (leucine, isoleucine, and valine) and deficient in methionine and aromatic amino acids (32).

Patients with hepatic encephalopathy who were given increased BCAA demonstrated significant improvement in psychometric tests as compared to patients receiving isonitrogenous casein supplements (33).

Renal Failure

Isolated renal failure is typically treated with protein restriction. The catabolic nature of severe trauma and sepsis, however, usually demands an increased protein intake to avoid severe acute protein malnutrition. The use of essential amino acids as a means to control the rate of BUN elevation has been reported to be advantageous (34); however, this approach remains controversial.

AXIOM Dialysis should be performed as often as needed to allow optimal nutritional support in patients with oliguric renal failure.

Continuous arteriovenous hemofiltration (CAVH) has also been shown to be a useful method for increasing nutritional intake in patients with oliguric renal failure (35). Standard or increased volumes of TPN may be infused into patients undergoing CAVH because excess extracellular fluid and urea nitrogen are continuously removed by ultrafiltration.

SPECIALIZED NUTRIENTS

Glutamine is a nonessential amino acid that has received much attention because it is thought to

1. Sustain intestinal mucosal barrier function, thereby decreasing bacterial translocation;
2. Inhibit skeletal muscle proteolysis;
3. Maintain proper lymphocyte proliferation; and (36)
4. Help form glutathione, an important free radical scavenger.

Biolo et al. (37) recently studied the effects of carnitine and alanyl-glutamine administration in severely traumatized patients and found that both the carnitine and the glutamine dipeptide reduced whole-body nitrogen loss without adversely affecting protein metabolism in skeletal muscle.

The amino acid *arginine* has been shown experimentally to improve protein synthesis, wound healing, and immune function when it is provided as a nutritional supplement (38). Arginine is normally considered to be a nonessential amino acid. Under conditions of severe stress, however, arginine becomes essential for adequate nitrogen balance. Arginine supplements to postoperative feeding programs improve nitrogen balance compared to isonitrogenous nonarginine-containing diets (39). Arginine enhances collagen synthesis and increases wound strength in human studies. It also improves host immunity as evidenced by less severe depression and earlier return to normal of peripheral T lymphocyte mitogen responses after trauma (39). Gennari and Alexander (40) found that feeding with diets supplemented with arginine and glutamine plus treatment with dehydroepiandrosterone reversed the susceptibility to infections caused by prednisone and burn injury.

Some studies have also shown that arginine stimulates secretion of growth hormone, prolactin, insulin-like growth factor 1 (IGF-1), insulin, and glucagon (39). Increased growth hormone, insulin, and IGF-1 could account for the anabolic responses to arginine administration. The increased secretion of prolactin, which has immune regulatory properties, could account for some of the immunostimulating actions of arginine.

Nucleic acids are another group of nutrients that may exert favorable immunomodulating effects upon the host (41). The specific elements that appear to be responsible for these effects include purine and pyrimidine bases of ribonucleic (RNA) and deoxyribonucleic acid (DNA).

COMPLICATIONS OF NUTRITIONAL SUPPORT IN TRAUMA

Intravenous Catheters

The major long-term complication of central venous catheterization is infection, and strict attention must be paid to sterile technique during insertion of the intravenous catheter and follow-up care. When possible, blood should not be drawn through these catheters.

Thrombosis of the catheter after several days is not unusual, but can be prevented or retarded by flushing with heparin or by adding some heparin to the intravenous solutions. If a symptomatic thrombosis of a subclavian or innominate vein occurs, local thrombolytic therapy may be effective.

Complications of Enteral Feeding

Feeding Catheters

Mechanical complications of enteral nutritional support are primarily related to placement of the feeding catheters and to aspiration of gastric contents into the lungs. Tubes placed nasally can be associated with excess pulmonary secretions, pharyngeal irritation, sinusitis, otitis media, and pressure ulcers of the nasal ala. These problems are more common with stiffer polyethylene nasogastric tubes, but occasionally also occur with soft feeding catheters.

The incidence of significant aspiration, which may be as high as 40% with gastric feedings, can be minimized by elevating the head of the bed at least 30 degrees at all times and by frequently checking for gastric distension and high gastric residuals.

Gastrointestinal Problems

The development of gastrointestinal symptoms, such as bloating or cramping as a result of enteral nutrition, are usually related primarily to a high osmolarity or to too rapid rates of administration. These problem can often be avoided by gradual increases in formula concentration and infusion rates. Chronic malnutrition with gut mucosal atrophy, short gut syndromes, and pancreatic insufficiency may also contribute to the problem.

Lactose intolerance or difficulties with osmolarity can often be corrected with a change in formula. Pancreatic insufficiency may respond to commercially available pancreatic enzymes given four times daily.

⊘ PITFALL

Assuming that diarrhea that develops when enteral feeding is begun is caused by the enteral feeding rather than more serious problems.

Diarrhea may complicate nutritional therapy in more than 25% of patients. In critically ill patients who have been given antibiotics, *pseudomembranous enterocolitis* caused by overgrowth of *C. difficile*, should be ruled out, particularly in patients who have received broad-spectrum antibiotics. The presence of fecal leukocytes on stool analysis suggests an infectious etiology and warrants evaluation, which should include stool cultures for pathogens, such as *C. difficile*, *Campylobacter*, and *Yersenia*. Serologic tests should also be done for *C. difficile* toxin. Sigmoidoscopy to identify pseudomembranous colitis may also be warranted.

AXIOM Constipating agents are contraindicated in patients who may have *C. difficile* colitis.

Fluid and Electrolyte Problems

Disturbances in water balance caused by intravenous feedings are most commonly due to excess free-water, as reflected by hyponatremia, hypoproteinemia, and anemia. Inadequate free water is reflected by hypernatremia, prerenal azotemia, and hemoconcentration. This is most commonly seen in patients who also have abnormal large fluid losses, such as in burns, large open wounds, or gastrointestinal problems.

Potassium needs are increased during TPN, particularly when glucose is the primary caloric source. Increased potassium is also needed during protein synthesis. Diuretics and high urinary outputs can cause severe potassium losses, usually with at least 30 to 40 mEq of potassium in each liter of urine.

Hypophosphatemia is one of the more common electrolyte abnormalities associated with intravenous feeding, and it occurs in up to 30% of patients on TPN. Without adequate phosphate supplementation, hypophosphatemia can develop within 48 hours of institution of TPN.

Hyperphosphatemia is most commonly associated with renal failure, but it may also be associated with the use of 10% solutions of intravenous fat as a result of the phosphorous content of the solution (42).

Magnesium deficiency can be precipitated by excess gastrointestinal losses, alcoholism, diuretic use, and rapid protein anabolism. Unfortunately, serum magnesium levels may be normal despite a reduced total body content (43). Hebert et al. (44) found, using a magnesium-loading test of 30 mmol (7.5 g) of magnesium sulfate intravenously daily for 3 days, that 63% of critically ill patients without renal insufficiency had magnesium deficiency, even though serum levels were normal.

AXIOM The total body magnesium may be quite low, and serum levels can still be normal.

Hyperglycemia in stressed patients is a common complication of parenteral nutritional support and is particularly apt to occur in patients who are septic. In trying to prevent or treat hyperglycemia, however, it is important to not cause hypoglycemia, which can have much more severe consequences.

Essential Fatty Acid Deficiencies

If no lipids are given, EFAD may develop in 2 to 4 weeks in starving patients (5). In stressed patients receiving large amounts of glucose, hyperinsulinemia tends to suppress lipolysis. This can prevent mobilization of endogenous essential fatty acids and can cause a clinical EFAD to develop in as little 10 days. Signs of EFAD include malabsorption, diarrhea, dry skin, coarse hair, brittle nails, impaired wound healing, thrombocytopenia, hemolytic anemia, and increased capillary permeability. Prevention of the problem involves administering lipids on a twice weekly basis.

Hepatobiliary Complications

The most common hepatic complication of parenteral nutritional support is hepatic steatosis (fatty infiltration of the liver) (5). Etiologic factors include infusion of carbohydrate as the sole source of calories, infusion of excess calories, EFAD, and carnitine deficiency. EFAD promotes fat accumulation in the liver as a result of decreased synthesis of phospholipids, which are required for lipid transport. Carnitine deficiency, although unusual, may also lead to impaired transport and reduced mitochondrial oxidation of lipids.

Hepatobiliary complications of nutritional support are usually diagnosed because of blood chemistry changes. Elevation in amino transferase is suggestive of hepatocellular injury and usually reflects fatty infiltration or triaditis, whereas hyperbilirubinemia and elevation of alkaline phosphatase are more suggestive of cholestasis. Progressive liver dysfunction despite dietary changes may reflect toxic manifestations of other disease processes, such as sepsis or drug toxicity.

AXIOM Mild alterations in hepatic function that resolve with dietary maneuvers usually reflect a relatively benign cholestatic process.

EXPERIMENTAL DRUGS

Meyer et al. recently reported that protein catabolism can be reversed to some extent by anabolic agents, such as human growth hormone and IGF-1 (45). The administration of parenteral human growth hormone reduces nitrogen excretion under a variety of clinical conditions, but especially in burn patients.

Cioffi et al. recently reported on the effect of IGF-1 on energy expenditure and protein and glucose metabolism in patients with thermal injury (46). Although the REE was not altered by IGF-1, glucose uptake was promoted and protein oxidation was decreased significantly. IGF-1 appears to preserve lean body mass during severe stress by minimizing the oxidation of amino acids.

⊘ FREQUENT ERRORS

1. ***Underestimation or overestimation of the metabolic requirements in severely injured patients.***
2. ***Delay in providing nutritional therapy in poorly nourished or hypermetabolic trauma patients.***
3. ***Inadequate monitoring of nutritional parameters, especially in severely injured or severely malnourished trauma patients.***
4. ***Inadequate attention to organ function during nutritional therapy, thereby delaying recognition of organ failure.***
5. ***Reliance only on gross clinical estimates of nutritional needs in severely injured or malnourished patients.***

6. ***Allowing patients with head injuries to have blood glucose levels higher than 150 to 200 mg/dL.***
7. ***Failure to begin enteral nutrition as soon as possible in malnourished or hypermetabolic patients.***
8. ***Assuming that diarrhea in patients on enteral nutrition is due to the nutritional therapy.***
9. ***Failure to keep the stomach decompressed in patients who are unable to protect their airway.***
10. ***Administration of intravenous lipids without adequately monitoring triglyceride clearance.***
11. ***Failure to look for or diagnose early hepatic steatosis on long-term intravenous feeding.***

SUMMARY POINTS

1. Stress carbohydrate metabolism is characterized by increased glycogenolysis and gluconeogenesis that is poorly suppressed by the exogenous administration of glucose.

2. Blood ketone levels tend to be high during starvation and very low during stress.

3. UUN losses are usually less than 5 g/day in nonstressed starvation but may exceed 15 to 30 g/day in severe stress.

4. The net effect of the "primary stress hormones" (cortisol, glucagon, and catecholamines) is to provide increased glucose to injured tissues and to promote the retention of salt and water to support the intravascular volume and central circulation.

5. The postinjury and septic catabolic response is due largely to the combined influences of stress hormones and cytokines.

6. Evidence of persistent hypermetabolism or acute organ failure should stimulate a diligent search for an uncontrolled focus of infection.

7. Following major trauma, tissue perfusion and oxygen transport should probably be maintained at levels 25% to 50% greater than normal.

8. The increased caloric energy expenditure occurring after trauma should be provided from external sources to minimize the use of endogenous protein for fuel.

9. If indirect calorimetry is not available, it is probably wise to provide about 35 kcal/kg/day to severely hypercatabolic patients because the needs of up to 90% of such patients can be met by this level of caloric support.

10. Improperly timed indirect calorimetry studies may lead to underfeeding or overfeeding, which may have a detrimental effect on survival.

11. If the trauma patient was severely malnourished before injury, nutritional therapy should be begun as soon as the vital signs are stable.

12. EFAD can cause skin scaling, impaired wound healing, increased susceptibility to infection, capillary fragility, thrombocytopenia, fatty infiltration of the liver, and alterations in mental status.

13. EFAD can be prevented by administering 1% to 4% of the total caloric need as intravenous fat (i.e., 500 mL of 10% lipids intravenously once or twice a week)

14. Triglyceride concentrations exceeding 300 to 350 mg/dL 6 hours after infusion of 50 g of lipids over a period of 6 to 12 hours suggests that the use of intravenous fat should be limited.

15. The primary advantages of TPN is that its use does not depend on a functional gastrointestinal tract, it can be begun early, and it is reliable in the sense that whatever is given will appear in the bloodstream.

16. TPN lacks the ability of enteral nutrition to improve gut trophic factors and gastrointestinal barrier function.

17. The earlier enteral nutrition is begun after trauma, the more likely it is to be of benefit.

18. Critically injured patients who are able, by themselves, to maintain hemoglobin levels above 10.0 to 12.0 g/dL and albumin levels above 2.8 g/dL tend to do better than those who require repeated transfusions or have serum albumin levels less than 1.8 g/dL, even with comparable degrees of injury.
19. Anergy to recall skin test antigens can be caused by a wide variety of problems, but can be prevented or corrected best by prompt control of sepsis and early provision of adequate nutrition.
20. Dialysis should be performed in renal failure patients as often as needed to allow optimal nutritional support.
21. Aspiration of enteral feedings, especially in neurologically impaired patients, can be greatly reduced by keeping the patient's head up and feeding through jejunostomy catheters.
22. Constipating agents are contraindicated in patients who may have *C. difficile* colitis.
23. Total body magnesium may be quite low despite normal serum levels.
24. RQ values greater than 1.0 usually indicate an excessive carbohydrate intake and conversion of carbohydrate into fat, which eventually can cause hepatic steatosis.

REFERENCES

1. Dahn MS, Wilson RF. Metabolic and nutritional considerations in trauma. In: Wilson RF, Walt AJ, eds. *Management of trauma—pitfalls and practices,* 2nd ed. Philadelphia: Williams & Wilkins, 1996:796.
2. Dahn MS, Jacobs LA, Smith S, Hans B, Lange MP, Mitchell RA. The relationship of insulin production to glucose metabolism in severe sepsis. *Arch Surg* 1985;120:166–172.
3. Dahn MS, Kirkpatrick JR, Blasier R. Alterations in the metabolism of exogenous lipid associated with sepsis. *J Parenter Enteral Nutr* 1984;8:169.
4. Hasselgren PO, Pederson P, Sax HC, et al. Current concepts of protein turnover and amino acid transport in liver and skeletal muscle during sepsis. *Arch Surg* 1988;123:992.
5. Barton RG, Cerra FB. Metabolic and nutritional support. Moore EE, Feliciano DV, Mattox KL, eds. *Trauma,* 2nd ed. Norwalk, CT: Appleton & Lange. 1991:965.
6. Klasing KC. Nutritional aspects of leukocytic cytokines. *J Nutr* 1988;118:1436.
7. Nuytinck JRS, Goris RJA, Weerts JG, et al. Acute generalized microvascular injury by activated complement and hypoxia: the basis of the adult respiratory distress syndrome and multiple organ failure? *Br J Exp Pathol* 1986;67:537.
8. Long CL, Schaffel N, Geiger JW, et al. Metabolic response to injury and illness: estimation of energy and protein needs from indirect calorimetry and nitrogen balance. *J Parenter Enteral Nutr* 1979;3:452.
9. Jeevanandam M, Young DH, Schiller WR. Influence of parenteral nutrition on rates of net substrate oxidation in severe trauma patients. *Crit Care Med* 1990;18:467.
10. Alexander JW, Gonce SJ, Miskell PW, et al. A new model for studying nutrition in peritonitis. The adverse effect of overfeeding. *Ann Surg* 1989;209:334.
11. Verameij CG, Feenstra BWA, Van Lanschot JJB, et al. Day-to-day variability of energy expenditure in critically ill surgical patients. *Crit Care Med* 1989;17:623.
12. Moore EE, Jones TN. Benefits of immediate jejunostomy feeding after major abdominal trauma: a randomized prospective study. *J Trauma* 1986;26:874.
13. Bartlett RH, Dechert RE, Mault JR, et al. Measurement of metabolism in multiple organ failure. *Surgery* 1982;92:771.
14. Long CL. Fuel preferences in the septic patient: glucose or lipid? *J Parenter Enteral Nutr* 1987;11:333.
15. Nordenstrom J, Askanazi J, Elwyn D, et al. Nitrogen balance during total parenteral nutrition: glucose vs fat. *Ann Surg* 1983;197:27.
16. Shaw JHF, Wolfe RR. Response to glucose and lipid infusions in sepsis: a kinetic analysis. *Metabolism* 1985;34:442.
17. Nugent KM. Intralipid effects on reticulo-endothelial function. *J Leukoc Biol* 1984;36:123.

18. Wan JMF, Teo TC, Babayan VK, Blackburn GL. Invited comment: lipids and the development of immune dysfunction and infection. *J Parenter Enteral Nutr* 1988;2:435.
19. Skeie B, Askanazi J, Rothkopf MM, et al. Intravenous fat emulsions and lung function: a review. *Crit Care Med* 1988;6:193.
20. Bower RH, Cerra FB, Bershadsky B, et al. Early enteral administration of formula (IMPACT[R]) supplemented with arginine, nucleotides, and fish oil in intensive care unit patients: results of a multicenter, prospective, randomized, clinical trial. *Crit Care Med* 1995;23:436.
21. Kemen M, Senkal M, Homann HH, et al. Early postoperative enteral nutrition with arginine-W-3 fatty acids and ribonucleic acid-supplemented diet versus placebo in cancer patients: an immunologic evaluation of IMPACT. *Crit Care Med* 1995;23:652.
22. Bower RH, Muggin-Sullam M, Fisher J. Branched chain amino acid-enriched solutions in the septic patient. *Ann Surg* 1986;203:13.
23. von Meyenfeldt MF, Soeters PB, Vente JP, et al. Effect of branched chain amino acid enrichment of total parenteral nutrition on nitrogen sparing and clinical outcome of sepsis and trauma: a prospective randomized double blind trial. *Br J Surg* 1990;77:924.
24. Zaloga GP, Knowles R, Black KW, et al. Total parenteral nutrition increases mortality after hemorrhage. *Crit Care Med* 1991;19:54.
25. Moore EE, Jones TN. Benefits of immediate jejunostomy feeding after major abdominal trauma: a prospective randomized study. *J Trauma* 1986;26:874.
26. Kudsk KA, Minard G, Wojtysiak SL, et al. Visceral protein response to enteral versus parenteral nutrition and sepsis in patients with trauma. *Surgery* 1994;116:516.
27. Eyer SD, Micon LT, Konstatinides FN. Early enteral feeding does not attenuate metabolic responses after blunt trauma. *J Trauma* 1993;34:639.
28. Konstantinides FN, Cerra FB. Can urinary urea nitrogen be substituted for total urinary nitrogen when calculating nitrogen balance in clinical nutrition. *J Parenter Enteral Nutr* 1988;11:18S.
29. Girvent M, Maestro S, Hernandez R, et al. Euthyroid sick syndrome, associated endocrine abnormalities, and outcome in elderly patients undergoing emergency operation. *Surgery* 1998;123:560.
30. Meakins JL, Pietch JB, Burenick O, et al. Delayed hypersensitivity: indicator of acquired failure of host defenses in sepsis and trauma. *Ann Surg* 1977;186:241.
31. Fischer JE. Branched-chain enriched amino acid solutions in patients with liver failure: an early example of nutritional pharmacology. *J Parenter Enteral Nutr* 1990;14:249S.
32. Cerra FB, Cheung NK, Fischer JE, et al. Disease-specific amino acid infusion (FO80) in hepatic encephalopathy: a prospective, randomized, double-blind, controlled trial. *J Parenter Enteral Nutr* 1985;93:288.
33. Egberts EH, Schomerus H, Hamster W, et al. Branched chain amino acids in the treatment of latent portosystemic encephalopathy: a double-blind placebo-controlled crossover study. *Gastroenterology* 1985;88:887.
34. Cerra FB, Blackburn B, Hirsch J, et al. The effect of stress level, amino acid formula, and nitrogen dose on nitrogen retention in traumatic and septic stress. *Ann Surg* 1987;205:282.
35. Barlett RH, Mault JR, Dechert RE, et al. Continuous arteriovenous hemofiltration: improved survival in surgical acute renal failure. *Surgery* 1986;100:400.
36. Souba WW, Herskowitz K, Austgen TR, et al. Glutamine nutrition: theoretical considerations and therapeutic impact. *J Parenter Enteral Nutr* 1990;14:237S.
37. Biolo G, Toigo G, Ciocchi B, et al. Metabolic response to injury and sepsis: changes in protein metabolism. *Nutrition* 1997;13[9 Suppl]:52S.
38. Kirk SJ, Barbul A. Role of arginine in trauma, sepsis and immunity. *J Parenter Enteral Nutr* 1990;14:226S.
39. Daly JM, Reynolds J, Thom A, et al. Immune and metabolic effects of arginine in the surgical patient. *Ann Surg* 1988;208:512.
40. Gennari R, Alexander JW. Arginine, glutamine, and dehydroepiandrosterone

reverse the immunosuppressive effect of prednisone during gut-derived sepsis. *Crit Care Med* 1997;25:1207.
41. Rudolph FB, Kulkarni AD, Fanslow WC, et al. Role of RNA as a dietary source of pyrimidines and purines in immune function. *Nutrition* 1990;61:45.
42. Cerra FB, Lehman S, Konstantinides N, et al. Effect of enteral nutrients on in vitro tests of immune function in ICU patients: a preliminary report. *Nutrition* 1990;6:84.
43. Chernow B, Smith S, Rainet TG, et al. Hypomagnesemia: implications for critical care specialists. *Crit Care Med* 1983;10:193.
44. Hebert P, Mehta N, Wang J, et al. Functional magnesium deficiency in critically ill patients identified using a magnesium-loading test. *Crit Care Med* 1997; 25:749.
45. Meyer NA, Mueller MJ, Hendon DN. Nutrient support of the healing wound. *New Horiz* 1994:2:202.
46. Cioffi WG, Gore DC, Rue LW 3rd, et al. Insulin-like growth factor-1 lowers protein oxidation in patients with thermal injury. *Ann Surg* 1994;220:310.

39. SEPSIS IN TRAUMA[1]

INTRODUCTION

Incidence of Infection

In patients with major trauma, the incidence of infection following a laparotomy is at least 15% to 20% (2,3) and the incidence of bacteremia is at least 10%. Stab wounds of the abdomen are usually associated with a 1% to 2% incidence of abdominal infection, whereas gunshot wounds tend to have an incidence of abdominal infection rate that is 5 to 10 times higher. Colon injuries, especially those requiring a colostomy, may be associated with abdominal infection rates exceeding 20%.

AXIOM In patients surviving for at least 48 hours, sepsis is the single most frequent cause of later morbidity and mortality.

Up to 80% of late, nonneurologic deaths following trauma are a result of infection and resultant multiple organ failure (MOF). In one study of patients surviving at least 48 hours after major abdominal vascular trauma, serious infections developed in one-half, causing death or at least 14 days of hospitalization.

Definitions

Infection is defined as invasion of pathogenic microorganisms into body tissues. *Bacteremia* is the presence of bacteria in the bloodstream documented by positive blood cultures. The systemic inflammatory response syndrome is characterized by

1. Hypothermia (temperature less than 95°F) or hyperthermia (temperature greater than 101°F);
2. Tachycardia (heart rate greater than 90);
3. Tachypnea (respiratory rate greater than 20) or a low P_{aCO_2}; and
4. Clinical evidence of infection.

The "sepsis syndrome" includes all of the criteria for sepsis, along with evidence of abnormal end-organ function, such as altered cerebral function, oliguria (urine output less than 0.5 mL/kg/h), hypoxemia (PaO_2/FIO_2 ratio less than 300), or elevated lactate levels.

Septic shock has all of the criteria for the sepsis syndrome, plus hypotension (systolic blood pressure 90 mm Hg or a 40-mm Hg decrease from baseline for greater than 1 hour despite adequate volume resuscitation).

FACTORS INCREASING THE RISK OF INFECTION

Bacterial Factors

The *virulence* or ability of bacteria to invade and cause infection varies tremendously. Some of the best studied virulence factors are the various toxins or enzymes that these organisms can release.

Endotoxin (the lipopolysaccharides in the outer membrane of the cell wall of gram-negative bacteria) can cause a wide variety of systemic changes, including fever, tachycardia, hyperventilation, hypotension, intravascular coagulation, and death. The endotoxins of so-called "smooth" bacteria (bacteria that form smooth colonies when cultured in the laboratory) are macromolecules composed of three main regions:

1. Inner layer of lipid A;
2. Intermediate layer of core polysaccharides; and

3. Outer layer of "O" antigens made up of repeating oligosaccharide units.

Absence of "O" antigens makes bacterial colonies "rough" on culture media.

Bacterial capsules can also greatly increase their virulence. These gelatinous coverings of mixed polysaccharides impede phagocytosis. Some gram-negative bacilli, such as certain *Klebsiella* species, have extremely thick capsules.

The incidence and degree of infection developing in any wound correlate directly with the number of contaminating organisms. The number of bacteria necessary to cause infection is often referred to as the *critical inoculum*. Foreign bodies, blood, and dead space in a wound can reduce the critical inoculum of bacteria needed to cause infection from 10^6 to 10^2.

Certain *combinations of organisms* may have much more virulence than the sum of their individual virulences, thus, they are synergistic and greatly increase the likelihood of infection. For example, aerobic bacteria in a wound may consume the oxygen that is present, thereby improving the environment for the growth and multiplication of anaerobic bacteria. Anaerobic bacteria may help the aerobic bacteria by elaborating various toxins that reduce the ability of phagocytes to remove the aerobes.

A bacterial population may become resistant to an antimicrobial agent either by spontaneous mutation or by transfer of genetic material between bacteria. The organisms most frequently causing sepsis in hospitalized patients are not the classic high-virulence organisms, such as alpha- or beta-hemolytic streptococci, but rather organisms such as *Pseudomonas* species, which, although they are usually of relatively low virulence, have great genetic versatility and can quickly become resistant to most antibiotics.

Most bacteria that cause infection in humans can replicate by binary fission every 20 minutes. Therefore, if the proper nutrients and temperature are available, one organism can produce more than 10 billion (10^9) other organisms within 10 hours. With such large numbers of bacteria, the mutation rate, which is usually about 1 in 10 million (10^7), is more than adequate for mutant organisms to be seen regularly.

One way to "select out" the mutant is to administer antibiotics to which the mutant strain is resistant but the others are sensitive. When the mutant is the only organism capable of replicating in the presence of the antibiotics, it can replace the current microbial population with descendants of the antibiotic-resistant mutants within 24 to 48 hours.

A great deal of evidence has accumulated to show that bacteria can directly transmit antibiotic resistance to other bacteria. The genetic information controlling antibiotic resistance is frequently contained in extrachromosomal deoxyribonucleic acid (DNA) molecules called plasmids. These special DNA molecules, which are also called resistance (R) factors, are self-replicating and are passed on to or exchanged with adjacent bacteria by physical contact.

HOST DEFENSES

Epithelial Defenses

The usual first line of defense against external pathogens is provided by epithelial cells and tissue macrophages lining the body's surfaces. These epithelial surfaces can be damaged directly by trauma or by attempts at treatment, such as inserting intravenous lines. Hypoxia and hypoperfusion can also damage epithelial surfaces, including the gastrointestinal tract, thereby allowing bacteria or their toxins to enter the body.

Intravenous Catheters

Intravenous catheters left in place longer than 2 to 3 days can be an important cause of sepsis in critically ill patients. About 20% to 40% of intravenous catheters eventually become colonized with bacteria or fungi, and about 10% to 20% of the infected catheter cause bacteremia or septicemia (4). Catheters inserted via a cutdown are even more likely to become infected.

AXIOM Fever developing 2 to 3 days after surgery or trauma is often a result of infected intravenous catheters.

Intravenous catheters placed in the emergency department are often inserted with less than ideal sterile conditions and should be replaced within 12 to 24 hours. When any catheter that may be infected is being removed, a blood culture should be drawn through it and the catheter tip and the intracutaneous portion should be cultured separately.

AXIOM Any patient who becomes septic without another obvious cause should be considered to have an infected intravenous line until proven otherwise.

To reduce the risk of infection with intravenous plastic catheters, there appears to be some value in having increased distance between the puncture site or incision in the skin and the point at which the catheter enters the vein. When permanent Hickman or other types of catheters are inserted, the subcutaneous tunnel between the skin incision and vein should generally be at least 2 to 3 inches long.

Urethral Catheters

Urethral catheters and/or cystoscopy in patients with infected urine is a frequent source of serious infection, particularly by gram-negative rods, such as *Escherichia coli.* When a Foley catheter is in place for more than 5 days, bacterial counts in the urine often exceed 100,000 (10^5) per milliliter of urine. Most physicians consider this to be evidence of a urinary tract infection; however, others believe that increased numbers of polymorphonuclear leukocytes (PMNs) in the urine help to differentiate between colonization and actual infection. In some series, urinary tract infections account for up to 40% of hospital-acquired infections, and most of these infections are associated with indwelling urethral catheters.

Maintenance of a closed-drainage system with Foley catheters is extremely important for preventing urinary tract infections. A high rate of urine flow and careful cleansing of the catheter at the urethral meatus once or twice daily are also important.

AXIOM The longer that ventilatory assistance is required, the more likely it is that pneumonia will develop.

Endotracheal Tubes

Freedland et al. reported that when a ventilator was required on patients with a flail chest for more than seven days, 100% of them developed pneumonia (5). If an endotracheal tube is likely to be required for more than 7 to 10 days, an early tracheostomy should be considered. Rodriguez et al. showed that when long-term ventilatory support is required, performing a tracheostomy by the fourth or fifth day results in a shortened hospital stay (6).

Gastric pH

A low gastric pH is a physiologic barrier to microorganisms that enter the upper gastrointestinal tract. Decreased gastric acidity allows a greatly increased number of bacteria to survive and multiply there. This could theoretically cause higher pneumonia rates and increased translocation of bacteria in the distal bowel. Consequently, the routine use of H_2 blockers for the prevention of stress gastritis has been challenged, and cytoprotective agents, such as sucralfate, have been recommended to decrease lung infection rates; however, the benefits of such a program are controversial (7).

The Inflammatory Response

Inflammation is the tissue response to injury or infection. Several processes are involved, including vasodilation, increased capillary permeability, and chemotaxis (i.e., attraction of various cells, especially neutrophils and macrophages to an inflamed area). Vasodilatation results in an increased supply of blood, bringing more PMNs, macrophages, and antibodies to the involved area. The increased local capillary permeability allows the PMNs and macrophages plus large quantities of fluid and protein to leak into the involved tissues to help fight or localize the microorganisms.

AXIOM Early eradication of all underlying infection is the best way to stop the downward spiral of organ dysfunction in sepsis.

Complement Activation

Complement refers to a group of at least 11 proteins in serum that can be activated in a proteolytic cascade fashion to destroy or assist in the destruction of bacteria, abnormal cells, or particulate matter. The complement cascade can be initiated by the classic pathway via C_1 activation by antigen–antibody reactions or via the alternative pathway by activation of C_3 by endotoxin, natural antibody, or several other substances.

Complement acts to enhance standard antigen–antibody immune reactions by promoting chemotaxis, immune adherence, and phagocytosis and by liberating anaphylotoxins, especially C_{3a} and C_{5a}, which appear to be important in the development of the adult respiratory distress syndrome (ARDS). The C_{3a} and C_{5a} stimulate PMN chemotaxis and cause them to stick to pulmonary capillary endothelium. Liberation of lysosomal enzymes and superoxides from these PMNs is generally the major cause of ARDS.

Spleen

The spleen is a major site of antibody and complement production and is the major filter for removing microorganisms from the bloodstream. Thus, asplenic individuals can have greatly impaired host defenses, particularly for removing encapsulated organisms entering the body through the respiratory tract. Asplenic patients also have decreased levels of IgM, properdin, and tuftsin and have decreased activation of the complement system.

Fibronectin

Fibronectin is a high-molecular weight (440,000 to 450,000) glycoprotein that occurs in two forms (8). The soluble form functions in blood and tissue fluids as a nonspecific opsonin, and the insoluble form is located near the basement membrane of small vessels and is important in vascular integrity.

Macrophages

AXIOM In addition to providing cell-mediated immunity and activating antibody production, macrophages secrete multiple cytokines that influence the immune response.

Macrophage activation is a complex process, and cytokines produced by tissue macrophages, circulating monocytes, or T (thymus-derived) lymphocytes are generally believed to be the principal mediators of cell-mediated immunity. Upon activation by the proper cytokine, macrophages exhibit increased phagocytosis, enhanced oxidative metabolism with generation of microbicidal oxygen radicals, increased production of hydrolytic enzymes, and augmented killing of a wide variety of intracellular organisms.

Macrophages also stimulate specific lymphocytes by processing and presenting antigens to them. Activation of T lymphocytes produces the cellular immune response, and the activation of B lymphocytes causes them to produce specific antibodies against invading microorganisms.

Polymorphonuclear Leukocytes

Once an epithelial barrier has been breached, PMNs are generally the first cells that attempt to prevent the spread of invasive organisms. For PMNs to perform properly, they must be capable of carrying out a number of activities including margination on (sticking to) the vascular endothelium in the involved area, migration through the capillary wall, directed movement toward the chemical stimulus of the bacteria that are present (by a process called chemotaxis), phagocytosis (ingestion), and finally intracellular killing.

AXIOM Tissue oxygen tension is an important variable influencing the risk of infection because PMNs require oxygen to kill bacteria (9).

Specific Immune Functions

The immune system may be divided arbitrarily into nonspecific and specific response systems. Nonspecific systems include anatomic and physiologic barriers, such as the inflammatory response, which includes the complement cascade and nonspecific cellular responses by macrophages and neutrophils. The specific response system includes the humoral (antibody) response of B lymphocytes and the cell-mediated response of T lymphocytes.

AXIOM Specific immune responses are divided into two broad categories: cell-mediated (against intracellular pathogens, such as viruses) and humoral or antibody-producing (primarily against extracellular pathogens, such as bacteria).

Lymphocyte Activation

In the specific immune response (10), an antigen presenting cell, often a macrophage, presents antigen to T-helper lymphocytes (which are identified by a surface protein designated as CD-4). The T-helper cells become activated when the antigen is presented along with various costimulatory factors, including interleukin-1 (IL-1), which is produced by activated macrophages. Only T-helper cells with the specific receptor for the presented antigen are activated. The T-helper cells then activate the cell-mediated or humoral (or both) arms of the immune system. Which specific arm is turned on depends on the mixture of cytokines presented and produced. The end result is production of either (1) cytotoxic (CD-8) lymphocytes capable of killing diseased cells or (2) plasma cells, which produce soluble antibody against the antigen.

Humoral Immunity

Antibodies are specific proteins that are made to destroy or inactivate a specific antigen or enhance its phagocytosis. Almost all antibodies are formed in plasma cells, which are found primarily in lymph nodes, spleen, and bone marrow. Severe trauma can cause significant reductions in the quantity and quality of antibodies produced, particularly in the presence of shock or multiple blood transfusions (11).

Cytokines and Other Chemical Responses

AXIOM The main substances involved in the host response to trauma and infection include tumor necrosis factor (TNF), various ILs (especially IL-1), platelet-activating factor (PAF), and various arachidonic acid metabolites.

TNF, also known as cachectin, is produced by macrophages and multiple other cells. Infusion of endotoxin initially stimulates the release of TNF, which can cause virtually every symptom and sign of infection. TNF is a pyrogen, as well as a stimulant for release of IL-1, IL-6, and IL-8, platelet-activating factor, leukotrienes, thromboxane A_2, and prostaglandins. It induces expression of adhesion molecules, which promote margination (the attachment of neutrophils to endothelial cells). It also activates complement and the coagulation cascade.

Interleukin-1 (IL-1, endogenous pyrogen), causes proteolysis and is capable of enhancing T-cell responsiveness to almost any activating stimulus. Together with *IL-2*, a lymphokine produced by T-helper cells, IL-1 participates in the activation of T lymphocytes. IL-2 also activates neutrophils and T and B lymphocytes.

Interleukin-6 stimulates acute-phase protein production by the liver, and its level in the bloodstream tend to correlate with the severity of infection.

Interleukin-8 has strong chemotactic factors and appears to be important in the development of ARDS.

Interleukin-10 (IL-10) markedly inhibits the production of TNF, IL-1, and IL-8, and potentiates the release of the inflammatory mediator IL-Ira. Neidhardt et al. (12) noted that injured patients (n=417) showed elevated IL-10 levels throughout an observation period of 21 days compared with healthy volunteers (n=137). Patients with severe injury (injury severity score >25) (especially those who had MOF or died), demonstrated significantly increased IL-10 levels compared with other patients. Parsons (13), however, noted in animals that IL-10 infusion decreased mortality rate, but it did not predict the development of ARDS in patients at risk for this problem.

PAF is an important phospholipid mediator of the sepsis cascade (14). It is released from many cells (including endothelial cells, neutrophils, pneumocytes, and platelets) when they are stimulated by a number of compounds including TNF, leukotrienes, and histamine. PAF has been shown to produce hypotension and increase vascular permeability, particularly in the lung, and has been implicated as a causative agent of ARDS. It also decreases cardiac output and causes coronary vasoconstriction.

Arachidonic acid metabolites include thromboxane A_2, leukotrienes, and prostaglandins (14). Thromboxane A_2 is a potent vasoconstrictor and bronchoconstrictor. It also increases vascular permeability and increases platelet aggregation. Various leukotrienes can also cause vasoconstriction, bronchoconstriction, or increased vascular permeability.

Prostaglandin E_2 (PGE_2) causes vasodilatation and may have a protective effect on the microvasculature. It has a direct pyrogenic effect on the hypothalamus, and depending on the dose, it may either stimulate or inhibit TNF release. Prostaglandin E_2 also tends be immunosuppressive.

Opsonins

AXIOM Opsonins refer to substances that attach themselves to the surface of antigens (usually microorganisms or particulate matter) and thereby enhance the ability of phagocytes to recognize and engulf the antigens.

The three main types of opsonins are antibodies, complement, and fibronectin. Immunoglobulin G (IgG) and immunoglobulin M (IgM) antibodies to specific microorganisms are the most common immunoglobulins that can function as opsonins. IgM is about five times as large as IgG and tends to respond earlier but has a more transient effect than IgG. Complement and fibronectin are relatively nonspecific opsonins that can react immediately to invading microorganisms or foreign substances.

Other Factors That Can Impair Host Defenses

Other factors that may impinge on the host's ability to defend himself or herself against microorganisms include various drugs that may be administered, extremes of age, and severe metabolic problems.

Drugs

Immunosuppressive drugs (to prevent transplant rejection) and cytotoxic drugs (for treating malignancies) can profoundly depress bone marrow and the reticuloendothelial system (RES). Cytotoxic drugs also tend to injure rapidly growing cells, such as intestinal mucosa, thereby creating additional portals of entry for various microorganisms.

Glucocorticoids depress the inflammatory response and can induce lysis of mononuclear cells. Corticosteroids also redistribute T cells from the circulation, thereby impairing their access to inflammatory sites.

Almost all antibiotics in therapeutic doses cause changes in gastrointestinal, oropharyngeal, and skin flora, replacing susceptible microorganisms with others that are more antibiotic resistant.

Extremes of Age

Host resistance is most likely to be impaired in individuals who are younger than the age of 3 months or older than 70 years (15). In addition to impaired host defenses, aged patients are more likely to have cardiovascular, pulmonary, and other organ dysfunction. Infections in older patients are also particularly likely to be caused by gram-negative bacilli.

Metabolic Problems

Patients with uncontrolled *diabetes mellitus* can have an incidence of infections up to several times higher than nondiabetic patients (16). Although increased blood glucose levels play only a minor role, ketoacidosis can cause defective inflammatory responses with sluggish PMN migration, ineffective phagocytosis, and decreased killing and fibroblast proliferation.

Uremia can have a number of effects on host defense including the following:

- Impaired early phases of the acute inflammatory response
- Reduced immune responses to antigenic stimuli
- Impaired delayed cellular hypersensitivity
- Altered production of all types of immunoglobulins
- Defective cell division

Patients with severe cirrhosis have a greatly reduced resistance to infection, and fatal septic shock can develop from relatively mild infections. In addition to the impaired liver metabolism and the reduced hepatic RES function, there is shunting of portal venous blood—which may contain enteric bacilli or endotoxin—around the hepatic RES directly into the systemic circulation.

Severe, acute protein or calorie malnutrition can markedly reduce the number and functional capability of T lymphocytes (17). Severe nutritional deficiencies also interfere with lymphokine production by T lymphocytes and may increase the number of suppressor cells. Prolonged fasting or total parenteral nutrition also reduces intestinal mucosal thickness and increases the tendency to bacterial translocation.

Ethanol

Gentilello et al. (18) reported that intoxicating levels of alcohol are associated with a higher risk of trauma-related infections after penetrating injury. Tamura and colleagues (19) recently found that acute ETOH intoxication inhibits several arms of immune defense, causing attenuation of T-cell function and decreased bacterial clearance from both the lungs and the RES because of impaired macrophage bactericidal activity.

DIAGNOSIS OF INFECTION

Diagnosis involves not only determining that an infection is present, but also finding its source and determining the organisms involved.

AXIOM Infections in patients with severe trauma may develop without pain, fever, or leukocytosis.

History

The most frequent symptoms of infection after trauma include chills and fever, pain, cough, dysuria, and night sweats. Pain and tenderness may help to localize the probable site of infection. Although fever is one of the classic signs or symptoms of infection, fever may be present without an infection, especially during the first 3 to 4 days after major trauma, and significant sepsis can occur without fever. Some of the worst infections, especially those caused by gram-negative organisms, may cause hypothermia.

With fever in the first 24 to 28 hours, one should look for atelectasis and intravenous catheter infections; however, β-hemolytic streptococci and *Clostridium perfringens* infections can also cause severe sepsis within 24 to 48 hours.

A new or increased cough in a septic patient generally indicates a tracheobronchial or pulmonary infection of some type, particularly when copious or purulent sputum is produced. It may also indicate that aspiration has occurred. Copious amounts of foul sputum are typically associated with anaerobic organisms in lung abscesses or bronchiectasis. Sharp chest pain with cough or deep breaths generally indicates pleuritic involvement.

Acute cystitis is characterized by frequency of urination, dysuria, and urgency. Such symptoms are common in injured patients who have had a urinary catheter for more than 3 or 4 days, even if the urine is sterile.

Physical Examination

The classic signs of inflammation are pain, redness, heat, and swelling. If the involved area is also indurated and has fluctuation in its center, this is strongly indicative of an abscess. Swelling of the lower leg, especially at the calf, may indicate thrombophlebitis or phlebothrombosis. Rales in the lungs may be associated with pneumonia, atelectasis, or congestion. Flank tenderness may indicate infection in the kidney or subphrenic space. A pelvic abscess is often first noted as lower abdominal tenderness and severe cervical motion tenderness on vaginal examination.

AXIOM If daily rectal examinations are not performed on patients in whom a pelvic abscess may develop, severe systemic toxicity may develop before the diagnosis is made.

Septic Patterns after Trauma

Failure to Thrive

In older patients, recovery from trauma or surgery may be extremely slow, often because of preexisting organ dysfunction. Failure to recuperate properly in any patient, (i.e., "failure to thrive") may be the result of unsuspected sepsis. Host defenses in older patients with severe trauma are often so impaired that, even with severe sepsis, few objective signs of infection may be evident, except for increasing confusion.

The patient with failure to thrive as a result of sepsis tends to be lethargic. Although blood gases may be relatively good, the patient is often too weak to be extubated. The blood urea nitrogen and serum creatinine also tend to be normal, but the measured creatinine clearance is often less than 40 mL/min. The abdomen tends to be somewhat distended, and the patient may not pass gas per rectum for many days. Hepatic enzymes are often at least two to three times normal.

Typical Sepsis

Although fever is seen in most typical cases of sepsis without shock or organ failure, up to 13% of septic patients have temperatures less than 36.4°C (less than 96.6°F) and another 5% to 20% are afebrile (20). Hyperventilation is often an early clinical finding, and a sudden onset of tachypnea should make one suspect sepsis or a pulmonary embolus.

AXIOM Septic patients tend to be restless, anxious, and confused.

Frequently, increasing confusion or restlessness is the first sign that a patient is becoming septic; however, some patients with gram-negative sepsis are remarkably awake and alert until just before death. Tachycardia is also common, and tachyarrhythmias may be the first clinical sign of sepsis.

In septic patients, ileus tends to develop early, even without an abdominal focus of infection. If abdominal or renal sepsis is present, the ileus can rapidly become much more severe.

The skin in early sepsis is typically warm and dry with a flushed or pink color. Occasionally, acrocyanosis may develop as a result of intravascular clotting. A characteristic skin lesion, ecthyma gangrenosum, occurs in up to 25% of patients with *Pseudomonas* bacteremia, but it may occasionally be caused by *E. coli.*

Multiple Organ Failure

AXIOM Once MOF syndrome has developed, the process becomes self-perpetuating, and the patient's prognosis is poor, even if initiating factors, such as abscesses, are finally controlled.

Increasing MOF is usually caused by persistent, inadequately treated sepsis. Although up to 50% of patients with MOF have repeated negative blood cultures, evidence of advanced sepsis can be found eventually in up to 90% of these patients (21).

Polk and Shields noted that organ failure, especially if it involves the lungs and kidneys in postoperative trauma victims, often indicates the presence of occult intraabdominal infection (22). Fry et al., in a study of 38 patients with MOF and a mortality rate of 74%, found that MOF was primarily due to infection, and MOF was the most common fatal evidence of uncontrolled infection (23).

Hyperdynamic (Warm) Septic Shock

AXIOM Characteristically, patients in early septic shock are vasodilated, have a normal or increased cardiac output, and have warm, dry, pink, or flushed skin (24).

It may be difficult at times to determine precisely when severe sepsis with a slightly low blood pressure becomes hyperdynamic septic shock; however, shock is generally considered to be present if

1. Systolic blood pressure decreases to less than 90 mm Hg or decreases by more than 25%;
2. Urine output decreases to less than 0.4 mL/kg/h;
3. Metabolic (lactic) acidosis develops; and
4. VO_2 is less than 100 mL/min/m^2.

Even with a normal oxygen delivery (DO_2), oxygen extraction in sepsis may be less than 15%. A low or decreasing VO_2 often indicates that shock is developing before there is a significant decrease in blood pressure. Furthermore, failure of the VO_2 to increase to normal or higher levels with treatment is a grave prognostic sign.

Even if hypotension becomes severe, the cardiac index in early sepsis tends to be normal or high, particularly if the blood volume is adequately maintained or increased; however, there is also evidence of some myocardial failure as evidenced by a reduced ejection fraction.

Hypodynamic (Cold) Septic Shock

A low cardiac output is characteristic of late septic shock. Oxygen delivery is generally reduced, and oxygen consumption is often less than half of normal. With increasing vasoconstriction, the skin becomes cold, clammy, mottled, or cyanotic, and severe oliguria tends to develop.

The main causes of the low cardiac output of late septic shock are cardiac failure and hypovolemia. In a study of 48 septic shock patients, Parker et al. reported that right and left ventricular ejection fractions were decreased (25). These changes are believed to be a result of a myocardial depressant factor (14). Similar results have been obtained when TNF, IL-2, or endotoxin is given to human volunteers (26).

As sepsis progresses, capillaries and small veins throughout the body develop increasing permeability, causing increasing amounts of fluid to leave the vascular space and become sequestered in the interstitial spaces. In a period of 12 to 24 hours, more than 10 L of extra fluid may be required to replace this loss.

Water, sodium, and calcium also tend to move into cells that have impaired metabolism. Consequently, even though the total body water may be much greater than normal and the patient appears to be overhydrated, an increasing tendency exists for the development of absolute or relative hypovolemia.

Laboratory Studies

White Blood Cell Count

In most septic patients, the white blood cell (WBC) count is elevated to 15,000/mm^3 or more, usually with a "shift to the left" (i.e., greater than 80% PMNs or more than 5% immature [band] forms). In some patients, the total WBC count may be normal, and the only evidence of sepsis may be a shift to the left. In severe, advanced sepsis, particularly that caused by gram-negative bacilli, the WBC count may be low (less than 4,000/mm^3), and this is often an ominous prognostic sign.

Blood Chemistries

Blood glucose levels tend to be elevated in sepsis, and the response to insulin is impaired.

In septic patients, plasma-ionized calcium levels can rapidly decrease to values much less than the normal of 2.1 to 2.4 mEq/L (1.05 to 1.20 mmol/L). Because the extracellular fluid–ionized calcium is about 10^{-3} molar and the intracellular fluid–ionized calcium levels may be as low as 10^{-7}, the gradient across many cell membranes is about 10,000 to 1 (27). When cell metabolism becomes impaired, increased amounts of ionized calcium move into the cytoplasm, and the plasma-ionized calcium can rapidly decrease to levels of less than 0.9 mmol/L. If ionized calcium levels decrease to less than 0.7 mmol/L, cardiovascular performance is often impaired, and the prognosis is usually poor.

Coagulation Studies

In sepsis, increasing activation of platelets and the coagulation cascade results in a progressive reduction in the platelet count and the concentrations of most clotting factors. Neame et al., using sensitive tests for detecting thrombin and plasmin activation, found evidence of disseminated intravascular coagulation (DIC) in almost all patients with bacteremia who had platelet counts of less than 50,000/mm^3 (28). Wilson et al. were able to predict early sepsis by very low or decreasing plasma antithrombin III levels in patients at risk for developing infection (29).

Blood Gases

Blood gas analyses in patients in early septic shock generally reveal a $Pa{CO_2}$ less than 30 to 35 mm Hg, normal bicarbonate levels (21 to 26 mEq/L), and pH greater than 7.45. Early hyperventilation so frequently accompanies sepsis that, if a patient with other evidence of infection is not hyperventilating, one should suspect that the patient has metabolic alkalosis or respiratory failure is developing. As shock becomes more severe, anaerobic metabolism increases, eventually producing an increasing lactic acidosis.

Bacteriologic Studies

Smears

⊘ PITFALL

If smears and cultures are not obtained before antibiotic therapy is begun, proper bacteriologic diagnostic and sensitivity studies are often delayed or impossible.

Whenever possible, pus or exudate from any infected or contaminated areas should be smeared and Gram stained and cultured before beginning antibiotic therapy. Frequently, various factors or technical errors may cause no organisms or the wrong organisms to grow on culture. Under such circumstances, the information obtained from examination of the initial smear may be especially valuable.

Quantification of the number of PMNs and bacteria on sputum smears may help to differentiate between positive sputum cultures resulting from colonization, tracheobronchitis, or pneumonitis. With colonization, few, if any, PMNs are present and only a small number of organisms (10^1 to 10^2/mL) are present. Tracheobronchitis is characterized by sputum with more bacteria (10^3 to 10^4/mL) and moderate numbers of PMNs. In pneumonitis, many bacteria (greater than 10^5/mL) and many PMNs are usually seen. Bronchial secretions obtained during bronchoscopy by bronchoalveolar lavage or protected brush specimens are generally more reliable than induced sputum or tracheal aspirates.

Obtaining a good urine specimen can be a problem in some patients with suspected urinary tract infection. Some clinicians believe that, if the patient is catheterized, the specimen should be obtained by aspirating the Foley catheter tubing with a needle rather than by disconnecting the tube and breaking the closed drainage system. If the patient is not catheterized, a clean, midstream catch in a man is usually a fairly accurate specimen.

AXIOM Even when urine contains more than 10^5/mL microorganisms, pyuria should also be present to warrant diagnosis and treatment of a urinary tract infection.

Culture and Sensitivity Studies

As with smears, the accuracy of culture studies depends primarily on how representative the material submitted is of the involved fluid or organ. It also depends on how rapidly and carefully the specimen is handled. Pus taken from a variety of abscesses show "no growth" in about 50% of cases if more than 2 hours pass before the specimen is taken to the laboratory. If the specimen is taken directly to the laboratory and is plated almost immediately, bacteria grow in almost 100% of cases.

AXIOM The ideal specimen for detecting the microorganisms responsible for an abscess is a tissue biopsy from the wall of the abscess.

Whenever possible, both aerobic and anaerobic cultures should be made of all infected or contaminated material recovered from tissue abscesses. Anaerobic cultures must be taken with the same precautions as arterial blood gases and then placed immediately into tubes containing carbon dioxide and no oxygen. The material should then be placed into appropriate media and incubated as soon as possible.

AXIOM False-negative anaerobic cultures are common, and this should be considered when choosing antibiotic therapy based on laboratory studies.

If rapid information on aerobic bacteria is desired, a direct smear of infected material onto blood agar plates may yield characteristic colonies within a few hours. If this is done with antibiotic discs already on the agar plate, helpful information on sensitivities may also be available within 24 hours.

Blood Cultures

In patients with bacteremias, at least two to three blood cultures should be obtained from uncatheterized veins at intervals of at least 20 to 30 minutes because one or more of these blood cultures are often negative, and a single positive blood culture may be due to a contaminant. Ideally, blood cultures should be drawn just before a patient spikes a fever.

If the patient is on antibiotics, inoculation of at least one hypertonic blood culture bottle or one resin-containing bottle should be done to remove the antibiotics.

Getting positive blood cultures can be a special problem in patients with gram-negative bacteremia because these are often relatively low-grade infections, and the bacteremia may be transient.

AXIOM The "rule of threes" for blood cultures states that three blood cultures per day for 3 days will generally detect gram-negative bacteremia in untreated cases.

If an intravenous catheter infection is suspected, blood cultures should be drawn through that catheter and directly from another vein. The tip and intracutaneous portion of the catheter should also be cultured. Intravenous catheter tips must be cultured carefully because of the high incidence of contamination as the catheter is removed.

Burn Wound Infections

Quantitative cultures of potentially infected tissue can be extremely useful. Colony counts greater than 10^5/g of burned tissue generally indicate invasive infection. Furthermore, open wounds containing more than this concentration of organisms usually cannot be skin grafted successfully.

Problems with Culture Results

The most rapidly growing organisms, rather than the ones responsible for the infection, may grow out on culture. When the culture result correlates with what is found on the Gram stain, the results are usually reliable. If the results do not correlate, one must use clinical judgment or obtain further cultures and smears.

If the patient has been receiving antibiotics but continues to have evidence of sepsis and the cultures keep showing "no growth" or "normal flora," a special effort should be made to culture anaerobic organisms and fungi, especially candida.

Temporarily Discontinuing Antibiotics

In some instances, antibiotics do not control the infection, but they can make it extremely difficult to locate and prevent the responsible organisms from growing in culture. If the infection is not controlled after one or more changes of antibiotics or if the location of the infection causing the sepsis cannot be determined, it may be advisable to stop all antibiotics for 24 to 48 hours. After that time, cultures are more likely to be positive, and the abscess or site of infection can be identified. The decision to stop antibiotics in critically ill or injured patients must be individualized because the patient's infection may get considerably worse while the antibiotics are discontinued.

In some instances, a relatively high, spiking fever disappears after antibiotics have been discontinued. When the fever does not reappear in 48 to 72 hours, it can generally be assumed that the patient had antibiotic (drug) fever.

Radiologic Procedures

Plain Films

Plain radiographs can be very helpful for diagnosing infections in the chest and are occasionally of some help in the abdomen. Air in the wall of intestines or gallbladder often indicates necrosis. Free intraabdominal air in a patient who has not had abdominal surgery generally indicates a bowel perforation. Air-fluid levels outside the bowel, such as between the liver and diaphragm, are highly suggestive of a subphrenic abscess. Displacement of bowel loops or other abdominal organs may also be evidence of an abscess.

Ultrasonography

Ultrasonographic examination of the abdomen can be performed quickly, is relatively inexpensive, and can be done in the emergency department, operating room, or intensive care unit (ICU). Even under ideal circumstances, however, ultrasound is not very accurate for abdominal abscesses. Nevertheless, ultrasonography is occasionally helpful in screening for acute acalculous cholecystitis by demonstrating progressive gallbladder dilatation, increasing wall edema, and pericystic fluid.

Computed Tomography

Computed tomography (CT) scans are generally considered the most accurate, noninvasive technique for diagnosing abscesses or other fluid collections in the abdomen or chest. In some reports, it has had 98% sensitivity and 95% specificity (30); however, CT is expensive, and the patient may be too unstable to move to the CT scan suite.

AXIOM CT scans are the ideal tests for detecting intraabdominal abscesses, but they are relatively unreliable during the first 5 to 6 days after trauma.

INFECTIONS CAUSED BY VARIOUS MICROORGANISMS

Staphylococci

The typical lesion produced by (coagulase-positive) *Staphylococcus aureus* is usually well localized and consists of an indurated area that undergoes central necrosis and abscess formation with the development of a thick, creamy, odorless pus. Fever and leukocytosis are usually present. Bacteremia or septicemia can be dangerous because of the high frequency with which metastatic abscesses can develop, especially with bloodstream infections.

Coagulase-negative staphylococci are being recognized increasingly in intravenous catheter infections and following operations on the cardiovascular system. Because of the concern that a positive blood culture with *S. epidermidis* may be a contaminant, at least two separate positive cultures of this organism are usually required for diagnosis.

Streptococci

The lesions caused by *Streptococcus pyogenes* are characterized by a rapid progression of cellulitis, lymphangitis, lymphadenitis, and extension of the inflammation along fascial planes. The pus tends to thin and watery. Bacteremia occurs frequently and may result in septic shock within 24 hours of infection. It is characterized by chills, high fever, a rapid thready pulse, and general signs of toxemia.

Streptococcal gangrene, usually caused by group A beta-hemolytic streptococci (GAS), is a rapidly spreading, invasive, fascial, and subcutaneous infection that may be associated with thrombosis of nutrient vessels, resulting in necrosis and slough of the overlying skin.

Enterococcus

Infections containing *Enterococcus* organisms typically develop relatively late (7 or more days after trauma) and usually only in combination with gram-negative aerobes or anaerobes in debilitated individuals who had been receiving broad-spectrum antibiotics. An *Enterococcus* is usually not considered to be the cause of infection unless it is the only organism found.

Gram-Negative Bacilli

Gram-negative bacilli are involved in most infections associated with injury to the gastrointestinal or genitourinary tracts. These infections are usually polymicrobial and typically involve both anaerobic and aerobic organisms. Wound infections caused by gram-negative aerobes generally have a longer incubation period than those caused by staphylococci or streptococci, and often cause less systemic toxicity, at least initially.

After several days or weeks of treatment with broad-spectrum antibiotics, the likelihood of antibiotic-resistant gram-negative aerobes, especially *Pseudomonas*, being cultured from many parts of the body increases greatly, particularly in the tracheobronchial tree.

Anaerobes

Anaerobic organisms are recognized increasingly as a cause of infections following trauma or surgery. The three clinically important groups of anaerobic bacteria include the following:

1. Gram-negative nonsporulating rods, such as *Bacteroides* and *Fusobacteria*;
2. Large gram-positive sporulating rods, such as clostridial organisms; and
3. Gram-positive cocci, such as the peptostreptococci (31).

Bacteroides

Various *Bacteroides* species are, by far, the most frequent organisms in the colon. Because these organisms may cause only minimal local inflammatory changes, at least initially, infections by these organisms may be difficult to identify or localize. Although *Bacteroides fragilis* subspecies *fragilis* organisms are the only *Bacteroides* organisms with a capsule and although they make up only 7% of the *Bacteroides* organisms found in normal colons, its capsule increases its virulence so much that they are cultured in more than 40% of infections in which *Bacteroides* species are found.

Peptostreptococci

Peptostreptococcus is the most important anaerobic gram-positive coccus. It is often associated with anaerobic myositis, joint infection, breast abscess, septic abortion, liver abscesses, and empyema.

Clostridia

The clostridial infections most likely to occur in injured patients include clostridial cellulitis, clostridial myositis, and tetanus.

AXIOM Most gangrenous infections with gas in the tissues are not gas gangrene, but should be treated as such until proven otherwise.

Gangrene, even when associated with gas in the tissue, is often due to nonclostridial organisms, and even if clostridial organisms are present, they are not all of the same seriousness. For example, although clostridial cellulitis may be extremely painful and have an ominous appearance, it is seldom fatal unless the patient is debilitated and the treatment is inadequate.

Clostridial Cellulitis

Clostridial cellulitis can be caused by several *Clostridium* species, but *Clostridium welchii* is the most frequent (32). This infection of the skin, subcutaneous tissue, and connective tissue is a crepitant cellulitis, which spreads rapidly along fascial planes and typically produces a gray or reddish-brown discharge, plus necrosis and sloughing of the involved superficial fascia, subcutaneous tissue, and skin.

Gas Gangrene

Gas gangrene, which is also known as clostridial myositis, is usually caused by *Clostridium welchii*; however, *Clostridium novyi*, *Clostridium septicum*, and *Clostridium sordellii* may also cause this problem (32). This dreaded complication should be anticipated in any wound in which there is extensive destruction of muscle or deep contamination with soil or feces.

Gas gangrene is characterized by rapidly spreading gangrene of muscle and a profound toxemia. Swelling and pain occur early, often within the first 24 hours after injury. Gas formation with crepitation within the muscle and along fascial planes is usually found, but may be absent in some patients.

The prostration of the patient with gas gangrene is often far out of proportion to the fever. Early diagnosis is facilitated by examination of the wound discharge, which may contain many large gram-positive rods, usually without spores, and relatively few or no PMNs.

Tetanus

Tetanus, caused by *Clostridium tetani*, is an extremely serious anaerobic infection, which is uncommon in the United States because most citizens have had at least partial immunization. Although this infection is most likely to occur with deep and dirty wounds, it is occasionally seen in patients with relatively small, innocuous-appearing lacerations (33). After an incubation period of about 4 to 12 days, the patient typically begins to experience restlessness, headache, stiffness of the jaw muscles, and intermittent tetanic muscle contractions near the wound. Tachycardia, excessive sweating, and salivation are also often present. Generalized tonic contractions may follow within 12 to 24 hours, producing a classic facial distortion (risus sardonicus), opisthotonos, and rigidity. Severe clonic muscle contractions may result from even the slightest stimulation.

Mixed Aerobic and Anaerobic Infections

Intraabdominal infections occurring after injury to the distal small bowel or colon typically involve at least two to three aerobes and two to three anaerobes. Soft-tissue infections caused by mixed gram-positive and gram-negative organisms are characterized by necrosis of subcutaneous and fascial tissues with progressive gangrene from thrombosis of local nutrient vessels. A wide variety of etiologic agents have been associated with this condition, including *Bacteroides*, anaerobic streptococci, and various coliforms (Table 39-1).

Fungal Infections

Within the past few years, the incidence of fungal infections, particularly by *Candida* species, has increased sharply, especially in patients receiving intravenous hyperalimentation and those with diminished host resistance from severe debilitation or prolonged therapy with steroids or antirejection or antineoplastic agents. *Candida* superinfection is always a threat in severely injured patients who have been receiving broad-spectrum antibiotics for 1 week or longer.

⊘ PITFALL

One should suspect a fungal infection when bacterial cultures are repeatedly negative in a septic patient who has been on broad-spectrum antibiotics.

Systemic *Candida* infections can closely resemble those caused by gram-negative organisms. Fungal infections should be suspected when cultures from patients with clinical infections have repeatedly negative cultures for aerobic and anaerobic bacte-

Table 39-1. *Differential Diagnosis of Crepitant Soft-Tissue Wounds*

Parameter	Clostridial Cellulitis	Nonclostridial Anaerobic Cellulitis	Gas Gangrene	Streptococcal Myositis	Necrotizing Fasciitis	Infected Vascular Gangrene
Predisposing conditions	Local trauma or surgery	Diabetes mellitus; preexisting localized infection	Local trauma or surgery; colon cancer	Local trauma	Diabetes mellitus, abdominal surgery, perineal infection, drug addiction	Peripheral arterial insufficiency
Skin appearance	Minimal discoloration	Minimal discoloration	Yellow-bronze; dark bullae; green-black necrosis[a]	Erthema	Erythematous cellulitis	Discolored or black
Exudate	Thin, dark	Dark pus	Serosanguineous	Abundant seropurulent	Seropurulent	0
Gas	++++	++++	++	±	++ to ++++	0 to +++
Odor	Sometimes foul	Foul	Variable; slightly foul or peculiarly sweet	Slight; sour	Foul	0 to foul
Systemic toxicity	Minimal	Moderate	Marked	Only late in course	Moderate or marked	Minimal
Muscle involvement	0	0	++++	+++	0	Variable

[a]Early changes are minimal; these are late findings.
0, none; ±, mild; ++, moderate; +++, severe; ++++, very severe.
Revised from: ref. 34.

ria. Even when they cannot be cultured from the blood, the presence of *Candida* organisms should be suspected when they are found in large quantities in the mouth, urine, or feces.

Infection with Human Immunodeficiency Virus

Sloan et al. (35) found that young urban trauma patients were 15.3 to 17.6 times more likely to be positive for human immunodeficiency virus (HIV) than the trauma population overall. Other demographic factors associated with an increased risk of HIV infection in urban trauma patients included penetrating trauma, non-white race, male gender, positive drug or positive alcohol screens, and city residence (36). For example, 10% of the trauma patients seen at Johns Hopkins Hospital in Baltimore have tested positive for HIV. The percentage increases to 19% for male victims of penetrating trauma between the ages of 25 and 34 years.

Ankney et al. (37) in a review of aggregate data for HIV infection in rural trauma patients in the United States found that only 28 (0.6%) of 4,639 patients tested were HIV positive. Thus, the cost-effectiveness of HIV testing for rural trauma patients is questionable.

PREVENTING INFECTION

Rapid Control of Bleeding and Hypotension

Bleeding should be controlled as soon as possible. If 15 units or more of blood are needed for transfusion, the incidence of serious infections after major trauma can exceed 85% (38). Hypotension should not be allowed to persist for more than 15 to 30 minutes. Maintaining normal or increased blood flow to injured areas is particularly important.

Optimizing Oxygen Delivery (DO_2)

AXIOM Increasing the oxygen delivery index (DO_2I) to 600 mL/min/m^2 or more and the oxygen consumption index (VO_2I) to 150 to 170 mL/min/m^2 within 12 hours of injury may reduce the incidence of infection and MOF.

Shoemaker et al. showed that a DO_2I greater than 600 mL/min/m^2 and a VO_2I greater than 170 mL/min/m^2 in a variety of high-risk surgical patients reduced organ failure rates and mortality rates (39). Moore et al. showed that patients in whom a VO_2I of greater than 150 mL/min/m^2 was achieved within 12 hours of trauma had a decreased incidence of later MOF (4 of 24 [17%] versus 12 of 15 [80%]) (40).

Hayes et al. (41) have found survivors of sepsis syndrome or septic shock are characterized by an ability to increase both DO_2 and VO_2. In contrast, nonsurvivors typically failed to increase VO_2 following resuscitation, and when delivery was enhanced with aggressive inotropic support, oxygen extraction declined.

Wound Care

Wounds with increased amounts of blood or serum are at greater risk for infection than dry wounds, and a subcutaneous hematoma with its iron and protein can greatly increase the incidence and severity of infection. Nevertheless, the placement of additional sutures, (which also act as foreign bodies) in wounds in an attempt to eliminate dead space, may have the paradoxical effect of increasing infection (42). Leaving drains, especially of the open (Penrose) type, also increases the risk of infection.

AXIOM In heavily contaminated wounds or when all foreign material or devitalized tissue cannot be satisfactorily removed, the wound should be left open.

Prophylactic Antibiotics

Antibiotics given at the time the trauma victim is first seen are usually not "prophylactic" because some degree of local contamination is present if any mucosal or skin barrier has been damaged. Antibiotics are most likely to be effective when given within 2 hours of injury.

Antibiotics are generally recommended for the following:

1. All contaminated or dirty wounds;
2. All surgical procedures or wounds involving bowel, lungs, or urinary tract;
3. Clean wounds in which infection would be particularly dangerous, including neurosurgical and cardiovascular procedures, especially if prosthetic materials are implanted; and
4. Immunosuppressed patients.

Abdominal Trauma

AXIOM Antibiotics effective against anaerobic gastrointestinal bacteria and gram-negative aerobes should be administered as soon as possible to patients with abdominal trauma that may involve the gastrointestinal tract.

Proper use of prophylactic antibiotics can reduce infection rates in patients with trauma to the distal small bowel or colon. If the patient is bleeding massively, the antibiotics should be given again after the bleeding is controlled.

Lung Infection

Most prospective double-blind studies indicate that antibiotics are beneficial in patients who require chest tubes for trauma (43). Overall, the incidence of lung infection or empyema is reduced by antibiotics from 16.2% (47 of 290) to 2.3% (7 of 301) ($p<.001$). The only questions still being debated are (1) what are the best antibiotics to be used and (2) what is the duration required? For most types of trauma, giving a dose just before inserting the chest tube may be all that is needed (44).

Basilar Skull Fractures

Prophylactic antibiotics for uncomplicated traumatic cerebrospinal fluid leaks do not reduce the incidence of infection, but they do increase the likelihood of infection by an antibiotic-resistant organism.

Timing of Antibiotics

Several investigations have shown that maximum protection from infection in wounds is achieved when antibiotics are administered within 2 hours of bacterial tissue contamination. The optimal duration of prophylactic antibiotics is still unclear. In virtually all studies, the shorter durations of therapy have consistently been as effective as those given for several more days (45).

Choice of Antibiotics

The main organisms likely to cause wound infections are staphylococci and streptococci. The staphylococci are generally sensitive to penicillase-resistant penicillins (such as nafcillin and oxacillin) or first-generation cephalosporins, such as cefazolin (Ancef). β-Hemolytic streptococci are usually sensitive to penicillin.

With trauma to the face causing fractures of the skull, jaws, and other facial bones, antibiotics such as a penicillinase-resistant penicillin are usually effective. Major surgical procedures involving oral or pharyngeal mucosa should probably have a more broad-spectrum coverage to include the oral anaerobes.

The most common pathogens causing pulmonary infections after thoracic trauma include *S. aureus*, coagulase-negative staphylococci, *Streptococcus pneumoniae*, group A streptococci, and *Enterobacteriaceae*. Late infections are typically caused by *Pseudomonas* species or other gram-negative bacilli. Cefazolin is adequate for the gram-positive organisms likely to be involved. For more severe injuries that also involve the digestive tract or for injuries that involve the lungs of patients with chronic bronchitis, broader coverage is indicated. *Pseudomonas* and *Enterobacter* pneumonias developed in the hospital should be treated with piperacillin plus an aminoglycoside.

Antibiotic trials for abdominal trauma show that a variety of expanded-spectrum single agents (when compared with aminoglycoside-based combinations, such as gentamicin plus clindamycin) show similar efficacy. In addition, short-duration prophylaxis (12 hours) appears to be as effective as prolonged coverage (45).

The use of antibiotic irrigation at laparotomy for gastrointestinal perforation is controversial (46). Some authors have reported clinical benefits with antibiotic irrigation, but most authors believe that it provides no benefit over that obtained with systemic antibiotics plus irrigation with plain saline.

Single agents, such as cefazolin, with activity against *S. aureus* have been used with success to help prevent infections in open fractures. The addition of an aminoglycoside has been recommended in larger, more complex wounds that may also be contaminated with gram-negative aerobes (47).

Penicillin G is often recommended for human and animal bites because it covers most of the aerobic and anaerobic organisms contaminating such injuries; however, it is ineffective against *S. aureus*, which should also be covered. Consequently, with bites in which the risk of infection is high, a combination of a penicillin and a β-lactamase inhibitor (e.g., ticarcillin-clavulanate, ampicillin-sulbactam), may be more effective. For individuals taking oral antibiotics at home, amoxicillin-clavulanate is usually adequate.

TREATMENT OF INFECTIONS

AXIOM Early, adequate drainage and debridement is the most important treatment of localized infections.

Draining Abdominal Abscesses

Drainage of abdominal abscesses should be as complete as possible without spreading the infected material into uninvolved areas. Postoperative catheter drainage should be dependent, when possible. When drainage of the abdomen can only be accomplished anteriorly, soft sump tubes should be used.

With any gastrointestinal leak, the involved bowel should be excised or exteriorized, as soon as possible. Nasogastric suction alone is usually not adequate to prevent continued leakage from injured bowel.

AXIOM An abscess cavity, which continues to drain large quantities of pus or fluid for several days after surgical drainage, is usually inadequately drained or is associated with a fistula.

Increasing reports have described percutaneous catheter drainage of abdominal abscesses using ultrasonography or CT radiologic guidance. Although this technique can be safe and effective, some clinicians believe that percutaneous drainage should probably not be done if (48)

1. Three or more abscesses are present;
2. Bowel or pleura would have to be traversed to provide drainage;
3. The source of the infection has not been controlled (i.e., a bowel leak is present); and
4. A fungal abscess is present (i.e., pus is too thick and peel must be removed surgically).

Failure of the patient to improve within 48 to 72 hours after percutaneous drainage is an indication for better drainage, often via a laparotomy.

"Blind" Laparotomy

In a study of 77 patients with intraabdominal infections by Pitcher and Musher in 1982, a clear preoperative diagnosis was possible in only about one-half of the patients (49). Because the overall mortality rate was 64%, the authors believed that, in the absence of a clear diagnosis, failure to respond to 4 to 5 days of antibiotic therapy may be an indication for exploratory laparotomy. Polk and Shields also believed that MOF may be an indication for abdominal exploration (22).

When a surgical patient becomes increasingly septic after surgery or trauma involving the abdomen and no other obvious infected site can be found, the abdomen is often the source. Consequently, if such a patient's condition is deteriorating despite all other therapy, it may be wise to perform a "blind" laparotomy (i.e., a laparotomy without objective evidence of peritonitis or abdominal abscess).

In our experience, an infectious process requiring surgical drainage is found in about 50% of blind laparotomies. Many patients with MOF who have abdominal abscesses drained via a blind laparotomy do not survive because their general condition has already deteriorated too far.

Leaving the Abdomen Open

When severe, generalized peritonitis is found, it may be wise to leave the abdomen open and reexplore it on a daily basis until there is no further evidence of infection. If the abdomen is to be left open, the peritoneal cavity should be cleaned and irrigated thoroughly with 5 to 10 L of saline upon completion of the procedure. Fibrin that is firmly adherent is left undisturbed. A final rinse with an antibiotic solution (either 1.0 g of cefazolin or a combination of 500 mg of neomycin plus 500,000 units of polymyxin/L) can be used, but the irrigant should then be removed as completely as possible. The bowel loops are then covered with a rayon or nylon dressing (to prevent bowel adhesing to the abdominal wall) followed by moist fluff gauzes. Two binders are then applied over the abdomen.

Postoperatively, the patient is sedated, kept on a ventilator in the ICU, and brought to the operating room every 24 to 48 hours. The packs are removed and any fluid collections or debris accumulating since the previous exploration are cultured and removed. For 2 to 3 days, most of these patients have pockets of infected, cloudy fluid from which organisms can often be cultured. When the peritoneal cavity looks clean, often by the fifth day, the abdominal fascia can generally be closed safely. If the fascia cannot be approximated without too much tension, prosthetic mesh can be used to close the abdomen. The skin and subcutaneous tissue should be left open.

AXIOM Even when a surgeon does not believe in leaving the abdomen open in patients with severe, diffuse peritonitis, any later deterioration or failure to recover properly should be an indication for prompt reexploration.

Bronchoscopy

Bronchoscopy can be helpful in the treatment of lobar atelectasis and some pulmonary infections. The incidence of arrhythmias, which are the most frequent complication of therapeutic bronchoscopies, can be reduced by ensuring adequate ventilation and oxygenation during the procedure. This is best accomplished by performing bronchoscopy through a T-piece on an endotracheal tube while the patient is ventilated with 100% O_2. Protected brush specimens are generally more accurate than simple sputum samples.

AXIOM Repeated bronchoscopies for toilet should be strongly considered in patients with excess secretions plus severe atelectasis or pneumonia not responding promptly to other therapy, including tracheal suctioning.

Removal of Intravenous Catheters

Fever beginning 2 to 3 days after surgery is particularly likely to be the result of an infection of an intravenous catheter. When even a vague possibility exists that an intravenous catheter is infected and other veins are available, the intravenous catheter sites should be changed and the catheter tips cultured. Changing the catheter over a wire may be useful in patients who have no other venous access.

Removal of Urinary Catheters

Catheterization of the urinary tract should be avoided whenever possible. If the urine is infected and the urinary tract is even partially obstructed, it is usually impossible to correct the infection without adequate drainage.

Administration of Antimicrobial Agents

AXIOM No antibiotic, or combination of antibiotics, "covers everything."

When possible, only one or, at the most, two antibiotics should be used at a time. In addition, the antibiotics should not have a spectrum extending beyond that necessary to control the organisms involved. "Shotgun" therapy with three or more broad-spectrum antibiotics should be discouraged, except in the presence of life-threatening infections in which the involved microorganisms and their sensitivities are unknown.

If the patient has renal or hepatic failure, the choice and dose of antibiotics may be greatly altered. If possible, aminoglycosides and vancomycin should be avoided in patients with severe renal dysfunction. If such agents are used, it is essential to get peak and trough levels every 24 to 72 hours to determine whether the levels are high enough to adequately treat the infection and low enough to prevent toxic side effects.

The incidence of nephrotoxicity or ototoxicity with aminoglycosides may be as high as 11% to 16%, with the ototoxicity often being irreversible (50). Nevertheless, doses that are 50% to 100% higher than normal are often needed to achieve adequate peak levels in patients who have had severe trauma and have much third-spacing of fluid. Under such circumstances, the interdose interval must be increased to reduce the incidence and severity of toxic side effects. The best way to ensure the effectiveness and safety of aminoglycosides in critically ill patients is to serially monitor peak and trough levels at least every 2 to 3 days.

In the absence of preexisting renal insufficiency, a single daily dose regimen is being increasingly recommended for aminoglycosides. The targeted peak concentrations are twice as high as traditional regimens in order to take advantage of the concentration-dependent bactericidal activity of these agents. The long interdose interval takes advantage of the postantibiotic effect and minimizes exposure to toxic effects.

If a patient continues to have fever or leukocytosis after 48 to 72 hours of antibiotic therapy, one should suspect that a continuing or recurrent infection is still present and one should consider discontinuing the antibiotics and obtaining more cultures. One should also look for noninfectious causes of fever, such as deep venous thrombosis or drug fever.

Antibiotic Choices for Various Sites of Infection

Wound Infections

Once they are adequately drained, wound infections do not require antibiotics, but if there is residual cellulitis or continuing fever or leukocytosis, they may be warranted.

Wound infections developing outside the hospital in patients who have had no involvement of the gastrointestinal or female genitourinary tracts are usually caused by penicillin-sensitive staphylococci and streptococci. They can also be treated well by a first-generation cephalosporin. The staphylococci causing wound infections in the hospital are often coagulase-positive organisms that are resistant to penicillin; however, many are responsive to β-lactamase-resistant penicillins, such as methicillin or first-generation cephalosporins. If the patient is allergic to penicillin, drugs such as erythromycin or clindamycin, which are relatively nontoxic, may be used effectively. Methicillin-resistant *S. aureus* (MRSA) requiring antibiotic therapy is treated with vancomycin.

AXIOM Wound infections developing in patients who have had intraabdominal injury or have been receiving broad-spectrum antibiotics are often caused by gram-negative bacilli.

Pulmonary Infections

The generally accepted clinical criteria for making a diagnosis of pneumonia include a new or changing infiltrate on chest radiography, in addition to fever (temperature greater than 101.5°F), purulent sputum, many bacteria on Gram stain, and one or more positive sputum cultures. A WBC count greater than 15,000/mm^3 or with more than 10% immature forms is also often present. A wide variety of organisms may cause pulmonary infections after trauma, and Gram stains and cultures of the sputum are essential. Protected brush specimens and bronchoalveolar lavage probably improve diagnostic accuracy (9).

Gram stains of tracheal aspirates may correlate poorly with cultures of the same specimens, especially if there are relatively few bacteria or PMNs present. Indeed, Namias et al. (51) suggest that surgical ICU patients in whom pneumonia is developing should be given gram-negative rod coverage even if gram-positive cocci are seen on the smear.

AXIOM Although about one-third of positive sputum cultures in ICU patients are due to colonization, one should consider treating for the organism found, especially *Pseudomonas*, if the patient is severely immunodepressed.

When the patient has a community-acquired pneumonia, *S. pneumoniae* or *Haemophilus influenzae* is likely to be the causative agent, and erythromycin with or without cefuroxine is recommended (59). Gram-positive cocci in chains (streptococci) are usually sensitive to penicillin. Gram-positive cocci in clusters (staphylococci) are usually responsive to cephalosporins or penicillinase-resistant penicillins.

AXIOM Before treating pneumonia with antibiotics, great efforts should be made to perform Gram stains and culture and sensitivity testing on good sputum or bronchoscopic specimens.

Mild to moderate pulmonary infections caused by gram-negative bacilli may be treated with extended-spectrum penicillins, cephalosporins, a fluoroquinolone, or a beta-lactamase inhibitor combination. Severe gram-negative pulmonary infections developing after several days of antibiotic therapy are often caused by *Pseudomonas*, which should be treated with an aminoglycoside plus an extended-spectrum penicillin, such as piperacillin. This combination is preferred because it has synergistic bactericidal effects against *Pseudomonas* and other gram-negative aerobes.

Pulmonary abscesses caused by aspiration are generally caused initially by aerobic gram-positive cocci and mouth anaerobes, including the fusospirochetes. A growing number of these organisms are resistant to penicillin, and clindamycin is increasingly the initial drug of choice for pulmonary infections that may be caused by aspiration.

Empyema of the pleural space can occur after pneumonia or chest trauma with a hemothorax. Diagnosis is made by Gram stain and culture of the pleural fluid. If clinical sepsis persists despite the insertion of a thoracostomy tube and specific antibiotic therapy within 48 to 72 hours, another chest tube, open drainage, or a thoracotomy for decortication of the lung should be considered.

Peritonitis

The organisms most likely to cause intraperitoneal infections after trauma are of the family Enterobacteriaceae (including *Escherichia*, *Klebsiella*, *Enterobacter*, and *Proteus* species). Other organisms also likely to be present are streptococci, enterococci, and various anaerobic organisms, particularly *Bacteroides* species.

For mild to moderate peritoneal contamination, the best studied and documented antibiotic regimen is an aminoglycoside combined with either clindamycin or metronidazole (9). Alternatives to aminoglycosides include third-generation cephalosporins, ciprofloxacin, or aztreonam. If aztreonam is used, it should be combined with clindamycin because neither metronidazole nor aztreonam has significant activity against gram-positive aerobes.

Single-agent regimens with appropriate activity for empiric treatment of intraabdominal infections include Unasyn, Timentin, Zosyn and imipenem-cilastatin. For severe peritoneal contamination, especially by colon or distal small bowel injuries, triple antibiotics (ampicillin, an aminoglycoside, and metronidazole) can be used.

Urinary Tract Infections

Ampicillin, Bactrim, or ciprofloxacin may be effective against the gram-negative organisms that are involved in most urinary tract infections, but gentamicin is the antibiotic of choice for the most severe kidney infections. Ampicillin plus gentamicin is indicated in infections caused by enterococci.

Infected Vascular Prostheses

AXIOM Any inflammation in the groin following femoral vascular surgery, even months later, should be considered evidence of an infected vascular prosthesis until proven otherwise.

Early vascular graft infections are often caused by *S. aureus*, whereas late infections (after 3 months) tend to be caused by mucin-producing strains of *S. epidermidis*, which apparently show increased adherence to prosthetic material (52).

Infections around patent vascular prostheses can sometimes be managed with drainage, debridement, and intensive systemic and local antibiotic therapy, but infected, occluded grafts require resection of the graft. Parenteral antibiotics are administered for at least 2 to 4 weeks after resection of an infected graft. If a superficially infected graft is left in place, parenteral and then oral antibiotics should be continued for 3 to 6 months or longer.

Septic Phlebitis

Septic phlebitis has become much more common since the introduction of plastic intravenous cannulas. Infection is particularly common when cutdowns are performed and after emergency placement of intravenous lines. Multiple lumen lines and prolonged cannulation (more than 48 to 72 hours) are also associated with an increased rate of infection. Intravenous device infections caused by *S. aureus* are more likely to require surgical drainage of an associated abscess or a septic thrombophlebitis.

AXIOM Removal of the catheter is usually enough to "cure" most intravenous catheter infections, but intravenous antibiotics are needed for at least 10 to 14 days if *S. aureus* bacteremia occurs or if fever persists.

Interferon-γ

Dries et al. (53) in 1994 showed that interferon (INF)-γ can reduce infection-related deaths in patients with severe injuries; Wasserman et al. (54), however, in a double-blind placebo-controlled study, found that INF-γ did not protect burn patients from infections or decrease the mortality rate from infection.

TREATMENT FOR SPECIFIC MICROORGANISMS

Staphylococcus

Community-acquired *S. aureus* usually responds well to nafcillin, oxacillin, or first-generation cephalosporins; however, an increasing number of MRSA are being found, especially in intravenous drug abusers. In such patients, vancomycin is usually effective. Although *S. epidermidis* is usually sensitive to first-generation cephalosporins or antistaphylococcal penicillins, an increasing number are becoming resistant to such agents and require vancomycin for effective therapy.

Streptococci

Most streptococci are sensitive to penicillin; however, necrotizing infections caused by streptococci also require radical excision and drainage.

Enterococci

The enterococci generally respond well to a combination of ampicillin or vancomycin plus aminoglycoside; however, increasing resistance to vancomycin, especially by *Enterococcus faecium*, is being found.

Gram-Negative Aerobes

Gram-negative aerobic bacilli, such as *E. coli* and *Klebsiella*, generally respond well to aminoglycosides; however, these bacilli typically become increasingly resistant to whatever antibiotics are being used most frequently.

⊘ PITFALL

If the sensitivities of bacteria found within hospitals are not checked on a regular basis, the initial empiric antibiotic choices made by physicians are likely to be increasingly incorrect.

For the most severe *Pseudomonas* infections, combinations of aminoglycosides plus an extended-spectrum penicillin, such as piperacillin, are recommended. Alternatives include third-generation cephalosporins, such as ceftazidime, or the fluoroquinolones.

Tetanus

Although tetanus could be almost eliminated by universal active immunization during childhood, approximately 100 patients with clinical tetanus are reported in the United States each year (33). If the patient has a clean wound and has been properly immunized, a tetanus toxoid booster is needed only if the patient has not had a booster shot in the past 10 years. If prior tetanus immunization is uncertain, tetanus toxoid should be given along with a schedule for complete immunization (Table 39-2).

With a "dirty" (tetanus-prone) wound in a patient who has been properly immunized, a tetanus toxoid booster is all that is required if the patient has had a booster in the past 5 to 10 years. If a properly immunized patient with a tetanus-prone wound has not had a booster in the past 10 years or if prior immunization is uncertain, tetanus toxoid plus human tetanus immune globulin (TIG-H) should be given along with a complete immunization schedule if needed. Patients older than 65 years of age, even with a history of complete tetanus immunization, are less likely than young individuals to have adequate immunity against tetanus (55).

Hyperbaric oxygenation (HBO) can be extremely helpful in controlling severe infections caused by anaerobic organisms; however, the clinical results have often been inconclusive and, unless HBO facilities are readily available, the risks of moving critically ill patients may outweigh the potential benefits.

Table 39-2. *Tetanus Prophylaxis*

Tetanus immunization history	Clean wound	"Tetanus-prone" wound[a]
Fully immunized; last booster injection:		
<5 years	None	None
5–10 years	None	Toxoid booster
>10 years	Toxoid booster	Toxoid booster + TIG-H
Incompletely immunized or uncertain history	Toxoid + completion of immunization	Toxoid + TIG-H + completion of immunization

[a]Such as, but not limited to, wounds contaminated with dirt or feces, puncture wounds, deep avulsions, and wounds resulting from missiles or crushing.
TIG-H, tetanus immune globulin-human.
From Brand DA, et al: Adequacy of antitetanus prophylaxis in six hospital emergency rooms. *N Engl J Med* 1983;309:636.

Clostridial Cellulitis and Myositis

Surgical treatment of clostridial cellulitis or myositis (gas gangrene) must be prompt with extensive decompression and thorough debridement of all involved tissue. High doses of intravenous antibiotics, particularly penicillin (2,000,000 units every 2 hours), with or without concomitant cephalosporins, chloramphenicol, or clindamycin, should also be started immediately. In patients not responding to antibiotics and surgical debridement and drainage, HBO should be used when available. If HBO is not readily available, early amputation may be the only hope of cure.

Human Bite Infections

Human bite wounds should be promptly explored and debrided in the operating room. The antibiotics used increasingly are the newer beta-lactamase inhibitor combinations (ticarcillin-clavulanate, ampicillin-sulbactam, or piperacillin-tazobactam).

Necrotizing Fasciitis

Necrotizing fasciitis requires prompt opening of the involved area, excision of all involved tissues, and adequate drainage. Reinspection and debridement of the wound should be performed again within 24 to 48 hours (56). Antibiotic coverage should be effective against aerobic gram-positive cocci, aerobic gram-negative rods, and anaerobes.

Candida Infections

AXIOM Fungal infection should be suspected in septic ICU patients who have received broad-spectrum antibiotics for 7 to 10 days and have no obvious sites of infection, particularly if multiple cultures of all possible infected foci are negative for bacteria.

Amphotericin B or fluconazole should also be given to patients with two or more sites (e.g., mouth, sputum, urine, drain sites) positive for *Candida albicans* (57). One should not wait for positive blood cultures to begin therapy. Short-term, limited dosing with amphotericin B (total dose: 6 to 8 mg/kg at 0.25-0.5 mg/kg/day) appears to be adequate for many patients, but fluconazole is just as effective and is generally safer. In some instances, swish and swallow administration of nystatin (1,000,000 units every 4 hours) may help to reduce the tendency for *Candida* overgrowth in the gastrointestinal tract of patients receiving prolonged, broad-spectrum antibiotics.

OTHER TREATMENT

Improved Nutrition

Early adequate nutrition, particularly via the enteral route in severely malnourished individuals, can help to restore phagocytosis toward normal levels. This is particularly important if the patient has albumin levels less than 2.2 g/dL and an absolute lymphocyte count less than 800/mm^3. These patients may require more than 35 non-protein calories and 1.5 to 2.5 g of protein per kg body weight daily to restore immunologic competence.

Early enteral administration of Impact, which has arginine, nucleotides, and fish oil, may also improve host defenses.

Antithrombin III

Sepsis is associated with activation of thrombin and consumption of the physiologic inhibitors of the coagulation cascade, especially antithrombin. This imbalance can lead to an overactivation of the coagulation system with resultant occlusion of nutrient capillaries in vital organs, thereby causing MOF (58).

Based on these considerations, antithrombin III (AT-III) has been used to treat coagulation disorders and organ dysfunction in experimental and clinical sepsis (58). Inthorn et al. (59) found that 14 days of AT-III supplementation in patients with severe sepsis corrected DIC in all patients with that problem. It also caused a progressive increase in the PaO_2/FIO_2 ratio, a decrease in pulmonary hypertension index (mean pulmonary artery pressure/mean systemic arterial pressure (PAP/MAP) ratio), and reduced the incidence and severity of hepatic and renal failure.

Pentoxifylline

Bacher et al. (60) found that 5 mg/kg of pentoxifylline (diluted in 300 mL of physiologic saline administered intravenously over a period of 180 minutes at a rate of 100 mL/h to septic patients) resulted in a significant improvement in hemodynamic performance, with an increased DO_2 and VO_2 and an unchanged oxygen extraction ratio.

Granulocyte Colony-Stimulating Factor

Granulocyte colony-stimulating factor (G-CSF) promotes mitosis, differentiation, and survival of primitive stem cells, and can rapidly improve the WBC count in severely leukopenic patients. It also enhances phagocytosis, oxidant release, antibody-dependent cellular cytotoxicity, migration, and chemotaxis of mature granulocytes and macrophages (61).

The principle Food and Drug Administration–approved indication for G-CSF is treatment of chemotherapy-induced myelosuppresion, in which it reduces the duration of severe neutropenia and the incidence of febrile neutropenic episodes. This allows for optimization and intensification of chemotherapy (61).

Patton et al. (62) found that G-CSF given during resuscitation improves host defense in shock and polymicrobial sepsis in swine. It increased PMN proliferation and function without potentiating PMN-mediated lung reperfusion injury.

⊘ FREQUENT ERRORS

1. ***Dependence on prophylactic antibiotics instead of sound surgical principles.***
2. ***Prolonged use of prophylactic antibiotics.***
3. ***Masking the presence of fever with antipyretics.***
4. ***Beginning antibiotics without appropriate cultures and smears.***
5. ***Improper collection and handling of material for cultures, particularly for anaerobes.***
6. ***Administration of an agent with broad-spectrum coverage when specific therapy is possible.***
7. ***Selection of antibiotic doses that are inappropriate for the clinical status of the patient or preexisting organ system failure.***

8. ***Failure to check antibiotic sensitivities in the hospital at frequent intervals.***
9. ***Assuming that the cause of persistent fever is an antibiotic-resistant organism.***
10. ***Failing to consider unusual organisms, especially candida, when bacterial cultures are repeatedly negative in a patient who is septic, despite 7 to 10 days of broad-spectum antibiotics.***

SUMMARY POINTS

1. In patients surviving for at least 48 hours, sepsis is the single, most frequent cause of later morbidity and mortality.
2. Foreign bodies, blood, and dead space in a wound can reduce the critical inoculum of bacteria needed to cause an infection from 10^6 for many wounds to 10^2 (i.e. 10,000 less organisms per milliliter).
3. Fever developing 2 to 3 days after surgery or trauma is often due to an infected intravenous catheter.
4. Any patient who becomes septic without another obvious cause should be considered to have an infected intravenous line until proven otherwise.
5. The longer ventilatory assistance is required, the more likely it is that pneumonia will develop.
6. Early eradication of all underlying infected or necrotic tissue is the best way to stop the downward spiral of organ dysfunction in sepsis.
7. Tissue-oxygen tension is an important variable influencing the risk of infection because PMNs require oxygen to kill bacteria.
8. Infections in patients with severe trauma may sometimes develop without pain, fever, or leukocytosis.
9. Soft-tissue infections caused by either β-hemolytic streptococci or *C. perfringens* can cause striking systemic signs of sepsis within the first 24 to 48 hours after injury.
10. Once MOF syndrome has developed, the process becomes self-perpetuating, and the patient's prognosis is poor, even if the initiating infection is finally controlled.
11. Patients with jaundice developing 8 or more days after trauma should be assumed to be septic until proven otherwise.
12. If the VO_2, in patients with sepsis decreases to levels persistently less than 100 mL/min/m^2, the mortality rate is extremely high.
13. Characteristically, patients in early septic shock are vasodilated, have a normal or increased cardiac output, and have warm, dry, pink, or flushed skin.
14. Hypodynamic (cold) septic shock usually occurs late in sepsis and indicates that increased cardiac failure and some element of hypovolemia are present.
15. A progressive decrease in plasma-ionized calcium levels should make one look for sepsis or impaired tissue perfusion.
16. Very low antithrombin levels (<50% of normal) (in the absence of extensive clotting or severe liver disease) generally indicate that infection is present.
17. If one cannot rapidly correct high lactate levels, the patient will almost invariably die.
18. Bronchial secretions obtained by bronchoalveolar lavage or protected brush specimens are more reliable than induced sputum or tracheal aspirates.
19. Even when urine contains greater than 10^5/mL of microorganisms, pyuria should also be present to warrant the diagnosis and treatment of a urinary tract infection.
20. The ideal specimen for detecting the microorganisms responsible for an abscess is to submit a tissue biopsy from its wall.
21. False-negative anaerobic cultures are common and should be considered when choosing antibiotic therapy based on laboratory studies.
22. The "rule of threes" for blood cultures states that three blood cultures taken on 3 consecutive days will usually document a gram-negative bacteremia in untreated patients.

23. Smears and cultures should be obtained, when possible, before antibiotic therapy is begun.
24. The location and extent of an infection and the bacteria involved may be masked if the patient is receiving antibiotics.
25. Gallium or indium scans are of little value for detecting acute infections in trauma patients.
26. CT scans are the ideal test for detecting intraabdominal abscesses, but they are relatively unreliable during the first 5 to 6 days after trauma.
27. Most gangrenous infections with gas in the tissues are not gas gangrene, but they should be approached as if they may be.
28. Because of clostridial leukocidin, relatively few WBCs are found in the exudate from gas gangrene.
29. Increasing the oxygen delivery index (DO_2I) to 600 mL/min/m^2 or more and the oxygen consumption index (VO_2I) to 150 to 170 mL/min/m^2 within 12 hours of injury may reduce the incidence of infection and MOF.
30. In heavily contaminated wounds or when all foreign material or devitalized tissue cannot be satisfactorily removed, the wound should be left open.
31. Antibiotics effective against gastrointestinal anaerobes and gram-negative aerobes should be administered as soon as possible to patients with abdominal trauma that may involve the gastrointestinal tract.
32. Although controversial, data from five of seven prospective double-blind studies support using prophylactic antibiotics when chest tubes are inserted for traumatic pneumothorax or hemothorax.
33. Prophylactic antibiotics for uncomplicated traumatic cerebrospinal fluid leaks do not reduce the incidence of infection, but they do increase the likelihood that any infection that develops will be caused by an antibiotic-resistant organism.
34. In settings in which the risk of infection continues over an extended period of time, antibiotics have uniformly failed to prevent subsequent infection; furthermore, if infection develops, the bacteria involved are more likely to be antibiotic-resistant (9).
35. Although extremely controversial, antibiotic irrigation of heavily contaminated areas of the peritoneal cavity may be of some value in selected patients.
36. One should assume that all human bites are contaminated with a large number of virulent mouth aerobes and anaerobes.
37. Prompt, adequate drainage and debridement is the most important treatment of localized abdominal infections.
38. An abscess cavity, which continues to drain large quantities of pus or fluid for several days after surgical drainage, is usually inadequately drained or is associated with a fistula.
39. In patients who are, despite all other therapy, progressively deteriorating with sepsis after abdominal trauma, an exploratory laparotomy should be considered, even if all diagnostic tests for abscess or peritonitis are negative.
40. Even when a surgeon does not believe in leaving the abdomen open in severely septic patients with diffuse peritonitis, later deterioration should be an indication for prompt reexploration.
41. Repeated bronchoscopies for toilet should be strongly considered in patients with severe atelectasis or pneumonia not responding promptly to other therapy, including tracheal suctioning.
42. No antibiotic, or combination of antibiotics, "covers everything."
43. In critically injured patients, antibiotics should be given intravenously.
44. The best way to ensure maximum effectiveness and safety with aminoglycosides in critically ill patients is to give them only once a day, limit the duration of usage to less than 6 to 7 days if possible, and serially monitor peak and trough levels at least every 2 to 3 days.
45. Once treatment of an infection is begun with a carefully selected antibiotic, it should be continued for at least 48 to 72 hours before empirically adding or changing to another agent.
46. An infection in an abdominal incision that drains increased fluid or exhibits signs of fascial necrosis may be evidence of an underlying intraabdominal infection or anastomotic leak.

47. Although about one-third of positive sputum cultures in ICU patients are the result of colonization, one should consider treating for that organism, especially if it is *Pseudomonas* and the patient is severely immunodepressed.
48. Before treating pneumonia with an antibiotic, great efforts should be made to obtain good sputum or bronchoscopic specimens for Gram stains and culture and sensitivity testing.
49. Any inflammation in the groin following femoral vascular surgery, even months later, should be considered evidence of an infected vascular prosthesis until proved otherwise.
50. Intravenous catheter infection with a positive *S. aureus* culture requires at least 10 to 14 days of intravenous antibiotics.
51. Any finding suggesting the presence of an anaerobic infection is an indication for early, aggressive exploration, incision, and debridement.
52. Fungal infection should be suspected in septic ICU patients who have received broad-spectrum antibiotics for 7 to 10 days and have no obvious sites of infection, particularly if multiple cultures of all possible infected foci are negative for bacteria.

REFERENCES

1. Wilson RF, Tyburski JG, Janning SW. Sepsis in Trauma. In: Wilson RF, Walt AJ, eds. *Management of trauma—pitfalls and practices,* 2nd ed. Philadelphia: Williams & Wilkins, 1996:828–866.
2. Nichols RL, Smith JW, Klein DB, et al. Risk of infection after penetrating abdominal trauma. *N Engl J Med* 1984;311:1065.
3. Dellinger EP, Oreskovich MR, Wertz MJ, et al. Risk of infection following laparotomy for penetrating abdominal injury. *Arch Surg* 1984;119:20.
4. Collignon P, Suni N, Pearson I, et al. Sepsis associated with central venous catheters in critically ill patients. *Intensive Care Med* 1988;14:227.
5. Freedland M, Wilson RF, Bender JS, Levison MA. The management of flail chest injury: factors affecting outcome. *J Trauma* 1990;30:1460.
6. Rodriguez JL, Gibbons KJ, Bitzer LG. Pneumonia: incidence, risk factors, and outcome in injured patients. *J Trauma* 1991;31:907.
7. Fabian TC, Boucher BA, Croce MA, et al. Pneumonia and stress ulceration in severely injured patients. *Arch Surg* 1993;128:11.
8. Saba TM, Blumestock FA, Scovill WA, Bernard H. Cryoprecipitate reversal of opsonic glycoprotein deficiency in septic surgical and trauma patients. *Ann Surg* 1981;195:177.
9. Dellinger EP. Prevention and management of infections. In: Moore EE, Mattox KL, Feliciano DV, eds. *Trauma,* 2nd ed. Norwalk, CT: Appleton & Lange, 1991: 231–244.
10. Goodman JW. The immune response. In: Stites DP, Terr AI, Parslow TG, eds. Basic & clinical immunology. Norwalk, CT: Appleton & Lange, 1994:45–46.
11. Schneider RP, Christou NV, Meakins JL, Nohr C. Humoral immunity in surgical patients with and without trauma. *Arch Surg* 1991;126:143.
12. Neidhardt R, Keel M, Steckholzer U, et al. Relationship of interleukin-10 plasma levels to severity of injury and clinical outcome in injured patients. *J Trauma* 1997;42:863.
13. Parsons PE. Interleukin-10: The ambiguity in sepsis continues [editorial]. *Crit Care Med* 1998;26:818.
14. Fabian TC, Minard G. Sepsis. In: Mattox KL, ed. *Complications of trauma.* New York: Churchill Livingstone, 1994:61–79.
15. Cruse PJE. Wound infections: epidemiology and clinical characteristics. In: Howard RJ, Simmons RL, eds. *Surgical infectious diseases,* 2nd ed. Norwalk, CT: Appleton & Lange, 1988:319–329.
16. Allen JC. The diabetic as a compromised host. In: Allen JC, ed. *Infection and the compromised host. Clinical correlations and therapeutic approaches*, 2nd ed. Baltimore: Williams & Wilkins, 1981:229.
17. Alexander JW. Nutrition and infection*f*-new perspectives for an old problem. *Arch Surg* 1986;121:966.
18. Gentilello LM, Cobean RA, Walker AP, et al. Acute ethanol intoxication increases

the risk of infection following penetrating abdominal trauma. *J Trauma* 1993;34: 669.
19. Tamura DY, Moore EE, Patrick DA, et al. Clinically relevant concentrations of ethanol attenuate primed neutrophil bactericidal activity. *J Trauma* 1998;44: 320.
20. Musher DM, Fainstein V, Young EJ, et al. Fever patterns, their lack of clinical significance. *Arch Intern Med* 1979;139:1225.
21. Fry DE, Pearlstein L, Fulton RL, Polk HC Jr. Multiple system organ failure. *Arch Surg* 1980;115:136.
22. Polk HC Jr, Shields CL. Remote organ failure: a valid sign of occult intra-abdominal infection. *Surgery* 1977;81:310.
23. Fry DE, Garrison N, Heitsch RC, et al. Determinants of death in patients with intra-abdominal abscess. *Surgery* 1980;88:517.
24. Wilson RF, Thal AP, Kindling PH, et al. Hemodynamic measurements in septic shock. *Arch Surg* 1965;91:121.
25. Parker MM, Shelhamer JH, Natanson C, et al. Serial cardiovascular variables in survivors and nonsurvivors of human septic shock: heart rate as an early predictor of prognosis. *Crit Care Med* 1987;15:923.
26. Parrillo JE, Burch C, Shelhamer JH, et al. A circulating myocardial depressant substance in humans with septic shock. *J Clin Invest* 1985;76:1539.
27. White BC, Winegar CD, Wilson RF, Trombley JH. The possible role of calcium blockers in cerebral resuscitation: a review of the literature and synthesis for future studies. *Crit Care Med* 1983;11:202.
28. Neame PB, Kelton JG, Walker IR, et al. Thrombocytopenia in septicemia: the role of DIC. *Blood* 1980;56:88.
29. Wilson RF, Farag A, Mammen EF, Fujii Y. Sepsis and antithrombin III, prekallikrein and fibronectin levels in surgical patients. *Am Surg* 1989;55:450.
30. Aeder MI, Wellman JL, Haaga JR, Hau T. Role of surgical and percutaneous drainage in the treatment of abdominal abscess. *Arch Surg* 1983;118:273.
31. Finegold SM. Anaerobic bacteria. In: Howard RJ, Simmons RL, eds. *Surgical infectious diseases,* 2nd ed. Norwalk, CT: Appleton & Lange, 1988:49–62.
32. Simmons RL, Ahrenholz DH. Infections of the skin and soft tissues. In: Howard RJ, Simmons RL, eds. *Surgical infectious diseases,* 2nd ed. Norwalk, CT: Appleton & Lange, 1988:377–441.
33. Furste W, Aguirre A, Lutter K. Tetanus. In: Howard RJ, Simmons RL, eds. *Surgical infectious diseases,* 2nd ed. Norwalk, CT: Appleton & Lange, 1988: 837–847.
34. Ahrenholz DH, Simmons RL. Mixed and synergistic infections. In: Howard RJ, Simmons RL, eds. *Surgical infectious diseases,* 2nd ed. Norwalk, CT: Appleton & Lange, 1988:87–99.
35. Sloan EP, McGill BA, Zalenski R, et al. Human immunodeficiency virus and hepatitis B virus seroprevalence in an urban trauma population. *J Trauma* 1995; 38:736.
36. Kelen GD, Fritz S, Qaquish B, et al. Substantial increase in human immunodeficiency virus (HIV-1) infection in critically ill emergency patients: 1986 and 1987 compared. *Ann Emerg Med* 1989;18:378.
37. Ankney RN, Kurek SJ, Miller SL, et al. HIV infection among rural trauma patients: a blind serosurvey and literature review. *Am Surg* 1998;64:447.
38. Wilson RF, Wiencek R, Balog M. Predicting and preventing infection after abdominal vascular injuries. *J Trauma* 1989;29:1371.
39. Shoemaker WC, Appel PL, Kram HB, et al. Prospective trial of supranormal values of survivors as therapeutic goals in high-risk surgical patients. *Chest* 1988; 94:1176.
40. Moore FA, Haenel JB, Moore EE, Whitehill TA. Incommensurate oxygen consumption in response to maximal oxygen availability predicts postinjury multiple organ failure. *J Trauma* 1992;33:58.
41. Hayes MA, Timmins AC, Yau EHS, et al. Oxygen transport patterns in patients with sepsis syndrome or septic shock: influence of treatment and relationship to outcome. *Crit Care Med* 1997;25:926.

42. deHoll D, Rodeheaver G, Edgerton MT, Edlich RF. Potentiation of infection by suture closure of dead space. *Am J Surg* 1974;127:716.
43. Nichols RL, Smith JW, Muzik AC, et al. Preventive antibiotic usage in traumatic thoracic injuries requiring closed tube thoracostomy. *Chest* 1994;106:1493.
44. Demetriades D, Breckon V, Breckon C, et al. Antibiotic prophylaxis in penetrating injuries of the chest. *Ann R Coll Surg Engl* 1991;73:348.
45. Dellinger EP, Wertz MJ, Lennard ES, et al. Efficacy of short-course antibiotic prophylaxis after penetrating intestinal injury: a prospective randomized trial. *Arch Surg* 1986;121:23.
46. Lord JW Jr, LaRaja RD, Daliana M, Gordon MT. Prophylactic antibiotic wound irrigation in gastric, biliary, and colonic surgery. *Am J Surg* 1983;145:209.
47. Dellinger EP. Antibiotic prophylaxis in trauma: penetrating abdominal injuries and open fractures. *Rev Infect Dis* 1991;13(Suppl 10):S847.
48. Gerzof SG, Robbins AH, Johnson WC, et al. Percutaneous catheter drainage of abdominal abscess. *J Med* 1981;305:653.
49. Pitcher WD, Musher DM. Critical importance of early diagnosis and treatment of intra-abdominal infection. *Arch Surg* 1982;117:328.
50. Moore RD, Smith CR, Lietman PS. Risk factors for the development of auditory toxicity in patients receiving aminoglycosides. *J Infect Dis* 1984;149:23.
51. Namias N, et al. A reappraisal of the role of Gram's stains of tracheal aspirates in guiding antibiotic selection in the surgical intensive care unit. *J Trauma* 1998; 44:102.
52. Schmitt DD, Brandyk DF, Pequet AJ, et al. Mucin production by *Staphylococcus epidermidis:* a virulence factor promoting adherence to vascular grafts. *Arch Surg* 1986;121:89.
53. Dries DJ, Jurkovich J, Maier RV, et al. Effect of interferon gamma on infection-related death in patients with severe injuries. *Arch Surg* 1994;129:1031–1042.
54. Wasserman D, Ioannovich JD, Hinzmann RD, et al. Interferon-γ in the prevention of severe burn-related infections: a European phase III multicenter trail. *Crit Care Med* 1998;26:434.
55. Alagappan K, Rennie W, Kwiatkowski T, et al. Seroprevalence of tetanus antibodies among adults older than 65 years. *Ann Emerg Med* 1996;28:18–21.
56. Harmonson JK, Tobar MY, Harkless LB. Necrotizing fasciitis. *Clin Podiatr Med Surg* 1996;13:635–647.
57. Slotman GJ, Shapiro E, Moffa SM. Fungal sepsis: multisite colonization versus fungemia. *Am Surg* 1994;60:107.
58. Okajima K, Uchiba M, Murakami K. Antithrombin replacement in DIC and MOF. In: Vincent JL, ed. *Yearbook of intensive care and emergency medicine.* Berlin Heidelberg: Springer-Verlag, 1995:457–464.
59. Inthorn D, Hoffmann JN, Hartl WH, et al. Antithrombin III supplementation in severe sepsis: beneficial effects on organ dysfunction. *Shock* 1997;8:328.
60. Bacher A, Mayer N, Kimscha W, et al. Effects of pentoxifylline on hemodynamics and oxygenation in septic and nonseptic patients. *Crit Care Med* 1997;25:795.
61. Morstyn G, Goote M, Perkins D, et al. The clinical utility of granulocyte colony-stimulating factor: early achievements and future promise. *Stem Cells* 1994;12(Suppl 1):213 and 227.
62. Patton JH Jr, Lyden SP, Ragsdale DN, et al. Granulocyte colony-stimulating factor improves host defense to resuscitated shock and polymicrobial sepsis without provoking generalized neutrophil-mediated damage. *J Trauma* 1998;44:750.

40. POSTTRAUMATIC PULMONARY INSUFFICIENCY(1)

INTRODUCTION

Definition

Pulmonary insufficiency can be defined as a clinical state in which the gas exchange in the lungs is inadequate to maintain body function without mechanical support. This term may also refer to pathophysiologic changes that cause a patient to have a PO_2 less than 60 mm Hg on room air or a PCO_2 of more than 45 mm Hg with a normal or low pH.

Atelectasis or pneumonia frequently develop in critically injured patients as a result of chest pain or injury. In addition, there are less direct causes of pulmonary malfunction, such as fat emboli, severe sepsis, or thromboembolism (2,3). Of special interest, particularly in the patients who become septic, is the condition referred to as the adult respiratory distress syndrome (ARDS), which continues to have a mortality rate of at least 30% to 40% in most centers.

Incidence

In an analysis of 3,289 trauma patients, Hoyt et al. found that pulmonary complications developed in 368 (11.2%). These complications included pneumonia, 7.5%; atelectasis, 3.4%; respiratory failure/ARDS, 2.8%; aspiration, 1.5%; and pulmonary embolus, 0.7%.

The most important predictors of pulmonary complications included the following:

1. Injury severity score (ISS) greater than or equal to 16;
2. Blunt trauma;
3. Shock on admission;
4. Trauma score less than 13 of 16;
5. Chest surgery;
6. Pedestrian-motor vehicle accident;
7. Head injury (abbreviated injury scale greater than or equal to 3); and
8. Age greater than 55 years.

CAUSES OF PULMONARY INSUFFICIENCY

Shock

Inadequate blood flow to the lungs can cause a decrease in mucociliary clearance and surfactant production. Surfactant, a phospholipid produced in the lungs by type II alveolar cells, decreases surface tension in alveoli and thereby helps to prevent atelectasis. Surfactant activity is also reduced by various proteins and fluid leaking into the alveoli.

AXIOM Hemorrhagic hypotension by itself seldom produces ARDS; significant tissue damage or inflammation must usually also be present.

Fluid Overload

Any increase in pulmonary capillary pressure can greatly increase the rate at which fluid leaves the pulmonary capillaries and enters the pulmonary interstitial spaces; however, this increased lung water can develop in septic patients even if cardiac filling pressures are kept quite low.

Massive Blood Transfusions

Although massive blood transfusions can cause transient abnormalities of pulmonary function, the evidence that it causes pulmonary insufficiency is controversial. Our studies suggest that the main problem with massive blood transfusions is the increased incidence of infection in patients who receive them.

Pulmonary Contusion

Pulmonary contusion is usually diagnosed on the basis of infiltrates seen on radiography within 24 hours of chest trauma. The contusions generally get worse for the next 24 to 48 hours and then begin to clear. In patients with flail chest injuries, the hypoxemia is primarily due to the underlying pulmonary contusion rather than the mechanical chest wall defect. In addition, severe contusions increase the likelihood that pneumonia will develop in patients with a flail chest and that they will require prolonged ventilatory support (16).

Fat Emboli

AXIOM One should assume that all patients with pelvic or large bone fractures will have some degree of fat embolism, which is most easily quantified by the decrease in platelet count and the increased alveolar-arterial oxygen difference.

"Fat embolism" is the name given to a clinical syndrome characterized by cerebral and respiratory dysfunction following long bone fractures. A relatively asymptomatic interval of 12 to 48 hours occurs after injury, following which the patient begins to demonstrate increasing tachypnea, restlessness, and confusion (10). If this progresses to the full-blown syndrome of severe hypoxemia and coma, the mortality rate may exceed 10% to 20%.

Fat emboli come primarily from the fractured bones, but some fat emboli may also develop in blood because of increased lipolysis. Activated platelets adhere to these particles so that, characteristically, the platelet count decreases and petechiae may appear transiently on the chest and conjunctivae or in the axillae.

Continued motion at fracture sites increases the incidence and severity of pulmonary failure following trauma. Consequently, early reduction and fixation is important. In addition, early fixation of lower extremity fractures allows patients to be mobilized out of bed sooner, thereby reducing the incidence of pneumonia and deep venous thrombosis (DVT).

Central Nervous System Injuries

Patients with central nervous system (CNS) injuries have a greatly increased risk of development of pulmonary complications because of aspiration, atelectasis, and prolonged ventilatory support. In addition, neurogenic pulmonary edema may be a factor.

Neurogenic pulmonary edema is a poorly defined syndrome that is seen most frequently in patients who die soon after massive head or spinal cord injury (8). Increased pulmonary venous tone caused by the head injury elevates pulmonary capillary hydrostatic pressure and dilates intercellular clefts, thereby increasing the leak of capillary fluid into the pulmonary interstitial and alveolar spaces.

Pneumonitis

AXIOM Making an accurate diagnosis of pneumonia in intensive care unit (ICU) patients can be difficult; however, most trauma patients on a ventilator for more than 7 to 14 days probably have some pneumonitis and atelectasis.

It can be difficult to make an accurate diagnosis of pneumonia in the presence of ARDS. The major distinguishing features of pneumonia are

1. Fever (temperature greater than 101°F);
2. Leukocytosis (greater than 12,000/mm^3);
3. New pulmonary infiltrate;
4. Sputum with increased numbers of polymorphonuclear leukocytes (PMNs); and
5. Bacteria on Gram stain and culture.

Alkalinization of the stomach for stress ulcer prophylaxis use has been considered an important factor influencing the incidence of nosocomial pneumonia in mechanically ventilated patients. Thomason et al. (9) found no difference in the incidence of nosocomial pneumonia in mechanically ventilated trauma patients whether the stress ulcer prophylaxis was sucralfate, antacids, or ranitidine.

Sepsis

AXIOM The most serious pulmonary problem apt to develop in infected patients is ARDS.

ARDS is unusual in patients who are not septic, but it is quite common in patients with severe persistent infections, especially if the peritoneal cavity is involved.

Pulmonary Embolism

Pulmonary embolism (PE) is a relatively frequent finding in patients with severe trauma who die after several days in the hospital. Coon, for example, found a 14.3% incidence of PE in autopsies of 224 patients who died after trauma (10).

Risk Factors

A risk assessment profile for thromboembolism (RAPT) score was developed by Greenfield et al. (11) (Table 40-1). A RAPT score of 5 or more, out of a maximum of 14, was used to define a group of patients whose risk of DVT was at least three times greater than that of the average trauma patient.

Diagnosis

Arterial hypoxemia occurs in 80% to 90% of patients with PE. Even when the partial pressure of oxygen in arterial blood (Pa_{O_2}) is normal in patients with a PE (because of hyperventilation), the alveolar-arterial oxygen gradient is generally increased.

AXIOM Any sudden decrease in end-tidal carbon dioxide (ET-P_{CO_2}) or increase in $P(a\text{-}ET)_{CO_2}$ differences 1 to 2 weeks after major trauma should make one suspect a pulmonary embolus.

With a pulmonary embolus, the Pa_{CO_2} is usually decreased as a result of hyperventilation, but the $ETCO_2$ decreases even more because of increased dead space in the lungs. Normally, the $P(A\text{-}a)_{CO_2}$ is only 2 to 6 mm Hg in a supine individual, but a PE, by greatly increasing pulmonary dead space, can abruptly increase this to more than 15 to 20 mm Hg.

AXIOM A normal lung scan rules out a significant pulmonary embolus.

If a V/Q scan shows "unmatched" perfusion defects involving an area as big as two segments, such a finding is considered a "high-probability" scan and in a clinical high-risk individual allows a PE to be diagnosed with 85% to 90% accuracy (12). Nevertheless, a few patients with PE have low-probability scans (i.e., with defects on

Table 40-1. ***Risk Assessment Profile for Thromboembolism***

	Weight
Underlying conditions	
Obese (>120% Metropolitan Life Table)	2
Malignancy	2
Abnormal coagulation factors at admission	2
History of thromboembolism	3
Iatrogenic factors	
Central femoral line >24 h	2
Four or more transfusions during first 24 h	2
Surgical procedures >2 h	2
Repair or ligation of major venous injury	3
Injury-related factors	
AIS >2 for the chest	2
AIS >2 for the abdomen	2
Spinal fractures	2
AIS >2 for the head	3
Coma (GCS score <8 for >4 h)	3
Complex lower extremity fracture	4
Pelvic fracture	4
Spinal cord injury with paraplegia or quadriplegia	4
Age (yr)	
≥40 but <60	2
≥60 but <75	3
≥75	4

AIS, Abbreviated Injury Score; GCS, Glasgow Coma Scale

both the ventilation and perfusion scans). When a strong clinical suspicion of PE exists but the lung scan is not helpful, pulmonary angiography should be done.

Treatment

If the patients with thigh or higher DVT or with a PE cannot be adequately heparinized, a vena cava filter should be inserted promptly.

Smoke Inhalation

Clinical manifestations of an inhalation injury during the first 36 hours include bronchospasm, tracheobronchitis, atelectasis, coughing episodes, and upper airway edema (2). After 2 to 6 days, there also may be increasing pulmonary edema (3). During the next 1 to 2 weeks, the patient may have increasing mucus casts in the bronchi and bronchopneumonia may develop.

Ventilator-Induced Lung Injury (Volutrauma)

As alveoli are inflated to the limit of their distensibility, the elastic forces diminish and the contiguous epithelial, interstitial, and endothelial structures are subject to mechanical distortions that can cause increasing lung injury (13). Ventilator-induced lung injury can be produced in mice with normal lungs if they are persistently ventilated at tidal volumes that cause alveolar overexpansion and pressures greater than 35 cm H_2O. If the same high-inflation pressures are applied to alveoli that cannot be overdistended because of an artificial restriction to chest wall expansion, lung injury usually does not occur.

AXIOM Ventilator-induced lung injury appears to be due to overdistension of alveoli (i.e., volutrauma) rather than just exposure of the alveoli to high pressures (i.e., barotrauma).

PATHOPHYSIOLOGY OF ACUTE RESPIRATORY DISTRESS SYNDROME

Acute respiratory distress syndrome usually follows a rather predictable course characterized by overlapping phases, which include

1. Acute or exudative phase—0 to 6 days;
2. Proliferative phase—4 to 10 days; and
3. Chronic or fibrotic phase after 8 to 14 days (14).

Phases of Acute Respiratory Distress Syndrome

Exudative Phase

The initial or "exudative" phase—0 to 6 days—is characterized by "leaking" pulmonary capillary endothelium and increasing numbers of PMNs. After 24 to 36 hours, increasing numbers of lymphocytes and other mononuclear cells move into the interstitium and alveoli, and there is increasing fluid in the interstitial and alveolar spaces. There is also progressive destruction of the thin, flat, type I alveolar cells that are involved in gas exchange, leaving a denuded basement membrane, except for the cuboidal type II pneumocytes (that make surfactant) (Fig. 40-1).

Proliferative Phase

The proliferative stage of ARDS usually begins on the third or fourth day and may progress for 7 to 14 days. It is characterized by proliferation of the type II pneumocytes to line the alveoli (2,3). The inflammatory cells that infiltrate the lung during this stage are primarily mononuclear cells, especially lymphocytes, macrophages, and

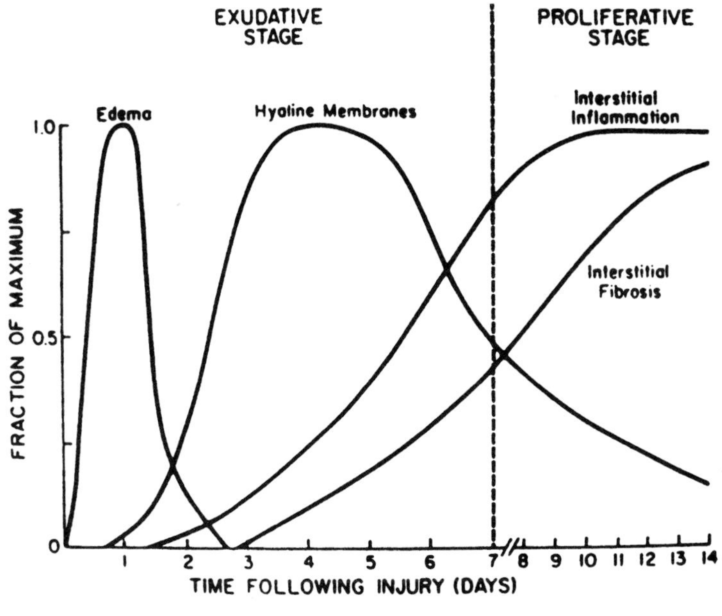

FIG. 40-1. A schematic representation of the time course of the evolution of adult respiratory distress syndrome. During the early or exudative phase, the lesion is characterized by a pulmonary capillary leak with edema. Within a few days, the proliferative phase may appear, with marked interstitial inflammation, followed by increasing fibrosis. (From Hall JB, Schmidt GA, Wood LDH, eds. *Principles of critical care.* New York: McGraw-Hill, 1992:1638).

plasma cells. After a few days, there are also increased numbers of proliferating fibroblasts.

Chronic Phase

In the final or chronic stage of ARDS, usually beginning 10 to 20 days after the process is initiated, there is evidence of increasing lung destruction, with progressive fibrosis of the interstitium and intraalveolar spaces (2,3).

Mediators of Acute Lung Injury

Vasoactive Substances

A large number of vasoactive substances, including catecholamines, serotonin, histamine, and polypeptides, are released during shock, sepsis, and trauma. Studies on isolated perfused dog lungs demonstrated that these substances can initiate and greatly accelerate the development of congestive atelectasis and pulmonary edema.

Leukocyte Activation

A great deal of experimental evidence suggests that the lung injury of ARDS is initiated by trapping of PMNs on pulmonary capillary endothelium and their subsequent release of free radicals (initially) and lysosomal enzymes (later). The margination and chemotaxis of the PMNs in the lung is thought to be largely due to C_{3a}, C_{5a}, and interleukin (IL)-8.

Toxic Oxygen Radicals

Activated PMNs can release highly reactive free radicals, including superoxide anion (O_2^-), hydrogen peroxide (H_2O_2), hydroxyl radicals (HO^-), and peroxide radicals (ROO^-) (15). Superoxide anion (O_2^-) is moderately unstable and, with the addition of an electron and two H^+ ions, it can be converted to H_2O_2, which is freely diffusible across capillary and cell membranes. In the presence of Fe^{2+}, superoxide anions produce the extremely unstable $HO\cdot$ radical. H_2O_2, in the presence of Cl^- ion and the lysosomal enzyme myeloperoxidase, may be converted to hypochlorous acid (HOCl), another powerful oxidant, which is important for killing bacteria in phagolysosomes (15).

Normally, the free radicals produced in tissues are neutralized rapidly by endogenous free-radical scavengers. These include superoxide dismutase (for oxygen free radicals), catalases (to convert hydrogen peroxide to H_2O and O_2), and glutathione peroxidase and glutathione reductase, which alter cellular susceptibility to oxidants. When free radicals are released in massive amounts, intracellular defenses may be overcome, and the toxic radicals may enter the extracellular space and cause extensive tissue damage.

Oxygen radicals usually cause damage to biologic membranes by lipid peroxidation. As a consequence, important membrane-bound enzymes (such as Na-K ATPase, adenylate cyclase, and cytochrome oxidase) may be inactivated. Lipid peroxidation also increases the production of reactive fatty acid hydroperoxides that are also toxic to plasma membranes.

Neutrophil Proteases

Release of various proteases (such as elastase, β-glucuronidase, cathepsin G, and collagenase) from granules in the lysosomes of neutrophils can also cause severe lung damage (16). Some of these enzymes, particularly elastase, have been found in significant quantities in bronchoalveolar lavage fluid from patients with ARDS.

Arachidonic Acid Metabolites

When any injury to the cell membrane occurs, such as by free radicals or lysosomal enzymes, an increase in intracellular calcium occurs and this activates phospholipase. This causes release of arachidonic acid from the cell membrane (2). The arachidonic acid is then acted on by cyclooxygenase and lipooxygenase.

The cyclooxygenase pathway leads to the production of various prostaglandins, such as PGE_2, and PGI_2, and thromboxane (T_xA_2). Thromboxane is a vasoconstrictor, and it enhances platelet aggregation. The prostaglandins also increase PMN influx into the lung.

The lipoxygenase pathway produces hydroperoxyeicosatetraenoic acid (HPETE), which is rapidly converted to hydroxyeicosatetraenoic acid (HETE) and leukotriene A4 (LTA4). HETE is chemotactic, and leukotriene B4 aggregates white cells and stimulates them to release lysosomal free radicals and enzymes. The leukotrienes also constrict smooth muscle, increase vascular permeability, and can contribute to the edema associated with lung injury (17).

Complement Activation

Complement, especially C_{3a} and C_{5a}, cause PMN sequestration in the lungs (24). C_{5a} des arginine, a low-molecular weight cleavage product of complement, appears to be particularly important for pulmonary vascular leukosequestration (3). This substance can also initiate the respiratory burst in PMNs that results in production of superoxide anion and selective release of lysosomal contents.

AXIOM ARDS can occur in animals and patients with neutropenia and complement deficiencies, but the presence of complement and activated PMNs greatly accelerates and intensifies the process.

Platelets

A wide variety of physiologic process can cause extensive platelet aggregation and embolization to the lungs. When pulmonary reticuloendothelial and fibrinolytic activities are normal, platelets and large amounts of procoagulants may be cleared from the pulmonary microcirculation with minimal morbidity. In patients with severe trauma or sepsis, they can greatly aggravate the situation.

Platelet-Activating Factor

Platelet-activating factor (PAF) is a phospholipid mediator of inflammation that is produced by platelets, PMNs, monocytes, and alveolar macrophages (3). It exerts at least some of its effects through stimulation of prostaglandin and leukotriene synthesis. It can cause protein-rich pulmonary edema, increased pulmonary vascular resistance, and decreased pulmonary compliance when infused into experimental animals.

Cytokines

AXIOM Of the various cytokines released by inflammatory processes, tumor necrosis factor, IL-1, and IL-8 appear most likely to have a role in ARDS.

Tumor necrosis factor (TNF) is produced by monocytes exposed to various types of stimulation, including bacterial endotoxins (3). When it is injected into experimental animals, TNF can produce acute injury in the lungs and other tissues similar to that produced by infusion of endotoxin. TNF causes pulmonary margination of PMNs and also directly increases pulmonary capillary permeability.

Interleukin-1 (IL-1), which is derived from several different cells, including macrophages and endothelial cells, amplifies the inflammatory response to a wide variety of stimuli, including TNF. The biologic activities of IL-1 and TNF overlap considerably and include activation of fibroblasts and augmentation of endothelial cell production of a leukocyte-adherence-promoting glycoprotein.

Interleukin-8 (IL-8) is a potent neutrophil chemoattractant and can induce neutrophil superoxide anion production. Rodriguez et al. found that the amount of IL-8 in the lungs was significantly increased in patients with multiple injuries, pulmonary dysfunction, and need for more prolonged ventilatory support (18).

Pulmonary Capillary Endothelium

The pulmonary capillary endothelial surface provides about one-fourth of the total capillary surface area of the body and accounts for 40% of the cells in the lungs (3). Tight gap junctions are normally found between pulmonary endothelial cells, and these restrict the passage of water-soluble macromolecules into the interstitial space. When the lung is injured by endotoxin, the gap junctions become wider and allow increased extravasation of fluid and protein into the interstitium.

Vascular Occlusion

In addition to capillary endothelial lesions, ARDS is characterized by occlusion of capillaries and other small pulmonary vessels. Polymorphonuclear leukocytes, platelets, and fibrin contribute to occlusion of pulmonary capillaries, via the action of inflammatory mediators that cause them to adhere to endothelium. As a general rule, at least 75% to 80% of the pulmonary vascular tree must be occluded before there is an increase in pulmonary artery pressures to the levels seen in moderate-severe ARDS.

Pathophysiologic Changes

The three main pathophysiologic changes seen with ARDS include

1. Gas exchange abnormalities;
2. Pulmonary hypertension; and
3. Decreased pulmonary compliance.

Gas Exchange Abnormalities

Hypoxemia

AXIOM The most prominent laboratory abnormality in severe ARDS is hypoxemia, which responds relatively poorly to increases in FIO_2.

V/Q abnormalities in ARDS are believed to be caused principally by atelectasis and alveolar flooding. This, in turn, results in shunting of venous blood through the lungs into the arterial circulation without being completely oxygenated. This is best quantified by the PaO_2/FIO_2 ratio and the amount of physiologic shunting in the lungs (Q_{sp}/Q_t).

AXIOM A PaO_2/FIO_2 ratio (PFR) of less than 200 or a physiologic shunt in the lungs (Qsp/Qt) exceeding 20% and developing more than 2 or 3 days after trauma usually indicates ARDS.

Because arterial oxygen tension (PaO_2) varies directly with the fraction of inspired oxygen (FIO_2), it is convenient to express oxygenation as the ratio of the PaO_2 to the FIO_2 (PaO_2/FIO_2 ratio). Normal values are about 600, which is equivalent to a shunt (Q_{sp}/Q_t) of about 3% to 5% (Table 40-2). If the ratio were to decrease acutely to 200 in a patient with previously normal lungs, the Q_{sp}/Q_t usually would be about 20%, and the patient generally would need mechanical ventilatory assistance (see Table 40-2).

AXIOM Physiologic shunting in the lung is usually the most sensitive test for diagnosing impending or early respiratory failure.

Increased Dead Space

AXIOM The need for increased minute ventilation to maintain normal levels of $PaCO_2$ in ARDS is primarily due to an increased dead space fraction (V_d/V_t).

Table 40-2. *Interpretation of Pa_{O_2}/Fi_{O_2} Ratio*

Pa_{O_2}	Fi_{O_2}	Ratio	Q_s/Q_t (%)	Abnormality
240	0.4	600	5	None
120	0.4	300	10	Minimal
100	0.4	250	15	Mild
80	0.4	200	20	Moderate
60	0.4	150	30	Severe
40	0.4	100	40	Very severe

Although most physicians believe that CO_2 exchange in the lungs is relatively normal until late in ARDS, it is frequently altered almost as early as oxygen exchange. When the dead space fraction is normal (i.e., about 30%), minute ventilation (V_e) in a male adult is generally 5 to 6 L/min. When the dead space fraction increases to 60% to 70% as a result of large numbers of nonperfused alveoli, the minute ventilation (V_e) must increase to at least 12 to 15 L/min or more to maintain a eucapnic state.

AXIOM V_d/V_t exceeding 0.60 to 0.65 usually indicates a severe degree of ventilation-perfusion mismatch.

End-tidal CO_2 tends to decrease and the arterial–ET-CO_2 difference tends to increase as dead space increases, often because of inadequate blood flow to functional alveoli. In a recent study of ET-CO_2 changes during emergency surgery in 100 critically ill or injured patients, Domsky et al. found that the ET-CO_2 and the arterial end-tidal P_{CO_2} difference (P[a-ET]CO_2), could provide important prognostic information (19). The patients who survived generally had an ET-PCO_2 of 28 mm Hg or more and a P(a-ET)CO_2 difference of less than 10 mm Hg.

Pulmonary Hypertension

AXIOM Increasing pulmonary hypertension is probably the most frequent and consistent hemodynamic evidence of a poor prognosis following trauma.

In the early stages of ARDS, pulmonary hypertension is primarily the result of neurohumoral activity, including increased thromboxane A_2, leukotrienes, and serotonin. In the later stages of ARDS, various types of microemboli and interstitial edema are probably more important.

Decreased Pulmonary Compliance

The increased stiffness of the lung in ARDS, which is primarily caused by interstitial and alveolar edema, makes it more difficult to inflate the lung, reduces lung volumes, and increases the work of breathing. Tachypnea is usually the first clinical indication of increased lung stiffness in ARDS.

AXIOM If a low and decreasing static and dynamic pulmonary compliance cannot be corrected, the prognosis with ARDS is poor.

The compliance of the lung and chest wall can be quantitated relatively easily when the patient is intubated. Dynamic compliance (C_D) is obtained by dividing the tidal volume by the peak inspiratory pressure (PIP) minus the positive end-expiratory pressure (PEEP). Static compliance (C_S) is equal to the tidal volume divided by the inspiratory plateau pressure (IPP) (obtained during a 0.5-second respiratory hold) minus the PEEP. Thus, if the PIP is 40 cm H_2O, the IPP is 30 cm H_2O, the PEEP is 10 cm H_20, and the V_t 1000 mL:

$$C_D = V_t/PIP - PEEP = 1000/40 - 10 = 33 \text{ mL/cm } H_2O$$
$$C_S = V_t/IPP - PEEP = 1000/30 - 10 = 50 \text{ mL/cm } H_2O$$

Normal values are 60 to 100 mL/cm H_2O for C_D and 100 to 200 mL/cm H_20 for C_S. With ARDS, C_S values less than 50 mL/cm H_2O are commonly seen, and in severe cases, they may be less than 30 mL/cm H_2O.

AXIOM In general, tidal volumes and PEEP should be adjusted, as needed, to provide the best static compliance for ventilated patients.

CLINICAL PROGRESSION

The clinical progression of ARDS can be described as occurring in four stages (3). In the first stage, some dyspnea and tachypnea can be noted, but generally no changes are seen on chest radiography. In the second stage, hypoxemia begins to develop along with a decrease in the functional residual capacity, an increase in the dead space ventilation, and an increase in pulmonary vascular resistance.

The third stage of ARDS is marked by a progressive clinical pulmonary insufficiency that usually requires ventilatory support. At this stage, patients often require an FIO_2 in excess of 0.6 and a V_E of 12 L/min or more. This stage is often also recognizable by the appearance of diffuse, pulmonary infiltrates on chest radiography.

In the fourth stage, patients become increasingly refractory to ventilatory support and PEEP. Terminally, hypercapnia also develops. A complete white-out of the lungs may develop on chest radiography in this stage. In these patients, increasing right ventricular failure with progressively lower ejection fractions also develops.

DIAGNOSIS

The criteria for diagnosis of ARDS vary somewhat from author to author, but generally include:

1. An inciting problem, such as sepsis;
2. Normal pulmonary arterial wedge pressure (PAWP) of less than 12 to 18 mm Hg;
3. Hypoxemia with a PaO_2/FIO_2 ratio (PFR) of less than 200;
4. Presence of diffuse, patchy infiltrates on chest radiography; and
5. Absence of any other conditions that could cause these changes.

Clinical Criteria for Diagnosis

Increasing tachypnea is often the first sign of posttraumatic pulmonary insufficiency, but it is nonspecific. Examination of the lungs at this time usually reveals nothing more than some basilar rales and a decrease in breath sounds. Although the clinical response to a low PaO_2 is undoubtedly responsible for some of the signs of ARDS, most ARDS patients continue to hyperventilate even after administration of enough oxygen to correct the hypoxemia.

AXIOM Restlessness should be considered to be due to hypoxemia until proven otherwise.

If restlessness is due to hypoxia, the patient's movements tend to be purposeless, abrupt, and irregular, whereas the actions of a patient who is restless because of pain but who is adequately oxygenated are generally directed to reducing a particular irritant and are slower and more repetitive. When in doubt, it is best to assume that a restless patient is hypoxic until proven otherwise.

Cyanosis is a late sign of respiratory failure and generally does not develop in patients with hemoglobin levels less than 10.0 g/dL until or unless severe impairment of blood flow to the skin or mucous membranes occurs. It usually takes a minimum of 5.0 g of reduced hemoglobin in the capillaries of the skin or lips before a patient looks cyanotic.

Laboratory Studies

AXIOM With suspected ARDS, one should follow not only the P_{AO_2} and Pa_{CO_2}, but also the Pa_{O_2}/F_{IO_2} ratio, the $P(A\text{-}a)_{O_2}$, P_{VO_2}, S_{VO_2}, and Q_{SP}/Q_t.

In general, the ventilatory compensation for a metabolic acidosis should result in a $P_{CO_2} = [(HCO_3)(1.5) + 8 \pm 4]$. Thus, if the HCO_3 is 12 mEq/L, the Pa_{CO_2} should be $[(12)(1.5) + 8 \pm 4]$ or 26 ± 4 mm Hg. Thus, a P_{CO_2} exceeding 30 mm Hg in a patient with HCO_3 of 12 mm Hg indicates an inadequate ventilatory response.

If the Pa_{O_2}/F_{IO_2} ratio decreases to less than 200 (such as with a Pa_{O_2} less than 80 mm Hg on an F_{IO_2} greater than or equal to 0.4), this generally indicates moderate to severe pulmonary changes requiring ventilatory support.

Static Compliance

If the static lung compliance (C_s), which is normally at least 100 mL/cm H_20, is less than 50 mL/cm H_2O, then one should suspect that ARDS may be developing. A static compliance of less than 25 to 30 mL/cm H_2O is usually evidence of severe ARDS. Although a gradual increase in lung stiffness is characteristic of ARDS, a sudden increase in airway pressure should make one suspect a pneumothorax or major airway obstruction.

Radiologic Changes

Lung infiltrates seen immediately after trauma are usually due to pulmonary contusions. Localized infiltrates appearing after 24 to 48 hours are often due to aspiration, and diffuse infiltrates at that time are often due to fat emboli. Diffuse infiltrates appearing after 48 to 72 hours tend to be due to ARDS.

AXIOM It cannot be assumed that pulmonary function is satisfactory if the lungs appear relatively normal on chest radiography.

The earliest changes noted on chest radiography in ARDS usually include (1) scattered areas of mild platelike atelectasis, particularly at the lung bases posteriorly, and (2) signs of vascular congestion with increased prominence of perihilar vascular markings. In many of these patients, scattered, fluffy, irregular areas of increased density then develop. These pulmonary infiltrates may then enlarge and coalesce. Eventually, both lung fields may be completely "whited out" on chest radiography.

Computed tomography (CT) scans of the chest generally reveal the extent of the parenchymal involvement in ARDS much better than chest radiographs. The typical appearance of ARDS on CT scans includes ground-glass opacities with air bronchograms, with increasingly dense areas of consolidation in the dependent portions of the lungs.

TREATMENT

Eradicate All Underlying Infection

AXIOM If ARDS is developing or getting worse, it usually implies that an inadequately treated infection is present.

The primary goal in the treatment of ARDS is to control the underlying sepsis, which is generally present. This is particularly important in patients with peritonitis; however, it may be extremely difficult to find the source of sepsis in many of these patients. It has been hypothesized that ARDS in some patients without apparent infection may be a result of bacterial translocation from the gastrointestinal tract. Although this has been well documented in experimental animals, the frequency and importance of bacterial translocation in the gut in humans is questionable.

General Supportive Measures

Frequent position changes, elevation of the head and chest, chest physiotherapy, and encouraging the patient to cough and take deep breaths may dramatically reduce pulmonary complications in severely injured patients.

Distended bowel and increased ascitic fluid may elevate the diaphragm markedly, thereby reducing tidal volume and increasing the work of breathing. This should be prevented or corrected with early nasogastric suction or paracentesis as needed.

One of the greatest deterrents to effective breathing and coughing following trauma is pain from an injury or surgical incision involving the chest or upper abdomen. Such pain can be controlled with multiple small doses of intravenous morphine, but these narcotics can also depress the cough reflex and ventilation markedly. Epidural analgesia is especially helpful in these patients.

AXIOM Controlling pain so that the patient can take deep breaths and cough effectively is probably the single best way to prevent atelectasis or pneumonia following trauma.

When the patient has a high fever or is agitated, oxygen requirements may be greatly increased. To reduce increased VO_2, one should reduce the patient's temperature with drugs, sponging, or induced hypothermia. If the patient is in pain, this is generally best corrected by epidural analgesia. Sedatives or muscle relaxants may also be used, but with caution, especially if the patient is not on a ventilator.

AXIOM When restlessness is due to pain, analgesics may be indicated; however, when restlessness is due to hypoxia, such agents may be lethal.

Fluid Therapy

Although rapid restoration of the blood volume after bleeding has been controlled and maintenance of a high-oxygen delivery to tissues is important to survival, once an adequate perfusion has been attained, the continued administration of fluid must be done carefully, with close attention to vital signs, central venous pressure (CVP), PAWP, urine output, and tissue perfusion.

AXIOM Excess fluid can greatly aggravate the tendency to develop ARDS.

Although the use of colloids to resuscitate trauma patients is extremely controversial, some value may exist in maintaining a colloid osmotic pressure that is at least one-half to two-thirds of the normal value of 22 to 28 mm Hg.

Although the optimal hemoglobin in critically injured patients is debated and is believed by many physicians to be about 10 g/dL with a hematocrit of about 30%, hemoglobin levels of 12.0 g/dL or higher tend to be associated with better survival rates.

In my experience, even when the initial hematocrit was about 30%, each unit of packed red blood cells given increased oxygen content 7% to 10% and increased oxygen delivery (DO_2) 4% to 6%.

AXIOM Increased oxygen-carrying capacity of the blood is particularly important in patients who have cardiac or pulmonary dysfunction.

Achieving Optimal DO_2 and VO_2

Numerous studies have shown the benefit of early "optimal" (supranormal) levels of DO_2 and VO_2 in preventing organ failure after surgery or trauma. Shoemaker et al. showed that increasing the DO_2 to greater than 600 mL/min/m^2 and the VO_2 to greater than or equal to 170 mL/min/m^2 reduced the incidence of pulmonary complications in high-risk surgical patients from 27% (16 of 60) to 4% (1 of 28) (20).

Fleming et al., in a prospective study of resuscitation in 67 patients with severe trauma (mean ISS = 27), found that *early* postinjury attainment of supranormal cardiac index (at least 4.5 L/min/m^2), DO_2 (at least 670 mL/min/m^2), and VO_2 (at least 160 mL/min/m^2) resulted in fewer deaths (14% versus 44%) and a lower incidence of respiratory failure (39% versus 68%) (21).

Nutritional Support

AXIOM Early, aggressive enteral nutrition appears to reduce complications after trauma.

Moore and Moore showed that early, aggressive enteral feeding of trauma patients is feasible despite major intraabdominal injuries and is preferable to parenteral nutrition because of the reduced incidence of septic complications (22). There also may be increased benefits from using arginine, dietary nucleotides, lipids from fish oil, and glutamine (23).

Commonly Used Drugs

Although it is not usually a prominent feature in respiratory failure following trauma, bronchospasm or wheezing should be treated aggressively if it occurs. Inotropic agents can be used to improve cardiac output and oxygen delivery if they are not optimal after fluid loading. Intravenous diuretics may help correct pulmonary insufficiency in patients with evidence of fluid overloading; however, great care must be taken to prevent hypovolemia as a result of excessive diuresis.

Oxygen

Unless an FIO_2 (fraction of inspired oxygen) exceeding 0.6 is required, the arterial PO_2 should be kept at 70 to 80 mm Hg in patients who have had recent, severe trauma. Concern about oxygen toxicity should not prevent the administration of FIO_2 of 0.60 or more if this is the only way to maintain a PaO_2 of at least 50 mm Hg in patients with severe ARDS.

Ventilatory Support

Indications

A ventilator should be used in trauma patients whenever the clinical situation or laboratory studies suggest that the patient has inadequate ventilation or respiratory failure is likely to develop.

Some of the more frequent clinical indications for early ventilatory assistance in injured patients include the following:

1. Flail chest, particularly if bilateral or involving seven or more ribs;
2. Severe pulmonary contusion with hypoxemia;
3. Severe CNS depression caused by trauma, drugs, or infection;
4. Injury to three or more major organs requiring surgery;
5. Previous severe pulmonary disease;
6. Severe, prolonged shock; and

7. Massive smoke inhalation or aspiration of vomitus.

Some of the laboratory values that suggest a need for ventilatory assistance in injured patients include

1. Arterial Po_2 less than 60 mm Hg on room air or Pao_2 less than 80 mm Hg on 40% or more oxygen;
2. Arterial Pco_2 greater than 50 mm Hg (in the absence of metabolic alkalosis);
3. Alveolar-arterial oxygen difference greater than 55 mm Hg on room air or greater than 350 to 400 mm Hg on 100% O_2;
4. Physiologic shunting in the lung greater than 20%; and
5. Pao_2:$F\text{IO}_2$ ratio less than 200.

Endotracheal Intubation

If there is any question about the adequacy of the upper airway or minute ventilation in a severely injured patient, the patient should be intubated and ventilatory support provided promptly.

Ordering Ventilatory Care

Orders for ventilatory assistance should include

1. The type of ventilatory support to be used;
2. The gases to be delivered;
3. The tidal volume;
4. The ventilatory pressure range;
5. The ventilatory rate;
6. The amount of PEEP; and
7. The frequency of sighing.

Type of Ventilatory Support

Ventilators. A pressure-cycled ventilator delivers gas until the pressure limit selected is reached, at which point the exhalation valve opens. Delivery of a specific volume of gas with each breath may be difficult; however, by assessing the airway resistance encountered and the dynamic compliance of the patient's lungs, the flow rates and pressure limits can usually be adjusted to provide adequate tidal volumes.

Volume-cycled ventilators, in which inspiration is terminated by delivery of a preset volume, are more suitable than pressure-cycled machines for patients with "stiff" lungs caused by ARDS, but the higher pressures generated may cause increased lung damage. Volume-cycled ventilators have a pressure-limit control that can be adjusted to a level slightly higher than the peak airway pressure generated by delivery of a preset tidal volume; however, one may have to lower inspiratory flow rates or tidal volumes or prolong the time for inspiration if the inspiratory pressure gets too high.

With high-frequency ventilation (HFV), the lung is ventilated at a frequency exceeding 60 cycles/min. Compared to conventional ventilatory modes, HFV reduces mean airway pressure (P_{aw}) and PIP. It is of most use in patients with a bronchopulmonary fistula. The tracheal mucosa can be seriously damaged by the low humidity of the gases often used.

Level of Ventilatory Support

With full ventilatory support, all of the work of breathing required to maintain eucapnia is provided by the ventilator. This may be provided by controlled ventilation or with assist-control ventilation.

The control mode of ventilation is used if one wants the patient's breathing rate to be completely determined by the ventilator. In this mode, the patient is not able to trigger inspiration independently, but receives breaths at a predetermined rate. To use this mode, one must usually paralyze or heavily sedate the patient.

The assist-control mode of ventilatory support allows patients to initiate inspiration as directed by their intrinsic respiratory drive. In this mode, the machine is triggered to deliver a breath after an inspiratory effort of the patient, which is sensed at the ventilator as slight negative pressure. A preset tidal volume is then delivered. If the patient does not initiate any breaths, the ventilator is set to deliver preset tidal volumes at a preset rate.

Partial Ventilatory Support. **Intermittent mandatory ventilation** (IMV) has been proposed as a technique to help wean adults from mechanical ventilatory support. IMV consists basically of two independent circuits connected to the patient. In one circuit, patients can breathe spontaneously from a reservoir bag, at whatever rate and depth is desired. The other circuit is connected to the ventilator, which delivers mandatory inspirations of a preset volume at a set rate. This allows the patient to breathe spontaneously as much as desired with mechanical inflations supplied at regular preset intervals.

One of the main physiologic advantages of IMV is the lower inspiratory intrapleural pressures during spontaneous breathing. This results in increased right ventricular filling and cardiac output. Spontaneous breathing with IMV also promotes more normal matching of ventilation to perfusion.

Synchronized intermittent mandatory ventilation (SIMV) allows spontaneous breathing between mechanically delivered ventilator breaths, but the mandatory ventilator breaths are synchronized to begin with the patient's next spontaneous inspiratory effort. This technique was introduced because of concern that a mechanical breath might "stack" with a spontaneous breath, causing a great increase in peak inspiratory and alveolar pressures.

Pressure-support ventilation (PSV) is a form of mechanical ventilation in which the patient's spontaneous inspiratory efforts are augmented with a previously selected level of positive pressure so that airway pressure is held constant at an increased level throughout the inspiratory period (24). The inspiratory pressure support in PSV is usually in the range of 5 to 15 cm H_2O. This pressure is held constant until the patient's inspiratory flow demand decreases to a preselected percentage of the initial peak mechanical inspiratory flow. Following this, passive exhalation occurs. PSV is different from conventional volume-cycled ventilation in that, with PSV, the clinician selects only the inspiratory pressure; the patient controls the ventilatory timing and interacts with the delivered pressure to determine the inspiratory flow and tidal volume.

When 3 to 8 cm H_2O-pressure support is incorporated with SIMV, the work of breathing imposed by the endotracheal tube, ventilator circuit, and demand valve system is reduced to that of a continuous flow system. With levels exceeding 10 cm H_2O, pressure support may be considered an independent mode of ventilation. Pressure support is generally superior to IMV or SIMV as a partial support mode because the work of breathing is assisted with every breath, and most patients are more comfortable.

Severe unilateral lung injury may best be managed with a double-lumen endobronchial catheter and **synchronous independent lung ventilation**. In these patients, the standard forms of mechanical ventilation can make the ventilation-perfusion abnormality worse by overexpanding the more normal lung and underventilating the damaged lung.

Total Ventilatory Support. In patients with high ventilatory pressures, especially if the plateau (alveolar) pressure exceeds 30 to 35 cm H_20, one should use lower tidal volumes or **pressure-controlled ventilation** (PCV). PCV begins inspiration at preset time intervals, rapidly achieves the preset circuit pressure, maintains the preset inspiratory pressure, and ends the inspiratory cycle at a preset time interval. Assuming an adequate inspiratory time, the delivered tidal volume is determined by the preset airway pressure and pulmonary compliance.

With PCV, tidal volumes and minute ventilation may be so low that the P_{CO_2} increases above normal. This "**permissive hypercapnia**" does not seem to cause problems as long as the arterial pH does not decrease too abruptly. Hickling et al. managed 50 patients with severe ARDS by limiting the peak inspiratory pressure and disregarding the resultant hypercapnia (25). Tidal volumes were reduced to as low as 5 mL/kg. The mean maximum Pa_{CO_2} was 62 torr and the highest Pa_{CO_2} was 129 torr. No specific treatment was given for the respiratory acidosis that developed, and no statistical difference was found in the maximum Pa_{CO_2} of survivors and nonsurvivors. The group mortality rate of 16% was significantly lower than the 40% mortality rate predicted by the Acute Physiology and Chronic Health Evaluation II (APACHE II) scoring system, and only a single death was attributed to respiratory failure.

Inverse ratio ventilation (IRV) should be considered in patients requiring an F_{IO_2} of more than 0.6 to maintain a Pa_{O_2} of at least 60 mm Hg. Normally, the ratio of the inspiratory time (I) to expiratory time (E) is 1:2, 1:3, or 1:4. Positive-pressure ventilation with the inspiratory time (I) equal to or less than the expiratory time (E) is referred to as IRV, which improves gas exchange by a progressive alveolar recruitment, but it may take several hours for such recruitment to be fully accomplished. IRV can be provided with PCV and has been used successfully to treat a number of cases of severe respiratory failure in infants and adults whose cases did not respond to other types of ventilatory support (26).

Gases to be Delivered

The gases most frequently used in mechanical ventilation are oxygen and compressed air. Whenever possible, the oxygen concentration is limited to the minimum required to provide reasonable oxygenation of the blood (i.e., an arterial oxygen saturation of at least 90%), particularly if an F_{IO_2} greater than 0.5 is required to do that. When high ventilatory pressures are required, one may have to be satisfied with a Pa_{O_2} of 50 to 59 mm Hg (i.e., "permissive" hypoxemia).

AXIOM In most situations in which a ventilator is used, the injured patient needs mechanical assistance, and providing additional oxygen is often only a secondary consideration.

When initially ventilating the patient, it may be wise to use 100% oxygen (F_{IO_2} = 1.0) for at least 20 minutes, and then obtain a set of blood gases. This allows one to determine what F_{IO_2} is probably needed to maintain a Pa_{O_2} of about 70 to 80 mm Hg.

Tidal Volume

The tidal volume in patients with relatively normal lungs is generally started at about 10 to 12 mL/kg. Using a ventilatory rate of 10 to 16/min, the V_t is usually adjusted to provide a Pa_{CO_2} of 35 to 40 mm Hg. There is an increasing tendency to use tidal volumes as low as 5 to 7 mL/kg to keep ventilatory pressures low so as to prevent volutrauma (overdistension of alveoli).

Ventilatory Pressure

The airway pressure required to inflate the lungs properly varies greatly from patient to patient and is largely dependent on the tidal volume used, the inspiratory flow rate, and the resistance of the airway, lungs, and chest wall. In general, plateau pressures (during an inspiratory hold of 0.5 second) less than 30 to 35 cm H_2O are relatively safe.

If a certain tidal volume seems to be needed but the ventilatory pressures are too high, one can reduce the inflation pressures by decreasing the inspiratory flow rate, prolonging the inspiratory time, or using PCV; however, such maneuvers also increase the tendency to auto-PEEP.

AXIOM Patients with high ventilatory pressures may have increased pleural fluid that may not be detected clinically or radiographically but that will benefit from chest tube drainage.

Ventilatory Rate

Normally, a ventilatory rate of 8 to 16 per minute with an inspiration-to-expiratory time ratio (I/E) of 1:2 is used. In patients with either acute or chronic restrictive lung disease, requiring use of low tidal volumes, ventilatory rates exceeding 20/min may be necessary, depending on the desired V_E and targeted $Pa{CO_2}$.

Positive End-Expiratory Pressure

PEEP can be very effective for treating ARDS (27). The major pulmonary effects of continuous positive airway pressure (CPAP)/PEEP therapy are redistribution of extravascular lung water from the less compliant interstitial spaces (between the alveolar epithelium and capillary endothelium where gas exchange occurs) to the more compliant interstitial spaces (toward the peribronchial and hilar areas). Recruitment of collapsed alveoli also occurs. This redistribution of extravascular lung water also usually results in improved oxygen diffusion and improved lung compliance, especially if any alveolar fluid is present.

AXIOM The main functions of PEEP are to keep alveoli expanded during expiration and increase the patient's functional residual capacity back toward normal.

PEEP tends to "splint" the lung in an inflated state by keeping unstable alveoli open at end-expiration. PEEP acting on alveoli that contain fluid tends to "spread the fluid out" over a larger area so that the distance for oxygen to diffuse from alveoli into capillaries is reduced.

The major problem with PEEP is its tendency to reduce venous return and cardiac output, especially with levels greater than 10 to 15 cm H_2O; consequently, monitoring of PAWP and DO_2I is important in patients with more than 10 cm H_2O PEEP.

The reduced preload seen with PEEP can be offset to some extent by increasing intravascular volume or using inotropes. PEEP also increases pulmonary vascular resistance and right ventricular afterload. With an intact pericardium, the resultant right ventricular dilation can also decrease left ventricular filling.

PEEP is usually applied in 2.5- to 5.0-cm H_2O increments, and it takes at least 20 to 30 minutes for it to exert its full effect on oxygenation. Simultaneous monitoring of SaO_2 by pulse oximeter and of $Sv{O_2}$ by continuous, mixed venous oximetry catheter may expedite estimation of intrapulmonary shunt (Q_{sp}/Q_t), oxygen utilization, and oxygen extraction to help determine the optimal levels of PEEP.

Although PEEP has been used for more than 25 years since it was first described by Ashbaugh and Petty (28), the "optimal" level of PEEP is still controversial. Initially, optimal PEEP was believed to be the level that provided the best static lung compliance. Later, "best PEEP" was believed to be the level of PEEP that achieved the lowest Q_{sp}/Q_t without a physiologically significant decrease in cardiac output (27). The term "rational PEEP" has been used by some to indicate the level of PEEP that maintains an adequate DO_2 but allows the $F{IO_2}$ to be reduced to less than 0.5 to 0.6.

Auto-PEEP. In patients with high minute ventilation or any tendency to bronchoconstriction, increasing end-expiratory lung volumes can develop if expiration is interrupted by the next inspiratory effort. The resulting increased end-expiratory lung volume is termed *dynamic hyperinflation, auto-PEEP,* or *intrinsic PEEP.*

Adverse effects of excessive auto-PEEP are that (1) the respiratory muscles operate at an unfavorable position on their length-tension curve and (2) breathing takes place at a higher, less compliant portion of the pressure-volume curve of the lung. In addition, a much greater reduction in alveolar pressure may be required to trigger the ventilator.

AXIOM If increases in minute ventilation cause an increase in the $Pa{CO_2}$, one should suspect that significant auto-PEEP is present.

To measure the amount of auto-PEEP present, one can occlude the expiratory port of the ventilator circuit immediately before the onset of the next breath. The pressure in the lungs and ventilator circuit equilibrate, and the level of auto-PEEP is displayed on the ventilator manometer. The level of auto-PEEP can also be estimated from continuous recordings of air flow during mechanical ventilation.

Therapeutic measures to reduce the level of auto-PEEP include bronchodilators, a larger diameter endotracheal tube, decreased minute ventilation by controlling fever and pain, and increasing expiratory time ratio by increasing the inspiratory flow rate.

Continuous Positive Airway Pressure

In patients who are breathing spontaneously, CPAP and spontaneous PEEP (sPEEP) can be used to prevent airway and alveolar collapse during expiration. With CPAP, both the inspiratory and expiratory pressures are positive, although the inspiratory level may be less. With sPEEP, airway pressure is zero or negative (subambient) during inspiration, but it is increased at the end of expiration to a predetermined positive pressure.

Sighing

AXIOM Intermittent sighing is an important method for preventing atelectasis in patients taking frequent, small, spontaneous, or ventilator breaths.

Under normal circumstances, individuals spontaneously take at least four to six deep breaths (sighs) each hour. These sighs inflate many of the alveoli that are not opened with the usual tidal volumes. With patients who are weaning and taking only small rapid breaths, it is important to hyperinflate the lungs at least two to three times each hour with a tidal volume 1.5 to 2 times greater than normal, as long as the peak inflation pressures do not exceed 45 to 50 cm H_2O. The optimal frequency of sighing varies among patients but four to six times per hour appears to be satisfactory for most patients.

Nebulization and Humidification

In general, one should provide the maximum humidity possible to patients on a ventilator because of the drying effect that most ventilators have on the tracheobronchial tree. However, in small patients, particularly those with heart disease, some of the newer machines can provide so much moisture that the quantity of fluid absorbed through the alveoli and bronchial mucosa may overload the circulation and cause congestive heart failure.

Monitoring Ventilatory Support

Ventilatory parameters requiring frequent monitoring are tidal volume, respiratory rate, PIP, plateau pressure (during an inspiratory hold), PEEP, FIO_2, and minute ventilation. The patient and the ventilatory equipment should be monitored at least every 1 to 2 hours.

A rapid increase in PIP may be the result of a mucous plug, pneumothorax, kinking of the endotracheal tube, or slipping into a mainstem bronchus. A slow progressive increase in airway pressure is usually an indication of increasing lung stiffness and deteriorating pulmonary function. A rapid decrease in pressure usually indicates a ventilator or circuit disconnection or an endotracheal cuff leak.

Blood Gases

AXIOM The patient who is awake, alert, comfortable, and cooperative, and has normal vital signs on a ventilator is generally doing well, even if arterial blood gases (ABGs) do not appear to be optimal.

The arterial PO_2 should be kept at 60 mm Hg or higher, and preferably at 70 to 80 mm Hg, unless one would have to increase the FIO_2 above 0.5 or use high-ventilatory pressures. Although the $PaCO_2$ has traditionally been kept at about 35 to 40 mm Hg in most trauma patients on a ventilator, there is an increasing tendency to use lower tidal volumes to keep alveolar pressures low and allow some (permissive) hypercapnea to develop.

AXIOM In critically injured patients in the ICU, obtaining venous blood gases at the same time as ABGs provides a great deal more physiologic information.

Several pulmonary artery catheters have been developed to continuously monitor mixed venous oxygen saturation (SvO_2). The normal SvO_2 is about 70% to 75%. When DO_2 decreases (because of a decrease in cardiac output, arterial oxygen content, or oxygen delivery), SvO_2 tends to decrease. Thus, changes in the SvO_2 can provide early warning of problems with the lungs or cardiovascular system.

AXIOM If the SvO_2 increases to greater than or equal to 80%, the catheter tip may have wedged into a small pulmonary artery so that pulmonary capillary (oxygenated) blood is being analyzed.

A decrease in SvO_2 to less than 50% to 60% is usually the result of a significant decrease in cardiac output so that oxygen delivery to the tissues is inadequate. This could also be caused by an increase in oxygen consumption. Although a sudden decrease in SvO_2 often indicates important physiologic changes, the patient's condition can deteriorate seriously sometimes without any change in SvO_2.

⊘ PITFALL

Assuming that a patient's cardiovascular and pulmonary systems are stable because the SvO_2 has not changed.

Pulse Oximetry

Continuous monitoring of oxygen saturation and pulse amplitude in the fingers, toes, or ears with pulse oximetry can provide early warning of pulmonary or cardiovascular deterioration before it becomes clinically apparent; however, impaired local perfusion or a high PO_2 can limit its accuracy and usefulness. It is also not unusual for a pulse oximeter to indicate an arterial oxygen saturation that is 2% to 3% higher than the values seen on ABG analysis.

Capnography

Capnography, by monitoring the PCO_2 in expired gases, can provide a real-time estimate of $PaCO_2$. This can help assess ventilatory adequacy and the cardiovascular status of the patient. Although the measurement of end-tidal carbon dioxide (ET CO_2) underestimates $PaCO_2$ by at least 2 to 6 mm Hg in patients on a ventilator, the difference is constant for a given patient provided the dead space to tidal volume ratio (V_d/V_t) and airway resistance do not change.

AXIOM If dead space in the lung increases, as with a pulmonary embolus or hypovolemia, the ET-CO_2 tends to decrease and arterial-ET CO_2 differences increase.

Efforts should be made with fluid resuscitation or adjustment of ventilator settings to get the arterial-ET P_{CO_2} difference to 10 mm Hg or less (19).

VENTILATORY WEANING

Criteria for Weaning

General Condition of the Patient

One should not attempt to wean patients from a ventilator if they are hemodynamically unstable or if the problem that initially required the mechanical support has not been corrected. The patient to be weaned should not be septic, and chest radiography should be improving or at least "stable."

AXIOM Rapid, shallow breathing, respiratory alternans, or abdominal paradox during attempts at spontaneous breathing generally indicate that the patient is not ready to be weaned from the ventilator.

Weaning Parameters

Tests to help determine whether a patient is ready for withdrawal from ventilatory support can be separated into three areas of assessment:

1. Ability to oxygenate;
2. Resting ventilatory needs; and
3. Ventilatory mechanical capability.

Young, cooperative, otherwise healthy patients can often be weaned successfully even though they do not meet the aforementioned criteria.

AXIOM In elderly and uncooperative individuals, particularly those with other organ system dysfunction, even the presence of optimal criteria does not guarantee successful weaning.

In general, the F_{IO_2} to maintain a Pa_{O_2} of at least 80 mm Hg should be less than 0.35 to 0.40. A P_{CO_2} higher than one would expect from the pH or bicarbonate levels generally indicates that one should not attempt weaning, unless the patient has chronic obstructive pulmonary disease (COPD) with chronic hypercarbia. As a general rule, the arterial P_aCO_2 should not be higher than $[(HCO_3)(1.5) + 8 \pm 4]$. As a corollary, the minute ventilation (V_E) in a typical male adult should generally be less than 10 to 12 L/min (5.8 to 7.0 L/min/m^2) before the patient can be weaned from the ventilator.

The respiratory rate (machine breaths plus spontaneous breaths) ideally should be less than 20 per minute and, preferably, less than 30 per minute before attempting weaning. It was found, for example, that if, after a minute of spontaneous breathing, the respiratory rate (RR) increased to 38 per minute or more, the weaning failure rate was 80% (12 of 15). In contrast, if the RR stayed at 25 per minute or less after 1 minute, the failure rate was only 13% (2 of 15).

Yang and Tobin (29) did a retrospective study of indices used to try to predict when weaning from mechanical ventilation was possible. They found that rapid, shallow breathing, as reflected by respiration rate/tidal volume ratio (RR/V_t) after 1 minute of spontaneous breathing, was the most accurate predictor of weaning failure (29). If the RR/V_t ratio was greater than or equal to 100 breaths per minute per liter (i.e., RR ≥ 30 with a $V_t \leq 0.3$ L), 95% (19 of 20) of the patients failed the weaning attempt. At an RR/V_t ratio of 80 to 100 breaths/min/L, the failure rate was 50% (6 of 12), and with an RR/V_t ratio less than 80, the weaning failure rate was 9% (3 of 32).

The two mechanical ventilatory parameters that have been used most frequently to evaluate a patient's ability to be weaned are the forced vital capacity (FVC) and the negative inspiratory force (NIF). The FVC in young adults is normally about 65 to 70 mL/kg, and patients usually need an FVC of at least 10 mL/kg and, preferably

15 mL/kg, before they are ready to be taken off the ventilator. In normal individuals, NIF can be greater than 100 to 150 cm H_2O, but a patient usually only has to have NIF of at least 25 to 30 cm H_2O to be weaned successfully.

Techniques of Weaning

The three most frequent methods used for weaning patients from mechanical ventilatory support are the traditional T-piece trials, IMV, and PSV.

T-Piece Trials

With T-piece weaning, one can either use an abrupt "sink-or-swim" trial or gradually increase the periods of spontaneous ventilation on the T-piece. If the duration of the intubation was brief in a relatively healthy individual, the patient can generally assume the work of breathing fairly abruptly. The trial period can extend from a few minutes to several hours before extubation. If the patient becomes anxious or restless, or becomes tachycardic or tachypneic, the trial is ended, and one can try again 6 to 12 hours later, or switch to a more gradual withdrawal technique.

In patients who have been on a ventilator for more than a few days or who have severe muscle weakness, gradually prolonged trial periods of spontaneous ventilation are more likely to be successful. During these periods, the patient breathes a humidified gas mixture with enough O_2 to maintain an SaO_2 of at least 90%.

AXIOM In weaning patients from prolonged ventilatory support, it is essential to provide adequate rest between periods of "stress."

Intermittent Mechanical Ventilation Technique

With the IMV technique of weaning, the patient is allowed to assume the work of breathing progressively by gradually decreasing the number of ventilator breaths between the patient's spontaneous efforts. The number of ventilator breaths per minute can generally be reduced if the following criteria are met:

1. pH is greater than or equal to 7.35;
2. PCO_2 is less than or equal to 45 mm Hg; and
3. Ventilator rate plus spontaneous breaths is less than or equal to 30 per minute.

If the patient remains clinically stable at an IMV rate of 2 to 4 breaths per minute, one can usually discontinue mechanical ventilation successfully. If the patient is unable to progress beyond an IMV of 2 to 4 per minute, further weaning on 5 to 10 cm H_2O CPAP or PSV can be tried.

Pressure-Support Ventilation Technique

Pressure support ventilation is increasingly used to gradually decrease the level of ventilator support. The level of PSV is gradually decreased to the level that compensates for the resistance of the endotracheal tube and ventilatory circuit (usually 3 to 5 cm H_20). The patient can often then be extubated at that level of PSV if he or she meets the weaning criteria.

Improving the Chances of Weaning

When there is failure to wean, despite all efforts to improve ventilation, one should consider doing the following:

1. Improve nutrition, especially protein, but reduce the carbohydrate load.
2. Correct any potassium, calcium, phosphorus, thyroid, or adrenal deficiencies.
3. Discontinue all sedatives and muscle relaxants.
4. Consider epidural analgesia for continued chest or abdominal pain.
5. Search for organic neuromuscular disease.
6. Consider methylprednisolone in COPD patients or in those with evidence of pulmonary fibrosis (0.5 mg/kg/day and then gradually withdrawn over 1 to 2 weeks).
7. Vitamin B_{12}, 1,000 μg intramuscularly to improve muscle strength, especially in elderly individuals.

Other Therapy

Corticosteroids

In patients who have ARDS but who cannot be weaned from the ventilator after 2 to 3 weeks in an ICU, despite eradication of all infection, methylprednisolone has been of some help in selected patients who have evidence of increasing pulmonary fibrosis. The dose of methylprednisolone used by Ashbaugh and Maier under such circumstances was 125 mg intravenously every 6 hours (plus antacids and H_2-blockers) until evidence of improvement occurred (30). The dose was then gradually tapered. They used this regimen successfully in eight of ten selected surgical patients. Previously, similar patients of theirs had a mortality rate exceeding 85%.

Nitric Oxide

Inhaled nitric oxide (NO) had been reported to be a helpful selective pulmonary vasodilator. The ability of NO to dilate blood vessels, block platelet aggregation, inhibit leukocyte adhesion, and scavenge superoxide suggests that NO can play a role in endothelium protection and maintenance of microvascular blood flow during sepsis (31). Rossaint et al. reported on 16 patients with severe ARDS who were given inhaled NO (32). The NO reduced the mean pulmonary artery pressure, decreased the physiologic shunt, and increased the $Pa{O_2}/F{IO_2}$ ratio from 152 ± 15 mm Hg to 199 ± 23 mm Hg (p=.008).

Johannigman et al. (33) and Dellinger et al. (34) found that inhaled NO was successful in increasing the $Pa{O_2}/F{IO_2}$ ratio or pulmonary artery pressures. However, a trial of inhaled NO at a dose of less than 10 ppm may be helpful in determining which ARDS patients are most apt to benefit from NO.

Freeman et al. (31), in a review of the literature on NO, have also noted that use of this endogenous vasodilator is associated with hypotension, catecholamine hyporesponsiveness, and myocardial depression in septic shock. Furthermore, NO is cytotoxic and can cause direct tissue injury and contribute to sepsis-induced multiple organ failure. Thus, like many other endogenous mediators of sepsis, NO appears to have both harmful and beneficial effects.

Triiodothyronine

The “sick euthyroid syndrome” with low circulating levels of free triiodothyronine (T_3) is frequently seen in critically ill or injured patients. Noting that lung function, growth, and repair are dependent on thyroid hormonal stimulation, Dulchavsky and Bailey experimentally demonstrated improved lung compliance, histologic integrity, and surfactant availability with T_3 administration during sepsis-induced hypothyroidism (35). They also showed that administration of T_3 to septic animals helps to restore pulmonary vascular permeability and compliance to normal without affecting cellular metabolic rates (36).

Extracorporeal Membrane Oxygenator

Extracorporeal membrane oxygenation (ECMO) is the term used to describe prolonged cardiopulmonary bypass using a membrane lung to exchange oxygen and carbon dioxide. Despite the initial dismal results with ECMO, Anderson et al. reported on the use of extracorporeal life support (ECLS) for severe ARDS in 17 multiply injured adults who were considered moribund despite conventional mechanical ventilation (37). Eleven patients were successfully weaned off ECLS and nine were discharged from the hospital (53% survival rate). Delay in beginning ECLS reduces its benefits. Pranikoff et al. (38) noted in 36 patients treated with ECLS that the mortality rates increased about 10% for each day the patient had ventilatory support before going on ECLS.

Extracorporeal carbon dioxide removal ($ECCO_2R$) is a venovenous technique introduced in 1980 to provide carbon dioxide removal in adults (39). This technique may decrease mortality rate in adults with severe, acute respiratory failure by allowing adequate carbon dioxide removal with significantly reduced tidal volumes and thereby reduced airway pressures. In a randomized, controlled, clinical trial by Morris et al., however, no survival advantage was demonstrated for the $ECCO_2R$ (40).

OUTCOME

The mortality rate with ARDS after trauma still averages about 30% to 40%. The overwhelming majority of these deaths are caused by MOF, usually because of persistent sepsis or some other inflammatory problem.

After 1 year, most survivors of ARDS are not restricted in their activities; however, in some of the patients who had a prolonged need for oxygen concentrations exceeding 60%, permanent restrictive changes and pulmonary hypertension develop.

⊘ FREQUENT ERRORS

1. ***Delay of ventilatory assistance until obvious clinical evidence of severe respiratory failure exists.***
2. ***Assuming that a patient's lungs are functioning well if the patient is not in obvious distress, has "good color," and has relatively normal chest radiographs.***
3. ***Failure to realize that if severely injured or septic patients are not hyperventilating, "something is wrong."***
4. ***Failure to realize that an injured patient with only a mild to moderate reduction in arterial PO_2 but a very low $PaCO_2$ actually has a severe alveolar-arterial O_2 difference associated with significant pulmonary changes.***
5. ***Reliance on absolute values rather than on trends in the patient's ventilatory parameters and blood gases.***
6. ***Increasing the FIO_2 to more than 0.5 to 0.6 rather than using improved ventilation and PEEP to elevate the arterial PO_2.***
7. ***Failure to keep ventilatory pressures low to reduce or prevent the development of "volutrauma."***
8. ***Failure to adequately monitor DO_2 and VO_2 when increasing PEEP to more than 10 cm H_2O.***
9. ***Failure to look hard enough for infections or pulmonary emboli in patients whose lungs are getting progressively worse.***

SUMMARY POINTS

1. The most important predisposing factor for ARDS is inadequately treated sepsis.

2. Giving excess fluids to a patient in whom ARDS is developing greatly accelerates the pulmonary dysfunction.

3. Patients who receive massive blood transfusions have an increased chance of developing ARDS, primarily because of the increased chance of becoming septic.

4. An increase in the $P(A\text{-}a)O_2$ and a decrease in the platelet count occurs in virtually all patients with major fractures.

5. Many more pulmonary emboli occur than are ever suspected antemortem. Any sudden increase in the $P(a\text{-}ET)CO_2$ difference should make one suspect a pulmonary embolus.

6. A normal lung scan effectively rules out a significant pulmonary embolus.

7. Ventilator-induced lung injury appears to be due to overdistension of alveoli (i.e., volutrauma), rather than just exposure of the alveoli to high pressures (i.e., barotrauma).

8. Intraalveolar distending pressures (as reflected by the "plateau pressure" during an inspiratory hold) should be kept less than 30 to 35 cm H_2O.

9. Toxic oxygen radicals released from neutrophils attached to pulmonary capillary endothelium are probably the most important cause of the early changes in ARDS.

10. Pathologically, ARDS is characterized by congestive atelectasis, which is usually worse in the dependent portion of the lungs.

11. A PaO_2/FIO_2 ratio less than 200 or a physiologic shunt in the lungs (Q_{sp}/Q_t) greater than 20% developing more than 2 to 3 days after trauma usually indicates that ARDS is developing.

12. The need for an increased minute ventilation to maintain a normal Pa_{CO_2} in ARDS is primarily due to increased dead space (V_d/V_t).
13. An $ETCO_2$ persistently less than 28 mm Hg or an arterial ET-CO_2 difference of 10 mm Hg or more following resuscitation is associated with a poor prognosis.
14. Increasing pulmonary hypertension is probably the most frequent and consistent hemodynamic evidence of a poor prognosis following trauma.
15. Tidal volumes and PEEP should be adjusted to provide the best static compliance for ventilated patients.
16. Restlessness should be considered to be due to hypoxemia until proven otherwise.
17. With suspected ARDS, one should document not only the Pa_{O_2} and Pa_{CO_2}, but also the Pa_{O_2}/F_{IO_2} ratio, $P(A\text{-}a)_{O_2}$, Pv_{O_2}, and Sv_{O_2}.
18. With a normal ventilatory response to a metabolic acidosis, the P_{CO_2} should be equal to $[(HCO_3)(1.5) + 8 \pm 4]$.
19. Decreasing static lung compliance in a patient after trauma, in the absence of hemopneumothorax or abdominal distension, is usually caused by increased lung water and may indicate increasing ARDS.
20. The amount of lung damage seen initially on plain chest radiography usually greatly underestimates the severity and extent of ARDS.
21. If ARDS is getting worse, it usually implies that an inadequately treated infection is present.
22. Controlling pain so that the patient can take deep breaths and cough effectively is probably the single best way to prevent atelectasis or pneumonia following truncal trauma or surgery.
23. When restlessness is due to pain, analgesics may be indicated; however, when restlessness is due to hypoxia, such agents may be lethal.
24. In attempting to find the ideal cardiac-filling volume, one should use the hemodynamic response to fluid challenges rather than isolated PAWP or CVP levels.
25. Although controversial, patients with severe ARDS or other cardiopulmonary dysfunction tend to have a better prognosis if the hemoglobin level is kept at 12.0 g/dL or more.
26. Achieving optimal (supernormal) DO_2 and VO_2 levels in the first 12 to 24 hours after trauma or surgery in high-risk patients seems to reduce the incidence and severity of organ failure and death.
27. Early enteral nutrition can reduce complications after trauma.
28. Concern about oxygen toxicity should not prevent the administration of a high F_{IO_2} of 0.60 or more if this is the only way to maintain Pa_{O_2} of at least 50 mm Hg in patients with severe ARDS.
29. If a patient requires long-term ventilation or protection of the upper airway, early tracheostomy appears to reduce the time spent on a ventilator.
30. Physiologic advantages of IMV include increased venous return and better V/Q relationships during spontaneous breaths. IMV also improves weaning from the ventilator in some patients.
31. Lower tidal volumes or PCV should be used as needed to keep PIP from exceeding 45 to 50 cm H_2O and the inspiratory plateau (alveolar) pressure (PP) from exceeding 30 to 35 cm H_2O.
32. Patients with high ventilatory pressures may have increased pleural fluid that may not be detected clinically or radiologically on supine chest radiograph, but which will benefit from chest tube drainage.
33. The main functions of PEEP are to keep alveoli expanded during expiration and increase the patient's functional residual capacity back toward normal.
34. The major problems with PEEP occur because of its tendency to reduce venous return and cardiac output, especially when levels greater than 10 to 15 cm H_2O are used.
35. When optimizing the level of PEEP in a patient, it is essential to also maintain optimal DO_2 and VO_2 levels by giving fluids, blood, or inotropes as needed.
36. If increases in minute ventilation cause an increase in Pa_{CO_2}, one should suspect that significant auto-PEEP is present.

37. When the patient's ventilatory flow rate tracing indicates that the next inspiration interrupts an expiratory effort, auto-PEEP is present.
38. Intermittent sighing is an important method for preventing atelectasis in patients taking frequent, small breaths.
39. The patient who is awake, alert, comfortable, and cooperative, and has normal vital signs on a ventilator is generally doing well, even if ABGs do not appear to be optimal.
40. The main value of pulse oximetry is its ability to provide early warning of potentially dangerous trends in pulmonary or cardiovascular function.
41. If dead space in the lung increases, as with a pulmonary embolus or hypovolemia, the ET CO_2 tends to decrease and arterial-ET PCO_2 differences increase.
42. Efforts should be made with fluid resuscitation or ventilator settings to get the arterial ET-P_{CO_2} difference to 9 mm Hg or less.
43. Rapid, shallow breathing, respiratory alternans, or abdominal paradox during attempts at spontaneous breathing generally indicate that the patient is not ready to be weaned from the ventilator.
44. An FVC less than 10 mL/kg or NIF less than 25 cm H_2O usually indicates that the patient is not ready for weaning.
45. Patients on T-piece weaning trials tend to have fixed, low-tidal volumes and should be "sighed" at least four to six times per hour.
46. In weaning patients from prolonged ventilatory support, it is essential to provide adequate rest between periods of stress.
47. Few patients actually die of ARDS; they usually die of MOF, often with inadequately controlled infection.

REFERENCES

1. Wilson RF. Post traumatic pulmonary insufficiency. In: Wilson RF, Walt AJ, eds. *Management of trauma—pitfalls and practice,* 2nd ed. Philadelphia: Williams & Wilkins, 1996:867–905.
2. Nacht A, Kahn RC, Miller SM. Adult respiratory distress syndrome and its management. In: Capan LM, Miller SM, Turndorf H, eds. *Trauma: anesthesia and intensive care.* Philadelphia: JB Lippincott, 1991:725–753.
3. Horn JK, Lewis FR Jr. Respiratory insufficiency. In: Moore EE, Mattox KL, Feliciano CV, eds. *Trauma,* 2nd ed. Norwalk, CT: Appleton & Lange, 1992:909–926.
4. Bernard GR, Artigas A, Brigham KL, et al. The American European Consensus Conference on ARDS: definitions, mechanisms, relevant outcome, and clinical trial coordination. *Am J Respir Crit Care Med* 1994;149:818.
5. Hoyt DB, Simons RK, Winchell RJ, et al. A risk analysis of pulmonary complications following major trauma. *J Trauma* 1993;35:524.
6. Freedland M, Wilson RF, Bender JS, et al. The management of flail chest injury: factors affecting outcome. *J Trauma* 1990;30:1460.
7. Shier MR, Wilson RF. Fat embolism syndromes: traumatic coagulopathy with respiratory distress. *Surg Ann* 1980;12:139.
8. Colice GL. Neurogenic pulmonary edema. *Clin Chest Med* 1985;6:473.
9. Thomason MH, Payseur ES, Hakenewerth AM, Norton J, et al. Nosocomial pneumonia in ventilated trauma patients during stress ulcer prophylaxis with sucralfate, antacid, and ranitidine. *J Trauma* 1996;41:503–508.
10. Coon WW. Risk factors of pulmonary embolism. *Surg Gynecol Obstet* 1976;143: 385.
11. Greenfield LJ, Proctor MC, Rodriguez JL, et al. Posttrauma thromboembolism prophylaxis. *J Trauma* 1997;42:100.
12. Hull RD, Hirsh J, Carter CJ, et al. Diagnostic value of ventilation-perfusion lung scanning in patients with suspected pulmonary embolism. *Chest* 1985;88:819.
13. Parker JC, Hernandez LA, Peevy KJ. Mechanics of ventilator-induced lung injury. *Crit Care Med* 1993;21:131.
14. Meyrick BO. Pathology of the adult respiratory distress syndrome. *Crit Care Clin* 1986;2:405.

15. Fantone JC, Feltner DE, Brieland JK, et al. Phagocytic cell-derived inflammatory mediators and lung disease. *Chest* 1987;91:428.
16. Westaby S. Mechanism of membrane damage and surfactant depletion in acute lung injury. *Intensive Care Med* 1986;12:2.
17. Gadaleta D, Davis JM. Pulmonary failure and the production of leukotrienes. *J Am Coll Surg* 1994;178:309.
18. Rodriguez JL, Miller CG, DeForge LE, et al. Local production of interleukin-8 is associated with nosocomial pneumonia. *J Trauma* 1992;33:74.
19. Domsky M, Wilson RF, Hines J. Intraoperative end-tidal carbon dioxide values and derived calculations correlated with outcome: prognosis and capnography. *Crit Care Med* 1995;23:1497.
20. Shoemaker WC, Appel PL, Kram HB, et al. Prospective trial of supranormal values as therapeutic goals in high-risk surgical patients. *Chest* 1988;94:1176.
21. Fleming A, Bishop M, Shoemaker W, et al. Prospective trial of supranormal values as goals of resuscitation in severe trauma. *Arch Surg* 1992;127:1175.
22. Moore EE, Moore FA. Aggressive enteral feeding reduces sepsis and multiple organ failure? A review of recent studies. *J Crit Care Nutr* 1993;1:5.
23. Alexander JW. Immunonutrition: an emerging strategy in the ICU. *J Crit Care Nutr* 1993;1:21.
24. MacIntyre NR, Leatherman NE. Ventilatory muscle loads and the frequency-tidal volume pattern during inspiratory pressure assisted (pressure supported) ventilation. *Am Rev Respir Dis* 1990;141:327.
25. Hickling KG, Henderson SJ, Jackson R. Low mortality associated with low volume pressure limited ventilation with permissive hypercapnia in severe adult respiratory distress syndrome. *Intensive Care Med* 1990;16:372.
26. Greaves TH, Cramolini GM, Waler DH, et al. Inverse ratio ventilation in a 6 year old with severe post-traumatic adult respiratory distress syndrome. *Crit Care Med* 1989;17:588.
27. Shapiro BA. General principles of airway pressure therapy. In: Shoemaker WC, Ayres S, Grenvik A, et al, eds. *Textbook of critical care.* Philadelphia: WB Saunders, 1989:505.
28. Asbaugh DG, Petty Tl. PEEP: physiology indications and contraindications. *J Thorac Cardiovasc Surg* 1973;65:195.
29. Yang KL, Tobin MJ. A prospective study of indexes predicting the outcome of trials of weaning from mechanical ventilation. *N Engl J Med* 1991;324:1445.
30. Ashbaugh DG, Maier RV. Idiopathic pulmonary fibrosis in adult respiratory distress syndrome. Diagnosis and treatment. *Arch Surg* 1985;120:530.
31. Freeman BD, Zeni F, Banks SM, et al. Response of the septic vasculature to prolonged vasopressor therapy with N^{w}-monomethyl-L-arginine and epinephrine in canines. *Crit Care Med* 1998;26:877.
32. Rossaint R, Falke KJ, Lopez F, et al. Inhaled nitric oxide for the adult respiratory distress syndrome. *N Engl J Med* 1993;328:399.
33. Johannigman JA, Davis K Jr, Campbell RS, et al. Inhaled nitric oxide in acute respiratory distress syndrome. *J Trauma* 1997;43:904.
34. Dellinger RP, Zimmerman JL, Taylor RW, et al. Effects of inhaled nitric oxide in patients with acute respiratory distress syndrome: results of a randomized phase II trial. *Crit Care Med* 1998;26:15.
35. Dulchavsky SA, Bailey J. T_3 maintains surfactant synthesis in sepsis. *Surgery* 1992;112:475.
36. Dulchavsky SA, Hendrick HR, Dutta S. Pulmonary biophysical effects of triiodothyronine augmentation during sepsis-induced hypothyroidism. *Crit Care Med* 1993;35:104.
37. Anderson HL, Shapiro MB, Steimle CN, et al. Extracorporeal life support for respiratory failure due to traumaƒ-a viable alternative. *J Trauma* 1993;35:158.
38. Pranikoff T, Hirschl RB, Steimle CN, Anderson HL, Barlett RH. Mortality is directly related to the duration of mechanical ventilation before the initiation of extracorporeal life support for severe respiratory failure. *Crit Care Med* 1997;25: 28–32.

39. Gattinoni L, Agnostomi A, Pesenti A, et al. Treatment of acute respiratory failure with low frequency positive pressure ventilation and extracorporeal CO_2 removal. Lancet 1980;2:292.
40. Morris AH, Wallace J, Menlove RL, et al. Randomized clinical trial of pressure-controlled inverse ratio ventilation and extracorporeal CO_2 removal for adult respiratory distress syndrome. *Am J Respir* 1994;149:295.

41. CARDIOVASCULAR FAILURE FOLLOWING TRAUMA[1]

INCIDENCE

Although some heart failure seen after trauma is due to prolonged, severe hypotension, much of it is related to preexisting cardiac disease. It is estimated that 2.4 million Americans suffer from heart failure, and approximately 400,000 new cases are added each year (2). The prevalence rate is about 1% to 2% at age 50 years; at 80 years and older, about 10% to 15% have heart failure. A diagnosis of heart failure carries a grim prognosis, with up to 35% to 50% of patients dying within the following 2 years.

MYOCARDIAL FUNCTION

During the early phase of ventricular diastole, blood flows passively from the atria into the ventricles, but in the last phase of diastole, the atria contract, pumping in about 20% to 30% of the total end-diastolic volume of the ventricles (Fig. 41-1). Loss of atrial systole in a normal heart has only minimal effect, but with any impediment to left ventricular (LV) filling, such as with mitral stenosis, left atrial systole may account for more than 50% of LV filling. Consequently, if atrial fibrillation develops in a patient with severe mitral stenosis, the patient may go into acute pulmonary edema (3).

The normal right ventricle usually cannot achieve a mean pulmonary artery pressure greater than 40 mm Hg unless there is preexisting right ventricular hypertrophy. In like manner, the normal left ventricle often cannot achieve a systolic pressure greater than 180 mm Hg, such as with thoracic aortic cross-clamping, without dilating and developing some dysfunction.

Physiology of Muscle Contraction

All striated muscle, including skeletal and cardiac muscle, consists of numerous muscle fibers about 10 to 100 microns in diameter, which, in turn, consist of several hundred to several thousand myofibrils (3). Myocardial cells are separated from each other by sarcolemma and intercalated disks. Each cell contains (1) an energy generation system (the mitochondria), (2) an intracellular transportation and storage system for calcium and other ions (the transverse tubular system and sarcoplasmic reticulum), and (3) an electromechanical apparatus (the myofibrils) that converts chemical energy into mechanical work. Each myofibril contains about 1,500 myosin and about 3,000 actin filaments, which lay parallel to each other. Depolarization is initiated by a short-duration increase in the permeability of the cell membrane to Na^+ and Ca^{2+}.

Factors Affecting Cardiac Function

The main factors that affect cardiac function and cardiac output include

1. Preload (filling of the heart during diastole);
2. Afterload (resistance against which the heart must pump);
3. Contractility of the heart;
4. Coordinated pattern of contractions; and
5. Heart rate.

Preload

Preload refers to the tension on a muscle fiber as it begins to contract. In the heart, this is determined by the quantity of blood in the ventricle at the end of diastole. As a general rule, the greater the tension in the myocardium during systole, the stronger the contraction will be.

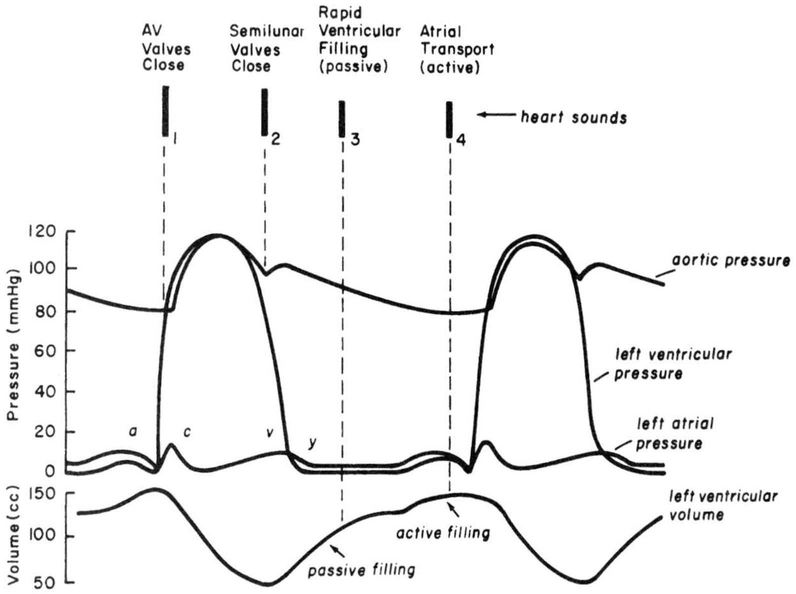

FIG. 41-1. The phases of the cardiac cycle correlated with the occurrence of heart sounds and changes in aortic, left ventricular, and left atrial pressures. (From Shatz IJ, Wilson RF. Cardiovascular failure. Walt AJ, Wilson RF, eds. *Management of trauma: pitfalls and practice.* Philadelphia: Lea & Febiger, 1975:537).

The intrinsic autoregulation of the heart (in which the size of the ventricular chamber determines its contractility) has been referred to as heterometric autoregulation (3). In contrast, homeometric autoregulation refers to changes in increased contractility resulting from an increased heart rate (Bowditch effect) or increased aortic pressure (Anrep effect) without any change in diastolic ventricular fiber length.

Increased blood volume, by increasing atrial distension, causes increased secretion of atrial natriuretic peptide (ANP), primarily by the left atrium. ANP reduces cardiac filling by increasing the loss of salt and water in the urine and by dilating blood vessels. Patients with congestive heart failure usually have significantly elevated plasma levels of ANP.

Afterload

Afterload for a ventricle can be defined as its wall tension during ejection. The two principal determinants of this tension are the end-diastolic volume (radius) and the systolic blood pressure (BP), which is related to the impedance to blood flow in the aorta (i.e., the systemic vascular resistance [SVR]).

The formula for calculating SVR is as follows:

$$SVR = [(MAP - CVP)/CO] \times 80$$

where MAP = mean arterial pressure, CVP = central venous pressure, and CO = cardiac output. Thus, if MAP = 95 mm Hg, CVP = 5 mm Hg, and CO = 6 L/min, SVR = $[(95 - 5)/6] \times 80 = 1{,}200$. Normal SVR = 900 to 1,400 dyne·sec·cm^{-5}.

In the failing heart, an increase in SVR, as with use of vasopressors to correct hypotension, can cause a severe decline in cardiac output.

⊘ PITFALL

Failure to recognize that drugs that increase BP also increase MVO_2 and reduce cardiac output, tissue perfusion, and oxygen delivery (DO_2).

In its most strict sense, afterload for a heart chamber refers to the difference between the pressures inside and outside the chamber being studied. Thus, if one adds a great deal of positive end-expiratory pressure (PEEP), the pulmonary artery pressures usually increase more than the intrathoracic pressures, and consequently, the afterload for the right ventricle increases; however, if aortic pressure stays constant, the afterload for the left ventricle decreases.

Cardiac Contractility

The rate of generation of cross-linkings between actin and myosin determines the state of myocardial contractility, which, in turn, controls stroke volume if preload and afterload are kept constant. Until recently, there was no readily available way to quantify cardiac contractility. With special pulmonary artery (RIF) catheters, one can determine right ventricular ejection fraction (RVEF) (4).

Coordinated Contractions

Even when all individual muscle units in the heart are functioning properly, failure of these units to beat in a coordinated fashion can greatly impair cardiac function (3). Some of the more frequent causes of uncoordinated myocardial contraction include the following:

1. Bundle-branch blocks as a result of ischemia or trauma;
2. Ischemia or trauma to portions of the myocardium causing slower or weaker contraction than normal; and
3. Arrhythmias.

Heart Rate

When stroke volume remains constant, an increased heart rate up to about 150 to 180 beats/min tends to increase cardiac output (3). Cardiac output in very young and very old individuals (who tend to have a relatively fixed stroke volume) is rate-dependent; however, in patients with coronary artery disease (CAD), the benefits of improving cardiac output by increasing heart rate must be weighed against the increase in myocardial oxygen consumption that occurs with tachycardia.

If the heart rate is less than 50 or greater than 150 per minute in older nonathletic patients, cardiac output often decreases and the tendency to arrhythmias increases.

Heart Rate Variability

It is normal for the heart rate to vary somewhat with the ventilatory cycle and with the various factors that alter preload and afterload. Following an acute myocardial infarction, 44% of the patients who had decreased heart rate variability in one study had overt signs of heart failure, compared with only 8% of the patients who maintained a high heart rate variability (5).

Other Factors Affecting Cardiac Function

Hypoxia

Mild to moderate hypoxia tends to cause a moderate increase in sympathetic stimulation, which, in turn, increases cardiac contractility. Severe hypoxia, however, impairs myocardial function.

Anemia

Anemia decreases the viscosity of blood, which, in turn, decreases the afterload for the heart and increases cardiac output. Cardiac output tends to increase in an almost linear fashion as hematocrit decreases; however, with hematocrit levels less than 15% to 20%, blood flow may be too fast to unload O_2 in the capillaries adequately, and cardiac output may have to increase geometrically to keep the tissues supplied with O_2 properly.

Electrolyte Abnormalities

With hyperkalemia or hypocalcemia, contraction of the heart becomes progressively weaker and slower. Similar problems may also occur with severe hypophosphatemia or hypermagnesemia.

Factors Affecting Myocardial Oxygen Consumption (MVO_2)

Systolic Tension-Time Index

Sarnoff, in his studies on isolated hearts, showed that myocardial oxygen consumption (MVO_2) correlates well with the calculated systolic tension-time index (STTI) (6). STTI is equal to the average tension developed by the left ventricle during systole multiplied by the duration of systole per minute. Because the tension developed in the ventricular wall during systole is a function of systolic pressure and ventricular volume, if the systolic pressure and the volume (radius) of the ventricle both doubled, the MVO_2 should increase almost fourfold. As the pulse rate increases, the amount of time that the heart is in systole each minute also increases, causing the MVO_2 to increase even more.

Pulse-Pressure Product

Changes in the pulse-pressure product (PPP), which is equal to the systolic BP multiplied by the heart rate, can be used to estimate changes in MVO_2. For example, if the BP is 120/80 and the pulse rate is 70/min, the PPP is 120×70, or 8,400. If the BP were to increase to 140/90 and the pulse rate to 120/min, the new PPP would be 16,800 and the MVO_2 would also double. Reducing the PPP with calcium-channel blockers after aortic surgery appears to reduce the incidence of myocardial ischemia (7).

Increases in heart rate and contractility can increase cardiac output, but they can also greatly increase MVO_2. In contrast, increases in preload can increase cardiac output with a relatively small increase in MVO_2 (8).

AXIOM The best relationship between cardiac output and MVO_2 is achieved by increasing preload and decreasing afterload rather than by inotropic or chronotropic stimulation.

DEFINING HEART FAILURE

To most clinicians, "cardiac failure" refers to signs and symptoms related to venous hypertension, pulmonary congestion, or reduced cardiac output. However, in some patients with heart failure, cardiac output is normal or even elevated. From the physiologist's viewpoint, cardiac failure is defined as a diminished work output of the heart in relation to its filling volume.

The pumping ability or contractility of the heart may be defined more accurately by cardiac function curves that correlate the stroke work of the heart (mean BP multiplied by stroke volume index) with the filling pressure or diastolic volume of the heart. Under these circumstances, left heart failure is considered to be present when a low LV stroke work index is present despite a high pulmonary artery wedge pressure (PAWP). Right heart failure would be reflected by a low RV stroke work index despite a high central venous pressure (CVP).

Right and Left Heart Failure

With "right" heart failure, the main signs and symptoms are pedal edema, hepatomegaly, and distended neck veins. With "left" heart failure, the usual problems

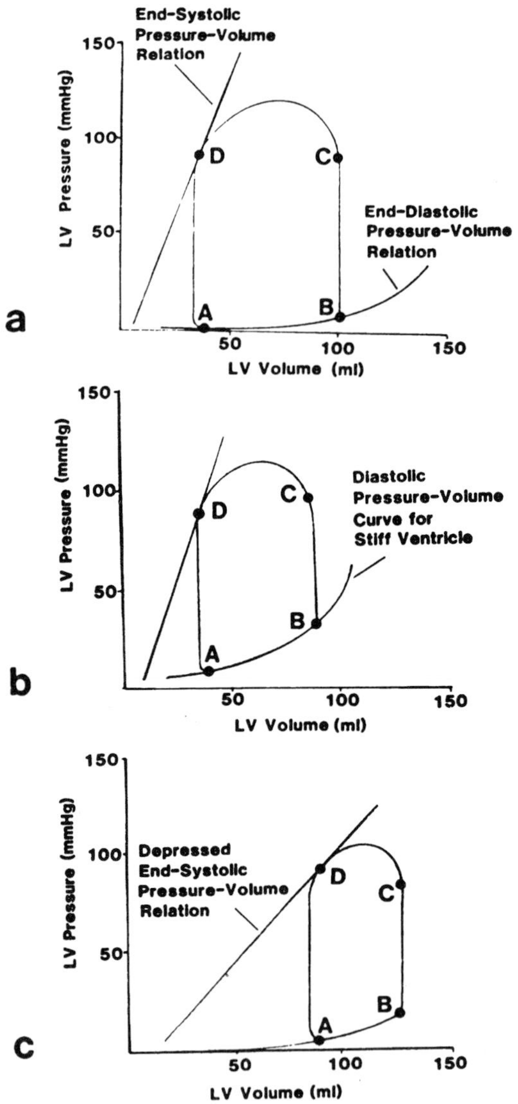

FIG. 41-2. Left ventricular pressure-volume loops in **(A)** a normal heart, **(B)** in a heart with diastolic dysfunction, and **(C)** in a heart with systolic dysfunction. The pressure-volume curve in diastolic dysfunction differs from the normal curve in that the end-diastolic pressure is elevated (*point B*) without a concomitant increase in end-diastolic volume. In systolic dysfunction, there is a depressed end-systolic pressure-volume relationship resulting in a decreased ejection fraction (EF) (from ref. 9, with permission).

are pulmonary congestion and dyspnea, often with weakness or fatigue and lightheadedness.

The most frequent causes of heart failure, such as myocardial infarction, hypertension, or valvular heart disease, often affect only the left ventricle initially. Right heart failure is usually a result of left heart failure, and right heart failure, in turn, can impair LV filling.

Isolated right heart failure as a result of pulmonary disease or RV infarction is much less common than left heart failure; however, when one side of the heart becomes weakened or fails, a sequence of events begins that eventually causes the opposite side to also fail.

Systolic and Diastolic Dysfunction

Heart failure can mechanistically also be considered as diastolic dysfunction or systolic dysfunction (Fig. 41-2) (9). Diastolic dysfunction is characterized by high filling pressures at normal or low diastolic volumes. This may be caused by severe LV hypertrophy resulting from hypertension, aortic stenosis, or hypertrophic cardiomyopathy. Systolic dysfunction is characterized by a reduced EF. This typically occurs when ventricular contractility diminishes because of myocardial ischemia or degeneration (myocarditis or cardiomyopathy).

CAUSES OF HEART FAILURE

Primary Myocardial Failure

Impaired Myocardium

Myocardial Infarction

AXIOM The most frequent cause of primary myocardial failure is a myocardial infarction.

A linear correlation exists between the extent of LV damage after an acute myocardial infarction and the amount of systolic dysfunction that develops (8). Clinical heart failure generally develops when 20% to 35% of the ventricular myocardium develops hypokinesis, akinesis, or dyskinesia. Loss of more than 40% of the ventricular myocardium usually results in cardiogenic shock, and loss of function of more than 60% to 70% of the left ventricle is usually rapidly fatal.

Cardiomyopathy

Cardiomyopathy can be divided into three types: congestive (dilated), restrictive (nondilated), and hypertrophic. The most common causes of dilated cardiomyopathy are idiopathic (the most frequent type), alcoholic, ischemic, diabetic, viral, and drug-related (e.g., adriamycin). Restrictive cardiomyopathy (impaired ventricular distensibility during diastole in the presence of relatively normal systolic function) is usually secondary to specific diseases, such as amyloidosis, sarcoidosis, hemochromatosis, glycogen storage disease, and endomyocardial fibrosis. Hypertrophic cardiomyopathy includes severe asymmetric LV hypertrophy plus microscopic myocardial fiber disarray without an identifiable cause.

Severe Shock or Cardiac Arrest

AXIOM The most frequent cause of severe cardiovascular failure after trauma in young, previously healthy patients is severe, prolonged shock or cardiac arrest.

Inadequate blood flow to the myocardium eventually causes the membrane integrity of a large number of cells to be destroyed. As a consequence, sodium, calcium, and water tend to enter the cell, and potassium leaves it. As the adenosine triphosphate is consumed, cyclic adenosine monophosphate (cAMP) concentrations decrease, and lactate production increases. Histologically, these "sick cells" begin to swell and progressive cellular disruption develops.

Myocardial Contusion

Significant myocardial damage can be caused by the impact of the heart against the decelerating chest wall or by crushing the chest and has been implicated as the cause of death in at least 5% of fatal motor vehicle accidents.

The diagnosis of mild to moderate myocardial contusions can be difficult. The most common arrhythmias (sinus tachycardia and premature atrial or ventricular beats) are nonspecific (10). New S-T segment, T-wave, or conduction abnormalities are less common but are considered much more specific for myocardial damage.

Some investigators believe that increased blood levels of CPK-MB isoenzymes or troponin are more reliable criteria for diagnosing myocardial contusions (10). The CPK-MB isoenzyme is usually expressed as a percentage of the total serum CPK concentration, and a CPK-MB concentration greater than 5% of the total CPK is believed to be sensitive and specific for the diagnosis of myocardial injury (10). The CPK-MB fraction in the myocardium of young, healthy people, however, may be less than 1%.

AXIOM Patients with a suspected myocardial contusion do not require intensive care unit (ICU) monitoring unless they have arrhythmias, heart failure, other severe injuries, or preexisting cardiac disease.

Echocardiography is a noninvasive and relatively inexpensive means of evaluating patients with a possible myocardial contusion (10). The most common finding is abnormal wall motion, such as hypokinesis or dyskinesis. It also can detect acute valvular injury, pericardial effusions, and intracavitary clots.

Radionuclide angiography can also be used to detect wall-motion abnormalities, decreased EFs, and depressed Starling function curves (10).

AXIOM Patients with wall-motion abnormalities from myocardial contusion have an increased risk of shock or arrhythmias during general anesthesia until up to 1 month later (11).

Electrolyte and Acid-Base Abnormalities

Severe hypokalemia is often associated with arrhythmias and conduction defects, but many of these problems may actually be due to the hypomagnesia that is also often present (12).

Causes of magnesium depletion in patients with chronic heart failure (CHF) include diuretics, liver disease, and poor intake (13). Magnesium deficiencies should be suspected in any patient who has an arrhythmia of unknown etiology; however, serum magnesium levels may be normal in individuals with moderate-to-severe tissue magnesium depletion.

Cardiac failure also tends to occur in patients with severe hypocalcemia, but giving calcium may only provide temporary help. The cause of the hypocalcemia must also be corrected. Some of the more frequent causes of hypocalcemic myocardial dysfunction include hypoparathyroidism, hypocalcemia associated with end-stage renal disease, and hypocalcemia attributed to rapid transfusion of citrated blood. The electrocardiographic (ECG) effects of hypocalcemia include prolongation of the ST segment and QT interval.

Normal phosphorous metabolism is required for adequate utilization of high-energy compounds. Severe hypophosphatemia (less than 1.0 mg/dL) may be associated with a constellation of clinical findings, including ventricular dysfunction (13).

AXIOM Acidosis can depress cardiac contractility, but the increased catecholamine release it stimulates tends to override the depression unless the pH is less than 7.00 to 7.10.

Pulmonary Hypertension

AXIOM The hemodynamic change most significantly associated with an increased mortality rate more than 48 hours after trauma is pulmonary hypertension (14).

Pulmonary hypertension resulting from hypoxia is usually reversible by giving enough oxygen or providing ventilator support. Pulmonary hypertension resulting from fat emboli, catecholamines, or cytokines is difficult to control except by relieving the underlying causes.

Circulatory Overload

In healthy individuals, the difference in blood volume between hypovolemic shock and heart failure may exceed 4 to 5 L. Patients who have preexisting cardiac disease or myocardial dysfunction caused by prolonged shock may progress from hypovolemic hypotension to pulmonary edema with fluid infusions of as little as 1,000 mL.

Although fluid overloading may occur during the initial resuscitation from shock or trauma, it is much more likely to occur during the fluid mobilization phase, which usually begins 48 to 72 hours after acute injury or surgery. Patients with renal or hepatic failure are particularly likely to accumulate extracellular fluid (ECF) and have an increased tendency to develop hypertension and heart failure at that time.

Myocardial Depressant Factors

Even though sepsis tends to be associated with a normal or increased cardiac output, the EF tends to be reduced because of one or more myocardial depressant factors that may be liberated from ischemic tissues, especially the pancreas.

Myocardial depressant factors have been detected in hemorrhagic, endotoxin, traumatic, and burn shock from various species. Most of these agents are small peptides with molecular weights of 250 to 1,000 daltons (15). They usually arise from ischemic or damaged splanchnic organs, especially the pancreas, and exert a negative inotropic effect.

COMPENSATORY CHANGES IN HEART FAILURE

Acute Cardiovascular Changes

Normally, the carotid sinus is stimulated by an increase in BP, which then inhibits the vasomotor center and causes a lowering of BP to more normal levels. In CHF, however, the ability of cardiac and arterial baroreceptors to suppress sympathetic activity in the presence of an increased BP is impaired (16).

If the sympathetic stimulation is severe and prolonged, some adaptation to the prolonged sympathetic stimulation occurs. This includes a reduced responsiveness to catecholamines because of an intracellular deficiency of cAMP, which, in turn, is associated with a decrease in the density of β-adrenergic receptors. The failing myocardium also becomes depleted of catecholamines because of defects in the myocardial synthesis and uptake of norepinephrine.

Subacute Compensatory Changes

The subacute compensatory changes in heart failure are due primarily to increased secretion of vasopressin and aldosterone (8). Working together, they can increase extracellular fluid because of retention of salt and water by the kidneys. This fluid retention may increase blood volume by 15% or more, and the resultant increased diastolic filling of the heart may restore cardiac output to relatively normal levels.

Another cause of increased blood volume in patients with cardiac failure is increased production of red blood cells because of reduced oxygen delivery to tissues (8); however, if the hematocrit increases above 55%, the increased viscosity can increase cardiac work and decrease cardiac output, further aggravating the tendency to heart failure.

Chronic Compensatory Changes

Left Ventricular Hypertrophy

The principal chronic hemodynamic adjustment to heart failure is hypertrophy of the LV myocardium; however, although LV hypertrophy allows the left ventricle to maintain proper wall stress in the presence of an increasing afterload and preload, it also makes the heart more susceptible to ischemia.

Drugs designed to prevent excess LV hypertrophy in heart failure may be helpful. In the SAVE trial, the early use of captopril after myocardial infarction attenuated subsequent LV remodeling and improved survival rates in patients with LVEFs less than or equal to 40% (17). Inhibition of LV dilation was also observed with enalapril, which tended to reduce LV mass and ventricular sphericity (18).

Increased Atrial Natriuretic Factor

Dilation of the atria in CHF results in increased excretion of atrial natriuretic factor (ANF) (19) (sometimes also called atrial natiuretic peptide, or ANP). The main effects of ANF are increased water and sodium excretion by the kidneys, and dilation of arteries and veins. There is also enhanced baroreceptor sensitivity (thereby reducing central activation of the sympathetic nervous system) plus suppressed formation of renin, angiotensin II, aldosterone, and vasopressin.

Increased Prostaglandin Production

In the final phases of heart failure, ANF has less and less renal effect, and prostaglandins increasingly assume the role of antagonizing the renal effects of systemic vasoconstrictor hormones (20). As a consequence, use of nonsteroidal antiinflammatory drugs (NSAIDs) or other prostaglandin synthesis inhibitors at this stage increases the tendency to renal failure.

ORGAN CHANGES IN HEART FAILURE

Heart

AXIOM Myocardial oxygen consumption increases in heart failure, but coronary blood flow tends to decrease.

In ventricular failure, end-diastolic volume and fiber length tend to increase so that each fiber must develop more tension (T) at a given intraventricular pressure (P) to eject blood from the heart. This, plus the LV hypertrophy, results in a substantial increase in myocardial oxygen requirements; however, the reduced cardiac output, tachycardia, and high LV diastolic pressures of CHF tend to reduce coronary blood flow, thereby making the myocardium more ischemic.

Lungs

AXIOM One of the most sensitive indicators of increasing cardiac failure is a decrease in the arterial Po_2.

In cardiac failure, the vital capacity and functional residual capacity in the lungs are decreased because of increased blood in the pulmonary vessels and increased fluid in the pulmonary interstitial spaces. This increases the work of breathing and the tendency toward atelectasis. When fluid accumulates in the alveoli, oxygen diffusion is impaired. When pleural effusions develop, ventilation is further impaired.

With increasing water retention, the colloid osmotic pressure (COP) decreases and PAWP increases. As a consequence, the COP-PAWP gradient, which is normally 15 to 20 mm Hg, may decline to less than 5 mm Hg. Patients with COP-PAWP gradients of less than 5 mm Hg have an increased tendency to development of pulmonary edema.

Liver, Spleen, and Intestines

The increased right atrial pressure present in heart failure tends to reduce venous return from the splanchnic circulation, and this causes increasing congestion in the liver, spleen, and intestines. Occasionally, the pain and tenderness of an acutely congested liver can closely resemble acute cholecystitis. If cardiac failure is severe and persistent, the reduction in liver blood flow can eventually cause cardiac fibrosis (cirrhosis).

Kidneys

Severe cardiac failure decreases glomerular filtration and urinary output and can produce a prerenal azotemia with an elevated blood urea nitrogen (BUN) (13). If NSAIDs are given, thereby reducing the renal vasodilation caused by prostaglandins, oliguric renal failure may develop rapidly.

DIAGNOSIS OF CARDIAC FAILURE

History

Patients with left-sided heart failure typically complain of easily becoming "short of breath" (caused by congestion of the lungs) or weakness and fatigue (caused by inadequate cardiac output).

Orthopnea and paroxysmal nocturnal dyspnea (PND) are particularly interesting symptoms of left heart failure (8). When the patient lies down, the blood that progressively pooled in the legs during the day while the patient was up can return to the heart, causing increased congestion in the lungs. When shortness of breath occurs as soon as the patient lies down, the patient is said to have orthopnea. Patients who are relatively comfortable when they first lie down but awaken suddenly with severe dyspnea several hours later are said to have PND (8).

Physical Examination

Sinus tachycardia, although a nonspecific sign, is almost invariably present with cardiovascular failure. Pulsus alternans, in which only every other heartbeat produces a palpable peripheral pulse, although uncommon, is a reliable sign of severe LV failure. Cardiac dilatation may occur rapidly, but muscle hypertrophy usually requires at least several weeks or months to develop.

AXIOM A third heart sound during diastole in adults is an important sign of LV failure, but it is easily overlooked.

Unless heart failure is severe, the systemic BP tends to be elevated or at high-normal levels. A return toward normal of an elevated BP sometimes indicates increasing cardiovascular failure. A low pulse pressure, in particular, tends to suggest the presence of hypovolemia, aortic stenosis, tamponade, or very cardiac failure.

In early LV failure, rales may be present only at the lung bases; however, as heart failure worsens, rales become higher and more generalized. Wheezing is usually considered to be due to bronchial asthma. However, it may also occur with cardiac failure (in the absence of pulmonary disease) because of swelling and congestion of the mucosa in smaller bronchioles. The mucosal edema can also cause coughing.

AXIOM Pleural effusions resulting from heart failure tend to occur slightly more frequently on the right, whereas a left hydrothorax is said to be more characteristic of a pulmonary embolus.

One of the most obvious signs of heart failure is neck vein distension to at least 3.0 cm above the sternal notch when the patient is sitting up at a 45-degree angle (8). Severe, acute heart failure may also cause annular dilatation of the tricuspid valve with enough tricuspid regurgitation to cause neck vein pulsations.

Hepatomegaly and a positive hepatojugular reflux (pushing on the liver, producing increased neck vein distension) are important corroborative signs of congestive heart failure. If severe cardiac failure causes tricuspid insufficiency, the liver may pulsate.

Swelling of the feet and ankles is frequently caused by chronically increased venous pressure in the legs resulting from right heart failure. In the bedridden patient with heart failure, sacral edema is usually more prominent. Consequently, this is the area that should be examined for edema in such individuals.

Laboratory Evaluation

In acute heart failure, usually some hemodilution occurs because of increased plasma water. With CHF, increased bone marrow production of red blood cells as a compensatory response to chronic hypoxemia, may cause hemoglobin and hematocrit values to increase above normal, thereby increasing blood viscosity and afterload.

Increasing renal ischemia may cause a progressively increasing BUN. Later, with further reduction in arterial inflow and increased venous congestion, progressive renal and hepatic dysfunction may also cause increasing plasma creatinine and bilirubin levels. Chronic use of diuretics and a low-salt diet tend to cause hyponatremia and hypokalemia and these, in turn, can also increase the tendency for renal dysfunction.

A progressively decreasing PaO_2 usually indicates that heart failure is getting worse.

AXIOM A relatively sudden decrease in arterial PO_2 in a patient with heart failure should make one look carefully for pulmonary emboli.

Radiographic Changes

Plain Films

On upright chest radiography, transverse lines of increased density, particularly near the hilum (Kerley's A lines) or near the costophrenic angles in the lung bases (Kerley's B lines), are often the first radiographic signs of increased lung water (8). Increased prominence and dilatation of central lung vessels are usually detected somewhat later.

An enlarged heart suggests a chronic, underlying cardiac problem. When the cardiac silhouette enlarges rapidly, CHF with a superimposed, severe, acute process is usually present.

Pulmonary Arteriography

The most frequent cause of heart failure of unknown etiology in adults is recurrent undiagnosed pulmonary emboli, and the gold standard for diagnosing pulmonary emboli is pulmonary arteriography.

Radionuclide Angiography

First-pass, gated radionuclide angiography can be used to find early reductions in RVEFs and LVEFs and regional wall-motion (plus increased end-diastolic volumes) (21). By the time that LVEFs decrease to less than 40%, heart failure resulting from systolic dysfunction is usually clinically evident. Changes in end-systolic and end-diastolic volumes also provide much more accurate estimates of the functional capabilities of the right and left heart than do the CVP and PAWP.

Electrocardiography

ECG findings do not indicate the presence or absence of CHF. However, RV or LV hypertrophy tends to indicate a chronic strain, usually resulting from increased afterload. Evidence of ischemia, infarction, conduction disturbances, tachyarrhythmias, or bradyarrhythmias may also provide important clues to the origin of heart failure.

Hemodynamic Monitoring

For uncomplicated trauma patients, sophisticated monitoring is not required, and one can manage fluids by balancing outputs with intake and by following the BP, heart rate, respiratory rate, and urine output. If the hemodynamic picture becomes confusing, it may be necessary to monitor cardiac function more closely, with a central venous or pulmonary artery catheter.

Central Venous Pressure

A CVP of less than 4 to 6 cm H_2O in critically injured patients usually indicates hypovolemia. In contrast, a CVP exceeding 16 cm H_2O may indicate an excessive blood volume; however, the responses of the CVP or PAWP to fluid challenges are much more informative than absolute values.

Pulmonary Artery Catheterization

Because of the poor correlation between CVP and LV filling pressures in patients with sepsis, respiratory failure, or myocardial ischemia, PAWP can be extremely helpful. Staudinger et al. (22) recently showed in 149 consecutive patients undergoing right heart catheterization that a pulmonary artery catheter can add valuable, clinically relevant information to the clinical assessment in approximately 50% of cases. Consequently, its use should not be withheld in patients with unclear hemodynamic and metabolic profiles.

A patient with an elevated PAWP that increases abruptly with a standard fluid challenge (3.0 mL/kg of a balanced electrolyte in 10 minutes) without an increase in cardiac output or LV stroke work index, is said to have a flat ventricular function curve; this indicates that one should not push further intravenous fluids at this time.

Left heart failure is usually associated with a PAWP exceeding 18 to 22 mm Hg. Studies with right ventricular end-diastolic volume indices, however, indicate that about one-third of the patients with "high" PAWPs can still respond favorably to fluid loading (4).

One can also use a sensor on the pulmonary artery catheter tip to continuously monitor mixed venous (pulmonary artery) oxygen saturation (Svo_2) (Table 41-1). An Svo_2 of 60% to 65% often indicates decreased oxygen delivery (DO_2) relative to the oxygen consumption (VO_2), and an Svo_2 less than 60% is often indicative of impending shock or severe heart failure.

AXIOM A declining or low mixed venous oxygen saturation (Svo_2) can provide early warning of cardiopulmonary dysfunction; however, one cannot completely rely on a stable Svo_2 to exclude such problems.

Right Ventricular End-Diastolic Volume Index

AXIOM End-diastolic volumes are a more accurate guide for fluid resuscitation of critically ill patients than are PAWP or CVP levels.

Table 41-1. *Pressure and Oxygen Saturation in Various Chambers of the Heart*

	Pressure (mm Hg)	O_2 Saturation (%)
Superior vena cava	0–5	70–75
Inferior vena cava	0–5	75–80
Coronary sinus	—	30–40
Right atrium	0–5	70–75
Right ventricle	12–25/0–5	70–75
Pulmonary artery	12–25/5–10 (8–15)[a]	70–75
Pulmonary capillaries	6–12	98–100
Left atrium	5–10	95–98
Left ventricle	120/0–5	95–98
Aorta	120/80 (92)	95–97

[a]Parentheses refer to mean pressure
From Wilson RF. Cardiovascular physiology. Wilson RF, ed. *Critical care manual: applied physiology and principles of therapy*, 2nd ed. Philadelphia: FA Davis Co, 1992:6.

Comparisons of PAWP and right ventricular end-diastolic volume index (RVEDVI) have shown that misleading information concerning filling volume was provided by the PAWP at some time in 15 (52%) of 29 ICU patients evaluated with both techniques before and after fluid challenges (4). Of 15 patients given 22 fluid challenges, seven patients with high PAWPs (≥18 mm Hg) but an RVEDVI less than 139 mL/m^2 "responded" with an increase in cardiac index. All fluid challenges in patients with a RVEDVI less than 90 mL/m^2 responded with an increase in cardiac index. Chang et al. (23) also found that there was a statistically better correlation between right ventricular volume and cardiac index than there was with PAWP. This again demonstrates the problems of using only the PAWP to guide fluid therapy.

AXIOM RVEDVI more accurately predicts preload recruitable increases in cardiac output than do PAWP levels.

Miller et al. (24) found that trauma patients who are resuscitated to an increased preload rather than using inotropes have significantly better visceral perfusion as reflected by gastric tonometry.

Gastric Mucosal pH

Guzman et al. (25) have found that the gastric mucosal pH (pH_i) (measured with a tonometric catheter) can indicate systemic hypoperfusion before systemic oxygen delivery reaches the critical level at which oxygen consumption becomes supply dependent. Knudson et al. (26) have also described the persistence of gut hypoxia (as measured directly in a swine model with hemorrhage) even when global systemic indices of perfusion appeared to be restored.

ET CO2 Monitoring

Wilson et al. (27) found that inadequate pulmonary blood flow can exist despite a normal BP and base deficit and is reflected by a low ET CO2 and increased $P(a\text{-}ET)CO_2$ differences. They found that an end-tidal CO_2 of 22 mm Hg or less in the operating room following resuscitation was associated with a mortality rate of 53% (16 of 30) versus a 24% mortality rate (14 of 59) in patients with an end-tidal CO_2 of 23 mm Hg or more (p =.011). An arterial to end-tidal P_{CO_2} difference of 13 mm Hg or more after resuscitation was also associated with an increased mortality rate (50% versus 18%).

Echocardiography

Using M-mode and two-dimensional ECG, the majority of cardiac structural abnormalities can be diagnosed. ECG studies can also be used to determine the mean velocity of circumferential fiber shortening and the EF.

Cardiac Catheterization

When the patient has progressive heart failure of unknown cause and is not responding to standard treatment, cardiac catheterization may provide extremely useful diagnostic information, particularly if pressures and oxygen contents are studied in each chamber. Cardiac catheterization can also be used to detect lesions that may be corrected surgically. When surgical management of CAD is contemplated, coronary angiography is also performed.

TREATMENT

AXIOM The best way to prevent cardiac dysfunction after trauma is to keep hypotension and hypoxemia to a minimum and to prevent cardiac fluid and pressure overloads.

Optimizing Preload

Pericardial tamponade, tension pneumothorax, and any other causes of hypotension should be corrected promptly. Hypovolemia should also be corrected promptly, but some care must be taken to not overload the heart with fluids or cause an excessive afterload on the left or right ventricle. For the left ventricle, this involves keeping the use of vasoconstrictor agents or aortic clamping to a minimum. For the right ventricle, this involves avoiding high pulmonary inflation pressures and preventing ARDS and pulmonary emboli.

AXIOM Continuing hypotension in trauma patients is usually caused by continued bleeding or inadequate volume replacement.

Volume expansion generally has little detrimental effect on myocardial oxygen consumption, but it can cause a dramatic improvement in BP and cardiac output in patients who are hypovolemic.

Positive-pressure ventilation, especially with PEEP, can dramatically reduce venous return to the heart in hypovolemic patients; however, in patients with acute pulmonary edema, increased PEEP may be the most rapid and effective way to reduce preload to proper levels and restore a normal arterial P_{O_2}. Venous return can also be reduced rapidly be elevating the head and chest and applying rotating tourniquets to the extremities.

Correcting Core Temperature and Lab Abnormalities

AXIOM The hypothermic heart (<34°C–35°C) does not function well and it is difficult to resuscitate.

Severe acidosis with arterial pH less than 7.00 to 7.10 should be corrected to a pH of at least 7.20 as soon as possible, preferably by improving tissue perfusion. If bicarbonate is to be given, one must be certain that the minute ventilation and lung function are adequate to keep the P_{CO_2} within proper limits $[(1.5 \times HCO_3) + 8 \pm 4]$; otherwise, the bicarbonate can cause a "paradoxical" cellular acidosis because the increased CO_2 released from the HCO_3 can rapidly enter cells, but HCO_3 cannot.

Severe electrolyte abnormalities, particularly hypomagnesemia, can cause severe arrhythmias, especially in the operating room. Such abnormalities are particularly likely to develop during massive blood transfusions to hypothermic individuals. Prolonged aortic clamping can cause a severe washout acidosis and hyperkalemia after the clamp is released.

Inotropic Support

AXIOM Once preload is optimized, the next step in improving hemodynamic function and oxygen delivery generally includes inotropes or vasodilators.

Digitalis Glycosides

In patients with heart failure and atrial fibrillation with a rapid ventricular response, digoxin can be extremely effective for slowing the ventricular heart rate, improving diastolic filling, and augmenting ventricular systolic function.

For rapid digitalization of a patient (as in patients with atrial fibrillation with a fast ventricular responses), digoxin 0.75 to 1.0 mg can be given by slow intravenous injection (8). Additional doses of 0.125 to 0.25 mg may be needed in the following 4 to 6 hours. Alternatively, 0.75 to 1.50 mg of digoxin can be given in 250 mL of 5% dextrose by intravenous infusion over a period of 2 hours.

AXIOM Digoxin levels should not be checked sooner than 6 hours after the last dose.

Normal digoxin levels are 1 to 2 μg/mL, determined 6 hours after the last dose. Values greater than 2 to 3 μg/mL are frequently associated with signs and symptoms of toxicity; however, toxicity can occur at much lower levels in the presence of hypokalemia or hypercalcemia.

AXIOM Any arrhythmia that develops in a patient receiving digitalis should be considered a result of the digitalis until proven otherwise.

Dopamine

Dopamine is an inotrope given frequently to patients who have a low BP and cardiac output despite fluid loading. The effects of dopamine, however, depend on the dose given. Low-dose dopamine (1 to 3 μg/kg/min) tends to dilate renal and mesenteric vessels and often increases urine output; however, even in very small doses of 0.5 to 1.0 g/kg/min, it may profoundly improve BP and cardiac output in patients with a chronic failing myocardium that has been depleted of its catecholamine stores. As doses are elevated to 5 to 15 μg/kg/min, they increase myocardial contractility by acting directly on β-adrenergic receptors in the myocardium. This increase in contractility is often accompanied by an even greater increase in heart rate and myocardial oxygen consumption (14). With doses of dopamine above 20 to 30 μg/kg/min, α-adrenergic vasoconstriction tends to predominate, and this can decrease renal and mesenteric blood flow. It may also cause cardiac output to decrease.

Dobutamine

Dobutamine is a synthetic catecholamine with minimal β-adrenergic effects. At doses of 5 to 10 μg/kg/min, it selectively stimulates β_1-receptors, producing an increase in cardiac contractility with relatively minor increases in heart rate. Because of its vasodilating effects, dobutamine may also decrease CVP, pulmonary artery pressure, and PAWP.

AXIOM Dobutamine is most useful when an inotropic agent is indicated and the BP is high-normal or increased.

Dopamine Plus Dobutamine

A favored inotropic combination in critically ill elderly patients with a slightly low BP and quite low cardiac outputs is "cardiac vitamin D," which is dopamine at 5 μg/kg/min and dobutamine at 5 to 10 μg/kg/min.

Isoproterenol

AXIOM Isoproterenol should probably be used only in patients who have a slow, weak heart and a good coronary blood flow.

In patients with bradycardia and a low cardiac output, such as may occur after cardiac surgery, isoproterenol in doses of 1.0 to 2.0 μg/min (0.015 to 0.030 μg/kg/min) may dramatically improve cardiac output. It may be particularly helpful for patients with an increased pulmonary vascular resistance. However, if the pulse rate is greater than 120/min, isoproterenol tends to increase the heart rate much more and also reduces diastolic aortic pressure and coronary blood flow while greatly increasing myocardial oxygen consumption. This may be particularly detrimental in patients with myocardial ischemia or pulmonary embolism.

Epinephrine

Epinephrine in doses of 1 to 2 μg/min (0.015 to 0.030 μg/kg/min) may dramatically increase BP and cardiac output in patients who are unresponsive to dopamine or dobutamine. The lower doses have a relatively greater inotropic effect, whereas large doses are more vasoconstrictive. Large doses also increase the tendency for severe tachycardia and ventricular arrhythmias.

Amrinone and Milrinone

Amrinone is an excellent inotrope for improving cardiac function in patients with pulmonary hypertension, but its long half-life can be a major problem if an undesirable response occurs. Amrinone is believed to act through inhibition of phosphodiesterase, which cleaves cAMP. Because increases in intracellular cAMP cause vascular smooth muscle to relax, phosphodiesterase inhibitors are also potent vasodilators. Although amrinone and milrinone decrease systemic, pulmonary, and coronary vascular resistance, the heart rate and BP usually do not change significantly (28).

Amrinone requires a loading dose of 0.75 mg/kg over 2 to 3 minutes, and then a maintenance infusion of 5 to 10 μg/kg/min. Another bolus of 0.75 μg/kg may be given in 30 minutes as needed. An alternative approach is to give it at 40 μg/kg/min for 1 hour, followed by 10 μg/kg/min as a maintenance infusion.

Adverse effects of amrinone include nausea and vomiting (0.5% to 2.0%), thrombocytopenia (2% to 4%), and increased ventricular dysrhythmogenicity. Although hypotension is rare, amrinone can cause a sudden, severe decrease in BP in patients who are hypovolemic.

Milrinone is similar to amrinone, and a bolus of 50 μg/kg over 10 minutes followed by 0.5 μg/kg/min appears to be more effective and have fewer adverse effects (28). In many patients with a low cardiac output that is unresponsive to all other medications, milrinone can produce rather dramatic effects.

Calcium

Ionized calcium levels less than 0.7 to 0.8 mmol/L (normal is 1.05 to 1.2 mmol/L) can impair cardiac contractility. Hypocalcemia can develop rapidly in patients with shock, sepsis, or congestive failure, particularly if they are getting massive blood transfusions at a rate faster than one unit every 5 minutes (29).

Calcium should not be given to improve cardiac function, except possibly in patients with shock or heart failure after multiple rapid blood transfusions, after calcium-blockers, or in patients with severe hyperkalemia.

Glucagon

Glucagon is a polypeptide hormone produced by the alpha cells of the pancreatic islets. It helps to maintain plasma glucose levels during fasting and stress by increasing hepatic glycogenolysis. Glucagon also has inotropic and chronotropic effects that are independent of the β-adrenergic receptors (30). Consequently, glucagon may be effective in restoring proper cardiovascular function in some patients who have been on β-blockers or calcium-channel blockers.

The dosage of glucagon used is variable. Boluses of 1 to 5 mg intravenously every 30 to 60 minutes may be effective. An infusion of 10 mg/h may also be effective in some patients. Disturbing side effects may include severe hyperglycemia and nausea and vomiting.

Vasodilators

Vasodilators may be used to reduce afterload or preload. Afterload reduction is particularly important when cardiac output remains low because of an elevated SVR.

AXIOM Vasodilators can cause sudden severe hypotension in patients with unrecognized hypovolemia.

Nitrates

Nitroprusside

Sodium nitroprusside is considered a "balanced" vasodilator because it dilates both venous capacitance and arterial resistance vessels, thereby causing a decrease in both preload and afterload. In patients with a normal blood volume, the venous pooling may cause a relative hypovolemia and this, combined with a decreased afterload, can cause BP and cardiac output to decrease abruptly. In contrast, when preload is very high, venous return is still adequate following nitroprusside, and the decrease in afterload caused by nitroprusside can cause a substantial increase in cardiac output. Pulmonary vascular resistance generally decreases during nitroprusside infusions.

The dose of sodium nitroprusside required to produce a satisfactory reduction of afterload in cardiac failure varies from 15 to 400 μg/min (0.2 to 6.0 μg/kg/min), averaging approximately 50 μg/min (0.7 μg/kg/min). One should start at the lower doses.

Other than hypotension, the major side effects of nitroprusside include thiocyanate/cyanide toxicity. Thiocyanate toxicity, which usually only occurs in patients with renal failure, is manifested by confusion, hyperreflexia, and convulsions. Cyanide toxicity is usually first manifested by metabolic acidosis caused by cyanide combining with cytochromes and inhibiting aerobic cellular metabolism. Thiocyanate or cyanide toxicity generally occurs only in patients receiving more than 3 μg/kg/min for more than 72 hours.

Nitroglycerin

In addition to its ability to dilate coronary arteries and relieve ischemic myocardial pain, nitroglycerin also dilates systemic vessels, usually with a greater reduction in venous return than arterial resistance. If nitroglycerin is administered to patients with only mild heart failure, cardiac output may decrease. However, in severe heart failure with a more than adequate preload, the arterial dilating effect of nitroglycerin is usually enough to produce an increase in cardiac output. Nitroglycerin also tends to reduce pulmonary arterial pressure, and this may be helpful in patients with COPD or severe ARDS.

Intravenous nitroglycerin can be started in doses of 0.3 μg/kg/min and gradually increased to about 3.0 μg/kg/min. One of the main drawbacks to continued intravenous nitroglycerin therapy is the rapid development of tolerance and the occasional development of methemoglobinemia (31).

Calcium-Channel Blockers

Calcium-channel blocking agents interfere with muscular excitation-contraction coupling by reducing the movement of calcium into cells via the so-called "slow channels." This results in peripheral and coronary artery vasodilation and a negative inotropic effect. If the decreased contractility is offset by a decreased LV afterload, there may be a favorable net effect on LV function.

Nifedipine

Nifedipine has been widely used in the treatment of angina pectoris, and in patients with severe LV failure, nifedipine tends to cause an increase in cardiac output and a decrease in SVR. Nevertheless, many clinicians are reluctant to use calcium-channel blockers in heart failure because of their depressant effect on the myocardium.

Verapamil

Verapamil is a vasodilator, but its direct myocardial depressant effect is more profound, and this may seriously aggravate myocardial dysfunction in patients with heart failure. It may, however, be of value in treating tachyarrhythmias, which may be contributing to the heart failure.

Hydralazine

Hydralazine is a potent, direct dilator of vascular smooth muscle, especially in arterioles. Consequently, its main effect is to reduce afterload. In patients with severe heart failure and a high SVR, hydralazine can produce impressive increases in stroke volume and renal blood flow, thereby promoting a diuresis (14).

Administration is usually started by giving 5 to 10 mg by a slow intravenous drip over at least 20 to 30 minutes. The maximal effect occurs 25 to 45 minutes after injection and the effect may last 4 to 24 hours. Subsequent doses of up to 20 mg can be administered intravenously every 6 hours. In some patients, a severe tachycardia develops after hydralazine, and this can exacerbate angina pectoris in patients with CAD.

Oxygen

AXIOM Oxygen can be a very effective pulmonary vasodilator.

Because hypoxia can cause pulmonary artery vasoconstriction, giving oxygen to a hypoxic individual can significantly reduce the afterload on the right ventricle. Severe hypoxia may also impair myocardial function. Consequently, patients with CHF often benefit from the administration of sufficient oxygen to maintain an arterial Po_2 of at least 80 mm Hg.

TREATMENT OF ARRHYTHMIAS

Need for Treatment

AXIOM If an arrhythmia is asymptomatic and may be chronic, one should think twice or obtain cardiology consultation before treating it.

Pain, anxiety, hypovolemia, anemia, acidosis, and hypoxia are major causes of tachycardia in acute trauma victims and should be treated aggressively. However, if severe tachycardia persists despite all other therapy in a patient with an adequate cardiac output and BP, a short-acting β-adrenergic blocking agent may be given very cautiously (9).

AXIOM Magnesium depletion can be an important cause of arrhythmias, and serum Mg levels may be normal despite serious Mg tissue depletion.

Classification of Antiarrhythmic Drugs

Group I drugs, such as quinidine and procainamide, act by depressing sodium conductance. This results in decreased conduction velocity, increased refractoriness of myocardial muscle, decreased automaticity of the myocardium, and direct suppression of conduction in the atrioventricular (AV) node, His bundle, and ventricular muscle. They are most effective in supraventricular and ventricular arrhythmias that are caused by either an automatic focus or reentry. These agents can cause prolongation of the PR interval and QRS complex. Toxic levels of group I agents may result in complete heart block.

Group II drugs, such as phenytoin and lidocaine, have little effect on the conduction velocity of normal tissue, but they can selectively decrease conduction velocity through ischemic myocardium. These agents are frequently used to treat reentry ventricular arrhythmias. Phenytoin (Dilantin) may be of particular benefit in patients with tachyarrhythmias resulting from digitalis toxicity.

Group III drugs have β-adrenergic blocking capability and some group I and group II effects. They are commonly used to treat supraventricular and ventricular arrhythmias, but in high doses they can cause AV nodal block and suppress lower pacemaker function, which may result in asystole. They can also be used to treat excessive sinus tachycardia.

Group IV drugs, such as bretylium, are Quaternary ammonium compounds whose major action is to reduce the disparity in duration of action potential between normal and ischemic myocardium. Bretylium is as effective as lidocaine in controlling ventricular fibrillation, but it can cause severe hypertension initially and then severe hypotension.

Group V drugs, such as verapamil, act by blocking or reducing calcium influx into myocardial cells. They depress activity in the sinoatrial node, AV node, and in diseased myocardial fibers, which have slow channel-dependent properties. They have a mild, negative inotropic effect, but can often provide excellent control of supraventricular tachycardias that are resistant to group I, II, and IV agents.

Group VI antiarrhythmic drugs may be considered for the therapy of bradycardia. Patients with symptomatic bradycardia, particularly when associated with a second- or third-degree heart block, may respond dramatically to atropine, isoproterenol, or a pacemaker.

Treatment of Specific Arrhythmias

AXIOM If an arrhythmia causes hemodynamic instability, the patient should be electrically cardioverted.

Tachyarrhythmias

AXIOM The most frequent cause of persistent sinus tachycardia in trauma patients is inadequate volume resuscitation.

If a beta-blocker is used to treat severe, persistent sinus tachycardia in a patient with heart failure, esmolol is an excellent choice because it has a half-life of only 9 minutes; therefore, if hypotension develops, it is usually of short duration (9).

A verapamil dose of 5 to 10 mg given over 1-3 min i.v. is used in patients with supraventricular tachycardia (SVT); however, if atrial fibrillation or flutter is due to an accessory conduction pathway (e.g., Wolff-Parkinson-White [WPW] syndrome), agents such as verapamil, beta-blockers, or lidocaine may cause a ventricular fibrillation that is difficult to reverse. With atrial fibrillation or flutter that may be due to an accessory pathway, procainamide is the drug of choice.

AXIOM Verapamil should not be used to treat atrial fibrillation or flutter in a patient with WPW syndrome.

Bradyarrhythmias

Bradyarrhythmias may be caused by direct trauma to the heart, head, spinal cord, neck, or eyes. Increased intracranial pressure (ICP) may result in sinus bradycardia associated with hypertension (Cushing's reflex). Acute compression of the spinal cord may also result in bradyarrhythmias and even sinus arrest.

When bradycardia results from causes other than severe hemorrhage, atropine (0.5 to 1.0 mg) is the drug of choice. Occasionally, an initial 0.5-mg dose of atropine, paradoxically, causes a more severe bradycardia, but this is generally reversed by giving another 0.5 mg promptly.

AXIOM Administration of atropine in the presence of hypovolemic bradycardia can cause ventricular fibrillation (8).

Isoproterenol or epinephrine (1 to 2 μg/min intravenously) may be tried if atropine fails; however, if the patient is hypovolemic, isoproterenol can cause severe hypotension. If the heart rate fails to respond to these measures, external pacing or insertion of a temporary transvenous pacemaker is indicated.

Conduction Defects

AXIOM Conduction defects can be caused by trauma to the head, eyes, spine, or heart.

If the AV node is blocked, the QRS complexes are narrow and the heart rate is often only 45 to 55 beats/min. If the block occurs below the AV node, the QRS complexes are wide and the heart rate is usually 30 to 40 beats/min. A left bundle-branch block (LBBB) or bifascicular block with unstable vital signs despite adequate fluid loading is an indication for a pacemaker (9). Complete heart block is also an indication for pacemaker insertion.

Ectopic Beats

Premature atrial contractions are usually of no significance and do not require treatment. Premature junctional contractions usually do not require treatment unless the patient is hemodynamically unstable or requires a faster heart rate to maintain a reasonable cardiac output.

Premature ventricular contractions (PVCs) arise from an ectopic focus below the AV node. The QRS complex is wide and often bizarre in appearance. PVCs in trauma patients are usually associated with hypokalemia, hypomagnesemia, myocardial ischemia, hypoxia, hypercapnia, or cardiac contusion (9). Treatment should be started if the PVCs are multifocal in origin, if more than five occur per minute, or if they occur on the ascending limb of the prior T-wave. Lidocaine is the drug of choice.

AXIOM If the patient has PVCs and a slow heart rate, the "PVCs" are probably escape beats and should not be suppressed.

Electrical-Mechanical Dissociation

Electrical-mechanical dissociation (EMD) or pulseless electrical activity is characterized by normal cardiac electrical activity but no mechanically effective heartbeat (9). This problem may be caused by trauma, massive bleeding, hypocalcemia, tension pneumothorax, acute pericardial tamponade, or inhalation anesthetic overdose. Insertion of an arterial catheter may reveal some mechanical cardiac function that is not apparent clinically.

AXIOM If EMD develops in a trauma patient, one should look carefully for pericardial tamponade, pneumothorax, or hypovolemia.

TREATMENT OF ACUTE PULMONARY EDEMA

AXIOM The most rapid and effective method for treating severe acute pulmonary edema is positive-pressure ventilation with increased oxygen.

1. If the pulmonary edema is mild, oxygen may be given by nasal catheter, mask, or intermittent positive-pressure breathing. Positive-pressure ventilation with an endotracheal tube is indicated in the more severe cases and may help to retard the development of pulmonary edema fluid by increasing intraalveolar pressure and reducing venous return.
2. Elevation of the patient's head and chest to an upright sitting position can improve ventilation and reduce venous return.
3. Morphine sulfate, 2 to 5 mg, may be given slowly intravenously, depending on the patient's BP, with careful observation for respiratory depression or hypotension.

AXIOM Morphine may be contraindicated in patients with pulmonary edema if the patient has (1) ICP, (2) severe pulmonary disease, or (3) severe lethargy or semicoma.

4. Furosemide, 40 to 80 mg intravenously, is given and repeated as needed to obtain a urine output of at least 200 to 500 mL in the next 1 to 2 hours.
5. Tourniquets can be applied to three extremities and rotated every 15 minutes to decrease venous return. Vasodilators may also be used in particularly severe cases to reduce venous return, but should not be used in hypotensive patients.
6. In undigitalized patients, 0.5 to 1.0 mg digoxin may be given intravenously followed by additional increments of 0.25 mg every 4 to 6 hours for three to four doses as indicated. The dose must be lowered if renal function is impaired or if the patient is hypokalemic or hypercalcemic.
7. Cardioversion should be used if the patient has a supraventricular or ventricular tachycardia that does not respond rapidly to the usual antiarrhythmic drugs. It is generally preferable to try cardioversion before a patient is given digitalis.

AXIOM If a patient has been digitalized, attempts at cardioversion may precipitate severe ventricular arrhythmias.

MECHANICAL SUPPORT OF CARDIAC FUNCTION

Criteria for considering use of mechanical support for a failing heart include hypotension (mean BP less than 60 mm Hg) or a low cardiac index (less than 1.5 to 2.0 L/min/m^2), which persists despite a more than adequate preload (determined by CVP or PAWP responses to fluid challenges) and maximal drug therapy.

Intraaortic Balloon Pump

Although relatively few exclusion criteria exist for intraaortic balloon pump (IABP) support for acute cardiac failure or cardiogenic shock, long-term mechanical support is generally not advocated if the patient has irreversible renal, hepatic, or pulmonary failure, severe peripheral vascular disease, symptomatic cerebrovascular disease, incurable cancer, coagulopathies, blood dyscrasias, or severe persisting infection. Other contraindications to IABP (relative to its insertion) include aortic regurgitation, aortic aneurysm, and severe peripheral vascular disease (8). Tachydysrhythmias or irregular heart rhythms are also relative contraindications.

The major use of IABP support has been in cardiac surgery patients unable to come off cardiopulmonary bypass. It has also been used extensively in patients with acute LV failure or cardiogenic shock resulting from an acute myocardial infarction. IABP also permits relatively safe performance of cardiac catheterization and angiography so that patients can be evaluated for possible emergency surgical intervention.

Complications of IABP support include damage or perforation of the aortic wall, leg ischemia distal to the femoral artery catheter, peripheral arterial embolization, thrombocytopenia, and hemolysis (8).

Extracorporeal Membrane Oxygenation

Extracorporeal membrane oxygenation (ECMO) systems have generally not been used for periods of support longer than 48 hours, but it can be of help in patients not responding well to IABP. ECMO systems require continuous heparin for anticoagulation and provide incomplete biventricular support.

Left Ventricular Assist Devices

In some centers, left ventricular assist devices (LVADs) are available to support severe LV failure, but they are primarily used as a bridge to cardiac transplantation.

CARDIAC TRANSPLANTATION

Cardiac transplantation provides the only effective therapy for meaningful long-term survival in patients who have EFs persistently less than 15% to 25% despite all other therapy.

⊘ FREQUENT ERRORS

1. ***Delayed or inadequate correction of hypovolemia in a trauma patient because of a fear of overloading the patient with fluid.***
2. ***Failure to consider hypovolemia as a possible cause of continued severe tachycardia in older trauma patients with a history of heart failure.***
3. ***Delay in detecting or treating acid-base, potassium, magnesium, or calcium abnormalities in a patient with heart failure.***
4. ***Failing to provide an adequate preload in a patient with diastolic cardiac dysfunction because the CVP or PAWP is already high.***
5. ***Assuming that bronchospasm or coughing in an elderly patient is due to a pulmonary problem.***
6. ***Attempts to increase BP with vasoconstrictor drugs in a patient with cardiac systolic dysfunction.***
7. ***Failure to keep pulse rate and systolic BP at relatively normal levels if CAD is present.***
8. ***Using a vasodilator without ensuring a continuing adequate preload and without monitoring filling pressure and BP closely.***
9. ***Delay in providing ventilatory support to patients with pulmonary edema.***

SUMMARY POINTS

1. If the aortic systolic pressure exceeds 180 mm Hg in a previously normotensive patient, the LVEDP, even in a normal heart, often doubles, and the left ventricle may dilate and go into failure.

2. Because myocardial oxygen extraction is already maximal, if increased oxygen is required by the heart, it can only be provided by increasing coronary blood flow.
3. Use of PEEP reduces the net distending pressure of the atria, thereby reducing ANF secretion and urine output; PEEP also reduces urine output by reducing venous return.
4. Increased afterload, such as with vasoconstrictor drugs, decreases stroke volume and increases myocardial oxygen consumption (MVO_2).
5. The best relationships between cardiac output and MVO_2 are achieved by increasing preload and decreasing afterload rather than by inotropic or chronotropic stimulation.
6. Cardiac failure can be defined as an inability of the heart to pump enough blood to meet the metabolic demands of the body; however, it is usually diagnosed clinically from evidence of pulmonary or systemic venous overload.
7. Right heart failure is occasionally due to chronic pulmonary disease or occult recurrent pulmonary emboli, but is usually due to left heart failure.
8. Systolic cardiac dysfunction is characterized by reduced EF and need for higher end-diastolic volumes. Diastolic dysfunction is characterized by a poorly relaxing heart requiring higher filling pressures.
9. The most frequent cause of severe cardiovascular failure after trauma in young, previously healthy patients is severe prolonged shock or a cardiac arrest.
10. Although tachycardia up to 180 beats/min can improve cardiac output in young individuals, it can severely limit myocardial blood flow if CAD is present.
11. Patients with a suspected myocardial contusion do not require ICU monitoring unless they have arrhythmias, heart failure, other severe injuries or preexisting cardiac disease, or will require general anesthesia.
12. Patients with wall-motion abnormalities from myocardial contusion have an increased risk of shock or arrhythmias if general anesthesia is given within the following 30 days.
13. Most arrhythmias in patients with hypokalemia are actually due to the hypomagnesemia, which is usually also present.
14. Acidosis tends to depress cardiac contractility, but the increased catecholamine release it stimulates tends to override the depression unless the pH is less than 7.00 to 7.10.
15. The hemodynamic change most significantly associated with an increased mortality rate more than 48 hours after trauma is pulmonary hypertension.
16. Volume overloads (such as those resulting from aortic insufficiency) are tolerated better than pressure overloads (as may occur with aortic stenosis).
17. Progressively decreasing serum sodium levels (usually caused by a progressive expansion of the ECF) is a bad prognostic sign in patients with CHF.
18. Use of prostaglandin synthesis inhibitors (such as NSAIDs) in patients with severe CHF increases the tendency to renal failure in such patients.
19. Myocardial oxygen consumption increases in heart failure, but coronary blood flow tends to decrease.
20. One of the most sensitive indicators of increasing cardiac failure is a decrease in the arterial Po_2.
21. The most frequent cause of heart failure of unknown etiology in adults is recurrent undiagnosed pulmonary emboli
22. A gallop rhythm in an adult should be considered a sign of LV failure until proven otherwise.
23. All that wheezes is not asthma; congestion of bronchial mucosa by CHF can also cause wheezing and coughing.
24. A sudden decrease in the Pao_2 without apparent cause is often due to pulmonary emboli.
25. The response of CVP or PAWP to fluid challenges is much more important than the absolute values.
26. Mixed venous oxygen saturation can provide early warning of cardiopulmonary dysfunction, but one cannot completely rely on a stable Svo_2 to exclude such problems.

27. RVEDVI more accurately predicts preload recruitable increases in cardiac output than does the PAWP level.
28. ECG, especially if done transesophageally, is an excellent technique for evaluating the heart, pericardium, and thoracic aorta after trauma.
29. The increased catecholamine release associated with stress, pain, and anxiety can cause heart failure to worsen despite all other therapy.
30. Continuing hypotension in trauma patients is usually due to continued bleeding or inadequate volume replacement.
31. Once preload is optimized, the next step in improving hemodynamic function and oxygen delivery generally includes inotropes or vasodilators.
32. Digoxin levels should not be checked sooner than 6 hours after the last dose.
33. Any arrhythmia that develops in a patient receiving a digitalis preparation should be considered to result from that drug until proven otherwise.
34. Dopamine should be considered in patients who have a low BP and cardiac output despite optimal fluid loading.
35. Isoproterenol should probably only be used in patients who have a slow, weak heart.
36. Amrinone or milrinone can improve cardiac function in patients with pulmonary hypertension, but its long half-life can be a problem if undesirable responses occur.
37. Calcium should not be given to improve cardiac function except perhaps in patients with shock or heart failure after multiple, rapid blood transfusions, after calcium-channel blockers, or in patients with severe hyperkalemia.
38. Glucagon can be helpful in some patients with a poor cardiac output resulting from beta-blockers or calcium-channel blockers.
39. Vasodilators should not be given to patients who are hypovolemic or hypotensive.
40. Nitroprusside should not be used in high doses (>3.0 μg/kg/min) for more than 72 hours.
41. Intravenous nitroglycerin by slow infusion may be the vasodilator of choice in patients with heart failure when a high preload is the main problem or the patient has moderate to severe ischemic heart disease.
42. Oxygen can be a very effective pulmonary vasodilator.
43. If an arrhythmia is asymptomatic and may be chronic, one should obtain cardiology consultation before treating it.
44. Magnesium depletion can be an important cause of arrhythmias, but serum Mg levels may be normal despite serious Mg tissue depletion.
45. The most frequent cause of persistent sinus tachycardia in trauma patients is inadequate volume resuscitation.
46. If an arrhythmia results in hemodynamic instability, the patient should be electrically cardioverted.
47. Verapamil should not be used to treat atrial fibrillation or flutter in a patient who may have WPW syndrome.
48. Administration of atropine in the presence of hypovolemic bradycardia can cause ventricular fibrillation.
49. If the patient has PVCs and a slow heart rate, the "PVCs" are probably escape beats and should not be suppressed.
50. If EMD occurs in a trauma patient, one should look carefully for pericardial tamponade, pneumothorax, or hypovolemia.
51. The most rapid and effective method for treating severe acute pulmonary edema is positive-pressure ventilation with increased oxygen.
52. If a patient has been fully digitalized, attempts at cardioversion may precipitate severe ventricular arrhythmias.
53. IABP therapy should be considered in patients with cardiogenic shock or acute severe left heart failure persisting despite other therapy.

REFERENCES

1. Wilson RF. Cardiovascular failure following trauma. In: Wilson RF, Walt AJ, eds. *Management of trauma—pitfalls and practice,* 2nd ed. Philadelphia: Williams & Wilkins, 1996:906–944.

2. Furburg CD, Yusuf S, Thom TJ. Potential for altering the natural history of congestive heart failure: need for large clinical trials. *Am J Cardiol* 1985;55:45A.
3. Schlant RC. Normal anatomy and function of the cardiovascular system. Hurst JW, Logue RB, eds. *The heart.* New York: McGraw Hill, 1966:28–30.
4. Diebel LN, Wilson RF, Taggett MG, et al. End-diastolic volume: a better indicator of preload in the critically ill. *Arch Surg* 1992;127:817.
5. Tuninninga YS, van Veldhuisen DJ, Brouwer J, et al. Heart rate variability in left ventricular dysfunction and heart failure: effects and implications of drug treatment. *Br Heart J* 1994;72:509.
6. Sarnoff SJ. Hemodynamic determinants of oxygen consumption of the heart with special reference to the tension-time index. *Am J Physiol* 1958;192:148.
7. Dahn MS, Wilson RF, Lange MP, et al. Hemodynamic benefits of verapamil after aortic reconstruction. *J Vasc Surg* 1989;9:806.
8. Majid PA, Roberts R. Heart failure. In: Civetta JM, Taylor RW, Kirby RR, eds. *Critical care.* Philadelphia: JB Lippincott, 1988:945–974.
9. Grande CM, Tissot M, Bhatt VP, et al. Preexisting compromising conditions. In: Capan LM, Miller SM, Turndorf H, eds. *Trauma: anesthesia and intensive care.* Philadelphia: JB Lippincott, 1991:240–251.
10. Tenzer ML. The spectrum of myocardial contusion: a review. *J Trauma* 1985; 25:620.
11. Frazee RD, Mucha P, Farnell MB, et al. Objective evaluation of blunt cardiac trauma. *J Trauma* 1986;26:510.
12. Geheb MA, Desai TK. Clinical disorders of calcium and magnesium metabolism in critically ill patients. In: Carlson RW, Geheb MA, eds. *Principles and practice of medical intensive care.* Philadelphia: WB Saunders, 1993:1196–1212.
13. Oster JR, Preston RA, Materson BJ. Fluid and electrolyte disorders in congestive heart failure. *Semin Nephrol* 1994;14:485.
14. Weigelt JA, Stanford GG. Cardiovascular failure. In: Moore EE, Mattox KL, Feliciano DV, eds. *Trauma,* 2nd ed. Norwalk: Appleton & Lange, 1991:941–964.
15. Reilly JM, Cunnion RE, Burch-Whitman C, et al. A circulating myocardial depressant substance is associated with cardiac dysfunction and peripheral hypoperfusion (lactic acidemia) in patients with septic shock. *Chest* 1989;95: 1072.
16. Harris P. Congestive cardiac failure: central role of the arterial blood pressure. *Br Heart J* 1987;58:190.
17. Sutton JSJ, Pfeffer MA, Plappert T, et al. Quantitative two-dimensional echocardiographic measurements are major predictors of adverse cardiovascular events after acute myocardial infarction. The protective effects of captopril. *Circulation* 1994;89:68.
18. Konstam MA, Kronenberg MW, Rousseau, et al. Effects of the angiotensin converting enzyme inhibitor enalapril on the long-term progression of left ventricular dilatation in patients with asymptomatic systolic dysfunction. *Circulation* 1993;88:2277.
19. Giles TD. Defining the role of atrial natriuretic factor in health and disease. *J Am Coll Cardiol* 1990;15:1331.
20. Dzau VJ, Packer M, Lilly LS, et al. Prostaglandins in severe congestive heart failure. *N Engl J Med* 1984;310:347.
21. Berger HJ, Zaret BL. Nuclear cardiology. *N Engl J Med* 1981;305:855.
22. Staudinger T, Locker GJ, Laczika K, et al. Diagnostic validity of pulmonary artery catheterization for residents at an intensive care unit. *J Trauma* 1998; 44:902.
23. Chang MC, Blinman T, Rutherford EJ, et al. Preload assessment in trauma patients during large-volume shock resuscitation. *Arch Surg* 1996;131:728.
24. Miller PR, et al. Randomized, prospective comparison of increased preload versus inotropes in the resuscitation of trauma patients: effects on cardiopulmonary function and visceral perfusion. *J Trauma* 1998;44:107.
25. Guzman JA, Lacoma FJ, Kruse JA. Relationship between systemic oxygen supply dependency and gastric intramucosal PCO_2 during progressive hemorrhage. *J Trauma* 1998;44:696.

26. Knudson MM, Bermudez KM, Doyle CA, et al. Use of tissue oxygen tension measurements during resuscitation from hemorrhagic shock. *J Trauma* 1997;42:608.
27. Wilson RF, Tyburski JG, Kubinec SM, et al. Intraoperative end-tidal carbon dioxide levels and derived calculations correlated with outcome in trauma patients. *J Trauma* 1996;41:606.
28. Prielipp RC, MacGregor DA, Butterworth JF IV, et al. Pharmacodynamics and pharmacokinetics of milrinone administration to increase oxygen delivery in critically ill patients. *Chest* 1996;109:1291.
29. Wilson RF, Binkley LE, Sabo FM, et al. Electrolyte and acid base changes with massive blood transfusions. *Am Surg* 1992;58:535.
30. Zaritsky AL, Horowitz M, Chernow B. Glucagon antagonism of calcium channel blocker-induced myocardial dysfunction. *Crit Care Med* 1988;16:246–251.
31. Bojar RM, Rastegar H, Payne DD. Methemoglobinemia from intravenous nitroglycerin: a word of caution. *Ann Thorac Surg* 1987;43:332.

42. RENAL RESPONSE TO SEVERE INJURY AND HYPOVOLEMIC SHOCK[1]

PHYSIOLOGY IN NORMAL STATE

Renal Blood Flow

The kidneys receive 20% to 25% of the cardiac output so that renal blood flow (RBF) averages about 1,250 to 1,500 mL/min in adults (2,3). This is equivalent to a mean renal plasma flow (RPF) averaging about 600 to 650 mL/minute. About 85% of the RBF perfuses the outer cortical (component I) glomeruli, and the remaining 15% of the RBF enters the juxtamedullary glomeruli located in the inner cortex and outer medulla (component II). Only a tiny fraction enters the inner medulla (component III) (Fig. 42-1) (2,3).

Glomerular Filtration

The normal glomeruli permit about 20% of the plasma to be filtered as a cell-free and protein-free filtrate. Thus, the normal glomerular filtration rate (GFR) averages about 125 mL/min or about 180 L/day. GFR can be determined by calculating the renal clearance of exogenously administered inulin. Inulin is completely filtered and is neither secreted nor reabsorbed by the tubules. "Clearance" is calculated as UV/P or the ratio of the urine (U) and plasma (P) concentrations of the substance being "cleared" multiplied by the urine volume (V) in mL/min.

Creatinine is almost completely filtered and relatively little is secreted by the tubules except in severe renal disease so that creatinine clearance can be used to estimate the GFR.

Proximal Convoluted Tubule

Normally, about 60% to 80% of the filtered water, sodium, chloride, potassium, and bicarbonate are reabsorbed in the proximal convoluted tubules. Virtually all of the filtered glucose and amino acids are also reabsorbed.

Loops of Henle

Each loop of Henle has a thin descending, thin ascending, and thick ascending segment. About 20% of the filtered water is reabsorbed in the descending limb. The ascending segments are impermeable to water. The thin ascending limb does very little, but the thick ascending segment reabsorbs about 25% of the filtered sodium, chloride, and potassium, as well as large amounts of calcium, bicarbonate, and magnesium. This segment also secretes hydrogen ions into the lumen.

The active sodium reabsorption against a gradient causes the inner medullary interstitium to become hypertonic, and this hypertonicity facilitates the subsequent concentration of filtrate with preservation of salt and water.

Following hemorrhagic shock, a redistribution of RBF to C_{III}, may "wash out" the osmoles in the medulla, thereby causing a transient "paralysis" of the renal concentrating mechanisms. Hypovolemic shock may also cause ischemia to the tubular cells, further impeding sodium reabsorption and disrupting medullary hypertonicity.

AXIOM Prolonged shock can interfere with the ability of the kidney to preserve water and sodium after renal perfusion is reestablished.

Distal Convoluted Tubule

The 20% of the glomerular filtrate (25 mL/min or 36 L/day) not reabsorbed in the proximal convoluted tubules enters the distal convoluting tubules where additional salt

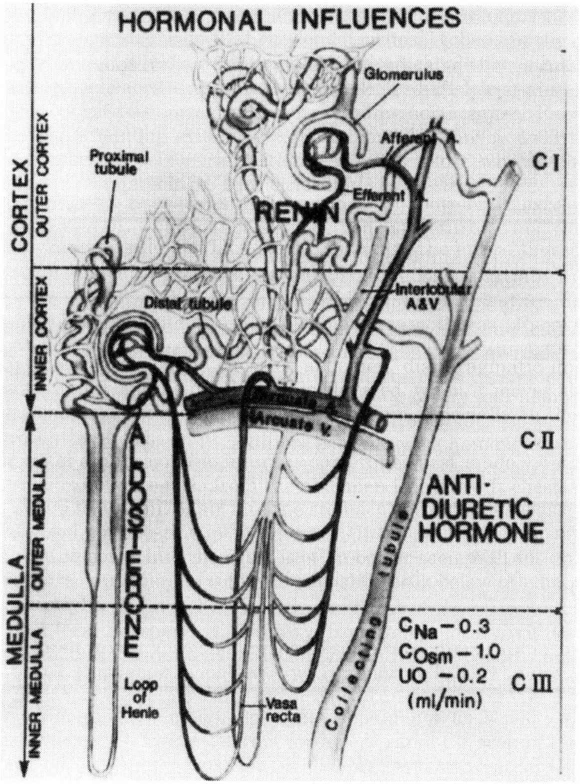

FIG. 42-1. Component I (CI) is outer cortex with greatest blood flow. Component II (CII) is inner cortex/outer medulla, which contains the juxtamedullary glomeruli, which have, within their nephrons, loops of Henle that extend into component III (CIII), the inner medulla, which helps to regulate the countercurrent mechanism.

and water are reabsorbed under the influence of aldosterone. The distal tubules also exchange sodium for potassium or hydrogen depending on pH and potassium delivery.

Each distal tubule passes near its glomerulus at a special site where the macula densa and Polkissen body combine to form the juxtaglomerular apparatus (JGA), which functions as a feedback loop affecting sodium and water balance.

Renin is released from the JGA in response to renal sympathetic nerve stimulation, increased renal arterial catecholamines, decreased afferent arteriolar perfusion, and reduced tubular sodium delivery. Once secreted, renin cleaves an α-2-globulin to produce angiotensin I, a decapeptide, which is a weak vasoconstrictor. This is converted in the lung to its highly active form, angiotensin II, which is an octapeptide. In addition to its renal effects, angiotensin II also stimulates adrenal secretion of aldosterone, which augments sodium reabsorption in the distal convoluting tubules.

Collecting Ducts

After exiting the distal tubules, the remaining hypotonic filtrate (15 mL/min or 20 L/day) enters the collecting ducts where water reabsorption occurs as the filtrate passes through the hypertonic inner medulla. Water reabsorption is regulated by antidiuretic hormone (ADH), which, in turn, is released from the posterior pituitary in response to baroreceptor (hypotension) and osmolar (increased tonicity) stimuli. Because of these concentrating mechanisms, urine osmolality may be as high as 1,400 mOsm/L in young healthy dehydrated individuals.

RENAL PHYSIOLOGY AFTER TRAUMA

During a class I hemorrhage (loss of 10% to 15% of blood volume), autoregulation allows GFR to be rather well maintained even when RBF is decreased to 70% of normal. To accomplish this, the filtration fraction (ratio of glomerular filtration to effective renal plasma flow [GFR/ERPF]) is increased from a normal of about 20% to more than 30%.

Class II hemorrhage (15% to 30% of the blood volume) exceeds the autoregulatory capacity of the kidney, and there is vasoconstriction at both the preglomerular and postglomerular arterioles (3). This causes a reduction in RBF to about 30% of normal and the GFR decreases to about 50% to 60% of normal. Blood flow is also shifted to juxtamedullary glomeruli, which have much longer loops of Henle and can absorb much more water and sodium. Even if urine volume is relatively well maintained, urine sodium tends to decrease below 10 to 20 mEq/L.

During a class III hemorrhage (30% to 40% of blood volume), RBF decreases to about 10% of normal and GFR decreases to less than 20% of normal.

After adequate resuscitation has restored the plasma volume and cardiac output, renal vasoconstriction subsides slowly over a number of hours or days, first in the afferent arterioles and later in the efferent arterioles.

INITIAL MANAGEMENT

Oliguria

AXIOM Oliguria immediately following trauma is generally due to hypovolemia and should not be treated with diuretics.

The treatment of oliguria after trauma should be directed toward rapid replenishment of the circulatory volume and cardiac output. The volume of balanced electrolyte solution (BES) replacement generally should be at least 3 L for every 1 L of estimated blood loss. Consequently, a patient with an acute 2.5-L hemorrhagic insult will have severe hypotension and require about 7.5 L of BES plus some restoration of the lost red cell mass.

If the hypovolemic trauma patient also has a general anesthetic, the renal autoregulatory response to the plasma volume deficit is altered. The protective preoperative renal vasoconstriction and the systemic vasoconstriction are inhibited by the anesthetic agents, and these changes can cause a marked reduction in cardiac output and RBF.

AXIOM Protection of the kidney during emergency surgery after acute trauma is best provided by administering enough fluid before and during surgery to achieve a urine output of at least 2 mL/min without diuretics.

After the mean arterial pressure and cardiac output have been restored to normal or higher levels by fluid and blood therapy, there may be continued oliguria for at least several hours as a result of persistent renal vasoconstriction and continued movement of fluid from the plasma volume (PV) into the interstitial fluid space, which becomes markedly depleted during the period of hypotension and hypovolemia.

Transient Postoperative Polyuria

A potentially hazardous renal response to severe hemorrhagic shock is a transient period of polyuria that may occur immediately after resuscitation. This increased urine output usually is not excessive, and it seldom exceeds 250 mL over a period of 30 minutes and seldom persists for more than 3 hours after the conclusion of surgery.

The purported mechanism for the polyuria is a "wash out" of osmoles from the inner medullary interstitium during the period of hypovolemic shock when the RBF was moved from the outer cortex to the inner medulla. Following resuscitation from hemorrhagic shock, the high urine volume should be ignored while addressing the resuscitation needs of the patient according to changes in blood pressure, pulse, pulse pressure, and the function of other organs.

Postoperative Obligatory Extravascular Fluid Sequestration

Following control of the bleeding and fluid resuscitation in the operating room, there is a period of obligatory extravascular fluid sequestration, sometimes referred to as phase II (4). The hallmarks of this postoperative fluid uptake phase, which usually lasts about 12 to 36 hours, include tachycardia, decreased blood pressure (BP), reduced pulse pressure, oliguria, weight gain, increased central venous pressures, and some degree of respiratory insufficiency.

If fluid administration is restricted or diuretics are given at this time because it is mistakenly believed that the patient is overloaded with fluid, the unrecognized plasma-volume deficit worsens, and the likelihood of acute renal failure (ARF) and death increases.

AXIOM Restriction of fluids or use of diuretics during the first 24 to 72 hours after traumatic shock while the patient is oliguric but looks overloaded with fluid can greatly increase morbidity and mortality rates.

Fluid Mobilization Phase

Following the period of extravascular fluid sequestration, the patient enters a period of fluid mobilization and diuresis, which is sometimes referred to as phase III (4). During the fluid mobilization phase, water may be added to the plasma volume faster than it can be excreted in the urine. Consequently, the BP may increase above 150/100 mm Hg, producing what has been referred to as "postresuscitation hypertension." Despite the combination of hypertension, expanded PV, increased total body water, and elevated cardiac index, the renal vascular resistance remains elevated, and the RBF tends to remain decreased. Use of diuretics at this point may successfully reduce the BP to less than 150/100 mm Hg, but an excessive diuresis may cause hypovolemia with progressive oliguria and renal dysfunction, which occasionally is fatal.

If antihypertensive agents are used during the fluid mobilization phase to control severely elevated BP, cardiovascular function should be monitored carefully to avoid hypotension. Hypotension is usually much more dangerous than mild to moderate postresuscitation hypertension. Slow, careful incremental intravenous (5 to 20 mg) doses of labetalol (to a total dose of 60 to 80 mg) can often provide adequate BP and heart rate control without causing hypotension.

Effects of Artificial Ventilation on Fluid Therapy

Varying degrees of pulmonary insufficiency that require ventilatory support may later develop in patients who have had severe hemorrhage (5). Controlled mechanical ventilation, even with zero end-expiratory pressure, has been shown to reduce renal perfusion. With the addition of positive end-expiratory pressure (PEEP), renal perfusion is reduced even more. As a consequence, additional fluid often has to be given to maintain an adequate RBF and urine output.

Acid-Base Balance after Hemorrhagic Shock

Severe hemorrhagic shock tends to cause an increasing lactic acidosis. Even after intravascular volume is repleted, metabolic acidosis may persist for several hours because the improvement in cell metabolism may be quite slow as a result of impaired renal excretion of the acids that were formed.

The renal mechanisms of acid excretion include tubular reabsorption of sodium bicarbonate and the excretion of acid with phosphate and ammonia, and these enable adults to normally excrete 70 to 80 mEq of acid per day through the kidneys. Even though acid excretion may be increased fourfold to fivefold by the kidneys in the presence of severe metabolic acidosis, these mechanisms require a reasonably normal GFR and RBF and intact renal tubules, which are disrupted by hemorrhagic shock. Consequently, a persistent metabolic acidosis can often be corrected more quickly by giving additional fluid and increasing the urine output.

Renal Response to Sepsis

Hyperdynamic Sepsis

In many septic patients, a hyperdynamic state develops, which is associated with increased cardiac output, increased RBF, decreased systemic vascular resistance, expanded extracellular fluid (ECF) volume, and increased urine output, which may persist even if the ECF becomes reduced. The mechanisms for this "inappropriate polyuria" may be related to the vasodilators that are present in hyperdynamic sepsis or a juxtamedullary "wash out." If fluid intake is restricted because it is thought that the polyuria is a result of fluid overloading, oliguric renal failure may develop. Careful monitoring of intake and output, vital signs, and urine sodium concentrations can help prevent development of severe hypovolemia and a resultant oliguric renal failure.

AXIOM A high urine output with a urine sodium concentration less than 10 mEq/L in septic patients indicates that the polyuria is present despite significant hypovolemia.

Hypodynamic Sepsis

In the later stages of severe sepsis, the patient often develops a hypodynamic state with decreased cardiac output and increased systemic vascular resistance despite aggressive fluid replacement. These patients also tend to have a decreased total RBF and GFR. This is best treated with aggressive fluid resuscitation. If oliguria persists despite adequate fluid resuscitation, blood pressure, and cardiac output, cautious loop diuretic therapy may be helpful.

ACUTE RENAL FAILURE

AXIOM Acute oliguric renal failure in sepsis or after trauma requiring hemodialysis is almost invariably fatal.

The mortality rate of ARF in the posttrauma patient averages about 50% to 60% (2,3). If it is an oliguric renal failure requiring hemodialysis, the mortality rate may exceed 90%. In contrast, nonoliguric ARF is usually associated with a mortality rate of less than 20%.

Terminology

Acute renal failure, which some physicians have also called acute vasomotor nephropathy, refers to a sudden, severe deterioration in renal function occurring from any cause (3). The term *acute tubular necrosis* (ATN) refers to a specific form of ARF occurring after shock or certain nephrotoxic agents.

Oliguria is defined as a urine output less than 400 mL/day. This represents the minimal amount of urine in which the normal daily solute load of 500 mOsm can be excreted when the urine is concentrated to 1,200 mOsm/kg of H_2O (3).

Anuria is defined as a urine volume less than 50 mL/day. Mechanical blockage of the bladder drainage system is the most common cause of sudden complete anuria.

Nonoliguric renal failure is defined as progressive azotemia despite a urine output exceeding 400 mL/day. High-output renal failure is defined as acute renal insufficiency developing in patients with urine volumes greater than 4,000 mL/day.

Causes

The most common cause of renal dysfunction within the first few days after trauma is severe, prolonged hypotension. Renal dysfunction that develops 1 to 2 weeks after trauma is usually caused by drug or radiocontrast dye-induced ischemia, drug-induced acute tubular interstitial nephritis (ATIN), or postinfectious glomerulonephritis. Other conditions associated with an increased risk of posttraumatic ATN include aortic cross-clamping, extensive muscle damage with myoglobinuria, major blood transfusion reactions, and severe persistent sepsis. Additional contributing factors include advanced age and preexisting renal vascular disease or hypertension.

Myoglobinuria and Hemoglobinuria

Severe myoglobinuria from muscle necrosis or hemoglobinuria from red blood cell destruction from hemolytic transfusion reactions may cause ATN in trauma patients even if renal perfusion is fairly well maintained. Each kilogram of skeletal muscle contains approximately 40 to 45 mEq of potassium, 730 mL of H_2O 23 mmol (2.25 g) of phosphate, and 4 g of myoglobin. Thus, severe crush injury can cause hyperkalemia, hyperphosphatemia, azotemia, hypocalcemia, disseminated intravascular coagulation, systemic hypotension, and myoglobinuria. Myoglobin concentrations exceeding 100 to 150 mg/dL discolors the plasma and urine. Myoglobin or hemoglobin nephrotoxicity is largely due to the toxic effects of ferrihemate and is dose dependent.

AXIOM ARF caused by hemoglobinuria or myoglobinuria is much more likely to occur if the patient is hypotensive and has an acid urine.

Myoglobinuria and hemoglobinuria are treated with fluids, loop diuretics, and mannitol to maintain a urine output of at least 100 to 200 mL/h and with sodium bicarbonate to keep urine pH above 6.5 (6). The alkalinity also reduces the formation of ferrihemate (6).

Drug-Induced Acute Renal Failure

The pathogenesis of ARF secondary to drugs varies with the specific agent (2,3). Important predisposing nephrotoxicity factors include preexisting renal disease, advanced age, volume depletion, prolonged therapy, and use of other nephrotoxic agents.

The most widely publicized drugs causing direct tubular toxicity are aminoglycosides; however, low trough levels and use of the aminoglycosides for only a few days greatly reduces the risk of nephrotoxicity. Nevertheless, simultaneous therapy with cephalosporins or clindamycin can potentiate aminoglycoside nephrotoxicity.

Azotemia, with serum creatinine levels increasing to more than 1.3 mg/dL, has occurred in up to 11% of hospitalized patients receiving aminoglycoside therapy (7). Clinically significant ARF (i.e., serum creatinine exceeding 2.0 mg/dL) occurs in only 3% to 5% of patients. The nephrotoxicity of aminoglycosides is increased in elderly patients, especially if the aminoglycosides are given concurrently with diuretics, radiographic contrast media, or amphotericin. The usual problem seen is a nonoliguric azotemia.

AXIOM Renal function, especially creatinine clearance, should be monitored closely in patients receiving prolonged courses or high doses of aminoglycosides.

Other antimicrobials that can produce ATN include amphotericin B and polymyxin B and E (3). The penicillin class of antibiotics, in particular methicillin, can cause a hypersensitivity reaction, resulting in acute interstitial nephritis, which is usually rapidly reversible once the offending drug is discontinued. Furosemide, thiazide, and allopurinol can also cause an allergic interstitial nephritis.

AXIOM Nonsteroidal antiinflammatory drugs should not be used in patients who may have renal impairment resulting from hypotension or nephrotoxic drugs.

A reversible decline in GFR has been reported after the administration of aspirin or nonsteroidal antiinflammatory agents, such as indomethacin, that inhibit prostaglandin synthesis. These agents appear to have no deleterious effect on renal function in healthy persons, but in patients with hypovolemia, preexisting hepatic or renal disease, or advanced congestive heart failure (CHF), they may produce a severe, persistent renal vasoconstriction. Gentamicin, amphotericin, and heavy metals can also cause excessive renal vasoconstriction.

Radiocontrast-Induced Nephropathy

The incidence of ARF after administration of radiocontrast agents may be as high as 13%. The possible mechanisms of the renal damage include direct tubular toxicity, renal ischemia, intratubular obstruction, and immunologic abnormalities. Changes in red blood cell morphology and function have also been implicated.

Contrast medium-induced nephropathy is characterized by serum creatinine levels beginning to increase about 24 hours after dye injection and peaking between the 3rd and 5th day. Renal function usually returns to normal in about 10 days unless the patient is allowed to become oliguric. Hemodialysis is seldom needed (8).

AXIOM In patients who are at risk for development of a contrast medium-induced nephrotoxicity, a high urine output should be maintained before and for 12 to 24 hours after the procedure.

Low-dose dopamine to improve RBF and urine output may be of some value. Hans et al. (9) prospectively studied 55 patients with chronic renal insufficiency (serum creatinine of 1.4–3.5 mg/dL) who underwent abdominal aortography and arteriography of the lower extremities. Group 1 (28 patients) received dopamine 2.5 μg/kg/min beginning 1 hour before arteriography and continuing for 12 hours. Group 2 received an equal volume of saline for the same period of time. Creatinine clearance did not change significantly from baseline after arteriography in the dopamine group; however, the control group showed a significant linear decrease in creatinine clearance by the 4th day (p=.016).

Classification of Acute Renal Failure

Prerenal Azotemia

Prerenal azotemia refers to acute renal insufficiency caused by inadequate renal perfusion. This is usually due to hypovolemia and hypotension, but it may also be caused by the low cardiac output of cardiac failure or renal artery stenosis. Initially at least, the prerenal oliguria is characterized by a low urine sodium and relatively high urine creatinine levels. Prerenal azotemia becomes irreversible if RBF is reduced so severely that oxygen and substrate delivery to the renal tubular cells is inadequate to keep them functional (3).

Postrenal Azotemia

Complete or almost complete anuria is rare in the absence of bilateral ureteral or lower urinary tract obstruction. Continued obstruction of the lower urinary tract results in a reduced GFR and concomitant increases in urea reabsorption. Prolonged obstruction to urine flow also causes renal vasoconstriction with further reduction in RBF, which may be severe enough to cause ischemic injury.

AXIOM Prompt recognition and therapy of urinary tract obstruction are necessary to prevent severe renal parenchymal damage.

Acute Tubular Interstitial Nephritis

In trauma patients, ATIN is almost invariably drug induced (10). The drugs that most commonly cause this entity are antibiotics (especially penicillins, sulfadiazines, and cephalosporins), nonsteroidal antiinflammatory agents (with the possible exception of Sulindac), diuretics, cimetidine, allopurinol, and diphenylhydantoin.

The classic features of ATIN are rash, arthralgias, fever, and eosinophilia in association with ARF. Peripheral blood eosinophilia and elevated serum IgE concentrations help to confirm the diagnosis of ATIN, but their absence does not exclude this disorder. Improvement in urine output and renal function within several days of removing the offending drug or agent is strongly suggestive of the diagnosis. The diagnosis of ATIN can be made by renal biopsy, if necessary. Although most patients make good recoveries from ATIN after withdrawal of the offending agents, some conditions may continue to deteriorate and severe renal failure may develop, requiring dialysis.

Pathophysiology of Acute Renal Failure

Some of the pathophysiologic changes believed to occur in kidneys developing ARF include the following:

- Tubular obstruction
- Passive backflow of glomerular filtrate
- Preglomerular arterial vasoconstriction causing decreased glomerular plasma flow
- Ultrastructural changes in the glomerular capillary bed resulting in decreased glomerular permeability (3)

Several investigators have noted that renal vasomotor abnormalities caused by toxins and ischemia are the main cause of oliguria in ATN and have suggested the name "acute vasomotor nephropathy." Indeed, studies using dye dilution techniques and radioactive microspheres have shown a pattern of renal cortical ischemia in patients with ARF of a magnitude severe enough to depress glomerular filtration.

Clinical Changes

AXIOM Characteristic electrolyte and acid-base changes in ARF include hyponatremia, hyperkalemia, metabolic acidosis, hyperphosphatemia, hypermagnesemia, and hypocalcemia.

The increase in serum creatinine in ARF is a direct result of decreasing rates of glomerular filtration. In the patient with near cessation of glomerular filtration, serum creatinine can be expected to increase at a rate of about 1.0 to 1.5 mg/dL/day (2).

Blood urea nitrogen (BUN) levels increase as GFR decreases. In contrast to creatinine, however, urea is partially reabsorbed in the tubules. Nevertheless, in hypercatabolic states associated with dehydration, the increases in BUN may exceed 25 mg/dL/day (3).

Hyponatremia is present in most patients with ARF as a result of intake of salt-poor fluids, an increased production of endogenous water, and increased loss of sodium in the urine resulting from decreased reabsorption of sodium by the damaged tubular epithelium.

The marked reduction of urinary potassium excretion in ARF results from decreased GFR and the impaired ability of renal tubules to secrete potassium into the tubular fluid (3). In the presence of continuing breakdown of muscle protein as a result of trauma or ischemia, potassium levels in the ECF can increase abruptly in oliguric patients.

AXIOM Hyperkalemia can become a life-threatening problem rapidly in hypercatabolic patients who are oliguric, particularly if they are also acidotic.

Accelerated protein catabolism caused by trauma, when combined with the declining ability of the kidney to excrete an acid load, also results in the rapid accumulation of sulfuric, phosphoric, and organic acids (3). Lactic acidosis may also contribute to this metabolic acidosis, which can become severe enough to require dialysis.

Plasma phosphorus and magnesium levels tend to increase and calcium levels decrease in trauma patients with acute oliguric renal failure.

Differential Diagnosis

Urinary Tract Obstruction (Postrenal Azotemia)

AXIOM Obstruction of the urinary tract (resulting from an occluded Foley catheter, or prostatic hyperplasia or urethral stricture in men) is the most common cause of sudden, complete cessation of urine output (3).

Trauma patients who are completely anuric should be examined promptly for bladder distension. In a patient without an indwelling catheter, the bladder should be catheterized. Ultrasonography may be used to evaluate upper urinary tract obstruction. If this study is equivocal, it may be helpful to obtain a computed tomography scan, radionuclide scanning, or retrograde pyelography.

Hypovolemia (Prerenal Oliguria)

Normal kidneys respond to a decreased RBF by conserving water and Na^+; however, in ARF, the GFR is severely decreased and the ability of the kidneys to concentrate urine and conserve Na^+ is impaired. The low GFR in ARF causes decreased urea and creatinine excretion, and the usual daily plasma BUN and creatinine increase is 5 to 10 and 0.5 to 1.0 mg/dL, respectively. After severe trauma, serum BUN and creatinine levels may increase more than 20 to 25 and 2.0 to 2.5 mg/dL/day, respectively; however, because the body's creatinine production may decrease from 1,000 to 1,500 mg/day to less than 300 to 600 mg/day, serum creatinine levels may not reflect the severe decrease in creatinine clearance or GFR for some time after the renal dysfunction has developed.

Normally, the BUN-to-plasma creatinine ratio is 10 to 15: With accelerated tissue catabolism, this ratio increases. Conversely, with rhabdomyolysis, the ratio tends to decrease because muscle creatine is converted to creatinine (10).

As GFRs decrease, tubular excretion of creatinine by the damaged tubular epithelium tends to increase. Consequently, creatinine clearance in these instances may overestimate GFR by up to 100%. For example, if the actual (inulin) GFR is 15 mL/min, creatinine clearance may be 30 mL/min or more, a value that is still below the normal range of 80 to 125 mL/min.

Normally, the concentration of creatinine in the urine is approximately 80 to 150 times that of plasma; in renal failure, the ratio usually declines to less than 20 to 40. Normally, the urea nitrogen in urine is about 50 to 80 times that of plasma; in renal failure, the ratio often declines to less than 5 to 10.

The "renal failure index" in which the urinary sodium concentration is divided by the U_{cr}/P_{cr} ratio may provide an accurate differential diagnosis between prerenal oliguria and ARF. A value greater than 1.0 suggests ATN, whereas a value less than 1.0 usually indicates prerenal azotemia.

The fractional excretion of sodium (FE_{Na}) is an index of tubular Na^+ reabsorption and glomerular filtration. This index is calculated according to the following equation:

$$FE_{Na}\ (\%) = [(U_{Na}/P_{Na})/(U_{cr}/P_{cr})] \times 100\%$$

An FE_{Na} value in an oliguric patient less than 1% is consistent with prerenal azotemia, whereas values exceeding 2% to 3% suggest renal parenchymal damage. This test requires only simultaneously collected "spot urine" and blood samples. Occasionally, however, the FE_{Na} is less than 1% in patients with ARF, especially after burn injury.

AXIOM FE_{Na} may not detect renal dysfunction in nonoliguric patients.

Impairment of water reabsorption by the tubular epithelium in ARF results in isosthenuric urine (specific gravity less than 1.010). The amount of plasma containing the solutes excreted in the urine per minute is referred to as osmolar clearance (C_{osm}). The free water clearance is equal to the urine volume (V) minus the osmolar clearance. In other words,

$$C_{osm} = U_{osm}/P_{osm} \times V$$
$$C_{H_2O} = V - C_{osm}$$

where U_{osm} is the urinary osmolality, C_{H_2O} is the free water clearance, V is the urinary flow in mL/min, and P_{osm} is the plasma osmolality. C_{H_2O} has a negative value when the urine is hypertonic, and a positive value when the urine is hypotonic. Thus, the normal C_{H_2O} is −15 to − 50 mL/h. In ARF, the C_{H_2O} is much less negative and usually ranges from −15 to + 15 mL/h. Thus, a decreasing urine osmolality and less negative free water clearance can be used to help diagnose ARF, but they are much more accurate when used in conjunction with creatinine clearance.

Urinalysis

AXIOM Urine in prerenal azotemia and obstructive uropathy is usually unremarkable except for hyaline casts.

Heavy proteinuria is suggestive of glomerular disease. With acute allergic interstitial nephritis, sterile pyuria is frequently present, and the demonstration of eosinophils in the urinary sediment is almost diagnostic.

In patients with ATN, it is common for urine to contain granular casts, white blood cells, tubular cells, and some protein, especially if oliguria is present. Gross hematuria is unusual in ATN and suggests bilateral renal arterial occlusion or obstruction. A positive dipstick for heme or red-brown pigmentation of the urine in the absence of red blood cells suggests renal failure secondary to hemoglobinuria or myoglobinuria.

Response to a Fluid Challenge

AXIOM Before making a diagnosis of ARF, a fluid bolus should be given to eliminate hypovolemia.

If renal failure is developing and the patient is not already overloaded with fluid, an intravenous fluid challenge of 500 to 1,000 mL of normal saline should be administered over 15 to 30 minutes. If the urine output fails to increase, a central venous pressure (CVP) or Swan-Ganz catheter should be inserted to monitor additional fluid challenges.

Treatment of Acute Renal Failure

Diuretics

AXIOM Indiscriminate use of diuretics in trauma patients with oliguria may precipitate the development of ATN; however, if hypovolemia has definitely been ruled out as the cause, diuretics may have both a diagnostic and therapeutic value.

If hypovolemia has been corrected, diuretics given soon after the onset of oliguria may convert the renal dysfunction to a nonoliguric type, which has a much better prognosis.

Mannitol is an osmotic diuretic that decreases proximal tubular sodium reabsorption. Beneficial effects may include an increase in GFR, a decrease in renin secretion, and a washout of any tubular casts. A 25-g intravenous bolus may be beneficial if given during the onset of oliguric renal failure after circulatory insufficiency has been eliminated, especially in patients with muscle injury, mismatched transfusions, intravascular hemolysis, or acute hyperuricemia.

Furosemide is a loop diuretic that acts primarily by inhibiting active sodium and chloride transport in the thick ascending limb of the loop of Henle (3). It has also been reported that it can increase RBF and decrease renin secretion by the macula densa. Furosemide is given as a 20- to 40-mg bolus in patients with persistent oliguria, and the dose is doubled every 15 to 30 minutes if no diuresis results. The recommended maximum cumulative dose to reverse impending oliguric renal failure is 500 to 1,000 mg.

Dopamine, when infused intravenously at doses of 1 to 3 μg/kg/min, is reported to increase RBF and shift blood flow from the renal medulla to the cortex. The diuresis and natriuresis seen after low-dose dopamine infusion is at least partially caused by the effects of dopamine on ADH.

Sodium and Water Balance

AXIOM Fluid restriction is an important part of the treatment of established acute oliguric renal failure, but adequate perfusion of vital organs must still be maintained.

The daily fluid requirement for a patient with acute oliguric renal failure is equivalent to measured losses from the gastrointestinal (GI) tract and kidneys plus 500 to 600 mL/day (3). Provision of water in excess of this amount can lead rapidly to fluid overload and hyponatremia. Accurate daily weights and measurement of intake and output are essential. Sodium intake should be limited to measured losses.

Metabolic Acidosis

In normal adults who consume an average diet, approximately 1 mEq/kg of nonvolatile acid is produced daily by a variety of metabolic processes. Hypercatabolic patients with trauma may generate much larger acid loads so that serum HCO_3 levels decline more rapidly. The specific cations released during catabolism include sulfate, phosphate, and a number of organic acids, including lactic acid. The accumulation of these ions in the body results in the development of an anion gap acidosis.

AXIOM The severe metabolic acidosis of established acute oliguric renal failure is best treated by reducing catabolism or with dialysis, not with sodium bicarbonate.

Medication Adjustments in Renal Failure

Loss of renal function requires dosage adjustment of all drugs that are excreted by the kidneys; however, if hemodialysis or peritoneal dialysis is being used, plasma levels must be followed closely.

Antithrombin III

Data suggest that the low antithrombin III (AT-III) levels seen in sepsis may contribute to renal and other organ failure by allowing intravascular coagulation to occur in nutrient capillaries. Indeed, Inthorn et al. (11) have noted that long-term AT-III supplementation in patients with severe sepsis improved pulmonary function and prevented the development of septic hepatic and renal failure.

Bedside Ultrafiltration

Continuous arteriovenous hemofiltration, using small hollow-fiber hemofilters without pumps, is an alternative to conventional acute dialysis methods (12). Arterial blood, usually from the radial artery, passes through an ultrafiltration apparatus by the force of the patient's BP and then returns to the patient usually via a cephalic or brachial vein line.

Continuous arteriovenous hemofiltration (CAVH) causes little or no hemodynamic change and is particularly useful in acute renal failure patients in whom hypotension develops during standard hemodialysis. Another important advantage of this method is that filtrate removal of up to 500 to 800 mL/h permits administration of the large volumes of parenteral nutrition solutions that are often needed by hypercatabolic oliguric patients. This system, however, requires continuous heparinization and constant supervision.

Hemodialysis

Indications

Hemodialysis, the mainstay of therapy for oliguric ARF, is urgently needed in patients who have

- Refractory pulmonary edema
- Hyperkalemic crises
- Uremic complications, such as pericarditis or encephalopathy
- Severe metabolic acidosis (13)

Benefits

AXIOM Hemodialysis, done prophylactically, can be extremely beneficial in hemodynamically stable patients with severe ARF.

Hemodialysis rapidly corrects uremia, fluid and electrolyte disturbances, and acidosis. Routine "prophylactic" dialysis simplifies the management of most patients by liberalizing water and electrolyte management. It also enhances the well-being of the patient by keeping the levels of urea and other nitrogenous substances at more normal levels (3). Perhaps the greatest benefit of aggressive or prophylactic hemodialysis is that it makes it possible to provide adequate calories and nutrition so as to minimize catabolism and promote improved wound healing.

Side Effects

Hemodialysis can cause a wide array of physiologic problems that can eventually be fatal in critically ill patients. It can cause transient hypoxemia caused by complement activation, which causes an increased adherence of platelets and polymorphonuclear leukocytes to pulmonary capillary endothelium. The hypoxemia and decreased white blood cell count usually return to baseline within 2 hours of the completion of the dialysis, but occasionally it can greatly aggravate a tendency for the development of adult respiratory distress syndrome.

Other complications of hemodialysis may include hypotension, hypoxemia, hemorrhage, arrhythmias, and problems related to technical errors (e.g., air embolism, dialysate contamination). "Disequilibrium syndrome," manifested by headache, nausea, vomiting, disorientation, tremors, and increased cerebrospinal fluid (CSF) pressure, may also occur with hemodialysis. These symptoms are probably caused by cerebral edema caused by sudden changes in the osmotic gradient between the brain and blood during hemodialysis. Paradoxical acidosis may also develop in the CSF during hemodialysis and cause similar symptoms. Elevation of intracranial pressure (ICP) has also been described in head-injured patients during dialysis (32).

AXIOM Even mild hypovolemia can cause severe hypotension when hemodialysis is started.

Bleeding from heparin anticoagulation during hemodialysis can be reduced by using a constant low-dose heparin infusion to maintain the activated clotting time or partial thromboplastin time at twice normal. Occasionally, it may be necessary to use protamine in the venous return channel of the dialysis system. Other dangers with hemodialysis include infected or thrombosed arteriovenous shunts or grafts.

Peritoneal Dialysis

Peritoneal dialysis, although much slower than hemodialysis, has the advantages of widespread availability, technical simplicity, and a low incidence of complications; however, hypercatabolic patients cannot be adequately dialyzed by this technique.

Peritoneal dialysis is the treatment of choice in children with ARF and in patients with gastrointestinal bleeding, shock, acute myocardial infarction, or acute pancreatitis. Contraindications include abdominal sepsis or recent laparotomy for abdominal trauma. Complications of peritoneal dialysis include peritonitis and compromised pulmonary function.

Complications of Renal Failure

Stress gastric ulcers develop in more than 20% of ARF patients. They may result from a number of factors, including elevated gastrin levels. Aluminum hydroxide antacids not only decrease gastric acidity and the risk of peptic ulcer disease but can also help to control the hyperphosphatemia that is often seen in ARF. Constipation caused by aluminum-containing antacids may be minimized by administering them with sorbitol.

Magnesium-containing antacids should not be given because of their potential for causing magnesium toxicity. Cimetidine can also prevent stress ulceration; however, it can cause mental confusion and encephalopathy, especially in elderly patients with ARF (24).

Hyperkalemia

AXIOM Hyperkalemia is the most rapidly fatal complication of acute oliguric renal failure.

Hyperkalemia is a frequent cause of death in patients with ARF, especially if tissue breakdown and metabolic acidosis are present. Blood transfusions add to this hazard. Acidosis increases the hyperkalemia. For each 0.1-unit decrease in pH, there is an increase of about 0.5 mEq/L in the serum K^+ levels.

Hyperosmolemia also causes hyperkalemia. Thus, hyperkalemia tends to be worse in oliguric patients with acute head injury treated with mannitol. Other factors that may cause an increased tendency to hyperkalemia include β-adrenergic receptor blockers, salt substitutes, captopril, and nonsteroidal antiinflammatory drugs.

Hyperkalemia with levels greater than 6.0 to 6.5 mEq/L can cause peaked T waves, prolongation of PR interval, and loss of the P wave on the electrocardiogram.

AXIOM Hyponatremia, hypocalcemia, and acidosis increase the cardiotoxic effects of hyperkalemia and should be corrected promptly.

The treatment of hyperkalemia is directed at

- Antagonizing the effect of K^+ on the cardiac conduction system
- Shifting K^+ intracellularly
- Removing K^+ from the body

An infusion of 1 to 2 ampules of 10% calcium gluconate (or $CaCl_2$ if the hyperkalemia is severe) over 10 to 30 minutes moderates the effects of K^+ on the heart without lowering its serum levels.

Potassium can be shifted into cells by intravenous administration of bicarbonate (50 to 100 mL of 8.4% $NaHCO_3$ given over 20 to 60 minutes), which elevates pH. Each 0.1-pH increase decreases serum potassium levels about 0.5 mEq/L. If the $NaHCO_3$ is given too rapidly, however, the resulting hyperosmolarity may transiently cause a hyperkalemia. Serum K^+ can also be reduced by inducing respiratory alkalosis.

The hypokalemic effect of glucose and insulin is concentration dependent; therefore, intermittent bolus insulin injections (plus glucose) every few hours is more effective than a continuous infusion.

Kayexalate (50 g) given orally or rectally every 2 to 3 hours decreases the total body potassium pool. Because the resin releases sodium in exchange for potassium, one must monitor the effects of sodium on central volume, especially if the patient is fluid overloaded.

AXIOM Kayexelate must be used carefully in hypervolemic patients.

Hemodialysis can extract 100 to 200 mEq of K^+ in 4 hours, and if done every other day, can maintain appropriate K^+ concentrations in most patients. Hypercatabolic and acidotic patients may require more frequent dialysis.

Anemia

Anemia develops in ARF because of reduced serum erythropoietin levels (10). Other factors, such as gastrointestinal bleeding and hemolysis, may be contributing factors. Consequently, the hematocrit should be measured frequently, and the anemia should be corrected with packed red blood cell transfusions as needed. With the recent introduction of erythropoietin as therapy for the anemia of chronic renal failure, there is much less need for blood transfusions in these patients.

Platelet Dysfunction

Bleeding secondary to platelet dysfunction is common in acute renal failure, but this can be corrected with dialysis. The prolonged bleeding time can also be corrected with cryoprecipitate or with 1-deamino-8-D-arginine vasopressin (DDAVP) given as a 0.3-μg/kg bolus in 50 mL of normal saline for 30 minutes before a procedure (14). Some success has also been reported with the use of intravenous conjugated estrogens, which have a longer half-life than DDAVP.

AXIOM Even if the platelet count is normal, bleeding time should be measured before any invasive or surgical procedure is undertaken in a patient with renal failure.

Pericarditis

Pericarditis, with or without pleuritis or pleural effusion, occasionally develops in patients with ARF. Pleuritic chest pain and pericardial friction rub are the most common clinical findings, but they often disappear as the effusion increases in size. Some fever with or without leukocytosis is also often present.

AXIOM If cardiac failure or hypotension develops in a patient with chronic renal failure, one should suspect pericardial effusion with tamponade.

Treatment of uremic pericarditis is directed toward treating the uremia with dialysis; however, hypovolemia after dialysis or ultrafiltration is a potential hazard. If true cardiac tamponade with hypotension or heart failure occurs, a pericardial window may be required.

Calcium Abnormalities in Acute Renal Failure

Shortly after the onset of ARF, plasma phosphate levels start to increase, and ionized calcium levels decline. Calcitonin and parathyroid hormone concentrations also increase. Tetany rarely occurs in ARF patients with hypocalcemia (unless total serum calcium levels decrease to less than 6.0 mg/dL) because the associated metabolic acidosis increases ionized calcium levels.

Nutritional Support

Providing proper nutrition in patients with ARF may be very difficult because of the high-energy requirements, insulin resistance, and negligible free water and urea clearance. Supplemental glucose is provided to minimize protein breakdown, and fluid overload is prevented by infusing the glucose as a 35% solution. These hypertonic solutions often have a caloric-nitrogen ratio exceeding 450-to-1. Administration of increased amounts of essential amino acids may also be helpful.

Each 6.25 g of protein or amino acids contains 1 g of nitrogen. Thus, patients with severe ARF receiving hyperalimentation may rapidly accumulate significant amounts of nitrogenous waste products. Amino acid loss during hemodialysis averages 10 to 15 g per run. CAVH can also be used to get rid of nitrogenous wastes, and it can remove up to 6 to 12 g every 24 hours. Because the water-soluble vitamins are also lost into the dialysate, they must be replaced after each dialysis.

OUTCOMES OF ACUTE RENAL FAILURE

Diuretic Phase of Oliguric Acute Tubular Necrosis

Most patients who survive acute oliguric ARF can expect return of adequate renal function in 3 weeks (13). Once the oliguric phase has passed and the patient enters the diuretic phase, the likelihood for survival is greatly increased, but one must still be careful to prevent recurrent hypotension, hypokalemia, or hyponatremia resulting from persistent impaired tubular reabsorption of free water and electrolytes.

The duration of dialysis for ARF does not appear to correlate with the degree of functional recovery, but older patients progress to chronic renal failure much more often and rarely make a complete recovery.

Nonoliguric Acute Renal Failure

The incidence of nonoliguric ATN is increasing. This increase is probably related to earlier and more aggressive fluid resuscitation and to an increased incidence of nephrotoxin-induced ATN. With more frequent monitoring of blood levels of nephrotoxic substances, milder forms of nonoliguric ARF are diagnosed with greater accuracy. The use of diuretics may also convert some cases of early oliguric ATN to a nonoliguric form.

Generally, management of nonoliguric patients is easier than of those with oliguric ARF because they have fewer fluid, electrolyte, and acid-base abnormalities. Only a few of the nonoliguric patients require dialysis, and nonoliguric ATN has a much lower mortality rate.

⊘ FREQUENT ERRORS

1. ***Assuming that oliguria is the result of renal failure without adequately ruling out hypovolemia and mechanical obstruction.***
2. ***Assuming that an elevated central venous pressure indicates adequate or excessive blood volume.***
3. ***Failure to recognize that polyuria resulting from sepsis or diuretics without adequate fluid replacement may result in severe plasma volume deficits, which can then cause acute oliguric vasomotor nephropathy.***
4. ***Failure to maintain high-volume urine flow during prolonged general anesthetics.***
5. ***Administration of potassium-containing fluids before ascertaining that renal function is adequate and hyperkalemia is not developing.***
6. ***Restriction of fluids to prevent pulmonary insufficiency in an oliguric patient.***
7. ***Failure to carefully monitor fluid and electrolyte balance during the recovery (diuretic) phase of acute vasomotor nephropathy.***

SUMMARY POINTS

1. Prolonged shock can interfere with the ability of the kidney to preserve water and sodium for hours or even days after renal perfusion is reestablished.

2. Oliguria immediately following trauma is generally caused by hypovolemia and should not be treated with diuretics.

3. Protection of the kidney during emergency surgery is best provided by administering enough fluid before and during surgery to achieve a urine output of at least 2 mL/min without diuretics.

4. Postoperative polyuria after hemorrhagic shock may mimic fluid overload and can cause the patient to become hypovolemic rapidly if fluids are restricted.

5. Glucose should generally not be present in the resuscitation fluids for severe trauma because of the hyperglycemia and osmotic diuresis that can result.

6. Following shock and resuscitation, there is often a period of obligatory extravascular fluid sequestration, which may cause the patient to appear overloaded with fluid even though the blood volume may be quite low.

7. Even with adequate fluid resuscitation, urine flow may be somewhat reduced for 24 to 48 hours following severe shock because of persistent renal vasoconstriction.

8. Current therapeutic guidelines for postresuscitative hypertension include fluid restriction and avoidance of colloids but not aggressive diuresis.

9. Hypotension caused by diuresis and fluid restriction is usually much more dangerous than moderate degrees of postresuscitation hypertension.

10. Positive-pressure ventilation, especially with PEEP, can greatly reduce RBF and urine output.

11. Metabolic acidosis may persist to some degree for up to several hours after shock has been corrected by adequate fluid resuscitation.

12. The polyuria of sepsis can cause severe hypovolemia if fluid intake is restricted because it is thought that the "inappropriate" polyuria is due to fluid overloading.

13. A "normal" urine output of 0.5 mL/kg/hour is inadequate in severely septic patients.

14. A high urine output with a urine sodium concentration less than 10 meq/L in a septic patient generally indicates that an inappropriate polyuria is present.

15. Hypodynamic sepsis with oliguria is best treated with aggressive fluid resuscitation.

16. If oliguria persists despite an adequate fluid resuscitation, BP, and cardiac output, then cautious loop diuretic therapy might be helpful; one should also look for the abdominal compartment syndrome.

17. Acute oliguric renal failure in sepsis or after trauma requiring hemodialysis is frequently fatal; nonoliguric renal failure has a much better prognosis.

18. ARF resulting from hemoglobinuria or myoglobinuria is much more likely to occur if the patient is also hypotensive and has an acid urine.
19. Renal function, especially creatinine clearance, should be monitored closely in patients receiving prolonged high doses of aminoglycosides.
20. Nonsteroidal antiinflammatory drugs should not be used in patients who may have renal impairment because of hypotension, drugs, or chronic heart failure.
21. Salt-loading and a high urine output should be maintained in patients who may be at risk for development of a contrast-medium-induced nephrotoxicity.
22. Prerenal oliguria should not be allowed to progress to acute oliguric renal failure because of inadequate fluids or inappropriate use of loop diuretics.
23. Prompt recognition and therapy of urinary tract obstruction is necessary to prevent severe renal parenchymal damage.
24. The classic features of ATIN are rash, arthralgias, fever, and eosinophilia in association with ARF.
25. Characteristic electrolyte and acid-base changes in ARF include hyponatremia, hyperkalemia, metabolic acidosis, hyperphosphatemia, hypermagnesemia, and hypocalcemia.
26. Hyperkalemia can rapidly become a life-threatening problem in hypercatabolic patients who are oliguric, particularly if they are also acidotic.
27. Obstruction of the urinary tract is the most frequent cause of sudden, complete cessation of urine output.
28. FE_{Na} is the best test for differentiating between pre-renal and renal oliguria.
29. A decreasing urine osmolality and less negative free-water clearance can be used to help predict the onset of ARF, but they are more accurate when used in conjunction with measured creatinine clearance.
30. Before making a diagnosis of ARF, a fluid bolus should be given to eliminate hypovolemia.
31. Indiscriminate use of diuretics in trauma patients with oliguria may precipitate the development of ATN; however, if hypovolemia has definitely been ruled out as the cause, diuretics may have both a diagnostic and therapeutic value.
32. Fluid restriction is an important part of the treatment of established acute oliguric renal failure, but maintaining adequate tissue perfusion is more important.
33. The severe metabolic acidosis of established acute oliguric renal failure is best treated with dialysis, not sodium bicarbonate.
34. Hyperkalemia is the most rapidly fatal complication of acute oliguric renal failure.
35. Hyponatremia, hypocalcemia, and acidosis increase the cardiotoxic effects of hyperkalemia and should be corrected promptly.
36. The treatment of hyperkalemia is directed at (1) antagonizing the effect of K^+ on the cardiac conduction system, (2) shifting K^+ intracellularly, or (3) removing K^+ from the body.
37. Kayexelate must be used cautiously in patients with congestive heart failure.
38. Throughout the period of renal failure and during the subsequent recovery phase, the drugs given must be selected and doses administered with great care to provide maximum benefit without aggravating renal dysfunction.
39. Even if the platelet count is normal, bleeding time should be measured before any invasive or surgical procedure is undertaken in a patient with renal failure.
40. If cardiac failure or hypotension develops in a patient with chronic renal failure, one should suspect pericardial effusion with tamponade.
41. When oliguria and impaired renal function develop in injured patients, fluid and electrolyte abnormalities can often be treated by bedside CAVH.
42. If nutritional protein causes the BUN to increase rapidly, dialysis or CAVH should be used to control the BUN.
43. Hemodialysis must be performed with extreme caution in patients with an elevated ICP.
44. Even mild hypovolemia can cause severe hypotension when hemodialysis is started.
45. Peritoneal dialysis, although slower than hemodialysis, has the advantages of widespread availability, technical simplicity, and a low incidence of complications.

REFERENCES

1. Lucas CE, Ledgerwood AM. Renal response to severe injury and hypovolemic shock. In: Wilson RF, Walt AJ, eds. *Management of trauma—pitfalls and practice,* 2nd ed. Philadelphia: William & Wilkins, 1996:945.
2. Etheredge EE, Hruska KA. Acute renal failure in the surgical patient. In: Zuidema GD, Rutherford RB, Ballinger WF, eds. *The management of trauma,* 4th ed. Philadelphia: WB Saunders, 1985:169.
3. Sirinek KR, Hura CE. Renal failure. In: Moore EE, Mattox KL, Feliciano DV, eds. *Trauma,* 2nd ed. Norwalk, CT: Appleton & Lange, 1991:927–939.
4. Lucas CE. Resuscitation of the injured patient: the three phases of treatment. *Surg Clin North Am* 1977;57:3.
5. Lucas CE, Ledgerwood AM. Hemodynamic management of the injured. In: Capan LM, Miller SM, Turndorf H, eds. *Anesthesia and intensive care.* Philadelphia: JB Lippincott, 1991:83–113.
6. Knochel JP. Rhabdomyolysis and myoglobinuria. *Semin Nephrol* 1981;1:75.
7. Bennett WM. Aminoglycoside nephrotoxicity. Nephron 1983;35:73.
8. Schwab SJ, Hlatky MA, Pieper KS, et al. Contrast nephrotoxicity: a randomized controlled trial of a nonionic and an ionic radiographic contrast agent. *N Engl J Med* 1989;320:149.
9. Hans SS, Hans BA, Dhillon R, et al. Effect of dopamine on renal function after arteriography in patients with pre-existing renal insufficiency. *Am Surg* 1998;64:432.
10. McGoldrick MD, Capan LM. Acute renal failure in the injured. In: Capan LM, Miller SM, Turndorf H, eds. *Anesthesia and intensive care.* Philadelphia: JB Lippincott, 1991:755–785.
11. Inthorn D, Hoffmann JN, Hartl WH, et al. Antithrombin III supplementation in severe sepsis: beneficial effects on organ dysfunction. *Shock* 1997;8:328.
12. Kaplan AA, Longnecker RE, Folkert VW. Continuous arteriovenous hemofiltration. *Ann Intern Med* 1984;100:358.
13. Hakim R, Lazarus M. Hemodialysis in acute renal failure. In: Brenner BM, Lazarus MJ, eds. *Acute renal failure.* Philadelphia: WB Saunders, 1983:643.
14. Mannucci PM, Remuzzi G, Pusineri F, et al. Deamino-8-D arginine vasopressin shortens the bleeding time in uremia. *N Engl J Med* 1983;308:8.

43. GASTROINTESTINAL COMPLICATIONS FOLLOWING TRAUMA[1]

PSEUDOMEMBRANOUS COLITIS

Pseudomembranous or antibiotic-associated colitis is an acute exudative infection of the large intestine caused by *Clostridium difficile*. This organism is an anaerobic, spore-forming, gram-positive bacillus that produces at least four toxins:

1. Toxin A (or enterotoxin, which is the most active one);
2. Toxin B (or cytotoxin);
3. A heat labile toxin; and
4. A motility-altering factor (2).

C. difficile colitis has been reported to follow almost all commonly used antibiotics.

AXIOM Diarrhea in a patient who has been on antibiotics should be considered the result of pseudomembranous colitis until proven otherwise.

C. difficile colitis is also referred to as pseudomembranous colitis because, in the advanced form, necrotic membranes adhere to the mucosal surface. The clinical presentation is variable and ranges from a mild, self-limited diarrhea to toxic megacolon. Patients who are immunosuppressed because of infection with human immunodeficiency virus, cancer chemotherapy, or antitransplant rejection drugs should also be suspected of having cytomegalovirus colitis (3).

The time of onset of symptoms from pseudomembranous colitis is extremely variable. Symptoms may begin in 2 to 3 days or develop as late as 3 to 4 weeks after antibiotics are started. Multiple liquid bowel movements are common, but bloody diarrhea or colonic perforation are rare. The responsible organism (*C. difficile*) and its toxin are found frequently in the feces of affected patients, especially those with the more severe involvement. Diagnosis is usually made by examining the feces for toxin, but the toxin may not be detected in mild-moderate cases. Fiberoptic sigmoidoscopy can also miss mild lesions.

The current treatment of choice for pseudomembranous colitis is oral metronidazole. If the patient cannot take oral medication, intravenous metronidazole may control the problem. Vancomycin tends to be more effective, but its use is being restricted to discourage growth of vancomycin-resistant enterococci.

⊘ PITFALL

Antidiarrheal drugs are contraindicated in patients who may have pseudomembranous colitis.

Antidiarrheal medications, such as Lomotil (diphenoxylate), are contraindicated in patients who may have *C. difficile* colitis because they would allow the *C. difficile* toxin to stay in the bowel longer, producing more systemic toxicity and possible perforation. In rare circumstances, a subtotal colectomy with a temporary ileostomy may be necessary for bowel necrosis or perforation.

COMPLICATIONS FROM TRAUMA

Stress Gastric Ulcerations

Etiology

Stress ulcers are a manifestation of mucosal ischemia and severe underlying illness. Lasky et al. (4) have recently noted that the factors that increase the risk of stress ulcers in trauma patients include mechanical ventilation longer than 48 hours, head injury, extensive burns, acute renal failure, acid-base disorders, coagulopathy, multiple operative procedures, coma, hypotension for longer than 1 hour, and sepsis. Gastric lesions in the body and fundus of the stomach occur in virtually 100% of patients with severe shock or trauma and in up to 85% of patients with severe burns (>35% body surface area). The antrum is usually either spared or only minimally involved.

Areas of superficial mucosal necrosis, referred to as erosions, often appear within 24 to 48 hours. When they extend beyond the muscularis mucosa, these erosions are referred to as ulcers, which may develop by 48 to 96 hours.

A large amount of data in experimental animals suggest that any process that decreases gastric mucosal blood flow, when combined with gastric acid, can cause stress gastritis (5). As the acid from the gastric lumen diffuses back into the mucosa and submucosa, the development of the gastritis and ulcerations is related to an imbalance between the amount of diffusing acid and the ability of the mucosa to neutralize acid.

Diagnosis

Stress ulcers are painless unless perforation occurs. Although some bleeding may be encountered within hours of injury, it generally takes 4 to 5 days for significant bleeding to occur; this is more likely to occur in the presence of sepsis.

The clinical diagnosis of stress gastritis is generally made after blood begins to appear in the nasogastric aspirate of an intensive care unit (ICU) patient; however, a hazard exists in assuming that such blood is caused by stress ulcer and not some other condition, such as a bleeding peptic ulcer or missed injury. Definitive diagnosis is established by esophagogastroduodenoscopy (EGD).

Prophylaxis

AXIOM Antacids, H2-receptor antagonists, or sucralfate can usually prevent severe stress gastritis, as long as severe shock and sepsis are controlled and the gastric pH is kept higher than 4.5.

An effective prophylactic regimen for most patients with stress gastritis involves instillation of 30 mL of antacid into the stomach via a nasogastric tube which is then clamped. The tube is aspirated at the end of one hour, and the pH of the aspirate is measured using pH paper. If the pH exceeds 4.5, 30 mL of antacid are reinstalled again for one hour; however, if pH is less than 4.5, 60 mL of antacid are given. This sequence is repeated hourly or every two hours. Unfortunately, use of antacids is quite labor-intensive, and diarrhea can accompany the treatment.

A continuous intravenous drip of an H_2-receptor antagonists is as good as antacids and requires much less work by the nurses; however, if bleeding occurs while using one of these agents, adding an antacid or Carafate (sucralfate) often causes the bleeding to cease.

Sucralfate in doses of 1 gram every 6 hours is though to be equally effective, and since the gastric acidity is not altered, some feel there is less risk of bacteria multiplying in the stomach and causing pneumonia if gastric contents are aspirated.

Cook et al. (6) in a recent study of 1200 mechanically ventilated patients found clinically important gastrointestinal bleeding in 10 of 596 (1.7 percent) of the patients receiving ranitidine, as compared with 23 of 604 (3.8 percent) of those receiving sucralfate. In the ranitidine group, 114 of 596 patients (19.1 percent) had ventilator-associated pneumonia, as compared with 98 of 604 (16.2 percent) in the sucralfate group. There was, however, no significant difference between the groups in mortality in the intensive care unit (23.5% versus 22.8%).

Treatment

Once stress gastric bleeding begins, the stomach should be irrigated with warm (not cold) saline. Iced saline may inhibit clotting and may reduce gastric mucosal blood flow.

If stress gastric bleeding continues, one can try an intravenous infusion of vasopressin at 0.1 to 0.4 units/min. This can cause severe vasoconstriction of gastrointestinal vessels and is anecdotally successful, as long as the gastric luminal contents remain continuously neutralized with antacid. The adverse effects of vasopressin (e.g., hypertension, coronary artery constriction, cardiac arrhythmia, congestive heart failure, and water retention) can be reduced by simultaneous intravenous nitroglycerin or nitroglycerin paste on the skin. The patient should be on a cardiac monitor because arrhythmias can occur. Intravenous somatostatin analogue (octreotide 100-mg bolus intravenous followed by 25 mg 1 h ¥ 24 h) is considered safer and more effective than vasopressin (7).

Most bleeding from stress ulcers tends to occur within the distribution of the left gastric artery. If this is confirmed by arteriography, the left gastric artery can be occluded by the injection of autologous clot; this has been successful in some patients.

Although it is a major procedure in these critically ill patients, total gastrectomy is probably the procedure of choice if severe bleeding persists despite rigorous control of gastric pH and suturing of the major mucosal bleeding points.

Cushing's Ulcer

In 1933, Harvey Cushing described several patients with head trauma or brain surgery in whom deep gastric, duodenal, or esophageal ulcers developed. The gastric mucosal changes caused by stress are similar to those associated with intracranial pathology; however, patients with typical Cushing's ulcers tend to have high gastrin levels and secrete more acid, and the ulcers are usually deeper and more likely to perforate.

Curling's Ulcer

Acute *duodenal* ulcerations associated with burns were reported in 1923 by a London surgeon, Joseph Swan, who called them Curling's ulcers after the 1843 report by Thomas Blizard Curling (1811–1888) (8). Most physicians also refer to *gastric* ulcers occurring in burn patients as Curling's ulcers.

Enterocutaneous Fistulas

Causes

Although most enterocutaneous fistulas are the result of an operative injury to the intestine or an anastomotic disruption, a few enterocutaneous fistulas that develop after trauma are due to failure to detect the bowel injury at the time of surgery or to inadequately debride the injury (11). Small perforations can easily be missed at the initial operation, especially if the patient had multiple other injuries and the operation was completed quickly because of continuing hypotension, acidosis, or coagulopathy. Forcing distended bowel into the peritoneal cavity without decompressing the lumen can also cause delayed iatrogenic leaks. Bowel may also be eroded by drains or exposed fascial sutures used to close a large abdominal wall defect under some tension.

Pathophysiology

Fistulas involving any part of the small intestine have a higher mortality rate than those of the stomach or colon. Mortality rates range from 7% to 21% and tend to be higher with high-output proximal fistulas (9). Definitions of a high-output fistula ranges from 200 or more mL/day to greater than 1,000 mL/day during the first 48 hours. The increased mortality rate from high-output fistulas is usually due to the increased risk of developing intraabdominal infection and the significantly lower rate of spontaneous closure.

Several other variables also affect the outcome of a patient with an enterocutaneous fistula. These include obstruction of distal bowel, foreign bodies (such as sutures), carcinoma, Crohn's disease, prior radiation therapy, short tract between the bowel and skin, adjacent infection, or large abdominal wall defect.

Treatment

General Principles

The essential principles in managing most intestinal fistulas include control of the fistula, control of any associated sepsis, and nutritional support. Control of the fistula means that the effluent is well drained from the peritoneal cavity, the skin or surface wound is protected from enzymatic digestion, and fluid and electrolyte balance is maintained. In some instances, early surgery may be required to achieve control of the fistula output.

Although sump tubes or closed-drainage systems can generally provide effective drainage, they are easily plugged by debris. Consequently, if an operation is performed to place sump tubes near a fistula, it may be advisable to place additional drains in the area in case the sump tubes should fail.

Placing a sump tube directly into a small bowel fistula may protect the skin, but additional measures, such as the use of karaya powder or protective skin wafers and ointments are often necessary. If the fistula opening on the skin is far enough away from the incision and bony prominences, application of a disposable ileostomy appliance can be helpful.

AXIOM Metabolic support with adequate calories and protein plus accurate replacement of the fistula output of water and electrolytes are essential for obtaining optimal healing of the fistula.

A "drain me/feed me" arrangement can occasionally be made with a proximal and distal tube in the lumen, thereby conserving fluid and electrolyte losses. This approach often requires a great deal of time and effort to function properly.

Sepsis is the most frequent complication associated with intestinal fistulas. Although antibiotics are of little value until the fistula contents are well drained, they should be used whenever there is evidence of sepsis. Furthermore, antibiotics are not a substitute for drainage of intraabdominal abscesses. If the patient is septic and no other source is evident, exploration of the abdominal cavity is indicated, even if an intraabdominal abscess cannot be localized preoperatively with radiologic studies.

When control of the fistula and any associated sepsis is achieved, radiography with contrast may be helpful for determining the site of origin of the fistula, the continuity of the proximal and distal bowel, and the presence or absence of a distal obstruction. This information is useful for planning the next phase of management, which involves provision of adequate enteral nutrition when possible; however, attempts to provide adequate nutrition are of little value if severe sepsis persists.

Enteral nutrition is usually much more effective and much less expensive than total parenteral nutrition (TPN), and it provides a convenient portal for refeeding proximal fistula effluent. In some instances, a feeding tube can be passed beyond a proximal fistula or a feeding jejunostomy can be constructed distal to the fistula. It is generally unnecessary to resort to parenteral nutrition for small, well-drained distal ileal or colonic fistulas, which are no different in principle from an ileostomy or colostomy.

AXIOM Spontaneous closure of a fistula should not be expected to occur until adequate control of the fistula, eradication of the sepsis, and nutritional repletion occur.

The overall figures for spontaneous closure of small bowel fistulas vary from 30% to 70%. Longer fistula tracts are more likely to heal. Only 17% of the fistulas with tracts less than 2 cm in length close spontaneously (9). Of the intestinal fistulas that close spontaneously, about 90% do so within 1 month of the eradication of infection. If the fistula output continues to decrease after 1 month of nonoperative treatment, such therapy should be continued as long as there appears to be a reasonable hope of spontaneous healing.

AXIOM If the output of an intestinal fistula has not significantly decreased within 1 month of proper control of infection and provision of adequate nutrition, definitive surgical correction is often required.

Intestinal fistulas associated with large abdominal wall defects rarely close spontaneously. Consequently, it is advisable to provide soft-tissue coverage of the abdominal cavity at the time of the definitive operative procedure. Reconstruction of the abdominal wall with polypropylene mesh is inadvisable if omentum cannot be placed between the bowel and the mesh. If the bowel and mesh are in direct contact, the mesh eventually becomes incorporated into the bowel wall, and this can cause new enterocutaneous fistulas. An additional problem in using prosthetic mesh is that it can become contaminated by the fistula and be a nidus for later persistent infection.

AXIOM The most successful operative approach for an enterocutaneous fistula is resection of the involved segment of bowel with reanastomosis of normal tissue.

Lateral Duodenal Fistulas

The treatment of lateral duodenal fistulas is extremely controversial with spontaneous closure rates ranging from 27% to more than 90% (9). Many authors advocate a Billroth II gastrectomy or "diverticularization" of the duodenum with closure of the pylorus and construction of a gastrojejunostomy. This converts the lateral or "side-fistula" to an "end-fistula," which has much less bowel content running by it and is more likely to close spontaneously. Other measures helpful in the control of a lateral or side duodenal fistula include a feeding jejunostomy and insertion of a tube into the fistula itself, which results in more rapid formation of an established tract.

If surgery is required to treat a persistent duodenal fistula, the simplest and most effective approach is to drain it with a Roux-en-Y loop of jejunum.

Enteroenteric Fistulas

Etiology

Most enteroenteric fistulas (in the absence of Crohn's disease) occur following an operation involving a colonic anastomosis or resection. Most of these fistulas occur as a result of a bowel leak causing an abscess, which then erodes into an adjacent segment of bowel (or vice versa). Such fistulas are usually diagnosed several days after the initial surgery or trauma.

AXIOM A fistula between the small intestine and colon frequently presents with diarrhea, which is usually caused by reflux of colonic organisms into the small bowel, causing malabsorption.

Treatment

In some instances, the diarrhea associated with enteroenteric fistulas is incapacitating and difficult to treat without surgery; however, definitive repair may be inadvisable for some time because of debility of the patient or the local inflammatory reaction. In such circumstances, a colostomy proximal to the fistula is often a simple, effective procedure because the bacterial reflux into the small intestine is stopped or at least is greatly reduced.

AXIOM Enteroenteric fistulas rarely heal spontaneously, but definitive repair is undertaken only if the patient is symptomatic and is in optimal condition for the operation.

Anastomotic Disruptions

Diagnosis

Because about half of the disruptions of bowel anastomoses occur on the second through the fourth postoperative days, the clinical picture may be difficult to differentiate from routine postoperative changes.

AXIOM Patients with persistent fever plus ileus or delayed gastric emptying following small bowel repairs should be considered to have an anastomotic disruption until proven otherwise.

Early diagnosis of anastomotic leaks can be extremely difficult, but satisfactory radiographic demonstration of all suture lines is essential if suspicion of an anastomotic disruption exists. Water-soluble contrast media should be used (instead of barium) to diagnose proximal leaks when possible because barium is irritating to the peritoneal cavity and can act as an adjuvant to increase the seriousness of intraperitoneal infection. Nevertheless, barium is usually needed to demonstrate distal small bowel leaks.

Treatment

By the time the diagnosis of an anastomotic disruption is made, peritonitis is often present, and the involved bowel is generally edematous and inflamed. The safest approach usually is to exteriorize the anastomotic disruption either as a loop stoma or as a proximal stoma and distal mucous fistula. Although a proximal small bowel stoma can pose additional morbidity for the patient, it should not be repaired surgically until the patient has regained his or her normal state of health.

AXIOM An intestinal leak that is contained and is not causing sepsis does not need to be drained, as long as it has good communication with the lumen.

Delayed Colon Perforation

Delayed perforation of the colon may not occur until days or weeks after the initial trauma. Most colon serosal tears and intramural hematomas heal without complication; however, a few of these seemingly innocuous injuries can lead to complications, such as delayed perforation or stricture as a result of (1) liquefaction of a hematoma within a pseudocapsule and subsequent osmotic expansion of the contained fluid, causing compression of the intestinal blood supply, or (2) intramural abscess formation. In addition, omentum or small bowel may initially wall off an acute perforation, only to subsequently break down.

AXIOM Evidence of sepsis or multiple organ failure after abdominal trauma should be considered the result of an intraabdominal infection until proven otherwise.

Development of increasing signs of peritonitis prompts immediate operation. In less obvious situations, laparotomy may be indicated for the patient in whom an ileus develops more than 12 hours after injury or in the patient who has an initial ileus that fails to resolve after 3 to 4 days. Most postoperative septic complications reported after intraperitoneal repair of colonic injuries are not the result of suture line disruption; however, confirmation of an intact suture line is essential.

BOWEL OBSTRUCTION

Etiology

Adhesions are the most common cause of small intestinal obstruction, particularly following trauma or surgery. Many of these adhesions appear to be related to foreign body reactions, and the most frequent foreign materials are glove powder, lint or threads off sponges, and sutures. Another mechanism involves serosal injury from trauma, operative manipulation, or drying during operative exposure. If the trauma patient did not have abdominal surgery, one should also look for hernias or a preexisting malignancy.

Diagnosis

AXIOM Increasing abdominal distension after the fourth postoperative day should be considered a result of bowel obstruction until proven otherwise.

Most patients with bowel obstruction have cramping, intermittent abdominal pain, distension, and absence of flatus or stool. A distinction should be made between the crampy lower abdominal pain that patients frequently experience before first passing flatus and the periumbilical cramping pain characteristic of small bowel obstruction, which tends to get progressively worse. Making the diagnosis early is much more difficult if flatus or stool is initially passed before the bowel obstruction became complete.

AXIOM A feculent odor or appearance of nasogastric aspirate or vomitus is often a sign of complete small bowel obstruction.

When small bowel is completely obstructed, the bacterial count in the proximal lumen increases rapidly. Once the number of anaerobes exceeds 10^8/g, the intestinal contents increasingly look and smell like feces.

AXIOM High-volume gastric aspirates after abdominal trauma should make one suspicious of a bowel obstruction or peritonitis.

Although the presence of high-pitched tinkling bowel sounds coincident with crampy abdominal pain is characteristic of a mechanical small bowel obstruction, the presence or absence of bowel sounds or the type of bowel sounds heard are frequently of little help in differentiating between ileus and mechanical obstruction, especially in the early postoperative period.

With small bowel obstructions, upright films of the abdomen typically show dilated small bowel loops with differential air-fluid levels and little or no gas in the colon; however, occasionally an ileus can cause a similar x-ray picture. Serial radiography may be particularly helpful for differentiating between complete and incomplete bowel obstructions.

Contrast studies can sometimes help clarify confusing situations; however, a distal obstruction may not be evident with water-soluble contrast material because it becomes too diluted by the time it reaches that area. Nevertheless, diarrhea resulting from the hyperosmotic effect of water-soluble contrast medium may occasionally occur if only a partial obstruction is present. Barium can outline distal bowel fairly well, even when it is diluted, and follow-through radiography with this material may be helpful in distinguishing between partial and complete obstructions. If it is not clear whether a loop of bowel is dilated small bowel or colon, a contrast enema should be performed.

Treatment

If the patient has relatively little pain and is not at all toxic, a partial small bowel obstruction can be treated with nasogastric suction for at least 5 to 7 days. At that time, TPN should be considered and, unless the patient is known to have severe adhesions, an exploratory laparotomy should be strongly considered. Although a partial small bowel obstruction does not usually require surgery, a complete small bowel obstruction with no passage of gas or feces should be relieved surgically within 24 to 48 hours.

STRANGULATION OF BOWEL

Diagnosis

If possible, bowel obstruction should be diagnosed before strangulation occurs; however, this can be extremely difficult at times. After placement of a functioning nasogastric tube and restitution of plasma volume losses, the patient may feel somewhat better, even if strangulated bowel is present. The observation that the patient has had a bowel movement or passed flatus can also be deceptive because the stool and gas may have been present in the colon at the time that the more proximal obstruction developed.

An onset of constant severe abdominal pain localized to one abdominal quadrant should make one suspicious of bowel strangulation. Localized peritoneal signs should also make one suspicious of this diagnosis. Increasing arterial lactate levels may occasionally be the first evidence of strangulated bowel.

One study indicated that, if one of four signs (pulse greater than 96/minute, oral temperature more than 37°C, abdominal tenderness, or white blood cell count greater than 10,000/mm^3) was present, there was a 7% incidence of strangulation. If two or three of those findings were present, the incidence of gangrenous bowel increased to 24%, and if all four findings were present, the incidence reached 67%. Although these data may be different at other centers, they do offer some guidelines for managing these patients.

Strangulating bowel obstruction can be confused with acute pancreatitis because both may present with relatively constant pain and elevated serum amylase levels. If the differential diagnosis between strangulation and pancreatitis is unclear, it is safer to operate. A diagnosis of strangulation on plain abdominal radiography can be made if gas is seen in the portal vein or in the wall of the involved intestine, but these are infrequent and late radiographic signs that are usually not seen until other grave clinical signs are present.

Treatment

AXIOM One of the main reasons to operate early on what is probably a simple intestinal obstruction is the difficulty in excluding the presence of strangulation.

Following reduction of a strangulating bowel obstruction, it can be difficult to determine whether the bowel is viable. Criteria such as mesenteric pulsations, color of the bowel wall, bleeding from a superficial incision in the bowel, and presence of peristalsis are not always reliable indicators. Other methods that have been proposed for determining bowel viability include fluorescent dyes and Doppler ultrasound. Another problem with intraoperative assessment in borderline cases is that bowel perfusion is directly related to cardiac output, which may not be optimal at the time that the bowel is being examined.

When only a small portion of the small bowel is questionably viable, it is usually safer to resect the area in question rather than to procrastinate. If the viability of a majority of the small intestine is in question, however, it is usually safer to observe it and perform a "second-look" operation within 24 hours. Rarely, a patient may even require a third look to ensure viability.

PITFALL

Failure to perform a second-look operation on marginally viable bowel greatly increases the risk of nonviable bowel being left in place and causing fatal peritonitis.

COMPLICATIONS FROM TREATMENT

Improperly Functioning Ileostomy

Creation of an imperfect, albeit temporary, ileostomy can generate inordinate morbidity for a patient. Some of the more common technical errors include

1. Improper location of the ostomy so that it is difficult to place an appliance;
2. Too short an ileostomy bud;
3. Inadequate fascial apertures;
4. Tension;
5. Stripping of mesentery from the end of the stoma; and
6. Failure to close the intraperitoneal space around the bowel leading to the stoma.

Timing of ileostomy closure should not be at a fixed, arbitrary interval. It is safest to do it electively after all of the patient's wounds have healed and good nutritional balance and the usual state of health have returned.

Tube Jejunostomy Feedings

Although early jejunostomy feedings can be beneficial to severely injured patients who are not likely to eat for 7 days or longer, they can be associated with a number of complications. A dislodged jejunostomy tube can rapidly cause severe peritonitis, which may not be detected promptly in the immediate postoperative period, especially after severe trauma. Needle catheter jejunostomies are more likely to occlude and usually cannot be replaced if they were dislodged prematurely. A catheter jejunostomy, however, may also have problems. With the Witzel technique, partial small bowel obstruction may occur if too much jejunum is plicated over the catheter. In addition, successful replacement may be impossible if dislodgement occurs within 48 to 72 hours. If a dislodged catheter is promptly reinserted along what seems to be a well-established tract, it is essential to confirm proper replacement of the catheter by obtaining a radiograph while flushing water-soluble contrast material through the new catheter.

AXIOM The position of the jejunostomy feeding tube within the bowel lumen should be confirmed after any manipulation or replacement prior to beginning or resuming feedings.

Colostomy Complications

A colostomy that is brought out to the skin under tension invites major problems because retraction into the subcutaneous tissues can lead to a devastating necrotizing infection of the abdominal wall or severe peritonitis. Thus, any retraction of the stoma in the early postoperative period is an indication for prompt operative revision. Suturing the colon wall to the abdominal fascia does little to prevent such retraction because the bowel will still pull away from the fascia if enough tension is present. Indeed, such sutures can pull through the bowel wall as it retracts and cause prestomal fistulas.

Stripping more than 5 to 10 mm of mesentery away from the colostomy stoma so that it can come through the hole in the abdominal wall easier is not advised because it increases the risk of necrosis developing in the protruding colon. The abdominal wall aperture should not constrict the colon, and fascial stenosis is best avoided by an adequate cruciate incision. If any change in the color of the exposed bowel occurs, one should assume that the viability of the bowel is threatened; however, if careful endoscopy or examination through a glass or clear plastic tube placed in the lumen shows darkening of only a few millimeters of distal mucosa, one can continue to carefully observe the stoma.

Internal Hernias

Internal hernias can develop for a variety of reasons following a celiotomy for abdominal trauma. Mesenteric defects may not be closed completely, particularly if the patient was unstable and efforts were being made to complete the operation as rapidly as possible. Such defects are notorious for trapping small bowel and causing later bowel obstruction. Failure to close the space between a colostomy or ileostomy and the lateral peritoneum may also allow an internal hernia to develop. Occasionally, the remaining bowel twists around the bowel leading up to the ostomy site.

Wound Complications

Wound Dehiscence

Postoperative dehiscence (separation of the fascial closure, while the skin closure remains intact) is often manifested by the discharge of serosanguinous fluid ("red pop") from the incision after 3 to 4 days. Bowel in the subcutaneous tissues may be palpable in thin patients, but can be extremely difficult to detect in obese patients. A cross-table radiograph or computed tomography scan of the abdomen can help to confirm the diagnosis in questionable circumstances.

AXIOM Drainage of serosanguinous fluid from an abdominal incision postoperatively is due to a fascial dehiscence until proven otherwise.

As a general rule, fascial dehiscences are corrected promptly in the operating room. In patients who are extremely ill, however, one may elect to apply moist dressings to keep the bowel beneath the plane of the fascia until everything seals or the patient can tolerate surgery.

Eviscerations

Repair of an evisceration should generally be performed as an emergency procedure to minimize the risk of bowel damage and resultant peritonitis. Preparation of the abdominal wall before repair must be done with care because soaps or detergents can harm exposed bowel.

Attempts to reclose the abdomen by merely resuturing the fascia is prone to failure, and the safest approach is to use full thickness abdominal wall retention sutures. When omentum is not available to cover the underlying bowel, the sutures should be placed through the properitoneal fat so that they will not contact underlying distended intestine. Retention sutures are generally left in place for at least 3 weeks. Even then, a 30% chance of development of a ventral hernia exists.

Necrotizing Fasciitis

If the patient develops an infection with necrotic superficial fascia, adequate debridement generally requires removal of most, if not all, of the sutures used to close the abdomen. The debridement should continue all around the wound until normal, uninfected fascia is identified. Even though the bowel may appear to be adherent to either the parietal peritoneum or to omentum covering it, the bowel may eviscerate later. This is best prevented with packs to keep the bowel below the plane of the fascia, but danger still exists that bowel may work its way up between the compressive dressing and the skin and necrose there.

AXIOM Bowel that appears to be adherent to the peritoneum can still eviscerate out an open abdominal incision or develop fistulas unless the bowel is carefully kept below the plane of the peritoneum of the anterior abdominal wall by suitable dressings.

ACALCULOUS CHOLECYSTITIS

Acalculous cholecystitis develops most frequently in severely traumatized patients who become septic and receive prolonged parenteral nutrition with no enteral feedings. Dehydration and poor tissue perfusion may also be predisposing factors.

The clinical manifestations of acute acalculous cholecystitis can be variable and may be subtle. The actual time of onset of acalculous cholecystitis after trauma is varied, but it typically develops after 2 to 3 weeks of parenteral nutrition.

AXIOM Unless one has a high index of suspicion for the development of acalculous cholecystitis in critically ill patients who are on prolonged parenteral nutrition, the diagnosis may be greatly delayed.

On ultrasound, acalculous cholecystitis typically reveals a dilated gallbladder with a thickened wall, sludge, and some surrounding fluid. Air in the wall of the gallbladder usually indicates the presence of severe infection or necrosis. A hepatoiminodiacetic acid scan visualizing the gallbladder rules out the diagnosis, but increased viscosity of bile from prolonged fasting may prevent sufficient isotopic entry into a normal gallbladder to visualize it.

Periodic administration of oral fat or cholecystokinin to critically ill patients, especially those on TPN, has been suggested as a means of preventing acalculous cholecystitis. Although fat in the duodenum releases cholecystokinin, which should cause the gallbladder to contract, the efficacy of such a regimen has not been proven.

If acute acalculous cholecystitis is diagnosed, the gallbladder should be resected as soon as possible. Depending on how early the diagnosis is made, the operative findings may vary from mild edema of the gallbladder wall to gangrene with perforation. Although it may be tempting to perform a cholecystostomy in some very high-risk patients, multiple scattered areas of gangrene are present in at least 40% of these gallbladders, and these local areas of necrosis could leak and cause later peritonitis.

The mortality rate for acute acalculous cholecystitis can be as high 60% (10), with the highest death rates generally being the result of the severe underlying problems and multiple organ failure.

⊘ FREQUENT ERRORS

1. ***Failure to consider* C. difficile *colitis as a cause of posttraumatic diarrhea if the patient has been receiving antibiotics.***
2. ***Failure to monitor gastric pH and its response to therapy in critically ill posttraumatic patients.***
3. ***Providing inadequate attention to nutrition and peritoneal drainage in patients with posttraumatic enterocutaneous fistulas.***
4. ***Failure to consider the possibility of mechanical bowel obstruction in patients who have prolonged ileus or excessive gastric aspirate.***
5. ***Reluctance to perform second-look operations in patients with bowel of questionable viability.***
6. ***Failure to consider the possibility of acute acalculous cholecystitis in patients receiving TPN for more than 2 to 3 weeks.***

SUMMARY POINTS

1. One should look carefully for *Candida* infections in trauma patients who are septic despite 7 to 14 days of broad-spectrum antibiotics.

2. Diarrhea, in a patient who has been on broad-spectrum antibiotics, should be considered to be due to pseudomembranous colitis until proven otherwise.

3. All patients with prolonged stress, particularly when caused by severe sepsis, have some degree of stress gastritis.
4. Antacids, H_2-receptor antagonists, or sucralfate can usually prevent severe stress gastritis, as long as severe shock and sepsis are controlled and the gastric luminal pH is kept greater than 4.5.
5. Surgical intervention is rarely necessary for stress gastritis, but it may be indicated if nonsurgical methods fail to control severe bleeding.
6. Cushing's ulcers (versus the usual stress ulcers) tend to be associated with secretion of more gastrin and acid and are more apt to have fewer ulcers, which are deeper and more likely to perforate.
7. Patients with severe burns should have gastric luminal pH monitored while nasogastric tubes are present, and antacids, H_2 blockers, or sucralfate should be given until the burns are completely healed.
8. The increased mortality rate of high-output fistulas is usually due to increased incidence of intraabdominal infections and a lower rate of spontaneous closure.
9. Although many factors tend to make an intestinal fistula persist, the most important is a distal obstruction.
10. Metabolic support with adequate calories and protein plus accurate replacement of the fistula output of water and electrolytes are essential for obtaining optimal healing of enterocutaneous fistulas.
11. Definitive surgical treatment of a gastrointestinal fistulas should usually not be attempted at the same time that an abscess is drained.
12. Enteral feeding is preferred over parenteral nutrition whenever possible.
13. Spontaneous closure of a fistula should not be expected until there is control of the fistula, eradication of sepsis, and provision of adequate nutrition.
14. If the output of an intestinal fistula has not significantly decreased within 1 month of proper control of infection and provision of adequate nutrition, definitive surgical correction is usually required.
15. The most successful operative approach for enterocutaneous fistulas is resection of the involved segment of bowel with reanastomosis of normal tissue.
16. Most persistent upper gastrointestinal fistulas can be controlled with a Roux-en-Y limb of jejunum.
17. A fistula between the small intestine and colon frequently presents with diarrhea, which is usually due to reflux of colonic organisms into the small bowel, causing malabsorption.
18. Enteroenteric fistulas rarely heal spontaneously, but definitive repair is undertaken only if the patient is symptomatic and is in optimal condition for the operation.
19. Before an anastomotic disruption is repaired surgically, its anatomy should be outlined and confirmed with a radiographic contrast study.
20. Patients with persistent fever plus ileus or delayed gastric emptying following small bowel repairs should be considered to have an anastomotic disruption or peritoneal sepsis until proven otherwise.
21. An intestinal leak that is contained and is not causing sepsis does not need be drained, especially if it is a colonic fistula.
22. Although they cannot be completely prevented, peritoneal adhesions can often be reduced by careful surgical technique.
23. Abdominal distension developing after the fourth postoperative day should be considered to be due to bowel obstruction until proven otherwise.
24. A feculent odor or appearance of nasogastric aspirate or vomitus is often a sign of a complete small bowel obstruction.
25. High-volume gastric aspirates after abdominal trauma should make one suspicious of a bowel obstruction or peritonitis.
26. Absence of intermittent cramping, abdominal pain, or high-pitched tinkling bowel sounds does not exclude a postoperative mechanical bowel obstruction.
27. A tendency for the patient to require increased intravenous fluids after the third day postoperatively should make one suspect complications, such as bowel obstruction or infection.
28. If it is not clear whether a loop of bowel is dilated small bowel or colon, a contrast enema should be performed.

29. Bowel obstruction associated with constant abdominal pain, fever, leukocytosis, or localized tenderness is an indication for an exploratory laparotomy for possible strangulated bowel.
30. When the patient continues to have flatus, indicating that a suspected bowel obstruction is probably only partial, there is much less risk that strangulated bowel is present.
31. Failure to perform a second-look operation on marginally viable bowel greatly increases the risk of nonviable bowel being left in place and causing fatal peritonitis.
32. If any spill of the contents of obstructed bowel occurs, the skin and subcutaneous tissues should not be closed.
33. Diarrhea associated with small bowel distension frequently is due to partial obstruction.
34. Intussusception usually presents as a partial small bowel obstruction.
35. Any intussuscepted bowel that cannot be readily reduced at surgery should be resected.
36. Early enteral feeding can be beneficial in patients with severe trauma, but careful construction of the feeding jejunostomy and monitoring of intestinal acceptance of the diet are extremely important.
37. The position of a jejunostomy feeding tube within the bowel lumen should be confirmed after any manipulation or replacement before beginning or resuming feedings.
38. Excessive distension of bowel by enteral feeding should be suspected if the patient has increasing abdominal pain or distension.
39. Suturing colon to abdominal fascia to prevent a colostomy from retracting is likely to cause more complications than it prevents.
40. A colostomy stoma that becomes progressively more dusky demands immediate revision.
41. One should look carefully for hernias in any patient in whom signs or symptoms suggestive of postoperative bowel obstruction develop.
42. Drainage of serosanguinous fluid from an abdominal incision postoperatively is due to a fascial dehiscence until proven otherwise.
43. Bowel that appears to be adherent to the peritoneum can still eviscerate out an open abdominal incision or develop fistulas unless the bowel is carefully kept below the plane of the peritoneum of the anterior abdominal wall by appropriate dressings.
44. Eviscerations should generally be closed with full thickness retention sutures.
45. Unless one has a high index of suspicion for the development of acalculous cholecystitis in critically ill patients who are on prolonged parenteral nutrition, the diagnosis is usually greatly delayed.

REFERENCES

1. Fromm D. Gastrointestinal complications following trauma. In: Wilson RF, Walt AJ, eds. *Management of trauma—pitfalls and practice,* 2nd ed. Philadelphia: Williams & Wilkins, 1996:966.
2. Guandalini S, Fasano A, Migliavacca M, et al. Pathogenesis of postantibiotic diarrhea caused by *Clostridium difficile: an in vitro study in the rabbit intestine.* Gut 1988;29:598.
3. Machens A, Bloechle C, Achilles EG, et al: Toxic magacolon caused by cytomegalovirus colitis in a multiply injured patient. *J Trauma* 1996;40:644.
4. Lasky MR, Metzler MH, Phillips JO. A prospective study of omeprazole suspension to prevent clinically significant gastrointestinal bleeding from stress ulcers in mechanically ventilated trauma patients. *J Trauma* 1998;44:527.
5. Fromm D. Gastric mucosal "barrier." In: Johnson LR, ed. Physiology of the digestive tract. Vol I. New York: Raven Press, 1981:733.
6. Cook D, Guyatt G, Marshall J, et al. A comparison of sucralfate and ranitidine for the prevention of upper gastrointestinal bleeding in patients requiring mechanical ventilation. *N Engl J Med* 1998;338:791.
7. Imperiale TF, Teran JC, McCullough AJ. A meta-analysis of somatostatin versus vasopressin in the management of acute esophageal variceal bleeding. *Gastroenterology* 1995;109:1289.

8. Czaja AJ, McAlhany JC, Pruitt BA Jr. Acute gastroduodenal disease after thermal injury: an endoscopic evaluation of incidence and natural history. *N Engl J Med* 1974;291:925.
9. Reber HA, Roberts C, Way LW, et al. Management of external gastrointestinal fistulas. *Ann Surg* 1978:188:460.
10. Flancbaum L, Majerus TC, Cox EF. Acute posttraumatic acalculous cholecystitis. *Am J Surg* 1985;150:252.

44. LIVER FAILURE AFTER TRAUMA[1]

The liver is the largest organ in the body; it weighs about 1,500 g in men and 1,200 g in women (2). The liver parenchymal cells or hepatocytes are arranged in plates that are distributed in the form of lobules. Between the lobules are the portal triads, which contain branches of the portal vein, hepatic artery, and bile ducts. The branches of the portal vein and hepatic artery divide and subdivide, and then empty directly into dilated hepatic capillaries or sinusoids.

The hepatic sinusoids are lined by endothelium, which is much more permeable to large molecules than are systemic capillaries. This allows large nutrient particles to get to the liver cells. Within each lobule is a small central vein that drains into sublobular veins, which drain finally into the major hepatic veins entering the inferior vena cava.

The bile canaliculi drain into small cholangioles known as the canals of Hering, which empty into intralobular ductules. These, in turn, empty into larger and larger ducts, which finally unite to form segmental ducts and then the right and left hepatic bile ducts.

PHYSIOLOGY

Carbohydrate Metabolism

Glucose absorbed from the intestine is converted by the liver into glycogen, the main storage form for carbohydrates. The liver has the largest readily available store of glycogen (about 150 g) for rapid glucose production during acute stress; however, the amount of liver glycogen present in patients with have severe diabetes mellitus or cirrhosis may be greatly reduced.

Protein Metabolism

Large quantities of nitrogenous compounds are synthesized, changed, or broken down in the liver daily. The liver is the body's major source of plasma proteins. It produces all of the albumin and α-globulins and some of the β-globulins found in the blood.

Chemical tests used to assess hepatic protein synthesis include serum or plasma levels of albumin, transferrin, thyroxine-binding prealbumin, and retinol-binding protein (3). These tests can be reasonably reliable as nutritional indices, but they are affected by a number of variables other than nutritional status, such as hydration, sepsis, and abnormal gastrointestinal or urinary losses.

Albumin is contained in a large body pool (4 to 5 g/kg), and it has a long half-life (20 to 22 days) (3). As a result, it is relatively insensitive to acute changes and responds slowly to therapy. Plasma levels are decreased by sepsis, malnutrition, hepatic failure, dialysis, uremia, and acute volume expansion. Plasma albumin levels may be increased in patients who are dehydrated and those who have increased levels of cortisol, growth hormone, insulin, or estrogen.

Transferrin is contained in a smaller body pool than albumin (3). It has a shorter half-life (8 to 10 days) and, therefore, is a more sensitive indicator of the patient's current nutritional status. Its concentrations (which are normally 250 to 300 mg/dL) are adversely affected as a nutritional indicator by the same variables as albumin. Iron deficiency leads to elevations in transferrin, and iron overload depresses transferrin levels.

Thyroxin-binding prealbumin is involved in the transport of thyroid hormone (3). Its normal serum level is 22 ± 7 mg/dL, and it has a short half-life (2 days). It can be a sensitive indicator of nutritional status, but it is affected by the same variables that affect albumin and transferrin. In addition, low levels are seen in hyperthyroidism, cystic fibrosis, chronic illness, and acute stress.

Retinol-binding protein is a specific carrier involved in vitamin A transport (3). Normal serum levels are 5.1 ± 2.5 mg/dL. It has a very short half-life (12 hours) and is very sensitive to synthesis and utilization changes. Levels increase in renal disease and with excess vitamin A, but are reduced in liver disease, cystic fibrosis, hyperthyroidism, and vitamin A deficiency.

Urea Formation
The ammonia formed from the breakdown of protein and amino acids is largely converted into urea by the liver. In severe liver failure, blood urea nitrogen (BUN) levels may decrease to less than 5 mg/dL.

Acute Phase Protein Synthesis
Following trauma or during sepsis, the liver reorients protein synthesis to favor the production of acute phase reactants, such as α_1-antitrypsin, lactoferrin, C-reactive protein, fibrinogen, and ceruloplasmin (3). Simultaneously, proteolysis of skeletal muscle increases, and the resulting amino acids are transported to the liver to be used for energy production (alanine) or new protein synthesis.

Hepatic acute phase protein production is stimulated by tumor necrosis factor, interleukin (IL)-1, and especially IL-6. Maximal production also requires increased glucocorticoids (4).

Fat Metabolism
The liver can synthesize fatty acids and triglycerides or it can break them down into glycerol and fatty acids. Glycerol is usually then converted to acetyl coenzyme A (CoA). Fatty acids are converted to either acetyl-CoA or ketone bodies. The liver is also the major source of cholesterol, cholesterol esters, and phospholipids. The ability of the liver to metabolize triglycerides and fatty acids is one of the last metabolic liver functions to fail in hepatic failure.

AXIOM Increasing serum triglyceride levels in patients with sepsis are often a sign of terminal liver failure.

Production of Coagulation Factors
Most coagulation factors are made in the liver. These include

- Factor I fibrinogen
- Factor II prothrombin
- Factor V proaccelerin
- Factor VII proconvertin
- Factor IX plasma thromboplastin component
- Factor XI plasma thromboplastin antecedent
- Factor XII Hageman factor

Some factor VIII (antihemophilic globulin) is also made in the liver, but it is formed primarily by endothelial cells outside the liver.

Vitamin Metabolism
All vitamins, particularly A, D, E, K, and B_{12}, are stored in the liver and either used there or released as needed by other parts of the body.

Detoxification
A large variety of endogenous and exogenous chemicals are rendered harmless by the liver and then released into the blood (for excretion in the urine) or into the bile (for excretion through the bowel). With decreasing hepatic function, the capacity of the liver to conjugate lipid-soluble drugs is also impaired. Consequently, drugs such as thiopental, propranolol, and diazepam tend to have a prolonged increase in concentration and reduced dose requirement in the elderly (Table 44-1).

Table 44-1. ***Drugs that Should Be Used with Caution or Not at All in Liver Disease Patients***

Group I:	Drugs capable of causing hepatic damage
	Acetaminophen
	Acetylsalicylic acid
	Chlorpromazine
	Erythromycin estolate
	Methotrexate
	Methyldopa
Group II:	Drugs that can compromise liver function
	Anabolic and contraceptive steroids
	Prednisone
	Tetracycline
Group III:	Drugs that may make complications of liver disease worse
	Cyclooxygenase inhibitors (indomethacin)
	Diuretics
	Meperidine and other CNS depressants
	Morphine
	Pentazocine
	Phenylbutazone

From Kubisty CA, Arns PA, Wedlund PJ, et al. Adjustment of medications in liver failure. Chernow B, ed. *The pharmacologic approach to the critically ill patient,* 3rd ed. Baltimore: Williams & Wilkins, 1994:98.

Reticuloendothelial System Functions

The liver is the initial filter for whatever bacteria and bacterial products are absorbed from the intestine into the portal venous system (2). More than 60% of the cells of the reticuloendothelial system (RES) are present in the liver.

AXIOM In severe hepatic failure, increased quantities of bacteria and bacterial products from the gut can traverse the liver and get into the systemic circulation.

Bile Formation and Secretion

The hepatocytes of the normal man secrete about 500 to 1,000 mL of bile per day (2). This is an active process that depends on functioning hepatocytes and bile ducts and an adequate hepatic blood flow (HBF) and oxygen supply.

Bile secretion is responsive to neurogenic, humoral, and chemical controls. Vagal stimulation increases bile secretion and flow, whereas stimulation of the splanchnic (sympathetic) nervous system decreases bile flow and causes stasis of bile in the gallbladder. The main hormonal stimulus for bile formation is secretin. Bile salts absorbed from the gut are particularly effective choleretics and can greatly increase the rate of bile formation and secretion by the liver.

The most important compounds in bile are bilirubin, bile salts, cholesterol, and phospholipids (especially lecithin).

Bilirubin

Bilirubin is formed in the RES as the end product of the breakdown of hemoglobin from destroyed red blood cells (2). Under normal circumstances, 6 to 35 g of hemoglobin are broken down daily and 30 to 300 mg of bilirubin are formed. The initial step involves release of biliverdin from hemoglobin. Biliverdin is reduced to unconjugated bilirubin in the extrahepatic RES, then bound to albumin and transported to the liver. In the liver, unconjugated (indirect) bilirubin is conjugated by the enzyme uridine diphosphate glucuronyl transferase to form bilirubin diglucuronide (direct bilirubin), which is excreted in the bile and gives bile its pale green color. In the bowel, bacteria convert conjugated bilirubin into urobilinogen, about 40% of which is reabsorbed and excreted again in the bile. The urobilinogen that escapes the liver is excreted in the urine.

Bile Salts and Acids

Bile salts are essential for fat digestion because they can emulsify triglycerides and thereby lower the surface tension of fat droplets. Phospholipids in the bile greatly increase the ability of bile salts to form micelles, which are necessary for effective absorption of lipids.

In individuals on a normal diet, the liver secretes an average of 24 g (16 to 72 g) of bile acids per day. These combine with cations, particularly sodium, to form bile salts. Although only about 3 to 6 g of bile acids are present in the body at any one time, this bile acid pool is circulated about eight times per day. More than 95% of the bile acids secreted in bile are normally reabsorbed in the distal ileum, which actively absorbs bile acids, particularly those conjugated with taurine or glycine.

The enterohepatic circulation refers to the circulation of bile acids from the liver through the bile ducts to the intestine, reabsorption from the terminal ileum into the portal vein, and then back to the liver.

AXIOM Resection or severe disease of the distal ileum can cause bile salt deficiencies.

Two major types of bile acids are recognized. The *primary bile acids* are those synthesized by the liver; they include cholic acid and chenodeoxycholic acid. Within the bowel, these primary bile acids may be converted by bacteria to the *secondary bile acids*, which are deoxycholic and lithocholic acid. When they are absorbed and returned to the liver in the portal blood, the secondary bile acids are secreted into bile along with the primary bile acids.

Normally, about 50 mg of bile acids are lost in the feces and replaced daily by the liver. Although the liver can temporarily increase its synthesis of new bile acids to about 3 g/day, any factor that interferes with their absorption in the distal ileum can eventually deplete the bile acid pool.

If bile salt malabsorption occurs, the resulting high concentration of bile salts in the colon may interfere with the absorption of sodium and water, and a severe watery diarrhea may develop. Excess production of gastric acid, such as with the Zollinger-Ellison syndrome, may also cause diarrhea because excess acid reaching the small intestine interferes with bile salt absorption.

Cholesterol

Cholesterol is generally present in bile in concentrations similar to those found in plasma. Although high-fat diets tend to elevate blood cholesterol levels, most of the cholesterol in the blood is formed in the liver.

Much attention has been directed to the solubility of cholesterol in bile because cholesterol crystals appear to be the nidus of many gallstones. Low ratios of bile salts and lecithin to cholesterol in the bile increase the likelihood of cholesterol crystals forming, and this predisposes to the formation of gallstones.

Lecithin

Lecithin, formed in the liver, is the principal phospholipid in the bile. Low levels of lecithin increase the tendency to gallstone formation.

Hepatic Hemodynamics

The liver receives about 25% to 30% of the cardiac output or about 1,250 to 1,500 mL/min (2). The hepatic artery carries fully oxygenated blood and provides approximately 25% of the HBF and about 50% of its oxygen. The portal vein drains the splanchnic circulation, has an oxygen saturation of about 80%, and provides the remaining 75% of the HBF. A reciprocal relationship exists between hepatic artery and portal vein flow. If, for some reason, the flow in one is reduced, the flow in the other tends to increase.

AXIOM Patients with cirrhosis or any other intrahepatic obstruction to portal venous blood flow are particularly sensitive to any reduction in cardiac output or hepatic artery blood flow.

The pressure in the portal vein is normally 7 to 10 mm Hg (100 to 140 mm H_2O). In the hepatic sinusoids, where blood from the hepatic artery and portal veins joins, the pressure is about 2 to 6 mm Hg. Hepatic venous pressure is normally 1 to 5 mm Hg.

AXIOM A portal vein pressure exceeding 15 mm Hg (200 mm H_2O) is considered to be portal hypertension (2).

DISORDERS OF THE LIVER

Jaundice

Jaundice (icterus) is a yellow discoloration of tissue caused by staining with bilirubin. It is best observed in tissues containing elastic tissue, such as the sclerae and the skin of the face and neck. Jaundice can usually be detected when the concentration of conjugated bilirubin is greater than 3 mg/dL or the concentration of unconjugated bilirubin is greater than 4 mg/dL.

To facilitate diagnosis, the causes of jaundice are often divided into prehepatic, hepatic, and posthepatic (bile duct) disorders.

Prehepatic Disorders

The most important prehepatic cause of jaundice is excessive hemolysis of red blood cells. Indeed, following major trauma, large hematomas or massive transfusions may be associated with elevations of bilirubin for several days.

It is estimated that about 10% of the erythrocytes in transfused blood that is 14 days old undergo hemolysis daily during the first few days (5). Thus, 1 unit of whole blood (with a hemoglobin concentration of 15 g/100 mL) would liberate about 7.5 g of hemoglobin per day for several days. This amount of hemoglobin (7.5 g) results in the formation of about 250 mg of bilirubin following phagocytosis by the RES. This equals the usual daily physiologic bilirubin load of 250 mg resulting from the breakdown of senescent red cells, which approximates 1% of the circulating red cell mass. Similarly, resolving hematomas liberate a pigment load in direct relation to the amount of sequestered hemoglobin and serve as an additional source of bilirubin.

Damaged muscle (releasing myoglobin and cytochromes) also causes increased pigment loads to be handled by the liver. Flint estimated that the heme pigment load with a closed femur fracture may exceed 1,000 mg, whereas a major pelvic fracture with hemorrhage may result in an excess pigment load of 7,500 mg to be converted to bilirubin (6).

Prehepatic jaundice is often associated with a relatively high fraction of indirect (unconjugated bilirubin) and relatively normal liver enzymes (aspartate aminotransferase [AST] and alkaline phosphatase).

Hepatic Disorders

The most common hepatic problems causing jaundice are the various types of hepatitis, cirrhosis, and congenital hepatic disorders. Following accidental trauma, the most frequent causes of hepatocyte damage or dysfunction include direct trauma, shock, (causing ischemic injury of the liver), drugs, and sepsis.

AXIOM Shock can rapidly cause ischemic injury to the liver, especially if the patient has preexisting liver disease.

Jaundice resulting from ischemic liver damage usually becomes apparent by the third to fourth postoperative day and is generally associated with mild elevations in alkaline phosphatase and AST.

Sepsis resulting in impaired hepatocellular function is the most common cause of persistent jaundice developing 8 or more days after major abdominal operations.

Major hepatic resections may also contribute to liver failure (6). Right hepatic lobectomy is regularly followed by an early increase in bilirubin to greater than 5 mg/dL, but usually for only a few days. Similar findings of jaundice and elevation of hepatic enzymes are common if hepatic artery ligation or portal vein ligation is used to achieve hemostasis in patients with liver injury.

AXIOM Packing a liver after ligation of a major hepatic artery branch may cause severe hepatic lobar necrosis because the packing will also interfere with portal venous flow.

Deficient hepatic uptake of bilirubin is seen in many types of acquired liver disease. This may also be seen in Gilbert's disease, which is a fairly common congenital disorder characterized by a normal liver biopsy and intermittent low-grade hyperbilirubinemia (less than 5 mg/dL) consisting mainly of unconjugated bilirubin.

Some degree of deficient conjugation of bilirubin is seen with virtually all types of acquired liver disease (2). It is also seen, but much less frequently, with the following:

1. Inadequate glucuronyl transferase, as in physiologic jaundice of the newborn and in Crigler-Najjar syndrome;
2. Inhibition of glucuronyl transferase by large doses of vitamin K analogues (in premature infants) or by increased blood levels of pregnanediol; and
3. Competitive inhibition of glucuronyl transferase by drugs that are detoxified as glucuronides.

Deficient liver-cell (hepatocyte) secretion of bilirubin in the adult is usually the result of acquired liver disease. In infants and children, it may be due to immaturity of the liver or the congenital disorders known as Dubin-Johnson syndrome or Rotor syndrome. Dubin-Johnson syndrome characteristically produces a slate-gray or black liver (caused by excess bilirubin pigment). The Rotor syndrome is similar physiologically, but does not result in pigment deposition in the liver.

Intrahepatic bile duct obstructions are characterized by elevated levels of conjugated bilirubin and alkaline phosphatase and may occur at the level of the canaliculi, in the large intrahepatic bile ducts, or in the extrahepatic bile ducts. Many acquired liver disorders, particularly viral hepatitis and sepsis, produce some canalicular or intrahepatic bile duct obstruction, which may be difficult at times to differentiate from extrahepatic (posthepatic) obstruction.

Posthepatic Disorders

AXIOM In patients with increasing jaundice after trauma, one should make a special effort to rule out extrahepatic biliary obstruction.

The most likely cause of posthepatic jaundice in an injured patient is a common bile duct injury. Endoscopic retrograde cholangiopancreatography or percutaneous transhepatic catheterization can be used to diagnose or relieve posttraumatic obstructive jaundice.

Acute Hepatocellular Diseases

Of the acute hepatic diseases, the one most frequently seen is viral hepatitis. Less frequent causes of acute liver problems include toxic (drug-induced) hepatitis, alcoholic hepatitis, "septic jaundice," and postanoxic (shock) changes.

Viral Hepatitis

Epidemiologic studies have demonstrated five relatively distinct types of viral hepatitis: A, B, C, D, and E. Hepatitis E is rarely seen except in recent travelers or immigrants from outside the United States.

Infectious hepatitis (IH), or type A, is primarily an enteric disease. It is usually transmitted by the fecal-oral route, but it can also be transmitted parenterally. It has a relatively short incubation period (15 to 40 days).

Serum hepatitis (SH) is usually transmitted via contaminated needles or blood. Hepatitis B (and probably hepatitis C) can also be acquired sexually. The incubation period for SH is much longer (60 to 90 days) than for IH. The virus is found in the serum, but it has not been demonstrated in feces. It should be considered highly infectious via blood or bloody secretions. The severity and mortality rate of SH is usually somewhat higher than for IH. Use of a vaccine against hepatitis seems to be protective in health care workers.

Relatively little is known about non-A, non-B hepatitis (hepatitis C), but its incidence is becoming increasingly recognized. It appears to be the most common cause of viral hepatitis following blood transfusions. The use of screening tests to eliminate donors at increased risk of transmitting non-A, non-B hepatitis have reduced the risk of transmission to as low as 1% to 2%. Recent isolation of a hepatitis C virus and the characterization of hepatitis C virus antibody in both blood donors and recipients has further decreased the likelihood of this complication (7).

Acute symptoms from hepatitis C may be noted 1 to 3 months after transfusions. They are characteristically mild and easily mistaken for a nondescript viral syndrome. Jaundice is unusual, and severe illness from overwhelming hepatic necrosis is uncommon. Thus, unless one carefully screens transfusion recipients with serial liver function tests (particularly AST levels), the majority of non-A, non-B hepatitis cases will be overlooked.

AXIOM Chronic liver disease subsequently develops in up to half of the patients in whom posttransfusion hepatitis develops.

Diagnosis of Hepatitis

Viral hepatitis is generally characterized by relatively persistent and extremely high AST levels (often exceeding 1,000 units). Bilirubin and alkaline phosphatase levels vary a great deal, but are usually also elevated. Serial viral hepatitis antigen and antibody studies are important to determine the diagnosis and prognosis. Patients with serum hepatitis often have positive hepatitis antigen in their blood for several days, weeks, or even months.

Management of Hepatitis

The management of viral hepatitis consists primarily of providing adequate physical rest and nutrition. In severe cases, steroids may be of some help, particularly if acute hepatic necrosis seems to be developing. Although steroids usually make the patients feel better, they probably have little effect on eventual mortality. In some of the most severe cases, exchange transfusions have been used to reduce the toxicity secondary to the severe chemical abnormalities that may develop.

Alcoholic Hepatitis

Acute alcoholic hepatitis is caused by excessive alcohol ingestion in a patient who usually already has a fatty or cirrhotic liver. The swollen, inflamed liver often causes some pain and tenderness. Enzyme changes, especially AST, are usually not as severe as those in viral hepatitis; however, the alkaline phosphatase may be somewhat higher. The stigmata of cirrhosis (ascites, spider nevi, and bleeding problems) may develop relatively rapidly in patients with alcoholic hepatitis.

HEPATIC DYSFUNCTION AFTER SHOCK AND TRAUMA

Phase I (during Shock)

During severe hepatic ischemia, there is a consistent increase in lipids in the hepatocytes with increased numbers of acute inflammatory cells in the central and midzonal areas of the hepatic lobule.

Phase II (Functional Impairment)

The functional impairment phase of hepatic dysfunction extends from the time of reestablishment of liver perfusion until hepatic function begins to improve (8). Lactate dehydrogenase (LDH) levels may increase to 400 to 500 units, and the AST may increase to 100 to 200 units within a few hours. These concentrations gradually return to normal over the next 3 to 4 days. With additional hepatic insults, such as the development of sepsis, a secondary increase in LDH and AST often precedes an increase in bilirubin by 3 to 5 days (9).

AXIOM Increasing jaundice with high alkaline phosphatase levels soon after trauma should be considered a result of extrahepatic biliary tract obstruction until proven otherwise.

Phase III: Recovery of Hepatic Function

During recovery of hepatic function, bilirubin, LDH, and AST gradually decline to normal. Alkaline phosphatase and gamma-glutamyl transpeptidase concentrations begin to decrease several days later.

Treatment of Hepatic Dysfunction

Therapy for postischemic hepatic dysfunction is directed primarily at correcting any other medical problems and supplying adequate blood flow, oxygen, and glucose to the liver. Eradication of necrotic tissue or areas of inflammation, especially in the abdomen, is also essential.

MULTIPLE ORGAN FAILURE AND SEPSIS

The incidence of hepatic dysfunction following trauma is only occasionally reported. Fry noted the development of liver failure in 50 (9%) of 553 patients requiring emergency operations, 61 (18%) of 337 patients with splenic trauma, 42 (43%) of 98 patients with *Bacteroides* bacteremia, and 66 (46%) of 143 patients with intraabdominal abscesses (10).

Pathophysiology

Gottlieb et al. measured splanchnic oxygen consumption and effective HBF in patients without sepsis who had episodes of systolic blood pressure (BP) less than 90 mm Hg following severe trauma (11). They found a significant elevation in splanchnic oxygen consumption despite a 50% decrease in effective HBF by 12 hours after injury. This decrease in effective hepatic perfusion persisted for about 4 to 5 days after injury.

In an effort to more accurately characterize the clinical hemodynamic response of the liver to sepsis, Dahn et al. measured HBF in ten control subjects and nine patients with sepsis (12). HBF was determined using two different indicators and three methods of analysis, including indocyanine green (ICG) dye clearance (HBF_{ICG}), galactose clearance (GC), and GC with splanchnic galactose gradient measurements (HBF_{GG}). Estimates based on peripheral venous sampling showed a decreased effective HBF in sepsis, even though total splanchnic blood flow was increased. As sepsis worsened, the total HBF tended to increase, but the effective HBF (galactose extraction) tended to decrease. Gottlieb et al. found that a decreased ICG clearance was a much earlier indication of hepatic failure after injury than was hyperbilirubinemia (11).

AXIOM The total HBF in hypermetabolic sepsis is generally increased, even though peripheral extraction studies usually indicate that effective HBF is reduced.

Treatment

All infections should be diagnosed and eradicated as soon as possible. Dahn et al. have noted that data from the Krogh-Erlang tissue model indicates that, despite an increase in oxygen delivery to the splanchnic bed during sepsis, portions of the liver are more likely to have hypoxic events than normal patients and patients with trauma (12).

AXIOM A higher than normal cardiac index and oxygen delivery is required to maintain adequate hepatic oxygenation after trauma and during sepsis.

Inthorn et al. (13) have noted that long-term antithrombin III supplementation in patients with severe sepsis improved lung function and prevented the development of septic liver and kidney failure.

LIVER FAILURE AFTER TRAUMA

Pathophysiology

Carbohydrate Metabolism

Carbohydrate stress metabolism is characterized by the following:

- Increased glucagon-to-insulin ratios
- Increased insulin resistance
- Increased glycogenolysis and gluconeogenesis despite exogenous glucose
- Hyperglycemia
- Increased lactate production

One of the responses of the liver to increased catecholamines and glucagon is increased glycogenolysis. A great increase in gluconeogenesis from lactate, alanine, glutamine, glycine, serine, and glycerol also occurs. In the presence of endotoxin, the hepatic conversion of lactate to glucose is no longer sensitive to stimulation from glucagon or norepinephrine. Therefore, although hepatic conversion of lactate to glucose continues, it may not be capable of coping with the greatly increased lactate production that can occur in sepsis. In the final stages of hepatic failure, serum glucose levels decrease and lactate levels increase.

The increased blood lactate levels seen in multiple organ failure may be due to several factors, including the following:

1. Increased substrate flow through glycolytic pathways;
2. Downregulation of the tricarboxylic acid cycle; and
3. Inadequate gluconeogenic pathways to handle lactate (14).

Because the conversion of pyruvate to lactate is not blocked in sepsis, the ratio of lactate to pyruvate remains normal. When the patient has an elevated lactate level in the presence of an increased lactate-to-pyruvate ratio, it generally indicates inadequate tissue perfusion.

Protein Metabolism

During the hypermetabolic response to sepsis, amino acids released from catabolism of proteins, especially in skeletal muscle, are an important precursor for gluconeogenesis.

Patients with sepsis or cirrhosis tend to have increased levels of aromatic amino acids (AAA) (phenylalanine, tyrosine, and tryptophan) and decreased levels of branched chain amino acids (BCAA). Increased concentrations of AAAs, particularly phenylalanine, correlate directly with increased degrees of hepatic dysfunction, elevated levels of bilirubin, reduced rates of amino acid clearance, worsening encephalopathy, and eventual death.

Fat Metabolism

Stress fat metabolism is characterized by the following:

- Increased lipolysis of fat
- Decreased lipogenesis
- Increased fatty acid oxidation
- Increased triglyceride turnover
- Decreased ketosis (15)

Stress hypermetabolism is accompanied by hypertriglyceridemia despite increased peripheral fat utilization relative to the starvation state. Although much of this increase is caused by release of triglycerides from adipocytes, increased hepatic lipolysis and lipogenesis also contribute to the hypertriglyceridemia.

When the liver is making fat, the respiratory quotient (RQ) tends to exceed 1.0. This can easily occur with overfeeding of carbohydrates. Terminally, in sepsis, triglyceride intolerance may develop so that a reduced ability to clear exogenous triglycerides and long-chain fatty acids occurs.

The usual metabolic response to injury peaks on days 2 and 3 and is usually gone by days 7 through 10 (16). Severe hypermetabolism persisting for more than 3 to 4 days is usually associated with some form of persisting injury or impaired perfusion, and serum bilirubin and serum creatinine levels begin to progressively increase.

AXIOM If severe hypermetabolism with hepatic dysfunction persists for more than 2 to 3 weeks, most patients eventually die.

Cholestatic jaundice with elevation of serum bilirubin and alkaline phosphatase levels is the most common manifestation of hepatic failure in sepsis. It is most commonly seen with severe, generalized peritonitis involving anaerobic organisms, particularly *Bacteroides fragilis* (8). Because hyperbilirubinemia is predominantly of the conjugated form, the problem is primarily impaired excretion rather than impaired hepatocellular uptake.

AXIOM Bilirubin concentrations greater than 5 mg/dL in the absence of biliary tract obstruction, transfusion reaction, or resolving hematomas are strongly suggestive of liver dysfunction caused by sepsis.

AST and ALT are often elevated in posttraumatic or septic liver failure, but seldom to concentrations more than two to three times normal. Plasma albumin levels are often very low, but the prothrombin time is usually normal until relatively late.

AXIOM If the cause of persistent jaundice in a patient who has had major abdominal surgery or trauma cannot be determined in any other manner, an exploratory celiotomy should be considered.

Treatment of Liver Failure

Control of the Source

If the primary process (usually sepsis) can be controlled, the patient's condition and the liver function tests soon begin to improve; however, the white blood cell count may continue to increase for several days before beginning to decline back toward a normal level (8).

Flint noted that persistent jaundice (i.e., bilirubin greater than 5 mg/dL lasting longer than 3 days) appearing 8 days after trauma was associated with intraperitoneal infection in 75% of patients (6). Although necrotizing pulmonary and soft-tissue infections causing jaundice are usually easy to diagnose, intraperitoneal sepsis can sometimes only be detected by exploratory laparotomy.

Optimal Oxygen Delivery

Rapid restoration and maintenance of optimal (supranormal) oxygen delivery is extremely important for preventing hepatic failure after trauma. Dahn et al. observed that resuscitation of patients was not complete until hyperdynamic splanchnic perfusion could be demonstrated (18). This may require the use of inotropes or vasodilators as well as large quantities of fluid.

Intraabdominal hypertension can impair mesenteric arterial and intestinal mucosal blood flow as well as hepatic arterial, portal venous, and hepatic microcirculatory blood flow. Nakatami et al. (17) found that at an intraabdominal pressure of 20 mm Hg, a slight decrease in hepatic sinusoidal flow. At 30 mm Hg, there was a much greater reduction in sunusoidal blood flow plus a reduced hepatic mitochondrial redox status and decreased energy level.

Early Enteral Nutrition

Metabolic support can be an important part of the treatment of hepatic failure (16). Early enteral nutrition may be particularly important for preserving intestinal mucosa and helping to prevent translocation of bacteria and bacterial products from the gut into intestinal lymphatics and portal venous blood.

Hepatobiliary Complications from Nutritional Support

A number of hepatobiliary complications of parenteral nutritional support have been reported and include hepatic steatosis, cholestasis, and nonspecific triaditis (19). Progression to chronic liver disease has been reported most frequently in premature infants, but it can also occur in adults.

Pathophysiology

Hepatic Steatosis

One of the more common complications of relatively short-term (2 to 3 weeks) parenteral nutrition support is some fatty infiltration of the liver, which is also known as hepatic steatosis. Factors associated with fatty infiltration of the liver include carbohydrate as the sole source of total parenteral nutrition (TPN) calories, infusion of excess calories, and deficiencies of essential fatty acids or carnitine. An RQ exceeding 1.0 indicates that carbohydrate nutrients are being converted into fat, and such fat is likely to accumulate in the liver.

AXIOM Indirect calorimetry to monitor RQ may be of great help in optimizing nutritional intake and preventing hepatic steatosis.

Essential fatty acid deficiency can be caused by inadequate intake and high insulin levels suppressing the mobilization of endogenous fatty acids. This promotes fat accumulation in the liver as a result of decreased synthesis of phospholipids, which are required for lipid transport. Carnitine deficiency, although unusual, may also lead to impaired fat transport and subsequent decreased mitochondrial oxidation of lipids.

Extensive fatty infiltration presents clinically with moderate elevations in AST and mild elevations of alkaline phosphatase. In the most severe cases, hepatic steatosis may present with hepatic enlargement, right upper quadrant pain, and marked elevations in hepatocellular enzymes and alkaline phosphatase.

Intrahepatic Cholestasis

Intrahepatic cholestasis tends to occur later than fatty infiltration and is not usually seen in liver biopsies until after at least 3 weeks of TPN (3). Clinically, intrahepatic cholestasis presents with elevated alkaline phosphatase and bilirubin levels. Jaundice is usually the only symptom. Histologically, the lesion presents as periportal canalicular bile plugging, bile staining of surrounding hepatocytes, and some degree of triaditis with a predominantly lymphocytic infiltration. This triaditis may persist for several weeks or months after discontinuation of TPN.

Nonspecific Triaditis

Although it is often associated with cholestasis, nonspecific triaditis associated with TPN can occur independent of this problem. Clinically, triaditis can appear early in the course of TPN, and it is characterized by moderate elevations of hepatocellular enzymes. In patients with high aminotransferase levels, bilirubin and alkaline phosphatase levels may also be elevated.

Treatment of Hepatobiliary Complications

Management of hepatobiliary complications of TPN are primarily aimed at prevention (3). Excess calories should be avoided. In most patients, except those with severe malnutrition or hypermetabolism, the total nonprotein caloric intake probably should only be about 25 kcal/kg/day.

AXIOM Using resting energy expenditures and RQs to adjust TPN should help to prevent hepatic complications caused by underfeeding or overfeeding.

Up to 20% to 30% of the nonprotein calories can be given as fat to provide essential long-chain fatty acids. Cyclic TPN, to allow mobilization of fat between periods of hyperinsulinemia, may also minimize the tendency toward steatosis.

Enteral nutrition, even when only partial, should be instituted as soon as possible to minimize biliary stasis (3). In our experience at the Detroit Receiving Hospital, 30 to 60 mL of isosmotic enteral feedings, rather than antacids, can be instilled into the stomach via a nasogastric tube every hour. Clamping the tube for 45 to 50 minutes and aspirating for 10 to 15 minutes prevents gastric accumulation of feedings, and, even if the gastric instillation and aspiration volumes are the same, at least 20% to 30% of the feedings reach the small bowel.

CIRRHOSIS AND PORTAL HYPERTENSION

Portal hypertension is usually a complication of liver disease that results in portal vein pressures exceeding 200 mm H_2O (15 mm Hg). Because portal vein pressures are partly dependent on inferior vena cava pressures, one can also consider portal hypertension to exist when the difference between the pressure in the portal vein and inferior vena cava exceeds 100-150 mm H_2O.

Etiology

Intrahepatic Causes

Intrahepatic disease causes about 95% of all portal hypertension. Of these liver diseases, nutritional cirrhosis, posthepatic (postnecrotic) cirrhosis, and biliary cirrhosis are the most common. Other hepatic diseases that can cause portal hypertension include toxic (drug) hepatitis, metabolic cirrhosis (including hemochromatosis, Wilson's disease, and galactosemia), intestinal bypass, alcoholic hepatitis, neoplasms, and schistosomiasis.

Nutritional cirrhosis–also referred to as Laennec's, alcoholic, or portal cirrhosis–is the underlying disorder in approximately two-thirds of patients with portal hypertension. It is usually caused by alcohol abuse and the associated malnutrition. Fibrosis and formation of nodules of regenerating liver distort the liver's architecture and impair its function. On gross examination, the liver has uniform, diffuse, small nodules. Microscopically, the nodules consist of proliferating liver cells and fibrosis, particularly around the portal triads.

The cirrhosis that follows severe viral or toxic hepatitis causes about 10% to 20% of portal hypertension. This postnecrotic cirrhosis tends to cause a small, shrunken liver with large, irregular nodules. Consequently, the liver in these patients is often called "macronodular" as opposed to the "micronodular" appearance typically seen with nutritional cirrhosis.

Extrahepatic Disease

The most frequent extrahepatic problems causing portal hypertension include portal vein obstruction, hepatic vein obstruction, and excessive portal venous blood flow.

Portal vein obstruction is most frequently a result of thrombosis, which, in children, is usually due to neonatal omphalitis. Cavernous transformation of the portal vein is probably due to recanalization of a previously thrombosed portal vein. In these patients, portal hypertension tends to develop in childhood or early adult life and liver function tends to be good. As a consequence, such patients usually tolerate surgery for portal hypertension well.

Extrahepatic obstruction of the hepatic venous outflow system is caused by a group of rare conditions and is often referred to as the Budd-Chiari syndrome. These problems include neoplastic and inflammatory disorders occluding the hepatic veins or adjacent inferior vena cava. The most striking clinical findings in the Budd-Chiari syndrome are marked hepatomegaly and ascites.

Pathophysiology of Portal Hypertension

With portal hypertension, continuing destruction of liver parenchyma can lead to excessive formation of scar tissue and regenerative nodules, which compresses the vessels inside the liver just distal to the hepatic sinusoids. This postsinusoidal obstruction results in increased portal vein pressure and decreased blood flow to the liver. As the portal venous pressure increases, increasing amounts of blood from the portal venous system use collateral channels to enter the systemic circulation.

The main collaterals between the systemic and portal venous systems include coronary (left gastric) vein to the lower esophageal veins and then to the azygous vein, periumbilical veins, and the hemorrhoidal venous system.

In severe portal hypertension, blood may flow retrograde from the liver back into the portal vein and then via collateral veins into the systemic circulation. In such individuals, any reduction in hepatic artery flow can rapidly cause lethal hepatic failure.

Natural Progression of Cirrhosis

Hepatic cirrhosis is the predominant cause of death in approximately 30,000 patients each year (20). Not only is cirrhosis the sixth leading cause of death in the United States, but after jaundice, ascites, or esophageal variceal bleeding develop, the 1-year survival rate is only 21% to 35% (21). Class C cirrhotic patients with jaundice or ascites who have sepsis or major trauma have an extremely high mortality rate (Table 44-2).

AXIOM Any surgery requiring a laparotomy poses a grave risk to patients with severe cirrhosis.

Arahna and Greenlee reported a mortality rate of 86% in patients with advanced cirrhosis who underwent emergency surgery (22). In another study of cirrhotic patients with trauma, the average mortality rate of 30% was significantly higher than the predicted mortality rate (7%) in otherwise normal patients with similar injury severity scores (23). Patients with blunt abdominal trauma with hemoperitoneum or visceral injury requiring a laparotomy had a mortality rate of 67%.

In a recent study of 92 cirrhotic patients having abdominal operations, Mansour et al. (24) noted a coagulopathy in 24 (27%) and sepsis in 15 (16%). The mortality rate after emergent operations was 50%, compared to 18% for elective cases (p=.001). Other factors that predicted mortality included the presence of ascites (p=.006), encephalopathy (p=.002), and elevated prothrombin time (p=.021). The mortality rate in Child's class A patients was 10%, compared to 30% in class B and 82% in class C patients.

Postoperative Complications in Cirrhotics

Excess Bleeding

Cirrhotic patients may have an increased bleeding tendency for a wide variety of reasons (25). The cirrhosis itself reduces the production of prothrombin (factor II), and

Table 44-2. ***Child's Classification of Patients with Laennec Cirrhosis***

Characteristic	Child's Class[a] A	B	C
Serum albumin (g/dL)	>3.5	3.0–3.5	<3.0
Serum bilirubin (mg/dL)	>2.0	2.0–3.0	>3.0
Ascites	None	Mild, easily correctable	Moderate-to-severe
Muscle wasting	None	Mild	Moderate-to-severe
Encephalopathy	None	None	Present
Mortality risk of elective shunt	2%	10%	50%

[a]Only one laboratory or clinical characteristic is needed to place a patient in a lower (high risk) class.

factors VII, IX, and X. Platelet counts also tend to be low because of a tendency to hypersplenism. There may also be increased fibrinolysis because the liver is unable to remove plasminogen activators.

Administration of fresh frozen plasma and platelets should be considered in any cirrhotic patient who is bleeding and has abnormal bleeding and coagulation studies. If possible, the prothrombin time should be less than 5 seconds (and preferably only 3 seconds) longer than control before any surgery is performed.

Hepatic Encephalopathy

Hepatic encephalopathy usually increases pari passu with hepatic failure. Although the central nervous system (CNS) changes often do not correlate well with blood ammonia levels, removal of blood from the gastrointestinal tract (to decrease the substrate for NH_3 production in the gut) and use of enteral antibiotics (to reduce the number of ammonia-forming organisms in the gut) can be of value (26).

Hepatic coma is often the result of decreased plasma levels of the BCAA (leucine, isoleucine, and valine) and increased levels of AAAs (phenylalanine and tyrosine) and methionine. A decreased BCAA/AAA ratio in the plasma of patients with encephalopathy tends to be associated with increased levels of false neurotransmitters, such as octopamine, in the brain (27).

Signs of hepatic encephalopathy include changes in personality progressing to confusion, obtundation, and finally coma. Asterixis or "liver flap" is a characteristic sign of hepatic failure. It consists of a flapping rough tremor of the hands that is best demonstrated when the patient extends the arms, dorsiflexes the wrists, and spreads the fingers.

It has been shown in a multicenter, prospective, double-blind, randomized trial of patients with hepatic decompensation that the provision of adequate glucose and amino acids in the form of a mixture enriched with BCAA and deficient in methionine and AAAs is superior to a diet containing adequate glucose calories alone in terms of improvement of hepatic encephalopathy (28).

Hepatorenal Syndrome

A special type of renal failure (often referred to as the hepatorenal syndrome) tends to occur coincidentally with hepatic failure and is characterized by increasing creatinine and BUN levels with little or no oliguria. The urine osmolality tends to be normal or high; urine sodium levels are usually low, and urine sediment tends to be normal. Diuretics may make the hepatorenal syndrome worse.

Ascites

The primary mechanism for the development of ascites in cirrhotic patients is high pressure in the liver sinusoids with greatly increased movement of fluid into the perisinusoidal space of Disse. Although increased thoracic duct flow can remove much of the excess fluid from the hepatic lymphatics, the remainder moves into the peritoneal cavity through the liver capsule. Fluid overload, hyponatremia, or hypoalbuminemia can contribute to this problem.

Keeping the patient "on the dry side" and limiting sodium intake may help to reduce the tendency to ascites. Diuretics, especially the antialdosterone types, can also be helpful. If a portosystemic shunt is needed in patients with ascites, especially those with hepatofugal portal venous blood flow, a side-to-side portacaval shunt is generally preferred over an end-to-side shunt. If there is any possibility of hepatic transplantation later, the shunt should probably be an H-graft away from the portal vein or a TIPS (transcutaneous intrahepatic portosystemic shunt) procedure.

In poor-risk patients with severe, intractable ascites, a peritoneovenous shunt may be helpful. The shunt apparatus, which connects the peritoneal cavity with the superior vena cava via the internal jugular vein, has a special valve that opens when intraperitoneal pressure is 3.0cm H_2O higher than central venous pressure. Diuretics are important following peritoneovenous shunts because one must be careful to not allow the patient to develop congestive heart failure because of a sudden influx of ascitic fluid into the circulation.

Other complications of peritoneovenous shunting include disseminated intravascular coagulation (especially if the ascitic fluid is infected), local infection, systemic sepsis, thrombosis of the vena cava, and air embolism. Many of these shunts eventually require reoperation because of a failure to continue to function properly.

⊘ FREQUENT ERRORS

1. ***Failure to optimize blood pressure and tissue perfusion promptly in trauma patients with preexisting liver disease.***
2. ***Failure to consider biliary tract obstruction as a possible cause of increasing bilirubin levels in the first 5 days after trauma.***
3. ***Failure to rule out sepsis as a cause of bilirubin levels increasing more than 7 days after trauma.***
4. ***Supplying too much carbohydrate so that the RQ exceeds 1.0, thereby increasing the tendency to hepatic steatosis.***
5. ***Allowing efforts to control ascites cause hepatic perfusion to be reduced to less than normal.***
6. ***Allowing obstructive jaundice (which itself can cause biliary cirrhosis) to persist longer than absolutely necessary.***
7. ***Inadequate or delayed removal of blood from the gastrointestinal tract of a patient in whom hepatic encephalopathy has a tendency to develop.***
8. ***Failure to maintain a good urine output and closely following renal function in patients with hepatic failure.***

SUMMARY POINTS

1. Inadequate glycogen stores in the liver can greatly reduce the ability of the patient to tolerate severe trauma.

2. Albumin, because of its long half-life and because its plasma levels are affected by so many factors, is generally not a good guide to the adequacy of nutritional support.

3. If the BUN is less than 5.0 mg/dL, one should suspect hepatic failure.

4. Increasing serum triglyceride levels in patients with sepsis are often a sign of terminal liver failure.

5. High serum concentrations of unconjugated bilirubin in adults during the first 4 to 5 days after trauma are often the result of hemolysis of red cells in hematomas or transfused blood.

6. Resection or severe disease of the distal ileum can cause bile salt deficiencies.
7. Patients with cirrhosis or any other intrahepatic obstruction to portal venous blood flow are particularly sensitive to any reduction in hepatic artery blood flow.
8. Sepsis resulting in impaired hepatocellular function is the most common cause of jaundice developing 1 week or more after major abdominal operations.
9. Packing over a portion of the liver which has had its major hepatic artery blood supply ligated may cause hepatic necrosis there.
10. In patients with increasing jaundice after trauma, one should make a special effort to rule out extrahepatic biliary obstruction.
11. Non-A, non-B hepatitis is the most frequent type of hepatitis transmitted by transfusion of blood or blood products.
12. Most cases of posttransfusion hepatitis are not detected unless liver function or serology tests are performed 3 months after transfusion of blood products.
13. Increasing jaundice with high alkaline phosphatase levels soon after trauma should be considered a result of extrahepatic biliary tract obstruction until proven otherwise.
14. The *total HBF* in hypermetabolic sepsis is generally increased even though peripheral extraction studies usually indicate that the *effective HBF* is reduced.
15. A higher than normal cardiac index and oxygen delivery is required to maintain adequate hepatic oxygenation after trauma and during sepsis.
16. Increased lactate in the presence of a normal lactate-to-pyruvate ratio suggests aerobic glycolysis or reduced hepatic clearance, which is often caused by sepsis.
17. Bilirubin levels greater than 5 mg/dL in the absence of biliary tract obstruction, transfusion reaction, or resolving hematomas is strongly suggestive of liver dysfunction caused by sepsis.
18. When the cause of persistent jaundice in a patient with major abdominal surgery or trauma cannot be determined in any other manner, an exploratory celiotomy should be considered.
19. Optimization of oxygen delivery with fluids and blood (and possibly inotropes) within the first 12 to 24 hours after trauma is particularly important in patients with severe liver injury or disease.
20. Early enteral nutrition, which may decrease bacterial translocation in the gut, may be an important part of reducing hepatic dysfunction in critically ill or injured patients.
21. Indirect calorimetry to monitor RQ may be of great help in optimizing nutrition and preventing hepatic steatosis.
22. Patients with prehepatic portal hypertension can tolerate trauma and surgery much better than patients with other causes of esophageal varices.
23. Cirrhotic patients with jaundice or ascites who have sepsis or major trauma have an extremely high mortality rate.
24. Shock persisting for more than 30 minutes in patients with severe cirrhosis is almost invariably fatal.
25. Cirrhotic patients often have an increased bleeding tendency because they tend to have reduced levels of all of the coagulation factors (except factor VIII) and platelets, and they may also have increased fibrinolysis.
26. Although blood levels of ammonia often do not correlate well with the presence or severity of encephalopathy in liver failure, efforts to reduce blood ammonia levels often improve the encephalopathy.
27. Patients in whom hepatic failure is developing, especially with encephalopathy, may benefit from diets high in BCAA and low in AAAs.
28. One should look carefully for early renal dysfunction in patients with hepatic failure.
29. When diuretics are used to reduce ascites resulting from hepatic failure, one must be careful not to cause prerenal oliguria.
30. End-to-side portacaval shunts may reduce portal venous pressure, but they tend to make ascites worse and can greatly interfere with later liver transplantation.
31. One must make every effort to prevent excessive cardiac filling pressures in patients with peritoneovenous shunts.

REFERENCES

1. Wilson RF. Liver failure after trauma. In: Wilson RF, Walt AJ, eds. *Management of trauma—pitfalls and practice,* 2nd ed. Philadelphia: Williams and Wilkins, 1995:988.
2. Sherlock S. Anatomy and function and assessment of liver function. In: Sherlock S, ed. *Diseases of the liver and biliary system,* 8th ed. Boston: Blackwell Scientific Publications, 1989:1–18.
3. Barton RG, Cerra FB. Metabolic and nutritional support. In: Moore EE, Mattox KL, Feliciano DV, eds. *Trauma,* 2nd ed. Norwalk: Appleton & Lange, 1991: 965–994.
4. Marinokovic S, Jahreis GP, Wong GG, Baumann H. IL-6 modulates the synthesis of a specific set of acute phase plasma proteins in vivo. *J Immunol* 1989; 142:808.
5. Hermreck AS, Proberts KS, Thomas JH. Severe jaundice after rupture of abdominal aortic aneurysm. *Am J Surg* 1977;134:745.
6. Flint LM. Liver failure. *Surg Clin North Am* 1982;62:157.
7. Alter HJ. Discovery of the non-A, non-B hepatitis virus: the end of the beginning or the beginning of the end. *Trans Med Rev* 1989;3:77.
8. Champion HR, Jones RT, Trump BF, et al. A clinicopathologic study of hepatic dysfunction following shock. *Surg Gynecol Obstet* 1976;142:657.
9. Chiarelli A, Casadei A, Pornaro E, et al. Alanine and aspartate aminotransferase serum levels in burned patients: a long-term study. *J Trauma* 1987;27:790.
10. Fry DE. Splanchnic perfusion and sepsis. In: Roth BL, Nielsen TB, McKee AE, eds. *Prog Clin Biol Res.* New York: Alan R. Liss, 1989;299:9–17.
11. Gottlieb ME, Sarfeh IJ, Stratton H, et al. Hepatic perfusion and splanchnic oxygen consumption in patients postinjury. *J Trauma* 1983;23:836.
12. Dahn MS, Lange MP, Wilson RF, et al. Hepatic blood flow and splanchnic oxygen consumption measurements in clinical sepsis. *Surgery* 1990;107:295.
13. Inthorn D, Hoffmann JN, Hartl WH, et al. Antithrombin III supplementation in severe sepsis: beneficial effects on organ dysfunction. *Shock* 1997;8:328.
14. Walvatne C, Cerra FB. Hepatic dysfunction in multiple organ failure. In: Deitch EA, ed. *Multiple organ failure: pathophysiology and basic concepts of therapy.* New York: Thieme Medical Publishers, 1990:241.
15. Cerra FB, Seigel JH, Border JR, et al. The hepatic failure of sepsis: cellular versus substrate. *Surgery* 1979;86:409.
16. Cerra FA, Mazuski JE, Bankey PE, et al. Role of monokines in altering hepatic metabolism in sepsis. In: Roth Bl, Nielsen TB, McKee AE, eds. *Prog Clin Biol Res* New York: Alan R. Liss, 1989;286:265–277.
17. Nakatami T, Sakamoto Y, Kaneko I, et al. Effects of intra-abdominal hypertension on hepatic energy metabolism in a rabbit model. *J Trauma* 1998;44:446.
18. Dahn MS, Lang P, Lobdell K, et al. Splanchnic and total body oxygen consumption differences in septic and injury patients. *Surgery* 1987;101:69.
19. Baker AL, Rosenberg IH. Hepatic complications of total parenteral nutrition. *Am J Med* 1987;82:489.
20. Reported Cirrhosis Mortality—United States, 1970-1980. *MMWR Morbid Mortal Wkly Rep* 1988;33:657-659.
21. Grant PG, DuFour MC, Hartford TC. Epidemiology of alcoholic liver disease. *Semin Liver Dis* 1988;8:12.
22. Arahna GV, Greenlee HB. Intra-abdominal surgery in patients with advanced cirrhosis. *Arch Surg* 1986;121:275.
23. Tinkoff G, Rhodes M, Diamond D, et al. Cirrhosis in the trauma victim: effect on mortality rates. *Ann Surg* 1990;211:172.
24. Mansour A, Watson W, Shayani V, et al. Abdominal operations in patients with cirrhosis: still a major surgical challenge. *Surgery* 1997;122:730.
25. Sherlock S. The haematology of liver disease. In: Sherlock S, ed. *Diseases of the liver and biliary system,* 8th ed. Boston: Blackwell Scientific, 1989:49.
26. Sherlock S. Hepatic encephalopathy. In: Sherlock S, ed. *Diseases of the liver and biliary system.* Boston: Blackwell Scientific, 1989:95–115.

27. Fisher JE, Baldessarini RJ. False neurotransmitters and hepatic failure. *Lancet* 1971;2:75.
28. Cerra FB, Cheung NK, Fisher JE, et al. Disease-specific amino acid infusion (F080) in hepatic encephalopathy: a prospective, randomized, double-blind, controlled trial. *JPEN J Parenter Enteral Nutr* 1985;9:3:288.

45. COAGULATION ABNORMALITIES IN TRAUMA[1]

HEMOSTASIS IN TRAUMA

Normally, hemostasis is initiated by the cooperative action of the endothelium, vasoconstriction, platelets, and coagulation factors in response to a disruption of the vascular endothelium surface. Abnormal hemostasis in the injured patient, unless recognized and treated promptly and appropriately, may lead not only to excessive bleeding and possible death but also to poor wound healing or thromboembolic complications (2).

AXIOM Even if a defect is found in bleeding and coagulation laboratory tests, intraoperative and postoperative bleeding is usually the result of inadequate surgical efforts.

Primary Hemostasis

Vasoconstriction

Following trauma, injured blood vessels respond promptly with local vasoconstriction which appears to be chiefly mediated by thromboxane, serotonin, catecholamines, and the sympathetic nervous system.

AXIOM Partial transection of a vessel, which prevents vascular occlusion by vasoconstriction, is more likely to lead to significant blood loss than is complete transection.

Platelets

The exposure of collagen fibers in injured vessels initiates "adhesion" of a single layer of platelets at the site of injury (2). This first step in the formation of the primary hemostatic plug requires von Willebrand factor (vWF), which is produced by endothelial cells and is found in both the vessel wall and in plasma. The vWF binds to specific glycoprotein receptors on the platelet surface (glycoproteins Ib and Ia-IIb).

The adhesion of platelets is followed by a "release reaction" in which adenosine diphosphate (ADP) and serotonin are released from the adhered platelets. These substances activate adjacent platelets, which then change shape and develop pseudopods. Another receptor (glycoprotein IIb-IIIa) is assembled on the platelet surface membrane, and fibrinogen and other adhesive proteins bind to this receptor causing platelet *aggregation*. This continuing platelet aggregation leads to the formation of a "first hemostatic plug" or "platelet plug," which facilitates "primary hemostasis" to close off vessels that are 50 microns or less in diameter.

Excessive or unwanted aggregation of platelets is inhibited by prostacyclin (PGI_2), which is produced by vascular endothelium; prostacyclin also acts as a vasodilator, thereby helping to maintain the fluidity of blood.

Secondary Hemostasis

Pathophysiology

Following the adhesion and aggregation of platelets at a disrupted vessel site, a series of enzymatic reactions is initiated by the release of phospholipids in micellar form (platelet factor 3) from platelet surfaces (2). Serial activation of the procoagulant proteins then results in the formation of thrombin, which stimulates platelets to release vasoactive products and ADP, which attract more platelets to the injured site.

In regions such as peripheral arteries, where blood flow is brisk, one is more likely to see a "white thrombus," which is composed predominately of platelets and fibrin. In areas of sluggish blood flow, such as large veins, the presence of abnormal surfaces activates clotting factors leading to formation of a "red thrombus," composed of red cells trapped in fibrin strands (3).

Phases of Fibrin Formation

The process of fibrin formation, also referred to as "secondary hemostasis," can be divided into three phases, which include the formation of activated factor X (factor Xa), then thrombin, and finally fibrin (Fig. 45-1). The proteolytic cascade that makes up the coagulation system amplifies the response at each step. In other words, each activated (factor) enzyme tends to activate many more molecules of the next enzyme (factor), and thus an initial, small stimulus can cause a much larger response (Fig. 45-1).

Formation of Activated Factor X (Factor Xa)

The formation of activated factor X (Xa) can be accomplished either by the intrinsic or extrinsic coagulation pathways.

Intrinsic Pathway. The intrinsic coagulation pathway, which can be monitored by the activated partial thromboplastin time (aPTT), begins when factor XII is activated

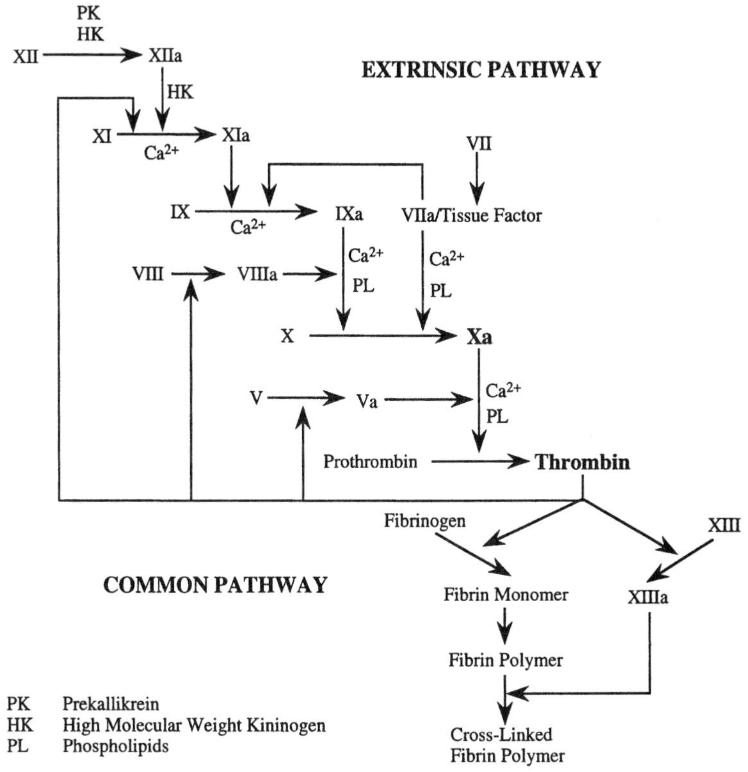

FIG. 45-1. Schematic representation of the entire clotting system involving the intrinsic, extrinsic, and common pathways.

to factor XIIa, usually on injured endothelium or platelet phospholipid surfaces. Factor XIIa, in turn, activates factor XI to factor XIa. Factor XIa then converts factor IX to factor IXa (2). A complex is formed between platelet phospholipids in micellar form serving as surfaces, calcium ions serving as binders, and factor IXa serving as the enzyme.

Extrinsic Pathway. The extrinsic coagulation pathway, which can be monitored with prothrombin time (PT), begins when a complex of factor VII, tissue factor, phospholipids, and calcium is formed. The extrinsic pathway is marked by the involvement of tissue thromboplastin (1). All tissues contain a clot-promoting factor called tissue thromboplastin (which has a phospholipid and a tissue factor [enzyme] component). The phospholipids act as surfaces for formation of a complex between factor VII (enzyme), tissue factor, and calcium ions (acting as binders).

Formation of Thrombin

Prothrombin is converted to thrombin by the prothrombinase complex, which includes phospholipid micelles (acting as surfaces), calcium ions (acting as binders), activated factor X (acting as an enzyme), and factor V (also known as AC-globulin).

Formation of Fibrin

Normally, 200 to 400 mg of clottable fibrinogen is present in every 100 mL of plasma. The formation of fibrin from the clottable fibrinogen can be divided into three phases: proteolytic phase, polymerization phase, and stabilization phase.

The *proteolytic phase* of fibrin formation is marked by the cleavage of a pair of A peptides and a pair of B peptides from the N-terminal end of the alpha and beta chains of fibrinogen by the proteolytic enzyme, thrombin, leaving behind a dimer called a "fibrin monomer" (2).

In the *polymerization phase,* the fibrin monomers combine to form an end-to-end and side-to-side polymerized fibrin network.

During the *stabilization phase*, the polymerized fibrin monomers are covalently bonded by activated factor XIII (1).

Coagulation Inhibitors

Inappropriate activation of coagulation in blood vessels is prevented by nonplasma proteinase inhibitors and plasma proteinase inhibitors. The nonplasma proteinase inhibitors block contact activation and fibrinolysis (4). The plasma proteinase inhibitors are serine proteases, which include antithrombin III and α_2-macroglobulin (which form inactive complexes with all coagulation enzymes) as well as protein C and its cofactor, protein S. Protein C is activated by thrombin when complexed with an endothelial cell surface bound receptor, called thrombomodulin. Activated protein C causes proteolytic degradation of factors Va and VIIIa.

AXIOM Recurrent venous thromboembolic disease in young individuals without apparent predisposing factors should make one suspect an inherited or acquired deficiency of antithrombin III, protein C, or protein S.

Clot Retraction

After fibrin fibers form, they begin to shorten, causing the clot to retract. This fibrin shortening is the result of thrombasthenin, a protein found in platelets. If there is a thrombocytopenia or platelet dysfunction, clots do not retract well and are not as firm and hemostatic.

Fibrinolysis

The fibrinolytic system is important in opposing any excess tendency toward blood coagulation and in maintaining the fluid characteristics of blood in the intravascular space (5). It is also important for allowing fibroblasts to come in contact with injured tissue to repair it.

Fibrinolysis is accomplished primarily by a proteolytic enzyme referred to as plasmin, which is formed from plasminogen by plasminogen activators.

The two primary plasminogen activators are the tissue type (t-PA) and the urokinase type (u-PA). Tissue plasminogen activator (t-PA) is the primary physiologic activator of intravascular plasminogen (5). t-PA is produced in endothelial cells. Urokinase is formed by endothelial cells throughout the body and by epithelial cells lining various excretory ducts of the body (e.g., renal tubules, mammary ducts). Urokinase is normally found in urine, and it has been used clinically to treat thromboembolic disease. Streptokinase, a bacterial product not normally found in the body, is a potent activator of plasminogen and can be used clinically to induce fibrinolysis therapeutically.

Plasmin

Plasmin acts not only on fibrin, but also on fibrinogen and factors II, V, VIII, IX, and XI (3). It also activates factor XII, which, in turn, can trigger the coagulation, complement, and kinin systems. Fibrin and fibrinogen are digested or broken down by plasmin into fibrinogen or fibrin split products (FSPs). The large-molecular weight split products produced initially are called fragments X and Y or "early split products."

Fibrin split products can block primary and secondary hemostasis by

1. Competing with fibrinogen for active-binding sites on the thrombin molecule;
2. Inhibiting the polymerization phase of fibrin formation;
3. Competitively inhibiting thrombin; and
4. Coating the surface of platelets, thereby rendering them unaggregable.

AXIOM Normal thrombin times plus normal fibrinogen levels exclude serious activation of the fibrinolytic system.

Laboratory evaluation of fibrinolysis as part of the assessment of thrombotic and bleeding disorders includes measurements of plasminogen, plasminogen activators, plasminogen activator inhibitors, thrombin time, circulating fibrinogen, and cross-linked fibrin degradation products (D-dimers).

Plasminogen Activator Inhibitors

Prevention of excessive fibrinolysis is largely achieved through the action of specific plasminogen activator inhibitors (PAIs) and α_2-antiplasmin. Endothelial cells produce type 1 PAI (PAI-1), the most important physiologic inhibitor of t-PA and u-PA. Elevated PAI-1 levels also appear to contribute to the development of postoperative deep venous thrombosis (DVT).

DIAGNOSIS OF BLEEDING DISORDERS

History

When seeking a history of possible hemostatic disorders, it is important to ask direct questions related to bruising tendency, spontaneous epistaxis, hemorrhage following minor trauma or operations, melena, hematuria, joint swellings, and prolonged menstrual periods or postpartum bleeding. A family history of any bleeding tendency is extremely important.

AXIOM Patients with primary hemostatic (platelet or vascular) defects tend to give a history of either prolonged oozing from cuts or mucous membranes or excessive bruising. In contrast, individuals with impaired secondary hemostasis (inadequate clotting factors) tend to have hemarthrosis and deep (intramuscular) hematomas.

All current medications must be known. A particular effort should always be made to determine whether the injured patient has been taking any "blood thinners" (anticoagulants), such as Coumadin, or "pain pills" containing acetylsalicylic acid, nonsteroidal antiinflammatory agents, or any other compounds that may interfere with platelet function (2). A history of excessive alcohol intake may point to hepatic dysfunction with impaired coagulation factor production.

Physical Examination

The physical examination of the trauma patient with a possible bleeding disorder should include several direct observations: Is the bleeding localized or diffuse? Is it related to a traumatic or surgical lesion? Is there mucosal bleeding? Are there signs of arterial or venous thrombosis?

AXIOM Prolonged or excessive bleeding from needle puncture sites or spontaneous bleeding from mucous membranes suggests a severe coagulopathy, such as disseminated intravascular coagulation (DIC).

The presence of an enlarged spleen in a thrombocytopenic patient suggests splenic sequestration. Hepatomegaly or other evidence of liver disease may indicate decreased factor synthesis as the cause of a prolonged PT or aPTT.

When evidence of an advanced malignancy exists, chronic DIC should be suspected as the cause of prolonged coagulation times, hypofibrinogenemia, and thrombocytopenia. Palpable purpura suggests capillary leak resulting from vasculitis, whereas purpura resulting from thrombocytopenia or platelet defects cannot usually be detected by touch. Venous telangiectasias may be seen in some patients with von Willebrand disease (vWD), and arterial telangiectasias may be seen in liver disease. When point pressure is centrally applied to an arterial telangiectasia, the lesion fades, whereas venous telangiectasia requires confluent pressure across the entire lesion (as with a glass slide) for blanching to occur.

Laboratory Evaluation

Excessive bleeding after severe trauma may occur if the concentration of coagulation factors is less than 50% of normal, but most of the laboratory coagulation tests are normal if 30% to 35% of the normal amount of each factor is present.

AXIOM Mild to moderate congenital or acquired bleeding disorders are easily overlooked by screening coagulation tests.

Six screening tests can document most of the disorders likely to be involved in excess hemorrhage not caused by mechanical problems. Platelet counts and bleeding times screen for most of the serious quantitative and qualitative platelet abnormalities. The PT and aPTT screen for virtually all serious clotting factor deficiencies. Fibrinogen determinations plus thrombin clotting times or FSP assays screen for the presence of increased fibrinolysis (2).

Platelet Count and Function

A platelet count less than 100,000/mm^3 can increase bleeding to some degree depending on how low it is. A platelet count less than 50,000/mm^3 can greatly increase bleeding from any skin or mucosal injury. A platelet count less than 10,000 to 20,000/mm^3 may be associated with spontaneous bleeding without trauma.

Bleeding time, preferably performed according to the procedure described by Ivy (2), is abnormal not only in patients with thrombocytopenia, but also with many forms of thrombocytopathy. Bleeding times should be normal when platelet counts are more than 100,000/mm^3, but they are always prolonged with counts less than 50,000/mm^3.

AXIOM Mild quantitative or qualitative platelet disorders are usually not discovered by performing a bleeding time (BT) (2).

Peterson et al. (6) recently reported (in a position paper for the College of American Pathologists and American Society of Clinical Pathologists) that (1) in the absence of a history of a bleeding disorder, the bleeding time is not a useful predictor of the risk of hemorrhage associated with surgical procedures, (2) a normal bleeding time does not exclude the possibility of excessive hemorrhage associated with invasive procedures, and (3) the bleeding time cannot be used to reliably identify patients who may have recently ingested aspirin or nonsteroidal antiinflammatory agents or those who have a platelet defect attributable to these drugs.

Coagulation Factors

The aPTT screens the activity of all of the coagulation factors involved in the formation of thrombin via the intrinsic and common pathways. Only factor VII activity is not measured by aPTT. Because the aPPT is not very sensitive, coagulation factors involved in the intrinsic pathway usually have to be reduced to less than 30% to 35% of normal before the aPTT is significantly prolonged (2).

PT screens for the activity of all coagulation factors involved in the extrinsic and common pathway of thrombin formation.

AXIOM A normal aPTT and PT effectively exclude any serious defects in the clotting system.

When fibrinogen levels are greater than 100 mg/dL and are not associated with other defects, hemostasis is generally normal.

Thrombin (clotting) times (TT) are most helpful in determining defects associated with the formation of fibrin from fibrinogen by thrombin. The TT is abnormal when the fibrinogen level is less than 50 mg/dL, when heparin is present, when abnormal plasma proteins (paraproteinemias) are present and, most importantly, when increased quantities of FSP are present. TTs, in the absence of heparin and in the presence of greater than 50 mg/dL fibrinogen, are highly sensitive to the presence of increased FSP as a result of increased fibrinolysis.

With the tube clotting test, 2 to 3 mL of blood are drawn into a single clean test tube, and the rate of clot formation is observed (3). The tube is tilted every minute or so to determine whether a clot has formed. Normal blood should clot within 10 minutes. It should then gradually retract and remain stable. Absence of clotting within 20 to 30 minutes indicates a major coagulopathy. Absence of retraction (after a clot has formed) indicates possible thrombocytopenia. When blood clots properly but subsequently lyses rapidly (within another 5 to 10 minutes), excess fibrinolysis should be suspected.

Reptilase time, when available, can be used to differentiate hyperheparinemia from increased split products. A normal reptilase time combined with a prolonged TT is seen with heparin therapy. In the presence of FSP, both tests are prolonged.

SPECIFIC BLEEDING AND COAGULATION DISORDERS

Congenital Disorders

Plasma concentrations of the involved coagulation factors in most congenital coagulation disorders tend to be extremely low, but an early accurate diagnosis, especially of the milder disorders, may still depend primarily on a careful history and physical examination. Laboratory tests, especially PT and aPTT, plus assay of plasma levels of specific factors, can confirm the clinical impressions.

Proper hematologic management of congenital coagulation disorders usually includes administration of a specific factor concentrate; however, in emergency situations, treatment can be started with fresh frozen plasma (FFP) or cryoprecipitate. In addition, meticulous intraoperative hemostasis and careful clinical and laboratory monitoring of blood coagulation during surgery and in the perioperative period are essential.

Hemophilias

Pathophysiology

Classic hemophilia, also called hemophilia A, is characterized by factor VIII deficiency and is inherited as a sex-linked, recessive disorder. It is manifested almost exclusively in male patients; women are the genetic carriers. Approximately one male patient in 10,000 is afflicted, making it one of the most common severe hereditary coagulation disorders (8). The factor VIII protein complex consists of procoagulant factor VIII:C (FVIII:C) and vWF. Patients with classic hemophilia lack FVIII:C.

Hemophilia B (Christmas disease), which is clinically and genetically indistinguishable from hemophilia A, occurs less frequently and is caused by hereditary deficiency of Christmas factor (factor IX) (7).

AXIOM In hemophiliacs, the first hemostatic plug develops promptly after trauma, but excessive bleeding tends to develop after a delay that may last several hours or days.

In hemophilia, fibrin formation is limited to deposition of thin strands at the wound periphery, preventing the central core of the thrombus from gaining proper consistency (7). Because primary hemostasis is unaffected in hemophilia, the onset of abnormal bleeding is characteristically somewhat delayed, but then may persist for several days or even weeks, if not treated.

Bleeding is unlikely in patients with FVIII:C concentrations more than 50% of normal even after major injury or surgery. The likelihood of bleeding with FVIII:C concentrations less than 50% is dependent on the severity of trauma; however, concentrations that are only 1% to 4% of normal predispose the patient to abnormal bleeding even after minor injury. Recurrent, spontaneous bleeding, usually into muscles or weight-bearing joints, generally occurs only in patients with FVIII:C levels that are less than 1% of normal.

Diagnosis

AXIOM The diagnosis of hemophilia should be suspected in male patients with a history of excessive bleeding since childhood.

The presence of excessive bleeding into muscles or joints after trauma or of prolonged oozing from wounds or sites of venipuncture should make one consider the possibility of a preexisting hemostatic defect.

In hemophilia, laboratory tests typically reveal normal platelet counts, BTs, and PTs with a prolonged aPTT (8). Severe trauma with prolonged shock or massive transfusions may result in decreased platelet counts and a prolonged PT, making diagnosis much more difficult. In hemodynamically stable patients in whom the diagnosis of hemophilia can be made by FVIII:C measurement, one should also look for a FVIII inhibitor as a cause of excessive bleeding.

AXIOM If normal blood is placed in a test tube with an equal amount of the hemophilia blood and the blood does not clot properly, an inhibitor is probably present.

Treatment

Treatment of hemophilia must be rapid and accurate, especially if the trauma involves intracranial, lingual, laryngeal, retropharyngeal, pericardial, or pleural spaces or tissues. Hematomas at these sites can expand rapidly and result in life-threatening displacement of intracranial, cervical, or thoracic organs (7). Although these conditions require immediate factor VIII replacement, emergency decompression of the brain or heart or establishment of airway patency may also be necessary.

AXIOM Intraoperative positioning of hemophiliacs should be done carefully to reduce the likelihood of bleeding into tissues at pressure points.

General guidelines for the treatment of congenital coagulopathies are

1. Determine the plasma level of the factor prior to surgery.
2. Exclude the presence of a possible inhibitor.
3. Infuse the factor in question and be certain that the plasma level increases appropriately.
4. Increase the concentration of the factor in plasma to its desired level immediately before surgery.
5. Maintain sufficient concentrations until wound healing is complete.

Most patients who have received replacement therapy either with factor VIII concentrates or with large amounts of cryoprecipitate have antibodies to the HIV causing acquired immunodeficiency syndrome (AIDS) (3). Because virus-inactivated factor VIII concentrates are available, only these products should be used. Recently, recombinant factor concentrates have also become available.

AXIOM The initial treatment of excessive bleeding in hemophiliacs is volume resuscitation with blood transfusions and FFP.

FFP, which contains all of the clotting factors, and blood should be used in the initial treatment of abnormal bleeding after trauma. This permits volume resuscitation in addition to providing factor VIII or IX. After the initial emergency has been corrected, more extensive evaluation is appropriate, including tests to determine the quantity of factor VIII or IX present in the blood. FFP, cryoprecipitate, or factor concentrates can then be given as needed to maintain factor levels at 50% to 100% of normal, depending on the severity of the trauma, until there is complete healing (7,8) (Table 45-1).

Although the amount of factor VIII in individual *cryoprecipitate* bags varies somewhat, a bag may be assumed to contain 80 units of factor VIII when calculating the number of bags needed for replacement therapy. In major surgical procedures, the plasma levels of factors VIII or IX should be increased to 50% to 100% of normal immediately before and during surgery and should be maintained at concentrations of at least 20% to 30% of normal in the postoperative period. This usually involves giving one-half of the initial dose every 8 to 12 hours for 7 to 14 days. The fibrinogen level should also be maintained at 100 mg/dL or more at all times.

AXIOM Each unit of factor VIII activity infused per kilogram of body weight should produce a 2% increase in plasma concentrations (2).

For *factor VIII concentrates*, dosage can be calculated by multiplying the patient's weight in kilograms by 44 and by the level in units desired. Thus, to increase the factor VIII level of a man who weighs 68 kg (150 lb) from a level of essentially zero to a level of 0.5 u/mL (i.e. 50%), the dosage needed would be $68 \times 44 \times 50\%$ or 1,496 (about 1,500) units.

Table 45-1. *Presence of Clotting Factors in Blood and Blood Components*

	Factors									
	I	II	V	VII	VIII	IX	X	XI	XII	XIII
Fresh whole blood	+	+	+	+	+	+	+	+	+	+
Bank blood (<5 days old)	+	+	–	+	–	+	+	+	+	+
Fresh frozen plasma	+	+	+	+	+	+	+	+	+	+
Cohn fraction I	+	–	+?	–	+?	–	–	–	–	+
Cryoprecipitate	+	–	+	–	+	–	–	+	+	+
Factor VIII concentrates	–	–	–	–	+	–	–	–	–	–
Factor IX concentrates	–	+	–	+	–	+	+	–	–	–
Fibrinogen concentrates	+	–	+?	–	+?	–	–	–	–	+

Giving factor VIII to patients who have factor VIII inhibitors stimulates further antibody production and increases the plasma titer of antibody within 3 to 4 days (9). In patients with serious bleeding and a low initial inhibitor antibody titer, a large dose of factor VIII, calculated to overcome the inhibitor and temporarily increase plasma factor VIII levels, may be given. If this does not control bleeding, further factor VIII infusions are useless because of the rapid increase in antibody induced.

Prothrombin complex concentrates can be used to manage serious bleeding in patients with high titers of factor VIII inhibitor. Special preparations of prothrombin complex concentrate are available for treating this problem, but they are very expensive. A porcine factor VIII preparation, which is insensitive to the inhibitor, has also been used with good results (9).

Replacement therapy for factor IX deficiencies requires an amount double that calculated as necessary. Each unit of *factor IX concentrate* infused per kilogram body weight should theoretically increase levels by 1%; however, only about one-half the factor IX units listed on each unit of prothrombin complex concentrate can be recovered after infusion (3).

AXIOM In patients receiving multiple units of factor IX concentrate, 5 to 10 units of heparin should be added to each milliliter of reconstituted prothrombin complex concentrate because of the activated clotting factors it contains.

The drug 1-deamino-8-D-arginine vasopressin, also known as desmopressin acetate or *DDAVP*, is useful for treating patients with factor VIII concentrations of 5% to 10% or more by mobilizing factor VIII from endothelial stores. Administration of DDAVP after minor trauma or before elective dental surgery may reduce or even obviate the need for factor VIII replacement therapy.

The antifibrinolytic agent, *epsilon aminocaproic acid* (EACA), in doses of 2.5 g four times daily for 1 week can be given to hemophiliac patients to prevent late bleeding after dental extraction or other types of oropharyngeal mucosal trauma (e.g., tongue lacerations); however, when giving prothrombin complex concentrates (which may contain activated clotting factors), EACA should not be given until 10 hours after the prothrombin complex.

von Willebrand's Disease

vWD, the most frequent congenital coagulopathy, is encountered more often than both hemophilias combined. It is an autosomal dominant disorder of variable severity (10). It results from a quantitative (type I) or qualitative (type II) abnormality of vWF. This plasma protein is secreted by endothelial cells and circulates in plasma in various subtypes with multimers of up to 14,000,000 daltons.

vWF has two known hemostatic functions:

1. Large multimers of vWF are required for platelets to adhere to collagen and other biologic surfaces; and
2. Multimers of all sizes form complexes in plasma with factor VIII:C. Formation of such complexes is required to maintain normal plasma factor VIII:C levels.

Bleeding manifestations in vWD are usually mild to moderate and include easy bruising, epistaxis, bleeding from small skin cuts (that may stop and start again over a period of several hours), increased menstrual bleeding (in some women), and abnormal bleeding after surgical procedures (e.g., tooth extraction and tonsillectomy).

In the laboratory, vWD is characterized by prolonged BTs because of abnormal platelet adhesion and prolonged APTTs resulting from an associated factor VIII:C deficiency; however, in persons with mild vWD, variations in plasma levels of factor VIII:C may cause screening tests to be normal on some occasions. A definitive diagnosis of vWD requires measurement of total plasma vWF activity and antigen and the ability of the plasma to support agglutination of normal platelets by ristocetin (11).

Type I or type II variants of vWD, although characterized by impaired platelet adhesion, should be treated with DDAVP, FFP, or cryoprecipitate and not platelet concentrates (10). The dosage of cryoprecipitate for treating vWD is often selected empirically and is typically one bag for each 10 kg of body weight every 8 to 12 hours just before and for several days after major surgery.

DDAVP may be helpful in type I vWD. Thirty minutes after intravenous administration of DDAVP in a dose of 0.3 to 0.4 μg/kg, one can expect a significant shortening in BTs and increased factor VIII:C and vWF activities. If possible, one should wait 48 hours for new endothelial stores of vWF to accumulate before trying a second injection of DDAVP.

Acquired Bleeding Disorders

AXIOM Acquired bleeding disorders are much more frequently encountered than those of congenital origin, particularly in adult trauma patients.

Acquired bleeding disorders such as hepatic or renal failure can usually be detected preoperatively by conducting a careful history and physical examination and by performing the screening tests.

Hepatic Failure

Because most coagulation factors, except vWF and FVIII:C, are synthesized in the liver, the blood levels of the various coagulation factors especially factor II, VII, IX, and X are decreased in patients with cirrhosis. Excess bleeding, however, is not likely to occur until the concentration of coagulation factors is less than 30% of normal.

Splenomegaly, which often develops because of the increased portal pressure present in cirrhosis, may cause thrombocytopenia; hyperbilirubinemia, if present, can also alter platelet function.

Heparin infusions in patients with severe liver disease have been shown to increase fibrinogen levels transiently, suggesting that a chronic low-grade DIC probably exists in those patients and may contribute to the decreased fibrinogen levels. In cirrhotic patients, hyperfibrinolysis may also develop because the diseased liver cannot remove fibrinolysius from the circulation properly.

The diagnosis of bleeding and coagulation problems caused by hepatic failure depends primarily on clinical evidence of hepatic dysfunction plus prolonged PTs (12). The TT may also be prolonged as a result of severe hypofibrinogenemia, abnormal or dysfunctional fibrinogen molecules, or elevated FSPs. Elevated D-dimer levels suggest the presence of DIC.

Treatment of the clotting problems in patients with hepatic dysfunction includes administration of vitamin K, but this may not cause any improvement in the PT in patients with severe liver disease, even after 24 to 48 hours (3). Therefore, severe, acute bleeding problems in patients with liver failure should be treated with FFP. Because factor VII has the shortest half-life (6 hours) of the various coagulation factors, the least amount of FFP necessary to restore and maintain levels of factor VII of at least 25% to 50% is at least 10 mL/kg every 6 hours. In severe liver disease with significant trauma or bleeding, an initial bolus of 4 to 8 units of FFP plus 2 units every 2 hours may be needed to maintain adequate coagulation factor levels.

If a bleeding cirrhotic patient is found to have hypofibrinogenemia plus fibrinolysis, therapy with EACA (Amicar) may be considered; however, this must be done with great care, and one must be sure that there is no evidence of ongoing intravascular clotting (i.e., D-dimer levels must not be elevated).

Renal Failure

Severe renal disease with blood urea nitrogen (BUN) levels exceeding 100 mg/dL can cause a reversible bleeding disorder largely related to platelet dysfunction (3). Although no reliable correlation exists between BUN levels and bleeding tendencies, prolonged bleeding times often return to normal following dialysis.

The precise mechanisms by which renal insufficiency causes thrombocytopathy are not known, but increased levels of phenol and guanidine derivatives can impair platelet aggregation and platelet adhesiveness (13). Cryoprecipitate infusions may improve platelet function in these patients.

Although hemodialysis eliminates the thrombocytopathy of uremia, this procedure cannot usually be done in the presence of severe, ongoing bleeding. In such circumstances, transfusion of platelet concentrates may be necessary as an emergency; DDAVP 0.4 μg/kg intravenously in uremic patients is also often helpful. Conjugated estrogen (Premarin) in doses of 10 to 50 mg/day has effects like DDAVP, but the duration of its effects may persist for several days.

Vitamin K Deficiency

AXIOM Vitamin K deficiency should be suspected in patients with chronic, severe biliary tract obstruction or malabsorption.

Vitamin K is necessary for carboxylase to attach carboxy groups to glutamic acids. When vitamin-K–dependent factors are synthesized in the absence of vitamin K, they lack carboxyglutamic acid residues and, consequently, cannot bind calcium properly (12).

Causes of vitamin K deficiency include inadequate dietary intake, malabsorption, lack of bile salts, obstructive jaundice, biliary fistulas, oral administration of antibiotics, and parenteral alimentation (3). A number of broad-spectrum antibiotics, including cefoperozone, moxalactam, cefamandole, and ceftizoxime, can also cause a vitamin-K–dependent coagulopathy.

AXIOM Coagulation defects caused by pure vitamin K deficiency can be partially corrected by intravenous vitamin K within 6 to 12 hours.

The initial treatment of vitamin K deficiency is 5 mg given slowly intravenously (<lmg/mm). Previous preparations of vitamin K were less purified than those used presently, and anaphylaxis and death were occasionally reported with intravenous administration of the older agents (3). The newer, more purified forms are less likely to cause complications, but intravenous vitamin K should still be given selectively. In acutely bleeding patients, administration of adequate quantities of FFP can generally correct the coagulation deficit rapidly and should be given in addition to vitamin K (12).

Coumarins

Coumarins prolong PTs but can also cause prolongation of the aPTTs by reducing the levels of prothrombin (factor II) and factors IX and X. Coumadin has a half-life of 40 hours. Such therapy should be stopped 48 to 96 hours before surgery, which should be performed only after the PT has returned to within 3.0 seconds of control. In acute situations, administration of both vitamin K and FFP can rapidly reverse the effects of coumarins, but it can also make the patient hypercoagulable. Consequently, a simultaneous heparin infusion may be warranted.

AXIOM Treatment of severe, active bleeding which is the result of Coumadin or vitamin K deficiency should include intravenous vitamin K and at least 4 to 8 units of FFP.

PROBLEMS WITH ANTICOAGULANT THERAPY

Coumadin

The effect of coumarins can be potentiated by a large number of drugs (e.g., acetaminophen, heparin, phenytoin, alcohol, metronidazole, and cimetidine) and a number of disease states (including congestive heart failure and liver disease), and may result in spontaneous or excessive bleeding. Some of the drugs that inhibit the effects of Coumadin on blood coagulation include barbiturates, corticosteroids, estrogen, and alcohol. Hypothyroidism also inhibits the effects of Coumadin.

Heparin

Heparin has multiple effects on hemostasis:

1. By combining with antithrombin III, it can rapidly inhibit the actions of thrombin and factor Xa.
2. In slightly larger doses, heparin can block other factors, especially factor XIIa.
3. In very large doses, heparin can decrease platelet adhesiveness and aggregation.

Heparin has a dose-dependent mean plasma half-life of 60 to 90 minutes. A dose of heparin is normally almost completely cleared from the blood in 6 hours, but this time can be greatly prolonged if a large dose was given or if the patient has hepatic dysfunction, hypothermia, or shock.

AXIOM Reduced plasma levels of antithrombin (because of liver disease or excessive clotting) can greatly increase the amount of heparin needed to prolong aPTT.

Protamine Neutralization

Because heparin is a strong, negatively charged anion, it can be neutralized with intravenous protamine sulfate, which is a strong, positively charged cation. Protamine (1.0 mg) can neutralize 100 units of heparin, which is equivalent to about 1.0 mg of heparin. The dose of protamine given should be approximately equal to the dose of heparin given, with allowance made for the half-life of heparin. For every 30 to 60 minutes after heparin has been given, the amount of protamine needed is reduced by about half. Because it can have significant vasodilator and negative inotropic effects, protamine should be given slowly, and the patient should be monitored carefully to avoid hypotension or an excessive dosage of protamine, which, by itself, can cause excessive bleeding.

Heparin-Induced Thrombocytopenia

Heparin tends to cause platelets to aggregate, and in some patients, large quantities of platelet antibodies are formed. These cause much more platelet aggregation and can rapidly cause severe thrombocytopenia, sometimes with large platelet clots occluding major vessels.

Heparin-induced thrombocytopenia (HIT) can be severe in up to 6% of patients. The likelihood of HIT is independent of the route of administration; however, severe thrombocytopenia is seen more frequently with large intravenous doses of bovine lung heparin.

AXIOM Platelet counts should be carefully monitored daily or every other day whenever heparin is given.

Platelet counts normally decrease about 1% to 2% per day while on heparin, but a 30% decrease in the platelet count or the development of an arterial vascular occlusion is strongly suggestive of HIT. This usually occurs about 6 to 12 days after the initiation of heparin therapy, but it may occur at any time throughout the course of its use, particularly with repeated courses of heparin. If heparin treatment is required, patients with HIT should avoid unfractionated heparin, and low-molecular weight heparin (LMWH) may be considered a possible alternative (14).

Low Molecular Weight Heparin

In a recent study, 1,021 patients with symptomatic DVT were prospectively randomized to fixed-dose subcutaneous LMWH or adjusted-dose intravenous unfractionated heparin. Both treatments were found to be equally safe and effective (15). Simmoneau et al. in the THESEE Study Group found, in a prospective, randomized trial of 612 patients, that subcutaneous therapy with LMWH was as safe and effective as intravenous unfractionated heparin in patients with acute pulmonary embolism (16).

Thrombocytopathies Resulting from Drugs

Many drugs can interfere with platelet function. The most common drugs that block platelet function are the prostaglandin inhibitors (particularly aspirin), and the nonsteroidal antiinflammatory drugs (NSAIDs). Aspirin blocks prostaglandin metabolism in platelets by permanently acetylating cyclooxygenase. Affected platelets remain dysfunctional throughout their 8- to 10-day lifespan. As little as 80 mg of aspirin can depress platelet aggregation and prolong BT (but usually by only 2 to 3 minutes) for at least 72 hours. Simultaneous alcohol ingestion can have a profound potentiating effect on the platelet dysfunction caused by aspirin. NSAIDs, such as ibuprofen have a similar, but reversible, effect (for about 6 to 12 hours) on platelet aggregation.

Patients who have ingested aspirin or NSAIDs within 72 hours of surgery should probably have BTs performed. If the BT is significantly abnormal, the urgency of the surgery dictates whether delay is advisable until the BT returns to normal; DDAVP, however, can sometimes normalize the prolonged BT caused by aspirin.

AXIOM Platelet transfusions are indicated in patients in whom abnormal bleeding develops as a result of thrombocytopenia or thrombocytopathy during emergency major surgery.

Paraproteinemias

Diseases, such as Waldenstrom's macroglobulinemia, cryoglobulinemia, multiple myeloma, and hypergammaglobulinemia, which cause the formation of abnormal proteins, occasionally cause defects in primary and secondary hemostasis (2). Coating of platelets by these abnormal proteins may interfere with aggregation and cause prolonged BT. Secondary hemostasis may also be impaired because of abnormal fibrin formation caused by disturbed polymerization of the fibrin monomers. Therapy is difficult, but platelet concentrates, FFP, or purified fibrinogen, when available, may be helpful.

Thrombocytopenias

Severe thrombocytopenias can cause spontaneous bleeding into the skin, manifested by petechiae, purpura, or confluent ecchymoses. It can also cause spontaneous mucosal bleeding (such as epistaxis or gastrointestinal, genitourinary, or vaginal bleeding) or excessive bleeding after trauma or during surgery.

Decreased platelet production may be caused by drugs, chemicals, or myeloproliferative diseases, whereas increased peripheral destruction may result from consumption coagulopathies, splenomegaly, autoantibodies, isoantibodies, anaphylactic reactions, drugs, and some infections. The drugs most likely to cause a thrombocytopenia include quinidine, sulfa preparations, oral antidiabetic agents, gold salts, rifampin, and heparin. Thrombocytopenia may also be caused by recent blood transfusions (e.g., posttransfusion purpura) or heavy alcohol consumption (causing alcohol-induced thrombocytopenia).

Patients with malignancies frequently have chronic DIC with thrombocytopenia, which may significantly worsen during or after surgery. Excessive bleeding may develop in patients with burns for a variety of reasons, including DIC, reduced concentrations of coagulation factors as a result of protein loss, thrombocytopenia caused by increased consumption, and thrombocytopathy related to antibiotics.

AXIOM Fever is usually present in thrombocytopenia, which is due to infection, active systemic lupus erythematosus, or thrombotic thrombocytopenic purpura (TTP); however, fever is usually absent in idiopathic thrombocytopenic purpura (ITP) and drug-related thrombocytopenias.

The spleen is not palpably enlarged in most thrombocytopenias because of the presence of antibodies (such as with ITP, drug-related immune thrombocytopenias, or TTP), whereas it often is palpably enlarged in patients with thrombocytopenia caused by hypersplenism, lymphoma, or myeloproliferative disorders.

Platelet size should be noted on blood smears. An increased proportion of large (young) platelets (determined by scanning the blood smear or by measuring mean platelet volume with an electronic blood counter) suggests a compensatory increased platelet production and early release from the marrow into the bloodstream. An increased proportion of large platelets is often found in thrombocytopenias secondary to increased destruction or utilization of platelets.

In addition to laboratory tests testing for primary and secondary hemostasis and clot retraction, a bone marrow aspirate may also be helpful for determining the cause of thrombocytopenia.

Treatment of thrombocytopenia secondary to decreased platelet production is directed toward attempting to correct its cause (e.g., discontinue various drugs, such as heparin). Platelet concentrates can be given to increase the platelet count temporarily; however, repeated platelet transfusions can cause increased production of platelet autoantibodies, which can greatly reduce the life expectancy of subsequently transfused platelets.

AXIOM One should avoid transfusing platelets in patients with thrombocytopenia associated with autoantibodies unless the patient has life-threatening bleeding.

Vascular Abnormalities

Bleeding disorders are rarely secondary to blood vessel abnormalities; however, severe infections, such as meningococcemia, typhoid fever, and subacute bacterial endocarditis can cause vascular defects and hemorrhage. Severe vitamin C deficiency or excessive endogenous or exogenous steroids can also cause breakdown of small blood vessels. In Henoch-Schönlein purpura, senile purpura, and hereditary hemorrhagic telangiectasia, the blood vessels are fragile and tissues throughout the body can bruise or bleed excessively with little or no trauma.

TRAUMA AND ITS EFFECT ON COAGULATION

With the widespread distribution of tissue thromboplastin in the body, one would expect tissue trauma to accelerate clotting. Although acidosis and ischemia tend to shorten clotting times, they can also cause a consumptive coagulopathy. Thus, it is not surprising that patients with only mild to moderate injury usually have normal PT and aPTT findings; however, in more severely injured patients, PT and aPTT are often prolonged, even without massive blood transfusions (3).

Blood levels of the plasma antiproteases, especially antithrombin III, decrease with trauma because of increased activation of the clotting system, and the extent of the decrease usually correlates with the severity of the injuries (17,18). The resulting low antithrombin levels cause an increased tendency for thrombosis, which can result in DVT or multiple organ failure (MOF) (19).

AXIOM Severe antithrombin deficiencies in sepsis increase the tendency for DIC and MOF.

Platelet Problems

Thrombocytopenia and platelet dysfunction are the major causes of microvascular (nonmechanical) bleeding (MVB) after massive transfusions.

Platelet Transfusions

AXIOM Routine prophylactic administration of FFP or platelets is not warranted in patients receiving massive blood transfusions unless there is clinical or laboratory evidence of a bleeding or clotting disorder.

Some general indications for platelet transfusion include the following:

1. Platelet counts less than 10,000 to 20,000/mm^3 (even if the patient is not bleeding);
2. Patients who are actively bleeding or are going to surgery and have platelet counts less than 50,000/mm^3 or bleeding times greater than 15 minutes; and
3. Red blood cell transfusions equivalent to more than a normal blood volume in a patient who has microvascular bleeding.

Depending on the clinical situation, the platelet count at 1 hour should have increased by at least 5,000 to 10,000/mm^3 for each unit of platelets transfused. Less than the expected increase suggests that the patient may have antibodies to platelets. If the patient is consuming platelets rapidly because of bleeding, sepsis, or DIC, the platelet count elevates as expected initially, but is then much lower after 12 to 24 hours.

AXIOM In general, platelet transfusions are contraindicated in patients with a diagnosis of TTP, posttransfusion purpura, or HIT.

Fresh Frozen Plasma

Due to increased consumption of clotting factors in patients who have head trauma, FFP has been advocated by some as a resuscitation fluid in such patients to prevent the development of abnormal coagulation (3). Although several studies have demonstrated that patients with traumatic brain injury have a tendency toward development of DIC because of the massive release of tissue thromboplastin, review of 149 head-injured patients with Glasgow Coma Scale scores of 9 or less showed no difference between patients receiving FFP and those who did not (20).

DDAVP

DDAVP may be especially useful in patients with isolated prolongation of BT with normal platelet counts and without exposure to antiplatelet agents (3). Uremia is one of the best established indications for the use of DDAVP. Hepatic cirrhosis and acquired platelet dysfunction are other indications for its use. It can be given intravenously, intranasally, or subcutaneously.

The BT often improves within 30 minutes following a DDAVP infusion; however, the compound is often ineffective in patients with thrombocytopenia or congenital platelet dysfunction (21).

Side effects with DDAVP (such as facial flushing, conjunctival erythema, increases in heart rate, or mild headache) are usually minor and usually occur only during the infusion. DDAVP should be given with caution to patients with atherosclerosis because of reports of thrombosis of severely diseased vessels (21).

Hypothermia

AXIOM Hypothermia is one of the most common causes of altered coagulation in trauma.

Shock, alcohol intoxication, massive fluid and blood infusions, exposure to cold, and prolonged surgery predispose trauma patients to hypothermia. In one study, hemorrhage accounted for 90% of deaths occurring within 48 hours of abdominal injury, and at least half of those deaths were associated with hypothermia (22).

The effects of decreased body temperature on clotting function include altered platelet number, morphology, function, and sequestration; increased fibrinolysis; and retardation of enzyme systems involved in the initiation and propagation of clot formation (23). These changes generally are reversible upon rewarming. Hypothermia may also induce DIC by producing cell injury and subsequent thromboplastin release and by causing tissue hypoxia because of a depressed cardiac output. Hypothermia may also cause hepatic dysfunction and increased blood citrate levels following massive transfusions.

In patients with nonmechanical bleeding associated with severe hypothermia, the best course to follow is to pack the bleeding areas as needed and to complete only those portions of the surgical procedure that are absolutely necessary. The patient is then taken to the intensive care unit and rewarmed as rapidly as possible, administering FFP, platelets, and other blood products as necessary.

Dextran and Hydroxyethyl Starch

AXIOM Administration of large volumes of dextran or hydroxyethyl starch (HES) (more than 20 mL/kg/day) can cause a bleeding tendency.

Of the many effects that dextran can have on hemostasis, perhaps the most important is its binding on platelet surfaces, thus causing defective platelet aggregation (2). When administered to replace blood losses, large volumes of dextran can also increase bleeding by causing dilution of fibrinogen and other coagulation factors. Dilutional coagulopathy may also occur after HES if more than 20 mL/kg is given in any 24-hour period. Lesser quantities of HES can cause prolongation of PT and aPTT, but seldom cause excessive clinical bleeding.

Massive Blood Transfusions

Bleeding diatheses associated with massive blood transfusions is primarily caused by thrombocytopathy, but thrombocytopenia, decreased clotting factors, and increased fibrinolytic activity may also be seen. Occasionally, because of shock and the massive tissue trauma that are also present, DIC may develop.

AXIOM The most frequent cause of excessive blood loss in patients receiving massive transfusions is inadequate surgical control of open vessels (24).

Indeed, if a coagulopathy is diagnosed clinically and by laboratory studies, one should make an increased effort to find and control major bleeding sites.

Although the number of platelets may not change significantly after 24 to 48 hours of storage in the blood bank, the ability of platelets to form a first hemostatic plug is greatly impaired (2). Blood that is older than 48 hours essentially has no effective platelets, and it has decreased levels of factor V and factor VIII:C; fibrinolysis also tends to be increased.

Factor V and factor VIII:C are often referred to as "labile factors" because they lose their biologic activity rapidly during storage. After 6 days, less than 50% of the original activity of factor V remains, and after 21 days, less than 10% of both their activities remains.

Although administration of massive blood transfusions and accompanying fluids may dilute clotting factors, severe shock appears to be the major factor causing depression of the coagulation factors. Shock not only causes consumption of platelets and coagulation factors, but it also decreases coagulation factor production and mobilization from tissue spaces.

Autotransfusions

Shed blood that is carefully washed and administered is relatively safe; however, administration of more than 6 units of autotransfused blood, even if it is washed, can contribute to development of a coagulopathy. The shed blood that is recovered is mostly red blood cells plus serum and procoagulants. Consequently, it is not surprising that autotransfusions can activate the clotting system, and DIC can occur if large quantities of shed blood are autotransfused.

It has been the impression of many of the surgical staff at Detroit Receiving Hospital that the use of 6 or more units of autotransfused blood in trauma patients increases the tendency toward development of a severe coagulopathy; as a consequence, autotransfusion tends to be avoided in such patients.

DISSEMINATED INTRAVASCULAR COAGULATION

Pathophysiology

In DIC, generalized activation of prothrombin to thrombin occurs with conversion of fibrinogen to fibrin. As the fibrinogen, prothrombin, platelets, factor V, and factor VIII are "consumed," their concentration in the blood can decrease to less than that needed for normal hemostasis, resulting in a "consumption coagulopathy" (2).

DIC can present in one of three forms:

1. Generalized intravascular activation of the clotting system with simultaneous activation of the fibrinolytic system (i.e., secondary fibrinolysis);
2. DIC without activation of the fibrinolytic system; and
3. Activation of the fibrinolytic system without intravascular clotting (i.e., primary fibrinolysis) (2).

Intravascular coagulation with secondary fibrinolysis is the most frequent type of DIC. Disseminated intravascular coagulation without secondary fibrinolysis is rare and has the poorest prognosis because fibrin, which is formed in DIC, is deposited in the microcirculation, causing occlusion of nutrient capillaries with resultant MOF.

Damage to organs, such as the prostate, placenta, lung, or liver, tends to release activators of the fibrinolytic system (t-PA) and can cause primary fibrinolysis. Severe hypoxia, as encountered during shock or improper anesthesia, can also be a powerful stimulus for activation of plasminogen to plasmin.

The FSPs that are formed can also inhibit coagulation (by delaying polymerization of fibrin monomers). FSPs may also interpose themselves between fibrin monomers, causing a weak fibrin clot to form.

Etiology

A wide variety of conditions may cause or predispose a patient to development of DIC. All types of tissue damage or necrosis, such as shock, sepsis, trauma, malignancy, or burns, can release thromboplastic substances (tissue factor) that may cause DIC. Septic shock may also cause intravascular platelet aggregation and tissue-factor release. Severe acidosis may also cause intravascular platelet breakdown, thus explaining the presence of DIC in some nonseptic shock conditions.

The body's defense mechanisms, especially the reticulendothelial system, can inhibit the development of DIC; however, poor liver function or prolonged shock greatly reduces the effectiveness of these defenses.

Diagnosis

Acute DIC is usually diagnosed by demonstrating the following:

1. Presence of an appropriate predisposing condition;
2. Clinical evidence of excessive bleeding or microthrombosis; and
3. Demonstration of laboratory changes consistent with consumptive coagulopathy.

The laboratory diagnosis of DIC usually requires a minimum of four tests:

1. Fibrinogen levels;
2. Platelet counts;
3. FSP; and
4. D-dimer levels.

Fibrinogen and platelets decrease because they are consumed, whereas FSP and D-dimer levels increase because of the increased intravascular clotting.

Although differentiating between the three forms of DIC may be difficult at times, accurate diagnosis is essential for proper treatment. Primary fibrinolysis is generally associated with a normal platelet count, low fibrinogens levels, elevated FSPs, and negative D-dimers; however, the platelet count may decrease as increased quantities for blood and fluid are given; consequently, this criterion is valid only early in the syndrome.

The most common form of DIC (clotting plus fibrinolysis) is characterized by low platelet counts and fibrinogen levels and by elevated FSPs and D-dimers. Rarely, patients have primary clotting (with little or no fibrinolysis), and these patients have low platelet counts and fibrinogen levels, but normal levels of FSP and D-dimers.

⊘ PITFALL

When blood for coagulation tests is drawn from an indwelling arterial or venous catheter, any heparin flush in the line can produce erroneous results.

Treatment

Patients with consumption coagulopathy are endangered by exsanguination resulting from the consumption coagulopathy or deposition of fibrin in the microvasculature leading to irreparable organ damage. The bleeding problem is present in all forms of DIC, but excess intravascular fibrin deposition occurs predominantly when fibrinolysis is absent or insufficiently present. Generally, a patient who has secondary fibrinolysis with FSP concentrations of more than 40 μg/mL is not likely to deposit fibrin, whereas a patient with FSP levels less than 10 μg/mL probably will.

Correction of the Primary Process

AXIOM The best way to treat consumption coagulopathy is to eliminate the underlying disease process.

Abruptio placentae serves as an appropriate example because at the moment the uterus is evacuated, either spontaneously or by cesarean section, the trigger for DIC is removed and consumption coagulopathy ceases. Rapid and aggressive treatment of shock or sepsis is also crucial to reduce both the immediate morbidity and the secondary mortality from organ failure.

Replacement of Platelets and Coagulation Factors

Although many authors stress that treatment of the underlying cause is the only therapy necessary to arrest DIC, patients who are injured or bleeding and require emergency surgery need vigorous replacement therapy with blood, FFP, and platelets to reverse the bleeding diathesis. Maintaining an adequate intravascular volume is extremely helpful because a major inciting factor of DIC in trauma patients is inadequate tissue perfusion. Because it also replaces depleted antithrombin (which is the most important endogenous anticoagulant), FFP may also help to control any tendency toward a hypercoagulable state.

Heparin

Heparin treatment is imperative in patients who have DIC without adequate fibrinolysis, and the earlier it is initiated, the better the prognosis. DIC can generally be interrupted in an adult by rapidly administering 2,000 to 3,000 units of heparin intravenously as a loading dose, followed by 700 to 1,000 units/hour given by continuous intravenous infusion. Any bleeding that is already present is not arrested by the heparin, but within hours, one will usually be able to measure an increase in fibrinogen levels and platelet counts. This restoration of the hemostatic mechanisms is aided by infusion of FFP with platelet concentrates.

Antifibrinolytic Drugs

Antifibrinolytic therapy with EACA or aprotinin should be considered only for patients in whom the diagnosis of primary fibrinolysis is established beyond any doubt (2).

⊘ FREQUENT ERRORS

1. ***Assuming that excessive intraoperative or postoperative bleeding is caused by a coagulation abnormality rather than realizing that such bleeding is often the result of inadequate surgical efforts to obtain hemostasis.***
2. ***Failure to obtain appropriate laboratory tests as soon as possible in patients with possible coagulation abnormalities.***
3. ***Assuming that a clinical coagulation disorder cannot be present if the coagulation tests are normal.***
4. ***Failure to obtain an adequate history concerning drugs with possible anticoagulant effects in preoperative patients or in patients who are bleeding excessively.***
5. ***Assuming that a platelet count greater than 50,000/mm^3 eliminates a bleeding disorder caused by platelet problems.***
6. ***Drawing blood for coagulation tests from indwelling venous or arterial catheters, particularly if those catheters have been flushed with any solution containing heparin.***
7. ***Failure to provide adequate quantities of FFP and platelets to patients in whom a coagulopathy developed after massive transfusions.***

SUMMARY POINTS

1. Even if a defect is found in bleeding and coagulation laboratory tests, intraoperative and postoperative bleeding is often due to inadequate surgical efforts.
2. Partial transection of a vessel, which prevents vascular occlusion by vasoconstriction, is more likely to lead to significant blood loss than is complete transection.
3. Recurrent venous thromboembolic disease in young individuals without apparent predisposing factors should make one suspect an inherited or acquired deficiency of antithrombin III, protein C, or protein S.
4. Increased levels of FSPs can block primary and secondary hemostasis.
5. Normal thrombin times plus normal fibrinogen levels exclude serious activation of the fibrinolytic system.
6. The diagnosis of hemostatic disturbances depends primarily on a careful history and physical examination.
7. A diligent effort must be made to determine whether a trauma or preoperative patient is taking any drugs that may have anticoagulant properties.
8. Patients with primary hemostatic defects tend to give a history of either prolonged oozing from cuts or mucous membranes or excessive bruising. In contrast, individuals with impaired secondary hemostasis tend to have hemarthrosis and deep (intramuscular) hematomas.
9. Prolonged or excessive bleeding from needle puncture sites or spontaneous bleeding from mucous membranes suggests a severe coagulopathy, such as DIC.
10. Excessive bleeding after severe trauma may occur if the concentration of coagulation factors is less than 50% to 100% of normal, but most of the coagulation tests are normal if only 30% to 35% of the normal amount of the factors is present.
11. Mild thrombocytopathies usually are not discovered by performing a bleeding time.

12. A normal aPTT and PT effectively exclude serious defects in the clotting system.
13. In hemophiliacs, the first hemostatic plug usually develops promptly after trauma, but excessive bleeding tends to develop after a delay that may last several hours or days.
14. The diagnosis of hemophilia should be suspected in male patients with a history of excessive bleeding since childhood.
15. Posttraumatic intracranial bleeding in hemophiliac patients may not be apparent for 24 to 48 hours.
16. Intraoperative positioning of hemophiliacs should be done carefully, and pressure points must be thickly padded to prevent hemorrhage into the involved tissues.
17. Whenever a blood product is used, the risk of subsequent hepatitis or AIDS should be considered.
18. The initial treatment of excessive bleeding in hemophiliacs is volume resuscitation with blood transfusions and FFP.
19. Each unit of factor VIII activity infused per kilogram of body weight should produce a 2% increase in plasma levels.
20. If the PT and aPTT can be returned to normal levels by adding an equal amount of normal plasma to the sample, the clotting problem is probably a deficiency of one or more clotting factors. If adding an equal amount of normal plasma to the sample does not correct the abnormal PT or aPTT, it is likely that an inhibitor or anticoagulant is present.
21. If possible, musculoskeletal bleeding in classic hemophiliacs with factor VIII inhibitors is managed without giving factor VIII.
22. In patients receiving multiple units of factor IX concentrate, 5 to 10 units of heparin should be added to each milliliter of reconstituted prothrombin complex concentrate given.
23. Even though the bleeding time may be prolonged, vWD should not be treated with platelet concentrates.
24. Severe liver disease can cause thrombocytopenia, increased fibrinolysis, and decreased production of most coagulation factors, except FVIII:C and vWF.
25. When coagulation tests are abnormal in patients with liver disease, little or no improvement may be evident after vitamin K injection, even after 24 to 48 hours.
26. In patients with severe liver dysfunction, large volumes of FFP may be required initially and every 2 to 6 hours to maintain reasonable factor levels.
27. The use of EACA in cirrhotic patients who are bleeding excessively should be discouraged because some of these patients also have a consumption coagulopathy, in which case EACA would be contraindicated.
28. Increased bleeding resulting from a qualitative platelet problem (thrombocytopathy) can be expected in most patients with severe uremia.
29. Coagulation defects resulting from pure vitamin K deficiency can be partially corrected by intravenous vitamin K within 6 to 12 hours unless coincident liver dysfunction exists.
30. Treatment of severe, active bleeding, which is due either to Coumadin administration or to vitamin K deficiency, should include intravenous vitamin K and at least 4 to 8 units of FFP.
31. Reduced plasma levels of antithrombin (because of liver disease or excessive clotting) can greatly increase the amount of heparin needed to prolong aPTT.
32. Rapid infusion of protamine can cause hypotension, and an excessive amount of protamine can anticoagulate the patient again.
33. Platelet counts should be carefully monitored daily or every other day whenever heparin is given.
34. When HIT syndrome develops in a patient requiring anticoagulation, oral anticoagulants should be begun and heparin stopped immediately.
35. Aspirin causes permanent impaired function of all platelets exposed to it (up to 8 to 10 days).
36. Platelet transfusions are indicated in patients in whom excessive bleeding develops as a result of thrombocytopenia or thrombocytopathy during emergency major surgery.

37. One should avoid transfusing platelets in patients with thrombocytopenia associated with autoantibodies (such as ITP, TTP, or posttransfusion purpura) unless the patient has life-threatening bleeding.
38. Severe antithrombin deficiencies in sepsis increase the tendency to DIC and MOF.
39. Trauma to the brain, which has the highest tissue thromboplastin concentration in the body, can cause multiple clotting abnormalities, including DIC.
40. Routine prophylactic administration of FFP or platelets is not warranted in patients receiving massive blood transfusions unless there is clinical or laboratory evidence of a bleeding or clotting disorder.
41. Hypothermia is one of the most common causes of altered coagulation in trauma.
42. Administration of dextran or HES in doses of more than 20 mL/kg/day can cause a significant bleeding tendency.
43. Hemostatic defects typically seen with massive blood transfusions include thrombocytopenia, thrombocytopathy, decreased factors V and VIII, and elevated FSP.
44. The most frequent cause of excessive blood loss in patients receiving massive transfusions is inadequate surgical control of open vessels.
45. The major causes of nonmechanical or MVB during or after massive transfusions are thrombocytopathy and thrombocytopenia.
46. Platelet transfusions should be considered if the patient has MVB after massive transfusions and has a platelet count less than 100,000/mm^3.
47. D-dimers are fragments derived from lysis of cross-linked fibrin and, therefore, increased D-dimer levels indicate that increased clotting has occurred.
48. The best way to treat a consumption coagulopathy is to eliminate the underlying disease process.
49. Heparin treatment should be strongly considered in patients who have DIC without adequate fibrinolysis.
50. Antifibrinolytic therapy should generally not be given to patients with DIC unless heparin is also administered.

REFERENCES

1. Mammen EF, Wilson RF. Coagulation abnormalities in trauma. In: Wilson RF, Walt AJ, eds. *Management of trauma—pitfalls and practice,* 2nd ed. Philadelphia: Williams and Wilkins, 1996:1012.
2. Mammen EF. Coagulation abnormalities in trauma. In: Walt AJ, Wilson RF, eds. *Management of trauma—pitfalls and practice.* Philadelphia: Lee & Febiger, 1975: 566.
3. Rutledge R, Sheldon GF. Bleeding and coagulation problems. In: Moore EE, Mattox KL, Feliciano, eds. *Trauma,* 2nd ed. Norwalk: Appleton & Lange, 1991: 891–908.
4. Bikfalvi A, Beress L. Natural proteinase inhibitors: blood coagulation inhibition and evolutionary relationships. *Comp Biochem Physiol B* 1987;87:435.
5. Rosenberg R, Rosenberg J. Natural anticoagulant mechanisms. *J Clin Invest* 1984;74:1.
6. Peterson P, Hayes TE, Arkin CF, et al. The preoperative bleeding time test lacks clinical benefit. *Arch Surg* 1998;133:134.
7. Mammen EF. Congenital coagulation protein disorders. In: Bick RL, Bennett JM, Brynes RK, et al, eds. *Hematology: clinical and laboratory practice.* Vol 2. St. Louis: Mosby, 1993:1391–1420.
8. Mammen EF. Laboratory evaluation of congenital coagulation protein disorders. In: Bick RL, Bennett JM, Bryns RK, et al, eds. *Hematology: clinical and laboratory practice.* Vol 2. St. Louis: Mosby, 1993:1421–1433.
9. Macik BG. Treatment of factor VIII inhibitors: products and strategies. *Semin Thromb Hemost* 1993;19:13.
10. Ruggeri ZM, Zimmerman TS. von Willebrand factor and von Willebrand disease. *Blood* 1987;70:895.
11. Zimmerman TS, Ruggeri ZM. Laboratory diagnosis of von Willebrand disease. In:

Bick RL, Bennett JM, Brynes RN, et al, eds. *Hematology: clinical and laboratory practice.* Vol 2. St. Louis: Mosby 1993:1441–1447.
12. Mammen EF. Coagulation abnormalities in liver disease. *Hematol Oncol Clin North Am* 1992;6:1247.
13. Mammen EF. Acquired coagulation protein disorders. In: Bick RL, Bennett JM, Brynes RD, et al, eds. *Hematology: clinical and laboratory practice.* Vol 2. St. Louis: Mosby, 1993:1449–1462.
14. Chong BH, Ismail F, Cada J, et al. Heparin-induced thrombocytopenia: studies with a low molecular weight heparinoid, ORG 10172. *Blood* 1989;73:1592.
15. The Columbus Investigators. Low-molecular-weight heparin in the treatment of patients with venous thromboembolism. *N Engl J Med* 1997;337:657.
16. Simmoneau G, Sors H, Carbonnier B, et al. A comparison of low-molecular-weight heparin with unfractionated heparin for acute pulmonary embolism. *N Engl J Med* 1997;337:663.
17. Wilson RF, Mammen EF, Robson MC, et al. Antithrombin, prekallikrein, and fibronectin levels in surgical patients. *Arch Surg* 1986;121:635–640.
18. Wilson RF, Farag A, Mammen EF, Fujii Y. Sepsis and antithrombin III, prekallikrein and fibronectin levels in surgical patients. *Am Surg* 1989;55: 450–456.
19. Owings JT, Bagley M, Gosseling R, et al. Effect of critical injury on plasma antithrombin activity: low antithrombin levels are associated with thromboembolic complications. *J Trauma* 1996;41:396.
20. Winter JP. Early fresh frozen plasma prophylaxis of abnormal coagulation parameters in the severely head injured patient is not effective. *Ann Emerg Med* 1989;18:553.
21. Salva KM, Kim H, Nahum K, Fallot PL. DDAVP in the treatment of bleeding disorders. *Pharmacotherapy* 1988;8:94.
22. Patt A, McCroskey BL, Moore EE. Hypothermia induced coagulopathy in trauma. *Surg Clin North Am* 1988;68:775.
23. Yoshihara H, Yamamoto T, Mihara H. Changes in coagulation and fibrinolysis occurring in dogs during hypothermia. *Thromb Res* 1985;37:503.
24. Wilson RF, Dulchavsky SA, Soullier G, Beckman B. Problems with 20 or more blood transfusions in 24 hours. *Am Surg* 1987;53:410.

46. ORGAN TRANSPLANTATION AND TRAUMA[1]

AXIOM The main obstacle to the transplantation of organs is, generally, lack of donor availability.

Refinements in organ preservation, surgical technique, and immunosuppression with cyclosporine and other new drugs have made transplantation of solid organs increasingly more successful; however, at least 12% to 15% of patients listed for heart or lung transplantation die before a suitable organ donor is found.

Legal Guidelines

Most states require that hospital physicians inform the families of potentially brain-dead patients of the possibility of organ donation (2). Indeed, several authorities have also advocated the concept of "presumed consent" (3).

Laws incorporating this type of consent state that, unless a person has explicitly indicated that he or she does not want his or her organs donated, the consent is assumed, and transplant surgeons may proceed with the procurement of organs.

Practical Guidelines

AXIOM The referral of an organ or tissue donor begins with recognition (by physicians, nurses, or other individuals) that a particular patient may be a suitable donor.

When an individual is identified as a potential donor, even before criteria for brain death have been met, the Organ Procurement Organization serving the area should be notified. The referral of the potential organ donor may be expedited by providing patient's height, weight, age, medical history, diagnosis, hemodynamic data, urinalysis, serum creatinine levels, culture results, and ABO blood group. The transplant coordinators may then begin evaluation of the suitability of the potential donor.

AXIOM Even if a patient does not meet criteria for whole organ transplantation, he or she is frequently a suitable donor for skin, cornea, or bone.

O'Brien et al. (4) were able to increase organ donor rates from 26% to 50% by a hospital development plan that included six steps:

1. Identification of key contact individuals;
2. Development and modification of relevant hospital policies;
3. Improvement in procurement agency visibility in hospital units;
4. Education of hospital staff regarding organ donation;
5. Institution of early on-site donor evaluations; and
6. Provision of feedback to hospital staff about the disposition of potential organ donors.

Another effort to improve donor availability involves the use of non–heart-beating trauma donors (5). Experience in Europe and Japan has demonstrated that the function of kidneys harvested from non–heart-beating donors approaches that of organs harvested from brain-dead, heart-beating donors as long as the warm ischemia time is minimized. The duration of warm ischemia time is probably less than 30 minutes.

GENERAL CRITERIA FOR ORGAN DONORS

The ideal candidate for solid organ donation is a young, previously healthy patient who has had irreversible brain injury caused by head trauma, subarachnoid hemorrhage, drug overdose, primary brain tumors, or cerebral ischemia; however, the chronologic age of donors is certainly less important than their physiologic age (6) (Table 46-1).

General exclusion criteria for organ donation include acute untreated or uncontrolled infections, positive serology for the human immunodeficiency virus (HIV) antigen, active tuberculosis, malignancies other than brain or skin, trauma or disease involving the organs considered for donation, prolonged hypotension, or severe diabetes mellitus, hypertension, or peripheral vascular disease (6).

Establishing Brain Death

The general criteria for determination of brain death require documentation that

1. Cerebral and brain stem functions are absent.
2. This condition is irreversible, which requires that the causes of the condition be known.
3. Cessation of all brain function persists after an appropriate period of observation and an adequate trial of therapy is accomplished (7).

AXIOM The ultimate determination of brain death of a potential donor remains the clinical judgment of the attending physician.

Despite some variations, all guidelines for determining brain death require a detailed neurologic evaluation, and many also require an electroencephalogram (7). If no brain function is found, a repeat confirmatory neurologic examination must be performed again in some centers after 6 to 12 hours; however, if a radioisotope or other perfusion study shows no blood flow to the brain, no other confirmatory test is

Table 46-1. ***Donor Criteria for Various Organ Harvesting***

General criteria
No cancer, except primary skin or brain
No systemic infections
No hepatitis
No history of tuberculosis or syphilis
No history of recent intravenous drug abuse
No prolonged episodes of hypotension or asystole
No acute or chronic renal failure
Criteria for specific organs
Serum creatinine under 1.8 mg/dL (K), BUN < 20 mg/dL (K)
No established hypertension (K)
No evidence of urinary tract infection by urinalysis (K)
No evidence of diabetes mellitus or abnormal pancreatic function (P)
No visible infiltrate or evidence of trauma on chest radiography (Lu, H/L)
Donor arterial oxygen tension exceeding 250 mm Hg on 100% O_2 (Lu, H/L)
Normal ECG and cardiac function; no evidence of cardiovascular disease (H, H/L)
Sputum obtained by bronchoscopy is free of organisms as demonstrated by Gram stain (Lu, H/L)
Normal liver function tests (Li)

K, kidney; P, pancreas; Lu, lung; H, heart; H/L, combined heart-lung; Li, liver.

required. Testing for the brain death in potential organ donors can be carried out by any physician who has no involvement in the proposed transplantation.

If there is a possibility of a drug effect or if there is uncertainty concerning the nature of the intracranial pathology, four-vessel cerebral angiography, radionuclide cerebral imaging, or a xenon-computed tomography cerebral blood flow scan may be necessary to establish the absence of cerebral circulation (7). Spinal cord reflexes are irrelevant in the diagnosis of brain death and, therefore, are not routinely tested.

AXIOM Brain death should be pronounced as soon as possible after it occurs.

Cardiac arrest usually occurs within 72 hours of the occurrence of brain death of a potential donor unless special efforts are taken to maintain adequate cardiopulmonary function.

⊘ PITFALL

Not considering a brain-dead patient for organ donation because it is a "medical examiner's case" can overlook many potential trauma donors.

In cases in which the medical examiner has jurisdiction, his or her permission along with the consent of the next of kin is required for removal of organs for transplantation. Jaynes and Springer (8) have pointed out that, with well-informed medical/legal personnel and demonstrated efforts to meet all parties' needs, protocols can be established to help reduce these barriers. This theoretically could result in the release of up to 73% more nonaccidental trauma, 51% more homicides (gunshot wound to the head), and 46% more suicides for donation each year.

Consent for Organ Donation

The Uniform Anatomical Gift Act (UAGA) has been enacted in all states to standardize methods for organ donation (9). Victims may carry uniform donor cards, which are legal documents; nevertheless, consent should also be obtained from next of kin before organ donation.

Pre-Retrieval Patient Management

Pre–Brain Death Management

AXIOM Consideration of patients as potential organ donors should in no way interfere with the treatment of their injuries or diseases.

Even when a patient has been identified as a potential organ donor, treatment should be given in the most appropriate way to aid in his or her recovery.

Post–Brain Death Management

AXIOM After pronouncement of brain death, oxygenation and perfusion should be optimally maintained until the donor surgery is completed.

Following the pronouncement of brain death, the potential donor should be hydrated rapidly with appropriate solutions so that blood pressure and blood volume can be maintained at levels that allow optimal perfusion of vital organs without vasoconstrictor drugs and a urinary output of at least 1.0 to 1.5 mL/kg/h.

Central venous pressure measurements and, in some instances, a pulmonary artery wedge pressure (PAWP) catheter may be helpful. If blood pressure cannot be maintained with a PAWP of 18 or more mm Hg, dopamine in doses that do not exceed 10 to 15 μg/kg/min may improve blood pressure without causing dangerous degrees of vasoconstriction.

If the patient has a cardiac arrest before or after pronouncement of brain death, he or she must be resuscitated rapidly, using internal cardiac massage if needed. External cardiac massage for more than a few minutes generally excludes a patient from becoming a heart or lung donor. Cardiac arrest or severe hypotension for more than 15 minutes also contraindicates intrathoracic and intraabdominal organ donation.

AXIOM Core temperature should be monitored constantly and maintained as close to 35°C to 37°C as possible.

After brain death has been declared, the Pa_{CO_2} should be gradually normalized. The Pa_{O_2} should be maintained at 80 to 100 mm Hg using the lowest F_{IO_2} possible and less than 10 cm H_2O positive end-expiratory pressure. Patients with neurogenic pulmonary edema should be monitored with a pulmonary artery catheter and efforts made to get the PAWP to less than 12 to 15 mm Hg.

AXIOM Diabetes insipidus in brain-dead potential organ donors should be corrected with aqueous Pitressin or desmopressin (DDAVP) as soon as possible.

With brain injury, especially if it involves the hypothalamus or posterior pituitary gland, diabetes insipidus may occur. The resultant output of very large volumes of urine with a low specific gravity can be extremely difficult to replace appropriately. Therefore, if the urinary output exceeds 200 mL/h and the patient is not overloaded with fluid, consideration should be given to the administration of aqueous Pitressin (10 units subcutaneously) or DDAVP.

Other tests that should be obtained by hospital or transplantation personnel include ABO blood group, blood urea nitrogen, serum creatinine, urinalysis, HIV, human T-cell leukemia virus, cytomegalovirus, hepatitis surface antigens, and blood and urine cultures. Organ specific tests include liver function tests on potential liver donors, electrocardiogram on potential heart donors, and blood gases and chest radiographs on potential lung donors. In patients with major fractures, bronchoalveolar lavage to rule out the presence of severe fat embolism may also be appropriate.

AXIOM The presence of an active systemic infection is a contraindication to solid organ donation.

The results of all predonation cultures should be known. In addition, cultures of blood, urine, and sputum should be drawn 30 minutes before any organs are removed. To help prevent bacteremia from intravenous lines, a first-generation cephalosporin is usually given immediately before operations for organ retrieval begin.

Blood and Tissue Typing

Before moving the patient to the operating room, blood is drawn for tissue typing and stored at room temperature. Tissue typing for all solid organs is similar, but it is generally not done in heart, liver, and pancreas donors (10).

Matching is based primarily on ABO compatibility, the absence of a lymphocytotoxic cross-match, and an appropriate size match of donor and recipient organs.

OPERATION

Multiple cadaveric procurement (heart, liver, kidneys) takes approximately 2 to 3 hours. At least two surgeons with special interest and expertise in transplantation surgery and organ retrieval should participate in multiorgan procurement operations.

⊘

1. ***Failure to consider every trauma victim, especially those with isolated head injuries, to be a possible donor of organs or tissues.***
2. ***Failure to optimally support a potential organ donor so as to make the tissue or organs more suitable for donation.***
3. ***Failure to promptly notify the local donor procurement agency of the presence of a potential organ donor.***
4. ***Failure to actively prevent or treat organ failure or infection in a potential organ donor.***

SUMMARY POINTS

1. The main obstacle to the transplantation of organs is, generally, donor availability.
2. The referral of an organ or tissue donor begins with recognition by physicians, nurses, or other individuals that a particular patient may be a suitable donor.
3. Even if a patient does not meet criteria for whole organ transplantation, he or she is frequently a suitable donor for skin, cornea, or bone.
4. The ultimate determination of brain death of a potential donor remains the clinical judgment of the attending physician.
5. Brain death should be pronounced as soon as possible after it occurs.
6. Consideration of patients as potential organ donors should in no way interfere with the treatment of their injuries or diseases.
7. After pronouncement of brain death, oxygenation and perfusion should be optimally maintained until the donor surgery is complete.
8. Vasoconstrictor drugs should be avoided or used only in low doses in brain-dead potential organ donors.
9. Core temperature should be monitored constantly and maintained as close to 36°C to 37°C as possible.
10. Diabetes insipidus in brain-dead potential organ donors should be corrected with aqueous Pitressin or DDAVP as soon as possible.
11. The presence of an active systemic infection is a contraindication to solid organ donation.

REFERENCES

1. United Network for Organ Sharing. *1994 Annual Report of the US Scientific Registry of Transplant Recipients and the Organ Procurement and Transplantation Network* (abstract). Richmond, VA: United Network for Organ Sharing, 1994.
2. Evans RW, Manninen DL, Garrison LP Jr, et al. Donor availability as the primary determinant of the future of heart transplantation. *JAMA* 1989;255:1892.
3. Starzl TE, Miller CM, Rapaport FT. Organ procurement. In: *American College of Surgeons Care of the Surgical Patient 2. Elective Care, Vol 1.* Scientific American Inc., NYC;1988:1.
4. O'Brien RL, Serbin MF, O'Brien KD, et al: Improvement in the organ donation rate at a large urban trauma center. *Arch Surg* 1996;131:153–159.
5. Wisner DH, Lo B. The feasibility of organ salvage from non-heart-beating trauma donors. *Arch Surg* 1996;131:929–934.
6. Soifer BE, Gelb AW. The multiple organ donor: identification and management. *Ann Intern Med* 1989;110:814.
7. Grenvik A. Brain death and permanently lost consciousness. In: Shoemaker WC,

Thompson WL, Holbrook PR, eds. *Textbook of critical care.* Philadelphia: WB Saunders, 1984:968.
8. Jaynes CL, Springer JW. Decreasing the organ donor shortage by increasing communication between coroners, medical examiners and organ procurement organizations. *Am J Forensic Med Pathol* 1994;15:156–159.
9. Lee PP, Kissner P. Organ donation and the Uniform Anatomical Gift Act. *Surgery* 1986;100:867.
10. Peitzman AB, Webster MN, Gordon RD. Organ procurement and transplantation. In: Moore EE, Feliciano DV, Mattox KL (eds). *Trauma,* 2nd ed. Norwalk, CT: Appleton & Lange, 1991:797–804.

SUBJECT INDEX

Page numbers followed by "f" indicate a figure; page numbers followed by "t" indicate a table

C

J

S